The Basic Science of Oncology

Notice

The Basic Science of Oncology

Fifth Edition

Editors

Ian F. Tannock, MD, PhD, DSc

Staff Physician and Senior Scientist
Princess Margaret Cancer Centre
University Health Network
Professor of Medicine and Medical Biophysics
University of Toronto
Toronto, Ontario

Richard P. Hill, PhD

Senior Scientist, Ontario Cancer Institute and
Campbell Family Institute for Cancer Research
Princess Margaret Cancer Centre
University Health Network
Professor of Medical Biophysics and
Radiation Oncology
University of Toronto
Toronto, Ontario

Robert G. Bristow, MD, PhD

Staff Physician and Senior Scientist
Ontario Cancer Institute and Campbell
Family Institute for Cancer Research
Princess Margaret Cancer Centre
University Health Network
Professor of Radiation Oncology
and Medical Biophysics
University of Toronto
Toronto, Ontario

Lea Harrington, PhD

IRIC-Institut de Recherché en Immunologie
et en Cancérologie
Professor, Faculty of Medicine
Université de Montréal
Montréal, Québec

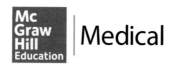

New York   Chicago   San Francisco   Lisbon   London   Madrid   Mexico City
Milan   New Delhi   San Juan   Seoul   Singapore   Sydney   Toronto

The Basic Science of Oncology, Fifth Edition

Copyright © 2013, 2005, 1998, 1992, 1987 by The McGraw-Hill Companies, Inc. All rights reserved. Printed in China. Except as permitted under the United States Copyright Act of 1976, no part of this publication may be reproduced or distributed in any form or by any means, or stored in a data base or retrieval system, without the prior written permission of the publisher.

2 3 4 5 6 7 8 9 0   DSS   18 17 16 15

ISBN 978-0-07-174520-8
MHID 0-07-174520-3

This book was set in Minion Pro by Thomson Digital.
The editors were James Shanahan and Regina Y. Brown.
The production supervisor was Sherri Souffrance.
Project management was provided by Kunal Mehrotra, Thomson Digital.
The cover designer was Pehrsson Design.
Cover Image: Telomeres. Image Credit: Hybrid Medical/Science Source.
China Translation & Printing Services, Ltd. was printer and binder.

This book is printed on acid-free paper.

Library of Congress Cataloging-in-Publication Data

The basic science of oncology / editors, Ian F. Tannock ... [et al.]. — 5th ed.
  p. ; cm.
  Includes bibliographical references and index.
  ISBN 978-0-07-174520-8 (alk. paper) — ISBN 0-07-174520-3
  I. Tannock, Ian.
  [DNLM: 1. Neoplasms. QZ 200]
  616.99′4—dc23

                                        2012038366

McGraw-Hill books are available at special quantity discounts to use as premiums and sales promotions, or for use in corporate training programs. To contact a representative please e-mail us at bulksales@mcgraw-hill.com.

International Edition ISBN 978-0-07-176732-3; MHID 0-07-176732-0. Copyright © 2013. Exclusive rights by The McGraw-Hill Companies, Inc., for manufacture and export. This book cannot be re-exported from the country to which it is consigned by McGraw-Hill. The International Edition is not available in North America.

Contents

Contributors

Eitan Amir, MB ChB, PhD
Staff Physician and Clinician Scientist
Ontario Cancer Institute and Princess Margaret
  Cancer Centre
University Health Network
Assistant Professor of Medicine
University of Toronto
Toronto, Ontario

Paul C. Boutros, PhD
Principal Investigator, Informatics and Biocomputing
Assistant Professor of Medical Biophysics
Assistant Professor of Pharmacology and Toxicology
University of Toronto
Toronto, Ontario

Robert G. Bristow, MD, PhD
Staff Physician and Senior Scientist
Ontario Cancer Institute and Campbell Family
  Institute for Cancer Research
Princess Margaret Cancer Centre
University Health Network
Professor of Radiation Oncology and
  Medical Biophysics
University of Toronto
Toronto, Ontario

Rob A. Cairns, PhD
Associate Scientist
Campbell Family Institute for Cancer Research
Ontario Cancer Institute and Princess Margaret
  Cancer Centre
University Health Network
Toronto, Ontario

Eric X. Chen, MD, PhD
Staff Physician
Ontario Cancer Institute and Princess Margaret
  Cancer Centre
University Health Network
Assistant Professor of Medicine
University of Toronto
Toronto, Ontario

Susan P.C. Cole, PhD, FRSC, FCAHS
Canada Research Chair and Bracken Chair in
  Genetics and Molecular Medicine
Professor of Pathology and Molecular Medicine
Queen's University
Kingston, Ontario

Previn Dutt, PhD
Postdoctoral Fellow
Ontario Cancer Institute and Princess Margaret
  Cancer Centre
University Health Network
Toronto, Ontario

Gord Fehringer, PhD
Scientific Associate
Prosserman Centre for Health Research
Samuel Lunenfeld Research Institute of Mount
  Sinai Hospital
Toronto, Ontario

Craig Gedye, MBChB, FRACP, PhD
Postdoctoral and Medical Oncology Fellow
Ontario Cancer Institute and Princess Margaret
  Cancer Centre
University Health Network
University of Toronto
Toronto, Ontario

Denis M. Grant, PhD
Professor
Department of Pharmacology and Toxicology
Faculty of Medicine and Department
  of Pharmaceutical Sciences
Leslie Dan Faculty of Pharmacy
University of Toronto
Toronto, Ontario

Razqallah Hakem, PhD
Senior Scientist
Ontario Cancer Institute and Princess Margaret
  Cancer Centre
University Health Network
Professor of Medical Biophysics and Immunology
University of Toronto
Toronto, Ontario

Shane M. Harding, PhD
Post-Doctoral Fellow
Department of Cancer Biology
University of Pennsylvania School of Medicine
Philadelphia, Pennsylvania

Lea Harrington, PhD
IRIC-Institut de Recherché en Immunologie
et en Cancérologie
Professor, Faculty of Medicine
Université de Montréal
Montréal, Québec

Richard P. Hill, PhD
Senior Scientist
Ontario Cancer Institute and Campbell Family Institute
for Cancer Research
Princess Margaret Cancer Centre
University Health Network
Professor of Medical Biophysics and Radiation Oncology
University of Toronto
Toronto, Ontario

Rayjean J. Hung, PhD, MS
Principal Investigator, Samuel Lunenfeld Research
Institute of Mount Sinai Hospital
Cancer Care Ontario Research Chair in
Population Studies
Division of Epidemiology
Dalla Lana School of Public Health
University of Toronto
Toronto, Ontario

David A. Jaffray, PhD, ABMP
Head
Radiation Physics, Radiation Medicine Program
Princess Margaret Cancer Centre
Director, Techna Institute
Senior Scientist
Ontario Cancer Institute
University Health Network
Professor of Radiation Oncology, Medical Biophysics,
and IBBME
University of Toronto
Toronto, Ontario

Paul Jorgensen, PhD
Senior Research Associate
Terrence Donnelly Centre for Cellular and
Biomolecular Research
University of Toronto
Toronto, Ontario

Anthony M. Joshua, MBBS, PhD, FRACP
Staff Physician and Associate Scientist
Ontario Cancer Institute and Princess Margaret
Cancer Centre
University Health Network
Assistant Professor of Medicine
University of Toronto
Toronto, Ontario

Rama Khokha, PhD
Senior Scientist
Ontario Cancer Institute and Campbell Family Institute
for Cancer Research
Princess Margaret Cancer Centre
University Health Network
Professor of Medical Biophysics
University of Toronto
Toronto, Ontario

Thomas Kislinger, PhD
Senior Scientist
Ontario Cancer Institute and Princess Margaret
Cancer Centre
University Health Network
Professor of Medical Biophysics
University of Toronto
Toronto, Ontario

Eric Leblanc, PhD
Research Associate
Urologic Sciences
The Vancouver Prostate Centre
University of British Columbia
Vancouver, British Columbia

Evan F. Lind, PhD
Postdoctoral Fellow
The Campbell Family Institute for Breast
Cancer Research
Ontario Cancer Institute and Princess Margaret
Cancer Centre
University Health Network
Toronto, Ontario

Fei-Fei Liu, MD, FRCPC
Chief
Radiation Medicine Program
Princess Margaret Cancer Centre
University Health Network
Professor of Radiation Oncology
University of Toronto
Toronto, Ontario

Geoffrey Liu, MD, FRCPC
Alan B. Brown Chair in Molecular Genomics and
Senior Scientist
Ontario Cancer Institute and Princess Margaret
Cancer Centre
University Health Network
Associate Professor of Medicine
Medical Biophysics and Epidemiology
University of Toronto and Dalla Lana School of
Public Health
Toronto, Ontario

C. Jane McGlade, PhD
Senior Scientist
Program in Cell Biology and the Arthur and Sonia
    Labatt Brain Tumour Research Centre
Hospital for Sick Children
Professor of Medical Biophysics
University of Toronto
Toronto, Ontario

Leigh C. Murphy, PhD
Chair
Breast Cancer Research Group at the
    University of Manitoba
Senior Scientist, Manitoba Institute for Cell Biology
Professor of Biochemistry and Medical Genetics
University of Manitoba
Winnipeg, Manitoba

Linh T. Nguyen, PhD
Head
Translational Immunotherapy Laboratory
Campbell Family Institute for Breast Cancer Research
Ontario Cancer Institute and Princess Margaret
    Cancer Centre
University Health Network
Toronto, Ontario

Pamela S. Ohashi, PhD
Director
Immune Therapy Program
Senior Scientist
Ontario Cancer Institute and Princess Margaret
    Cancer Centre
University Health Network
Professor of Immunology
University of Toronto
Toronto, Ontario

Janusz Rak, MD, PhD
Jack Cole Chair in Pediatric Hematology/Oncology
Professor, Department of Pediatrics
McGill University
Montreal Children's Hospital and The Research Institute
    of the McGill University Health Centre
Montreal, Quebec

Michael Reedijk, MD, PhD
Surgeon Scientist
Princess Margaret Cancer Centre
University Health Network
Associate Professor of Surgery and
    Medical Biophysics
University of Toronto
Toronto, Ontario

Paul S. Rennie, PhD, FCAHS
Director
Laboratory Research
The Vancouver Prostate Centre
Professor, Department of Urologic Sciences
University of British Columbia
Vancouver, British Columbia

Christopher D. Richardson, PhD
Professor and Canada Research Chair
Department of Microbiology and Immunology
Department of Pediatrics
Dalhousie University
Halifax
Nova Scotia

Aaron D. Schimmer, MD, PhD, FRCPC
Staff Physician and Senior Scientist
Ontario Cancer Institute and Princess Margaret
    Cancer Centre
University Health Network
Associate Professor of Medicine and Medical Biophysics
University of Toronto
Toronto, Ontario

Yang W. Shao, BSc
PhD Candidate
Ontario Cancer Institute and Princess Margaret
    Cancer Centre
University Health Network
Department of Medical Biophysics
University of Toronto
Toronto, Ontario

Vuk Stambolic, PhD
Senior Scientist
Ontario Cancer Institute and Princess Margaret
    Cancer Centre
Associate Professor of Medical Biophysics
University of Toronto
Toronto, Ontario

Ian F. Tannock, MD, PhD, DSc
Staff Physician and Senior Scientist
Princess Margaret Cancer Centre
University Health Network
Professor of Medicine and Medical Biophysics
University of Toronto
Toronto, Ontario

Bradly Wouters, PhD
Senior Scientist
Ontario Cancer Institute and Princess Margaret
    Cancer Centre
University Health Network
Professor of Radiation Oncology and Medical Biophysics
University of Toronto
Toronto, Ontario

Preface

Since the publication of the fourth edition of *The Basic Science of Oncology* there have been major advances in our knowledge about the molecular basis of cancer, largely as a result of the rapid development of powerful techniques to study the genome and epigenome and to the parallel advances in techniques to study the levels of gene expression and the proteins that are produced. Concurrent with understanding of the molecular pathways that drive the development and progression of cancer, and the heterogeneity of the changes in these pathways in individual cancers, new molecular-targeted agents have been developed and are being tested, with variable success, in attempts to treat cancers selectively. The 5th edition of *The Basic Science of Oncology* places the major advances that have occurred in the context of previous studies that have generated the important background to cancer biology. Many of the chapters have new authors and all have been extensively revised and rewritten to reflect our new knowledge. We have added new chapters on the emerging areas of the tumor microenvironment and metabolism (Chapter 12) and cancer stem cells (Chapter 13).

As in previous editions we have attempted to bring together the contributions of experts into a book that, we believe, is suitable for fellows, residents, nurses, medical students, graduate students, and senior undergraduates who are interested in the biology of cancer. We have maintained a format of using relatively short sections that allows the reader to investigate a particular interest selectively, and include references that can be used as a guide for those seeking information in greater depth. We believe that the book will be useful as a teaching aid and as a broad introduction for those interested in the study and treatment of cancer.

We are grateful to many people for their assistance in producing this fifth edition. To our authors, particularly the new ones, who have responded to our many requests for alterations with forbearance. To our publishers who have encouraged us and accepted with good grace our failure to meet our initial deadlines and whose artists have redrawn all the figures in keeping with the new color format. To our students and trainees who have provided us with helpful and constructive criticism. And to our families who have continued to provide support and encouragement during the several phases of writing, rewriting, and reviewing.

I.F. Tannock
R.P. Hill
R.G. Bristow
L. Harrington

Introduction to Cancer Biology

Lea Harrington, Robert G. Bristow,
Richard P. Hill, and Ian F. Tannock

1.1 PERSPECTIVE AND HISTORY

One of the first scientific investigations into the cause of cancer dates from 1775, when Sir Percival Pott carried out an epidemiological study and suggested that the causative agent of scrotal cancer in young chimney sweeps in the United Kingdom might be chimney soot (now known to be tar). Frequent washing and changing of clothing that trapped the soot was recommended so as to reduce exposure to the "carcinogen" (see Chap. 4). Not only did Pott's study identify a putative carcinogenic agent but it also demonstrated that a cancer may develop years after exposure. One other dramatic example is mesothelioma, which is a rare lung cancer that develops decades after exposure to asbestos. A third epidemiological example is the identification of tobacco smoke as a major environmental cause of cancer. Doll and Hill (1950) showed that cigarette smoking is causative in lung cancer: heavy smokers older than the age of 50 years have a 1 in 2 chance of dying from a smoking-related disease such as lung cancer (see Chap. 3). On the positive side, individuals who quit smoking exhibit a gradual return to a near-normal risk of lung cancer after a 10- to 15-year smoke-free period. These and other studies underscore the possibility that, with some types of cancer, a degree of prevention may be achieved via changes in lifestyle.

Early advances in understanding of the biological properties of cancer followed the development of the microscope, which allowed Virchow, a 19th-century pathologist, to declare: "Every cell is born from another cell." This property is true of both normal and cancer cells. Microscopic examination of tumors and normal tissues established many important properties, including the characteristics of the cell cycle; the hierarchical organization of cells within normal tissues and to a lesser extent in tumors; the requirement for angiogenesis for tumor growth; heterogeneity among tumor cell populations;

and relationships between histopathological characteristics of tumors and their prognosis. Development of methods to culture cells, and establishment of colony forming assays to reflect reproductive survival allowed quantitative studies of the response of cancer cells to radiation and drugs, and allowed therapeutic response of tumors to be related to the sensitivity of individual cells within them. The establishment of inbred (syngeneic) mice allowed tumors to be transplanted between them, while subsequent development of immune-deprived mice allowed further study of some human tumors, and of cell lines derived from them, in an *in vivo* environment. Together with large-scale cell cultures that allowed screening of drugs in a semiautomated way, these tools were instrumental in allowing agents to be evaluated for antitumor effects and led to the development of some of the drugs used in cancer therapy.

The 1980s ushered in the modern era of molecular biology that led to the discovery of genes involved in cancer development. Notably, dysregulation of endogenous genes encoded in normal cells, called *(proto)oncogenes*, and/or loss of function of genes that provided checks on processes such as cell proliferation, called *tumor-suppressor genes*, were found to be associated with cancer induction and progression (see Chap. 7). These findings helped to explain earlier observations that viruses can cause cancer as they had evolved to carry oncogenes that mimic cellular gene function and subvert normal cellular processes to promote viral replication, such as the Rous sarcoma virus that was first discovered to be a causative factor in the development of tumors in chickens (v-src). Viruses are now known to be causative in the development of some common human cancers, including hepatitis viruses (B and C) as precursors of hepatocellular carcinoma, and human papilloma viruses (HPVs) as a causative agent for cervical and oropharyngeal cancer (see Chap. 6). The development of vaccines against HPVs (Future II Study Group, 2007) and of vaccination programs against hepatitis B virus (HBV) and hepatitis C virus (HCV) in regions where these viruses are endemic (Luo and Ruan, 2012) holds promise for marked reduction in the incidence of these cancers.

Other historically important contributions to the understanding of cancer include an appreciation that cancer is heritable. Studies of geographically or socially isolated populations, such as the Mormons in Utah, and of changes in cancer incidence in migrant families, demonstrated that both genetic predisposition and environmental factors are important in cancer causation. Analysis of cancer-prone families have assisted in the identification of genetic abnormalities that can lead directly to malignancy, such as mutation of tumor-suppressor genes, including the retinoblastoma gene (*Rb*) in children, the *p53* gene in the Li-Fraumeni syndrome, and the *BRCA1* and *BRCA2* genes, which are associated with familial breast and ovarian cancer (see Chap. 7). Thus cancer has been established as a genetic disease.

1.2 RECENT ADVANCES IN ONCOLOGY

The underlying biology of cancer can perhaps be best conceptualized as a process of many small changes similar to evolution. Genetic changes that affect growth potential provide an environment permissive for further changes that are selected for (or against) by environmental conditions. Increasing knowledge of cellular signal-transduction pathways has revealed that many aspects of cellular function, including proliferation and death, are controlled by a balance of positive and negative signals received from inside and outside the cell (see Chaps. 8 and 9). Thus, a decreased or increased ability to respond to a specific signal may allow the cell to proliferate in the face of other signals that would normally prevent such proliferation. Interaction of cancer cells with their surrounding tissue (stroma) is also a key factor in cancer initiation, progression, and metastasis (see Chap. 10). For example, the development of the vascular networks in tumors (angiogenesis) is necessary for tumor growth, and the behavior of cancer cells is influenced by external signals from circulating molecules (hormones and growth factors) and from neighboring cells and the extracellular matrix (see Chap. 11). Furthermore, changes to the extracellular environment in tumors (such as poor oxygenation) can cause changes in gene expression that enhance the development of more aggressive tumor phenotypes (see Chap. 12). These investigations have led to a better understanding of how and why cancer cells can spread from the primary tumor to grow at other sites in the body; metastasis is the property of a malignant cancer, which makes it particularly difficult to treat successfully (see Chap. 10). Although cancers may originate from a single cell, they become heterogeneous in their cellular properties and cells within different regions of an established tumor may express different genes (Gerlinger et al, 2012). One aspect of heterogeneity may be retention of a limited number of cells with high proliferative potential that can regenerate the tumor after

treatment, known as cancer stem cells (CSCs; see Chap. 13). Surface markers have been identified, which appear to characterize CSCs, but the stability of these markers, and of the CSC phenotype is uncertain and may be heterogeneous within and between tumors. The plasticity of cancer cells allows them to develop or select for resistance to therapeutic agents, and this property will likely pose a major challenge to treating tumors by targeting specific genetic pathways (see Chap. 19).

The past 10 years has yielded a watershed in our molecular understanding of the genetic basis of cancer (see Chap. 2). The use of genetically modified mice has enabled researchers to demonstrate that loss-of-function or gain-of-function in tumor-suppressor genes and oncogenes are important changes that occur during the development of cancers. Such animal models, for example those deficient in *TP53* or harboring constitutively active cellular signaling factors (eg, the guanosine triphosphatase [GTPase] Ras), have provided key model systems in which to dissect the progression from normal cell growth to malignant transformation and metastasis. These studies have yielded a working model in which cancer acquisition and progression is believed to result from a series of successive mutations that destabilize the genome and permit unregulated cell growth, which, in turn, elicit further alterations in the surrounding tissue that permit growth and invasion (see Chap. 5). These genetic alterations may arise directly or indirectly from inherited gene mutations, chemical- or radiation-induced DNA damage and genetic instability, incorporation of certain viruses into the cell, or random errors during DNA synthesis (see Chaps. 3 and 15). The behavior of cancer cells is also determined by epigenetic modifications that influence the expression of genes, and which contribute to more transient changes in properties of cancer cells, including those that convey resistance to therapy (see Chap. 2).

Cancer treatment has evolved to employ a combination of traditional approaches, such as surgery, chemotherapy, and radiotherapy, increasingly in conjunction with each other and with drugs that target specific biological networks (see Chaps. 15–20). Some successful targeted biological therapies already in clinical use include the treatment of chronic myelogenous leukemia with a specific, competitive inhibitor (imatinib) of the binding site of the Bcr-Abl protein kinase, the protein that is aberrantly expressed as a result of the Philadelphia chromosome translocation. Another example is trastuzumab, a monoclonal antibody that recognizes the HER2/neu receptor expressed on the tumor cells of some patients with aggressive breast cancer; treatment with this agent has been shown to improve quality and duration of survival. A third example is vemurafenib, which improves survival by inhibiting the BRAF kinase in the approximately 50% of human melanomas that have a BRAF mutation. Although these therapies have improved outcome for patients, tumor cells can become resistant to them; for example, resistance to imatinib develops as a result of outgrowth of tumor cells bearing a drug-resistant mutation within Bcr-Abl, and resistance of metastatic disease to other targeted agents develops invariably after a few months of therapy. Thus, as with more traditional approaches, a combinatorial approach to cancer treatment is most likely to be successful, although combinations of targeted therapies have in some instances proven to be more toxic.

Traditional methods have also undergone substantial refinement and improvement. New methods for delivery of radiotherapy, such as image-guided and intensity-modulated radiotherapy and stereotactic body radiotherapy, have allowed higher doses to be delivered to the tumor with increased precision and at the same time, lower doses to normal tissue. These techniques have improved local control of primary tumors, such as those in the prostate and brain, and new combinations of radiation with surgery and chemotherapy are also improving patient survival. One instrument, called the Cyber-knife, is an example of stereotactic precision radiotherapy, which is already in use in cancer centers around the world, and is able to deliver a highly focused beam of irradiation (in 3 dimensions) to tumors in the brain. Development of these techniques has paralleled that of enhanced methods of imaging tumors in the body with high resolution including CT, MRI, and positron emission tomography (PET) (see Chap. 14).

1.3 THE FUTURE OF ONCOLOGY AND CANCER TREATMENT

The recent ability to sequence the DNA and RNA of cancer and normal tissue genomes has provided insights into the molecular signals that are associated with various types of cancers. Molecular profiling of key oncogenic factors has allowed many types of cancers to be subdivided into subcategories and is being validated for use in defining better treatments for subpopulations of patients to optimize survival (see Chaps. 2 and 22). For example, a breast tumor is now defined not just by "stage" (size of the primary tumor, and whether it has spread to lymph nodes) and grade (the extent to which it differs from normal breast tissue), but whether the tumor is estrogen-responsive (eg, estrogen receptor or ER-positive or ER-negative) and whether it expresses HER-2 (see Chap. 20). These data enable the clinician to recommend treatment with agents that inhibit stimulation of growth by estrogens (tamoxifen or aromatase inhibitors) and by agents such as trastuzumab (which targets the HER-2 receptor). More recently, larger scale genomic profiling with Oncotype DX or the "Amsterdam" 70-gene signature are aimed at defining patients whose outcome can be significantly improved by adjuvant chemotherapy, or those where it adds only toxicity and hormonal therapy should be instead used alone.

Another area where the last decade of research has shown considerable progress is immunotherapy (see Chap. 21). Research is leading to an understanding of how to promote an immune response against cancers as well as developing a detailed understanding of how the tumor microenvironment exerts a negative influence. Reagents have been developed that are directed against many molecules that have the potential to modulate immune responses and clinical trials have begun to demonstrate an impact in promoting patient survival. Novel immunotherapeutic approaches are starting to take their place in the cancer treatment armamentarium.

There is intense research in large cancer centers into "personalized medicine," where the goal is to provide treatment of an individual's cancer that will be tailored to the genetic profile of his or her cancer. The cost for sequencing an entire genome costs approximately $800 in 2012, and many genomes from tumor samples have been analyzed; however, the cancer genome is far more complex than many anticipated and still requires high costs for complex bioinformatic analysis in order to understand the results of such sequencing. For example, a recent study of the genomes of 100 breast cancer patients found that the genetic profiles of their cancers were extremely diverse and did not fit neatly into histopathological classifications (Stephens et al, 2012). Furthermore, the tumor microenvironment (eg, hypoxia) may further alter gene expression and tumor biology such that both microenvironmental and genetic heterogeneity may have to be addressed in providing a "true" state of an individual's cancer genome (see Chaps. 10 and 12). Also, several studies have confirmed that genetic sequencing of single cells or from small regions of primary cancers shows substantial heterogeneity. This implies that there is ongoing mutation of cancer cells after tumor induction, and that multiple targeted agents would be necessary to eradicate all of the cells within a tumor. Anecdotal instances have been reported in which an individual's tumor has been sequenced and the information used to obtain access to an early stage clinical drug. Although such patients may have a transient response, the inability to achieve a substantial extension in life span or quality of life may reflect the limitations of the early stage drug itself, or that we have much to learn about simplistically choosing a single therapy based on a cancer genotype.

A positive aspect arising from the sequencing of cancer genomes is the realization that each cancer may have an Achilles heel. In single-celled organisms, such as the budding yeast *Saccharomyces cerevisiae*, the concept of synthetic lethality is well established. This phenomenon is based on the observation that a mutation in a gene pathway "A," although not lethal on its own, becomes incompatible with survival when combined with another nonlethal mutation in a separate gene pathway "B." Because cancer genomes possess many mutations that differentiate them from surrounding normal tissue, it should be possible to exploit this unique complexity of the cancer cell. As one example, researchers discovered that mutations in *BRCA1* and *BRCA2* predispose cancer cells to cell death upon inhibition of members of the polyadenosine diphosphate (ADP) ribosyl polymerase (PARP) gene family (Farmer et al, 2005; see Chaps. 5 and 17). Treatment with PARP inhibitors elicits cell death with exquisite specificity in *BRCA*-deficient tumor cells, and several highly potent PARP inhibitors are now in clinical trial for *BRCA*-mutated ovarian cancers.

The notion of personalized medicine also raises several social and ethical questions. Should insurance companies have access (or be able to request) a person's genomic data? Will all people, regardless of socioeconomic status, have access to personalized medicine? Will people whose normal cells show a genetic predisposition to a particular cancer be subjected to prophylactic treatments, and is this option financially feasible? These are but a few of the many challenges that face our society in addition to the scientific challenges that remain to disentangle the tremendous complexity of cancer. In the face of this genetic complexity, it has become all the more important to pursue research into the fundamental principles of how cancer gene networks interact with one another and how they affect cell growth, signaling, and response to the environment. The goal of the chapters which follow is to provide a succinct but comprehensive summary of the basic science underlying oncology.

REFERENCES

Doll R, Hill AB. Smoking and carcinoma of the lung; preliminary report. *Br Med J* 1950; 2:739-748.

Farmer H, McCabe N, Lord CJ, et al. Targeting the DNA repair defect in BRCA mutant cells as a therapeutic strategy. *Nature* 2005;434:917-921.

Future II Study Group. Quadrivalent vaccine against human papillomavirus to prevent high-grade cervical lesions. *N Engl J Med* 2007;356:1915-1927.

Gerlinger M, Rowan AJ, Horswell S, et al. Intratumor heterogeneity and branched evolution revealed by multiregion sequencing. *N Engl J Med* 2012;366:883-892.

Luo Z, Ruan B. Impact of the implementation of a vaccination strategy on hepatitis B virus infections in China over a 20-year period. *Int J Infect Dis* 2012;16:e82-e88.

Stephens PJ, Tarpey PS, Davies H, et al. The landscape of cancer genes and mutational processes in breast cancer. *Nature* 2012;486:400-404.

Methods of Molecular Analysis

Anthony M. Joshua, Paul C. Boutros, and Thomas Kislinger

2.1 INTRODUCTION

Advances made over the last 10 years in understanding the biology of cancer have transformed the field of oncology. While genetic analysis was limited previously to gross chromosomal abnormalities in karyotypes, DNA in cells can now be analyzed to the individual base pair level. This intricate knowledge of the genetics of cancer increases the possibility that personalized treatment for individual cancers lies in the near future. To appreciate the relevance and nature of these technological advances, as well as their implications for function, an understanding of the modern tools of molecular

biology is essential. This chapter reviews the cytogenetic, nucleic, proteomic, and bioinformatics methods used to study the molecular basis of cancer, and highlights methods that are likely to affect in the future management of cancer.

2.2 PRINCIPAL TECHNIQUES FOR NUCLEIC ACID ANALYSIS

2.2.1 Cytogenetics and Karyotyping

Cancer arises as a result of the stepwise accumulation of genetic changes that confer a selective growth advantage to the involved cells (see Chap. 5, Sec. 5.2). These changes may consist of abnormalities in specific genes (such as amplification of oncogenes or deletion of tumor-suppressor genes). Although molecular techniques can identify specific DNA mutations, cytogenetics provides an overall description of chromosome number, structure, and the extent and nature of chromosomal abnormalities.

Several techniques can be used to obtain tumor cells for cytogenetic analysis. Leukemias and lymphomas from peripheral blood, bone marrow, or lymph node biopsies are easily dispersed into single cells suitable for chromosomal analysis. In contrast, cytogenetic analysis of solid tumors has several difficulties; the cells are tightly bound together and must be dispersed by mechanical means and/or by digestion with proteolytic enzymes (eg, collagenase) which can damage cells. Secondly, the mitotic index in solid tumors is often low (see Chap. 9, Sec. 9.2), making it difficult to find enough metaphase cells to obtain good-quality cytogenetic preparations. Finally, lymphoid and myeloid and other (normal) cells often infiltrate solid tumors and may be confused with the malignant cell population.

Chromosomes are usually examined in metaphase, when they become condensed and appear as 2 identical sister chromatids held together at the centromere as DNA replication has already occurred at that stage of mitosis. Exposure of the tumor cells to agents such as colcemid arrests them in metaphase by disrupting the mitotic spindle fibers that normally separate the chromatids. The cells are then swollen in a hypotonic solution, fixed in methanol-acetic acid, and metaphase "spreads" are prepared by physically dropping the fixed cells onto glass microscope slides.

Chromosomes can be recognized by their size and shape and by the pattern of light and dark "bands" observed after specific staining. The most popular way of generating banded chromosomes is proteolytic digestion with trypsin, followed by a Giemsa stain. A typical metaphase spread prepared using conventional methods has approximately 550 bands, whereas cells spread at prophase can have more than 800 bands; these bands can be analyzed using bright-field microscopy and digital photography. The result of cytogenetic analysis is a karyotype, which, in written form, describes the chromosomal abnormalities using the international consensus cytogenetic nomenclature (Brothman et al, 2009; see Fig. 2–1 and Table 2–1). Table 2–2 lists common chromosomal abnormalities in lymphoid and myeloid malignancies.

The study of solid tumors has been facilitated by new analytic approaches that combine elements of conventional cytogenetics with molecular methodologies. This new hybrid discipline is called *molecular cytogenetics,* and its application to tumor analysis usually involves the use of techniques based on *fluorescence in situ hybridization* or FISH (see Sec. 2.2.6).

2.2.2 Hybridization and Nucleic Acid Probes

DNA is composed of 2 complementary strands (the sense strand and the non-sense strand) of specific sequences of

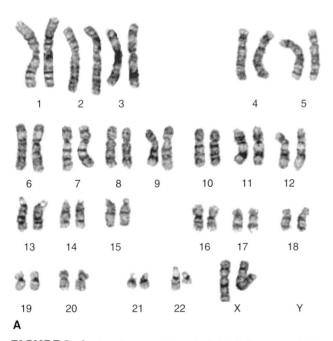

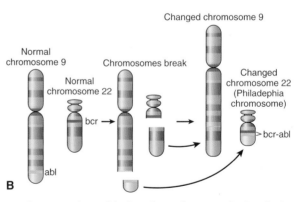

A   **B**

FIGURE 2–1   **The photograph on the left (A) shows a typical karyotype from a patient with chronic myelogenous leukemia.** By international agreement, the chromosomes are numbered according to their appearance following G-banding. Note the loss of material from the long arm of one copy of the chromosome 22 pair (*the chromosome on the right*) and its addition to the long arm of 1 copy of chromosome 9 (*also the chromosome on the right of the pair*). **B)** A schematic illustration of the accepted band pattern for this rearrangement. The green and red lines indicate the precise position of the break points that are involved. The karyotypic nomenclature for this particular chromosomal abnormality is t(9;22)(q34;q11). This description means that there is a reciprocal translocation between chromosomes 9 and 22 with break points at q34 on chromosome 9 and q11 on chromosome 22. The rearranged chromosome 22 is sometimes called the Philadelphia chromosome (or Ph chromosome), after the city of its discovery.

TABLE 2-1 Nomenclature for chromosomes and their abnormalities.

Description	Meaning
−1	Loss of one chromosome 1
+7	Gain of extra chromosome 7
2q⁻ or del (2q)	Deletion of part of long arm of chromosome 2
4p⁺	Addition of material to short arm of chromosome 4
t(9;22)(q34;q11)	Reciprocal translocation between chromosomes 9 and 22 with break points at q34 on chromosome 9 and q11 on chromosome 22
iso(6p)	Isochromosome with both arms derived from the short arm of chromosome 6
inv(16)(p13q22)	Part of chromosome 16 between p13 and q22 is inverted

4 nucleotide bases that make up the genetic alphabet. The association (via hydrogen bonds) between 2 bases on opposite complementary DNA or certain types of RNA strands that are connected via hydrogen bonds is called a *base pair* (often abbreviated bp). In the canonical Watson-Crick DNA base pair, adenine (A) forms a base pair with thymine (T) and guanine (G) forms a base pair with cytosine (C). In RNA, thymine is replaced by uracil (U). There are 2 processes that rely on this base pairing (Fig. 2–2). As DNA replicates during the S phase of the cell cycle, a part of the helical DNA molecule unwinds and the strands separate under the action of topoisomerase II (see Chap. 18, Fig. 18–13). DNA polymerase enzymes add nucleotides to the 3′-hydroxyl (3′-OH) end of an oligonucleotide that is hybridized to a template, thus leading to synthesis of a complementary new strand of DNA. Transcription of messenger RNA (mRNA) takes place through an analogous process under the action of RNA polymerase with one of the DNA strands (the non-sense strand) acting as a template; complementary bases (U, G, C, and A) are added to the mRNA through pairing with bases in the DNA strand so that the sequence of bases in the RNA is the same as in the "sense" strand of the DNA (except that U replaces T). During this process the DNA strand is separated temporarily from its partner through the action of topoisomerase I (see Chap. 18, Sec. 18.4). Only parts of the DNA in each gene are translated into polypeptides, and these coding regions are known as exons; non-coding regions (introns) are interspersed throughout the genes and are spliced out of the mRNA transcript during the RNA maturation process and before protein synthesis. Synthesis of polypeptides, the building blocks of proteins, are then directed by the mRNA in association with ribosomes, with each triplet of bases in the exons of the DNA encoding a specific amino acid that is added to the polypeptide chain.

To develop an understanding of the techniques now used in both clinical cancer care and research, it is necessary to understand the specificity of hybridization and the action and fidelity of DNA polymerases. When double-stranded DNA is heated, the complementary strands separate (denature) to

TABLE 2-2 Common chromosomal abnormalities in lymphoid and myeloid malignancies.

Malignancy	Chromosomal Aberration*	Molecular Lesion
Acute myeloid leukemia (AML)		
M1, M2 subtypes	t(8;21)(q22;q22)	*AML1-MTG8* fusion
M3 subtype	t(15;17)(q22;q11.2)	*PML-RARA* fusion
M4Eo subtype	inv(16)(p13;q22) or t(16;16)(p13;q22)	*MYH11-CBFB* fusion
M2 or M4 subtypes	t(6;9)(p23;q24)	*DEK-CAN* fusion
Therapy-related AML	~5/del(5q), ~7/del(7q)	
Chronic myeloid leukemia (CML)	t(9;22)(q34;q11) (Ph¹ chromosome)	*BCR-ABL* fusion encoding p210 protein
CML blast crisis	t(9;22)(q34;q11), 8, +Ph¹, 19, or i(17q)	*BCR-ABL* fusion encoding p210 protein, *TP53* mutation
Acute lymphocytic leukemia (ALL)	t(9;22)(q34;q11)	*BCR-ABL* fusion encoding p190 protein
Pre-B ALL	t(1;19)(q23;p13.3)	*E2A-PBX1* fusion
Pre-B ALL	t(17;19)(q22;p13.3)	*E2A-HLF* fusion
B-ALL, Burkitt lymphoma	t(8;14)(q24;q32) t(2;8)(p12;q24) t(8;22)(q24;q11)	Translocations between *myc* and *IgH, IgLκ* and *IgLλ* loci
B-Chronic lymphocytic leukemia	+12,t(14q32)	Translocations of *IgH* locus

*For an interpretation of the nomenclature of chromosomal rearrangements, see Table 2–1.

Source: Adapted from Sheer and Squire (1996).

form single-stranded DNA. Given suitable conditions, separated complementary regions of specific DNA sequences can join together to reform a double-stranded molecule. This renaturation process is called *hybridization.* This ability of single-stranded nucleic acids to hybridize with their complementary sequence is fundamental to the majority of techniques used in molecular genetic analysis. Using an appropriate reaction mixture containing the relevant nucleotides and DNA or RNA polymerase, a specific piece of DNA can be copied or transcribed. If radiolabeled or fluorescently labeled nucleotides are included in a reaction mixture, the complementary copy of the template can be used as a highly sensitive hybridization-dependent probe.

2.2.3 Restriction Enzymes and Manipulation of Genes

Restriction enzymes are endonucleases that have the ability to cut DNA only at sites of specific nucleotide sequences and always cut the DNA at exactly the same place within the designated sequence. Figure 2–3 illustrates some commonly used restriction enzymes together with the sequence of nucleotides that they recognize and the position at which they cut the sequence. Restriction enzymes are important because they allow DNA to be cut into reproducible segments that can be analyzed precisely. An important feature of many restriction enzymes is that they create sticky ends. These ends occur because the DNA is cut in a different place on the 2 strands. When the DNA molecule separates, the cut end has a small single-stranded portion that can hybridize to other fragments having compatible sequences (ie, fragments digested using the same restriction enzyme) thus allowing investigators to cut and paste pieces of DNA together.

Once a gene has been identified, the DNA segment of interest can be inserted into a bacterial virus or plasmid to facilitate its manipulation and propagation using restriction enzymes. A complementary DNA strand (cDNA) is first synthesized using mRNA as the template by a reverse transcriptase enzyme. This cDNA contains only the exons of the gene from which the mRNA was transcribed. Figure 2–4 presents a schematic of how a restriction fragment of DNA containing the coding sequence of a gene can be inserted into a bacterial plasmid conferring resistance against the drug ampicillin to the host bacterium. The plasmid or virus is referred to as a *vector* carrying the passenger DNA sequence of the gene of interest. The vector DNA is cut with the same restriction enzyme used to prepare the cloned gene, so that all the fragments will have compatible sticky ends and can be spliced back together. The spliced fragments can be sealed with the enzyme DNA ligase, and the reconstituted molecule can be introduced into bacterial cells. Because bacteria that take up the plasmid are resistant to the drug (eg, ampicillin), they can be isolated and propagated to large numbers. In this way, large quantities of a gene can be obtained (ie, cloned) and labeled with either radioactivity or biotin for use as a DNA probe for analysis in Southern or northern blots (see Sec. 2.2.4). Cloned DNA can

be used directly for nucleotide sequencing (see Sec. 2.2.10), or for transfer into other cells. Alternatively, the starting DNA may be a complex mixture of different restriction fragments derived from human cells. Such a mixture could contain enough DNA so that the entire human genome is represented in the passenger DNA inserted into the vectors. When a large number of different DNA fragments have been inserted into a vector population and then introduced into bacteria, the result is a *DNA library,* which can be plated out and screened by hybridization with a specific probe. In this way an individual *recombinant DNA clone* can be isolated from the library and used for most of the other applications described in the following sections.

2.2.4 Blotting Techniques

Southern blotting is a method for analyzing the structure of DNA (named after the scientist who developed it). Figure 2–5 outlines schematically the Southern blot technique. The DNA to be analyzed is cut into defined lengths using a restriction enzyme, and the fragments are separated by electrophoresis through an agarose gel. Under these conditions the DNA fragments are separated based on size, with the smallest fragments migrating farthest in the gel and the largest remaining near the origin. Pieces of DNA of known size are electrophoresed at the same time (in a separately loaded well) and act as a molecular mass marker. A piece of nylon membrane is then laid on top of the gel and a vacuum is applied to draw the DNA through the gel into the membrane, where it is immobilized. A common application of the Southern technique is to determine the size of the fragment of DNA that carries a particular gene. The nylon membrane containing all the fragments of DNA cut with a restriction enzyme is incubated in a solution containing a radioactive or fluorescently-labeled probe which is complementary to part of the gene (see Sec. 2.2.2). Under these conditions, the probe will anneal with homologous DNA sequences present on the DNA in the membrane. After gentle washing to remove the single-stranded, unbound probe, the only labeled probe remaining on the membrane will be bound to homologous sequences of the gene of interest. The location of the gene on the nylon membrane can then be detected either by the fluorescence or radioactivity associated with the probe. An almost identical procedure can be used to characterize mRNA separated by electrophoresis and transferred to a nylon membrane. The technique is called northern blotting and is used to evaluate the expression patterns of genes. An analogous procedure, called western blotting, is used to characterize proteins. Following separation by denaturing gel electrophoresis, the proteins are immobilized by transfer to a charged synthetic membrane. To identify specific proteins, the membrane is incubated in a solution containing a specific primary antibody either directly labeled with a fluorophore, or incubated with a secondary antibody that will bind to the primary antibody and is conjugated to horseradish peroxidase (HRP) or biotin. The primary antibody will

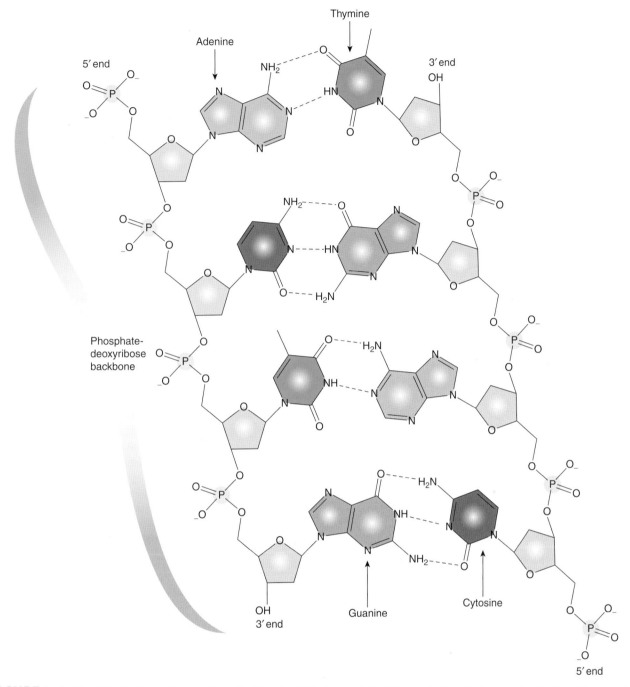

FIGURE 2–2 The DNA duplex molecule, also called the *double helix*, consists of 2 strands that wind around each other. The strands are held together by chemical attraction of the bases that comprise the DNA. A bonds to T and G bonds to C. The bases are linked together to form long strands by a "backbone" chemical structure. The DNA bases and backbone twist around to form a duplex spiral.

bind only to the region of the membrane containing the protein of interest and can be detected either directly by its fluorescence or by exposure to chemoluminescence detection reagents.

2.2.5 The Polymerase Chain Reaction

The polymerase chain reaction (PCR) allows rapid production of large quantities of specific pieces of DNA (usually about 200 to 1000 base pairs) using a DNA polymerase enzyme called *Taq* polymerase (which is isolated from a thermophilic bacterial species and is thus resistant to denaturation at high temperatures). Specific oligonucleotide primers complementary to the DNA at each end of (flanking) the region of interest are synthesized or obtained commercially, and are used as primers for *Taq* polymerase. All components of the reaction (the target DNA, primers, deoxynucleotides, and *Taq* polymerase) are placed in a small tube and

Enzyme

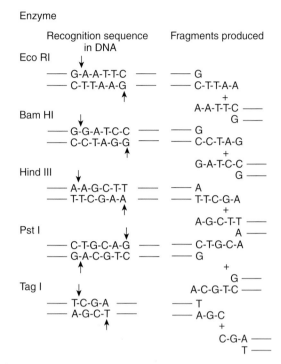

FIGURE 2–3 **The nucleotide sequences recognized by 5 different restriction endonucleases are shown.** On the left side, the sequence recognized by the enzyme is shown; the sites where the enzymes cut the DNA are shown by the arrows. On the right side, the 2 fragments produced following digestion with that restriction enzyme are shown. Note that each recognition sequence is a palindrome; ie, the first 2 or 3 bases are complementary to the last 2 or 3 bases. For example, for Eco R1, GAA is complementary to TTC. Also note that following digestion, each fragment has a single-stranded tail of DNA. This tail is useful in allowing fragments that contain complementary overhangs to anneal with each other.

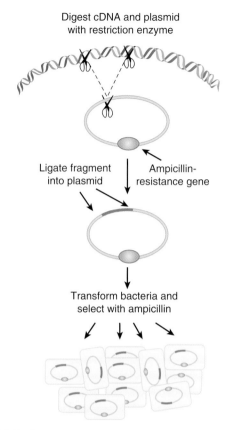

FIGURE 2–4 **Insertion of a gene into a bacterial plasmid.** The cDNA of interest (*pink line*) is digested with a restriction endonuclease (depicted by *scissors*) to generate a defined fragment of cDNA with "sticky ends." The circular plasmid DNA is cut with the same restriction endonuclease to generate single-stranded ends that will hybridize and to the cDNA fragment. The recombinant DNA plasmid can be selected for growth using antibiotics because the ampicillin-resistance gene (*hatched*) is included in the construct. In this way, large amounts of the human cDNA can be obtained for further purposes (eg, for use as a probe on a Southern blot).

the reaction sequence is accomplished by simply changing the temperature of the reaction mixture in a cyclical manner (Fig. 2–6*A*). A typical PCR reaction would involve: (a) Incubation at 94°C to denature (separate) the DNA duplex and create single-stranded DNA. (b) Incubation at 53°C to allow hybridization of the primers, which are in vast excess (this temperature may vary depending on the sequence of the primers). (c) Incubation at 72°C to allow *Taq* polymerase to synthesize new DNA from the primers. Repeating this cycle permits another round of amplification (Fig. 2–6*B*). Each cycle takes only a few minutes. Twenty cycles can theoretically produce a million-fold amplification of the DNA of interest. PCR products can then be sequenced or subjected to other methods of genetic analysis. Polymerase proteins with greater heat stability and copying fidelity can allow for long-range amplification using primers separated by as much as 15 to 30 kilobases of intervening target DNA (Ausubel and Waggoner, 2003). The PCR is exquisitely sensitive and its applications include the detection of minimal residual disease in hematopoietic malignancies and of circulating cancer cells from solid tumors.

PCR is widely used to study gene expression or screen for mutations in RNA. Reverse transcriptase is used to make a single-strand cDNA copy of an mRNA and the cDNA is used as a template for a PCR reaction as described above. This technique allows amplification of cDNA corresponding to both abundant and rare RNA transcripts. The development of real-time quantitative PCR has allowed improved quantitation of the DNA (or cDNA) template and has proven to be a sensitive method to detect low levels of mRNA (often obtained from small samples or microdissected tissues) and to quantify gene expression. Different chemistries are available for real time detection (Fig. 2–6*C, D*). There is a very specific 5′ nuclease assay, which uses a fluorogenic probe for the detection of reaction products after amplification, and there is a less specific but much less expensive assay, which uses a fluorescent dye (SYBR Green I) for the detection of double-stranded DNA products. In both methods, the fluorescence emission from each sample is collected by a charge-coupled device camera and the data

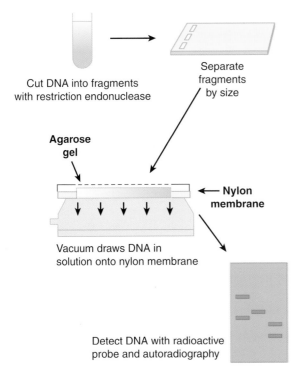

Cut DNA into fragments
with restriction endonuclease

Separate
fragments
by size

**Agarose
gel**

← **Nylon
membrane**

Vacuum draws DNA in
solution onto nylon membrane

Detect DNA with radioactive
probe and autoradiography

FIGURE 2–5 **Analysis of DNA by Southern blotting.** Schematic outline of the procedures involved in analyzing DNA fragments by the Southern blotting technique. The method is described in more detail in the text.

are automatically processed and analyzed by computer software. Quantitative real-time PCR using fluorogenic probes can analyze multiple genes simultaneously within the same reaction. The SYBR Green methodology involves individual analysis of each gene of interest but, using multiwell plates, both approaches provide high-throughput sample analysis with no need for post-PCR processing or gels.

2.2.6 Fluorescence in Situ Hybridization

To perform fluorescence in situ hybridization (FISH), DNA probes specific for a gene or particular chromosome region are labeled (usually by incorporation of biotin, digoxigenin, or directly with a fluorochrome) and then hybridized to (denatured) metaphase chromosomes. The DNA probe will reanneal to the denatured DNA at its precise location on the chromosome. After washing away the unbound probe, the hybridized sequences are detected using avidin directly (which binds strongly to biotin), or antibodies to digoxigenin that are coupled to fluorescent secondary antibodies, such as fluorescein isothiocyanate. The sites of hybridization are then detected using fluorescent microscopy. The main advantage of FISH for gene analyses is that information is obtained directly about the positions of the probes in relation to chromosome bands or to other previously or simultaneously mapped reference probes.

FISH can be performed on interphase nuclei from paraffin-embedded tumor biopsies or cultured tumor cells, which allows cytogenetic aberrations such as amplifications, deletions or other abnormalities of whole chromosomes to be visualized without the need for obtaining good-quality metaphase preparations. For example, FISH is a standard technique to determine the HER2 status of breast cancers and can be used to detect N-*myc* amplification in neuroblastoma (Fig. 2–7). Whole chromosome abnormalities can also be detected using specific centromere probes that lead to 2 signals from normal nuclei, 1 signal when there is only 1 copy of the chromosome (monosomy), or 3 signals when there is an extra copy (trisomy). Chromosome or gene deletions can also be detected with probes from the relevant regions. For example, if the probes used for FISH are close to specific translocation break points on different chromosomes, they will appear joined as a result of the translocation generating a "color fusion" signal or conversely, alternative probes can be designed to "break apart" in the event of a specific gene deletion or translocation. This technique is particularly useful for the detection of the *bcr-abl* rearrangement in chronic myeloid leukemia (Fig. 2–8) and the *tmprss2-erg* abnormalities in prostate cancer (Fig. 2–9).

2.2.7 Comparative Genomic Hybridization

If the cytogenetic abnormalities are unknown, it is not possible to select a suitable probe to clarify the abnormalities by FISH. *Comparative genomic hybridization* (CGH) has been developed to produce a detailed map of the differences between chromosomes in different cells by detecting increases (amplifications) or decreases (deletions) of segments of DNA.

For analysis of tumors by CGH, the DNA from malignant and normal cells is labeled with 2 different fluorochromes and then hybridized simultaneously to *normal* chromosome metaphase spreads. For example, tumor DNA is labeled with biotin and detected with fluorescein (green fluorescence) while the control DNA is labeled with digoxigenin and detected with rhodamine (red fluorescence). Regions of gain or loss of DNA, such as deletions, duplications, or amplifications, are seen as changes in the ratio of the intensities of the 2 fluorochromes along the target chromosomes. One disadvantage of CGH is that it can detect only large blocks (>5 Mb) of over- or underrepresented chromosomal DNA and balanced rearrangements (such as inversions or translocations) can escape detection. Improvements to the original CGH technique have used microarrays where CGH is applied to arrayed sequences of DNA bound to glass slides. The arrays are constructed using genomic clones of various types such as bacterial artificial chromosomes (a DNA construct that can be used to carry 150 to 350 kbp [kilobase pairs] of normal DNA) or synthetic oligonucleotides that are spaced across the entire genome. This technique has allowed the detection of genetic aberrations of smaller magnitude than was possible using metaphase chromosomes, although they have now been superseded by high density single-nucleotide polymorphism (SNP) arrays (see below).

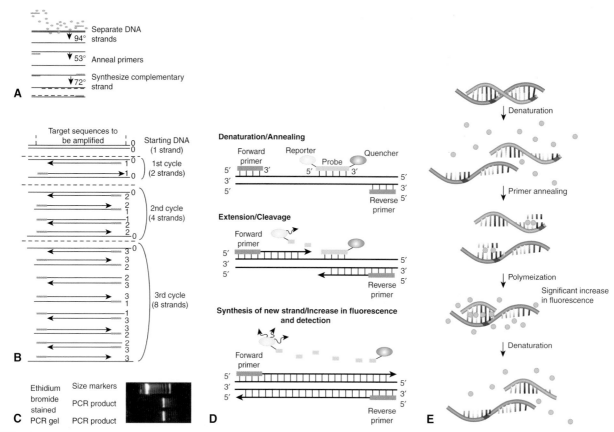

FIGURE 2–6 **A) Reaction sequence for 1 cycle of PCR.** Each line represents 1 strand of DNA; the small rectangles are primers and the circles are nucleotides. **B)** The first 3 cycles of PCR are shown schematically. **C)** Ethidium bromide-stained gel after 20 cycles of PCR. See text for further explanation. **D)** Real-time PCR using SYBR Green dye. SYBR Green dye binds preferentially to double-stranded DNA; therefore, an increase in the concentration of a double-stranded DNA product leads to an increase in fluorescence. During the polymerization step, several molecules of the dye bind to the newly synthesized DNA and a significant increase in fluorescence is detected and can be monitored in real time. **E)** Real-time PCR using fluorescent dyes and molecular beacons. During denaturation, both probe and primers are in solution and remain unbound from the DNA strand. During annealing, the probe specifically hybridizes to the target DNA between the primers (*top panel*) and the 5′-to-3′ exonuclease activity of the DNA polymerase cleaves the probe, thus dissociating the quencher molecule from the reporter molecule, which results in fluorescence of the reporters.

2.2.8 Spectral Karyotyping/Multifluor Fluorescence in Situ Hybridization

A deficiency of both array CGH and conventional cDNA microarrays is the lack of information about structural changes within the karyotype. For example, with an expression array, a particular gene may be overexpressed but it would be unclear whether this is secondary to a translocation placing the gene next to a strong promoter or an amplification. Universal chromosome painting techniques have been developed to assist in this determination with which it is possible to analyze all chromosomes simultaneously. Two commonly used techniques, spectral karyotyping (SKY) (Veldman et al, 1997) and multifluor fluorescence in situ hybridization (M-FISH) (Speicher et al, 1996), are based on the differential display of colored fluorescent chromosome-specific paints, which provide a complete analysis of the chromosomal complement in a given cell. Using this combination of 23 different colored paints as a "cocktail probe,"

subtle differences in fluorochrome labeling of chromosomes after hybridization allows a computer to assign a unique color to each chromosome pair. Abnormal chromosomes can be identified by the pattern of color distribution along them with chromosomal rearrangements leading to a distinct transition from one color to another at the position of the breakpoint (Fig. 2–10). In contrast to CGH, detection of such karyotype rearrangements using SKY and M-FISH is not dependent upon change in copy number. This technology is particularly suited to solid tumors where the complexity of the karyotypes may mask the presence of chromosomal aberrations.

2.2.9 Single-Nucleotide Polymorphisms

DNA sequences can differ at single nucleotide positions within the genome. These SNPs can occur as frequently as 1 in every 1000 base pairs and can occur in both introns and exons. In introns they generally have little effect, but in exons they can affect protein structure and function. For example, SNPs may

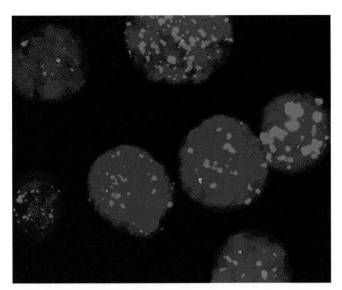

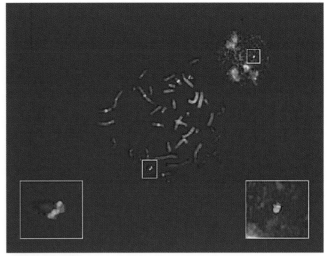

A

FIGURE 2–7 **MYCN amplification in nuclei from neuroblastoma detected by FISH with a MYCN probe (magenta speckling) and a deletion of the short arm of chromosome 1.** The signal (pale blue-green) from the remaining chromosome 1 is seen as a single spot in each nucleus.

be involved in altered drug metabolism because of their modifying effect on the cytochrome P450 metabolizing enzymes. They also contribute to disease (eg, SNPs that result in missense mutations) and disease predisposition. Most early methods to characterize SNPs required PCR amplification of the sample to be genotyped prior to sequence analysis; modern

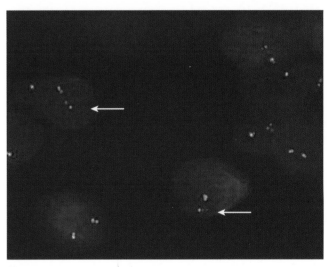

B

FIGURE 2–9 **FISH analysis showing rearrangement of TMPRSS2 and ERG genes in PCa. A)** FISH confirms the colocalization of Oregon Green-labeled 5 V ERG (*green signals*), AlexaFluor 594-labeled 3 V ERG (*red signals*), and Pacific Blue-labeled TMPRSS2 (*light blue signals*) in normal peripheral lymphocyte metaphase cells and in normal interphase cells. **B)** In PCa cells, break-apart FISH results in a split of the colocalized 5 V green/3 V red signals, in addition to a fused signal (comprising green, red, and blue signals) of the unaffected chromosome 21. Using the TMPRSS2/ERG set of probes on PCa frozen sections, TMPRSS2 (*blue signal*) remains juxtaposed to ERG 3 V (*red signal*; see *white arrows*), whereas colocalized 5 V ERG signal (*green*) is lost, indicating the presence of TMPRSS2/ERG fusion and concomitant deletion of 5 V ERG region. (Reproduced with permission from Yoshimoto et al, 2006.)

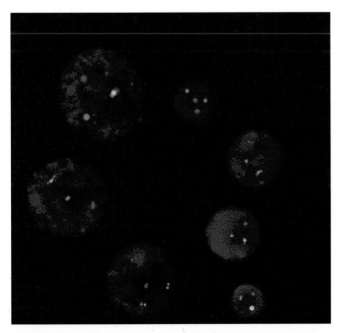

FIGURE 2–8 **Detection of the Philadelphia chromosome in interphase nuclei of leukemia cells.** All nuclei contain 1 green signal (BCR gene), 1 pink signal (ABL gene), and an intermediate fusion yellow signal because of the 9:22 chromosome translocation.

methods of gene sequencing and array analyses, however, have largely replaced this older technique. One application of SNPs in cancer medicine has been the use of SNP arrays in genomic analyses. These DNA microarrays, use tiled SNP probes to some of the 50 million SNPs in the human genome to interrogate genomic architecture. For example, SNP arrays can be

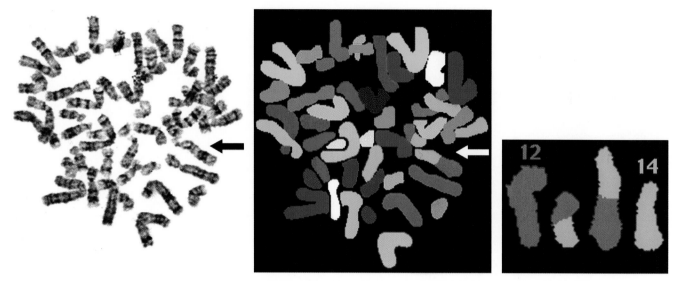

FIGURE 2–10 SKY and downstream analyses of a patient with a translocation. One of the aberrant chromosomes can initially be seen with G banding, the same metaphase spread has been subjected to SKY and then a 12;14 reciprocal translocation is identified.

used to study such phenomena as loss of heterozygosity (LOH) and amplifications. Indeed, the particular advantage of SNP arrays is that they can detect copy-neutral LOH (also known as uniparental disomy or gene conversion) whereby one allele or whole chromosome is missing and the other allele is duplicated with potential pathological consequences.

2.2.10 Sequencing of DNA

To characterize the primary structure of genes, and thus of the potential repertoire of proteins that they encode, it is necessary to determine the sequence of their DNA. Sanger sequencing (the classical method) relied on oligonucleotide primer extension and dideoxy-chain termination (dideoxy-nucleotides (ddNTPs) lack the 3′-OH group required for the phosphodiester bond between 2 nucleosides). DNA sequencing was carried out in 4 separate reactions each containing 1 of the 4 ddNTPs (ie, ddATP, ddCTP, ddGTP, or ddTTP) together with ddNTPs. In each reaction, the same primer was used to ensure DNA synthesis began at the same nucleotide. The extended primers therefore terminated at different sites whenever a specific ddNTP was incorporated. This method produced fragments of different sizes terminating at different 3′ nucleotides. The newly synthesized and labeled DNA fragments were heat-denatured, and then separated by size with gel electrophoresis and with each of the 4 reactions in individual adjacent lanes (lanes A, T, G, C); the DNA bands were then visualized by autoradiography or UV light, and the DNA sequence could be directly interpreted from the x-ray film or gel image (Fig. 2–11). Using this method it was possible to obtain a sequence of 200 to 500 bases in length from a single gel. The next development was automated Sanger sequencing which involved the development of fluorescently labeled-primers (dye primers) and –ddNTPs (dye terminators). With

the automated procedures the reactions are performed in a single tube containing all 4 ddNTPs, each labeled with a different fluorescent dye. Since the four dyes fluoresce at different wavelengths, a laser then reads the gel to determine the identity of each band according to the wavelengths at which it fluoresces. The results are then depicted in the form of a chromatogram, which is a diagram of colored peaks that correspond to the nucleotide in that location in the sequence. Then sequencing analysis software interprets the results, identifying the bases from the fluorescent intensities (Fig. 2–12).

So-called next-generation sequencing (NGS) uses a variety of approaches to automate the sequencing process by creating micro-PCR reactors and/or attaching the DNA molecules to be sequenced to solid surfaces or beads, allowing for millions of sequencing events to occur simultaneously. Although the analyzed sequences are generally much shorter (~21 to ~400 base pairs) than in previous sequencing technologies, they can be counted and quantified, allowing for the identification of mutations in a small subpopulation of cells which is part of a larger population with wild-type sequences. The recent introduction of approaches that allow for sequencing of both ends of a DNA molecule (ie, paired end massively parallel sequencing or mate-pair sequencing), make it possible to detect balanced and unbalanced somatic rearrangements (eg, fusion genes) in a genome-wide fashion.

There are several types of NGS machines in routine use that fall into 4 methodological categories; (a) Roche/454, Life/APG, (b) Illumina/Solexa, (c) Ion Torrent, and (d) Pacific Biosciences. It is beyond the scope of this chapter to describe these in detail or to foreshadow developing technologies, but an overview of the key differences is provided below.

Each technology includes a number of steps grouped as (a) template preparation, (b) sequencing/imaging, and (c) data analysis. Initially, all methods involve randomly

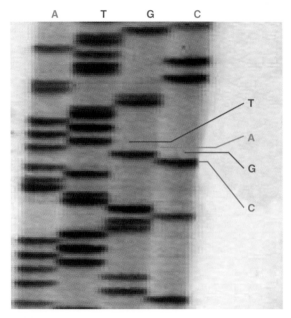

FIGURE 2–11 **Dideoxy-chain termination sequencing showing an extension reaction to read the position of the nucleotide guanidine (see text for details).** (Courtesy of Lilly Noble, University of Toronto, Toronto.)

breaking genomic DNA into small sizes from which either fragment templates (randomly sheared DNA usually <1 kbp in size) or mate-pair templates (linear DNA fragments originating from circularized sheared DNA of a particular size) are created.

There are 2 types of template preparation: clonally amplified templates and single-molecule templates. Clonally amplified templates rely on PCR techniques to amplify the DNA so that fluorescence is detectable when fluorescently labeled nucleotides are added. Emulsion PCR (Fig. 2–13) is used to prepare a library of fragment or mate-pair targets and then adaptors (short DNA segments) containing universal priming sites are ligated to the target ends, allowing complex genomes to be amplified with common PCR primers. After ligation, the DNA is separated into single strands and captured onto beads under conditions that favor 1 DNA molecule per bead. After the successful amplification of DNA, millions of molecules can be chemically cross-linked to an amino-coated glass surface (Life/APG; Ion Torrent) or deposited into individual PicoTiterPlate (PTP) wells (Roche/454). Solid-phase amplification (Fig. 2–14) used in the Illumina/Solexa platform produces randomly distributed, clonally amplified clusters from fragment or mate-pair templates on a glass slide. High-density forward and reverse primers are covalently attached to the slide and the DNA segments of interest and the ratio of the

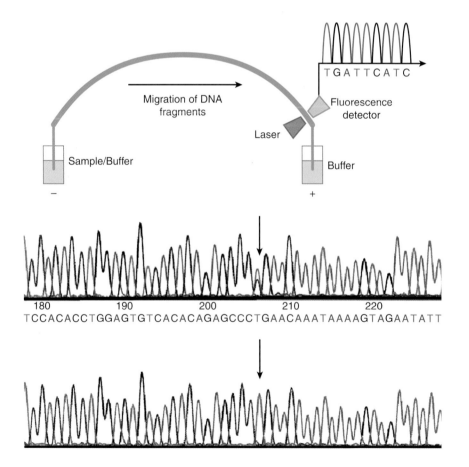

FIGURE 2–12 **Outline of automated sequencing and thereafter automated sequencing of *BRCA2*, the hereditary breast cancer predisposition gene.** Each colored peak represents a different nucleotide. The lower panel is the sequence of the wild-type DNA sample. The sequence of the mutation carrier in the upper panel contains a double peak (indicated by an *arrow*) in which nucleotide T in intron 17 located 2 bp downstream of the 5′ end of exon 18 is converted to a C. The mutation results in aberrant splicing of exon 18 of the *BRCA2* gene. The presence of the T nucleotide, in addition to the mutant C, implies that only 1 copy of the 2 *BRCA2* genes is mutated in this sample.

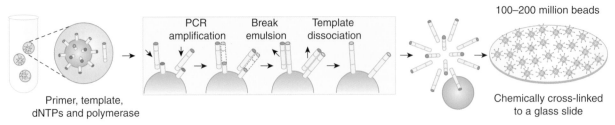

FIGURE 2–13 In emulsion PCR (emPCR), a reaction mixture is generated compromising an oil–aqueous emulsion to encapsulate bead–DNA complexes into single aqueous droplets. PCR amplification is subsequently carried out in these droplets to create beads containing thousands of copies of the same template sequence. EmPCR beads can then be chemically attached to a glass slide or a reaction plate. (From Metzker, 2010.)

primers to the template on the support define the surface density of the amplified clusters. These primers can also provide free ends to which a universal primer can be hybridized to initiate the NGS reaction.

In general, the preparation of single-molecule templates is more straightforward and requires less starting material (<1 μg) than emulsion PCR or solid-phase amplification. More importantly, these methods do not require PCR, which may create mutations and bias in amplified templates and regions. A variant of this (Pacific Biosciences; see below) uses spatially distributed single-polymerase molecules that are attached to a solid support that analyze circularized sheared DNA selected for a given size, such as 2 kbp, to which primed template molecules are bound.

Cyclic reversible termination (CRT) is currently used in the Illumina/Solexa platform. CRT uses reversible terminators in a cyclic method that comprises nucleotide incorporation, fluorescence imaging and cleavage. In the first step, a DNA polymerase, bound to the primed template, adds or incorporates only 1 fluorescently modified nucleotide, complementary to the template base. DNA synthesis is then terminated. Following incorporation, the remaining unincorporated nucleotides are washed away. Imaging is then performed to identify the incorporated nucleotide. This is followed by a cleavage step, which removes the terminating/inhibiting group and the fluorescent dye. Additional washing is performed before starting another incorporation step.

Another cyclic method is single-base ligation (SBL) used in the Life/APG platform, which uses a DNA ligase and either 1- or 2-base-encoded probes. In its simplest form, a fluorescently labeled probe hybridizes to its complementary sequence adjacent to the primed template. DNA ligase is then added which joins the dye-labeled probe to the primer. Nonligated probes are washed away, followed by fluorescence imaging to determine the identity of the ligated probe. The cycle can be repeated either by (a) using cleavable probes to remove the fluorescent dye and regenerate a 5′-PO4 group for subsequent ligation cycles or (b) by removing and hybridizing a new primer to the template.

Pyrosequencing (used in the Roche/454 platform) (Fig. 2–15) is a bioluminescence method that measures the incorporation of nucleotides by the release of inorganic pyrophosphate by proportionally converting it into visible light using serial enzymatic reactions. Following loading of the DNA-amplified beads into individual PTP wells, additional smaller beads, which are coupled with sulphurylase and luciferase are added. Nucleotides are then flowed sequentially in a fixed order across the PTP device. If a nucleotide complementary to the template strand appears, the polymerase extends the existing DNA strand by adding nucleotide(s). Addition of 1 (or more) nucleotide(s) results in a reaction that generates a light signal that is recorded. The signal strength is proportional to the number of nucleotides incorporated in a single nucleotide flow. The order and intensity of the light peaks are recorded to reveal the underlying DNA sequence.

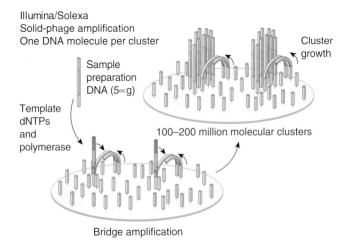

FIGURE 2–14 The 2 basic steps of solid-phase amplification are initial priming and extending of the single-stranded, single-molecule template, and then bridge amplification of the immobilized template with immediately adjacent primers to form clusters. (From Metzker, 2010.)

Roche/454 — Pyrosequencing

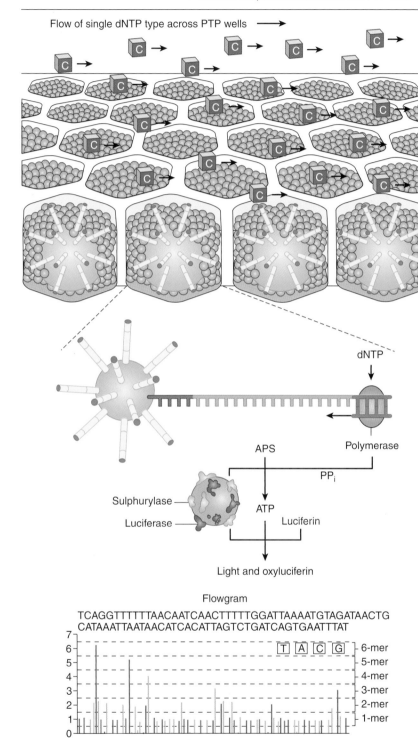

1–2 million template beads loaded into PTP wells

Flow of single dNTP type across PTP wells ⟶

dNTP

Polymerase

APS

PP_i

Sulphurylase

Luciferase

ATP

Luciferin

Light and oxyluciferin

Flowgram

TCAGGTTTTTTAACAATCAACTTTTTGGATTAAAATGTAGATAACTG
CATAAATTAATAACATCACATTAGTCTGATCAGTGAATTTAT

T A C G

6-mer
5-mer
4-mer
3-mer
2-mer
1-mer

FIGURE 2–15 Pyrosequencing.
After loading of the DNA-amplified beads into individual PicoTiterPlate (PTP) wells, additional beads, coupled with sulphurylase and luciferase, are added. The fiberoptic slide is mounted in a flow chamber, enabling the delivery of sequencing reagents to the bead-packed wells. The underneath of the fiberoptic slide is directly attached to a high-resolution camera, which allows detection of the light generated from each PTP well undergoing the pyrosequencing reaction. The light generated by the enzymatic cascade is recorded and is known as a flow gram. *PP*, Inorganic pyrophosphate. (From Metzker, 2010.)

The method of real-time sequencing (as used in the Pacific Biosciences platform, Fig. 2–16) involves imaging the continuous incorporation of dye-labeled nucleotides during DNA synthesis by attaching single DNA polymerase molecules to the bottom surface of individual wells known as "zero-mode waveguide detectors" that can detect the light from the fluorescent nucleotides as they are incorporated into the elongating primer strand.

The Ion Torrent sequencing relies on emulsion PCR amplified particles (ion sphere particles) to be deposited into an array of wells by a short centrifugation step. The sequencing is based on the detection of hydrogen ions that are released

Pacific Biosciences — Real-time sequencing

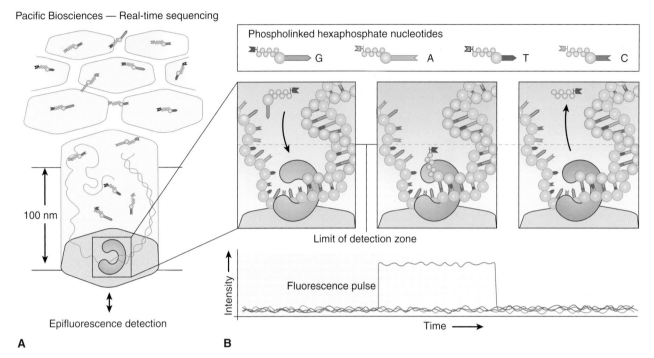

A   **B**

FIGURE 2–16 Pacific Biosciences' four-color real-time sequencing method. The zero-mode waveguide (ZMW) design reduces the observation volume, therefore reducing the number of stray fluorescently labeled molecules that enter the detection layer for a given period. The residence time of phospho linked nucleotides in the active site is governed by the rate of catalysis and is usually milliseconds. This corresponds to a recorded fluorescence pulse, because only the bound, dye-labeled nucleotide occupies the ZMW detection zone on this timescale. The released, dye-labeled pentaphosphate by-product quickly diffuses away, as does the fluorescence signal. (From Metzker, 2010.)

during the polymerization of DNA, as opposed to the optical methods used in other sequencing systems. A microwell containing a template DNA strand to be sequenced is flooded with a single type of nucleotide. If the introduced nucleotide is complementary to the leading template nucleotide it is incorporated into the growing complementary strand. This causes the release of a hydrogen ion that triggers a hypersensitive ion sensor, which indicates that a reaction has occurred. If homopolymer repeats are present in the template sequence multiple nucleotides will be incorporated in a single cycle. This leads to a corresponding number of released hydrogens and a proportionally higher electronic signal.

Despite the substantial cost reductions associated with next-generation technologies in comparison with the automated Sanger method, whole-genome sequencing is expensive but the costs are continuing to fall. In the interim, investigators are using the NGS platforms to target specific regions of interest. This strategy can be used to examine all of the exons in the genome, specific gene families that constitute known drug targets, or megabase-size regions that are implicated in disease or pharmacogenetic effects. Methods to perform the initial first step are known as genomic partitioning and broadly include methods involving PCR, or other hybridization methodologies. These are generally hybridized to target-specific probes either on a microarray surface or in solution.

The ability to sequence large amounts of DNA at low-cost makes the NGS platforms described above useful for many applications such as discovery of variant alleles through resequencing targeted regions of interest or whole genomes, de novo assembly of bacterial and lower eukaryotic genomes, cataloguing the mRNAs ("transcriptomes") present in cells, tissues and organisms (RNA–sequencing), and gene discovery.

2.2.11 Variation in Copy Number and Gene Sequence

The recent application of genome-wide analysis to human genomes has led to the discovery of extensive genomic structural variation, ranging from kilobase pairs to megabase pairs (Mbp) in size, that are not identifiable by conventional chromosomal banding. These changes are termed copy-number variations (CNVs) and can result from deletions, duplications, triplications, insertions, and translocations; they may account for up to 13% of the human genome (Redon et al, 2006).

Despite extensive studies, the total number, position, size, gene content, and population distribution of CNVs remain elusive. There has not been an accurate molecular method to study smaller rearrangements of 1 to 50 kbp on a genome-wide scale in different populations. Recent analyses revealed 11,700 CNVs involving more than 1000 genes (Redon et al, 2006;

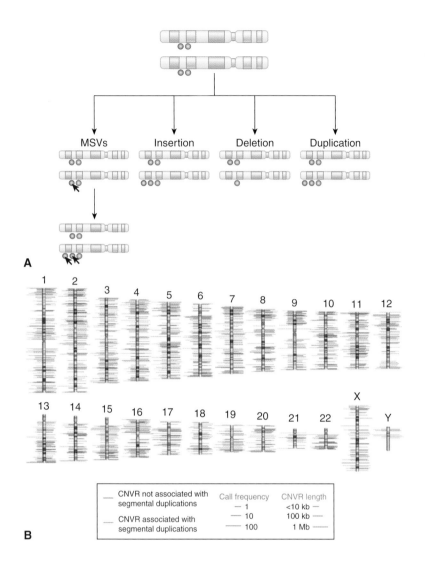

A

B

FIGURE 2-17 **A) Outline of the classes of CNVs in the human genome. B)** The chromosomal locations of 1447 copy number variation regions (a region covered by overlapping CNVs) are indicated by lines to either side of the ideograms. Green lines denote CNVRs associated with segmental duplications; blue lines denote CNVRs not associated with segmental duplications. The length of right-hand side lines represents the size of each CNVR. The length of left-hand side lines indicates the frequency with which a CNVR is detected (minor call frequency among 270 HapMap samples). When both platforms identify a CNVR, the maximum call frequency of the two is shown. For clarity, the dynamic range of length and frequency are log transformed (see scale bars). (From Redon et al, 2006.)

Conrad et al, 2010). Wider application of array CGH techniques and NGS is likely to reveal greater structural variation among different individuals and populations, as the majority of CNVs are beyond the resolving capability of current arrays. There are several different classes of CNVs (Fig. 2–17). Entire genes or genomic regions can undergo duplication, deletion and insertion events, whereas multisite variants (MSVs) refer to more complex genomic rearrangements, including concurrent CNVs and mutation or gene conversions (a process by which DNA sequence information is transferred from one DNA helix, which remains unchanged, to another DNA helix, whose sequence is altered). CNVs can be inherited or sporadic; both types may be involved in causing disease including cancer. However, the phenotypic effects of CNVs are unclear and depend on whether dosage-sensitive genes or regulatory sequences are influenced by the genomic rearrangement.

Use of high-resolution SNP arrays in cancer genomes has shown that CNVs are frequent contributors to the spectrum of mutations leading to cancer development. In adenocarcinoma of the lung, a total of 57 recurrent copy number changes were detected in a collection of 528 cases (Weir et al, 2007). In 206 cases of glioblastoma, somatic copy number alterations were also frequent, and concurrent gene expression analysis showed that 76% of genes affected by copy number alteration had expression patterns that correlated with gene copy number (Cerami et al, 2010). High-resolution analyses of copy number and nucleotide alterations have been carried out on breast and colorectal cancer (Leary et al, 2008). Individual colorectal and breast tumors had, on average, 7 and 18 copy number alterations, respectively, with 24 and 9 as the average number of protein-coding genes affected by amplification or homozygous deletions.

Heritable germline CNVs may also contribute to cancer. For example, a heritable CNV at chromosome 1q21.1 contains the NBPF23 gene for which copy number is implicated in the development of neuroblastoma (Diskin et al, 2009). Also, a germline deletion at chromosome 2p24.3 is more common in men with prostate cancer, with higher prevalence in patients with aggressive compared with nonaggressive prostate cancer (Liu et al, 2009). However, how CNVs, either somatic or germline, contribute to cancer development is still poorly understood. Possible explanations come from the Knudson's two-hit hypothesis (Knudson, 1971): tumor-suppressor genes can be lost as a consequence of a homozygous deletion leading directly to cancer susceptibility (see Chap. 7, Sec. 7.2.3). Alternatively, heterozygous deletions may harbor genes predisposing to cancer that become unmasked when a functional mutation arises in the other chromosome resulting in tumor development. Duplications or gains of chromosomal regions may result in increased expression levels of one or more oncogenes. Germline CNVs can provide a genetic basis for subsequent somatic chromosomal changes that arise in tumor DNA.

2.2.12 Microarrays and RNA Analysis

Microarray analysis has been developed to assess expression of the increasing number of genes identified by the Human Genome Project. There are several commercial kits designed to assist with RNA extraction from cells or tissues. The extracted RNA is then usually converted to cDNA with reverse transcriptase, and this may be combined with an RNA amplification step.

The principle of an expression array involves the production of DNA arrays or "chips" on solid supports for large-scale hybridization experiments. It consists of an arrayed series of thousands of microscopic spots of DNA oligonucleotides, called *features*, each containing specific DNA sequences, known as *probes* (or *reporters*). This approach allows for the simultaneous analysis of the differential expression of thousands of genes and has enhanced understanding of the dynamics of gene expression in cancer cells (Fig. 2–18).

There are a number of microarray platforms in common use. These platforms include: (a) Spotted arrays where DNA fragments (usually created by PCR) or oligonucleotides are immobilized on glass slides. The size of the fragment can be any length (usually 500 bp to 1 kbp) and the size of the oligonucleotides range from 20 to 100 nucleotides. These arrays can be created in individual laboratories using "affordable" equipment. (b) Affymetrix arrays, where the probes are synthesized using a light mask technology and are typically small (20 to 25 bp) oligonucleotides. (c) NimbleGen, the maskless array synthesizer technology that uses 786,000 tiny aluminum mirrors to direct light in specific patterns. Photo deposition chemistry allows single-nucleotide extensions with 380,000 or 2.1 million oligonucleotides/array as the light directs base pairing in specific sequences. (d) Agilent, which uses ink-jet printer technology to extend up to 60-mer bases through phosphoramidite chemistry. The capacity is 244,000 oligonucleotides/array. The analysis of microarrays is discussed in Section 2.7.1.

All the sequencing approaches described in Section 2.2.10 can be applied to RNA, in some cases by simply by converting the RNA to cDNA before analysis. It may also be necessary to remove the ribosomal RNA from the sample to increase the sensitivity of detection. This approach, known as RNA-Seq is becoming increasingly available, although it remains expensive. The technique possesses certain advantages when compared to expression microarrays in that it obviates the requirement for preexisting sequence information in order to detect and evaluate transcripts, and can detect fusion transcripts.

2.3 EPIGENETICS

Epigenetics relates to heritable changes in gene expression that are not encoded in the genome. These processes are mediated by the covalent attachment of chemical groups (eg, methyl or acetyl groups) to DNA and associated proteins, histones and chromatin (Fig. 2–19). Examples of epigenetic effects include imprinting, gene silencing, X chromosome inactivation, position effect, reprogramming, and regulation of histone modifications and heterochromatin. Importantly, epigenetic change is thought to be inherent in the carcinogenesis process. In general, cancer cells exhibit generalized, genome-wide hypomethylation and local hypermethylation of CpG islands associated with promoters (Novak, 2004). Although the significance of each epigenetic change is unclear, hundreds to thousands of genes can be epigenetically silenced by DNA methylation during carcinogenesis. Given these widespread effects, there are epigenetic modifier drugs in current clinical use and there is great potential for further therapeutic utility (see Chap. 17, Sec. 17.3). Additionally, because tumor-derived DNA is present in various, easily accessible body fluids, tumor specific epigenetic modifications such as methylated DNA could prove to be a useful biomarkers for cancer prediction or prognosis (Woodson et al, 2008).

2.3.1 Histone Modification

Histones are alkaline proteins found in eukaryotic cell nuclei that package and order DNA into structural units called *nucleosomes*. Core histones consist of a globular C-terminal domain and an unstructured N-terminal tail. The epigenetic-related modifications to the histone protein occur primarily on the N-terminal tail (Novak, 2004). These modifications appear to influence transcription, DNA repair, DNA replication and chromatin condensation. For example, acetylation of lysine is associated with transcriptionally active DNA, while the effects (ie, activation or repression of transcription) of lysine and arginine methylation vary by location of the amino acid, number of methyl groups, and proximity to a gene promoter (Turner, 2007).

2.3.2 DNA Methylation

DNA methylation involves the addition of a methyl group to the 5′ position of the cytosine pyrimidine ring or the number 6 nitrogen of the adenine purine ring in DNA. In humans, approximately 1% of DNA bases undergo methylation and 10% to 80% of 5′-CpG-3′ dinucleotides are methylated; non-CpG methylation is more prevalent in embryonic

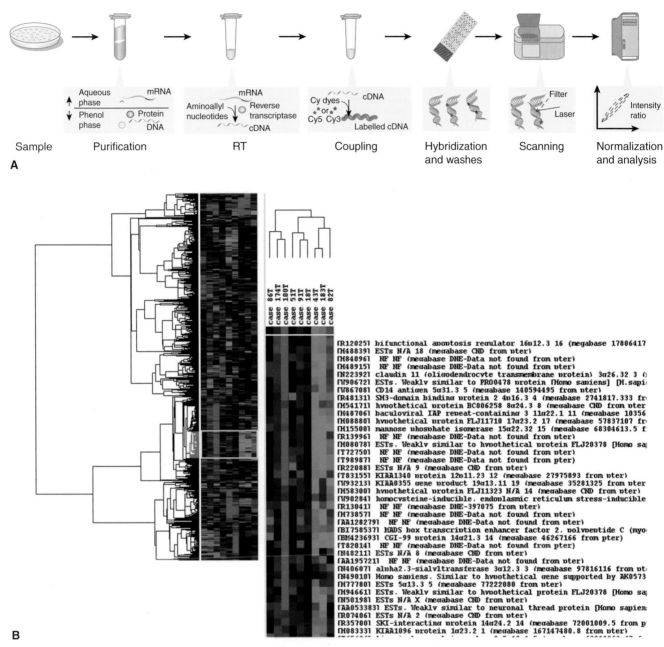

FIGURE 2–18 **A) The steps required in a microarray experiment from sample preparation to analyses.** *RT*, Reverse transcriptase. For details see text. Briefly, samples are prepared and cDNA is created through reverse transcriptase. The fluorescent label is added either in the RT step or in an additional step after amplification, if present. The labeled samples are then mixed with a hybridization solution that contains light detergents, blocking agents (such as COT1 DNA, salmon sperm DNA, calf thymus DNA, PolyA or PolyT), along with other stabilizers. The mix is denatured and added to a pinhole in a microarray, which can be a gene chip (holes in the back) or a glass microarray. The holes are sealed and the microarray hybridized, either in a hybridization oven, (mixed by rotation), or in a mixer, (mixed by alternating pressure at the pinholes). After an overnight hybridization, all nonspecific binding is washed off. The microarray is dried and scanned in a special machine where a laser excites the dye and a detector measures its emission. The intensities of the features (several pixels make a feature) are quantified and normalized (see text). (Reproduced with permission from Jacopo Werther/Wikimedia Commons.) **B)** The output from a typical microarray experiment, a hierarchical clustering of cDNA microarray data obtained from 9 primary laryngeal tumors. Results were visualized using Tree View software, and include the dendrogram (clustering of samples) and the clustering of gene expression, based on genomic similarity. Tree View represents the 946 genes that best distinguish these 2 groups of samples. Genes whose expression is higher in the tumor sample relative to the reference sample are shown in red; those whose expression is lower than the reference sample are shown in green; and no change in gene expression is shown in black. (Courtesy of Patricia Reis and Shilpi Arora, the Ontario Cancer Institute and Princess Margaret Hospital, Toronto.)

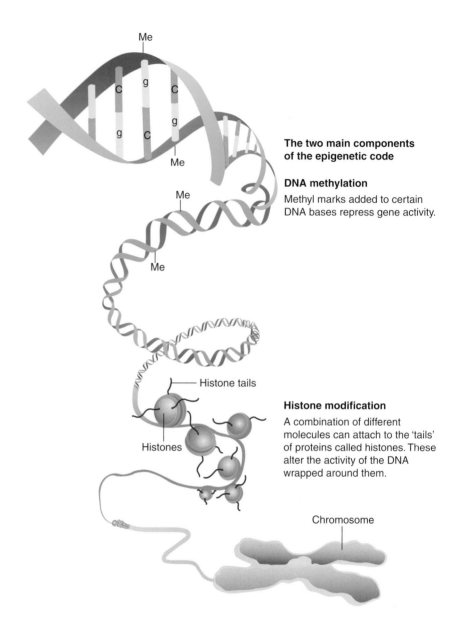

The two main components of the epigenetic code

DNA methylation
Methyl marks added to certain DNA bases repress gene activity.

Histone modification
A combination of different molecules can attach to the 'tails' of proteins called histones. These alter the activity of the DNA wrapped around them.

FIGURE 2–19 An overview of the major epigenetic mechanisms that affect gene expression. In addition, there are a number of varieties of histone modifications that are associated with alterations in gene expression or characteristic states, such as stem cells. (From http://embryology.med.unsw.edu.au/MolDev/Images/epigenetics.jpg.)

stem cells. Unmethylated CpGs are often grouped in clusters called *CpG islands*, which are present in the 5′ regulatory regions of many genes (Gardiner-Garden and Frommer, 1987). In cancer, for reasons that remain unclear, gene promoter CpG islands acquire abnormal hypermethylation, which results in transcriptional silencing that can be inherited by daughter cells following cell division. There are at least 2 important consequences of DNA methylation. First, the methylation of DNA may physically impede the binding of transcriptional activators to the promoter, and second, methylated DNA may be bound by proteins known as *methyl-CpG-binding domain proteins* (MBDs). These proteins can recruit additional proteins to the locus, such as histone deacetylases, thereby forming heterochromatin (tightly coiled and generally inactive) linking DNA methylation to chromatin structure.

2.3.3 Technologies for Studying Epigenetic Changes

Epigenetic research uses a wide range of techniques designed to determine DNA–protein interactions, including chromatin immunoprecipitation (ChIP) (together with ChIP-on-chip and ChIP-seq), histone-specific antibodies, methylation-sensitive restriction enzymes and bisulfite sequencing. Here, we focus on the main approaches for studying DNA methylation along with their relative advantages and disadvantages (Table 2–3). A few points are worth emphasizing; sodium bisulfite converts unmethylated cytosines to uracil, while methylated cytosines (mC) remain unchanged (Fig. 2–20). This technique can reveal the methylation status of every cytosine residue, and it is amenable to massively parallel sequencing methods. Affinity-based methods using methyl-specific

TABLE 2–3 Methods for analyzing DNA methylation.

Method	Description	Advantages	Disadvantages
Sodium bisulfite conversion	Treatment of denatured DNA (ie, single-stranded DNA) with sodium bisulfite leads to deamination of unmethylated cytosine residues to uracil, leaving 5-mC intact. The uracils are amplified as thymines, and 5-mC residues are amplified as cytosines in PCRs. Comparison of sequence information between the reference genome and bisulfite-treated DNA can provide single-nucleotide resolution information about cytosine methylation patterns.	Resolution at the nucleotide level Works on 5- methylated cytosines (mC)-containing DNA Automated analysis	Requires micrograms of DNA input Harsh chemical treatment of DNA can lead to its damage Potentially incomplete conversion of DNA Cannot distinguish 5-mC and 5-hmC Multistep protocol
Sequence-specific enzyme digestion	Restriction enzymes are used to generate DNA fragments for methylation analysis. Some restriction enzymes are methylation-sensitive (ie, digestion is impaired or blocked by methylated DNA). When used in conjunction with an isoschizomer that has the same recognition site but is methylation insensitive, information about methylation status can be obtained. Additionally, the use of methylation-dependent restriction enzymes (ie, requires methylated DNA for cleavage to occur) can be used to fragment DNA for sequencing analysis.	High enzyme turnover Well-studied Easy to use Availability of recombinant enzymes	Determination of methylation status is limited by the enzyme recognition site Overnight protocols Lower throughput
Methylated DNA	Fragmented genomic DNA (restriction enzyme digestion or sonication) is denatured and immunoprecipitated with antibodies specific for 5-mC. The enriched DNA fragments can be analyzed by PCR for locus-specific studies or by microarrays (MeDIP-chip) and massively parallel sequencing (MeDIP-seq) for whole genome studies.	Relatively fast Compatible with array-based analysis Applicable for high-throughput sequencing	Dependent on antibody specificity May require more than one 5-mC for antibody binding Requires DNA denaturation Resolution depends on the size of the immunoprecipitated DNA and for microarray experiments, depends on probe design Data from repeat sequences may be overrepresented
Methylated DNA-binding proteins	Instead of relying on antibodies for DNA enrichment, affinity-based assays use proteins that specifically bind methylated or unmethylated CpG sites in fragmented genomic DNA (restriction enzyme digestion or sonication). The enriched DNA fragments can be analyzed by PCR for locus-specific studies or by microarrays and massively parallel sequencing for whole genome studies.	Well-studied Does not require denaturation Compatible with array-based analysis Applicable for high-throughput sequencing	May require high DNA input May require a long protocol Requires salt elutions Does not give single-base methylation resolution data

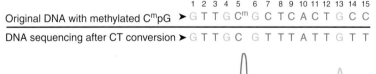

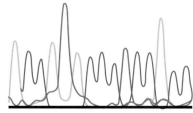

FIGURE 2–20 The most commonly used technique is sodium bisulfite conversion, the "gold standard" for methylation analysis. Incubation of the target DNA with sodium bisulfite results in conversion of all unmodified cytosines to uracils leaving the modified bases 5-methylcytosine or 5-hydroxymethylcytosine (5-mC or 5-hmC) intact. The most critical step in methylation analysis using bisulfite conversion is the complete conversion of unmodified cytosines. Generally, this is achieved by alternating cycles of thermal denaturation with incubation reactions. In this example, the DNA with methylated CpG at nucleotide position #5 was processed using a commercial kit. The recovered DNA was amplified by PCR and then sequenced directly. The methylated cytosine at position #5 remained intact, while the unmethylated cytosines at positions 7, 9, 11, 14, and 15 were completely converted into uracil following bisulfite treatment and detected as thymine following PCR.

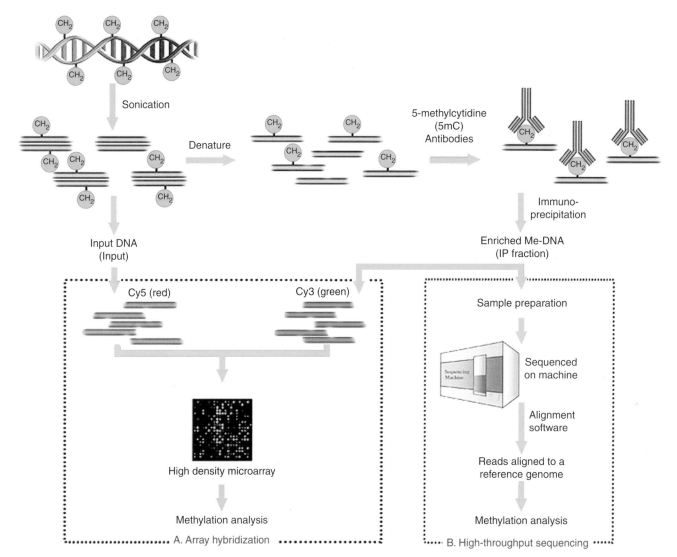

FIGURE 2–21 Schematic outline of MeDIP. Genomic DNA is sheared into approximately 400 to 700 bp using sonication and subsequently denatured. Incubation in 5-mC antibodies, along with standard immunoprecipitation (IP), enriches for fragments that are methylated (IP fraction). This IP fraction can become the input sample to 1 of 2 DNA detection methods: array hybridization using high-density microarrays (**A**) or high-throughput sequencing using the latest in sequencing technology (**B**). Output from these methods are then analyzed for methylation patterns to answer the biological question. (From http://en.wikipedia.org/wiki/Methylated_DNA_immunoprecipitation.)

antibodies (MeDIP) are becoming more popular for whole genome analyses as methyl-specific antibodies improve in sensitivity and specificity (Fig. 2–21).

A wide variety of analytical and enzymatic downstream methods can be used to characterize isolated genomic DNA of interest. Analytical methods, such as high-performance liquid chromatography (HPLC) and matrix-assisted laser desorption/ionization-time of flight mass spectrometry (MALDI-TOF MS; see also Sec. 2.4), have been used to quantify modified bases in complex DNAs. Although HPLC is highly reproducible, it requires large amounts of DNA and is often unsuitable for high-throughput applications. In contrast, MALDI-TOF MS provides relative quantification and is amenable to high-throughput applications.

Other methods to detect methylation include real-time PCR, blotting, microarrays (eg, ChIP on chip) and sequencing (eg, ChIP-Sequencing [ChIP-Seq]). ChIP-Seq combines ChIP with massively parallel DNA sequencing to identify the binding sequences for proteins of interest. Both ChIP techniques rely upon an antibody being available to an epigenetic modification of interest that is then used to "pull-down" the associated DNA via crosslinking so it can be subsequently analyzed. Previously, ChIP-on-chip was the most common technique utilized to study protein-DNA relations. This technique also utilizes ChIP initially, but the selected DNA fragments are ultimately released ("reverse crosslinked") and the DNA is purified. After an amplification and denaturation step, the single-stranded DNA fragments are identified by labeling with a fluorescent tag such as Cy5 or Alexa 647 and poured over the surface of a DNA microarray, which is spotted with short, single-stranded sequences that cover the genomic portion of interest.

2.4 CREATING AND MANIPULATING MODEL SYSTEMS

2.4.1 Cell Culture/Cancer Cell Lines

Cells that are cultured directly from a patient are known as *primary cells*. With the exception of tumor-derived cells, most primary cell cultures have a limited life span. After a certain number of population doublings (called the *Hayflick limit*) cells undergo senescence and cease dividing although generally retaining viability. However, established or immortalized cell lines have an ability to proliferate indefinitely either through random mutation or deliberate modification, such as enforced expression of the telomerase reverse transcriptase (see Chap. 5, Sec. 5.7). There are numerous well-established cell lines derived from particular cancer cell types such as LNCaP for hormone-sensitive prostate cancer; MCF-7 for hormone-sensitive breast cancer; U87, a human glioblastoma cell line; and SaOS-2 for osteosarcoma.

Despite cell lines often being used in preclinical experiments to explore cancer biology there are a number of caveats that limit their validity: (a) The number of cells per volume of culture medium plays a critical role for some cell types. For example, a lower cell concentration makes granulosa cells undergo estrogen production, whereas a higher concentration makes them appear as progesterone-producing theca lutein cells. (b) Cross-contamination of cell lines may occur frequently and is often caused by proximity (during culture) to rapidly proliferating cell lines such as HeLa cells. Because of their adaptation to growth in tissue culture plates, HeLa cells may spread in aerosol droplets to contaminate and overgrow other cell cultures in the same laboratory, interfering with the validity of data interpretation. The degree of contamination among cell types is unknown because few researchers test the identity or purity of already-established cell lines, although scientific journals are increasingly requiring such tests. (c) As cells continue to divide in culture, they generally grow to fill the available area or volume. This can lead to nutrient depletion in the growth media, accumulation of apoptotic/necrotic (dead) cells and cell-to-cell contact, which leads to contact inhibition or senescence. Furthermore, tumor cells grown continuously in culture may acquire further mutations and epigenetic alterations that can change their properties and may affect their ability to reinitiate tumor growth in vivo. (d) The extent to which cancer cell lines reflect the original neoplasm from which they are derived is variable. For example, the prostate cancer cell line DU145 was derived from a brain metastasis, which is unusual in prostate cancer. Furthermore, the line does not express prostate-specific antigen (PSA) and its hypotriploid

karyotype is uncommon in prostate cancer. The increasing recognition of the genetic heterogeneity both between and within individual cancers has raised further concerns about how well individual cell lines represent the cancer type from which they were derived.

2.4.2 Manipulating Genes in Cells

The function of a gene can often be studied by placing it into a cell different from the one from which it was isolated. For example, one may wish to place a mutated oncogene, isolated from a tumor cell, into a normal cell to determine whether it causes malignant transformation. The process of introducing DNA plasmids into cells is termed *transfection*. A number of transfection protocols have been developed for efficient introduction of foreign DNA into mammalian cells, including calcium phosphate or diethylaminoethyl (DEAE)-dextran precipitation, spheroplast fusion, lipofection, electroporation, and transfer using viral vectors (Ausubel and Waggoner, 2003). For all methods, the efficiency of transfer must be high enough for easy detection, and it must be possible to recognize and select for cells containing the newly introduced gene. Control over the expression of introduced genes can be achieved by the use of inducible expression vectors. These vectors allow the manipulation of a gene, most commonly when an exogenous agent (such as tetracycline or estrogen) is added or taken away from culture media: this is achieved with a specific repressor that responds to the exogenous agent, and is fused to domains that activate the gene of interest.

One method of transfection uses hydroxyethyl piperazine-ethanesulfonic acid (HEPES)-buffered saline solution (HeBS) containing phosphate ions combined with a calcium chloride solution containing the DNA to be transfected. When the 2 are combined, a fine precipitate of the positively charged calcium and the negatively charged phosphate of the DNA results in a fine solute, which is then added to the recipient cells. As a result of a process not completely understood, the cells take up the DNA-containing precipitate. A more efficient method is the inclusion of the DNA to be transfected in liposomes, which are small, membrane-bounded bodies that can fuse with the cell membrane, thereby releasing the DNA into the cell. For eukaryotic cells, transfection is better achieved using cationic liposomes (or mixtures). Popular agents are lipofectamine (Invitrogen, New York, USA) and UptiFectin (Interchim, Montiuçon Cedex, France). Another method uses cationic polymers such as DEAE-dextran or polyethylenimine: the negatively charged DNA binds to the polycation and the complex is absorbed via endocytosis.

Other methods require physical perturbation of cells (which may be detrimental to the study) to introduce DNA. Some examples include electroporation (application of an electric charge), sonoporation (sonic pulses), and optical (laser) transfection. Particle-based methods, such as the gene gun (where the DNA is coupled to a nanoparticle of an inert solid and "shot" directly into the target cell), magnetofection

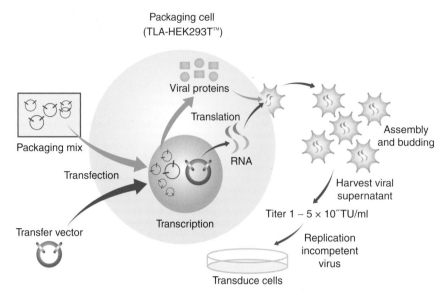

FIGURE 2–22 **Schematic outlining the process of lentiviral transfection.** Cotransfection of the packaging plasmids and transfer vector into the packaging cell line, HEK293T, allows efficient production of lentiviral supernatant. Virus can then be transduced into a wide range of cell types, including both dividing and nondividing mammalian cells. Note that the packaging mix is often separated into multiple plasmids, minimizing the threat of recombinant replication-competent virus production. Viral titers are measured in either transduction units (TU)/mL or multiplicity of infection (MOI), which is the number of transducing lentiviral particles per cell to which the following relationship applies under experimental conditions:
(Total number of cells per well) × (Desired MOI) = Total TU needed
(Total TU needed)/(TU/mL reported on certificate of authentication) = Total mL of lentiviral particles to add to each well

(utilizing magnetic forces to drive nucleic acid particle complexes into the target cell), and impalefection (impaling cells by elongated nanostructures such as carbon nanofibers or silicon nanowires which have been coated with plasmid DNA) are becoming less popular given the greater efficiency of viral transfection.

DNA can also be introduced into cells using viruses as carriers; the technique is called *viral transduction*, and the cells are *transduced*. Retroviruses are very stable, as their cDNA integrates into the host mammalian DNA, but only relatively small pieces of DNA (up to 10 kbp) can be transferred. Adenoviral-based vectors can accommodate larger inserts (~36 kbp) and have a very high efficiency of transfer (see Chap. 6, Sec. 6.2.2). However, with increasing frequency, lentiviruses (Fig. 2–22) are being used to introduce DNA into cells; they have the advantages of high-efficiency infection of dividing and nondividing cells, long-term stable expression of the transgene, and low immunogenicity.

Whichever method is used to introduce the DNA, it is usually necessary to select for retention of the transferred genes before assaying for expression. For this reason, a selectable gene, such as the gene encoding resistance to the antibiotics geneticin (G418), neomycin, or puromycin, can be introduced simultaneously.

2.4.3 RNA Interference

RNA interference (RNAi) is the process of mRNA degradation that is induced by double-stranded RNA in a sequence-specific manner. RNAi has been observed in all eukaryotes, from fission yeast to mammals. The power and utility of RNAi for specifically silencing the expression of any gene for which the sequence is available has driven its rapid adoption as a crucial tool for genetic analysis.

The RNAi pathway is thought to be an ancient mechanism for protecting the host and its genome against viruses that use double-stranded RNA (dsRNA) in their life cycles. RNAi is now recognized to be but one of a larger set of sequence-specific cellular responses to RNA, collectively called *RNA silencing*. RNA silencing plays a critical role in regulation of cell growth and differentiation using endogenous small RNAs called *microRNAs* (miRNAs). These miRNAs also play a role in carcinogenesis. For example, miR-15a and miR-16-1 act as putative tumor suppressors by targeting the oncogene BCL2. These miRNAs occur in a cluster at the chromosomal region 13q14, which is frequently deleted in cancer and is downregulated by genomic loss or mutations in CLL (Calin et al, 2005), prostate cancer (Bonci et al, 2008), and pituitary adenomas (Bottoni et al, 2005).

miRNAs are mostly transcribed from introns or other noncoding areas of the genome into primary transcripts of between 1 kb and 3 kb in length, called *pri-miRNAs* (Rodriguez et al, 2004) (Fig. 2–23). These transcripts are processed by the ribonucleases Drosha and DiGeorge syndrome critical region gene 8 (DGCR8) complex in the nucleus, resulting in a hairpin-shaped intermediate of approximately 70 to 100 nucleotides, called precursor miRNA (pre-miRNA) (Landthaler et al, 2004; Lee et al, 2003). The pre-miRNA is exported

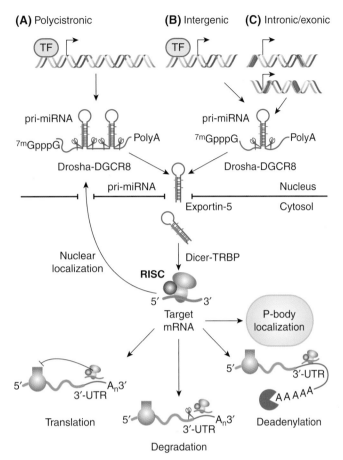

FIGURE 2–23 **miRNA genomic organization, biogenesis and function. Genomic distribution of miRNA genes. The sequence encoding miRNA is shown in red.** *TF*, Transcription factor. **A)** Clusters throughout the genome transcribed as polycistronic primary transcripts and subsequently cleaved into multiple miRNAs; **B)** intergenic regions transcribed as independent transcriptional units; **C)** intronic sequences (in gray) of protein-coding or protein-noncoding transcription units or exonic sequences (black cylinders) of noncoding genes. pri-miRNAs are transcribed and transiently receive a 7-methylguanosine (^{7m}GpppG) cap and a poly(A) tail. The pri-miRNA is processed into a precursor miRNA (pre-miRNA) stem-loop of approximately 60 nucleotides (nt) in length by the nuclear ribonuclease (RNase) III enzyme Drosha and its partner DiGeorge syndrome critical region gene 8 (DGCR8). Exportin-5 actively transports pre-miRNA into the cytosol, where it is processed by the Dicer RNase III enzyme, together with its partner TAR (HIV) RNA binding protein (TRBP), into mature, 22 nt-long double-strand miRNAs. The RNA strand (in *red*) is recruited as a single-stranded molecule into the RNA-induced silencing (RISC) effector complex and assembled through processes that are dependent on Dicer and other double-strand RNA-binding domain proteins, as well as on members of the argonaute family. Mature miRNAs then guide the RISC complex to the 3′ untranslated regions (3′-UTRs) of the complementary mRNA targets and repress their expression by several mechanisms: repression of mRNA translation, destabilization of mRNA transcripts through cleavage, deadenylation, and localization in the processing body (P-body), where the miRNA-targeted mRNA can be sequestered from the translational machinery and degraded or stored for subsequent use. Nuclear localization of mature miRNAs has been described as a novel mechanism of action for miRNAs. *Scissors* indicate the cleavage on pri-miRNA or mRNA. (From Fazi et al, 2008.)

from the nucleus to the cytoplasm by exportin 5 (Perron and Provost, 2009). Once in the cytoplasm, the pre-miRNA is processed by Dicer, another ribonuclease, into a mature double-stranded miRNA of approximately 18 to 25 nucleotides. After strand separation, the guide strand or mature miRNA is incorporated into an RNA-induced silencing complex (RISC) and the passenger strand is usually degraded. The RISC complex is comprised of miRNA, argonaute proteins (argonaute 1 to argonaute 4) and other protein factors. The argonaute proteins have a crucial role in miRNA biogenesis, maturation and miRNA effector functions (Hutvagner and Zamore, 2002; Chendrimada et al, 2005).

The discovery of the miRNAs suggested that RNAi might be triggered artificially in mammalian cells by synthetic genes that express mimics of endogenous triggers. Indeed, mimics of miRNAs in the form of short hairpin RNAs (shRNAs) have proven to be an invaluable research tool to further our understanding of many biological processes, including carcinogenesis. shRNAs contain a sense strand, antisense strand, and a short loop sequence between the sense and antisense fragments. Because of the complementarity of the sense and antisense fragments in their sequence, such RNA molecules tend to form hairpin-shaped dsRNA. shRNA can be cloned into a DNA expression vector and can be delivered to cells in the same ways devised for delivery of DNA. These constructs then allow ectopic mRNA expression by an associated pol III type promoter. The expressed shRNA is then exported into the cytoplasm where it is processed by dicer into short-interference RNA (siRNA), which then get incorporated into the siRNA RISC. A number of transfection methods are suitable, including transient transfection, stable transfection, and delivery using viruses, with both constitutive and inducible promoter systems.

2.4.4 Site-Directed Mutagenesis

Following the sequencing of the human genome (and that of other species), a plethora of genes are being identified without any knowledge of their function. Important clues concerning protein function may be provided through similarity in the amino acid sequence and secondary protein structure

to other proteins or protein domains of known function. For example, many transcription-factor proteins have a characteristic motif through which DNA-binding takes place (eg, leucine-zipper or zinc-finger domain; see Chap 8. Sec. 8.2). One way of testing the putative function of such a sequence is to see whether a mutation within the critical site causes loss of function. In the example of transcription factors, a single mutation might result in a protein that failed to bind DNA appropriately. Site-directed mutagenesis permits the introduction of mutations at a precise point in a cloned gene, resulting in specific changes in the amino acid sequence. By site-directed mutagenesis, amino acids can be deleted, altered, or inserted, but for most experiments, the changes do not alter the reading frame and disrupt protein continuity. There are two classical methods of introducing a mutation into a cloned gene (Ausubel and Waggoner, 2003). The first method (Fig. 2–24A) relies on the chance occurrence of a

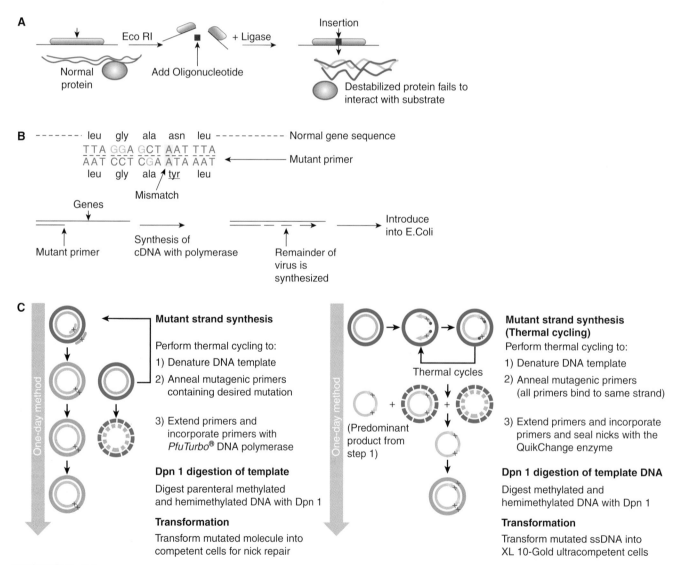

FIGURE 2–24 **Methods for site-directed mutagenesis. A)** Insertion of a new sequence at the site of action of a restriction enzyme by ligating a small oligonucleotide sequence within the reading frame of a gene. **B)** Use of a primer sequence that is synthesized to contain a mismatch at the desired site of mutagenesis. **C)** Outline of the PCR-based methodology. (From http://www.biocompare.com/Application-Notes/42126-Fast-And-Efficient-Mutagenesis/.)

restriction enzyme site in a region one wishes to alter. Typically, the gene is digested with the restriction endonuclease, and a few nucleotides may be inserted or deleted at this site by ligating a small oligonucleotide complementary to the cohesive DNA terminus that remains after enzyme digestion. The second method (Fig. 2–24B) is more versatile but requires more manipulation. The gene is first obtained in a single-stranded form by cloning into a vector such as M13 phage. First, a short oligonucleotide is synthesized containing the desired nucleotide change but otherwise complementary to the region to be mutated. The oligonucleotide will anneal to the single-stranded DNA but contains a mismatch at the site of mutation. The hybridized oligonucleotide-DNA duplex is then exposed to DNA polymerase I (plus the 4 nucleotides and buffers), which will synthesize and extend a complementary strand with perfect homology at every nucleotide except at the site of mismatch in the primer used to initiate DNA synthesis. The double-stranded DNA is then transfected into bacteria in the phage, and because of the semiconservative nature of DNA replication, 50% of the M13 phage produced will contain normal DNA and 50% will contain the DNA with the introduced mutation. Several methods allow easy identification of the mutant M13 virus. Using these techniques, the effects of artificially generated mutations can be studied in cell culture or in transgenic mice (see following section).

More recently, techniques such as whole plasmid mutagenesis that rely on PCR (see Sec. 2.2.5) are often used as this produces a fragment containing the desired mutation in sufficient quantity to be separated from the original, unmutated plasmid by gel electrophoresis, which may then be used with standard recombinant molecular biology techniques. Following plasmid amplification (usually in *Escherichia coli*), commercially available kits (see Fig. 2–24C) can be used that involve a pair of complementary mutagenic primers that are used to amplify the entire plasmid DNA in a thermocycling reaction using a high-fidelity non–strand-displacing DNA polymerase. The reaction generates a nicked, circular DNA. The template DNA is eliminated by enzymatic digestion with a restriction enzyme such as DpnI, which is specific for methylated DNA, as all the DNA produced from the *E. coli* vector is methylated; the template plasmid which is biosynthesized in *E. coli* will therefore be digested, whereas the mutated plasmid is generated in vitro and is therefore unmethylated and left undigested.

2.4.5 Transgenic and Knockout Mice

One way to investigate the effects of gene expression in specific cells on the function of the whole organism is to transfer genes directly into the germline and generate transgenic mice. For example, inappropriate expression of an oncogene in a particular tissue can provide clues about the possible role of that oncogene in normal development and in malignant transformation. Usually a cloned gene with the desired regulatory elements is microinjected into the male pronucleus of a single-cell embryo so that it can integrate

into a host chromosome and become part of the genome. If the introduced gene is incorporated into the germline, the resulting animal will become a founder for breeding a line of mice, all of which carry the newly introduced gene. Such mice are called *transgenic mice,* and the inserted foreign gene is called a *transgene.* Its expression can be studied in a variety of different cellular environments in a whole animal. Each transgene will have a unique integration site in a host chromosome and will be transmitted to offspring in the same way as a naturally occurring gene. However, the site of integration often influences the expression of a transgene, possibly because of the activity of genes in adjacent chromatin. Sometimes the integration event also alters the expression of endogenous genes (insertional mutation); this observation led to the development of gene-targeting approaches, so that specific genes could be inactivated or "knocked out." The effect of the inserted or "knocked out" gene can then be studied for phenotypic effects in the animal (unless it turns out to be lethal in the embryo).

In vivo site-directed mutagenesis (Fig. 2–25) is the method by which a mutation is targeted to a specific endogenous gene. Instead of introducing a modified cloned gene at a random position as described above, a cloned gene fragment is targeted to a particular site in the genome by *homologous recombination* (a type of genetic recombination in which nucleotide sequences are exchanged between 2 similar or identical molecules of DNA). This process relies on the ability of a cloned mammalian gene or DNA fragment to preferentially undergo homologous recombination in a normal somatic cell at its naturally occurring chromosomal position, thereby replacing the endogenous gene. The intent is for the introduced mutation to result in the disruption of expression of the endogenous gene, or to result in a prematurely truncated, nonfunctional protein product. In typical targeting experiments, a DNA construct is prepared with a gene encoding drug resistance (usually to G418) and the DNA of interest. Initially, the modified DNA is introduced into pluripotent stem cells derived from a murine embryonic stem (ES) cells. The frequency of homologous recombination is low (less than 1 in a million cells), but is greatly influenced by a variety of factors, such as the host vector, the method of DNA introduction, the length of the regions of homology, and whether the targeted gene is expressed in ES cells. ES cells that contain the correctly targeted gene disruption are selected by growth in medium containing G418, and these cells are cloned and tested with PCR for homologous recombination. Once an ES cell line with the desired modification has been isolated and purified, ES cells are injected into a normal embryo, where they often contribute to all the differentiated tissues of the chimeric adult mouse. If gametes are derived from the ES cells, then a *founder* line containing the modification of interest can be established.

Recent technologic advances in gene targeting by homologous recombination in mammalian systems enable the production of mutants in any desired gene. It is also possible to generate a *conditionally targeted mutation* within a mouse line using the *cre-loxP system.* This method takes advantage

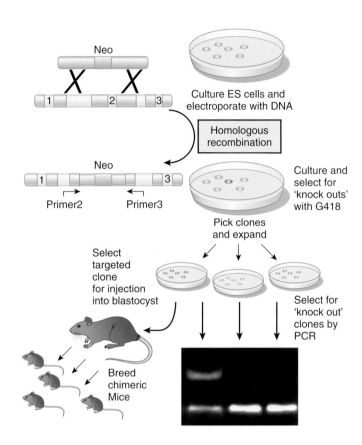

FIGURE 2–25 **Disruption of a gene by homologous recombination in embryonic stem (ES) cells.** Exogenous DNA is introduced into the ES cells by electroporation. The homologous region on the exogenous DNA is shown in gray, the selectable gene neomycin (*neo*) is speckled, and the target exons are black. The 2 recombination points are shown by Xs, and the exogenous DNA replaces some of the normal DNA of exon 2, thereby destroying its reading frame by inserting the small "neo" gene. ES cells that have undergone a successful homologous recombination are selected as colonies in G418 because of the stable presence of the neo gene. PCR primers for exons 2 and 3 are used to identify colonies in which a homologous recombination event has taken place. ES cells from such positive cells (*dark colony*) are injected into blastocysts, which are implanted into foster mothers (*white*). If germline transmission has been achieved, chimeric mice are bred to generate homozygotes for the "knocked out" gene.

of the properties of the Cre recombinase enzyme first identified in P1 bacteriophage. Cre recognizes a 34-base pair DNA sequence (*loxP*). When two *loxP* sites are oriented in the same direction, the Cre recombinase will excise the intervening sequence; when they are oriented in the reverse direction, Cre will invert the intervening sequence. This system can be applied to the transgenic mouse in a number of ways (for review, see Babinet and Cohen-Tannoudji, 2001); for example, using the technique of homologous recombination, it is possible to replace a murine genomic sequence with the same sequence containing *loxP* sites, thus flanking a desired region by *loxP* sites. The resulting mice are normal, until the Cre recombinase is introduced. The manner of introduction of the recombinase can be carefully chosen so that only a specific cell type may be affected, or only a particular phase of differentiation, or both, thus allowing for spatial and temporal control of gene mutation within the mouse genome. This system is particularly advantageous in examining the role of essential genes in the mouse, particularly when knockout of the gene of interest is embryonic lethal. A conditional knockout mouse utilizing the *cre-loxP* system may allow one to study the effects of turning the gene on or off in a living animal. The *cre-loxP* system may also be used to generate chromosomal aberrations in a cell type-specific manner, which can improve understanding of the biology of some human diseases, particularly leukemias (Fig. 2–26).

Other means of targeting genes for manipulation in vivo include zinc finger nucleases and transcription activator-like effector nucleases (TALENs). Zinc finger nucleases (ZFNs) are synthetic proteins consisting of an engineered zinc finger DNA-binding domain fused to the cleavage domain of the FokI restriction endonuclease. ZFNs can be used to induce double-stranded breaks (DSBs) in specific DNA sequences and thereby promote site-specific homologous recombination and targeted manipulation of genomic loci in a variety of different cell types. G-rich sequences are the natural preference of zinc fingers, which is currently a limitation to their use (Isalan, 2012). TALENs were discovered in plant pathogens but now have been modified to contain a TALEN DNA binding domain for sequence-specific recognition fused to the catalytic domain of the Fok1 nuclease that introduces DSBs. The DNA binding domain contains a highly conserved 33- to 34-amino acid sequence with the exception of the 12th and 13th amino acids. These 2 locations are highly variable (repeat variable diresidue [RVD]) and show a strong correlation with specific nucleotide recognition. This simple relationship between amino acid sequence and DNA recognition has allowed for the engineering of specific DNA binding domains by selecting a combination of repeat segments containing the appropriate RVDs. Therefore, the DNA binding domain of a TALEN is capable of targeting with high precision a large recognition site (for instance, 17 bp).

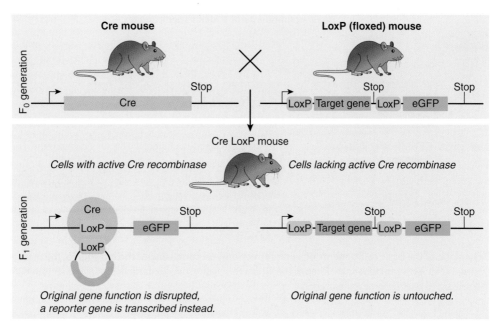

FIGURE 2–26 Illustration of a model experiment in genetics using the cre-lox system. The function of a target gene is disrupted by a conditional knockout. Typically, such an experiment would be performed with a tissue-specific promoter driving the expression of the cre-recombinase (or with a promoter only active during a distinct time in ontogeny). (From http://en.wikipedia.org/wiki/File:CreLoxP_experiment.png.)

2.5 PROTEOMICS

Proteomics refers to the systematic, large-scale analysis of proteins in a biological system. It is a fusion of traditional protein biochemistry, analytical chemistry, and computer science to obtain a systemwide understanding of biological questions. Table 2–4 summarizes the types of proteomic research.

TABLE 2–4 Types of Proteomics Studies.

Use	Application
Expression proteomics	Detection of all proteins present in a biological sample
Functional proteomics	Systematic detection of cellular protein–protein interactions
Quantitative proteomics	Quantify proteins on a relative or absolute scale
Posttranslational modification proteomics	Detection of the location of enzymatic and nonenzymatic posttranslational protein modifications (eg, phosphorylation, methylation, glycosylation, ubiquitination, sumoylation, oxidation, glycation, etc)
Chemical proteomics	Combining synthetic chemistry and proteomics to use defined chemical structures as molecular probes to isolate specific components of the proteome
Structural proteomics	Systematic determination of 3-dimensional structures for all proteins (ie, x-ray or nuclear magnetic resonance based).

Mass spectrometry (MS), x-ray crystallography, and nuclear magnetic resonance (NMR) spectroscopy are often employed in the systematic analysis of protein–protein interaction networks, with emerging high-throughput tools, such as protein and chemical microarrays, making an increasing contribution. However, there are other useful methods for interrogating protein–protein interaction networks that may be applied on a systematic, genome-wide scale, including the yeast 2-hybrid system (Colas and Brent, 1998; Fields, 2009) and protein complementation assays (PCA) (Michnick et al, 2011). Each technique tends to enrich for specific types of protein interactions; for example, the yeast 2-hybrid system is highly sensitive, but often assesses only direct interactions between bait protein and its interaction partner. Despite the obvious issues surrounding signal-to-noise ratio, MS and other similar proteomic approaches can interrogate all detectable proteins that bind a bait protein, or can interrogate complex protein mixtures that have not been otherwise enriched for a particular protein.

2.5.1 Mass Spectrometry

MS is an analytical tool used to determine the mass, structure, and/or elemental composition of a molecule. In simplistic terms, a mass spectrometer is a very sensitive "detector" that can be divided into 3 main components (Fig. 2–27): an *ion source*, used to transfer the molecules to be analyzed into the gaseous state/gas phase (mass spectrometers are under high vacuum and therefore ions need to be transferred to the gas phase); a *mass analyzer*, used to measure the mass-to-charge ratio (m/z) of the generated ions (the elemental composition

Basic components of a mass spectrometer

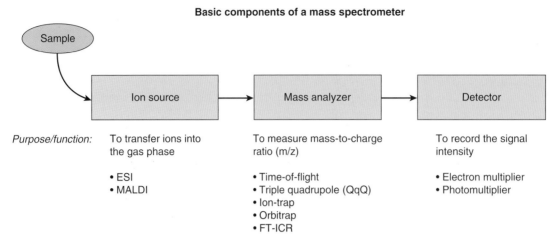

FIGURE 2–27   **Schematic of the basic components of a mass spectrometer consisting of the ion source, the mass analyzer, and the detector.** Individual examples for each component are listed in the figure. *ESI*, electrospray ionization; *FT-ICR*, fourier transform Ion cyclotron resonance; *MALDI*, matrix-assisted laser desorption/ionization.

of analyzed ions results in specific m/z values used for identification); and a *detector*, used to register the intensity of the generated ions. One of the major developments for MS-based proteomics was the introduction of mild ionization technologies (MALDI and ESI) capable of ionizing large, intact biomolecules such as proteins or peptides.

In MALDI (*matrix-assisted laser desorption/ionization*), molecules to be analyzed (the analyte) are mixed with an energy-absorbing matrix consisting of organic aromatic acids (eg, sinapinic acid) in a solvent mixture of water, acetonitrile, and trifluoroacetic acid. The analyte is then mixed with the matrix solution (large excess of matrix; ~1:1000) and spotted onto a stainless steel target plate, dried to generate a cocrystal of analyte and matrix molecules. Pulsed lasers are then fired onto the cocrystal of matrix and analyte. Matrix molecules are used to absorb the majority of the laser energy, thereby protecting the analyte (the proteins and peptides being analyzed) from destruction. The matrix molecules and the organic acids then transfer their charge to the peptide/protein molecules, resulting in the mild ionization of these labile biomolecules (Fig. 2–28A).

Electrospray ionization (ESI), involves analyte molecules being dissolved in the liquid phase and ionized by the application of a high voltage (2 to 4 kV) directly to the solvent, resulting in a fine aerosol at the tip of a chromatography column. The solvents used in MS-based proteomics are polar, volatile solvents (ie, water/acetonitrile containing trace amounts of formic acid). This ionization is ideally suited for coupling with high-resolution separation technologies such as liquid chromatography or capillary electrophoresis and is the most commonly used method of ionization in MS-based proteomics (see Fig. 2–28B).

A major challenge for comprehensive or large-scale, MS-based proteomics is the extreme complexity of the human proteome (Cox and Mann, 2007). Although there are only approximately 22,000 genes in the human genome, the human proteome is expected to be substantially larger,

as a result of splicing, posttranslational protein modifications, and/or protein processing. This problem is further amplified because proteins have a large range of physicochemical properties, complicating extraction and/or solubilization of individual proteins. For example, membrane proteins have been largely underrepresented in proteomics studies as their solubility in polar, aqueous buffers is poor. Additionally, proteins in the human proteome span a wide range of concentrations, and the detection of low abundance species in the presence of very highly abundant proteins is a challenge even for modern, highly sensitive mass spectrometers. As a result, whole proteome analyses are extremely challenging. To overcome these problems, a variety of different analytical fractionations are used, aimed at minimizing sample complexity, thereby increasing the ability of the mass spectrometer to detect less abundant proteins. Fractionation methods can be applied to the intact protein (ie, chromatographic or electrophoretic), or proteins can first be digested and resulting peptides fractionated by liquid chromatography. MS is then used for identification and quantification, as described below.

2.5.2 Top-Down or Bottom-Up Proteomics

Conceptually, there are 2 different strategies for the MS-based analysis of proteins. The most commonly used strategy for the analysis of complex proteomes is termed *bottom-up proteomics*. Proteins or even complex proteomes are first digested to smaller peptides using (polypeptide) sequence-specific enzymes (trypsin is used most commonly). Resulting peptides are then separated by liquid chromatography (LC) and analyzed by ESI-MS. This process is referred to as "LC-MS analysis." The resulting parent or precursor ions (ie, ions that have not undergone any collision-induced fragmentation) are consecutively selected for fragmentation by the MS, depending on their intensity. Fragmentation is

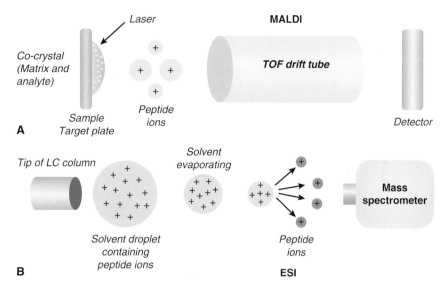

MALDI

Laser

Co-crystal
(Matrix and
analyte)

TOF drift tube

Peptide
ions

Detector

Sample
Target plate

A

Tip of LC column

Solvent
evaporating

Solvent droplet
containing
peptide ions

Peptide
ions

Mass
spectrometer

B

ESI

FIGURE 2-28 **Schematics of mild peptide ionizations used for proteomics analyses.** The 2 techniques used to ionize biological materials include matrix-assisted laser desorption/ionization (MALDI) and electrospray ionization (ESI). Both are soft ionization techniques allowing for the ionization of biomolecules such as proteins and peptides. **A)** In MALDI, ionization is triggered by a laser beam (normally a nitrogen laser). A matrix is used to protect the biomolecule from being destroyed by direct contact with the laser beam. This matrix-analyte solution is spotted onto a metal plate (target). The solvent vaporizes, leaving only the recrystallized matrix with proteins spread throughout the crystals. The laser is fired at the cocrystals on the MALDI target. The matrix material absorbs the energy and transfers part of its charge to the analyte and thus ionizing them. **B)** In ESI, a volatile liquid containing the analyte is passed through a microcapillary (ie, chromatography column). As the liquid is passed out of the capillary it forms an aerosol of small droplets. As the small droplets evaporate, the charged analyte molecules are forced closer together and the droplets disperse. The ions continue along to the mass analyzer of a mass spectrometer.

usually achieved using *collision-induced fragmentation* (CID) through collision with inert gas molecules such as helium. Alternative fragmentation mechanisms include *electron transfer dissociation* (ETD) (Mikesh et al, 2006) or *electron capture dissociation* (ECD) (Appella and Anderson, 2007; Chowdhury et al, 2007). The resulting MS/MS spectra (ie, tandem mass spectra) contain information regarding the peptide amino acid sequence of the fragmented parent ions. The fragmentation of a parent/precursor peptide ion to a sequence specific tandem mass spectrum used for identification is dependent on several parameters, including the energy used for fragmentation, the fragmentation mechanism, and the amino acid sequence of the peptide. Resulting fragment ions can be classified according to a defined nomenclature (Roepstorff and Fohlman, 1984) (Fig. 2–29). Under conditions of CID fragmentation, *b-ions* and *y-ions* (ions generated from the N- or C-terminus of the peptide) are observed most commonly. Figure 2–30 is a schematic of a LC-MS analysis using data recorded on an LTQ-Orbitrap mass analyzer.

Modern mass spectrometers are extremely fast scanning instruments, recording several hundred thousand spectra per day; computational spectral matching against available protein sequence databases is used for peptide/protein identification. To accomplish this task, several commercial (Sequest, Mascot) (Perkins et al, 1999) or open-source (X! Tandem,

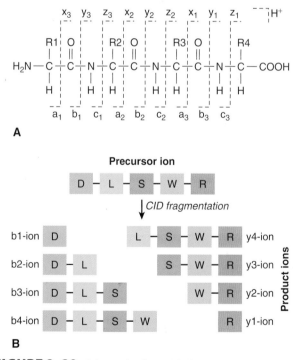

FIGURE 2-29 **Schematic of peptide fragmentation by CID.**
A) Nomenclature of peptide fragments generated by CID. **B)** Cartoon of typical b- and y-type ions generated by CID fragmentation of a pentapeptide.

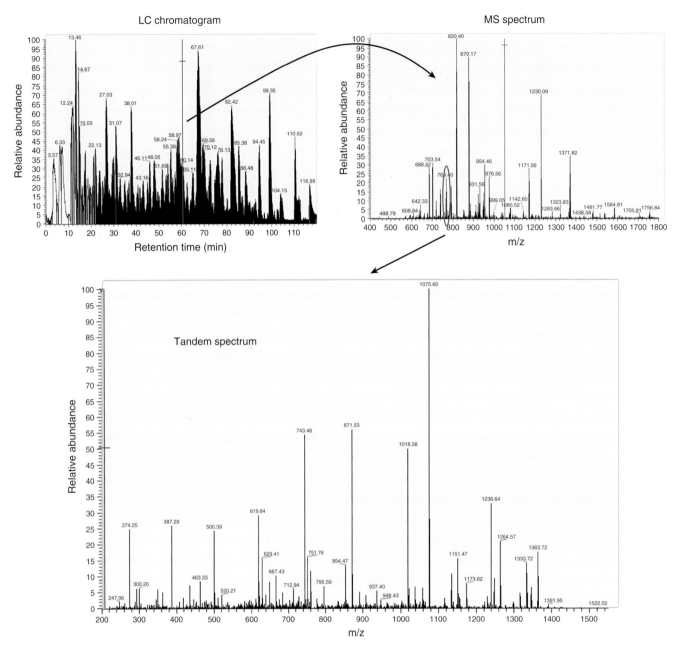

FIGURE 2–30 **Screen shots of a typical "data-dependent" LC-MS experiment.** Peptides are separated by nanoflow LC. Separated peptides are then analyzed by consecutive MS scans. First a MS spectrum of an intake parent ion is generated (ie, MS spectrum). An individual parent ion is then isolated by the mass analyzer and subjected to CID fragmentation resulting in a sequence specific tandem mass spectrum (ie, MS/MS spectrum).

OMSSA, MyriMatch) algorithms are available. Careful interpretation of the results is crucial to assure high data quality and minimize false-positive and false-negative identifications. This process of automated spectral matching is highly dependent on the availability of well-annotated protein sequence databases, that correlate experimentally recorded spectra to theoretically generated spectra from the protein sequence database. It also requires that any potential PTM (posttranslational modification) needs to be specified prior to database correlation. More recently, algorithms for direct spectral searching, such as SpectraST, have been introduced. The main

difference is that in spectral searching, experimental spectra are compared to experimental spectra that have been generated from the vast amount of proteomics data accumulated over the last decade.

Alternatively, proteins can be analyzed by *top-down proteomics* whereby intact proteins are directly ionized, fragmented by either ECD or ETD, and the resulting fragmentation pattern is used for protein identification (Kelleher, 2004). This strategy is less applicable to complex protein mixtures and is used mainly for the analysis of purified/enriched proteins. A potential advantage of top-down proteomics is that very high sequence coverage (ie, the majority of the protein's primary amino acid sequence is observed in the mass spectrum) can be obtained for the analyzed proteins. The accurate assignment of posttranslational protein modification is another advantage of top-down proteomics.

2.5.3 Gel-Based or Gel-Free Approaches

Two approaches are available to fractionate samples just prior to ionization. In the early years of proteome research, 2-dimensional gel electrophoresis (2-DE) was used routinely for protein separation. Proteins were separated according to their isoelectric point (pI) via isoelectric focusing in the first dimension and according to their molecular mass using sodium dodecyl sulfate-polyacrylamide gel electrophoresis (SDS-PAGE) in the second dimension, resulting in so-called 2D proteome maps that could be compared. Poor reproducibility and bias against proteins with extremes in pI, molecular mass, or membrane proteins were some of the major drawbacks of this technology. More recently, the use of computer-controlled image analysis software packages and fluorescence-based staining protocols (eg, difference gel electrophoresis [DIGE]) (Marouga et al, 2005) have improved 2-DE, because 2 samples are analyzed in the same gel. This is made possible by the labeling of 2 independent protein samples by 2 different fluorophores. Following labeling samples are combined and analyzed on the same gel and visualized based on their different excitation wavelengths. Separated protein spots are excised, in-gel digested, and eventually identified by MS. Alternatively, proteins are separated by molecular mass using 1-dimensional gel electrophoresis (1D SDS-PAGE) and the entire gel is cut into individual *gel blocks*, followed by in-gel digestion and extraction of the resulting peptides from the gel matrix (Shevchenko et al, 1996). These resultant peptide mixtures are separated by LC and eluting peptides are identified by MS. This method is routinely used in modern proteomics laboratories and is termed *gel-enhanced LC-MS* or *GeLC-MS*.

In recent years, methods have also been developed to eliminate the use of gel-based separation. In these *gel-free* approaches, complex protein mixtures are first digested in-solution, resulting in highly complex peptide mixtures, that are consecutively analyzed by LC-MS. In general, nano-bore LC columns (75- to 150-mm inner diameter and packed with reversed-phased chromatography resin) are used for peptide separation (termed *shotgun proteomics*) (Wolters et al, 2001). Peptides are separated and ions are directly electrosprayed into the mass spectrometer.

An alternative gel-free approach relies on a methodology termed *multidimensional protein identification technology (MudPIT)* (Washburn et al, 2001; Wolters et al, 2001), which is similar to 2-DE, and separates peptides by 2 orthogonal chromatographic resins: strong cationic exchange (SCX) and reversed phase (RP18). This 2D shotgun proteomics approach enables better peptide separation, ultimately resulting in the detection of lower abundance proteins.

2.5.4 Quantitative Proteomics

Quantifying proteins on a proteome level is a challenging analytical task, and not every protein identified can be accurately quantified. Some of the commonly used strategies for quantitative proteomics are based on the labeling of proteins with stable isotopes, similar to what has been used for quantitative MS of small molecules.

The 3 commonly used approaches to quantify proteins using isotope labeling are ICAT, SILAC, and iTRAQ. In the ICAT (*isotope-coded affinity tags*) approach, the relatively rare amino acid cysteine is chemically modified by the ICAT reagent. The ICAT label contains a chemical group that reacts specifically with cysteine moieties, and contains a linker region (which contains the light or heavy isotopes) and a biotin group for efficient affinity purification of labeled peptides. Briefly, protein lysates are either labeled with a light ICAT reagent (^{1}H or ^{12}C) or with the heavy analog (^{2}H or ^{13}C). The protein lysates are then combined (1:1 mixture), digested with trypsin, and labeled peptides purified by affinity chromatography using the biotin moiety (ie, streptavidin column). Resulting peptide mixtures are then analyzed by LC-MS to identify and quantify the relative levels of peptides/proteins in the mixture. Briefly, identification occurs as described above via spectral correlation of the resulting MS/MS spectra against protein sequence database using algorithms such as Sequest. Relative quantification requires the integration of the area under the curves for both the light and the heavy labeled peptides. This is accomplished by extraction parent ion intensities over time (ie, chromatographic retention time as these ions enter the MS). Because both the light and heavy isotopes have identical biophysical properties, they will coelute from the LC columns, but are separated by the MS as a result of their different mass. Comparison of the areas under the curves for both ions will provide relative quantification.

SILAC (*stable isotope labeling with amino acids in cell culture*) involves the addition of an essential amino acid (ie, light or heavy isotope version of lysine) to the cell culture medium, resulting in its metabolic incorporation into newly synthesized proteins (Ong et al, 2002). After complete labeling of the cellular proteome (ie, keeping cells in culture for several divisions), cells are lysed, combined at a 1:1 ratio and analyzed by MS as described above. Relative peptide quantification is accomplished by integration of the parent ion peak of either the light or heavy peptide ion. This procedure has been used recently for the relative quantification of tissue proteomes by metabolically labeling entire model organisms (Kruger et al, 2008).

iTRAQ (*isobaric tag for relative and absolute quantitation*) enables relative peptide quantification in the MS/MS mode (Ross et al, 2004). Primary amines (lysine side chains and/or the N-terminus) are covalently labeled by the iTRAQ reagent. Tryptic peptide mixtures, from 4 or 8 different experimental conditions, are individually labeled, combined, and analyzed by LC-MS. In contrast to the ICAT reagent, the individual iTRAQ labels have the same mass, resulting in the identical peptide mass for the same peptide isolated from individual experimental conditions. Upon fragmentation of a given parent ion via CID, the iTRAQ reagent will release a specific reporter ion for each experimental condition. The relative peak intensity of these reporter ions is used to quantify an individual peptide within the different experimental conditions (Fig. 2–31).

Some of the drawbacks of these reagents are the high cost, extensive data processing requirements (ie, integration of thousands of peptide ions), and the relatively low number of experimental conditions that can be compared (2 to 8 conditions depending on the reagent). To overcome some of these problems, label-free peptide/protein quantification was developed using spectral counting and label-free peak integration. Spectral counting uses the total, redundant number of tandem mass spectra (ie, spectral counts) recorded by MS/MS for each identified protein, as a semiquantitative measure of relative protein abundance (Liu et al, 2004) and is not limited by the number of analyzed samples. Thus, an unlimited number of experimental conditions could be compared.

Label-free peak integration is conceptually similar to the peptide quantification used by isotope labeling technologies but the major difference is that individual experimental

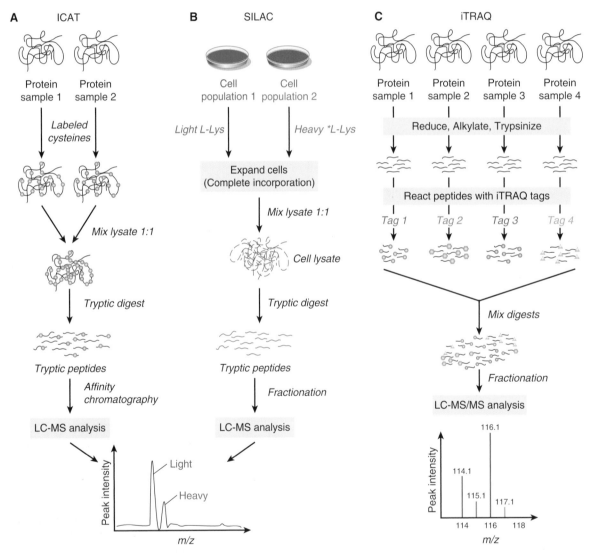

FIGURE 2–31 **Graphic demonstration of the workflow of 3 proteomic methodologies developed to utilize stable isotope technology for quantitative protein profiling by mass spectrometry. A)** ICAT can be used to label 2 protein samples with chemically identical tags that differ only in isotopic composition (heavy and light pairs). These tags contain a thiol-reactive group to covalently link to cysteine residues, and a biotin moiety. The ICAT-labeled fragments can be separated, and quantified by LC-MS analysis. **B)** SILAC is a similar approach to quantify proteins in mammalian cells. Isotopic labels are incorporated into proteins by metabolic labeling in the cell culture. Cell samples to be compared are grown separately in media containing either a heavy (*red*) or light (*blue*) form on an essential amino acid such as L-lysine that cannot be synthesized by the cell. **C)** iTRAQ is a unique approach that can be used to label protein samples with 4 independent tag reagents of the same mass that can give rise to 4 unique reporter ions (m/z = 114 to 117) upon fragmentation in MS/MS. This recorded data can be subsequently used to quantify the 4 different samples, respectively.

conditions are not combined (ie, light and heavy isotope), but analyzed individually by LC-MS. Therefore, chromatographic peaks need to be carefully aligned prior to integration/quantification, which is an extensive computational procedure.

2.5.5 Challenges for Biomarker Discovery with Proteomics

MS-based proteomics has the ability to identify and quantify hundreds to thousands of proteins in complex biological samples and has been used extensively for biomarker discovery (Faca et al, 2007; Jurisicova et al, 2008). Nonetheless, few such studies have been validated biologically and introduced into clinical practice. Some of the challenges of proteomics based biomarker discovery are: (a) extreme complexity of biological samples; (b) the heterogeneity of the disease and of the human population; (c) the difficulty to obtain accurate quantification for all proteins in the course of a discovery proteomics experiment; (d) the availability of adequate, well annotated human samples (tissue or body fluids); and (e) the expensive and very time-consuming process of proteomics-based biomarker discovery. Several analysis strategies were proposed and applied in recent years. The combination of extensive discovery-based proteomics on a limited number of patient samples, followed by the accurate quantification of putative biomarker candidates using targeted proteomics

approaches (ie, Selected Reaction Monitoring, SRM-MS) is considered the most promising strategy (Fig. 2–32).

2.5.6 X-Ray Crystallography

X-ray crystallography is a technique in which a high intensity x-ray beam is directed through the highly ordered crystalline phase of a pure protein. The regular array of electron density within the structure of the crystalline protein diffracts the x-rays so that the diffracted x-rays interfere constructively, giving rise to a unique diffraction pattern (detected on an x-ray imaging screen or film). From the diffraction pattern the distribution of electrons in the molecule (an electron density map) is calculated and a molecular model of the protein is then progressively built into the electron density map.

A critical step in this process is the generation of crystals of the protein of interest, which is a trial-and-error procedure in which a variety of solvent conditions are tested in multiple well plates with protein crystals almost always grown in solution. Crystal growth in solution is characterized by 2 steps: nucleation of a microscopic crystallite (possibly having only 100 molecules), followed by growth of that crystallite, ideally to a diffraction-quality crystal (Chernov, 2003). The solution conditions that favor the first step (nucleation) are not always the same conditions that favor the second step (subsequent

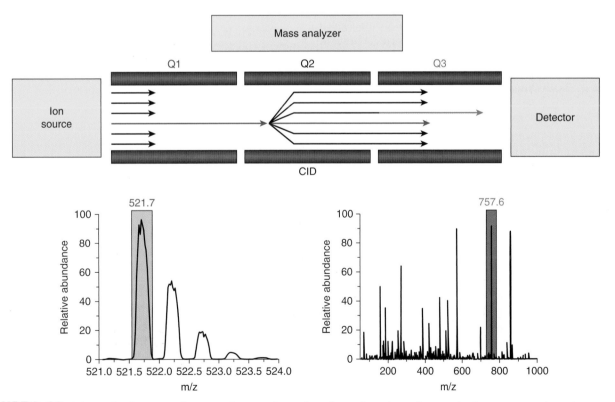

FIGURE 2–32 Schematic of a targeted proteomics experiment based on selected reaction monitoring-mass spectrometry (SRM-MS). Peptides that elute off an LC column are ionized by ESI and resulting ions are guided into the first quadrupole (Q1). This quadrupole works as a mass filter and transfers only peptide ions of interest (based on a predefined m/z value) into the second quadrupole (Q2), in which an inert gas induces fragmentation. All fragments are transferred into the third quadrupole (Q3), which, like Q1, acts as a mass filter, so that only few, select fragment ions will trigger a signal at the detector. The area under the curve of these ions can be used for quantification.

growth). Ideally, solution conditions should favor the development of a single, large crystal, as larger crystals offer improved resolution upon diffraction.

Generally, favorable conditions are identified by screening; a very large batch of the protein molecules is prepared, and a wide variety (up to thousands) of crystallization solutions are tested (Chayen, 2005). Thereafter, various conditions are used to lower the solubility of the molecule, including change in pH or temperature, adding salts or chemicals that lower the dielectric constant of the solution, or adding large polymers, such as polyethylene glycol, that drive the molecule out of solution. These methods require large amounts of the target molecule, as they use high concentration of the molecule(s) to be crystallized. Because of the difficulty in obtaining such large quantities (milligrams) of crystallization-grade protein, robots have been developed that can accurately dispense crystallization trial drops that are only approximately 100 nanoliters in volume (Stock et al, 2005). Highly pure protein (usually from recombinant sources) is divided into a series of small drops of aqueous buffers that often contain 1 or more cosolvents or precipitants. The drop is left to slowly evaporate or equilibrate with a reservoir solution (in the same well), and if conditions are favorable, the protein slowly comes out of solution in a crystalline form. This represents the limiting step in crystallography as the conditions may vary greatly from one protein to another, and it is impossible to know a priori under which conditions, if any, a given protein will crystallize. Indeed, not every protein will crystallize, and often researchers try individual domains or multiple domains within a given protein or homologous proteins from other species in order to find a combination of protein and conditions that will yield a well-diffracting crystal.

When a crystal is mounted and exposed to an intense beam of x-rays, it scatters the x-rays into a pattern of spots or reflections that can be observed on a screen behind the crystal. The relative intensities of these spots provide the required information to determine the arrangement of molecules within the crystal in atomic detail. The intensities of these reflections may be recorded with photographic film, an area detector or with a charge-coupled device (CCD) image sensor. The recorded series of 2-dimensional diffraction patterns, each corresponding to a different crystal orientation, is converted into a 3-dimensional model of the electron density. Each spot corresponds to a different type of variation in the electron density; the crystallographer must determine which variation corresponds to which spot (indexing), the relative strengths of the spots in different images (merging and scaling), and how the variations should be combined to yield the total electron density (phasing).

The final step of fitting the atoms of the protein into the electron density map requires the use of interactive computer graphics programs, or semiautomated programs if the data is of sufficient quality and resolution. Initially the electron density map contains many errors, but it can be improved through a process called *refinement* in which the atomic model is adjusted to improve the agreement with the measured diffraction data. The quality of an atomic model is judged through

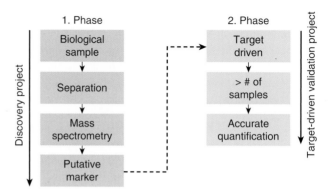

FIGURE 2–33 **Schematic of a typical biomarker experiment.** In the discovery project (*1. Phase*) a limited number of biological samples are separated to reduce sample complexity. Individual fractions are then analyzed by mass spectrometry to generate putative biomarkers for verification. In the target-driven validation project (*2. Phase*) targeted MS-assays (ie, SRM-MS) are developed for each putative candidate marker. This approach allows to significantly increase the sample throughput and provides accurate quantification in a multiplexed manner.

the standard crystallographic R-factor, which is a measure of how well the atomic model fits the experimental data.

The fine details revealed by high-resolution x-ray structures are useful to understand the principles of molecular recognition in protein-ligand complexes (Fig. 2–33). For example, the structure of imatinib bound to *c-Abl* kinase domain is an example of the application of this approach. Imatinib is a potent and selective inhibitor of the chronic myeloid leukemia-related translocation product *of bcr-abl*, making it an effective therapy for chronic myelogenous leukemia (CML; see Chap. 7, Sec. 7.5 and Chap. 17, Sec. 17.3). It was discovered by using high-throughput screening of compound libraries to identify the 2-phenylaminopyrimidine class of kinase inhibitors. The pharmaceutical properties of these compounds were then optimized through successive rounds of medicinal chemistry and evaluation of structure-activity relationships. Ultimately, the structural mechanism of the inhibition of *bcr-abl* by imatinib was shown by x-ray crystallography to involve binding by the inhibitor to inactive kinase structure of the enzyme (the kinase exists in active and inactive forms). The inactive form is the more unique conformation of the enzyme (relative to other similar kinases), thereby explaining its relatively few side effects (Schindler et al, 2000).

2.5.7 Nuclear Magnetic Resonance Spectroscopy

NMR spectroscopy takes advantage of a fundamental property of the nuclei of atoms called the nuclear spin (see Chap. 14, Sec. 14.3). When placed in a static magnetic field, nuclei with nonzero spin will align their magnetic dipoles with (low-energy state) or against (high-energy state) the magnetic field. Under normal circumstances there is a small difference in the population distribution between the 2 energy states, thereby creating a net magnetization, which is then manipulated using multiple electromagnetic pulses (and delays) which help to clarify the types of connections between nuclei. Each nucleus absorbs energy from these pulses at a characteristic frequency that is dependent on its chemical properties and the surrounding environment, including the conformation of the molecule and its nearest neighbor nuclei. Structures of noncrystalline proteins in aqueous solution are derived from a series of NMR experiments that reveal interactions of nuclei close together in 3-dimensional space, even though they are distant within the protein primary sequence. These data allow one to calculate an ensemble of protein conformations that satisfy a large number (hundreds to thousands) of experimental restraints. This necessitates extensive data collection (often more than 10 experiments lasting hours to days) and computer-assisted analysis of the spectra in order to calculate a structure.

The main nucleus observed by NMR is that of hydrogen (^{1}H). However, proteins have hundreds to thousands of ^{1}H signals, many with the same resonance frequency. This problem is solved by the use of multidimensional NMR, in which protein samples are labeled with the NMR-active stable isotopes,

^{15}N and ^{13}C. The incorporation of stable isotopes is required to resolve the large number of signals in 2, 3, or 4 dimensions, each dimension corresponding to ^{1}H, ^{15}N, and/or ^{13}C resonance frequencies. Because of the poor signal-to-noise ratio of the NMR signals in large proteins, the size of proteins amenable to high-resolution NMR structural studies is limited to approximately 30 kilodaltons (kDa) or less. Recent developments have made it possible to study larger molecules by using partial or full deuteration (ie, incorporation of heavy hydrogen) in combination with special NMR techniques, resulting in lower-resolution structural information. Samples typically need to be concentrated; this requirement makes it difficult to study proteins with low solubility or those that are prone to aggregation or precipitation. Much time is devoted in optimizing the stability and solubility of a protein prior to study by NMR spectroscopy.

2.5.8 Protein Arrays

A protein microarray provides an approach to characterize multiple proteins in a biological sample. There are 3 types of protein microarrays (Fig. 2–34). *Functional protein arrays* display

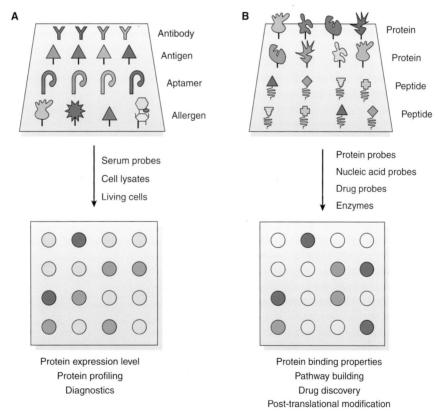

FIGURE 2–34 **A) Analytical protein microarray. Different types of ligands, including antibodies, antigens, DNA or RNA aptamers, carbohydrates, or small molecules, with high affinity and specificity, are spotted down.** These chips can be used for monitoring protein expression level, protein profiling, and clinical diagnostics. Similar to the procedure in DNA microarray experiments, protein samples from 2 biological states to be compared are separately labeled with red or green fluorescent dyes, mixed, and incubated with the chips. Spots in red or green color identify an excess of proteins from one state over the other. **B) Functional protein microarray.** Native proteins or peptides are individually purified or synthesized using high-throughput approaches and arrayed onto a suitable surface to form the functional protein microarrays. These chips are used to analyze protein activities, binding properties and posttranslational modifications. With the proper detection method, functional protein microarrays can be used to identify the substrates of enzymes of interest. Consequently, this class of chips is particularly useful in drug and drug-target identification and in building biological networks. (From Phizicky et al, 2003.)

folded and active proteins and are designed to assay functional properties (Zhu and Snyder, 2003). They are used for screening molecular interactions, studying protein pathways, identifying targets for protein-targeted molecules, and analyzing enzymatic activities. In *analytical* or *capture arrays*, affinity reagents (eg, antibodies) or antigens (that may be nonfolded) are arrayed for profiling the expression of proteins (Sanchez-Carbayo et al, 2006) or for the quantification of antibodies in complex samples such as serum. Applications of antibody arrays include biomarker discovery and monitoring of protein quantities and activity states in signaling pathways. Antigen arrays are applied for profiling antibody repertoires in autoimmunity, cancer, infection or following vaccination. Moreover, antigen arrays are tools for controlling the specificity of antibodies and related affinity reagents. *Reverse-phase arrays* comprise cell lysates or serum samples. Replicates of the array can then be probed with different antibodies. Reverse-phase arrays are particularly useful for studying changes in the expression of specific proteins and protein modifications during disease progression and, thus, are applied primarily for biomarker discovery.

2.6 TRANSLATIONAL APPLICATIONS WITH CELLS AND TISSUES

Genetic or epigenetic analysis of primary human tumors (or other tissues) requires access to appropriately handled material. Generally, human tumor or tissue samples are fixed in formalin and then embedded in paraffin wax to preserve cell and tissue morphology for histological analysis as part of diagnostic procedures. Formalin fixation is a rather erratic process with thick tissue sections requiring the formalin to diffuse into the tissue resulting in unequal protein preservation. Only seldom are tissues snap-frozen after an operation (or biopsy) so as to improve preservation of cellular antigens or mRNA. These limitations, as well as the presence of stroma, immune infiltrates, and other secreted proteins, create a number of difficulties for identifying genetic or epigenetic changes specifically associated with the tumor cells (or the stromal cell populations), emphasizing the need to develop better techniques to isolate individual cells from tissue sections for further study.

Fortunately, despite the fact that formalin crosslinks proteins, it has little effect on the structural integrity of DNA or miRNAs. Therefore, the ability to use FISH on paraffin-embedded archival specimens is dependent only on the accessibility of the target DNA within the cell nucleus, and can be enhanced by pretreatment that increases the efficiency of hybridization. Such protocols are now routinely used for the analysis of *HER2* in breast cancer tissues. Similarly, miRNAs can be retrieved from formalin-fixed tissue with reasonable success. Although there are protocols for extracting mRNA from archival formalin fixed tissue, its tendency to be degraded by ubiquitous RNases limits the performance of these assays.

Hematological malignancies aside, where it is much easier to retrieve the malignant cells, the development of a number of techniques over the last 10 years has enhanced substantially the ability of scientists to isolate and rapidly analyze cells and tissue from solid tumors.

2.6.1 Laser-Capture Microdissection

One problem associated with the molecular genetic analysis of small numbers of tumor cells is that substantial numbers of normal cells will often be present and can confound interpretation. Because these stromal and various infiltrating cells are scattered throughout a tumor section, it is rarely possible to dissect a pure population of tumor cells cleanly. This problem has been circumvented by the use of laser capture microdissection, in which sections (usually from frozen tissue) are coated with a clear ethylene vinyl acetate (EVA) polymer prior to microscopic examination (Emmert-Buck et al, 1996). Tumor cells can be captured for subsequent analysis by briefly pulsing the area of interest with an infrared laser. The EVA film becomes adherent and will selectively attach to the tumor cells directly in the laser path.

Laser capture microdissection

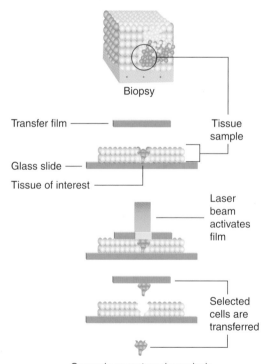

FIGURE 2−35 Outline of the process of laser-capture microdissection. Under a microscope–software interface, a tissue section (typically 5 to 50 μm thick) is assessed and cells are identified for the selection of targets for isolation. In general, collection technologies use an UV-pulsed laser for cutting the tissues directly, sometimes in combination with an infrared (IR) laser responsible for heating/melting a sticky polymer for cellular adhesion and isolation. After the collection, the tissue can be processed for protein, RNA, or DNA downstream analyses. (From http://www.cancer.gov/cancertopics/ understandingcancer/moleculardiagnostics/page29.)

When sufficient cells have been fused to the EVA film, it is placed into nucleic acid extraction buffers and used for PCR or other molecular analyses (Fig. 2–35). One application of laser capture microdissection is whole-genome amplification of captured cells, for example from a small number of tumor-derived cells. A variety of techniques including random PCR allow for the global amplification of all DNA sequences present in the microdissected samples, thereby increasing globally the amount of DNA for subsequent analysis. The method can also be adapted to generate representative amplification of the mRNA in a small number of cells. The technique has been useful in providing DNA for molecular genetic studies using microdissected DNA from paraffin blocks, cDNA from single-cell RT-PCR reactions, and chromosome band-specific probes derived for microdissected chromosomal DNA.

2.6.2 Tissue Microarrays

Tissue microarray (TMA) technology provides a method of relocating tissue from conventional histological paraffin blocks so that tissue from multiple patients (or multiple blocks from the same patient) can be analyzed on the same slide. The microarray technique (Kononen et al, 1998), introduced

a high-precision punching instrument that enabled the exact and reproducible placement and relocalization of distinct tissue samples. The construction of a TMA starts with the careful selection of donor tissues and precise recording of their localization. The slides must be reviewed so that suitable donor blocks can be selected and the region of interest defined on a selected paraffin wax block. Needles with varying diameters of 0.6 mm up to 2.0 mm are used to punch tissue cores from a predefined region of the tissue block embedded in paraffin wax. A hematoxylin and eosin stained slide arranged beside the donor block surface is used for orientation (Fig. 2–36). Tissue cores are transferred to a recipient paraffin wax block, into a ready-made hole, guided by a defined x–y position. This technique minimizes tissue damage and still allows sections to be cut from the donor paraffin wax block with all necessary diagnostic details, even after the removal of multiple cores. The number of cores in the recipient paraffin block varies, depending on the array design, with the current comfortable maximum using a 0.6-mm needle being approximately 600 cores per standard glass microscope slide. New techniques may allow as many as 2000 or more cores per slide. Using this method, an entire cohort of samples (eg, from different patients) can be analyzed by staining just 1 or 2 master array slides, instead of staining hundreds of conventional slides.

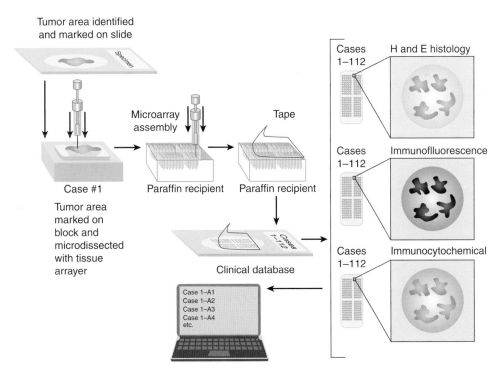

FIGURE 2–36 Outline of the process of TMA assembly. In the TMA technique, a hollow needle is used to remove tissue cores as small as 0.6 mm in diameter from regions of interest in paraffin-embedded tissues, such as clinical biopsies or tumor samples. These tissue cores are then inserted in a recipient paraffin block in a precisely spaced, array pattern, usually along with control samples. Sections from this block are cut using a microtome, mounted on a microscope slide and then analyzed by any method of standard histological analysis. Each microarray block can be cut into 100 to 500 sections, which can be subjected to independent tests. The number of spots on a single slide varies, depending on the array design, the current comfortable maximum with the 0.6-mm needle being about 600 spots per standard glass microscope slide. New technologies are under development that may allow as many as 2000 or more sections per slide. (Adapted from http://apps.pathology.jhu.edu/blogs/pathology/wp-content/uploads/2010/05/Tissue_Microarray_Process.jpg.)

Each core on the array is similar to a conventional slide in that complete demographic and outcome information is maintained for each patient contributing that core, so that rigorous statistical analysis can be performed when the arrays are analyzed.

The TMA approach has been criticized for its use of small punches of usually only a 0.6-mm diameter from tumors with much larger diameter (up to several centimeters) when there is considerable heterogeneity in the tissue sample or the marker of interest being studied. Several experimental and clinicopathological efforts have been made to reduce these concerns and they can be alleviated by including multiple cores from each patient block on the array (Rubin et al, 2002; Eckel-Passow et al, 2010). For example, the grading of breast cancer is dependent on the presence and number of mitoses. Because this important parameter of breast grading is evaluated mainly at the periphery of the tumor, breast cancer arrays focusing on proliferation markers should be mainly composed of punches taken from the periphery of the original tumor. Other studies show that the frequency of prognostically significant gene amplifications in a series of invasive breast cancers, such as erbB2 or cyclin D1, is similar after TMA analysis to frequencies described in the literature using other techniques (Kononen et al, 1998).

2.6.3 Flow Cytometry

Flow cytometry enables the analysis of multiple parameters of individual cells using a suspension of heterogeneous cells. The flow cytometer directs a beam of laser light of a single wavelength onto a hydrodynamically focused stream of saline solution, optimally of only 1 cell in diameter (Fig. 2–37). A number of fluorescent detectors are aimed at the point where the stream passes through the light beam: 1 in line with the light beam (forward scatter) and several beams perpendicular to it (side scatter). Each suspended cell passes through the beam and thus scatters the light. In addition, fluorescent chemicals found in the cell or attached to it may be excited and emit light at a longer wavelength than the light source. Forward scatter correlates with the cell size and side scatter depends on the inner complexity or granularity of the cell (ie, shape of the nucleus, the amount and type of cytoplasmic granules or the membrane roughness). By analyzing fluctuations in brightness at each detector (1 for each fluorescent emission peak), it is possible to derive various types of information about the physical and chemical properties of each individual particle. For example, fluorescently labeled antibodies can be applied to cells, or fluorescent proteins can be contained in cells. Modern flow cytometers are able to analyze several thousand cells every second, in "real time," and can separate, analyze, and isolate cells having specified properties. Acquisition of data is achieved by a computer using software that can adjust parameters (eg, voltage and compensation) for the sample being tested. Modern instruments usually have multiple lasers and fluorescence detectors. Increasing the number of lasers and detectors allows for multiple antibody labeling, and can more precisely identify a target population by their phenotypic markers. Some instruments can even take digital images of individual cells, allowing for the analysis of fluorescent signal location within or on the surface of the cell.

The applications of flow cytometry to research are constantly expanding but include the volume and morphological complexity of cells; total DNA content (cell-cycle analysis, see Chap. 12, Sec. 12.1.2); total RNA content; DNA copy number

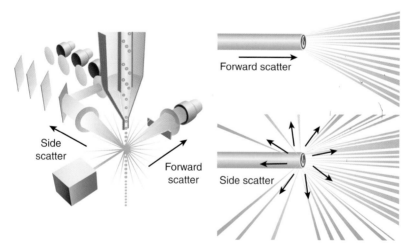

FIGURE 2–37 **In flow cytometry, lenses are used to shape and focus the excitation beam from a laser, directing the beam through the hydrodynamically focused sample stream.** Where the laser intersects the stream is the "interrogation zone," when the particle passes through the interrogation zone there is light scatter and possibly fluorescence; it is the detection and analysis of this light scatter and fluorescence that gives information about a particle. To detect the light scatter and fluorescent light, there are detectors—1 in line with the laser (to detect forward scatter) and 1 perpendicular to the laser (to detect side scatter). The intensity of the forward scatter is in relation to the particle size. The side scatter channel (SSC) detects light at a 90-degree angle to the laser source point; this scatter gives information on granularity and internal complexity. (Copyright © 2012 Life Technologies Corporation. Used under permission.)

variation (by Flow-FISH); chromosome analysis and sorting (library construction, chromosome paints); protein expression and localization; posttranslation protein modifications; fluorescent protein detection; detection of cell surface antigens (cell differentiation [CD] markers); intracellular antigens (various cytokines, secondary mediators, etc); nuclear antigens; apoptosis (quantification, measurement of DNA degradation, mitochondrial membrane potential, permeability changes, caspase activity; see Chap. 9, Sec. 9.4.2); cell viability; and multidrug resistance (see Chap. 19, Sec. 19.2.3) in cancer cells.

Fluorescence-activated cell sorting is a specialized type of flow cytometry that allows a heterogeneous cell population to be sorted into 2 or more containers, 1 cell at a time, based upon the light scattering and fluorescent properties of each cell. It utilizes a similar system of hydrodynamic focusing, but with a large separation between cells relative to cell diameter. A vibrating mechanism causes the stream of cells to break into individual droplets with a low probability of more than 1 cell per droplet. Just before the stream breaks into droplets, the flow passes through a fluorescence-measuring station where the fluorescent character of each cell is measured and an electrical charge is applied to the droplet, depending on the fluorescence-intensity measurement. The charged droplets then fall through an electrostatic deflection system that diverts droplets into different chambers based upon their charge.

2.7 BIOINFORMATICS AND OTHER TECHNIQUES OF DATA ANALYSIS

Bioinformatics employs a variety of computational techniques to analyze biological data and to integrate the data with publicly available resources. This section outlines some of the major biological problems that can be addressed using computational techniques, with a focus on 2 major areas particularly relevant to cancer biology and research: microarray analysis and pathway analysis.

2.7.1 Microarray Analysis

The first step in obtaining the most information from any large-scale experiment such as a microarray study is to consider its design. The statistical power of the analysis (called a *Type II* or *β error*) indicates the probability that a false-negative result will be avoided. There are several methods for analysis of power, based on trade-offs between the magnitude of the effect, the intersample variability, and the number of samples used, and these techniques can be extended to handle multidimensional datasets, like microarray data (Begun, 2008; Asare et al, 2009; Hackstadt and Hess, 2009).

The next step is to consider which types of samples should be processed for validation and quality control. For example, each sample can be hybridized once, or technical replicates can be used. A technical replicate occurs when the same RNA sample is split into 2 separate aliquots and each is hybridized separately to multiple microarray chips. The use of technical

replicates allows for the assessment of technical variability within the experiment but this comes with 2 costs. First, each sample is hybridized in duplicate, essentially doubling the price and sample requirements of the experiment. Second, more complex statistical models (called *repeated-measures models*) must be used to analyze this type of data. An alternative is to use multiple RNA samples from each biological sample. For example, different regions of a tumor can be isolated and RNA extracted from each and hybridized to independent microarrays. This type of experiment provides a highly informative assessment of intratumor heterogeneity, but requires the use of complex statistical techniques, such as mixed models (Bachtiary et al, 2006).

An important step in handling microarray data is the removal of spurious background signals. These signals can arise from pooling of samples during hybridization, from stochastic events, or from defects in array manufacture or scanning. Background signal almost always varies from 1 region of the array to another. A wide range of computational techniques have been developed to remove these background effects, but the most successful techniques model the fraction of bound probes in a given spot directly from the number of pixels available (Kooperberg et al, 2002). A very widely-used method for Affymetrix (ie, printed oligonucleotide) arrays, called *GCRMA*, takes into account the differential hybridization strengths of G:C and A:T base-pairings directly in the background correction procedure (Wu et al, 2004).

Normalization is the process of removing technical artifacts from a dataset. For example, successful normalization of a microarray experiment will remove variability caused by differential rates of dye incorporation, differential fluorescent efficiency of fluorophores, irregularities in the surface of a microarray, unequal sample loading, and differential sample quality or degradation. At the same time, biological factors like the inherent biological variability between replicate animals should be preserved. Normalization methods can be classified as either global or local. A global method considers the entire dataset, and excels at removing artifacts that are consistently present across multiple arrays in a study. By contrast, local methods focus on a subset of the data, usually a single array. These tend to be both more computationally efficient and to be more efficacious at removing nonsystematic (eg, stochastic) effects.

2.7.2 Statistical Analysis

Once microarray data has been preprocessed to remove or reduce nonbiological signals, statistical analysis is required to identify genes or features that have a specific pattern of interest. The most common question to arise from a microarray experiment is, "What differs between two prespecified groups?" This study design encompasses many common biological situations, such as treatment/vehicle, case/control, and genetic-perturbation/wild-type comparisons. A variety of novel statistical tests have been evaluated to address 2-group microarray questions, but it is common to apply t-tests, for example, to compare the mean expression of a gene between 2 groups, such as primary and metastatic tumors. First, the t-test assumes that the 2 groups have equivalent variability; this assumption is often violated, as some tumor types are more heterogeneous than others, and there is usually more variability in tumors than normal tissues, but corrections can be applied. Second, the t-test assumes that the data are drawn (sampled) from a population with a normal distribution, and it is difficult to verify this assumption—tests for the normality of a distribution are very insensitive. Third, the use of multiple t-tests assumes that each test is independent from the others. Microarray data often violate this assumption, as the expression of RNA from different genes can be highly correlated.

Often, queries related to translational oncology involve assessment of patient survival or tumor recurrence. It is rare that a clinical study is carried out until all patients have died, entered stable remission, or experienced a recurrence of their disease; instead, only a specified amount of follow-up will be available for each patient, and many will remain alive at the conclusion of the study. The analysis of survival is usually performed using log-rank analysis as described in Chapter 22, Section 22.2.5. An alternative, the Cox proportional hazards model, is analogous to a multiple regression model and enables the difference between survival times of particular groups of patients to be tested while allowing for other factors (covariates), each of which is likely to influence survival. These techniques have been widely applied in relating microarray data to survival or recurrence of disease in patients.

Independent of what statistical test is employed for a microarray analysis, the final set of p-values must be considered carefully. A p-value represents the chance of making a Type I (or α) error (a false-positive) for testing a *single* hypothesis. Consider an experiment where 20 primary colon cancers are analyzed by microarray to measure the mRNA abundance of 10,000 genes. These 20 samples are randomly split into 2 groups of 10 each, where there is no expectation that the groups are actually different. A simple t-test is used to compare the level of each of the 10,000 genes between groups, and a stringent p-value threshold of 0.01 is applied. In this case, we predict that there will be $10,000 \times 0.01 = 100$ false-positives; that is, 100 genes will be found different between the 2 groups by chance alone. There are several "multiple testing adjustments" that help alleviate this problem. One classic adjustment is called the *Bonferroni correction*, which involves dividing the threshold p-value by the number of tests to be performed. In the example above, we would use a threshold of $p < 0.01/10,000$, or $p < 10^{-6}$. This type of adjustment is very conservative, as it assumes that all of the comparisons are independent (whereas many are often correlated) and suggests that, across all 10,000 tests, we will have only a 1% chance of finding even 1 false-positive. An alternative approach is called the *false-discovery rate* (FDR) adjustment. This adjustment controls the percentage of tests that will be expected to be false-positives. For example, if there are 100 genes with an FDR <0.1 (eg, a FDR of 10%), then we anticipate that $100 \times 0.1 = 10$ genes from this list will be false-positives. Calculation of the FDR itself for any given experiment is complex (Storey and Tibshirani, 2003) but is easily performed in common statistical software packages, and the use of FDR-adjusted p-values (also called *q-values*) has become widespread in genomic studies.

2.7.3 Unsupervised Clustering

After differentially expressed genes have been identified using statistical techniques, as described above, there remains the major challenge of interpreting the biological relevance of these changes. A common technique is to group similar patterns of change in gene expression together. This may provide information about co-regulation of genes, and coregulated genes are well known to share biological functions (Boutros and Okey, 2005). Therefore patterns of similarity of differentially expressed genes might shed light into disease etiology or mechanisms.

The next step is to select an appropriate method to classify patterns (eg, of gene expression). If the biological question involves a characteristic of the samples—such as identifying novel tumor subtypes or predicting patient response—then supervised machine-learning methods (described below) are most appropriate. If the goals involve characteristics of individual genes, then an unsupervised method is more appropriate. These unsupervised methods are often called *clustering methods* (see also Chap. 22, Sec. 22.5), and there are a variety of available techniques that are distinguished by their mathematical characteristics and the assumptions that they make. For example, a commonly used method called *k-mean clustering* assumes that the number of "classes" of genes can be defined a priori but makes no other assumptions regarding the interrelationships between specific pairs of genes. Another very common method, called *hierarchical clustering*, makes no assumptions regarding the number of classes of genes (de Hoon et al, 2004). Instead, it assumes that genes are related to each other in a hierarchical way, where certain gene-pairs are more similar than others (Duda et al, 2001). A large number of clustering algorithms have been developed but there have been no comprehensive comparisons of them, so it is difficult to suggest optimal methods for particular experimental designs.

A common misconception about unsupervised methods such as clustering is that all genes within a single group share a common mechanism. However, although different genes may exhibit similar expression profiles, this does not necessarily indicate a single common mechanism. For example, the p53 response might be abrogated in tumors by multiple mechanisms, each producing the same resulting expression profile. Other causes may lead to sets of genes being coregulated, especially in genome-wide experiments where millions of gene-pairs are assessed. By definition, clustering methods only identify genes that are correlated. Mechanistic hypotheses can be framed from these data, but there is no necessity for a single underlying mechanism (Boutros and Okey, 2005; Boutros, 2006).

2.7.4 Gene Signatures

Increasingly microarray and other -omic datasets are being used to make predictions about clinical behavior. The approach is straightforward: Those features that are correlated with the presence of a specific clinical event are identified using an appropriate statistical methodology. These features are merged to construct a multifeature predictive signature. This signature is then evaluated in an independent group of patients to test and demonstrate its robustness. This general approach was first applied to demonstrate that acute myeloid and acute lymphoblastic leukemias could be distinguished with good accuracy, solely on the basis of their mRNA expression profiles (Golub et al, 1999). A large number of groups extended this initial work to demonstrate that many tumor subtypes could be distinguished and even discovered from microarray data (Bild et al, 2006; Chin et al, 2006; Neve et al, 2006).

The second major application of machine-learning techniques to -omic data has already substantially changed clinical practice. Rather than defining tumor subtypes, many investigators have sought to predict which patients might be under- or overtreated. The first major study, in breast cancer, identified a 70-gene signature that predicted survival of breast cancer patients (van 't Veer et al, 2002). Subsequent external validations have helped this predictor be developed into a tool that is used in clinical practice (van de Vijver et al, 2002; van 't Veer and Bernards, 2008). Similar efforts have led to the development of prognostic signatures for other tumor types, particularly non–small cell lung carcinoma (Beer et al, 2002; Chen et al, 2007; Lau et al, 2007; Boutros et al, 2009) and serous ovarian cancers (Mok et al, 2009). Nevertheless, the field has come under critical review recently for the proliferation of poorly validated and described signatures (Shedden et al, 2008; Subramanian and Simon, 2010), with evidence that current studies are under-powered (Ein-Dor et al, 2006). It therefore remains unclear if analogies to the promising breast cancer prognostic signatures can be found for other tumor types.

2.7.5 Pathway Analysis

Many -omic experiments result in a large list of genes. For example, the determination of genes that are amplified or deleted in cancer using array CGH (Li et al, 2009) can result in hundreds or thousands of genes present in copy-number altered regions. Similarly, a microarray analysis can identify hundreds or thousands of genes altered between cancerous and normal tissue or associated with prognosis. When presented with a gene-list of this size and scope, the most common question is, "What do all these genes have in common?" There is a reductionist tendency to search for a smaller number of underlying "driver" changes that drive or explain the

changes in all these genes. There are 2 primary approaches to this challenge: gene ontology enrichment analysis and protein-interaction network analysis.

Gene ontology (GO) is a systematic attempt to organize and categorize what is known about gene function and localization. GO defines functions first in a general, nonspecific manner and it is then refined into more specific statements. Each of these functions are given a specific GO identifier, and if a gene is assigned a specific function it automatically "inherits" all less-specific functions (Consortium, 2001). Different genes possess varying degrees of GO annotation. Some well-characterized genes will be annotated with dozens of different functions, whereas other less-characterized genes may possess little or no annotation. For example, a gene might first be described as involved in the general process of "metabolism," then the more specific process of "monosaccharide metabolism" (GO:0005996), then the more specific terms of "hexose metabolism" (GO:0019318), "fructose metabolism" (GO:0006000), and, ultimately, the most precise term, "fructose 1,6-bisphosphonate metabolism" (GO:0030388).

Numerous groups are working to annotate every gene with all specific functions that have been reported in the literature (Camon et al, 2003). Because information about gene-function is usually reported in the text of peer-reviewed journals this is a time-consuming and manual endeavor. More recently -omic studies have provided the capacity for more rapid assessment of gene function. GO stores both types of information, but allows users to distinguish them with "evidence codes." Every association of a gene and a function is supported by 1 or more codes that indicate their origin. The most common codes include IEA (inferred from electronic annotation, usually -omic datasets) and TAS (traceable author statement, usually published datapoints).

There are multiple online tools to associate each gene with its known GO annotation. Essentially, all these tools attempt to assign a statistical assessment of "GO enrichment": in other words, are there any specific GO terms that occur more often than expected by chance in this list of genes? The most common approach is to ignore the structure of the GO tree and to simply perform a large number of proportion tests—1 for every GO term. A proportion test essentially asks if a ratio differs between 2 conditions: It tests whether the fraction of genes in the gene list annotated with a given function is significantly different from the fraction of all genes with this function. The main challenges are the presence of unannotated genes, the statistical problems of performing parallel tests on correlated data, and the potential for error in existing annotations.

An alternative approach to using GO enrichment analysis to identify functions in a gene list is to analyze the data from the context of interacting networks of proteins. The rationale is that proteins that physically interact are highly likely to be involved in similar functions. There is substantial support for this concept, particularly from model organisms. Protein–protein interactions can be identified using several experimental techniques (see Sec. 2.5) however, the protein–protein interaction networks of humans and other mammals are less-well known than those of model organisms. Many groups have inferred mammalian protein–protein interactions from those of other organisms, under the assumption that they are likely to be evolutionarily conserved (Brown and Jurisica, 2005) or to manually curate protein–protein interactions in much the same way as GO annotations are annotated by manual review of the primary literature. Both approaches have problems, as the former biases against proteins with poor evolutionary conservation, while the latter biases toward well-studied proteins. Additional high-throughput screens will be needed to provide deeper coverage of human protein–protein interactions.

Once a database of protein–protein interactions has been identified, the most common approach is to superimpose a gene list upon the overall network. Each gene in the list, along with its nearest neighbors (ie, the direct interactions), is then be probed. The interaction network can be arranged in 2-dimensional space, and it can be determined if the genes on the gene list are more proximal to one another than would be expected by chance alone, thus suggesting that they encode components of common functional pathways. This type of approach has identified critical characteristics of cancer cells, including potential opportunities to exploit synthetic lethal interactions (Jonsson and Bates, 2006; Pujana et al, 2007; Rambaldi et al, 2008). Additionally, there is emerging evidence that lung cancer biomarkers may also be improved by addition of protein–protein interactions (Wachi et al, 2005; Lau et al, 2007).

SUMMARY

- Cytogenetics and karyotyping gave the initial insights into tumor genomics and pathophysiology; increasingly, however, these techniques have been replaced by newer techniques that rely on hybridization, which are increasingly fluorescence based.
- Techniques are available in the laboratory to examine the effects of DNA, RNA, and proteins within cellular systems. These include standard techniques of Southern, northern, and western blots, respectively, as well as functional manipulations, including the transfection of plasmids and siRNA into cells. Ultimately, xenograft or mouse models can be manipulated to provide in vivo assessments of cancer initiation, progression, and therapeutics.
- PCR-based techniques have allowed the assessment of (a) amplification of small volumes of DNA and cDNA, (b) quantification, both relative and absolute, of particular DNA or RNA sequences, and (c) assistance in next-generation sequencing.
- High throughput or "next-generation" sequencing approaches include a variety of techniques. Generally, these include an initial template preparation step (which may include a PCR amplification), followed by sequencing and imaging/detection steps. The latter 2 steps are often integrated and may rely on fluorescence, bioluminescence, or changes in pH to detect nucleotide sequence.

- Improved technologies have revealed the increasingly complex variation in the human genome at both the base-pair level (SNPs) and larger sequence levels (CNVs). The effect of these variations is still being explored but is already known to influence cancer predisposition, progression, and response to treatment.
- Epigenetics is the study of heritable changes in gene expression or cellular phenotype caused by mechanisms other than changes in the underlying DNA sequence. Epigenetic processes include (a) posttranslational modification of the amino acids that make up histone proteins such as acetylation, methylation, ubiquitination, phosphorylation, and sumoylation, and (b) the addition of methyl groups to the DNA.
- Established techniques for the assessment of human tissue samples for translational research include TMA construction (with subsequent downstream analyses for immunohistochemistry, immunofluorescence, or FISH), laser capture microdissection (for gene expression), and flow cytometry (for a variety of applications such as surface protein assessments).
- Proteome research provides a comprehensive description of the proteins present in a biological entity under specific conditions. With the recent advent of improved methods and the introduction of more sensitive and faster scanning mass spectrometers, the near-complete analyses of complex human proteomes is becoming feasible.
- Methodological advances enable the accurate relative quantification of thousands of proteins using stable isotope technology.
- Targeted proteomics approaches based on selected reaction monitoring (SRM) are currently the most commonly used approach for multiplex quantification in biomarker verification experiments.
- The data generated by high-throughput experiments can be subject to a number of biases. These can be mitigated by experimental techniques, imaging normalization and statistical assessments is analyzed using a series of bioinformatics processes that mitigate experimental and stochastic noise. In addition, the application of unsupervised and supervised learning shows promise to illuminate the unifying biological principles within a dataset.

REFERENCES

Appella E, Anderson CW. New prospects for proteomics—electron-capture (ECD) and electron-transfer dissociation (ETD) fragmentation techniques and combined fractional diagonal chromatography (COFRADIC). *FEBS J* 2007;274:6255.

Asare AL, Gao Z, Carey VJ, Wang R, Seyfert-Margolis V. Power enhancement via multivariate outlier testing with gene expression arrays. *Bioinformatics* 2009;25:48-53.

Ausubel JH, Waggoner PE. Assessing environmental changes in grasslands. *Science* 2003;299:1844-1845; author reply 1844-1845.

Babinet C, Cohen-Tannoudji M. Genome engineering via homologous recombination in mouse embryonic stem (ES) cells: an amazingly versatile tool for the study of mammalian biology. *An Acad Bras Cienc* 2001;73:365-383.

Bachtiary B, Boutros PC, Pintilie M, et al. Gene expression profiling in cervical cancer: an exploration of intratumor heterogeneity. *Clin Cancer Res* 2006;12:5632-5640.

Beer DG, Kardia SL, Huang CC, et al. Gene-expression profiles predict survival of patients with lung adenocarcinoma. *Nat Med* 2002;8:816-824.

Begun A. Power estimation of the t test for detecting differential gene expression. *Funct Integr Genomics* 2008;8:109-113.

Bild AH, Yao G, Chang JT, et al. Oncogenic pathway signatures in human cancers as a guide to targeted therapies. *Nature* 2006;439:353-357.

Bonci D, Coppola V, Musumeci M, et al. The miR-15a-miR-16-1 cluster controls prostate cancer by targeting multiple oncogenic activities. *Nat Med* 2008;14:1271-1277.

Bottoni A, Piccin D, Tagliati F, Luchin A, Zatelli MC, degli Uberti EC. miR-15a and miR-16-1 down-regulation in pituitary adenomas. *J Cell Physiol* 2005;204:280-285.

Boutros PC. To cluster or not to cluster: the uses and misuses of clustering algorithms. *Hypothesis (Tor)* 2006;4:28-32.

Boutros PC, Lau SK, Pintilie M, et al. Prognostic gene signatures for non-small-cell lung cancer. *Proc Natl Acad Sci U S A* 2009;106:2824-2828.

Boutros PC, Okey AB. Unsupervised pattern recognition: an introduction to the whys and wherefores of clustering microarray data. *Brief Bioinform* 2005;6:331-343.

Brothman AR, Persons DL, Shaffer LG. Nomenclature evolution: changes in the ISCN from the 2005 to the 2009 edition. *Cytogenet Genome Res* 2009;127:1-4.

Brown KR, Jurisica I. Online predicted human interaction database. *Bioinformatics* 2005;21:2076-2082.

Calin GA, Ferracin M, Cimmino A, et al. A microRNA signature associated with prognosis and progression in chronic lymphocytic leukemia. *N Engl J Med* 2005;353:1793-1801.

Camon E, Magrane M, Barrell D, et al. The Gene Ontology Annotation (GOA) project: implementation of GO in SWISS-PROT, TrEMBL, and InterPro. *Genome Res* 2003; 13:662-672.

Cerami E, Demir E, Schultz N, Taylor BS, Sander C. Automated network analysis identifies core pathways in glioblastoma. *PLoS One* 2010;5:e8918.

Chayen NE. Methods for separating nucleation and growth in protein crystallisation. *Prog Biophys Mol Biol* 2005;88:329-337.

Chen HY, Yu SL, Chen CH, et al. A five-gene signature and clinical outcome in non-small-cell lung cancer. *N Engl J Med* 2007;356: 11-20.

Chendrimada TP, Gregory RI, Kumaraswamy E, et al. TRBP recruits the Dicer complex to Ago2 for microRNA processing and gene silencing. *Nature* 2005;436:740-744.

Chernov AA. Protein crystals and their growth. *J Struct Biol* 2003;142:3-21.

Chin K, DeVries S, Fridlyand J, et al. Genomic and transcriptional aberrations linked to breast cancer pathophysiologies. *Cancer Cell* 2006;10:529-541.

Chowdhury SM, Munske GR, Ronald RC, Bruce JE. Evaluation of low energy CID and ECD fragmentation behavior of mono-oxidized thio-ether bonds in peptides. *J Am Soc Mass Spectrom* 2007;18:493-501.

Colas P, Brent R. The impact of two-hybrid and related methods on biotechnology. *Trends Biotechnol* 1998;16:355-363.

Conrad DF, Pinto D, Redon R, et al. Origins and functional impact of copy number variation in the human genome. *Nature* 2010; 464:704-712.

Consortium GO. Creating the gene ontology resource: design and implementation. *Genome Res* 2001;11:1425-1433.

Cox B, Kislinger T, Wigle DA, et al. Integrated proteomic and transcriptomic profiling of mouse lung development and Nmyc target genes. *Mol Syst Biol* 2007;3:109.

Cox J, Mann M. Is proteomics the new genomics? *Cell* 2007;130: 395-398.

de Hoon MJ, Imoto S, Nolan J, Miyano S. Open source clustering software. *Bioinformatics* 2004;20:1453-1454.

Diskin SJ, Hou C, Glessner JT, et al. Copy number variation at 1q21.1 associated with neuroblastoma. *Nature* 2009;459: 987-991.

Duda RO, Hart PE, Stork DG. *Pattern classification*, 2nd ed. New York, NY: Wiley; 2001.

Eckel-Passow JE, Lohse CM, Sheinin Y, Crispen PL, Krco CJ, Kwon ED. Tissue microarrays: one size does not fit all. *Diagn Pathol* 2010;5:48.

Ein-Dor L, Zuk O, Domany E. Thousands of samples are needed to generate a robust gene list for predicting outcome in cancer. *Proc Natl Acad Sci U S A* 2006;103:5923-5928.

Emmert-Buck MR, Bonner RF, Smith PD, et al. Laser capture microdissection. *Science* 1996; 274:998-1001.

Faca V, Krasnoselsky A, Hanash S. Innovative proteomic approaches for cancer biomarker discovery. *Biotechniques* 2007;43:279, 281-285.

Fazi F, Nervi C. MicroRNA: basic mechanisms and transcriptional regulatory networks for cell fate determination. *Cardiovasc Res* 2008;79:553-561.

Fields S. Interactive learning: lessons from two hybrids over two decades. *Proteomics* 2009;9:5209-5213.

Gardiner-Garden M, Frommer M. CpG islands in vertebrate genomes. *J Mol Biol* 1987;196:261-282.

Golub TR, Slonim DK, Tamayo P, et al. Molecular classification of cancer: class discovery and class prediction by gene expression monitoring. *Science* 1999;286:531-537.

Gramolini AO, Kislinger T, Alikhani-Koopaei R, et al. Comparative proteomics profiling of a phospholamban mutant mouse model of dilated cardiomyopathy reveals progressive intracellular stress responses. *Mol Cell Proteomics* 2008;7:519-533.

Grote T, Siwak DR, Fritsche HA, et al. Validation of reverse phase protein array for practical screening of potential biomarkers in serum and plasma: accurate detection of CA19-9 levels in pancreatic cancer. *Proteomics* 2008;8:3051-3060.

Hackstadt AJ, Hess AM. Filtering for increased power for microarray data analysis. *BMC Bioinformatics* 2009;10:11.

Hutvagner G, Zamore PD. A microRNA in a multiple-turnover RNAi enzyme complex. *Science* 2002;297:2056-2060.

Isalan M. Zinc-finger nucleases: how to play two good hands. *Nat Methods* 2012;9:32-34.

Jonsson PF, Bates PA. Global topological features of cancer proteins in the human interactome. *Bioinformatics* 2006;22: 2291-2297.

Jurisicova A, Jurisica I, Kislinger T. Advances in ovarian cancer proteomics: the quest for biomarkers and improved therapeutic interventions. *Expert Rev Proteomics* 2008;5:551-560.

Kelleher NL. Top-down proteomics. *Anal Chem* 2004;76:197A-203A.

Kislinger T, Cox B, Kannan A, et al. Global survey of organ and organelle protein expression in mouse: combined proteomic and transcriptomic profiling. *Cell* 2006;125:173-186.

Kislinger T, Gramolini AO, MacLennan DH, Emili A. Multidimensional protein identification technology (MudPIT): technical overview of a profiling method optimized for the comprehensive proteomic investigation of normal and diseased heart tissue. *J Am Soc Mass Spectrom* 2005;16:1207-1220.

Kislinger T, Gramolini AO, Pan Y, Rahman K, MacLennan DH, Emili A. Proteome dynamics during C2C12 myoblast differentiation. *Mol Cell Proteomics* 2005;4:887-901.

Kislinger T, Rahman K, Radulovic D, Cox B, Rossant J, Emili A. PRISM, a generic large scale proteomic investigation strategy for mammals. *Mol Cell Proteomics* 2003;2:96-106.

Knudson AG Jr. Mutation and cancer: statistical study of retinoblastoma. *Proc Natl Acad Sci U S A* 1971;68:820-823.

Kononen J, Bubendorf L, Kallioniemi A, et al. Tissue microarrays for high-throughput molecular profiling of tumor specimens. *Nat Med* 1998;4:844-847.

Kooperberg C, Fazzio TG, Delrow JJ, Tsukiyama T. Improved background correction for spotted DNA microarrays. *J Comput Biol* 2002;9:55-66.

Kruger M, Moser M, Ussar S, et al. SILAC mouse for quantitative proteomics uncovers kindlin-3 as an essential factor for red blood cell function. *Cell* 2008;134:353-364.

Landthaler M, Yalcin A, Tuschl T. The human DiGeorge syndrome critical region gene 8 and Its D. melanogaster homolog are required for miRNA biogenesis. *Curr Biol* 2004;14:2162-2167.

Lau SK, Boutros PC, Pintilie M, et al. Three-gene prognostic classifier for early-stage non small-cell lung cancer. *J Clin Oncol* 2007;25:5562-5569.

Leary RJ, Lin JC, Cummins J, et al. Integrated analysis of homozygous deletions, focal amplifications, and sequence alterations in breast and colorectal cancers. *Proc Natl Acad Sci U S A* 2008;105:16224-16229.

Lee Y, Ahn C, Han J, et al. The nuclear RNase III Drosha initiates microRNA processing. *Nature* 2003;425:415-419.

Li M, Lee KF, Lu Y, et al. Frequent amplification of a chr19q13.41 microRNA polycistron in aggressive primitive neuroectodermal brain tumors. *Cancer Cell* 2009;16:533-546.

Liu H, Sadygov RG, Yates JR 3rd. A model for random sampling and estimation of relative protein abundance in shotgun proteomics. *Anal Chem* 2004;76:4193-4201.

Liu W, Sun J, Li G, et al. Association of a germ-line copy number variation at 2p24.3 and risk for aggressive prostate cancer. *Cancer Res* 2009;69:2176-2179.

Marouga R, David S, Hawkins E. The development of the DIGE system: 2D fluorescence difference gel analysis technology. *Anal Bioanal Chem* 2005;382:669-678.

Metzker ML. Sequencing technologies—the next generation. *Nat Rev Genet* 2010;11:31-46.

Michnick SW, Ear PH, Landry C, Malleshaiah MK, Messier V. Protein-fragment complementation assays for large-scale analysis, functional dissection and dynamic studies of protein-protein interactions in living cells. *Methods Mol Biol* 2011; 756:395-425.

Mikesh LM, Ueberheide B, Chi A, et al. The utility of ETD mass spectrometry in proteomic analysis. *Biochim Biophys Acta* 2006;1764:1811-1822.

Mok SC, Bonome T, Vathipadiekal V, et al. A gene signature predictive for outcome in advanced ovarian cancer identifies a survival factor: microfibril-associated glycoprotein 2. *Cancer Cell* 2009;16:521-532.

Neve RM, Chin K, Fridlyand J, et al. A collection of breast cancer cell lines for the study of functionally distinct cancer subtypes. *Cancer Cell* 2006;10:515-527.

Novak K. Epigenetics changes in cancer cells. *MedGenMed* 2004;6:17.

Ong SE, Blagoev B, Kratchmarova I, et al. Stable isotope labeling by amino acids in cell culture, SILAC, as a simple and accurate approach to expression proteomics. *Mol Cell Proteomics* 2002;1:376-386.

Perkins DN, Pappin DJ, Creasy DM, Cottrell JS. Probability-based protein identification by searching sequence databases using mass spectrometry data. *Electrophoresis* 1999;20:3551-3567.

Perron MP, Provost P. Protein components of the microRNA pathway and human diseases. *Methods Mol Biol* 2009;487:369-385.

Phizicky E, Bastiaens PI, Zhu H, Snyder M, Fields S. Protein analysis on a proteomic scale. *Nature* 2003;422(6928):208-215.

Pujana MA, Han JD, Starita LM, et al. Network modeling links breast cancer susceptibility and centrosome dysfunction. *Nat Genet* 2007;39:1338-1349.

Rambaldi D, Giorgi FM, Capuani F, Ciliberto A, Ciccarelli FD. Low duplicability and network fragility of cancer genes. *Trends Genet* 2008;24:427-430.

Redon R, Ishikawa S, Fitch KR, et al. Global variation in copy number in the human genome. *Nature* 2006;444:444-454.

Rodriguez A, Griffiths-Jones S, Ashurst JL, Bradley A. Identification of mammalian microRNA host genes and transcription units. *Genome Res* 2004;14:1902-1910.

Roepstorff P, Fohlman J. Proposal for a common nomenclature for sequence ions in mass spectra of peptides. *Biomed Mass Spectrom* 1984;11:601.

Ross PL, Huang YN, Marchese JN, et al. Multiplexed protein quantitation in Saccharomyces cerevisiae using amine-reactive isobaric tagging reagents. *Mol Cell Proteomics* 2004;3:1154-1169.

Rubin MA, Dunn R, Strawderman M, Pienta KJ. Tissue microarray sampling strategy for prostate cancer biomarker analysis. *Am J Surg Pathol* 2002;26:312-319.

Sanchez-Carbayo M, Socci ND, Lozano JJ, Haab BB, Cordon-Cardo C. Profiling bladder cancer using targeted antibody arrays. *Am J Pathol* 2006;168:93-103.

Schindler T, Bornmann W, Pellicena P, et al. Structural metabolism of STI-571 inhibition of Abelson tyrosine kinase. *Science* 2000;289:1938-1942.

Shedden K, Taylor JM, Enkemann SA, et al. Gene expression-based survival prediction in lung adenocarcinoma: a multi-site, blinded validation study. *Nat Med* 2008;14:822-827.

Sheer D, Squire J. Clinical applications of genetic rearrangements in cancer. *Sem Cancer Biol* 1996;7:25-32.

Shevchenko A, Wilm M, Vorm O, Mann M. Mass spectrometric sequencing of proteins silver-stained polyacrylamide gels. *Anal Chem* 1996;68:850-858.

Speicher MR, Gwyn Ballard S, Ward DC. Karyotyping human chromosomes by combinatorial multi-fluor FISH. *Nat Genet* 1996;12:368-375.

Stock D, Perisic O, Lowe J. Robotic nanolitre protein crystallisation at the MRC Laboratory of Molecular Biology. *Prog Biophys Mol Biol* 2005;88:311-327.

Storey JD, Tibshirani R. Statistical significance for genomewide studies. *Proc Natl Acad Sci U S A* 2003;100:9440-9445.

Subramanian J, Simon R. Gene expression-based prognostic signatures in lung cancer: ready for clinical use? *J Natl Cancer Inst* 2010;102:464-474.

Turner BM. Defining an epigenetic code. *Nat Cell Biol* 2007;9:2-6.

van de Vijver MJ, He YD, van't Veer LJ, et al. A gene-expression signature as a predictor of survival in breast cancer. *N Engl J Med* 2002;347:1999-2009.

van 't Veer LJ, Bernards R. Enabling personalized cancer medicine through analysis of gene-expression patterns. *Nature* 2008; 452:564-570.

van 't Veer LJ, Dai H, van de Vijver MJ, et al. Gene expression profiling predicts clinical outcome of breast cancer. *Nature* 2002;415:530-536.

Veldman T, Vignon C, Schrock E, Rowley JD, Ried T. Hidden chromosome abnormalities in haematological malignancies detected by multicolour spectral karyotyping. *Nat Genet* 1997;15:406-410.

Wachi S, Yoneda K, Wu R. Interactome-transcriptome analysis reveals the high centrality of genes differentially expressed in lung cancer tissues. *Bioinformatics* 2005;21:4205-4208.

Washburn MP, Wolters D, Yates JR 3rd. Large-scale analysis of the yeast proteome by multidimensional protein identification technology. *Nat Biotechnol* 2001;19:242-247.

Weir BA, Woo MS, Getz G, et al. Characterizing the cancer genome in lung adenocarcinoma. *Nature* 2007;450:893-898.

Wolters DA, Washburn MP, Yates JR 3rd. An automated multidimensional protein identification technology for shotgun proteomics. *Anal Chem* 2001;73:5683-5690.

Woodson K, O'Reilly KJ, Hanson JC, Nelson D, Walk EL, Tangrea JA. The usefulness of the detection of GSTP1 methylation in urine as a biomarker in the diagnosis of prostate cancer. *J Urol* 2008;179:508-511; discussion 511-512.

Wu Z, Irizarry RA, Gentleman R, Murillo FM, Spencer R. A model based background adjustment for oligonucleotide expression arrays. *Johns Hopkins University, Dept of Biostatistics Working Papers* 2004;1.

Yoshimoto M, Joshua AM, Chilton-Macneill S, et al. Three color FISH analysis of TMPRSS2/ERG fusions in prostate cancer indicates that genomic microdeletion of chromosome 21 is associated with rearrangement. *Neoplasia* 2006;8: 465-469.

Zhu H, Snyder M. Protein chip technology. *Curr Opin Chem Biol* 2003;7:55-63.

3

Cancer Epidemiology

Gord Fehringer, Rayjean J. Hung, and Geoffrey Liu

3.1 INTRODUCTION AND TERMINOLOGY

3.1.1 Epidemiology: Definition and Scope

Epidemiology is the study of distribution and determinants of disease and disease outcomes in human populations. The primary research question for epidemiologists is why individuals, or different populations, have different risks of disease or disease outcomes. Epidemiology is broadly focused, examining a full spectrum of disease determinants. These encompass biological, environmental (including lifestyle), social, and economic factors. Consequently, concepts and methods from other disciplines, such as biological sciences and sociology, are critical to the design, conduct, and analysis of epidemiological studies. Important contributions are also made from the field of statistics. Epidemiology provides a critical link between clinical or laboratory results and observed health effects in populations. An observational approach is often the only way to examine risk between disease and a specific risk factor because, for example, it is unethical to assign individuals to an arm of a randomized trial that exposes them to a suspected carcinogen.

3.1.2 General Approach

Epidemiology is often dichotomized into 2 disciplines: descriptive and analytical. Descriptive epidemiology primarily describes rates of disease in populations, either over time or across geographic areas. Analytic epidemiology focuses on individuals in the population, comparing diseased to nondiseased members to determine what factors increase risk for disease. Measures commonly used in descriptive epidemiology are described in Section 3.2. Measures used in analytical epidemiology are described in Section 3.3.

3.1.3 Role of Epidemiology in Translational Medicine

Whereas in vitro and in vivo studies using cell lines and animal models can control for a multitude of experimental conditions, this is difficult in studies in humans. Ethical and feasibility considerations prevent deliberate repeated exposures of known carcinogens to human subjects and randomization of human groups to receive either inferior therapies or environmental exposures. Although some experiments in humans may utilize intermediate subclinical end points that are reversible following brief exposure to a potential carcinogen, these intermediate end points are often not a replacement for the clinical outcome of interest. An example of this type of intermediate end point is the measurement of carcinogen-adduct formation in humans after a single exposure to a putative carcinogen. Such results may support the role of such a carcinogen, but do not provide evidence of increased rates of cancer in individuals or groups of individuals exposed to the putative carcinogen. In general, the process of translating basic science discoveries into the clinical setting requires studies of humans, their biological specimens, and associated clinical data. Such studies require consideration of many factors that can affect the development of disease or its outcome. This is particularly important in the era of microarrays and gene sequencing, where a large number of biological parameters must be considered alongside clinical and epidemiological factors, all of which could affect risk of the disease or outcome of interest.

In the face of such analyses epidemiological principles become important. The majority of epidemiological studies involve observational data (whether aggregate or individual data) where, by definition, the investigator can only observe the characteristics of the population of interest, and cannot intervene to standardize exposures and other factors (such as confounders, see Sec. 3.2.4) that may affect the outcomes of interest. Thus, a key feature of epidemiology has been the development of methodological designs and tools to account for such confounders. These same tools can be adapted for analyses of biological parameters.

Epidemiological studies can serve not only to validate biological principles and translate findings into the clinical setting, but their findings can lead to new avenues of basic research. For example, long before the existence of an activating epidermal growth factor receptor (EGFR) mutation was found to drive certain lung tumors that are highly sensitive to small molecular inhibitors (see Chap. 7, Sec. 7.5.3) there were clinical and epidemiological clues to the existence of a biologically distinct subset of such patients. Patients with tumors that were highly sensitive to EGFR inhibitor drugs were more likely to be lifetime never-smokers, of Asian descent, who had developed the histological subtype of adenocarcinomas, and were (more often) female (Coate et al, 2009). In another example, there has been a dramatic increase since 2000 in the incidence of oropharyngeal cancers, an anatomic subset of head and neck squamous cancers. The patients in this subset were more likely to be younger, lifetime never-smokers, have lower rates of alcohol use, and be of higher socioeconomic status, when compared to the traditional head and neck cancer patient. As time went on, these oropharyngeal cancers were found to be associated with human papillomavirus infection (see Chap. 6, Sec. 6.2.3; Chung and Gillison, 2009). The relationship between alcohol and head and neck cancer is discussed in more detail in Section 3.5.3.

3.2 DESCRIPTIVE EPIDEMIOLOGY

3.2.1 Incidence, Mortality, Case Fatality, and Age-Standardized Incidence Rates

An *incidence rate* refers to the number of new cases of a disease observed in a defined population in a specific time period divided by the population size, whereas *mortality rate* refers to the number of deaths caused by the disease during a specific time period divided by the population size. A more precise definition would use the term *person time* instead of *population size*. For example, in a town with a population of 40,000 the number of new cases of cancer in a year can be thought of as being divided by 40,000 person-years, 1 year of person time per individual, with the assumption that everyone lived there for the entire year (births, deaths, and migration during the year are ignored). Similarly, the mortality rate would be calculated as the number of deaths from cancer in a year divided by 40,000 person-years.

A direct calculation of incidence rate, as determined in the above example, is termed the *crude incidence rate*, because the calculation is performed without consideration of other important factors that may differ across different populations. A major factor in the comparison of different populations is the difference in age-distribution across the different populations. Both cancer incidence and mortality generally increase markedly with age, and comparisons of populations with different age distributions using crude rates can therefore be misleading. One can statistically eliminate or reduce the effect of age in the calculation of the incidence of cancer (or of any other disease), and allow comparison of cancer incidence in communities or geographical regions with different age distributions or in the same community with changing age distribution. The procedure requires adjusting (or *standardizing*) rates so they are representative of the age distribution of some reference population. The reference populations can be chosen arbitrarily to have any age distribution, but typically, the standard population is often conveniently and practically chosen to be the age distribution at a particular census date of the relevant country (eg, U.S. year 2000 census). Different *age-standardized* rates can then be compared to each other, if they are adjusted to the same reference standard. Figures 3–1 and 3–2 show examples of age-standardized cancer incidence.

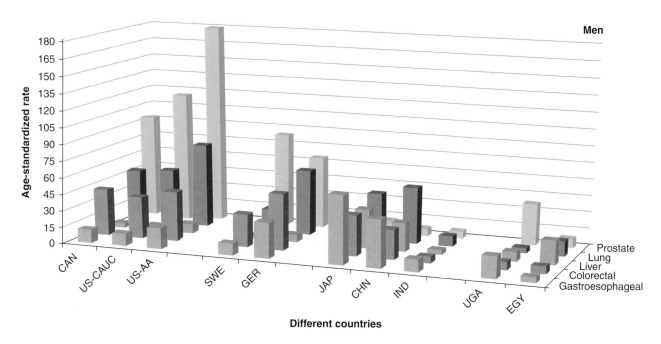

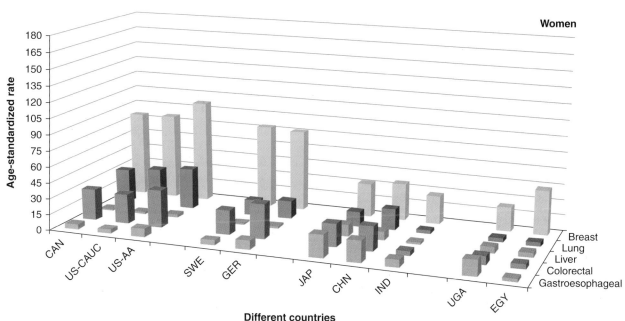

FIGURE 3-1 **Comparison of age-standardized incidence rate of selected cancers in selected countries, by sex, per 100,000 person-years.** X-axis is divided into different continents: *CAN*, Canada; *US-CAUC*, United States caucasians; *US-AA*, United States African American; *SWE*, Sweden; *GER*, Germany; *JAP*, Japan; *CHN*, China (Shanghai Registry); *IND*, India; *UGA*, Uganda; *EGY*, Egypt (Gharbiah Registry). Z-axis: *dark blue*, gastroesophageal cancer; *red*, colorectal cancer; *green*, liver cancer; *purple*, lung cancer; *light blue*, prostate cancer (men), breast cancer (women).

The age-standardized rate is commonly presented in publications as it accounts for differences in age between populations or changes in age within populations over time. However, such adjusted rates should be viewed as relative indices rather than actual measures of occurrence. Rates can also be compared within age groups.

The age-specific incidence rate is defined as the incidence of disease in a specific age group; typically, 5-year age groups (0 to 4, 5 to 9, 10 to 14, etc) are used. This method is informative about the disease pattern over the life course, but a

valid comparison across populations can only be made within age groups.

The *case fatality rate* is the number of deaths caused by a specific disease in a defined population divided by the number of individuals who have been diagnosed with that particular disease, in a fixed time interval. Only deaths among those diagnosed in the time interval are included in the numerator. An example of a case fatality rate is found with breast cancer, which in the Western world is around 25 individuals per 100, or 25%. This means that within a given year, of every

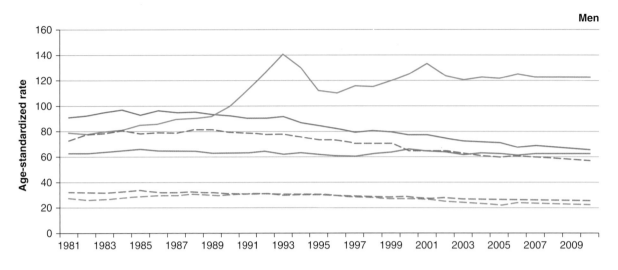

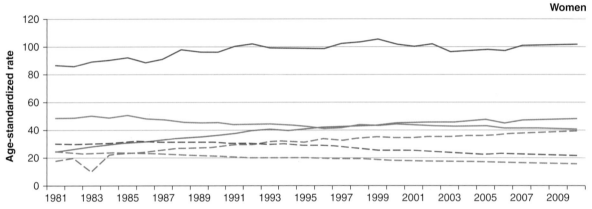

Estimated number of incident cases, deaths, and prevalent cases in Canada, 2000

	Incident cases		Deaths		No. of prevalent cases*	
	Males	Females	Males	Females	Males	Females
Colorectal	9200	7900	3500	3000	40,700	42,600
Lung	12,200	8400	10,700	7000	17,900	16,200
Prostate	16,900	–	4200	–	107,300	–
Breast	–	19,200	–	5500	–	151,100

FIGURE 3–2 Age-standardized incidence and mortality rates across 20 years, and incidence, death and prevalence estimates for the year 2000, Canada. (*Top*) Age-standardized incidence (*solid lines*) and mortality (*dashed lines*) rates for lung (*blue*), colorectal (*green*), breast (*dark red*), and prostate cancer (*bright red*) in Canada, per 100,000 person years for years 1981 to 2010. (*Bottom Table*) For the year 2000, incident cases, cancer-specific deaths, and number of prevalent cases. *One-year prevalence, 2000. (Data from *Canadian Cancer Statistics,* 2010.)

100 individuals carrying a diagnosis of breast cancer in a population, 25 individuals in the same population will have died of breast cancer. Contrast this result with pancreatic cancer, where the case fatality rate is more than 95%; that is, of 100 individuals carrying a diagnosis of pancreatic cancer, more than 95 patients will have died.

3.2.2 Prevalence

Prevalence is defined as the proportion of a population that has a disease at a specific time point (prevalent cases divided by population size), where prevalent cases include both new cases of disease and the number of previously diagnosed cases who are still alive in a population. Including all cases who are still alive as prevalent cases assumes that no cases can be considered cured. This raises the question of whether long-term survivors of cancer should be included in the prevalence group when calculating prevalence. Given the available data (which may not include treatment information), decisions should be made that ensures the prevalence calculation reasonably reflects the burden of disease in the population. For example, one can define prevalent cases as those diagnosed and still alive at the end of a specified time period (eg, the last 5 years).

Prevalence is a function of both cancer incidence and cancer survivorship (ie, how long the person lives with the disease or disease chronicity). As an example, although lung cancer ranks among the most common cancers in the Western world, its prevalence ranks lower than that of prostate cancer, breast cancer, and colorectal cancer, because lung cancer is such a lethal disease. Both cancer incidence and cancer prevalence are important measures. Cancer incidence reflects how commonly cancer develops in a population, and the impact of preventive measures and health service utilization related to initial diagnosis and treatment. In contrast, cancer prevalence may be important when considering the overall burden of a cancer on a global health system, and longer-term impact on survivors.

Figure 3–2 shows the relationship between incidence, mortality, and prevalence. In lung cancer, the dashed (mortality rate) line approaches the solid (incidence rate) lines, which represents a low survival rate (of approximately 10% to 20%). The low survival rate results in a low prevalence of disease in the population, as a high proportion of lung cancer patients die of their disease, resulting in few long-term survivors. For prostate, breast, and colorectal cancers, the age- standardized incidence rates are substantially higher than their corresponding mortality rates, as a result of high survival rates (all greater than 40%). In the figure, both the age-standardized incidence of prostate cancer and the incidence–mortality gap for prostate cancer in men was similar to the same indicators for breast cancer in women. Because prevalence is a function of incidence and survivorship, one would have expected a similar prevalence of prostate cancer and breast cancer patients in 2000. Yet there was approximately 50% more prevalence in breast cancer patients when compared to prostate cancer patients. The reasons for this finding are (a) women live longer than men, on average, and (b) the median age of diagnosis of breast cancer is lower than that of prostate cancer. Thus, in the year 2000, a breast cancer patient can expect to live longer, on average, than a prostate cancer patient, leading to a greater prevalence of breast cancer patients when compared to prostate cancer patients (see Fig. 3–2). This aspect of survivorship links incidence, mortality, case fatality rates, and survivorship characteristics with prevalence rates.

3.2.3 The Role of Sampling

A major focus of epidemiology is to identify associations that are true for an entire population. Optimally, one would collect exposure and disease status data from every member of that population. If the information collected is accurate, then any associations found would be true.

In the real world, it is not feasible to collect data from the entire population, and a subset of the population is studied. Even the most comprehensive national census data from countries that make completing a census mandatory will have certain individuals refusing to comply (typically the disenfranchised, those not in the country legally, and any groups that are suspicious of government oversight). In many cases, because of cost and feasibility, basic census data are collected from as many individuals as possible, while detailed comprehensive information

is collected from a subset of the population. Sampling is therefore a key component of epidemiological analyses. The goal of sampling is to evaluate a subset of the population where the exposure and disease status information is representative of the underlying population. In an ideal setting, the results found in the sample should fully reflect the true associations in the underlying population. When the results are different, bias and measurement errors may explain these discrepancies.

3.2.4 Types of Bias

A study is biased if the results are different than the truth. In epidemiology, bias can be viewed as a distortion of risk estimates from their true values. Bias can be related to the identification of cases, measurement of exposure, improper analysis of results, or systematic errors in data collection and entry. Many different kinds of biases have been described (Sackett, 1979; Szklo and Nieto, 2007). We describe the main types of bias found in observational studies, including confounding, selection, and information bias.

3.2.4.1 Bias Because of Confounding An important bias in observational studies comes from *confounding*, defined as the distortion of effect of an exposure on risk (of disease or outcome) that arises because of an association with other factors that affect such a risk. Confounding can lead to spurious associations, mask associations that are real, or distort the strength of an association. A variable is considered to be a confounder if it is associated with the potential disease-related factor under investigation (either causally or noncausally) and is causally related to the outcome of interest (either risk of disease or its outcome). An example of a confounder is smoking in lung cancer (Fig. 3–3A). Suppose we are studying the association between tooth loss and lung cancer risk. Tooth loss, a marker of poor hygiene, is strongly associated with heavy smoking. We may therefore find an association between tooth loss and lung cancer solely because both are associated with heavy smoking. In reality, tooth loss does not lead to lung cancer development, but its association with smoking makes it appear that it is related with lung cancer risk, while the true association is between smoking and lung cancer.

A variable is not considered to be a confounder if it lies in the same causal pathway as the potential disease-related factor under investigation. For example, bronchial dysplasia is an intermediary in the pathway between smoking and lung cancer, and is thus not a confounder (see Fig. 3–3B).

In summary, there are 3 criteria for a variable to be a confounder:

1. A confounding factor must be a risk factor for the disease;
2. A confounding factor must be associated with the exposure under study in the source population; and
3. A confounding factor should *not* be an intermediate factor in a causal path between exposure and disease.

Confounding can be dealt with in different ways. Individuals who have a disease (eg, cancer cases) and those without disease (eg, healthy controls) can be matched on potential confounding

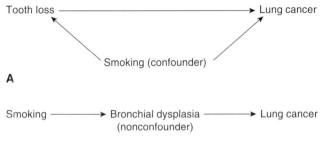

FIGURE 3–3 **Confounding in epidemiologic studies.** The confounder is related to both the exposure of interest and to either disease or outcome. Example **A** reflects confounding by smoking. Example **B** is not an example of confounding because bronchial dysplasia lies in the causal pathway leading to lung cancer.

exposure variables (eg, age and sex are commonly matched in a case-control study) to reduce or eliminate confounding by these variables, or data can be analyzed within specific strata of the confounding variable (eg, analyses stratified by ethnic group). In addition, one can control for confounding using multiple regression analysis, which is discussed in Section 3.3.3.

3.2.4.2 Selection and Information Bias Sometimes the results of analyses of a sample will differ from the true associations in the underlying population. This may be a result of sampling problems, whereby the sample selected does not represent the underlying population. *Selection bias* refers to systematic differences between those who participated in the study versus those who should be theoretically eligible for the study (including those who do not participate). An example of sampling bias results from recruiting cases from a surgical clinic to represent the entire population of stomach cancer. Because surgeons generally see more early stage patients (ie, those who are operable), the population will be skewed toward earlier stage patients, where as the whole population of patients with stomach cancer is eligible for the study.

Information bias occurs as a consequence of errors in obtaining the needed information, which is often termed *misclassification* or *classification error*. Sometimes these misclassifications can lead to results from studies that do not represent the true associations in the underlying population. An example of information bias occurs if lung cancer patients overestimate their exposures to asbestos (compared with healthy controls) while underestimating their own cigarette smoking history (perhaps as a means of reducing their own culpability in developing this disease). The resultant effect is a smaller-than-true risk associated with cumulative smoking, and an exaggerated risk associated with asbestos. This bias particularly affects case-control studies (see Sec. 3.4.3) where cases are recruited after their diagnosis, and is referred to as *recall bias*. Such a bias would be absent if individuals were asked for their exposure status prior to developing their cancer (as in the case of cohort studies; see Sec. 3.4.2). Another example of information bias may come from evaluating a molecular test. Assume that the

molecular test categorizes individuals into 3 levels: A, B, and C. However, because the test is inappropriately calibrated, a number of B test results are misclassified as C results, whereas B results are never misclassified as A results. The resultant error is directional in nature (ie, nonrandom).

Although systematic error such as selection bias and differential misclassification can generate biases in epidemiological studies, *random error* can also distort the results of epidemiological studies. Random error is the deviation that arises by chance between the observed value (in the sample) and its true value (in the underlying population). The greater the random error, the less precise the result.

Assessment of cancer diagnosis should be reasonably accurate as diagnosis is generally verified with a pathology report. The determination of cause of death can be more problematic if death certificates are used. Assessment of exposure can be particularly problematic, and misclassification of subjects with respect to their exposure can be extensive. Recall of certain past exposures, such as diet, may show considerable random error. Error in the measurement of biomarkers depends not only on the accuracy of the bioassay, but how well a single measurement may reflect long-term levels of the biomarker. The latency period for cancer can be many years and a single measurement of a biomarker during an individual's lifetime may not effectively represent long-term levels.

Generally, misclassification of a dichotomous (ie, positive or negative) exposure will lead to a bias toward the null (relative risk estimates will indicate a smaller association than actually exists or indicate no association when true association is present), and when the misclassification is extreme the result can go beyond null to the opposite direction. However, misclassification of a multilevel exposure could lead to errors in any direction. Efforts to increase the accuracy of assessment of exposure or use of large samples that can detect the attenuated associations are the only ways to address this problem. We discuss some of the newer strategies in Section 3.7.2. Table 3–1 defines and describes other common examples of selection and information biases.

3.2.4.3 Bias in Cancer Screening Two special causes of bias are related to cancer screening. These biases can affect incidence, prevalence, mortality, and survival rates. For example, as Figure 3–2 shows, prostate cancer incidence rates had 2 separate peaks (1993 and 2001). Each peak was related to the clinical adoption of a screening test based on the serum levels of prostate-specific antigen (PSA). The first peak followed initial adoption of the PSA test, while the second peak may be explained by increased PSA testing related to the publicity around a prominent Canadian politician's prostate cancer diagnosis (Canadian Cancer Society, 2010). New screening techniques may result in individuals with subclinical prostate cancer being diagnosed earlier than traditionally expected. In the absence of the screening, the prostate cancers would be detected at a later date, when the subclinical cancer grows large enough to produce symptoms and be detected using previous methods. At the time of clinical adoption of such screening,

TABLE 3–1 Types of selection and information biases in epidemiological studies.

Bias*	Study Design	Description
Selection Bias		
Admission rate (Berkson) bias	Hospital-based case-control studies	Admission rate of cancer patients differs with respect to exposure to potential disease-related factor under investigation. Exposed cases may be over- or underrepresented in sample.
Prevalence-incidence (or length or survival) bias	Cross-sectional studies, case-control studies of rapidly fatal cancers	Survival of cases is related to exposure. Exposed cases may be over- or underrepresented in sample.
Detection bias	Case-control studies	Detection of cases is related to exposure to potential disease-related factor, with cases in exposed group over- or underrepresented.
Bias related to selection of cases and controls from different catchment areas	Hospital-based case-control studies	Cancer patients that visit hospital arise from different region than controls selected among other patients. Distribution of potential disease-related factor may differ in the 2 underlying populations.
Sampling or ascertainment bias	All types	Some members of the population may be less likely to be included than others, resulting in a nonrandom sample.
Differential loss to follow-up	Cohort studies, survival analyses	Subjects with exposure are either more or less likely to be lost to follow-up (losses can be a result of mortality, migration, or refusal to continue with study).
Lead-time bias	Cohort studies, survival analyses	The appearance of prolonged survival as a result of earlier diagnoses because of earlier detection of the disease, without impacting actual outcome of treating the disease.
Overdiagnosis bias	All types	The appearance of increase in early stage disease with improved survival, because of new detection technologies that identify previously undiagnosed subclinical disease that would otherwise never have required treatment.
Information Bias		
Recall bias	Case-control studies (with interview/questionnaires)	Cases recall exposure differently than controls, either over- or underreporting exposure relative to controls.
Interviewer or experimenter's bias	Case-control studies	Interviewer/experimenter knows disease status of study subjects and over- or underreports exposure, either consciously or unconsciously affecting the results.

*All biases listed may lead to over- or underestimated risk estimates.

survival may be prolonged because there is a true benefit of screening and the cure rate has truly risen. However, 2 potential biases complicate the interpretation of findings. Lead-time bias and overdiagnosis bias may have accounted partly for these peaks.

Lead-time bias refers to the appearance of longer survival after diagnosis that is a result of diagnosis at an earlier time during the course of the disease, and thus a longer time that the patient is known to have the cancer rather than an improved treatment response. The fact that early detection may not necessarily benefit the patient clinically, because the patient may have died at the same time with or without screening, is an important consideration when evaluating cancer screening programs. In the context of screening, *length time bias* occurs when screened subjects with better prognosis are detected by a screening program. This can result from more rapidly growing (and more lethal) cancers being diagnosed outside of the screening program, thus leading to an impression of better survival among screened subjects (see Chap. 22, Sec. 22.3.3).

Screening can also lead to *overdiagnosis bias*. PSA screening may lead to the detection of subclinical cases of prostate

cancer that would never have become clinically diagnosed in individuals who would have eventually died from an unrelated cause. Nonetheless, overdiagnosis results in increase in cancer incidence, apparent prolonged survival after diagnosis (and, therefore, apparent decrease in case fatality rates), and greater prevalence of the disease, all as a result of the new detection of previously subclinical disease that has no real clinical relevance.

3.2.5 Geographic Variation

Geographic variations in cancer incidence can be a result of differences in prevalence of the underlying causes including environmental and ethnic (ie, genetic) differences, or to differences in diagnostic criteria. In addition, geographic comparison can be complicated by differences in screening, which, by detecting occult disease, usually has a much larger effect on the incidence of disease than on mortality (see Chap. 22, Sec. 22.3.3). Figure 3–1 shows the age-standardized incidence rate for selected cancer sites and countries. Some large variations can be observed across countries, and there may also be large variations within countries: for example, the rate of esophageal

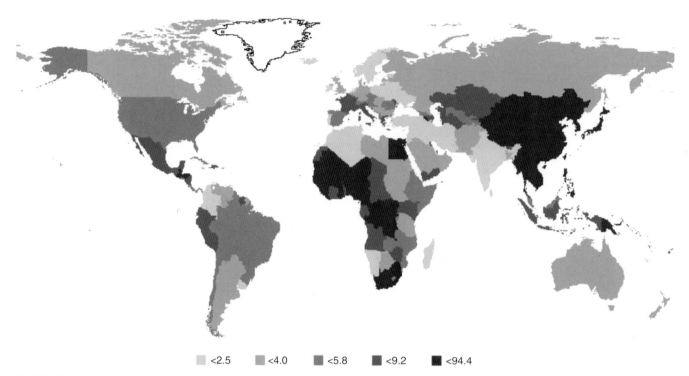

| ■ <2.5 | ■ <4.0 | ■ <5.8 | ■ <9.2 | ■ <94.4 |

FIGURE 3-4 **Global variation in incidence of liver cancer.** Annual age-standardized incidence rate, per 100,000 person years, across different countries of liver cancer. (From Ferlay et al, 2010 with permission.)

cancer varies by 10-fold within Iran (Saidi et al, 2000). In another example, shown in Figure 3-4, there is substantial geographic variation in incidence rates of liver cancer (Ferlay et al, 2010). The highest incidence rates are observed in sub-Sahara Africa and Asian countries such as China (~25 per 100,000 person years), Thailand (~30 per 100,000 person years), and Taiwan (~35 per 100,000 person years), whereas lower rates are observed in Europe and North America. This variation is partially accounted for by the prevalence of chronic infection with hepatitis B and C virus (HBV and HCV), which are causally associated with 80% to 95% of liver (hepatocellular) cancer (Maupas and Melnick, 1981). Similarly, the variation of cervical cancer can be partially accounted for by the prevalence of human papilloma virus (HPV), as we now know that cervical cancer is associated strongly with a few of the oncogenic genotypes of HPV (Munoz et al, 2003). Infection and cancer is described in more detail in Section 3.5.1 (see Chap. 6, Sec. 6.2.3).

3.2.6 Time Trends

Figure 3-2 shows the age-standardized incidence rate (ASIR) of the most common cancer sites in Canada for males and females in the last 20 years. Lung cancer incidence rates in men have been decreasing steadily since mid-1980s from approximately 90 to 65 per 100,000 person years in 2010, whereas the lung cancer incidence rate in women continues to rise from approximately 25 per 100,000 to 48 per 100,000 person years in 2010 (Canadian Cancer Society, 2010). The long-term projection suggests that this trend is beginning to level off. This pattern corresponds to the patterns of tobacco consumption

in men and women with a lag time of approximately 20 years. In contrast, colorectal cancer rates have remained relatively stable over the same period. Breast cancer incidence has slightly increased during this period. Changes over time for prostate cancer incidence rates have already been discussed in Section 3.2.4.3.

Worldwide, the incidence rate of stomach cancer in men has been decreasing in the last 30 to 40 years. Regardless of the steady decline, stomach cancer was still the fourth most common incident cancer worldwide in 2008 following cancer of lung, breast, and colorectum (Ferlay et al, 2010). In contrast, the incidence of thyroid cancer is increasing most rapidly among all cancers and it has doubled in women in the last 10 years, in both Europe and parts of the United States (Lundgren et al, 2003; Davies and Welch, 2006). The increase in incidence of thyroid cancer is mainly observed for papillary thyroid cancer and it may be a result of the change in the morphological recognition of this tumor (Lundgren et al, 2003). More frequent use of medical imaging may also contribute to the increased detection of early stage, asymptomatic cancers. The mortality of thyroid cancer did not show any increase during the same period of time.

In addition to adult cancers, recent publications based on the Automated Cancer Information System focused on childhood cancer have provided detailed statistics of major childhood cancer in Europe between 1978 and 1997 (Kaatsch et al, 2006). This analysis, based on 33 cancer registries in 15 European countries, showed an increased rate of childhood cancer in all regions for the majority of tumor types, including soft-tissue sarcoma (annual rate of increase 1.8%), brain tumors, tumors of the sympathetic nervous system, germ cell tumors, and leukemias (annual rate of increase 0.6%). Diagnostic methods can only partially explain the upward trend, and factors such as changing lifestyle and environmental exposures may be important.

3.3 ANALYTICAL EPIDEMIOLOGY

3.3.1 Basic Comparative Approaches: Relative Risk, Odds Ratio

The *relative risk* measures the risk in a group exposed to a potential disease-related factor and compares it to the risk in a group that is not exposed (or has lower exposure) to the factor. The risk itself may be to developing a specific cancer, or to a specific cancer outcome. In a population-based study of cancer risk, individuals who develop cancer and those who do not are classified into exposed and nonexposed groups according to their baseline measures, which are taken well before any individuals have developed cancer. In a population study of cancer outcome, individuals who develop a specific outcome (eg, response to therapy or drug toxicity) and those who do not are classified into exposed and nonexposed groups. In either example, the relative risk can then be calculated by dividing the risk of disease (or outcome) in the exposed group by the risk of disease (or outcome) in the unexposed group, as shown in Figure 3–5. Another related measure of relative risk is the *rate ratio*. It can be calculated when disease (eg, incidence) rates (Sec. 3.2.1) are available, by dividing the rate of a disease in a group exposed to a specific factor by the rate in a group that is unexposed or has lower exposure to the same factor. The rate ratio is useful in comparing populations in defined geographic areas with different exposures (eg, cigarette smoking or industrial pollution).

A relative risk of 1 (or more precisely a relative risk not statistically different than 1) indicates that there is no detectable increased risk of disease (or outcome) in the exposed group. A relative risk greater than 1 indicates risk is increased among the exposed, and a relative risk of less than 1 indicates lower risk in exposed verses unexposed groups. The farther away the value is from 1 (either very large numbers or very small numbers), the stronger the association.

Within either the entire population or a representative subset, the relative risk can be directly calculated because the size

Classification of exposure	Disease classification	
	Diseased	Nondiseased
Exposed	A	B
Unexposed	C	D

Risk of disease with exposure = A/(A + B)
Risk of disease with nonexposure = C/(C + D)
Relative risk as a result of exposure = A/(A + B) ÷ C/(C + D)

FIGURE 3–5 Calculation of relative risk of disease. (The letters *A, B, C,* and *D* refer to number of subjects in each group.)

Classification of exposure	Disease classification	
	Diseased (cases)	Nondiseased (controls)
Exposed	A	B
Unexposed	C	D

Odds of exposure in cases = A/C
Odds of exposure in controls = B/D
Odds ratio = A/C ÷ B/D = AD/BC

FIGURE 3–6 Calculation of the odds ratio. (The letters *A, B, C,* and *D* refer to number of subjects in each group.)

of both the exposed and unexposed groups from which cancer cases arose is known. In contrast, if a study selects cases from a population and then compares them to a selected set of controls, the size of the underlying exposed and unexposed groups in the population, and therefore the relative risk, cannot be directly calculated. Instead, the *odds ratio* must be calculated as outlined in Figure 3–6.

The odds ratio is generally presented as an approximate measure of relative risk. This approximation is valid if the prevalence of the disease is relatively low in the population, typically less than 10%. Although prevalence of all cancers together is relatively high in most Western populations, the prevalence of each individual cancer is quite low. This approximation can be demonstrated by starting with Equation 3.1 for the calculation of relative risk. If the disease is rare, then only a small change to the resulting estimate will be seen if both A (subjects with exposure and disease) and C (subjects with no exposure and disease) are removed from the denominator of the first and second parts of the equation (Eq. 3.2). The resulting equation can be rearranged so that it is identical to the equation for the odds ratio (Eq. 3.3).

$$\text{Relative Risk} = A/(A + B) \div C/(C + D) \qquad [\text{Eq. 3.1}]$$
$$\approx A/B \div C/D \text{ [A and C are removed from denominator]} \qquad [\text{Eq. 3.2}]$$
$$\approx A/C \div B/D \text{ or } AD/BC \qquad [\text{Eq. 3.3}]$$

The relative risk and odds ratio show strength of association, and are as applicable to analyses of relationships of biomarkers with disease as to clinicoepidemiological relationships.

3.3.2 Probability, Distributions, and Tests of Association

Let us assume that in the South Pacific there are exactly 1000 adult islanders (age 18 years and older) living on a remote atoll (Island A). On this island, 400 individuals have high blood pressure. If we are allowed to check for high blood pressure in 100 islanders (ie, sampling the population), we may obtain 40 with hypertension, but we may by chance, also obtain 39, 38, 37, or 41, 42, 43 individuals with high blood pressure, but it would be highly unlikely to obtain either no individuals with high blood pressure or all 100 individuals. If we repeated the experiment a million times, each time sampling

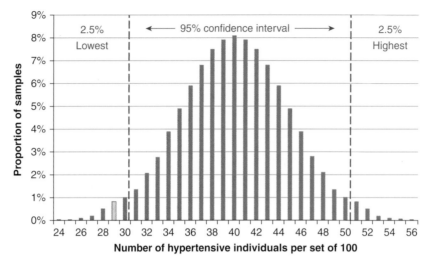

FIGURE 3-7   **Normal distribution approximation of binomial distribution for a 100-patient sample for a 40% proportion.** Assume that an underlying adult population has a 40% prevalence of hypertension. Researchers repeatedly and randomly sampled 100 individuals from this population (Island A), and reported the prevalence of hypertension in each sample. The X-axis shows the number of hypertensive individuals in each set of 100. The Y-axis shows the proportion of samples with that number of hypertensive individuals. The 95% confidence interval (within which 95% of these samples fall, around the median of 40) is shown in between the red dotted lines. The results in the yellow bar represent the proportion of samples that had 29 hypertensive patients (Island B).

100 individuals randomly, the most frequent result will be 40 individuals with high blood pressure, with other results farther away from 40 (in either direction) being less frequent. These results, if plotted, will form a shape similar to a normal distribution or probability curve (*note*: with two possible outcomes, hypertensive or not hypertensive, the distribution is in fact binomial but approximately equal to the normal distribution given the large number of data, thus leading to a bell-shaped [normal] curve; see Fig. 3–7). If we obtain a value from a sample that falls outside a certain range of values, then we might conclude it is highly unlikely that the value comes from a population similar to the Island A population. This range is conventionally chosen to be the 95% confidence interval, in which case the top and bottom 2.5% of values are considered to be too different to be likely to have come from the Island A population. Under different circumstances and depending on the experimental design of each study, different distributions or curves may be more appropriate, as would different ranges of confidence intervals.

If on a sister island (Island B) with 1000 people, we sample 100 individuals once and find that 29 of them have hypertension (Fig. 3–7, yellow bar), are the individuals on Island B similar to Island A? From Figure 3–7, the chance of this happening if the population of the 2 sets of islanders have the same risk of hypertension is found to be outside of the 95% confidence interval. We conclude that Island B's population has a different risk of hypertension than Island A's population.

A chi-squared (χ^2) and t-test are different tests for association. Each is based on an underlying distribution and compares the result of one group with that of another. The tests are considered significant when the 2 groups are thought to be too different from each other for the variable of interest to have come from the same underlying population.

Chi-squared tests evaluate variables that are discrete categorical values (ie, ex-smoker, current smoker, never smoker; or male, female), whereas *t-tests* evaluate continuous variables (eg, hormone levels, age).

3.3.3 Regression Approaches

Sometimes, one wants to compare more than one variable or factor (also known as a predictor or independent variable) with disease risk or outcome (the dependent variable) simultaneously. Chi-squared and t-tests can only evaluate 1 variable at a time. Regression techniques are statistical methods to examine the association of multiple potential disease-related factors with disease or disease outcome. Multivariate regression analysis also permits simultaneous inclusion of many covariates (ie, factors) that are essential in controlling for confounding. In essence, this allows for consideration (and adjustment) of multiple factors in the same analysis. Including multiple variables in the same model is the equivalent of asking what the true association of the factor of interest is when many other predictor variables are simultaneously considered together. In biomarker and biospecimen analyses, such factors of interest can involve protein levels, immunohistochemical staining patterns, serological levels, germline variation, somatic mutations, and epigenetic markers, while clinicoepidemiological factors may include, age, gender, patient comorbidities and general state of health, tumor grade and histological subtype, disease stage at diagnosis, and treatment.

Regression models generally follow a common pattern. Equation 3.4 represents a univariate analysis where the x represents the value of the independent (predictor) variable, while the y represents the dependent (outcome) variable. β_0 is a nominal constant, while β_1 represents the association between x and

TABLE 3–2 Different formats for the independent variable, x_n.

Types of Independent Variable, x_n	Examples of How Variable, x_n can be Incorporated into a Regression Model
Dichotomized (ie, two-level) (eg, Gender)	Male = 0; female = 1
Categorized (eg, smoking status)	Indicator Variables: Current smoker: Current = 1, Former = 0, Never = 0 Former smoker: Current = 0, Former = 1, Never = 0 Never smoker: Current = 0, Former = 0, Never = 1
Ordinal (ranked order) (eg, quartiles of intake of fruit, disease stages at diagnosis, germline variation)	Ordinal Categories (where Q1 to Q4 represents quartiles 1 to 4) Lowest quartile: Q1 = 0 Second lowest quartile: Q2 = 1 Third lowest quartile: Q3 = 2 Highest quartile: Q4 = 3 Indicator Variables: Lowest quartile: Q1 = 1, Q2 = 0, Q3 = 0, Q4 = 0 2nd Lowest quartile: Q1 = 0, Q2 = 1, Q3 = 0, Q4 = 0 3rd Lowest quartile: Q1 = 0, Q2 = 0, Q3 = 1, Q4 = 0 Highest quartile: Q1 = 0, Q2 = 0, Q3 = 0, Q4 = 1
Continuous (age, weight) (eg, age, weight)	Continuous: value (V) can range from 0 to infinity Dichotomized at median: Below median, V = 0 Median or above, V = 1 Divided into tertiles (T): Lowest tertile: T = 0 Second lowest tertile: T = 1 Highest tertile: T = 2

TABLE 3–3 The relationship between type of outcome variable and regression model.

Type of Outcome Variable (y)	Type of Regression Model
Continuous variable (eg, hormone levels; weight loss)	Linear regression
Dichotomous variable (eg, toxicity/no toxicity) Disease (case)/no disease (control)	Logistic regression
Ordinal variable (eg, nonsmoker, mild smoker, heavy smoker; disease response, disease stability, disease progression)	Polytomous ordinal logistic regression (3 or more nominal categories)
Survival outcome or time-to-event (with censoring) (see Chap. 22, Sec. 22.4.1)	Cox proportional hazards regression

Table 3–2 describes the various formats in which to incorporate the independent predictors, x_n, into a regression model. Table 3–3 summarizes the format of the outcome variable, y, which determines the type of regression.

All regression analyses must make assumptions about the nature of their underlying variables x_n and y. For instance, linear regression analyses assume that a continuous, independent x_n variable will have a linear relationship with the y outcome variable. If this is not true, then the x_n variable may need to be transformed to a format where a linear relationship between x_n and y exists; these may include taking the square root or taking the logarithmic function of x_n. In another example, the association between average adult weight and cancer risk may be the result of a threshold effect, in which case, dichotomizing weight at the threshold (rather than treating the variable as a continuous variable) would be more appropriate. In the case of a Cox proportional hazard model, the assumption is that the ratio of hazards (defined as the rate of dying in a short period of time) between the comparator arms remain constant. Many survival curves violate this assumption, most obviously when they cross each other. It is therefore critical that assumptions behind each of these models are checked, and any deviations from these assumptions lead to disclosure and use of alternative methods of analyses (see Chap. 22, Sec. 22.4.1).

A useful property of the logistic regression function is that the β estimates generated in the model are mathematically related to an odds ratio. This relationship is as follows:

$$\text{Odds Ratio of variable } x_n = e^{\beta n}, \text{ where } \beta_n \text{ is derived from an equation similar to Eqn. 3.5} \quad \text{[Eq. 3.6]}$$

3.3.4 Interaction

The term *interaction* has been used in the context of statistical, biological, and public health concepts. In general, interaction refers to 2 or more factors modifying the effect of one another with respect to outcome. Epidemiologists often refer to this as

y in the model, and its value is a constant that is generated as part of the regression analysis. The more the value of β_1 deviates from 0 (whether a large positive or large negative value), the stronger is the magnitude of association between x and y.

$$y = \beta_0 + \beta_1 x \quad \text{[Eq. 3.4]}$$

In Equation 3.5, a single model now incorporates multiple (n) independent variables altogether, as predictors of the outcome, y. This type of model is useful if all n variables are being evaluated as predictors of outcome, y. At other times, one is only interested in the association between y and a single predictor variable, x_1, while the other variables $x_2 \ldots x_n$, represent potential confounders. Data for each study participant (ie, values for x_1 through x_n and for y) are placed into the regression analysis, and values for β_0 through β_n are generated as part of the regression model.

$$y = \beta_0 + \beta_1 x_1 + \beta_2 x_2 + \beta_3 x_3 + \beta_4 x_4 + \ldots + \beta_n x_n \quad \text{[Eq. 3.5]}$$

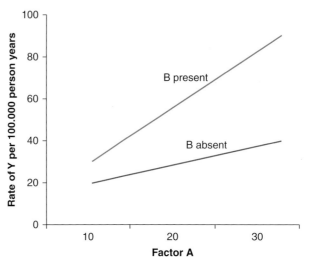

FIGURE 3–8 **Interaction between two independent predictors of disease or outcome.** In the example, an increase from 10 to 30 units for the factor of interest, A, results in the disease rate increasing from 20 per 1000 to 40 per 1000 when factor B is absent. In the presence of factor B the same increase in factor A results in a much greater increase in disease rate: from 30 per 1000 to 90 per 1000. Factor A interacts with factor B as factor A has a stronger effect on disease rates in the presence of factor B. Note that the examples in the table are not associated with the values given in the graph, which is presented for illustrative purposes.

Examples of possible variables for A, B, and Y

	A	B	Y
(i)	Cumulative smoking	Asbestos exposure	Lung cancer risk
(ii)	Cumulative smoking	Cumulative alcohol intake	Head and neck cancer risk
(iii)	Cisplatin chemotherapy	External-beam radiation	Proportion of cured lung cancer
(iv)	Tamoxifen	Estrogen receptor status	Proportion of cured breast cancer

effect modification. An interaction may arise when considering the relationship among multiple variables, and describes a situation in which the simultaneous influence of 2 variables on a third is synergistic or antagonistic. A classic example is the interaction between smoking and asbestos exposure. Each factor individually increases lung cancer risk, but exposure to asbestos increases the cancer risk in smokers much more than simply adding the 2 risks together.

In cancer, interaction analyses often focus on gene–environment interactions, where the goal has been to identify environmental factors that, in the presence of the right combination of genetic or host factors, substantially modify (typically increase) the risk of developing certain cancers. In the realm of pharmacogenetics and biomarker research, interaction analyses are increasingly important (see Sec. 3.7.1).

Interaction should not be confused with *confounding.* A confounder has a stable effect on the relationship of the exposure-to-risk and disease-to-outcome variables; proper analysis will "correct" such a confounder effect and produce an accurate estimate of risk for a potential disease-related factor. In an interaction, the risk estimate for the factor changes with different levels of the variable it interacts with, as illustrated in Figure 3–8. Interaction can be explored using regression techniques.

3.4 ANALYTICAL STUDY DESIGNS

3.4.1 Ecological Design

Ecological studies focus on groups of individuals (or populations) as the unit of observation. These groups may include people living in a defined geographic area, or people from different schools or workplaces. The outcome in these studies is generally the incidence rate (of cancer). For example, an ecological study may look at the association between use of alcohol and incidence of liver cancer in different countries. Measures of exposure to potential disease-related factors are based on aggregate data and can be classified into 3 subgroups:

1. Aggregate measures—characteristics of a group summarized as a mean or median of some putative exposure or the proportion exposed for the group (eg, median or mean income, proportion of smokers).
2. Environmental measures—physical characteristics of the defined area of interest (eg, measures of air pollution).
3. Global measures—characteristics of groups or locations for which there is no analog at the individual level (eg, laws or regulations that reduce exposure to second-hand smoke).

Relative to other study designs, ecological studies are generally inexpensive as data are often readily available. The availability of data can often permit comparisons where exposure differs markedly across populations, such as data representing intake of some foods or nutrients across countries, which may be critical in finding associations.

The most important bias related to ecological studies is known as the *ecological fallacy,* where associations between aggregate measures of exposure and disease may not represent associations at the individual level. Ecological studies generally assume that all members of a group exhibit characteristics of the group as a whole. When this assumption does not hold, the association for the ecological exposure measure will be flawed and can even be in the opposite direction than that of the individual measure. A commonly cited example is an ecological study that identified suicide rates to be positively correlated with the proportion of Protestants in Prussian communities. An obvious interpretation of this is that Protestants were more likely to commit suicide than other groups in these communities. However, because of the study design, it cannot be concluded that a greater proportion of Protestants were committing suicide. An alternative explanation is that differences in suicide rates between communities might be explained by other groups, such as Catholics, having a higher suicide rate in protestant communities, perhaps because of a feeling of social isolation (Szklo and Nieto, 2007). An ecological design does not allow one to confidently distinguish between these 2 opposing explanations because individual level measures (in this example, information on faith and cause of death for each of the study subjects) are not available.

3.4.2 Cohort Design

A cohort study follows a group of people over time comparing those exposed to a factor that may influence risk or outcome of disease to those not exposed to the factor. Individuals typically enter into a cohort because they meet clear-cut criteria using a defined sampling protocol. Cohorts can be prospective (also called concurrent) or retrospective (nonconcurrent or historical). In a prospective cohort, individual study subjects are recruited at a specific point or range in time. Measurements of potential disease-related factors (baseline measures) are made as individuals are recruited into the cohort, and study subjects are then followed over time with further measurements possible. Because exposed and nonexposed individuals within the study are followed over time, relative risk can be calculated directly (see Sec. 3.3.1 and Fig. 3–5). A retrospective cohort makes use of existing databases for information about disease (usually identifying incident cases or deaths) and the disease-related factor of interest. In specific circumstances, biological samples are also available for translational experiments from these retrospective cohorts, either because they were collected as part of a parallel biobanking process, or because such samples were stored long-term following original diagnostic biopsies. The quality of preservation, the quantity of usable material, and the completeness of collection across the entire cohort should be assessed critically, as should the quality of retrospectively collected clinical and epidemiological information.

Although a typical epidemiological cohort study begins with a healthy population (where risk of disease is the outcome being assessed), a growing number of observational cohorts follow individuals with disease (such as cancer), where the outcomes being assessed are treatment-related responses or toxicity, rates of disease relapse and progression, course of disease over time, and/or overall survival. Sometimes, these disease-specific cohorts are labeled *case series*. Case series may involve carefully collected sets of patients, but they may also consist of a convenient, haphazardly collected set of available cases. Use of the term *cohort* implies a well-defined set

of patients adhering to specific entry criteria, such as stage-specific, or geographic-specific sets of individuals.

Prospective cohorts have the advantage of allowing investigators to control subject selection, ascertainment of events, and follow-up, and to determine baseline measurements. In most modern large-scale cohort studies, subjects are chosen according to some defining criteria, such as occupation (eg, nurses in the Nurse Health Study) or residing in a particular area (eg, the Ontario Health Study). Generally, incidence of disease is the outcome of interest. Often, multiple diseases (including a variety of cancers and noncancer outcomes) are investigated in 1 study, to maximize its efficiency and cost-effectiveness. Assessments may involve interviews or mailed questionnaires or measures made at a clinic such as height and weight. Biological samples may be taken and stored for later assessment of molecular and genetic biomarkers. Similar to retrospective cohort studies, it is important to assure the quality of such biomaterials. In analyses of disease risk, the advantage of prospective cohort studies over other observational approaches is that exposure to a disease-related factor is measured prior to development of disease; it is this property that makes cohort studies so important in translational science. Assessing the exposure after development of disease can lead to bias. For example, biomarker levels in blood could be influenced by the presence of disease; thus, obtaining specimens well before diagnosis of cancer is important.

Ascertainment of outcome is critical in a cohort study. When the outcome is the development of cancer, a pathology report from a cancer registry is often used to identify the case and confirm the diagnosis. An accurate date of diagnosis is required so that prevalent cases are not counted, and is essential when one of the outcomes is survivorship after diagnosis. When the outcome of interest is response to treatment, toxicity, recurrence, and/or survival, careful standardization for measuring each outcome must take place, usually with systematic repeated evaluations (eg, standardizing a follow-up schedule). Many subjects can be lost to follow-up despite extensive efforts to track them. Losing subjects to follow-up can introduce bias if these losses are differential with respect to either the potential disease-related factor or the outcome of interest. Linkage to cancer registries and mortality databases can permit tracking of individuals so that disease occurrence and vital status can be ascertained even if subjects are lost to routine follow-up. Although overall survival requires a hard outcome measure (alive or dead), loss to follow-up and missing outcome may still require clinical interpretation, whereas other outcomes, such as disease-free survival and cancer-specific mortality may be subject to error or bias.

Prospective cohort studies designed to evaluate risk of disease are very expensive. For a disease such as cancer, many individuals will have to be recruited to ensure that a sufficient number of incident cases will occur for meaningful analyses. Also because cancer has a long latency period, researchers may have to wait for many years after recruitment before sufficient numbers of cases are available for analysis.

Cohort studies of outcomes after cancer diagnosis are also expensive, as a consequence of the costs of performing accurate and careful patient follow-up. In addition, heterogeneity in treatment and patient management is a substantial source of confounding in such studies. Thus, unlike cohort studies of disease risk, typically it is easier to analyze and interpret single-institution studies or studies involving a small number of institutions that follow similar treatment plans, compared to those studies in which treatments are heterogeneous. Yet single-institution studies can suffer because of inclusion of a highly selected subset of patients, limiting generalizability. In contrast, the analysis of cancer registry data for a geographic region, which represents an analysis of what is expected in the real world, may suffer from wide variability in patient management (eg, therapy, monitoring, and follow-up). In many ways, the single-institution observational study may mirror the clinical trial (rigorous entry criteria, uniform therapy, well-defined follow-up), whereas the registry and cohort data may mirror health outcomes research (real world analysis; see Chap. 22, Sec. 22.9).

3.4.3 Case-Control Design

In contrast to a cohort study where incidence of disease is compared in differently exposed groups, case-control studies recruit newly diagnosed cases and compare these to controls with respect to their exposure to a potential disease-related factor. The recruitment of incident cases means that there is no need to wait for disease to occur. This greatly reduces costs relative to cohort studies, particularly for rare diseases, because there is no need to recruit large number of subjects and wait for some to develop disease. In studies of disease outcome, a case-control study typically compares patients with certain outcomes (eg, cancer-free patients; patients without treatment toxicities) to patients with alternative outcomes (eg, patients who have relapsed from disease; patients with significant toxicities from a specific treatment). Relative risk cannot be calculated directly within a case-control analysis, but is estimated using the odds ratio (Sec. 3.3.1 and Fig. 3–6).

Various sampling strategies are employed for case-control studies. In hospital-based studies, patients diagnosed with the disease of interest are recruited, either as cases for an analysis of cancer risk, or as the basis of a nested case-control study of disease outcome (see below). Controls for analyses of cancer risk are obtained from groups of patients whose reason for attendance at an outpatient clinic or less frequently, admission to hospital, is expected to be unrelated to the potential disease-related factor of interest. Bias by confounding and selection can occur if clinic visits or hospitalization of controls are related to the disease-related factor or the cases and controls originate from geographic areas that do not entirely overlap (see Sec. 3.2.4 and Table 3–1). Selecting cancer cases and controls from a well-defined population, referred to as a *population-based case-control study*, addresses this bias. This can be accomplished by using cancer registries that register all cancers in a geographic region and with a scheme that randomly recruits control subjects from the same region.

A special form of case-control study is the *nested case-control study*, in which patients were recruited originally for a cohort study, but analyzed as if the study was of a case-control design. In such an analysis, cases with a specific disease that occurred in a defined cohort are identified. Controls, matched for the most important confounding variables (eg, age and gender) are selected from among those in the cohort who have not developed the disease. The Framingham Heart Study, the Nurses Health Study, and the Health Professional Study are examples of long-term cohort studies that originally recruited healthy individuals and followed them for a prolonged time period. Participants of these cohorts completed questionnaires that included detailed information about smoking exposures, medication use (eg, aspirin and metformin use), exercise patterns, and diet. During the follow-up of these studies, a number of cancer outcomes were reported. In one analysis, several researchers then used these cohorts to examine the association of various risk factors with the development of colorectal cancer. Individuals from these cohorts who were diagnosed with colorectal cancer were designated as cases. For each case, the researchers then selected 1 or more healthy controls (ie, healthy individuals without cancer) from the same cohort, matched for similar age and gender. The researchers then compared the risk exposures for cases and controls as they would in a case-control study. The word *nested* refers to performing a case-control analysis "nested" within a larger cohort study. Through these efforts, smoking, specific dietary patterns, aspirin and use of other medication, exercise, and energy balance were either discovered or confirmed to be associated with altered risks of colorectal (and other) cancers.

For many research questions, the nested case-control design offers reductions in costs and efforts of data collection and analysis compared with the full cohort approach, with relatively minor loss in statistical efficiency. This design is particularly useful when biological materials are being analyzed (as analysis of the biological material is often one of the more expensive components of such studies). Selection from a defined cohort has additional advantages in that information on exposure to the disease-related factor is collected prior to onset of disease instead of after diagnosis as in a population- or hospital-based study. This removes potential bias resulting from diseased subjects reporting exposures differently than controls (recall bias, Table 3–1), or blood-based measures of biomarkers being influenced by disease onset.

3.4.4 Cross-Sectional Design

In a cross-sectional study, sampling of individuals from an underlying population takes place at a specific time point. Disease status (ie, case or control status) and risk exposure data are collected for that particular time point. For example, we are interested in learning about the prevalence of diabetes in breast cancer patients. We randomly sample 10,000 women from an underlying population, and find that 300 individuals

| | Breast cancer | | |
	Yes	No	Total
Diabetes Yes	120 (A)	1880 (B)	2000
No	380 (C)	7620 (D)	8000
Total	500	9500	10,000

Odds ratio of the association between diabetes and breast cancer:
AD/BC = (120 × 7620)/(1880 × 380) ≈ 1.28

FIGURE 3–9 Results of a hypothetical cross-sectional study evaluating the relationship between the prevalence of diabetes and breast cancer.

have received a diagnosis of breast cancer by the date of sampling. We then find that 2000 women from our sample have a diagnosis of diabetes by the date of sampling. Figure 3–9 presents the data from this study. In this hypothetical scenario, the odds ratio of diabetes as a risk factor for breast cancer is AD/BC = (120/380)/(1880/7620) ≈ 1.28.

Because cases are not necessarily newly diagnosed and may include subjects who have had their disease for many years, cross-sectional studies are sometimes referred to as prevalence studies. The main drawback for this design is that it introduces survival (or prevalence) bias into the study. A factor found to be more prevalent in cases than controls may not be causally related to the onset of disease but instead may be related to living with the disease, its survival, its treatment, or other factors after diagnosis. In the example above, it is likely that having a diagnosis of breast cancer results in increased physical and emotional stress (eg, from surgical procedures, psychosocial stress, or stress that leads to an increase in poor eating habits). In this fashion, subclinical or borderline diabetic patients can become fully diabetic, as a result of these stressors. Second, patients who are diagnosed with breast cancer will see their doctors more often, and have more tests run, including standard blood work. This act can increase the detection of borderline or mild cases of diabetes disproportionate to the general healthy population. Third, some breast cancer chemotherapies are concomitantly administered with steroids (either to prevent anaphylactoid reactions or as a prophylactic antiemetic), which can further push a subclinical or borderline diabetic into being a clinically apparent diabetic.

In another example, the relationship of severe emphysema and early stage lung cancer is examined, using a cross-sectional study design. We may find, paradoxically, that emphysema appears to protect against development of early stage lung cancer. However, the reason for this finding may be a result of emphysema patients dying earlier after diagnosis of lung cancer, or as a result of suboptimal therapy (emphysema patients may not be able to tolerate standard lung resection, or may develop more life-threatening complications after resection). Alternatively, severe emphysema may be such a significant comorbidity that in the presence of a second cause of pulmonary compromise (eg, lung cancer), there is

an increase in pneumonia, bronchitis, or general debilitation, and a higher rate of death. Under these circumstances, in a prevalence or cross-sectional study, a substantial proportion of individuals who have lung cancer with severe emphysema may have died by the time of the cross-sectional sampling, and distort the relationship between lung cancer and emphysema, known as survival bias (see Table 3–1). In such circumstance, other study designs, such as case-control or cohort, which typically restrict cases to those who are newly diagnosed, are more appropriate.

Cross-sectional study designs are most useful when studying prevalence questions, such as with health and economic policy research (eg, How commonly are prostate cancer and dementia found together? How many breast cancer survivors are there who are overweight?). Many cross-sectional studies utilize routinely collected information for other reasons (eg, census data) and thus it can be of low cost to perform such secondary analyses. It is less common to have a prospectively designed cancer cross-sectional study, primarily because of the potential for the biases listed above, and the relatively large numbers of individuals (and associated expense) required for completing such a study.

3.4.5 Familial Design

Familial studies are commonly used to study the association of genetic factors with disease risk (Thomas, 2004). Initially family-based studies involved either using sibling pairs, generally one affected and one unaffected sibling, or a single affected offspring and 2 parents. The first can be analyzed using methods related to those used in case-control studies. The latter uses the *transmission disequilibrium test*, which compares parental alleles to those of the diseased offspring (case) and determines if there is excess transmission of specific alleles to the offspring. Newer statistical methods allow for analyses using families with affected individuals and 1 or more siblings, parents, or combinations of both (Thomas, 2004). The advantage of family based designs over a case-control design is that they are not subject to bias because of the presence of a systematic difference in allele frequencies between subpopulations as a result of different ancestry (known as *population stratification*). Bias occurs when such a systematic difference goes unrecognized, leading to potential genetic associations that are thought to be related to the disease of interest, but are, in reality, associated with genetic differences arising from individuals having different ethnic backgrounds.

A major difficulty of family based studies is recruitment of controls. If the diseased subject is older, parents may be deceased or not well enough to join a study. Recruitment of siblings can also be difficult as a subject must have a sibling willing to enroll in the study to be eligible. For these reasons familial study designs are rarely employed in cancer outside of a pediatric population. Instead, study designs in adult cancers generally rely on case-control studies where controls are matched to cases for ethnicity and statistical methods are employed to control for population stratification.

3.5 CANCER EPIDEMIOLOGY IN ACTION: SUCCESS STORIES

3.5.1 Infection and Cancer

There has been increasing recognition of the role of infection in cancer etiology. Specific examples include schistosomal infestations and bladder cancer, hepatitis viruses and hepatocellular carcinoma (HCC), and HPVs and cervical and head and neck cancer (see Chap. 6, Sec. 6.2.3). It has been estimated that attributable risk of all cancers worldwide to infections is approximately 18%, and that by reducing the effects of these infectious agents (through improved hygiene and public health measures, vaccination, and sometimes screening), cancer incidence might decrease by 8% and 26% in developed and developing countries, respectively (Parkin, 2006).

One of the most successful applications of analytical epidemiology in addressing infections and cancer is the research that helped establish a role for Epstein-Barr virus (EBV) in the etiology of Burkitt lymphoma (see Chap. 6, Sec. 6.2.4). Endemic Burkitt lymphoma occurs in children, primarily in equatorial Africa and Papua New Guinea. Its occurrence was first described by Dennis Burkitt in 1958 (Thompson and Kurzrock, 2004). The most frequent presentation of the tumor is a distinctive lesion of the jaw. In early ecological studies of this disease, this information was circulated to medical units in Africa and presence of the lesion was mapped to geographic location. Results indicated an association between the presence of Burkitt lymphoma and low-lying areas in tropical Africa (Burkitt, 1962a,b), suggesting that a virus transmitted by an insect vector might play a role in the etiology of this cancer. Laboratory-based studies by Epstein, Achong, and Barr implicated EBV as an etiological agent for this cancer and following further research, EBV became the first virus to be clearly implicated in the development of a human cancer (Thompson and Kurzrock, 2004). Additional research indicates that malarial infections, which correlate with the incidence of Burkitt lymphoma, may interact with EBV to increase risk of Burkitt lymphoma (Brady et al, 2007).

The evidence associating HBV and HCC was first observed in ecological studies, where a high prevalence of serum hepatitis B surface antigen (HBsAg) positivity was correlated with the high prevalence of HCC (Maupas and Melnick, 1981). Cohort studies also showed that populations receiving vaccination for HBV have much lower risk of developing HCC then those without vaccination (Lee et al, 1998). HCV was also identified as an etiological factor, both as a cofactor and an independent risk factor for HCC (Yu et al, 2005). Nowadays, HBV and HCV vaccination is routinely administered in high-prevalence regions, and has substantially reduced the incidence of HCC by 75% in school-age children in the last 2 decades (see Chap. 6, Sec. 6.2.5; Chien et al, 2006).

The association between HPV and cervical cancer was first proposed by zur Hausen in 1977 when he found HPV DNA in cervical cancer tissues (zur Hausen, 1977). In 1995, a large cross-sectional study by the International Agency for Research on Cancer (IARC) reported HPV DNA, predominantly HPV types 16 and 18, in 93% of the cervical tumor samples, thus providing strong epidemiological evidence of the association (Bosch et al, 1995). Now HPV is accepted as a necessary cause of cervical cancer; however, only a small portion of the HPV carriers develop cervical cancer, suggesting that other etiological factors are involved (Munoz et al, 2003). In 2006, the first HPV vaccine was approved by the U.S. Food and Drug Administration (FDA) (Markowitz et al, 2007) and HPV vaccine is now recommended in the United States and Canada for school-age girls to prevent cervical cancer (see Chap. 6, Sec. 6.2.3).

3.5.2 Tobacco and Cancer

Tobacco consumption is the most recognized risk factor for human cancer in Western countries. It accounts for approximately 30% of cancer death in the United States (CDC, 2002), and 16% worldwide (Parkin et al, 1999). Epidemiological studies have identified numerous detrimental health effects of tobacco consumption over the last 60 years, with the most striking example being Sir Richard Doll's British studies that established the association between tobacco smoking and lung cancer (Doll et al, 2004). Since then numerous epidemiological studies have been conducted for different cancer sites. In 2004, an IARC monograph stated that there is sufficient evidence to conclude that in humans tobacco smoking causes cancer of the lung, head and neck (including oral cavity, oropharynx, and larynx), esophagus, stomach, pancreas, liver, kidney, bladder, cervix, and myeloid leukemia (Fig. 3–10) (IARC, 2004). In addition to adult cancers, it is recognized that parental tobacco smoking in the time period just before conception or during pregnancy is associated with a higher risk of hepatoblastoma in the offspring (Secretan et al, 2009).

Data for lung cancer are overwhelming: 88% of male lung cancer and 72% of female lung cancer is attributable to tobacco use. Increasing intensity of cigarette smoking (ie, number of cigarettes per day) and increasing duration of smoking (ie, years) are both associated with increasing risk of lung cancer in a dose-dependent fashion. Increasing number of years since smoking cessation is associated with a fall in risk. Similar dose-dependent findings have been found for the risk of bladder, oral cavity, and other solid tumors. There have been more than 50 studies of second-hand smoking and lung cancer risk, many in lifetime never-smoking spouses. Most, especially those associated with higher second-hand smoking exposures, have shown significant increased lung cancer risks associated with inhaling smoke from others (IARC, 2004).

The understanding of the association between tobacco use and cancer risk (in addition to other nonmalignant diseases such as cardiovascular disease) through epidemiological studies have helped governments to implement policy for tobacco control, including banning smoking in public buildings, increasing tobacco taxes, and placing warning labels on the packaging. Government intervention and control policy have

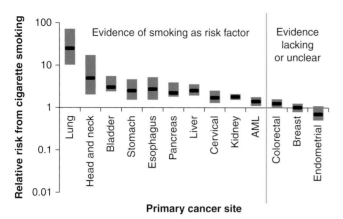

FIGURE 3–10 **Relative risks of cigarette smoking on risk of various cancers.** The approximate ranges of the relative risks of the heaviest cigarette smokers for developing various cancers, summarized from the tables of published studies reviewed by the International Association for Research in Cancer (IARC). The X-axis indicates various primary cancers. The Y-axis is the median relative risk on a logarithmic scale. The cancers to the left of the blue line were concluded by IARC to have an association with cigarette smoking, while the ones on the right did not. These ranges represent the majority of primary smoking data up to the year 2004. The heaviest smokers were defined variably by different studies. Outlier studies were not included in these ranges, but data for men and women were considered together. The median values are presented in black and the bars represent 25% and 75% quartiles. *AML*, Acute myelogenous leukemia. (Data from IARC *Monograph on Tobacco and Involuntary Smoking*, 2004.)

helped to reduce tobacco consumption at the population level substantially, and to reduce cancer deaths related to tobacco consumption.

3.5.3 Alcohol and Head and Neck Cancer

Epidemiological studies have found an association between alcohol consumption and cancer at various sites, including cancers of the oral cavity, pharynx, larynx, esophagus, liver, female breast, and colorectum (IARC, 2010). The role of alcohol as a causative factor for other cancers, such as lung cancer and non-Hodgkin lymphoma, is inconclusive. A systematic review estimated that alcohol accounts for 5.2% of overall cancer worldwide in males and 1.7% in females (Boffetta and Hashibe, 2006). Studies have also investigated the dose–response relationship between alcohol consumption and cancers, and the synergism between alcohol and tobacco smoking. Because alcohol is often consumed by tobacco smokers, there was a need to take tobacco smoking into account either by study design or statistical analysis to address potential confounding. The dose–response relationship between alcohol and head and neck cancers was shown to be linear with an approximately 2- to 3-fold increased risk per 50 g of alcohol per day, depending on the cancer site (IARC, 2004). The effect of smoking and alcohol consumption appear to be multiplicative for head and neck cancer, showing a synergistic interaction between these 2 factors (see Fig. 3–8).

3.6 EMERGING AREAS IN EPIDEMIOLOGY

3.6.1 Genomic Epidemiology

3.6.1.1 Genome-Wide Association Studies
Genome-wide association studies (GWAS, see Chap. 2, Sec. 2.7) aim to investigate the majority of genetic variations across the genome, and do not require prior knowledge of the functional significance of the variants studied. They are used increasingly to discover susceptibility genes in various health research domains. Genome-wide scans for cancer of the prostate, breast, colon, lung, kidney, bladder, and pancreas have been completed, and this approach has been successful in identifying cancer susceptibility loci. A catalog of published GWAS with complete references is maintained by the National Human Genome Research Institute (available at http://www.genome.gov/gwastudies/).

3.6.1.2 Addiction to Nicotine, and Risk of Lung Cancer
A previous linkage analysis of 52 high-risk pedigrees identified a lung cancer susceptibility locus at chromosome 6q23-25 (Bailey-Wilson et al, 2004), but specific genetic factors that influence lung cancer susceptibility were not defined until the GWAS findings were reported in 2008, when researchers identified the susceptibility loci at 15q25 and 5p15 (Hung et al, 2008). The Ch15q25 region is comprised of several nicotinic acetylcholine receptor genes and the 5p15 region includes the genes *hTERT* (see Chap. 5, Sec. 5.7) and *CLPTM1L*. The *hTERT* gene is the most likely candidate in this region. The Ch15q25 region was also shown to be associated with nicotine addiction and smoking behaviors (Thorgeirsson et al, 2008), although the association between 15q25 and smoking is not sufficient to explain its strong association with risk of lung cancer. Alternative hypotheses relating to potential roles in angiogenesis and in the repair of epithelium are being evaluated. This example illustrates how GWAS may contribute to the understanding of cancer etiology. As yet, none of the findings from GWAS is of strong enough magnitude to translate into the clinical setting; hence, GWAS is still a research tool used to identify novel biological pathways for further basic and translational research.

3.6.1.3 Alcohol, Alcohol Dehydrogenase, and Head and Neck Cancer
The metabolism of alcohol mainly involves two families of genes: alcohol dehydrogenases (*ADHs*) that oxidize ethanol to acetaldehyde, and acetaldehyde dehydrogenases (*ALDHs*) that further metabolize acetaldehyde to acetate. The genetic variation of *ADHs* and *ALDHs* that influences enzyme activity has been investigated for their association with head and neck cancer in several epidemiological studies (IARC, 2010). *ADH1B* (*1/*1, where *1/*1 is a genotype designation) and *ADH1C* are associated with increased risk of head and neck cancers, although the mechanism has not been elucidated. The *ALDH2 Glu487Lys* allele (*rs671*, also known as *2 variant allele) encodes an inactive form of the enzyme, and this Lys variant is prevalent in approximately 30% of Asian populations. The heterozygous

TABLE 3-4 Examples of cancer pharmacogenetic studies.

Disease	Candidate or GWAS	Environmental (Drug) Agent	Genetic Polymorphism	Result	Reference (n Cases/n Controls)
Hearing loss	Candidate (220 drug-metabolism genes)	Cisplatin chemotherapy	rs12201199 (*TPMT*) rs9332377 (*COMT*)	OR = 17 OR = 5.5	Ross et al, 2009 (33/20)
Severe neutropenia	Candidate	Irinotecan	−3156G>A (*UGT1A1*)	p = 0.007, no OR reported	Innocenti et al, 2004 (66 total)
Musculoskeletal adverse events	GWAS	Aromatase inhibitors	rs11849538 rs7158782 rs7159713 rs2369049	OR = 2.1–2.2	Ingle et al, 2010 (292/585)

GWAS, Genome-wide association studies; *OR*, odds ratio. Codes for genetic polymorphisms (rs followed by number) are established reference identification numbers for each polymorphism.

carriers have approximately 10% enzyme activity, and they accumulate acetaldehyde and have increased risks for alcohol-related esophageal and head and neck cancers compared with individuals with the common alleles. These findings have contributed to the understanding of alcohol as a carcinogen (IARC, 2010).

3.6.2 Pharmacogenomic Epidemiology and Pharmacoepidemiology

Pharmacogenomic epidemiology is focused on personalizing medicine through the evaluation of tumor and germline (heritable) genetic and genomic factors to select appropriate and individualized therapies, through the use of epidemiological tools. These factors, or biomarkers, are assessed for their association with pharmacokinetic and pharmacodynamic roles in affecting treatment response, recurrence, disease progression and survival, and toxicity of treatment (see Chap. 18, Sec. 18.1).

The classical example in cancer pharmacogenetics has been the genetic disorder that results in the complete absence of functional dihydropyrimidine dehydrogenase (DPD), or DPD deficiency, and the resultant severe hematological and gastrointestinal toxicities that affect such patients who receive fluoropyrimidines (eg, 5-fluorouracil), which are antimetabolites that inhibit thymidylate synthase and DNA synthesis (see Chap. 18, Sec. 18.1.3). DPD is the enzyme responsible for more than 85% of the inactivation and metabolism of 5-fluorouracil. However, the cause of this rare syndrome of DPD deficiency is multifactorial, including such factors as multiple functional genetic variants within the DPD gene, and both genetic and epigenetic regulation across other related pathway genes that secondarily alter DPD function. Pharmacological factors (drug–drug interactions) are also being evaluated. Thus, the original single defect in 1 gene leading to a single phenotype is too simplistic a model to explain sensitivity to fluoropyrimidines. Additional factors also explain the low positive predictive value of currently available tests; as such, routine clinical testing is generally not recommended. Because of the rarity of DPD deficiency,

pharmacoepidemiological (pharmacovigilance) studies have been used to identify potential cases, and these are matched, in a case-control design, to appropriate controls (patients receiving the drug who suffered no significant toxicity).

Several newer pharmacogenetic studies have identified promising associations between heritable genetic variations and either toxicity or efficacy of drugs (Table 3–4). Each of these studies has either used observational methods or involved secondary analyses of randomized clinical trials. Some have selected candidate polymorphisms (eg, of genes known to be important in metabolism of anticancer drugs), whereas others have utilized GWASs without a primary hypothesis. These studies have led to the discovery of unexpected genetic variants that have a biological rationale for their association with the pharmacogenetic effects. Validation studies are ongoing.

In addition to heritable genetic associations with drug therapy, molecular epidemiological studies and secondary analyses of randomized controlled trials are also demonstrating associations between tumor markers and treatment outcomes. Four examples are: estrogen receptor/progesterone receptor status and use of antiestrogen therapy (eg, tamoxifen or aromatase inhibitor; see Chap. 20, Sec. 20.4.1); KRAS mutation predicts lack of efficacy of monoclonal antibody therapy targeting EGFR in colorectal cancer (see Chap. 17, Sec. 17.3.1); Her2/neu overamplification predicts efficacy of monoclonal antibody therapy targeting Her2/neu (see Chap. 20, Sec. 20.3.3); and EGFR mutation predicts for response to small molecule inhibitors of EGFR (see Chap. 17, Sec. 17.3.1).

3.7 ISSUES AND CHALLENGES IN CANCER EPIDEMIOLOGY

3.7.1 Observational Studies Versus Clinical Trials, Predictive Versus Prognostic Biomarkers

Observational studies are the most common way to study the risk of disease, primarily because there are generally no other

TABLE 3–5 Comparing the advantages and disadvantages of using randomized trials versus observational studies as sources of epidemiological analyses.

Randomized Trials	Observational Studies
• Designed to measure survival differences, so good resource for secondary analyses of factors related to disease outcome (clinicoepidemiological and biological)	• Standard source for epidemiological studies of disease risk
• Not a good source for analyses of disease risk (because of highly selected case-entry criteria and lack of concurrent healthy controls in study)	• Evaluate rare and long-term toxicities
• Collect detailed treatment toxicity data	• Large, diverse populations
• Randomization should ensure equal distribution of confounding variables	• Follow-up can be extensive
• Accessible specimens for translational research	• Prone to selection and confounding bias
• Can incorporate collection of epidemiological data in study design	• Large number of drugs and drug combinations
• Efficient use of resources by tagging epidemiological study onto trial	• Include a wide range of comorbidities and past medication history
• Either the experimental or standard arm will become obsolete; thus, at least 1 arm may become irrelevant to clinical practice	• Can be utilized in rarer cancers where randomized trials are not available
	• Can study standard, approved drugs where no randomized trial data exist

approaches available. Observational studies are also a useful source of data for certain outcomes analyses.

Randomized clinical trials provide a convenient source of patients for analysis of disease outcome and may be linked to biospecimens. When available, they can be used sometimes for secondary analyses of factors other than the one that was randomized. Randomized clinical trials are a form of cohort study where subjects are assigned to 2 or more arms (eg, vitamin supplementation group and placebo group) and the cohort is followed over time. Unlike modern observational cohorts, randomized trials typically focus largely on a single factor. Their main advantage is that the researcher controls who is exposed to the potential disease-related factor, through random assignment. Randomized trials are most useful in clinical medicine for demonstrating effectiveness of a specific treatment intervention (see Chap. 22, Sec. 22.2.3).

When molecular factors are evaluated that might predict response, toxicity, or outcome related to the experimental therapy used in a randomized trial, a pharmacogenomic analysis takes place. A major benefit of performing a secondary analysis of a randomized trial is that one can determine whether the pharmacogenomic factor is predictive of treatment response or simply a general prognostic marker (see Chap. 22, Sec. 22.4). Predictive biomarkers are those that are associated with a specific therapy; in the absence of this therapy, the biomarker is either no longer associated with outcome, or is associated in a different manner. The absence of a differential effect by treatment implies that the specific biomarker is a general prognostic factor. Although prognostic factors may be helpful for improving our understanding of cancer biological pathways, they are less useful clinically than biomarkers that predict whether an outcome will change if a specific treatment is given. The predictive biomarker can then direct the choice of therapy, in essence, personalizing the treatment. Because the only way to determine whether a biomarker is predictive is to have a control arm, a randomized trial is optimal for identifying such predictive pharmacogenomic biomarkers.

The formal statistical method for determining whether a marker is predictive is to identify an interaction between a biomarker and a treatment arm. The presence of such an interaction implies that the biomarker has a different effect in the presence of the treatment than in the absence of treatment. Although observational studies may occasionally be used to study such interactions (Bradbury et al, 2009), randomized trials offer the best opportunity, partly because the choice of therapy is less confounded by other key prognostic variables such as patient co-morbidity.

Table 3–5 compares the use of randomized trials with observational studies. A randomized trial of the right set of patients may not be available (wrong patient subgroup, wrong therapy, rare cancer type where no such randomized trials are being conducted), and an observational study becomes the only option. Thus, both types of studies will continue to be important for epidemiological and translational research. Figure 3–11 details the long journey from biomarker discovery through to clinical adoption. Epidemiological studies are key to several of the steps in the biomarker developmental pipeline.

3.7.2 Exposure Misclassifications: The Example of Diet and Occupation

As discussed briefly in Section 3.2.4, misclassification of exposure has been a challenge for cancer epidemiology, and specific examples include assessment of dietary and occupational exposures. The general hypotheses are that certain micronutrients or specific chemical agents related to occupations can affect cancer risk. Proper assessments of these exposures require a comprehensive study protocol, thorough validation, and substantial resources.

For dietary exposures, specific instruments, such as 24-hour recall, have been developed to assist the validation of the self-reported dietary history. To validate a specific dietary exposure, biochemical indicators (if available) might be measured, such as serum level of vitamin B or folate. This approach,

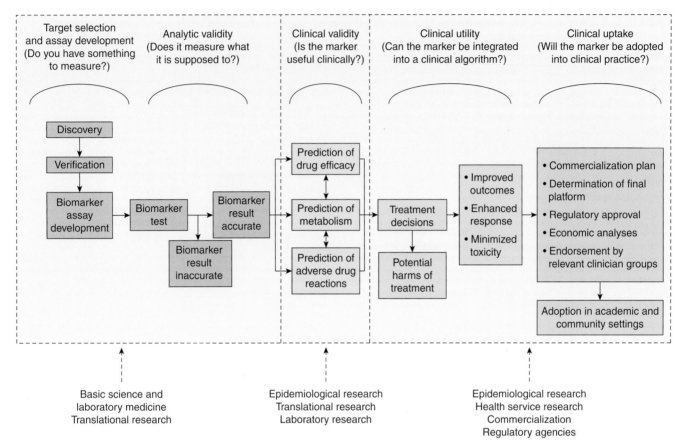

FIGURE 3–11 The long road from biomarker discovery to clinical use, and where epidemiological studies play a key role.

however, is subject to biomarker instability, laboratory measurement error, and when repeated samples are not available, the measurement at 1 time point does not reflect the long-term exposure history. Nevertheless, biomarkers can provide qualitative information regarding the validity of information obtained from questionnaires.

Perhaps the greatest challenge in evaluating exposure to putative risk factors is the problem with highly correlated exposures, where the challenge is to distinguish the independent effect of specific nutrients or foods, when food items are typically consumed in groups, and patterns of consumption are reflective of general lifestyle and socioeconomic status. An individual food item might be a better unit for analysis because it can be directly related to dietary recommendations and the same nutrients may exhibit different properties in different foods (eg, nitrates in smoked meat versus in green leafy vegetables). Analysis based on a specific nutrient can be more directly related to a biological mechanism and avoid the issues of interrelated dietary behavior patterns (eg, the tendency to eat certain foods together, such as milk and cereal, or certain habits together such as alcohol and tobacco consumption). In general, it has been suggested that maximum information can be obtained when analyses are performed using all of the data, including nutrient levels, food items, and food groups.

The approach of Mendelian randomization has also been proposed to address the issues of complex exposures (Smith and Ebrahim, 2003). The basic concept of Mendelian randomization is to analyze variants in genes (both as single genes or multiple genes) that determine metabolism of nutrients as instrumental (ie, surrogate) variables for the specific nutrients of interest, as genetic alleles are randomly assorted in the population based on Mendel's laws and their assortments are unrelated to other factors such as lifestyles or other food intake. Specific examples include ALDH (for alcohol consumption) and cardiovascular disease, or lactase persistence genotype (for milk consumption) and cancer (Smith and Ebrahim, 2003). The ideal instrumental variable needs to have very strong and specific correlations with the nutrient of interest, but for some nutrients, such an instrumental variable will not be found. Nevertheless, it provides a potential alternative solution to the issues of misclassification and high correlation in nutritional epidemiology.

3.7.3 High-Dimensionality Data and Multiple Comparisons

Biological and genetic data from cancer epidemiological studies typically involve tens or hundreds of thousands of variables related to genetics or biomarkers to be tested against a null hypothesis. If we conduct 100 independent tests each with 95% confidence interval (5% type I error rate, see Chap. 22, Sec. 22.2.5), we would expect to reject the null hypothesis for 5 tests as a result of chance. This is the result of *multiple comparisons*. The conventional approach to address the issue of multiple comparisons is to alter the level of significance by dividing it by the number of comparisons, known as the *Bonferroni* method. For example, one would use a type I error rate of $0.05/100 = 0.0005$ for 100 simultaneous comparisons. However this approach has various limitations, such as a naïve global null hypothesis that ignores prior knowledge about biological effects and low efficiency, and it is deemed to be too conservative for epidemiological investigation. Analogous to Bayesian statistical models that incorporate prior information (see Chap. 22, Sec. 22.3.5), modern approaches, such as hierarchical modeling or mixture modeling, can offer improved performance over the Bonferroni adjustment. These analytical approaches are being applied to the field of genomic and molecular epidemiology (Chen and Witte, 2007). The details of these modeling approaches are beyond the scope of this chapter, but the basic concept of hierarchical modeling is to incorporate prior knowledge of markers into analysis through a prior matrix of quantitative weighting factors (Hung et al, 2007) These weighted factors will be used to "adjust" for the biological and genetic results, thereby improving the potential for finding true positive associations.

3.7.4 Analyses across Multiple Studies

To integrate evidence from multiple studies, approaches such as pooled analysis and metaanalysis (see Chap. 22, Sec. 22.2.7) are being increasingly applied in cancer epidemiology. Metaanalysis is typically based on published results; thus, it is susceptible to publication bias, and then limited to results reported in the publication and subject to the definition of different variables and covariate adjustments. It is often impossible to conduct detailed analysis for specific subgroups using metaanalysis. Consequently, researchers have started to conduct pooled analysis to address the above limitations by combining individual-level data from different studies, analogous to patient-based metaanalysis of therapeutic trials. More detailed analysis can also be conducted for specific subgroups. The methodology of metaanalysis and pooled analysis is described elsewhere (van Houwelingen et al, 2002). To facilitate this type of pooled analysis, several cancer consortia have emerged, including the International Lung Cancer Consortium, the Breast Cancer Association Consortium, the Pancreatic Cancer Case-Control Consortium (Ioannidis et al, 2005). The growing list of cancer consortia can be found at http://epi.grants.cancer.gov/Consortia/. The same website lists consortia publications that replicate initial findings in the post-GWAS era, showing that such consortia are an efficient way to replicate an initial finding and provide further evidence for supporting or disputing an observed association.

SUMMARY

- Epidemiology is the study of the distribution and determinants of disease and disease outcomes in human populations. It is complementary to basic and translational research.
- Epidemiological methods can be descriptive or analytical:
  - Descriptive studies provide information about populations and their distributions, including distributions of disease determinants.
  - Analytical studies assess associations between disease determinants and disease and disease outcomes and include case-control, cohort, cross-sectional, and familial designs.
- Important epidemiological successes have demonstrated the relationships between various infections (HPV, viral hepatitis, EBV) and cancer risk, tobacco and cancers, and alcohol and head and neck cancer.
- Emerging areas in epidemiology include genomic epidemiology, and pharmacoepidemiology.
- Challenges for the future include:
  - Utilizing secondary analyses of clinical trials.
  - Novel analyses of exposure misclassifications.
  - High-dimensionality data and multiple comparisons, and analyses across multiple studies.

REFERENCES

Bailey-Wilson JE, Amos CI, Pinney SM, et al. A major lung cancer susceptibility locus maps to chromosome 6q23-25. *Am J Hum Genet* 2004;75:460-474.

Boffetta P, Hashibe M. Alcohol and cancer. *Lancet Oncol* 2006;7:149-156.

Bosch FX, Manos MM, Munoz N, et al. Prevalence of human papillomavirus in cervical cancer: a worldwide perspective. International biological study on cervical cancer (IBSCC) Study Group. *J Natl Cancer Inst* 1995;87:796-802.

Bradbury PA, Kulke MH, Heist RS, et al. Cisplatin pharmacogenetics, DNA repair polymorphisms, and esophageal cancer outcomes. *Pharmacogenet Genomics* 2009;19:613-625.

Brady G, MacArthur GJ, Farrell PJ. Epstein-Barr virus and Burkitt lymphoma. *J Clin Pathol* 2007;602:1397-1402.

Burkitt D. A "tumour safari" in East and Central Africa. *Br J Cancer* 1962a;16:379-386.

Burkitt D. Determining the climatic limitations of a children's cancer common in Africa. *Br Med J* 1962b;2:1019-1023.

Canadian Cancer Society. *Canadian Cancer Statistics 2010*. Toronto, Canada: Canadian Cancer Society; 2010.

Centers for Disease Control and Prevention (CDC). Annual smoking-attributable mortality, years of potential life lost, and economic costs—United States, 1995-1999. *MMWR Morb Mortal Wkly Rep* 2002;51:300-303.

Chen GK, Witte JS. Enriching the analysis of genomewide association studies with hierarchical modeling. *Am J Hum Genet* 2007;81:397-404.

Chien Y C, Jan CF, Kuo HS, et al. Nationwide hepatitis B vaccination program in Taiwan: effectiveness in the 20 years after it was launched. *Epidemiol Rev* 2006;28:126-135.

Chung CH, Gillison ML. Human papillomavirus in head and neck cancer: its role in pathogenesis and clinical implications. *Clin Cancer Res* 2009;15:6758-6762.

Coate LE, John T, Tsao MS, Shepherd FA. Molecular predictive and prognostic markers in non-small-cell lung cancer. *Lancet Oncol* 2009;10:1001-1010.

Davies L, Welch HG. Increasing incidence of thyroid cancer in the United States, 1973-2002. *JAMA* 2006;295:2164-2167.

Doll R, Peto R, Boreham J, Sutherland I. Mortality in relation to smoking: 50 years' observations on male British doctors. *BMJ* 2004;328:1519.

Ferlay J, Shin HR, Bray F, et al. Estimates of worldwide burden of cancer in 2008: GLOBOCAN 2008. *Int J Cancer* 2010;127(12): 2893-2917.

Hung RJ, Baragatti M, Thomas D, et al. Inherited predisposition of lung cancer: a hierarchical modeling approach to DNA repair and cell cycle control pathways. *Cancer Epidemiol Biomarkers Prev* 2007;16:2736-2744.

Hung RJ, McKay JD, Gaborieau V, et al. A susceptibility locus for lung cancer maps to nicotinic acetylcholine receptor subunit genes on 15q25. *Nature* 2008;452:633-637.

Ingle JN, Schaid DJ, Goss PE, et al. Genome-wide associations and functional genomic studies of musculoskeletal adverse events in women receiving aromatase inhibitors. *J Clin Oncol* 2010;28: 4674-4682.

Innocenti F, Undevia SD, Iyer L, et al. Genetic variants in the UDP-glucuronosyltransferase 1A1 gene predict the risk of severe neutropenia of irinotecan. *J Clin Oncol* 2004;22: 1382-1388.

International Agency of Research on Cancer. *Alcohol Consumption and Ethyl Carbamate. IARC Monographs on the Evaluation of the Carcinogenic Risk of Chemicals to Humans.* Lyon, France: IARC; 2010.

International Agency of Research on Cancer. *Tobacco Smoke and Involuntary Smoking. IARC Monographs on the Evaluation of the Carcinogenic Risk of Chemicals to Humans.* Volume 83. Lyon, France: IARC, 2004.

Ioannidis JP, Bernstein J, Boffetta P, et al. A network of investigator networks in human genome epidemiology. *Am J Epidemiol* 2005;162:302-304.

Kaatsch P, Steliarova-Foucher E, Crocetti E, et al. Time trends of cancer incidence in European children (1978-1997): report from the Automated Childhood Cancer Information System project. *Eur J Cancer* 2006;42:1961-1971.

Lee MS, Kim DH, Kim H, et al. Hepatitis B vaccination and reduced risk of primary liver cancer among male adults: a cohort study in Korea. *Int J Epidemiol* 1998;27:316-319.

Lundgren CI, Hall P, Ekbom A, et al. Incidence and survival of Swedish patients with differentiated thyroid cancer. *Int J Cancer* 2003;106:569-573.

Mahboubi E, Kmet J, Cook PJ, et al. Oesophageal cancer studies in the Caspian Littoral of Iran: the Caspian cancer registry. *Br J Cancer* 1973;28:197-214.

Markowitz LE, Dunne EF, Saraiya M, et al. Quadrivalent human papillomavirus vaccine: recommendations of the Advisory Committee on Immunization Practices (ACIP). *MMWR Recomm Rep* 2007;56:1-24.

Maupas P, Melnick JL: Hepatitis B infection and primary liver cancer. *Prog Med Virol* 1981;27:1-5.

Munoz N, Bosch FX, de Sanjose S, et al. Epidemiologic classification of human papillomavirus types associated with cervical cancer. *N Engl J Med* 2003;348:518-527.

Parkin DM. The global health burden of infection-associated cancers in the year 2002. *Int J Cancer* 2006;118:3030-3044.

Parkin DM, Pisani P, Ferlay J. Estimates of the worldwide incidence of 25 major cancers in 1990. *Int J Cancer* 1999; 80:827-841.

Ross CJ, Katzov-Eckert H, Dubé MP, et al. Genetic variants in TPMT and COMT are associated with hearing loss in children receiving cisplatin chemotherapy. *Nat Genet* 2009;41:1345-1349.

Sackett DL. Bias in analytic research. *J Chronic Dis* 1979;32:51-63.

Saidi F, Sepehr A, Fahimi S, et al. Oesophageal cancer among the Turkomans of northeast Iran. *Br J Cancer* 2000;83:1249-1254.

Secretan B, Straif K, Baan R, et al. A review of human carcinogens—part E: tobacco, areca nut, alcohol, coal smoke, and salted fish. *Lancet Oncol* 2009;10:1033-1034.

Smith GD, Ebrahim S. "Mendelian randomization": can genetic epidemiology contribute to understanding environmental determinants of disease? *Int J Epidemiol* 2003;32:1-2.

Szklo M, Nieto FJ. *Epidemiology: Beyond the Basics.* 2nd ed. Sudbury, MA: Jones and Bartlett; 2007.

Thomas DC. *Statistical Methods in Genetic Epidemiology.* New York, NY: Oxford University Press; 2004.

Thompson MP, Kurzrock R. Epstein-Barr virus and cancer. *Clin Cancer Res* 2004;10:803-821.

Thorgeirsson TE, Geller F, Sulem P, et al. A variant associated with nicotine dependence, lung cancer and peripheral arterial disease. *Nature* 2008;452:638-642.

van Houwelingen HC, Arends LR, Stijnen T. Advanced methods in meta-analysis: multivariate approach and meta-regression. *Stat Med* 2002;21:589-624.

Yu MW, Yeh SH, Chen PJ, et al. Hepatitis B virus genotype and DNA level and hepatocellular carcinoma: a prospective study in men. *J Natl Cancer Inst* 2005;97:265-272.

zur Hausen H. Human papillomaviruses and their possible role in squamous cell carcinomas. *Curr Top Microbiol Immunol* 1977; 78:1-30.

Chemical Carcinogenesis

Denis M. Grant

4.1 INTRODUCTION AND HISTORICAL PERSPECTIVE

Although many factors contribute to cancer causation, this chapter focuses on providing an overview of the mechanisms by which exogenous chemicals may influence the risk of cancer initiation and tumor growth, and how knowledge of these mechanisms might be exploited to improve human health through prevention or intervention. The reader is directed to the bibliography for a list of critical reviews that summarize the past history, current status, and future prospects for the field of chemical carcinogenesis. The relative importance of environmental chemical exposures to the total burden of cancer risk remains highly contentious and it has been estimated that chemical pollution of the environment accounts for no more than 1% to 3% of all human cancers. However, such estimates do not consider chemical exposures in the workplace (5%) or cigarette smoke (30%) to be environmental pollutants, and they tend to have a primary focus on genotoxic chemicals as causative agents. Thus they may underestimate the importance of the interplay between the permanent tumor-initiating effects of low-level carcinogen exposure, the

additional effects of nongenotoxic chemicals, and the potentially reversible modulating effects on tumor growth of diet, exercise, and other lifestyle factors.

Historically, epidemiological studies suggesting that chemicals can cause human cancer date to more than 230 years ago when Percival Pott observed that scrotal cancer was correlated with soot exposure in English chimney sweeps, and Butlin suggested subsequently that the better hygiene practices of European sweeps reduced their cancer risk. In 1895, Rehn reported a high rate of bladder cancer in German factory workers who were exposed to aniline-based azo dyes. The 20th century saw the identification of specific chemicals associated with increased risk of cancer, and provided methods for identifying cellular and molecular targets of the causative agents and for elucidating mechanisms involved in the conversion of normal cells to produce tumors. A seminal breakthrough was Yamagiwa's production of skin tumors in rabbits by the direct application of coal tar in 1915, which led to the isolation, identification, synthesis, and biological testing of polycyclic aromatic hydrocarbons (PAHs) as chemical carcinogens, including dibenz[a,h]anthracene and benzo[a]pyrene (Fig. 4–1). In 1938, Hueper followed up Rehn's observation

Direct-acting carcinogens

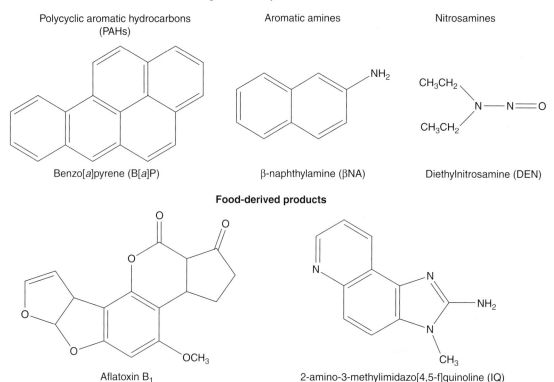

Dimethylcarbamoyl chloride   β-propiolactone   Nitrogen mustard

Procarcinogens that require metabolic activation

Polycyclic aromatic hydrocarbons (PAHs)   Aromatic amines   Nitrosamines

Benzo[*a*]pyrene (B[*a*]P)   β-naphthylamine (βNA)   Diethylnitrosamine (DEN)

Food-derived products

Aflatoxin B$_1$ 2-amino-3-methylimidazo[4,5-f]quinoline (IQ)

FIGURE 4–1   **Structures of some direct-acting carcinogens and procarcinogens that require metabolic activation.**

by demonstrating that the aromatic amine β-naphthylamine (Fig. 4–1), a reagent used in manufacturing azo dyes, caused bladder tumors in dogs.

With the establishment of DNA as the mediator of genetic inheritance in 1953, it became clear that carcinogen-induced DNA damage leading to fixed mutations that could be transmitted to progeny cells was a key event in the process by which exposure to carcinogens led to uncontrolled cell division and tumor growth. The concept that many carcinogens require enzymatic bioactivation into electrophilic metabolites that bind covalently with DNA was established by the Millers in the 1960s. This was followed by investigations that identified specific DNA adducts of various chemicals including benzo[*a*]pyrene and aflatoxin B1, and demonstrated their binding to human tissues. Finally, in the 1990s, key target genes for carcinogens were identified (ie, oncogenes and tumor-suppressor genes—see Chap. 7) whose functionally altered products are key in the initiation, promotion, or progression of tumor growth.

4.2 BIOLOGY OF CHEMICAL CARCINOGENESIS

4.2.1 Tumor Initiation, Promotion, and Progression

Human epidemiological and experimental laboratory studies have long indicated that a latent period (often decades in humans) exists between the exposure to a chemical and the appearance of cancer. This led to the formulation of a sequential model that divided the carcinogenic process into 3 stages termed tumor initiation, tumor promotion, and tumor progression.

Tumor initiation was regarded as involving the interaction of a reactive chemical species (often a procarcinogen metabolite, see Sec. 4.2.3) with DNA to produce damage which, if not repaired before the next cell division, would lead to erroneous DNA replication resulting in fixation of mutations within the genome of individual cells. Thus 3 cellular functions are

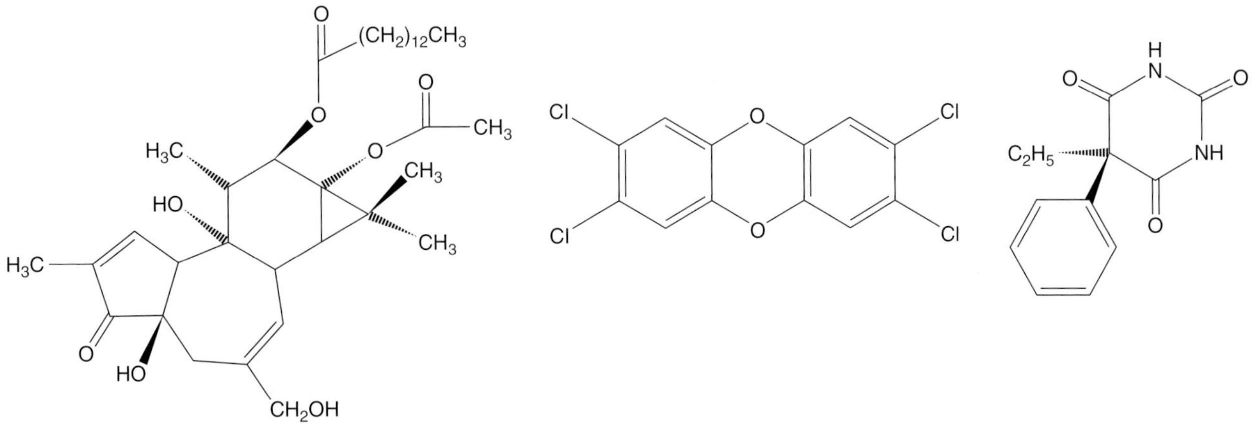

FIGURE 4–2   **Structures of some established tumor promoters.**

important in determining the likelihood of tumor initiation: the rate of procarcinogen activation, the efficiency and fidelity of DNA repair (see Chap. 5), and the capacity for cell proliferation. If a mutation disrupts the function of a gene whose product plays a role in maintaining the terminally differentiated function of the cell, the cell may acquire an altered (usually less differentiated) phenotype. Although initiation is irreversible, not all initiated cells will go on to establish a tumor, as many of these cells may die by apoptosis (see Chap. 9, Sec. 9.4), and further proliferation-enhancing signals are required for initiated cells to progress along the pathway to autonomous (cancerous) growth.

Tumor promotion was viewed as the clonal expansion of an initiated cell as a consequence of events that alter gene expression, so as to provide the cell with a selective proliferative advantage. Although there is no single unifying mechanistic feature of tumor-promoting agents, they tend to be nongenotoxic and to cause, directly or indirectly, cells to divide but not to terminally differentiate or die, resulting in the survival and proliferation of preneoplastic cells and the formation of benign lesions such as papillomas, nodules, or polyps. Many of these lesions may regress spontaneously, but a few cells may acquire additional mutations that allow them to progress to a malignant neoplasm. Figure 4–2 shows the structures of 3 established tumor promoters: tetradecanoyl phorbol acetate (TPA), 2,3,7,8-tetrachlorodibenzo-p-dioxin (TCDD), and phenobarbital. Early studies of mouse skin carcinogenesis illustrated the tumor-promoting activity of croton oil, which contains TPA, when applied following low doses of the tumor-initiator benzo[a]pyrene. Administration of benzo[a]pyrene led to skin tumors only when followed by repeated dosing with croton oil, even though croton oil alone was not carcinogenic.

Tumor progression described the stage whereby benign lesions acquire the ability to further grow, to invade adjacent tissues, and to establish distant metastases.

Although this simple 3-stage model can be a useful conceptual framework for understanding carcinogenesis, we now recognize that the process does not so neatly compartmentalize

within such stages: multiple sequential mutations in combination with epigenetic changes and prolonged alterations in the cellular microenvironment are required to convert a normal cell into a malignant tumor.

4.2.2 Genetic Instability and the Hallmarks of Cancer

Increased genetic instability and alterations in karyotype are often observed in tumor cells (see Chap. 5, Sec. 5.2). Inherited or acquired mutations in genes such as p53, retinoblastoma (Rb) or DNA mismatch repair genes can create a "mutator phenotype" of enhanced random mutation that accelerates the accumulation of further spontaneous or chemical-induced DNA damage that may be required for the development of cancer. This concept underlines the potential importance of DNA-damaging chemicals not only at the initiation stage but also at later stages of the carcinogenic process. The carcinogenic process requires that cells acquire Hanahan and Weinberg's (2000) "6 hallmarks" of cancer: self-sufficiency in growth signals; insensitivity to growth inhibitory signals; evasion of apoptosis; limitless replicative potential; sustained angiogenesis; and potential for metastatic/tissue invasion. Acquisition of each of these properties may be driven by both genetic and epigenetic changes, and they relate to 5 overlapping models of carcinogenesis: mutational; genomic instability; nongenotoxic clonal expansion; cell selection; and microenvironment. Key to the focus of the current chapter is the recognition that exogenous chemicals may contribute to the genetic, epigenetic, and microenvironment alterations that are required for the acquisition of these features, and thus for tumor growth to proceed.

4.2.3 Genotoxic Carcinogens, Metabolic Activation, and DNA-Damaging Species

Chemicals can contribute to the initiation, promotion, and progression stages of the carcinogenic process either through their ability to damage DNA and produce somatic mutations in cells, or as a consequence of their ability to establish a cellular microenvironment that provides initiated cells with a growth advantage via metabolic changes, local vascular alterations, and/or the ability to evade apoptosis, terminal differentiation and contact inhibition. The distinction between genotoxic carcinogens as tumor initiators and nongenotoxic carcinogens as tumor promoters is now considered overly simplistic as DNA damage in key genes may occur—and for most cancers is likely required—also at later stages of tumor development.

Genotoxic carcinogens have a wide diversity of chemical structures (see Fig. 4–1) but they share the property of either being directly electrophilic (electron-seeking) or being capable of conversion to electrophiles. These reactive electrophiles interact with nucleophilic (electron-rich) groups on intracellular molecules such as DNA and proteins, forming either covalent adducts or oxidative damage. These types of damage to DNA, if not repaired before the next cycle of DNA replication, may lead to errors in replication and hence to fixation of the damage as nucleotide substitutions. If the reactive electrophile damages key cellular proteins the result may be cytotoxicity and necrotic cell death, which can eliminate cells that also have damaged DNA, but which may also trigger the development of an inflammatory microenvironment that promotes the proliferation of any surviving initiated cells (Sec. 4.2.7).

Some genotoxic carcinogens, including carbamic acids, nitrosamides, epoxides, lactones, imines, and mustards (see Fig. 4–1), are "direct-acting" because they are either already electrophilic or are spontaneously hydrolyzed into electrophiles. However, the majority of genotoxic carcinogens require enzymatic bioactivation to electrophilic or electrophile-generating metabolites in order to damage DNA. These reactions are catalyzed largely by drug-metabolizing enzymes whose normal physiological role is protective, converting lipophilic chemicals into water-soluble metabolites that can be more readily eliminated from the body via the urine or bile. Drug-metabolizing enzymes have evolved both multiplicity and catalytic promiscuity to ensure that most potentially harmful environmental chemicals will undergo biotransformation, inactivation, and elimination. Chemicals that are carcinogenic, however, are those whose structures lead to their inadvertent biotransformation into reactive electrophiles with the potential to damage DNA. Because biotransformation can produce many metabolites from a single chemical via multiple cooperating and competing pathways, the net effect of exposure to a carcinogen in a particular individual will depend on the balance of activating versus detoxifying pathways, which may, in turn, be influenced by both genetic variation and by environmental factors, such as chemically-mediated enzyme induction or inhibition.

Among the many classes of drug-metabolizing enzymes that have been implicated in metabolic activation of carcinogens, members of the cytochrome P450 (CYP) mixed-function monooxygenase superfamily have been studied most intensively. These Phase I enzymes catalyze the hydroxylation of carbon, nitrogen and sulfur atoms on chemical molecules to produce metabolites that are more polar and either stable and excreted, reactive (ie, epoxides, nitroso compounds), or possess structures that make them suitable substrates for further metabolism by Phase II conjugating enzymes (see below). Oxidative procarcinogen bioactivation may also be catalyzed by other non-CYP Phase I enzymes such as nicotinamide adenine dinucleotide phosphate (NAD(P)H) quinone oxidoreductase, aldo-keto reductase, and various peroxidases (Shimada, 2006).

Phase II conjugating enzymes such as the uridine diphosphate (UDP)-glucuronosyltransferases (UGTs), sulfotransferases (SULTs), arylamine N-acetyltransferases (NATs), and glutathione S-transferases (GSTs) can also produce either stable conjugated metabolites or unstable conjugates that spontaneously decompose to reactive electrophiles. The likelihood of either protection against, or enhancement of DNA-damaging potential by the activity of Phase I and Phase II enzymes depends on a combination of the structure of the particular chemical in question, the chemical reactivity of the metabolites produced, and the relative levels of expression of the various enzymes that may compete or collaborate in the activation and detoxification processes in a given tissue. For example, potential carcinogen-bioactivating oxidases such as CYP1A2 show liver-selective expression, while others, such as CYP1A1 and cyclooxygenase, are present at high levels in extrahepatic target tissues, such as the lung and bladder, respectively.

Three of the most extensively studied classes of chemical carcinogens that require metabolic activation are the PAHs, such as benzo[a]pyrene (B[a]P; Fig. 4–3), the aromatic amines, such as β-naphthylamine (βNF; Fig. 4–4), and the nitrosamines, such as diethylnitrosamine (DEN; Fig. 4–5). PAHs, aromatic amines, and nitrosamines together comprise a substantial fraction of the total number of chemicals that are either known or reasonably anticipated to be carcinogenic in humans according to the U.S. National Toxicology Program's (NTP) *12th Report on Carcinogens* (2011). Although many of the chemicals on the NTP list are reagents or by-products of industrial processes, others are present in foodstuffs or in the natural environment. Notable examples of these include aflatoxin B_1, a potent liver carcinogen produced by *Aspergillus* fungi that contaminate improperly stored grains and nuts, and heterocyclic amines such as 2-amino-3-methylimidazo[4,5-f] quinoline (IQ), that form from the reaction of amino acids with creatine during high-temperature cooking of meat (Fig. 4–1). The single-step metabolic activation pathway of aflatoxin B_1 is shown in Figure 4–6.

The pathways shown in Figures 4–3 to 4–6 illustrate the following principles of metabolic activation: (a) a central role is played by oxidative metabolism—often mediated by one or more CYP isozymes whose identities depend on the structure of the chemical—in initiating the activation process; (b) multiple enzymes may participate in producing the

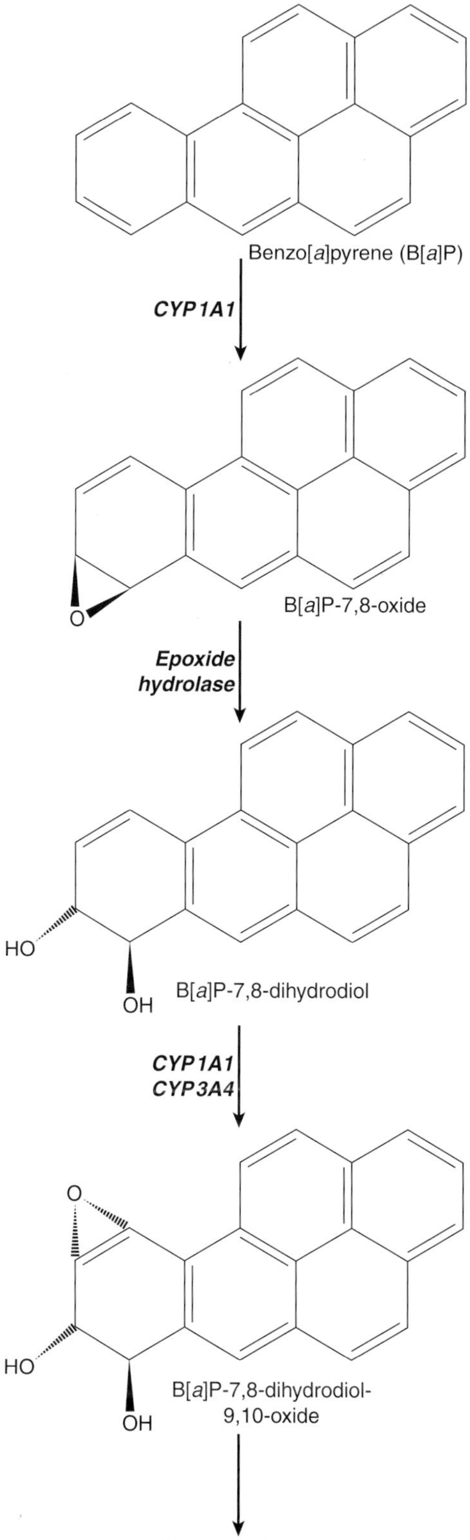

FIGURE 4–3 A proposed metabolic activation pathway for the polycyclic aromatic hydrocarbon Benzo[a]pyrene(B[a]P).

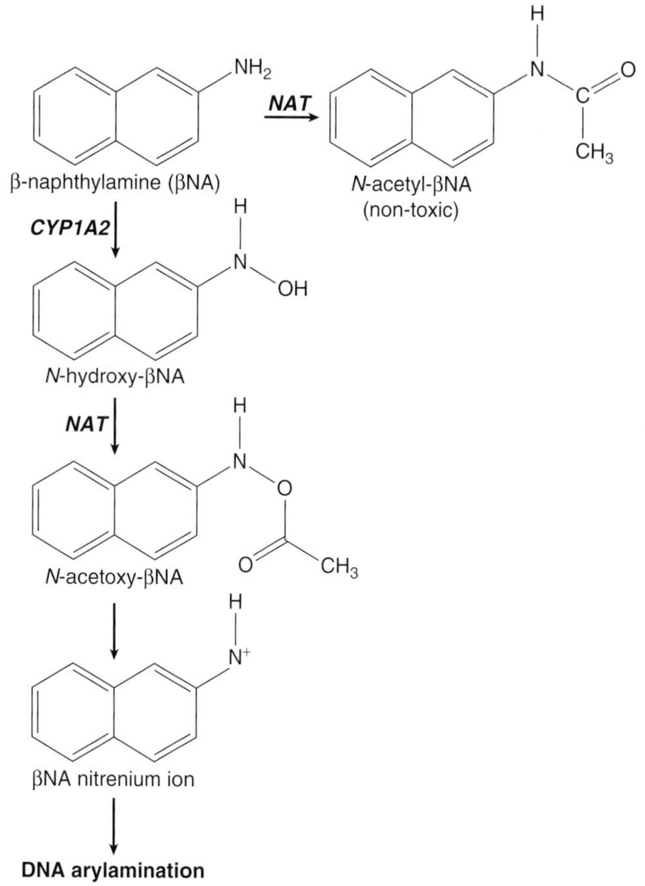

FIGURE 4–4 Proposed metabolic activation and detoxification pathways for the aromatic amine β-naphthylamine.

ultimate carcinogenic metabolite, either by acting sequentially on the chemical or by catalyzing the same reaction; and (c) the nonenzymatic, spontaneous chemical decomposition of unstable metabolites may contribute to activation. The pathways shown in Figures 4–3 to 4–6 represent only a subset of those that contribute to metabolic activation, and do not include many of the competing enzyme pathways that can produce stable, excretable metabolites and are thus protective. For example, although the initial step of βNA activation likely requires N-oxidation of its primary amino functional group into a hydroxylamine (Fig. 4–4), a competing reaction at the amino group is N-acetylation by NATs, which produces a stable and noncarcinogenic N-acetamide. This example also illustrates the potential duality of enzyme effects: the same NAT enzymes that may be protective by catalyzing N-acetylation on the parent molecule can participate in metabolic activation by catalyzing the O-acetylation of the hydroxylamine metabolite to the unstable acetoxy ester. Furthermore, O-conjugation of the hydroxylamine by either sulfotransferases or UDP-glucuronosyltransferases can also produce unstable oxy esters that ultimately generate the same nitrenium ion DNA-binding species.

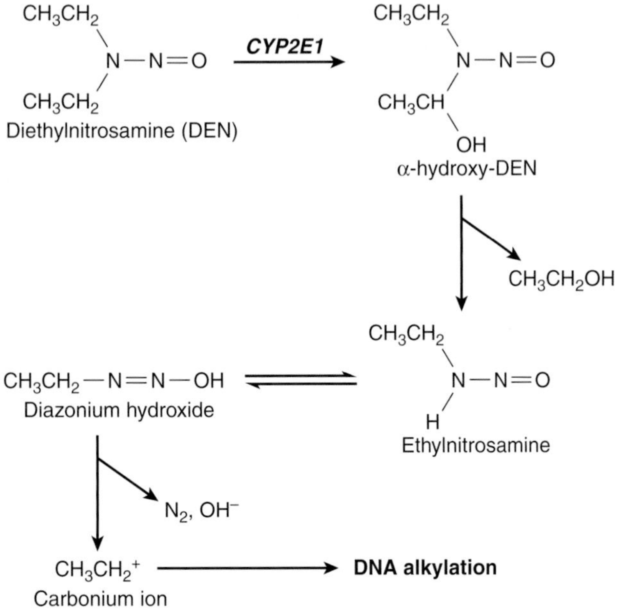

FIGURE 4–5 A proposed metabolic activation pathway for diethylnitrosamine.

The structures of the ultimate reactive electrophilic species that are produced by metabolic activation of carcinogens may vary widely. DNA damage may arise from the covalent interaction of its nucleotide bases with at least 11 different types of carbon, nitrogen and sulfur electrophiles on carcinogen molecules (Klaunig and Kamendulis, 2008). Of these, key examples are epoxides produced from the PAHs (see Fig. 4–3) and aflatoxin B$_1$ (see Fig. 4–6), nitrenium ions derived from aromatic amines (see Fig. 4–4), and carbonium ions derived from nitrosamines (see Fig. 4–5).

4.2.4 Nature and Consequences of DNA Damage

Different types of DNA-damaging chemicals tend to produce distinctive patterns of damage on the individual bases of DNA. In general, damage can consist of either a carcinogen adduct covalently bound to DNA, or of oxidative DNA damage. The site and type of adduct depends on the strength (charge) of the electrophile, the availability of nucleophilic sites (the unpaired O: and N: atoms) on DNA bases or the phosphodiester backbone, and the structure of the DNA relative to the size of the adduct. Strong electrophiles are capable of binding to a wide range of nucleophilic targets, whereas weaker electrophiles are only capable of binding to strong nucleophiles. Thus distinct chemical-selective patterns of nucleotide damage and the resulting mutations (see below) may be observed. However, it is likely that the persistence of particular adducts in particular genes is important in predicting carcinogenic risk, and the identification of these genes is important in monitoring DNA mutation profiles as biomarkers of either carcinogen exposure or cancer risk.

DNA may also be oxidized by hydroxylation of the nucleotide bases. Although there are a large number of possible oxidized forms of each of the 4 bases, 8-oxo-deoxyguanosine is one of the most prevalent, and it has been used extensively as a sensitive marker of overall oxidative DNA damage. Oxidative DNA damage can result from increased intracellular levels of reactive oxygen species, including hydrogen peroxide, hydroxyl radical, hydroperoxyl radical, and superoxide anions. These can be produced both by exogenous chemicals, often as a byproduct of CYP metabolism, and by endogenous processes. The latter include oxidative phosphorylation and inflammatory cell activation (Sec. 4.2.7).

Once DNA damage has occurred there are 2 possible cellular outcomes. Most probable is repair of the damage by DNA repair enzymes present in the cell, which have evolved to recognize a variety of types of DNA damage and replace damaged bases with intact ones (see Chap. 5, Sec. 5.2). If DNA repair has not taken place before the next cycle of DNA replication prior to cell division, 3 types of mutational events may take place: (a) error-prone replication resulting in a nucleotide substitution, whereby DNA polymerase incorporates the wrong complementary base (often adenine) in the nascent daughter strand opposite an adducted, apurinic, or apyrimidinic site; (b) frame-shift mutations (most commonly single-base deletions) that tend to occur when a carcinogen adduct is bound to a nucleotide base; and (c) DNA strand breaks resulting from either incomplete excision repair or alkylation and cleavage of the phosphodiester backbone.

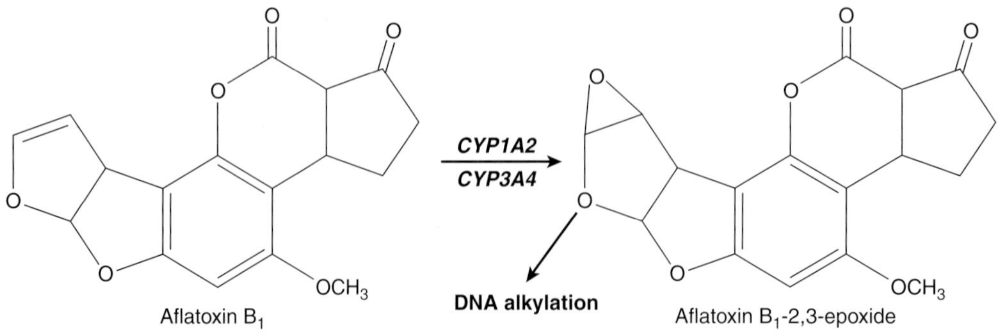

FIGURE 4–6 A proposed metabolic activation pathway for aflatoxin B$_1$.

Many of the relevant gene targets for mutagenesis by carcinogens include those classified as protooncogenes and tumor-suppressor genes, and mutations at specific sites in these genes have been detected in tumors. In general, when protooncogenes are activated by mutational events, signals for cell growth are increased, whereas for tumor-suppressor genes, which downregulate cell growth, loss of function abolishes this negative regulation (see Chap. 7). For example, in chemically induced rodent tumors, mutations commonly activate the *ras* family of oncogenes. Rat mammary tumors induced by exposure to nitrosomethylurea contain H-*ras* genes that have been activated by a single point mutation in codon 12 of the gene, while in mouse skin papillomas induced by 7,12-dimethylbenz[*a*]anthracene an activating mutation occurs in codon 61 of the same gene. The reasons for such DNA site selectivity are unclear, but they may include a combination of localized DNA accessibility in the context of chromatin packing, the nucleophilicity of particular bases within the exposed DNA region, the structure of the bioactivated chemical relative to the topography of the exposed DNA region, and the catalytic efficiencies (both substrate affinity and turnover rates) of DNA repair enzymes expressed within a given target tissue.

It has been estimated that mutations in the tumor-suppressor gene *p53* are present in more than 50% of human tumors. The sites of mutation are not random but occur at discrete hotspots (see Chap. 7, Sec. 7.6.1). Aside from the possible physical and biochemical mechanisms that may explain the occurrence of mutational hotspots, it is likely that selective growth and retention of function-altering mutations also occurs during tumor promotion and progression. Thus different carcinogens may leave distinct mutational signatures in *p53* and other genes. Lung tumors that develop in nonsmokers contain a different spectrum of *p53* mutations than those in smokers, while tumors in ex-smokers retain the smokers' pattern, indicating the persistence of molecular lesions that underlie the eventual manifestations of cancer (Hainaut and Pfeifer, 2001). Also, more than 50% of the liver tumors from aflatoxin B_1-exposed populations in Africa and China have a G-to-T transition at codon 249 of the *p53* gene, which is not present in tumors from patients with low aflatoxin B_1 exposure (Shen and Ong, 1996). This mutation produces an amino acid change from Arg to Ser that alters the binding properties of the p53 protein to a hepatitis B viral antigen and confers a subtle growth advantage to initiated cells. Thus the codon 249 mutation in *p53* is considered a molecular signature linking aflatoxin B_1 exposure to the eventual development of hepatocellular carcinoma by providing this selective growth advantage to cells rather than by an inherently greater frequency of its occurrence in DNA.

4.2.5 Exogenous Versus Endogenous Chemical Carcinogens

It is important to place the DNA damage produced by foreign electrophiles in the context of substantial damage that occurs within cells in the absence of exogenous chemical exposure. It has been estimated that more than 10,000 DNA-damaging events occur in every cell each day. This damage is produced not only by ambient ionizing radiation but also by reactive oxygen and nitrogen species and products of lipid peroxidation that are generated in the course of normal endogenous oxidative metabolism. Much of this high "background" damage may also be caused by continual exposure to low levels of the hundreds of natural and synthetic toxic chemicals and food constituents that enter the human body. The massive scale of this damage emphasizes the important role of cellular DNA repair pathways that ensure high efficiency, redundancy, and fidelity of repair for a broad range of DNA damage (see Chap. 5, Sec. 5.2). DNA damage that is detectable as a result of exposure to exogenous chemicals must be of sufficient magnitude to produce a signal above this high level of endogenous damage and very efficient repair. As discussed further in Section 4.3.2, this has important implications for the interpretation of dose–response relationships and thresholds for chemical exposure, as many tests for carcinogen potency make the assumption that cancer risk at low doses may be predicted by a linear extrapolation from experimental administration of high doses. Also, it is known that DNA damage may be necessary but not sufficient for tumor formation, and that additional tumor-promoting effects of chemicals on the cellular homeostasis and microenvironment of DNA-damaged cells contribute strongly to tumor formation (Secs. 4.2.6 and 4.2.7).

4.2.6 Chemicals as Modifiers of Cell Proliferation, Senescence and Death

Relative to normal cells, cancerous cells have impaired ability to control cell division, to age, and to undergo apoptotic (programmed) cell death. Thus any chemical agent that triggers or contributes to the impairment of these processes could promote progression to malignancy, tumor growth and metastasis, especially with chronic exposure. The nongenotoxic tumor promoters shown in Figure 4–2 are thought to function in this manner. TPA acts as a proinflammatory agent and inducer of oxidative stress to provide a microenvironment favoring the proliferation of initiated cells. TCDD appears to function by inhibiting the apoptosis of initiated cells (Schrenk et al., 2004). Phenobarbital influences both cellular proliferation and apoptosis by altering patterns of DNA methylation, thus modifying epigenetic control of gene expression (see Chap. 2, Sec. 2.3) in cancer cells (Phillips and Goodman, 2009). Chemicals may also promote the growth of initiated cells indirectly; for example, by producing acute cytotoxicity with resultant necrotic cell death in nearby cells that triggers the establishment of a chronic tumor-promoting inflammatory environment (Sec. 4.2.7).

4.2.7 Chemicals as Modulators of Inflammation

Epidemiological and experimental evidence supports the concept that inflammatory cells and the innate immune response (see Chap. 21, Sec. 21.2) may play pivotal roles in carcinogenesis by facilitating both tumor-initiating and tumor-promoting events. Some of the most consistently observed associations between chronic inflammation and risk of human cancer include those between colitis and colon cancer, gastric acid reflux and esophageal cancer, hepatitis B or C infection and liver cancer, papillomavirus infection and cervical and head and neck cancer, and schistosomiasis infection and urinary bladder cancer. Recognition of the key importance of inflammation in cancer is reflected in a recent suggestion by Hanahan and Weinberg that the 6 hallmarks of cancer described in Section 4.2.2 may now be supplemented with 2 emerging hallmarks—modified energy metabolism and immune escape—and 2 enabling mechanisms—genomic instability and inflammation (Hanahan and Weinberg 2011).

Acute inflammatory responses may be elicited by infections, metabolic stresses, generation of reactive oxygen species, hypoxia or tissue injury, which can act by producing necrotic or autophagic cell death as opposed to the generally noninflammatory apoptotic cell death. With the exception of infection, exogenous chemicals may trigger any of the events listed above. Contents released from dead cells, such as the chromatin-associated protein high mobility group box 1 (HMGB1) (Campana et al, 2008), can trigger the activation of nearby resident macrophages to release proinflammatory cytokines such as interleukin-6 (IL-6) and tumor necrosis factor alpha (TNF-α), as well as oxidant-generating enzymes such as nicotinamide adenine dinucleotide phosphate (NADPH) oxidase in a transient "respiratory burst" that produces high levels of free radicals and other reactive oxygen and nitrogen species. Although designed to quickly kill invading pathogens, the respiratory burst can damage the DNA, RNA, proteins and lipids of neighboring cells (Ohshima et al, 2003), and activate signal transduction pathways involving pro-inflammatory transcription factors such as nuclear factor-κB (NF-κB), which drives the expression of genes whose products can result in chronic inflammatory conditions (Karin and Greten, 2005).

Some chemicals may increase cancer risk by more than one mechanism, whereas others may play chemopreventive roles. For example, DEN (see Figs. 4–1 and 4–5) is a potent liver carcinogen that produces not only liver DNA damage in mice, but also an acute hepatic necrosis associated with increased levels of reactive oxygen species (ROS) and release of intracellular damage-associated molecular pattern molecules (DAMPs); the net effect is an elevation in proinflammatory IL-6 and TNF-α levels, subsequent activation of NF-κB, and a compensatory cellular proliferation that promotes tumor growth. This suggests that DEN can act as a "complete carcinogen" because it serves both tumor-initiating and tumor-promoting functions (Maeda et al, 2005; Naugler et al, 2007). In contrast, administration of the antioxidant butylated hydroxyanisole to DEN-treated mice reduces tumorigenicity by preventing the accumulation of ROS that can both damage DNA and activate *jun* kinase-mediated cellular proliferation pathways (see Chap. 12, Sec. 12.3.4). These examples illustrate that some chemicals may result in the occurrence of tumors by multiple mechanisms, whereas others may be chemoprotective, as discussed in the next section.

4.2.8 Cancer Chemoprevention

The largest cancer chemoprevention trials to date have employed hormonal agents against breast cancer, such as tamoxifen and raloxifene, as discussed in further detail in Chapter 20, Section 20.4.1. There is also great interest in blocking carcinogenesis by other pharmacological means, especially in high-risk groups. Because the process of carcinogenesis is complex and multistage, chemopreventive agents could act by many different mechanisms. However, any chemical worthy of consideration to prevent cancer must pose a very low health risk itself, because it would require long-term administration. Candidates for chemopreventive therapy fall into 2 main categories: (a) the general population; and (b) those who may be at elevated risk because of genetic predisposition or heightened levels of carcinogen exposure. Epidemiological studies show consistently that diets rich in fruits and vegetables, which contain high levels of antioxidants, reduce risk for cancers at many sites. Also, increasing evidence suggests that obesity resembles a chronic inflammatory state, which is known to be tumor-promoting (Longo and Fontana, 2010). Thus for the general population, the most logical chemoprevention strategy is to encourage a healthy lifestyle that includes exercise and caloric moderation to maintain a healthy body weight, and the intake of diets that are rich in fruits and vegetables. More specific chemical interventions are being investigated for individuals at higher risk, and these may be aimed either at preventing DNA damage or reducing the likelihood that DNA-damaged cells will proliferate to form a malignancy.

As described in Section 4.2.3, many procarcinogens are activated to their DNA-binding metabolites by isozymes of the CYP superfamily. Chemicals that inhibit particular CYPs and/or induce the Phase II conjugating enzymes that facilitate excretion of CYP-produced oxidized metabolites could reduce metabolic activation of carcinogens. There is support for this concept from the dietary associations between intake of fruits and vegetables containing enzyme inducers and cancer risk: in experimental animals certain chemicals found in cruciferous vegetables can reduce the metabolism and covalent binding of carcinogens to DNA and subsequent tumorigenesis (Srinivasan et al, 2008; Takemura et al, 2010).

Indiscriminate inhibition of CYP enzymes would not be a safe chemopreventive strategy because CYP enzymes constitute the major pathway for elimination of many potentially harmful chemicals, as well as therapeutically administered drugs. Moreover, the catalytic promiscuity of CYPs is such that even isoform-selective inhibition is likely to alter the disposition of many chemicals entering the body, including therapeutically useful drugs whose pharmacokinetics would be modified. Furthermore, a particular CYP isoform may play dual, competing roles in both carcinogen activation and carcinogen elimination that may not be apparent from in vitro investigations. For example, experimental evidence implicates the CYP isoform CYP1A2 as a key first step in the bioactivation of aromatic amines into DNA-binding electrophiles (see Fig. 4–4). This evidence includes cellular and molecular studies of CYP1A2-dependent production of reactive metabolites from aromatic amines such as the cigarette smoke component 4-aminobiphenyl, covalent DNA binding of these metabolites, production of DNA mutations, and transformation of cultured cells. However, in mice the absence of CYP1A2 (achieved by gene knockout) paradoxically does not protect against either DNA damage or the formation of liver tumors following 4-aminobiphenyl exposure. It is presumed that the protective effect resulting from CYP1A2's contribution to the efficient in vivo elimination of the chemical, hence reducing the overall exposure burden, outweighs its ability to produce DNA-damaging metabolites (Nebert et al, 2004).

A strategy of inducing expression of CYP enzymes so as to increase carcinogen elimination has similar challenges. High levels of Phase II drug-conjugating enzymes were thought to protect from chemical carcinogenesis. However, inhibition of a given Phase II enzyme may either be protective by preventing formation of an unstable metabolite (eg, acetylating, glucuronidating, and sulfonating enzymes can all produce very unstable oxyester metabolites of aromatic amines), or may be risk-enhancing if the enzyme's predominant function *in vivo* is to produce a stable and readily excretable metabolite.

Whether either Phase I or Phase II drug-metabolizing enzyme induction or inhibition is beneficial or harmful depends upon which chemical agent is the main threat. Unfortunately, exposure often occurs to mixtures of structurally unrelated chemicals (cigarette smoke contains several different PAHs, aromatic amines, and nitrosamines), and manipulations that protect from one class of carcinogen might increase the risk from another chemical class, or even between individual chemicals of the same class.

Chemicals that reduce either the levels of ROS, inflammatory mediators, or inflammation-inducing pathogens have the potential to protect against the development of tumors. For example, research is focusing on the identification of effective antioxidants, such as flavonoids, polyphenols, isothiocyanates and phytoalexins found in foods, that may reduce cellular oxidant burden and thus the levels of oxidative DNA and protein damage. Agents that inhibit inflammation, such as nonsteroidal antiinflammatory drugs that inhibit prostaglandin synthesis by blocking cyclooxygenase (COX) enzymes, have also been studied as potential cancer chemopreventive agents (Das et al, 2007; Lee et al, 2008). Although some randomized trials of selective COX-2 inhibitors have shown encouraging results, the possible cardiovascular side effects associated with large-scale use of these compounds limits their utility. Reducing the incidence of infection as a result of pathogens that cause chronic inflammatory conditions via immunization, such as papillomavirus vaccines for cervical cancer and hepatitis B/C virus vaccines for liver cancer, is effective in reducing cancer risk.

The relationships between exogenous chemicals and dietary/lifestyle factors to cancer risk and prevention are complex. For example, tumor production in rodents by potent genotoxic carcinogens such as aflatoxin B₁ may be drastically reduced, even after initiation has occurred, by dietary manipulations such as reducing the percentage or even the source (ie, animal vs. plant) of dietary protein. It is likely that lifestyle-based cancer prevention—comprised of a combination of exposure avoidance and dietary measures—promises greater potential for overall population impact than targeted, chemical-based chemoprevention.

4.3 ASSESSING RISK FROM CHEMICAL CARCINOGENS

Establishing that a chemical is a human carcinogen is a challenging and protracted process. Humans are exposed to chemicals in foods, medicines, and the environment, and there is a long latent period between exposure and tumor appearance. The most productive approach has involved astute clinical observation followed by carefully designed epidemiological and laboratory studies in vitro and in vivo. Reduction of risk first requires that the factors contributing to risk be identified. These factors may be external or they may be intrinsic to the population at risk. A systematic, stepwise approach is employed by regulatory agencies such as the Environmental Protection Agency (EPA) in the United States, which, in order to determine risk, attempts to integrate the multiple factors that interact in human carcinogenesis (Fig. 4–7). The assessment relies heavily on data from laboratory animals despite the numerous caveats that apply in any attempt to extrapolate data from animals to carcinogenesis in humans. The EPA's *2005 Guidelines for Cancer Risk Assessment* use the following set of criteria, based on an integrated assessment of all evidence, to categorize chemicals according to their risk: (a) carcinogenic to humans; (b) likely to be carcinogenic to humans; (c) suggestive evidence of carcinogenic potential; (d) inadequate information to assess carcinogenic potential; and (e) not likely to be carcinogenic in humans. A "mode of action framework" is applied to the analysis, which uses criteria that take into account the chemical's hypothesized mode of action and biological plausibility; identification of key events; the strength, specificity, and consistency of epidemiological associations; dose–response concordance and temporal relationship; consideration of other modes of action; support for the proposed mode of action in laboratory animals; relevance of the mode of action to humans; and population subgroups that may be particularly susceptible. Table 4–1 lists some of the methods that are used to determine the carcinogenicity of chemicals, which are described in further detail below.

4.3.1 Population Epidemiology of Chemical Carcinogens

Epidemiological observations provide the cornerstone for identifying cancer risk from chemicals (see Chap. 3, Sec. 3.5).

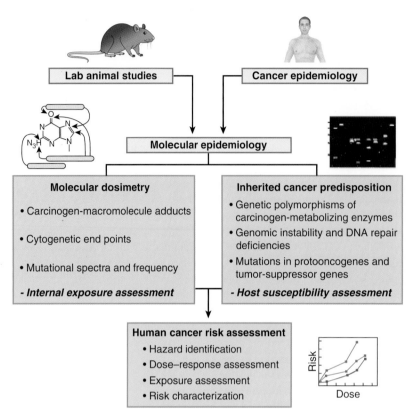

FIGURE 4–7 **Strategy for using multiple approaches to assess chemical carcinogens for their risk of causing human cancer.** (Adapted from Harris, 1993.)

Earliest observations were of associations between exposure to chemicals in industrial settings and the incidence of cancers at a variety of tissue sites. Some of these earlier observations led to drastic improvements in hygiene practices in the industrial workplace in the 20th century. The early associations were often striking because the exposure levels to particular chemicals were so high. Fortunately, such exposures and cancer clusters occur very rarely today, and it is much more challenging to establish unequivocally a causal association between cancer risk and exposure to chemicals at the low levels that occur in the environment or the cleaner workplace. Nonetheless, when evidence for a chemical–cancer association arises from epidemiological observations, it should prompt the conduct of dose–response and mechanistic studies using the experimental methods described below. These studies are then used to inform regulatory action designed to reduce exposure and risk where appropriate.

Even when epidemiological studies suggest that a particular chemical is carcinogenic, and it is shown to be DNA-damaging or mutagenic in laboratory animals or in vitro tests, several features of chemical carcinogens make it a challenge to establish unequivocally that a chemical does or does not cause cancer in humans. These are outlined in Table 4–2.

4.3.2 Animal Bioassays

Studies of carcinogenicity in rodents involve either the chronic repeated administration of high doses of a potential carcinogen, or the administration of the chemical at a particularly sensitive developmental stage. More recent developments include the use of genetically modified strains of mice that have been made more susceptible to carcinogens. Testing of putative carcinogens in animals is time-consuming, expensive,

TABLE 4–1 **Assays for carcinogens.**

Long-term assays
    Clinical observation and epidemiology
    Bioassays in laboratory animals, principally rodents

Short-term assays
    Detection of DNA damage
        Covalent adducts of the test compound with DNA after metabolic activation
        DNA strand breakage

    Detection of chromosomal damage
        Chromosomal abnormalities by cytogenetics
        Sister chromatid exchange
        Micronucleus frequency
        Sperm abnormalities

    Detection of mutational events
        Bacterial mutagenesis (Ames *Salmonella* assay, etc)
        Sex-linked mutations and reciprocal translocations in *Drosophila*
        Mutational spectra in transgenic mice

    Unscheduled DNA synthesis in cells in culture

    Neoplastic transformation of mammalian cells in culture

TABLE 4–2 Features of chemical carcinogens that cause difficulty in deciding that a chemical does or does not cause cancer in humans.

1. The time interval between exposure to a potential carcinogen and the clinical detection of a tumor may be 20 years or more in humans. This long latent period for many cancers makes it difficult to link current disease to exposures that may have occurred decades earlier.
2. The degree of cancer risk is driven by the level of carcinogen exposure, but it is often difficult to quantify the amount and type of exposure, especially when it may have occurred decades earlier. The use of biomarkers of exposure have limited utility as most have limited persistence after exposure ends.
3. Humans are exposed to a multitude of chemicals and other potentially carcinogenic agents (viruses, ionizing radiation, etc). These complex exposure patterns confound attempts to attribute the disease to a particular agent.
4. Individuals may vary widely from one another in their susceptibility to carcinogens as a result of genetic variation at key loci, such as those governing DNA repair capacity or pathways of carcinogen activation and detoxification.
5. Because of the generally low levels of exposure encountered today, the statistical power for detecting carcinogens is low unless the population studied is very large or unless there is a dramatic increase in tumor incidence at a particular site (see Chap. 3).

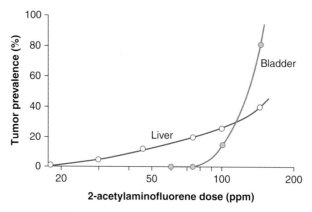

FIGURE 4–8 Dose–response curves for the production of liver and bladder tumors in female mice treated with 2-acetylaminofluorene. Tumors were observed after treatment for 18 to 33 months. *PPM*, Parts per million. (Data from Cohen and Ellwein, 1991.)

and requires relatively large numbers of animals to obtain valid results. Thus it is generally used to confirm results observed from short-term tests in bacteria or cell culture.

Studies in rodents are often criticized because they employ doses of suspected carcinogens that are far in excess of the probable human exposure. At high doses, acute cytotoxicity of the chemical (which would not be observed at lower doses) can cause necrosis, inflammation, and compensatory proliferation that contribute to tumor growth, and this might not occur at lower exposure levels. However, most chemicals that induce a high frequency of tumors at high doses will also induce some tumors at lower doses in studies using large numbers of animals. High doses are used for the practical reason of reducing the number of animals required, but such designs require the assumption that the dose–response relationship allows for valid extrapolation of risk from high doses to low doses. Most animal models can detect tumor incidence of approximately 5% but not as low as 1%, while in humans an increase in tumor incidence of 1% would be unacceptable.

The incidence of cancer in both rodents and humans caused by chemical agents generally increases with dose, but carcinogenic potency can differ between closely related compounds. Based on results from rodent studies, some generalizations concerning the quantitative relationship between exposure and response to carcinogens can be made:

1. A single exposure to some chemical carcinogens may be sufficient to induce tumors in a high proportion of animals. For example, a single dose of a polycyclic aromatic hydrocarbon can induce mammary carcinomas in more than 90% of female rats if the compound is administered as they are approaching sexual maturity. Similarly, 2 doses

of DEN or 4-aminobiphenyl can lead to a high frequency of liver tumors in mice if the doses are administered on days 8 and 15 after birth (the so-called neonatal carcinogenicity dosing protocol), when the liver is still actively proliferating.
2. Tumor production is often enhanced and the latency period reduced if chemical exposure is repeated. Mechanistically, repeated exposures may either enhance the likelihood that a required set of mutations in key genes has occurred, or it may produce prolonged changes in the microenvironment that promote the growth of initiated cells.
3. Tumor susceptibility varies widely among animal species and even between strains of the same species after exposure to the same dose of the same chemical. For example, rats are much more susceptible to aflatoxin B_1-induced liver tumors than mice, and hybrid offspring of inbred strains of mice (eg, the B6C3F1 offspring of a cross between C57BL/6 and C3H mice) are more susceptible to tumors than their inbred parents after exposure to many different chemicals.
4. Dose–response curves for carcinogenicity may vary in different tissues even within the same animals. For example, Figure 4–8 shows the results of a dose–response study of the aromatic amine-derived carcinogen 2-acetylaminofluorene. At lower doses liver tumors predominated, while at higher doses bladder tumors were more common, and the shapes of the dose–response curves in the 2 tissues differed markedly. The observed difference in tissue response is not related to differences in carcinogen pharmacokinetics, metabolism, or resultant DNA damage and mutation, but rather to increased rates of cell proliferation in bladder at higher doses of the chemical.
5. Not surprisingly, there is a very broad range of potencies among different chemical carcinogens. As shown in Figure 4–9, less than 1 µg/day of aflatoxin B_1 is sufficient

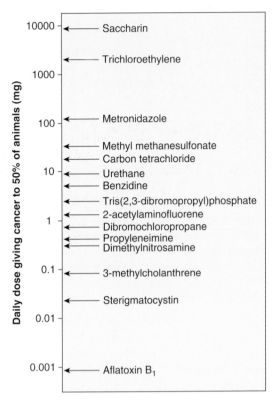

FIGURE 4–9   Range of carcinogenic potencies for various chemicals. (Data from Ames, as cited in Maugh, 1978.)

to produce tumors in 50% of rats after a lifetime of exposure, whereas compounds such as trichloroethylene or saccharin require more than 1 g/day to produce the same incidence of tumors. It is thus of key importance to relate tumor-producing doses of chemicals with the expected daily or lifetime exposures to the chemicals in humans.

4.3.3 Short-Term Assays

The main advantages of using in vitro assays to predict the carcinogenic activity of chemicals lies in the drastically shortened time to obtain results and reduced cost compared to animal testing. Table 4–1 lists several commonly used classes of short-term assays.

The covalent binding of carcinogenic chemicals to DNA may be measured directly using a variety of techniques. The simplest involves the measurement of covalently bound radioactivity following the in vitro incubation of purified DNA with radiolabeled carcinogen in the presence of an appropriate source of metabolic activating enzymes, such as subcellular fractions of liver. Another method that is more physiologically relevant, involves exposure of cultured cells or living animals to a carcinogen, isolation of DNA, radioactive postlabeling of the adducted DNA species, and their separation by silica gel chromatography. An advantage of this method is that it allows for the identification and quantification of multiple specific adducts, but a major drawback of both of the above methods is the requirement

for large quantities of potentially hazardous radioactivity. Technological advances now allow for DNA-carcinogen adducts to be detected and quantified, even in DNA isolated from humans exposed to carcinogens in the environment, using liquid chromatography coupled with mass spectrometry (see Chap. 2, Sec. 2.5). Finally, it is possible to raise antibodies that recognize particular DNA-adducted carcinogens, and these may be used in an immunoassay or with immunohistochemistry following exposure of animals or cultured cells to the carcinogen.

Other types of DNA damage may also be measured in short-term assays. Oxidative DNA damage following carcinogen exposure may be monitored by quantifying 8-oxo-deoxyguanosine as a marker of oxidative damage using either liquid chromatography or an immunoassay. The comet assay provides a general measure of overall DNA damage in individual cells using single-cell agarose gel electrophoresis of cell nuclei to visualize fragmented DNA (see Chap. 5, Table 5.2). Indirect methods for monitoring levels of DNA damage include immunoblotting and immunohistochemical assays for the phosphorylated form of the histone protein H2AX (γ-H2AX; see Chap. 5, Sec. 5.6), which is produced in the chromatin microenvironment surrounding DNA double-strand breaks, and an assay of unscheduled DNA synthesis, which is a marker for DNA repair occurring subsequent to carcinogen-induced DNA damage.

Various cytogenetic methods are also used for detecting gross chromosomal abnormalities caused by carcinogen exposure. These include breaks, terminal deletions, rearrangements and translocations; quantitation of damage-induced sister chromatid exchanges of differentially stained chromatids; and the frequency of micronuclei arising as a result of disruption of DNA distribution into nuclei during cell replication.

A potential drawback of many of the methods for detecting DNA damage is that they assume that DNA damage is correlated directly with DNA mutation—an assumption that does not take into account the importance of DNA repair. For this reason methods have evolved to measure the frequency of carcinogen-induced mutations in bacteria, mammalian cells, and whole animals. Perhaps the most widely used short-term mutagenesis assay is the Ames test (Fig. 4–10). It uses engineered strains of *Salmonella typhimurium* that have a mutation preventing them from synthesizing the amino acid histidine, thus they will grow only if histidine is added to the growth medium. Exposure of a culture of these bacteria to a mutagen can result in reversion of the mutation back to histidine-independent growth in a fraction of the cells, which can then grow on histidine-deficient agar plates. The number of revertant colonies that grow on these plates is a measure of the mutagenic potency of the test compound. Because most chemicals must be metabolically activated to be mutagenic or carcinogenic, these assays are usually conducted in the presence of a source of mammalian drug-metabolizing enzymes to generate the relevant reactive electrophile, or strains of *Salmonella* expressing particular recombinant human drug-metabolizing

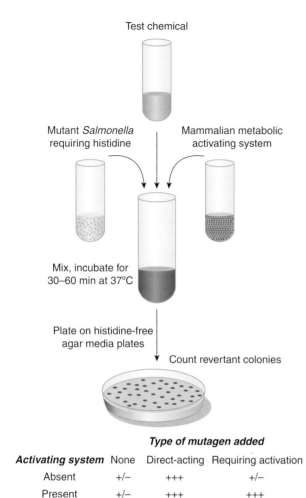

Type of mutagen added

Activating system	None	Direct-acting	Requiring activation
Absent	+/−	+++	+/−
Present	+/−	+++	+++

FIGURE 4–10 **Detection of mutagenic chemicals in** ***Salmonella typhimurium* (Ames test).** (Adapted from McCann, 1983.)

enzymes may be employed. An analogous method using mammalian splenic T cells monitors chemical-induced mutations in the endogenous hypoxanthine phosphoribosyltransferase (*hprt*) gene.

Transgenic animals carrying retrievable mutational target genes (eg, genes of viruses that infect bacteria—known as bacteriophages) have also been developed for in vivo testing of putative mutagens (Swiger et al, 1999). After in vivo exposure of the transgenic animal to a carcinogen and subsequent isolation of genomic DNA from a selected tissue, it is possible to retrieve the target transgene (such as the *cII* gene of a bacteriophage lambda) by in vitro packaging of the phage DNA contained in the mammalian host's genome. Bacteria are then exposed to such bacteriophages under conditions that select for growth of only those bacteria infected by viruses harboring mutated target transgenes. Thus the mutation frequency in the carcinogen-exposed animal is proportional to the number of bacteriophage plaques observed on bacterial lawns growing on agar plates. Although such systems can provide valuable predictive information regarding mutation potential and tissue specificity, the expense of the assay is such

that it is more commonly used following a primary screen in microorganisms.

The above assays that are used to detect potential carcinogens make the key assumption that rates of mutation are predictive of rates of tumor formation. Although most of the chemical agents that are carcinogenic in humans are also mutagenic in bacteria and cause cytogenetic changes in rodent bone marrow, a proportion of the chemicals that test positive in short-term assays or even in chronic rodent studies have not been shown to be carcinogenic in humans. Assessment of the carcinogenic potential of non-genotoxic carcinogens is even more challenging because there is no apparent common mechanism on which to base large-scale in vitro screening assays for chemicals that are not mutagenic.

4.3.4 Cellular Transformation Assays

Assays of malignant transformation in cell culture monitor the transformation of normal or immortalized cells into those that are capable of proliferating, independent of signals that would normally limit their growth, and that have tumor-forming potential. Although more time-consuming and expensive than the in vitro methods described above, these assays indicate whether cells exposed to a carcinogen exhibit an altered growth phenotype and can produce tumors when injected into recipient animals. Hence, cell transformation assays are probably the most relevant and predictive short-term tests for assessing risk of human cancer.

Conventional transformation assays may involve the plating of cells on soft agar plates and the counting of colonies that are able to grow after 3 to 4 weeks. Recent innovations allow assays to be performed in as little as 1 week with the use of microwell plates and intracellular dyes that permit automated colony counting using plate readers. One of the more widely used cell transformation assays is the Syrian hamster embryo (SHE) assay (Mauth et al, 2001), which counts the number of SHE cell colonies with an altered phenotype 7 to 8 days after carcinogen exposure based on distinctive morphological features such as cell piling, randomly oriented 3-dimensional growth, cell crisscrossing, and decreased cytoplasm/nucleus ratios. Advantages to this system are that SHE cells can be cryopreserved and that they maintain metabolic capabilities that eliminate the need for addition of an exogenous source of carcinogen-activating enzymes.

4.4 MOLECULAR EPIDEMIOLOGY OF CHEMICAL CARCINOGENESIS

Molecular epidemiology makes use of molecular markers that may relate quantitatively to either carcinogen exposure or to genetic markers of predisposition to cancer in human populations (see Fig. 4–7 and Chap. 3, Sec. 3.6). In estimating risk, molecular techniques allow for studies of human cancer incidence to be supplemented by surrogate markers and biological endpoints rather than only by cancer outcomes.

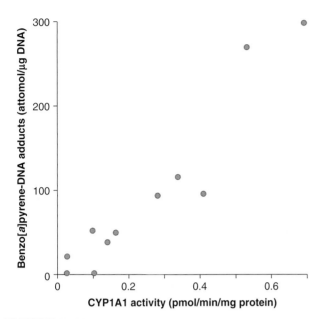

FIGURE 4–11 Correlation between cytochrome P450 isoform CYP1A1 activity and formation of benzo[a]pyrene DNA adducts in lung samples from human lung cancer patients.
(Adapted from Alexandrov et al, 1992.)

4.4.1 Biomarkers for Assessment of Carcinogen Exposure

The carcinogen dose received by individuals may be quantified by measuring biomarkers of exposure, such as carcinogen-DNA adduct levels or mutation frequencies in accessible cells. For example, Figure 4–11 illustrates a study showing that the level of B[a]P adducts in DNA samples from lungs of smokers was highly correlated with the activity of one of its key bioactivating enzymes, CYP1A1. CYP1A1 not only bioactivates B[a]P but its expression is also induced by it. In other studies induction of CYP1A1 has been correlated with the extent of exposure to cigarette smoke, which is a major source of B[a]P. Thus an increase in CYP1A1 activity may predict an increase in adduct formation and subsequent risk of lung cancer. Although this type of study is informative, it is limited by the requirement for lung biopsies to obtain tissue for analysis. In the Physicians Health Study, white blood cells were used as an easily accessible surrogate for lung tissue (Tang et al, 2001). It was found that current smokers who displayed elevated levels of carcinogen DNA adducts in their white blood cells were more likely to be diagnosed with lung cancer within 13 years than smokers who had lower adduct levels. Thus adduct levels in white blood cells of smokers appear to provide a predictive biomarker for risk of lung cancer.

4.4.2 Genetic Variation in Risk from Chemical Exposure

In populations where all members are exposed to the same carcinogens, some individuals develop cancer and others do not. For example, although cigarette smoking is a strong risk factor for lung cancer, some smokers develop lung cancer and a large number do not. One potential reason for this interindividual variation in risk for a given level of exposure is related to differences in the activities of the drug-metabolizing enzymes responsible for either detoxifying or activating procarcinogenic chemicals. Many epidemiological studies have provided evidence that genetic polymorphisms in drug-metabolizing enzymes may be associated (although usually weakly) with altered susceptibility to chemical carcinogens. For example, genetically based variations in the activity of arylamine N-acetyltransferase 2 (NAT2), which can play roles in either the detoxification or the metabolic activation of aromatic amines (see Fig. 4–4), are associated with altered risk for the occurrence of bladder cancer in populations that have been exposed to these agents (Hein et al, 2000). However, such associations are often inconsistent from study to study. For example, in one study individuals with an Ile462Val mutation in the PAH-metabolizing enzyme CYP1A1 were shown to have a 4.5-fold higher risk of lung cancer than those with the wild-type enzyme (San Jose et al, 2010), while other studies have shown no association between this variant and elevated risk of lung cancer. Such observations underline some of the challenges inherent in the conduct of epidemiological studies, particularly for genes related to risk of cancer that may be only weakly to moderately expressed.

In contrast, genetic variations in DNA repair enzymes are often associated with drastically increased predisposition to cancer. This is not surprising as cells repair a large amount of DNA damage on a daily basis. Thus any defect in the ability to repair DNA damage will result in the accumulation of mutations, and hence a greater probability that a cell will acquire mutations that drive its phenotype toward malignant growth. Examples of genetic defects in DNA repair that can significantly increase sensitivity to any DNA-damaging stimulus, including carcinogenic chemicals, include breast cancer (BRCA1/2), xeroderma pigmentosum (XP), Werner syndrome, ataxia-telangiectasis mutated (ATM), and Turcot syndrome (see also Chap. 5, Sec. 5.5). Each of these disorders has been studied extensively, and mutations in critical genes have been identified.

A major goal of molecular epidemiology is to identify individuals and populations who may have elevated cancer risk because of heritable predisposing factors so that preventive strategies can be implemented. In addition to mutations in DNA repair genes, mutation in other genes, such as the retinoblastoma gene, *Rb,* also confer a very high cancer risk in individuals who carry them (see Chap. 7, Sec. 7.6.4). However, such mutations are rare and thus do not constitute a major attributable risk to the population. A greater risk to the population may be caused by the common genetic traits that alter the balance of activation and detoxification of carcinogens. Particular combinations of polymorphisms can also act additively or synergistically to increase risk. For example, one study found no significant associations between risk for lung cancer and allelic variants in any of 10 postulated lung cancer susceptibility genes when considered individually, while a particular combination of 5 of these variants produced a highly significant 5.2-fold increase in overall risk, and an even higher 18-fold increased risk in females (Klinchid et al, 2009).

4.4.3 "Omics" Technologies and Molecular Signatures of Exposure and Risk

High throughput screening (see Chap. 2) can be used to study the structure and function of the genome (DNA sequences), the transcriptome (messenger ribonucleic acid [mRNA] expression levels), the proteome (proteins encoded by genes and transcripts), and the metabolome (small-molecule chemical fingerprints of intracellular processes) as they respond to toxic substances. The goal of such studies is to elucidate molecular mechanisms of toxicity and to derive molecular expression patterns that may better predict toxic events. Chemical carcinogenesis is particularly amenable to all of these approaches. Research has identified genomic signatures that associate with both risk for cancer (inherited alterations in DNA repair genes and carcinogen-metabolizing genes) as well as chemical-induced somatic mutations that are associated with tumor growth. Current research is studying the effects of exposures of experimental animals to genotoxic and nongenotoxic carcinogens on global gene expression profiles, protein expression patterns, epigenetic changes, and metabolic variables, and their consequences. For example, a recent study of the effect of chronic exposure of rats to the genotoxic carcinogen N-nitrosomorpholine demonstrated a concordance among altered gene, protein, and histopathological expression profiles for 8 candidate proteins in liver (Oberemm et al, 2009). Other proof-of-principle studies have compared the gene expression profiles of known genotoxic and nongenotoxic carcinogens to identify predictive multigene expression signatures for each class of chemical. Approaches to integrated systems biology that use computational modeling will be required to analyze the vast amount of data that can be generated by these techniques, and will ultimately contribute to enhancing our understanding of the complex impact of chemical carcinogens on the human genome and the cellular processes that it encodes.

SUMMARY

- Many chemical carcinogens form adducts with bases in DNA either directly or, more often, after metabolic activation.
- Cancers arise from multiple sequential unrepaired lesions that tend to accumulate at specific sites in oncogenes or tumor-suppressor genes that regulate cell cycle, proliferation, and cellular microenvironment.
- Genetic variation in the capacity to activate or detoxify carcinogens or to repair DNA damage also alters cancer risk.

- Many short-term methods to identify carcinogens rely on the assumption that most carcinogens are genotoxic, although this is now known to be overly simplistic.
- Nongenotoxic carcinogens may contribute to the provision of a selective growth advantage to DNA-damaged and initiated cells by a variety of mechanisms.
- Emerging toxicogenomic technologies allow for a better understanding of the mechanisms of contribution to cancer risk by both genotoxic and non-genotoxic chemicals.
- Based on knowledge of the mechanisms by which chemical carcinogens act, it may be possible to manipulate biochemical or cellular defense systems to reduce cancer risk, and clinical trials of chemoprevention have been completed or are underway, with mixed results.
- The most effective method to reduce the human cancer burden is likely to be through reduction of exposure to known carcinogens, especially to high-risk agents such as cigarette smoke, and by dietary and lifestyle interventions.

REFERENCES

Alexandrov K, Rohas M, Geneste O, et al. An improved fluorometric assay for dosimetry of benzo(*a*)pyrene diol-epoxide-DNA adducts in smokers' lung: comparisons with total bulky adducts and aryl hydrocarbon hydroxylase activity. *Cancer Res* 1992;52: 6248-6253.

Campana L, Bosurgi L, Rovere-Querini P. HMGB1: a two-headed signal regulating tumor progression and immunity. *Curr Opin Immunol* 2008;20:518-523.

Cohen SM, Ellwein LB. Genetic errors, cell proliferation, and carcinogenesis. *Cancer Res* 1991;51:6493-6505.

Das D, Arber N, Jankowski JA. Chemoprevention of colorectal cancer. *Digestion* 2007;76:51-67.

Environmental Protection Agency (U.S.) Guidelines for Carcinogen Risk Assessment, 2005. http://www.epa.gov/osa/mmoaframework/pdfs/CANCER-GUIDELINES-FINAL-3-25-05[1].pdf

Hainaut P, Pfeifer GP. Patterns of p53 G→ T transversions in lung cancers reflect the primary mutagenic signature of DNA-damage by tobacco smoke. *Carcinogenesis* 2001;22:367-374.

Hanahan D, Weinberg RA. The hallmarks of cancer. *Cell* 2000;100: 57-70.

Hanahan D, Weinberg RA. Hallmarks of cancer: the next generation. *Cell* 2011;144:646-674.

Harris CC. p53: at the crossroads of molecular carcinogenesis and risk assessment. *Science* 1993;262:1980-1981.

Hein DW, Doll MA, Fretland AJ, et al. Molecular genetics and epidemiology of the NAT1 and NAT2 acetylation polymorphisms. *Cancer Epidemiol Biomarkers Prev* 2000;9:29-42.

Karin M, Greten FR. NF-kappaB: linking inflammation and immunity to cancer development and progression. *Nat Rev Immunol* 2005;5:749-759.

Klaunig JE, Kamendulis LM. Chemical carcinogenesis. In: Klaassen CD, ed. *Casarett and Doull's Toxicology: The Basic Science of Poisons.* 7th ed. New York, NY: McGraw-Hill; 2008: 329-379.

Klinchid J, Chewaskulyoung B, Saeteng S, Lertprasertsuke N, Kasinrerk W, Cressey R. Effect of combined genetic polymorphisms on lung cancer risk in northern Thai women. *Cancer Genet Cytogenet* 2009;195:143-149.

Lee JM, Yanagawa J, Peebles KA, Sharma S, Mao JT, Dubinett SM. Inflammation in lung carcinogenesis: new targets for lung cancer chemoprevention and treatment. *Crit Rev Oncol Hematol* 2008;66: 208-217.

Longo VD Fontana L. Calorie restriction and cancer prevention: metabolic and molecular mechanisms. *Trends Pharmacol Sci* 2010;31:89-98.

Maeda S, Kamata H, Luo JL, Leffert H Karin M. IKKbeta couples hepatocyte death to cytokine-driven compensatory proliferation that promotes chemical hepatocarcinogenesis. *Cell* 2005;121: 977-990.

Maugh TH 2nd. Chemical carcinogens: how dangerous are low doses? *Science* 1978;202:37-41.

Mauth RJ, Gibson DP, Bunch RT, Custer L. The Syrian hamster embryo (SHE) cell transformation assay: review of the methods and results. *Toxicol Pathol* 2001;29 Suppl:138-146.

McCann J. In vitro testing for cancer-causing chemicals. *Hosp Pract* 1983;18(9):73-85.

Naugler WE, Sakurai T, Kim S, et al. Gender disparity in liver cancer due to sex differences in MyD88-dependent IL-6 production. *Science* 2007;317:121-124.

Nebert DW, Dalton TP, Okey AB, Gonzalez FJ. Role of aryl hydrocarbon receptor-mediated induction of the CYP1 enzymes in environmental toxicity and cancer. *J Biol Chem* 2004;279: 23847-23850.

Oberemm A, Ahr HJ, Bannasch P, et al. Toxicogenomic analysis of N-nitrosomorpholine induced changes in rat liver: comparison of genomic and proteomic responses and anchoring to histopathological parameters. *Toxicol Appl Pharmacol* 2009; 241:230-245.

Ohshima H, Tatemichi M, Sawa T. Chemical basis of inflammation-induced carcinogenesis. *Arch Biochem Biophys* 2003;417:3-11.

Phillips JM, Goodman JI. Multiple genes exhibit phenobarbital-induced constitutive active/androstane receptor-mediated DNA methylation changes during liver tumorigenesis and in liver tumors. *Toxicol Sci* 2009;108:273-289.

San Jose C, Cabanillas A, Benitez J, Carrillo JA, Jimenez M, Gervasini G. CYP1A1 gene polymorphisms increase lung cancer risk in a high-incidence region of Spain: a case control study. *BMC Cancer* 2010;10:463.

Schrenk D, Schmitz HJ, Bohnenberger S, Wagner B, Worner W. Tumor promoters as inhibitors of apoptosis in rat hepatocytes. *Toxicol Lett* 2004;149:43-50.

Shen HM, Ong CN. Mutations of the p53 tumor suppressor gene and ras oncogenes in aflatoxin hepatocarcinogenesis. *Mutat Res* 1996;366:23-44.

Shimada T. Xenobiotic-metabolizing enzymes involved in activation and detoxification of carcinogenic polycyclic aromatic hydrocarbons. *Drug Metab Pharmacokinet* 2006; 21:257-276.

Srinivasan P, Suchalatha S, Babu PV, et al. Chemopreventive and therapeutic modulation of green tea polyphenols on drug metabolizing enzymes in 4-nitroquinoline 1-oxide induced oral cancer. *Chem Biol Interact* 2008;172:224-234.

Swiger RR, Cosentino L, Shima N, Bielas JH, Cruz-Munoz W, Heddle JA. The cII locus in the MutaMouse system. *Environ Mol Mutagen* 1999;34:201-207.

Takemura H, Nagayoshi H, Matsuda T, et al. Inhibitory effects of chrysoeriol on DNA adduct formation with benzo[a]pyrene in MCF-7 breast cancer cells. *Toxicology* 2010;274:42-48.

Tang D, Phillips DH, Stampfer M, et al. Association between carcinogen-DNA adducts in white blood cells and lung cancer risk in the physicians health study. *Cancer Res* 2001; 61:6708-6712.

BIBLIOGRAPHY

Ames BN Gold LS. The causes and prevention of cancer: the role of environment. *Biotherapy* 1998;11:205-220.

Dipple A. DNA adducts of chemical carcinogens. *Carcinogenesis* 1995;16:437-441.

Gad SC. Carcinogenicity studies. In: Gad SC, ed. *Preclinical Development Handbook: Toxicology*. Hoboken, NJ: Wiley-Interscience; 2008:423-458.

Grivennikov SI, Greten FR, Karin M. Immunity, inflammation, and cancer. *Cell* 2010;140:883-899.

Guengerich FP. Forging the links between metabolism and carcinogenesis. *Mutat Res* 2001;488:195-209.

Hanahan D, Weinberg RA. The hallmarks of cancer. *Cell* 2000;100: 57-70.

Klaunig JE, Kamendulis LM. Chemical carcinogenesis. In: Klaassen CD, ed. *Casarett and Doull's Toxicology: The Basic Science of Poisons*. 7th ed. New York, NY: McGraw-Hill; 2008: 329-379.

Klaunig JE, Kamendulis LM, Xu Y. Epigenetic mechanisms of chemical carcinogenesis. *Hum Exp Toxicol* 2000;19:543-555.

Loeb LA, Harris CC. Advances in chemical carcinogenesis: a historical review and prospective. *Cancer Res* 2008;68:6863-6872.

National Toxicology Program, 12th Report on Carcinogens, 2011. http://ntp.niehs.nih.gov/?objectid=035E57E7-BDD9-2D9B-AFB9D1CADC8D09C1.

Nebert DW, Ingelman-Sundberg M, Daly AK. Genetic epidemiology of environmental toxicity and cancer susceptibility: human allelic polymorphisms in drug-metabolizing enzyme genes, their functional importance, and nomenclature issues. *Drug Metab Rev* 1999;31:467-487.

Okey AB, Harper PA. Chemical carcinogenesis. In: Kalant H, Grant DM, Mitchell J, eds. *Principles of Medical Pharmacology*, 7th ed. Toronto, Canada: Elsevier Canada; 2007:900-911.

Vineis P, Schatzkin A, Potter JD. Models of carcinogenesis: an overview. *Carcinogenesis* 2010;31:1703-1709.

Wogan GN, Hecht SS, Felton JS, Conney AH, Loeb LA. Environmental and chemical carcinogenesis. *Semin Cancer Biol* 2004;14:473-486.

Genomic Stability and DNA Repair

Shane M. Harding, Robert G. Bristow, and Lea Harrington

5.1 INTRODUCTION

There is overwhelming evidence that mutations can cause cancer. Major evidence for the genetic origin of cancer includes: (a) the observation of Ames (Ames et al, 1981) that many carcinogens are also mutagens, and (b), the finding that genetically determined traits associated with a deficiency in the enzymes necessary to repair lesions in DNA are associated with an increased risk of cancer. Mutations may occur in the germline of an individual and be represented in every cell in the body, or they may occur in a single somatic cell and be identified in a tumor following clonal proliferation. As described in Chapter 6, all species have numerous genes called *cellular oncogenes* (or *protooncogenes*), many of which are homologous to the transforming oncogenes carried by specific RNA retroviruses. Some human tumors have mutations in these oncogenes that may have led to their activation. However, there is no evidence for germline mutations in cellular oncogenes, perhaps because such mutations in the germline are lethal even in the heterozygous state. In contrast, there is good evidence for germline mutations affecting *tumor-suppressor genes*, which can lead to familial clustering of cancer or transmission of predisposition to tumors. In such cases, the loss-of-function of a tumor-suppressor gene is inherited in a mendelian manner.

The maintenance of genetic information is of paramount importance for prevention of genetic instability and accompanying carcinogenesis. In this chapter, intrinsic and extrinsic causes of genomic instability are discussed and the biochemical pathways that act to repair specific DNA lesions and the function of cell-cycle checkpoints following DNA damage are described. The methods used to evaluate DNA damage sensing and repair are detailed and human disorders that result in defective DNA damage sensing and repair are discussed. Finally, the importance of the appropriate maintenance of chromosomal length and telomerase activity is highlighted. Throughout the chapter, examples are given of the importance of each of these factors in the genesis, diagnosis, and treatment of human cancer.

5.2 GENETIC INSTABILITY AS THE BASIS FOR MALIGNANT TRANSFORMATION

5.2.1 Intrinsic Causes of Genetic Instability

Cellular carcinogenesis is known to require sequential mutations in DNA (see Chap. 4, Sec. 4.2.3). Damaged DNA is produced by a number of mechanisms, including (a) spontaneous reactions of DNA with the aqueous environment, (b) influence of metabolic byproducts such as reactive oxygen or nitrogen species, (c) action of environmental mutagens such as radon and chemical exposures, and (d) errors during DNA replication. Together these mechanisms can produce abasic sites, deamination, base alterations, single-strand DNA breaks and double-strand DNA breaks, which can amount to as many as 10^5 DNA lesions per cell per day (Ciccia and Elledge, 2010; Hoeijmakers, 2009). Unless the cell can protect and maintain the integrity of the genome, these genetic alterations may cause cancer by activating protooncogenes and/or inactivating tumor-suppressor genes. Natural mutation rates appear sufficient to drive the selection required for formation of many tumors (Bodmer et al, 2008). Some inactivating mutations occur in genes responsible for maintaining genomic integrity or DNA repair, which facilitate the development of a *mutator* cellular phenotype (Fig. 5–1; Loeb, 1991). Regardless of the

nature of the genotoxic insult, genomic instability is believed to be the main "enabler" of malignant transformation.

There are mechanisms other than mutation that lead to genetic instability, including *gene amplification,* and the epigenetic modification of chromatin-associated, transcriptional states through *gene methylation* and *gene acetylation* (see also Chap. 7, Sec. 7.4). In cells that display *gene amplification,* gene expression is aberrantly and constitutively enhanced above the level of physiologically normal levels. Gene-amplified cells can display discrete cytogenetic changes, such as *double-minute (DM) chromosomes* or *homogeneously staining regions (HSRs).* Cells may also acquire drug-resistance via mutation, gene amplification, or epigenetic changes (Otto et al, 1989; see Chap. 19). Consequently, the rate at which drug-resistant variants arise in a cell population is an indirect measure of genetic instability. Using specific markers of drug resistance, it has been observed that gene amplification occurs at a high frequency in transformed cells (10^{-3} to 10^{-7} events per cell

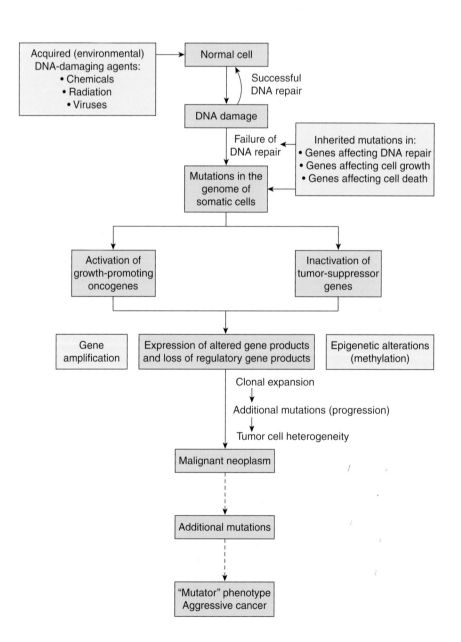

FIGURE 5–1   Genetic and epigenetic mechanisms of genetic instability.

per generation), yet is almost undetectable in normal diploid fibroblasts (a frequency of less than 10^{-8}; Tlsty, 1990).

If the amplified gene is a positive regulator of DNA replication or cell-cycle progression, gene overexpression may result in increased cellular proliferation leading to clonal selection and malignant transformation. Some amplified oncogenes, such as human epidermal growth receptor 2 (HER2) in breast cancer and the N-myc gene in neuroblastoma, are predictors of poor prognosis in those patients who harbor tumors containing them (see Chap. 7, Sec. 7.5 and Chap. 20, Sec. 20.3.3).

The structure and activity of chromatin can be altered by posttranslational modifications (eg, acetylation, phosphorylation, methylation, and ubiquitylation). *Methylation* of DNA is one of the main epigenetic modifications in humans and plays an important role in control of gene expression and normal cellular differentiation. It has been observed in more than half of the tumor-suppressor genes that cause familial cancers. In these tumors, there is methylation in normally unmethylated cytosine phosphate guanine (CpG) islands within the DNA. Methylation-induced transcriptional silencing begins early during the process of genetic instability and can affect many genes that are important in tumor progression. This includes methylation of genes involved in cell-cycle control (eg, p16^INK4a; see Chap. 9, Sec. 9.2), transcription, hormone biology (ie, estrogen and progesterone receptor genes; see Chap. 20, Sec. 20.2), intracellular signal transduction (see Chap. 8), apoptosis (see Chap. 9, Sec. 9.4), DNA repair and tumor-suppressor genes (eg, retinoblastoma [Rb]; see Chap. 7, Sec. 7.6.4). Given that methylation is a potentially reversible state, this creates a target for novel therapeutic strategies involving gene reactivation. For example, both retinoic acid and 5′-aza-deoxycytidine can reverse DNA methylation and reactivate gene expression of normal regulatory genes (eg, cyclin-dependent kinases), thereby leading to regression of some human leukemias.

Histones are the core protein components of chromatin and their acetylation status regulates, in part, gene expression. Two groups of enzymes, the histone deacetylases (HDACs) and the acetyl transferases, determine the level of histone acetylation. Deacetylated histones are generally tightly coiled with the DNA and are associated with silencing of gene expression; in contrast, the acetylation of histones leads to the uncoiling of chromatin and is generally associated with gene expression. HDAC inhibitors promote acetylation and are emerging as a new class of potential anticancer agents for the treatment of solid and hematological malignancies. Examples of these agents include short-chain fatty acids (sodium butyrate, valproic acid), hydroxyaminic acids (SAHA [suberoylanilide hydroxamic acid], Trichostatin A [TSA]), synthetic benzamide derivatives, and cyclic tetrapeptides (see Chap. 19, Sec. 19.2). Depending on the cell type, inhibition of HDACs in cancer cells can lead to transcriptional activation of approximately 2% of human genes, including tumor-suppressor genes. Treating cells with HDAC inhibitors increases cell-cycle arrest, induction of apoptosis, and differentiation in cancer cells, in vitro and in vivo, by promoting p21^WAF cdk-mediated cell cycle inhibition and downregulating proproliferative Raf/Mek/Erk cell signaling pathways (see Chap. 8, Sec. 8.2). Several HDAC

inhibitors have shown antitumor activity in vivo at nanomolar concentrations and are being evaluated in phase I-II clinical trials alone, or in combination with demethylating agents (Momparler, 2003).

Normal tissues may have different inherent abilities to maintain their genetic integrity when faced with similar exogenous or endogenous damaging stimuli. Comparison of primary stromal versus primary epithelial cell cultures suggests that normal epithelial cells may be predisposed to genetic instability. Stromal cells (eg, fibroblasts) eventually lose the ability to proliferate in culture (termed *cellular senescence*) as a result of loss of chromosomal telomere DNA (see Sec. 5.6). Other cell types, however, such as human mammary epithelial cultures (HMECs), exhibit genetic alterations caused by sequential loss of DNA repair and checkpoint control during cell proliferation that enable an increased number of population doublings; rare cells can then escape cellular senescence and become immortalized (Tlsty, 1990; Fig. 5–2). There are also

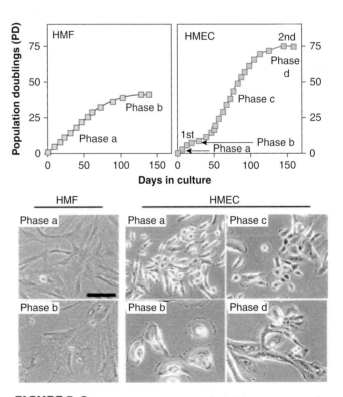

FIGURE 5–2 Genetic instability in epithelial tissues compared to stromal tissues. Data showing that human mammary fibroblasts (HMFs; left upper panel) undergo a limited number of cell divisions (phase a) before undergoing irreversible arrest, called *senescence* (phase b). In contrast, HMECs (upper right panel) exhibit an initial growth phase (phase a) that is followed by a transient growth plateau (termed *selection* or phase b), from which proliferative cells emerge to undergo further population doublings (phase c; approximately 20 to 70 doublings) before entering a second growth plateau (phase d). Seen in the panels below are representative cell images from each phase for each cell type. HMECs emerge from senescence, exhibit eroding telomeric sequences (see Sec. 5.6) and, ultimately, enter telomere-based crisis to generate the types of chromosomal abnormalities seen in the earliest lesions of breast cancer and point to differences between epithelial cells and fibroblasts during neoplastic transformation. (Data from Romanov et al, 2001.)

differences between stromal and epithelial cultures in their ability to initiate cell-cycle checkpoints following DNA damage. These and other observations may account for the higher incidence of epithelial-based compared to stromal-based tumors in humans. Importantly, recent studies have suggested that genetic stability is maintained in stem cells when compared to somatic cells, in part as a result of altered DNA repair pathways (Woodward and Bristow, 2009).

Multiple studies are attempting to document specific biomarkers of genetic instability in premalignant human tissues. This information can be used to ascertain whether an individual requires treatment with chemopreventive agents based on the biomarker panel, familial susceptibility, and carcinogenic insult. Tissue biomarkers can be related to mechanisms of DNA repair, cell-cycle checkpoint control, altered oncogenes or tumor-suppressor genes, or chromosomal aberrations. For example, biopsies have been obtained from tissues in high-risk patients (ie, bronchial biopsies from chronic smokers, oral or laryngeal biopsies from individuals with premalignancy) and examined for chromosome instability using in situ hybridization (Hittelman, 2001). Nearly all biopsy specimens show evidence for chromosome instability throughout the exposed tissue, often with multifocal clonal outgrowths that can persist for many years, perhaps accounting for continued risk of lung cancer following smoking cessation. Future investigations may lead to the discovery of new compounds that can reverse genetic instability in a given tissue, thereby preventing cancer.

5.2.2 Extrinsic Causes of Genetic Instability

In addition to reactions that occur spontaneously between DNA and the intercellular environment, many extracellular factors also place pressure on the genome. These extrinsic causes of genetic instability are produced by a myriad of sources including ultraviolet light (UV), ionizing radiation (IR), and chemical carcinogens (see Chap. 4).

5.2.2.1 Ultraviolet Radiation
There is a correlation between latitude (average sun exposure) and the incidence of malignant tumors of the skin, with the tumors tending to occur on sun-exposed areas, such as the face. Genetic background is also a determining factor, especially low skin pigmentation, as this contributes to an increase in the effective dose delivered to the cells at risk in the basal layer of the epidermis. Chronic exposure to sunlight is required for carcinogenesis, suggesting the need for multiple interactions of UV radiation with the target cells.

UV-induced tumors in mice demonstrate point mutations in the TP53 tumor-suppressor gene (see Chap. 7, Sec. 7.6.1) and these mutations are primarily C-to-T transitions (Kress et al, 1992). More than 50% of skin cancers in humans (both squamous and basal cell carcinomas) also have characteristic p53 mutations (Ziegler et al, 1993). Many of these mutations are CC-to-TT transitions and are characteristic of misrepair or lack of repair of pyrimidine dimers in the DNA induced

by the exposure to the UV radiation (Daya-Grosjean et al, 1995). Such dimers may be repaired by a number of processes, including nucleotide excision repair (see Sec. 5.3.3) and there is an increased risk of skin cancer in patients with xeroderma pigmentosum (XP), an inherited disease in which there is a deficiency in nucleotide excision repair (de Gruijl et al, 2001). The high incidence of p53 mutations found in preneoplastic lesions may cause genomic instability, which is consistent with the frequent loss of heterozygosity (LOH) seen in basal cell carcinoma (BCC; 9q) and squamous cell carcinoma (SCC; 3p, 9q, 13p, 17p, 17q), although LOH has also been observed in the absence of p53 mutations. The LOH at 9q also appears to be associated with deletion or mutation of the patched (PTCH) gene (see Chap. 8, Sec. 8.4.3) and 70% to 90% of BCC in XP patients have PTCH mutations (Daya-Grosjean and Sarasin, 2000). The PTCH gene is part of the Hedgehog (Hh) signaling pathway that can cause activation of the Gli transcription factors in human cells. One of the downstream targets of Gli is the Bcl2 gene, which acts to inhibit apoptosis (see Chap. 9, Sec. 9.4). Activation of this pathway may also override the G_1-arrest associated with the p21 (WAF1) gene (see Chap. 9, Sec. 9.3 and Sec. 5.4).

In familial cutaneous melanoma there are markers on 9p21 that map to the INK4a,b locus, which codes for the cyclin-dependent kinase inhibitors p16 and p15 (see Chap. 9, Sec. 9.2.2). This locus also codes for the p14[ARF] gene, which can stabilize p53 by binding to the HDM2 gene and interfering with degradation of p53 (see Chap. 7, Sec. 7.6.1). Loss of INK4a (p16) appears to be the most important defect in familial cutaneous melanoma, while, in sporadic disease, point mutations typical of UV irradiation can be observed in this gene. Additionally, up to 70% of melanomas exhibit BRAF mutations that are associated with UV-induced lesions (Besaratinia and Pfeifer, 2008). Thus skin cancers are clearly associated with UV damage to DNA (Cleaver and Crowley, 2002; de Gruijl et al, 2001).

5.2.2.2 Ionizing Radiation
The carcinogenic risks of radiation exposure have been derived from many sources, including occupational exposures (eg, radiologists and uranium miners), therapeutic exposures (eg, unavoidable treatment of normal tissues in cancer therapy, or treatment of ankylosing spondylitis), and accidental exposures (see Chap. 16, Sec. 16.8). Most information comes from studies of the A-bomb survivors in Hiroshima and Nagasaki, who were exposed in 1945, and from studies of exposures during medical x-ray examinations, particularly of pregnant women, which resulted in fetal exposure to irradiation. These groups of people were exposed to acute doses of radiation, and extrapolation of the risks from low levels of continuous exposure has relied on more limited information from occupational exposures and on experimental studies and modeling. Studies of radiation transformation in cultured cells point toward a high-frequency initial step followed by a rare second step (Little, 2000). The important initial effect of radiation appears to be the induction of genetic instability (Morgan et al, 2002; Syljuasen et al, 2001),

which then allows for a higher probability of "rare" mutations that lead to malignant transformation. The observations, that radiation tends to increase the incidence of the types of tumors that arise naturally in the population and that exposure at earlier ages leads to increased relative risk, are consistent with the concept that radiation acts to induce genetic instability.

The mechanism(s) by which genetic instability is induced by radiation and maintained in the population are uncertain, but probably include (a) mutations in genes involved in control of DNA synthesis or DNA repair, such as the mismatch repair system (see Sec. 5.3.1); (b) the induction of chromosome instability; and (c) persisting aberrant production of oxygen radicals that can damage DNA (Little, 2000; Morgan et al, 2002). Irradiated cells maintain a higher incidence of mutations and chromosome instability for many generations after the exposure both in vitro and in vivo (Morgan et al, 2002). These unstable cells may continually acquire further lesions such as point mutations, that may produce mutator phenotypes.

Hanahan and Weinberg (2010) proposed a model where the induction of genetic instability is a key driver of the subsequent mutagenic events that induce malignant transformation. Ionizing radiation induces deletions, translocations, or inversion of DNA sequences that may induce genetic instability secondary to DNA repair and cell-cycle checkpoint defects (Cox, 1994). Alternatively, chromosome breakage followed by faulty repair and translocation or amplification of DNA segments are also possible mechanisms for activation of genetic instability.

5.3 DNA REPAIR PATHWAYS

Recall that on the order of 10^5 DNA lesions are produced per cell per day (Sec. 5.2.1). Cells have evolved multiple mechanisms to detect and remove these lesions to prevent propagation to progenitor cells and, in the case of multicellular organisms, suppress tumorigenesis. An improved understanding of the mechanisms of DNA repair came from the isolation of repair-deficient rodent cells (ie, Chinese hamster ovary [CHO] mutants) with unusual sensitivity to different classes of DNA-damaging agents. Some mutants exhibited extreme sensitivity to UV light and crosslinking agents, such as mitomycin C, but little or no sensitivity to x-rays. Other cells exhibited sensitivity to x-rays and chemical agents known to cause DNA breakage, but little or no sensitivity to UV light or crosslinking agents. These various phenotypes, which are similar to those characterized previously in bacteria and yeast, indicate the involvement of several distinct DNA repair pathways and associated gene products. Some of these repair pathways are so highly conserved from yeast to humans that yeast proteins can substitute for human proteins and vice versa; this has been helpful in the cloning and functional characterization of the human homologs of yeast DNA repair genes.

Some frequent lesions, such as those formed by oxidation or DNA-reactive carcinogens, induce structurally distinct mutagenic and cytotoxic damage to the DNA (see Chap. 4, Sec. 4.3). Some of these adducts are recognized and repaired by a class of enzymes that are used only once. For example, induction of $O(6)$-methylguanine ($O(6)$-MeGua) by oxidation or N-nitroso compounds is recognized by $O(6)$-alkylguanine DNA *alkyltransferase,* which reverts the $O(6)$-MeGua back to guanine in a single-step irreversible reaction that inactivates the enzyme and prevents mutagenic G:C→A:T transitions.

An important property in DNA repair is the fidelity of the repair pathway leading to the concepts of error-prone, and error-resistant (or error-free), DNA repair. Many DNA lesions can block transcription of RNA, thereby inactivating the DNA damage-containing gene on the DNA strand that is being transcribed. Persistent blockage of RNA synthesis can lead to cell death so these lesions are often repaired through the *transcription-coupled repair* pathway (see Sec. 5.3.3 below); this pathway is designed to displace the stalled RNA polymerase and drive a high-priority repair mechanism. For lesions that block progression of the replication fork during DNA replication, several error-prone DNA polymerases have been described that have increased flexibility and low fidelity to allow for replicative bypass (ie, translesion DNA synthesis) of the base damage contained within DNA. These polymerases can be used temporarily by the cell during acute DNA replication damage and substituted by more accurate DNA polymerases at a later time. Use of these lower-fidelity bypass DNA polymerases can contribute to high error-rates during DNA replication and may lead to malignant transformation. This process is diagrammed in Figure 5–3 and is known as *translesion DNA synthesis.*

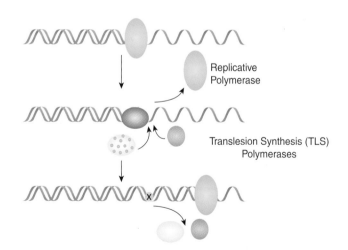

FIGURE 5–3 Translesion DNA synthesis. The "DNA polymerase switch model" for translesion synthesis and mutagenesis. This cartoon shows the replicative DNA polymerase (yellow sphere) blocked at a template lesion site. Cells contain several different DNA polymerases (other indicated spheres) that transiently replace the replicative DNA polymerase. After a short patch of synthesis in the vicinity of the lesion, the replicative DNA polymerase resumes high fidelity and processive synthesis. (Adapted from Cordonnier and Fuchs, 1999.)

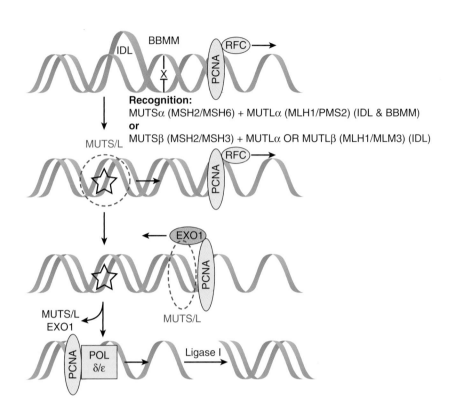

FIGURE 5–4 Mismatch repair (MMR).
The mismatch repair pathway is initiated
either when a base is misincorporated to
create a base–base mismatch (BBMM) or when
insertion–deletion loops (IDLs) are created
during replication in microsatellite regions.
These lesions are recognized by different
complexes: MSH2/MSH6 (MutSα) + MLH1/PMS2
(MutLα) recognize BBMMs and IDLs, whereas
MSH2/MSH3 (MutSβ) + MutLα or MLH1/MLH3
(MutLβ) can also recognize IDLs. Whichever
MutS/L complex is utilized, it translocates
along DNA until it reaches the proliferating cell
nuclear antigen (PCNA) associated with the
replication factor complex (RFC) at the site of
the replication fork. Next, the nuclease EXO1
is loaded and activated, which resects the fork
backward past the lesion, at which point MutS/L
and EXO1 are unloaded. The DNA polymerase δ
and ε(POL δ/ε) fills the gap and Ligase I seals the
nick if necessary. (Adapted from Jiricny, 2006.)

In the following sections, discrete biochemical pathways of
DNA repair are described. These pathways can be divided into
different classes depending on the specific DNA lesion they
are designed to repair, and include (a) mismatch repair, (b)
base excision repair, (c) nucleotide excision repair, (d) single-
strand break repair, and (e) homologous and nonhomologous
repair of DNA double-strand breaks.

5.3.1 Mismatch Repair

The mismatch repair (MMR) pathway is enacted when the
DNA-polymerase inserts an incorrect base during DNA replication or when the polymerase creates helical distortions by
inserting or deleting bases in short oligonucleotide repeats
(microsatellites) during replication. These helical distortions
are termed *insertion–deletion loops*. The protein products of
MMR genes form heterodimer complexes, and different protein pairs recognize specific mismatched nucleotides or inser-
tion-deletion loops in DNA (Fig. 5–4). For example, the MSH2
protein forms a heterodimer with an additional MMR protein, MSH6 or MSH3, and the resulting complexes are called
MutS-α or MutS-β, respectively. MUTS-α is required for the
recognition of DNA base–base mismatches, whereas MutS-α
and MutS-β have partially redundant functions for the recognition of DNA insertion–deletion loops. A second heterodimer forms between the MMR gene product MLH1 and PMS2
or MLH3 to form MutLα and MutLβ, respectively. The MutL
complexes coordinate the interplay between the initial mismatch recognition complex and subsequent protein interactions required to complete MMR. The latter proteins include
proliferating cell nuclear antigen (PCNA), DNA polymerases

δ and ε, and possibly DNA helicases that unwind the DNA
helix to facilitate DNA synthesis (Hoeijmakers, 2001). These
processes are diagrammed in Figure 5–4.

5.3.2 Base Excision Repair

Spontaneous oxidative damage is known to occur in cells
producing 10^4 to 10^5 oxidative residues, such as 8-oxo-
deoxyguanosine, per cell per day among the approximately
3×10^9 bases in the genome. DNA base damage, occurring as
a result of endogenous oxidative processes or exogenous DNA
damage (eg, from ionizing radiation) is repaired by the *base
excision repair pathway*. Base excision repair involves the enzymatic removal of the damaged DNA base by DNA glycosylases.
DNA glycosylases are a family of enzymes that cleave glyco-
sidic bonds and are specific to particular base lesions. There
are 2 classes of DNA glycosylases that differ in their reaction
mechanism: monofunctional enzymes leave the DNA strand
intact and bifunctional DNA glycosylases also cleave the
DNA backbone (Fig. 5–5). For example, the OGG_1 protein is
a bifunctional 8-oxoguanine DNA glycosylase that removes
spontaneous or ionizing radiation-induced lesions to prevent
cellular mutations. During base excision repair the initial base
removal step leaves an apurinic or apyrimidinic site that is
similar to single-strand DNA breaks. Such single-strand breaks
can be induced by free radicals or by ionizing radiation without
the action of DNA glycosylases, and repair of these 2 types of
lesions (base damage and single-strand breaks) converge into
this common pathway. Base excision repair and single-strand
break repair involve similar components and the processes are
shown in Figure 5–5. The major pathway is *short*-patch base

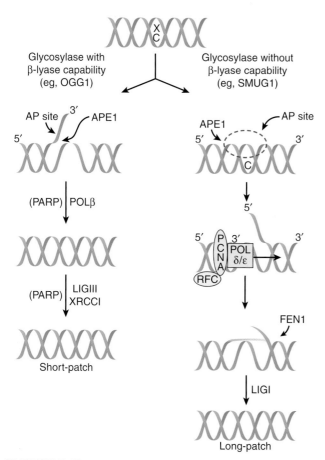

FIGURE 5–5 Mechanism of base excision repair (BER) and single-strand break repair (SSBR). Damaged bases are removed by the BER pathway and single-strand breaks are repaired by components of the same pathway. There are 2 subpathways, known as *short-* and *long-patch BER*, and pathway choice depends on the initial glycosylase enzyme that is required to recognize and remove the particular base lesion. When the enzyme includes β-lyase activity, the base is removed, leaving an apyrimidinic (AP)-site with a nick in the DNA backbone and a flap 3' to the removed base. The APE1 endonuclease removes this flap and the POLβ enzyme fills in the gap. Simultaneously the single-stranded DNA recruits the poly(ADP) ribose polymerase (PARP) enzyme that facilitates recruitment of ligase III and XRCC1 that seal the nick. Because only a single nucleotide is replaced, this is called *short-patch* BER. In the complementary long-patch BER pathway the recognition glycosylase does not contain β-lyase activity and leaves an AP site with an intact DNA backbone. The APE1 endonuclease catalyses the formation of a flap 5' to the removed base, and PCNA, POLδ/ε, and replication factor C (RFC) initiate synthesis and create a longer flap of 2 to 10 nucleotides. The FEN1 nuclease cleaves the overhang and the nick is sealed by ligase I. (Adapted from Sancar et al, 2004.)

knockout models for a variety of glycosylase genes have shown only mild increases in genetic mutations. This may be because of partial redundancy in the glycosylases and/or overlap with the transcription-coupled repair processes described below. However, base excision repair may be defective in cells that have mutations in p53 as the p53 protein can stimulate base excision repair by direct interactions with APE1 and DNA-Polβ (Offer et al, 2001). Indeed, the gene locus encoding the glycosylase 8-Oxoguanine glycosylase (OGG1) on chromosome 3p25-26 is frequently lost in lung cancers, consistent with a purported role in preventing carcinogenesis.

An exciting area of exploration is the clinical utility of poly(ADP)-ribose polymerase (PARP) inhibitors. As shown in Figure 5–5, PARP activity is required as an intermediate step preceding DNA synthesis during base excision repair or when single-stranded DNA regions are recognized. When PARP is inhibited by small molecule inhibitors, this causes the accumulation of single-stranded gaps that can cause collapse of replication forks during DNA replication. Under normal circumstances homologous recombination (see below) during DNA replication can rescue this and prevent double-strand break (DSB) formation. However, when homologous recombination is defective, such as in BRCA2-deficient breast cancers, these PARP inhibitors can lead to accumulation of DSBs and cell death (Helleday, 2010). This general concept of inhibiting compensatory pathways in tumor cells, while sparing normal tissues, is termed *synthetic lethality*, a common concept in yeast biology, and it has become an exciting area of research for novel cancer therapies (see Chap. 17, Sec. 17.3.2).

5.3.3 Nucleotide Excision Repair

In aqueous solution, DNA is susceptible to absorption of photons in the range of 200 to 300 nm, which increases reactivity of pyrimidine bases to produce 6-4 photoproducts (6-4PPs) and interstrand crosslinks in the form of cyclobutane pyrimidine dimers (CPDs; eg, thymine–thymine linkages). These lesions, and other bulky chemical adducts in DNA, are removed by nucleotide excision repair (NER), which is a complex DNA repair pathway involving more than 30 genes. Many of the NER genes were originally cloned from complementation analyses of cells from patients with XP and with cells from patients with Cockayne syndrome (CS), and are referred to as XPA-XPG or CSA or CSB in protein nomenclature. Patients with these syndromes have severe sensitivity to UV light and a much higher incidence of skin cancer (Fig. 5–6).

The process of NER is highly conserved in eukaryotes and consists of the following 4 steps: (a) recognition of the damaged DNA; (b) excision of an oligonucleotide of 24 to 32 residues containing the damaged DNA by dual incision of the damaged strand on each side of the lesion; (c) filling in of the resulting gap by DNA polymerase; and (d) ligation of the nick (Balajee and Bohr, 2000). In human cells, NER requires at least 6 core protein complexes for recognition of damage and dual incision (XPA, XPC-hHR23B (human homolog of RAD23B), RPA (replication protein A), TFIIH (transcription factor IIH),

excision repair and involves the replacement of a single nucleotide following DNA backbone cleavage at the base excision site. A minor pathway is the *long-patch* base excision-repair pathway, which exists for the repair of 2 to 13 damaged nucleotides.

No human disorders have been related directly to inherited deficiencies in base excision repair, and knockout mice engineered to lack core proteins in the pathway die as embryos, attesting to its important role in development. Genetic mouse

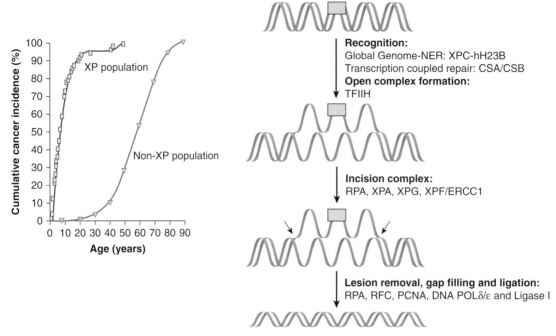

FIGURE 5–6 NER and XP. *Left:* Incidence of skin cancer in people with XP compared to the normal population with similar exposure to the sun. The 1000-fold excess risk of UV-induced skin cancer is secondary to defective repair of UV-induced DNA lesions in XP patients. *Right:* NER proceeds by initial recognition of the lesion by 1 of 2 different complexes, depending on whether "global genome"-nucleotide excision repair (GG-NER) or "transcription-coupled" repair (TCR) is used. In GG-NER helical distortions stimulate recognition by the xeroderma pigmentosum complementation group C (XPC)-hHR23B complex. Subsequently, XPA is recruited and transcription factor IIH (TFIIH) causes formation of an "open complex." The single-stranded regions of DNA are recognized by RPA. Two endonucleases, XPG and XPF/ERCC1, cut 3′ and 5′ to the lesion, respectively. The approximately 30-nucleotide gap is filled by POLδ/ε and the nick is sealed by ligase I. In TCR, the RNA polymerase II transcription machinery is thought to facilitate recognition of the lesion that, along with the CS proteins A and B (CSA/B), contribute to recognition of the lesion and induction of NER in a similar mechanism to GG-NER. The entire process of NER takes several minutes to complete.

XPG and ERCC1-XPF (excision repair cross complementation 1) and other factors for DNA synthesis and ligation to complete repair (PCNA, RFC [replication factor C], DNA polymerase δ or α, and DNA ligase I) (de Laat et al, 1999). The process of NER is diagrammed in Figure 5–6.

NER consists of 2 subpathways that differ in their mode of recognition of the helical distortions that the lesions produce. The first subpathway, termed *global genome repair* (GG-NER) is transcription-independent and surveys the entire genome for DNA lesions. The 6-4PPs, which distort the DNA more than CPDs, are removed rapidly, through recognition by the XPC-HH23B protein complex in GG-NER. In contrast, CPDs are repaired very slowly by GG-NER and are removed more efficiently from the transcribed strand of expressed genes by transcription-coupled repair (TCR). During TCR, the stalled RNA polymerase induces the recognition of the DNA lesions on the transcribed strand, and this process is facilitated by CSA and CSB proteins (Friedberg, 2001). The TCR and GG-NER pathways converge after this recognition step to form the open complex and removal of the damage as shown in Figure 5–6.

5.3.4 DNA Double-Strand Break Repair: Homologous Recombination

DSBs in DNA result from ionizing radiation and certain chemotherapeutic drugs, from endogenously generated reactive

oxygen species, and from mechanical stress on the chromosomes (Zhou et al, 1998). They can also be produced when DNA replication forks encounter DNA single-strand breaks, following defective replication of chromosome ends (ie, telomeres, see Sec. 5.6) or when topoisomerase enzymes are inhibited (eg, by etoposide) preventing the rejoining of the DSBs these enzymes induce. In addition, DNA DSBs are generated to initiate recombination between homologous chromosomes during meiosis and occur as intermediates during developmentally-regulated rearrangements, such as V(D) J recombination during the generation of immunoglobulins (see Chap. 21, Sec. 21.3.1).

In human cells, repair of DNA DSBs occurs either by *homologous recombination* (*HR;* Fig. 5–7) or *nonhomologous end-joining* (*NHEJ;* Fig. 5–8). The preferred pathway depends on tissue type, the extent of DNA damage, the cell-cycle phase in which the cell is damaged, and the relative need for repair fidelity. There may also be cooperation between the 2 pathways (Richardson and Jasin, 2000). Repair by HR requires homology between the broken DNA strand and the template strand used in repair. Typically, this is newly replicated sister chromatid and as a result HR is restricted to the S and G_2 cell-cycle phases (see Fig. 5–7). The HR pathway results in error-resistant repair of DNA DSBs because the intact undamaged template is used to pair new DNA bases between the damaged and undamaged strands during DNA synthesis.

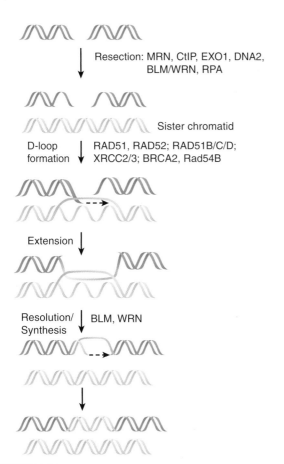

Resection: MRN, CtIP, EXO1, DNA2, BLM/WRN, RPA

Sister chromatid

D-loop formation   RAD51, RAD52; RAD51B/C/D; XRCC2/3; BRCA2, Rad54B

Extension

Resolution/ Synthesis   BLM, WRN

FIGURE 5–7 HR of DNA DSBs. HR is a major pathway for DSB repair and requires the presence of a sister chromatid. Here, single-stranded DNA overhangs are created and stabilized by nucleases (MRN [MRE11-RAD50-NBS1] complex, CtIP, EXOI, DNA2), helicases (BLM, WRN), and the single-strand DNA binding protein RPA. These RPA-coated overhangs are then exchanged to create RAD51-coated overhangs, a process facilitated by the RAD52 group of proteins (RAD52, RAD51B/C/D, XRCC2/3), BRCA2, and RAD54B, that also contributes to scanning for homologous DNA regions. This RAD51-filament can then invade the complementary DNA-duplex to form a D-loop. DNA polymerases then extend this invading strand and the corresponding strand on the opposite side of the DSB. (Adapted from Helleday et al, 2007.)

The HR pathway is highly conserved, likely owing to its ability to maintain the integrity of genetic information. Shown in Figure 5–7 is a general schematic of HR processes where a DSB is initially recognized by the MRN complex (MRE11-RAD50-NBS1). MRE11 possesses both single-stranded DNA (ssDNA) endonuclease and 3′ to 5′ exonuclease activities, which are enhanced by CtIP. Together with the 5′ to 3′ exonuclease EXO1 and endonuclease DNA2, these proteins collaborate with helicases (ie, BLM and WRN) to form resected ssDNA, which is rapidly coated with replication protein A (RPA). Exchange of RPA for the RAD51 protein is facilitated by the RAD52 epistasis group, XRCC2/3, BRCA1/2, and RAD54B, which also contributes to strand invasion of the sister chromatid forming a D-loop (Heyer et al, 2010; Svendsen and Harper, 2010). DNA synthesis extends the invading strand and the D-loop is

resolved by poorly understood mechanisms. There are actually several subpathways of HR that vary in their ability to prevent crossover of information from the strand acting as the template for DNA synthesis during the formation of so-called Holliday junctions (see Fig. 5–7; Helleday et al, 2007; Heyer et al, 2010).

The BRCA1/2 breast cancer-susceptibility proteins (see also Chap. 7, Sec. 7.6.3) also play a role in the homologous repair of DNA DSBs. Both BRCA1 and BRCA2 proteins form discrete nuclear foci during S-phase following exposure to DNA damaging agents at the sites of DNA damage. Although RAD51 colocalizes at subnuclear sites with BRCA1, their interaction is thought to be indirect, with only 1% to 5% of BRCA1 in somatic cells associating with RAD51 (Marmorstein et al, 1998). In contrast, the BRCA2 protein contains 8 BRC repeats, each of 30 to 40 residues, which are the major sites for the direct binding to RAD51 by a substantial fraction of the total intracellular pool of BRCA2 (Davies et al, 2001). As such, BRCA2-deficient cells have 10-fold lower levels of HR when compared to BRCA2-proficient cells (Moynahan et al, 2001). One model suggests that a BRCA2-RAD51 complex promotes the accurate assembly of DNA repair proteins required to offset DNA breaks that accumulate during DNA replication; these could otherwise lead to gross chromosomal rearrangements, LOH at tumor-suppressor gene loci, and carcinogenesis. In some instances, when a single-stranded gap is met by the replication machinery, a single DSB will be produced, which utilizes HR as a mechanism to restart replication forks if the delay is not prolonged.

Biochemical and genetic studies in yeast have been fundamental in the ability to clone human homologs of proteins involved in the HR pathway. In the yeast, *Saccharomyces cerevisiae*, the RAD52 group of genes are involved in HR including RAD50, RAD51, RAD52, RAD54B, RAD55, RAD57, RAD59, MRE11, and XRS2 (the latter retermed p95 or NBS1-nibrin in mammalian cells). RAD51[−/−] mice are embryonic lethal, attesting to the importance of this critical HR protein in meiosis and development. Careful observations during the initial stages of embryogenesis in RAD51[−/−] mice show that lethality is preceded by chromosomal rearrangements and deletions. It is thought that DNA replication errors and replication-associated DNA strand breaks are converted into DNA DSBs in HR-defective cells (Lim and Hasty, 1996). In cells derived from RAD54[−/−] mice (which are developmentally normal), there is also decreased HR and increased hypersensitivity to DNA crosslinking agents such as mitomycin C (Essers et al, 1997). Although in *S. cerevisiae* RAD52 is essential for DNA DSB repair, RAD52[−/−] mice are viable and fertile and do not show a DNA DSB repair deficiency. HR therefore appears to be more complex in mammalian cells than in yeast, possibly as a result of functional redundancy in many of the proteins.

A number of human cancers, including ovarian, breast, prostate, and pancreatic, have mutations or altered expression and function of the MRE11, RAD51/RAD52/RAD54, and BRCA1/2 genes. This observation suggests that tumorigenesis is associated with altered HR in sporadic tumors. Increased levels of RAD51 expression in certain cancer cell lines also has been associated with altered phosphorylation, ubiquitination and transcription of the RAD51 protein as a result of abnormal c-ABL– and STAT5-mediated tyrosine kinase signaling pathways in cancer cell lines (see Chap. 8). This can lead to acquired radioresistance and chemoresistance (Daboussi et al, 2002).

5.3.5 DNA Double-Strand Break Repair: Nonhomologous End-Joining

The NHEJ pathway is outlined in Figure 5–8. The recognition step of NHEJ is initiated by high-affinity binding of the KU70/80 heterodimer to the DNA ends, which causes a conformational change that recruits DNA-dependent protein-kinase catalytic subunit (DNA-PKcs). Autophosphorylation of DNA-PKcs at multiple sites is essential for NHEJ to occur and

appears to mediate DNA-PKcs dissociation from the break site (Dobbs et al, 2010). Many DNA DSBs have damaged ends that need to be processed to restore their ability to be ligated; for example, if 5'-phosphates are not present and/or 3'-phosphate groups need to be removed to create blunt ends. These structures are repaired by "end processors" that are partially dependent on the activity of the kinase mutated in ataxia telangiectasia (ATM [ataxia-telangiectasia mutated]) and include the Artemis protein, CtIP and MRN complexes, which are nucleases, PNKP which is both a 5' kinase and 3'-phosphatase and Polμ/λ. Once ends are restored the XRCC4-ligase IV complex, stimulated by XRCC4-like factor (XLF), rejoins the ends (Hiom, 2010). MMEJ and single-strand annealing (SSA), are minor subpathways of NHEJ that require end resection to reveal short (5 to 25) and longer (>30) homologous stretches of DNA, respectively (see Fig. 5–8). Although this pathway

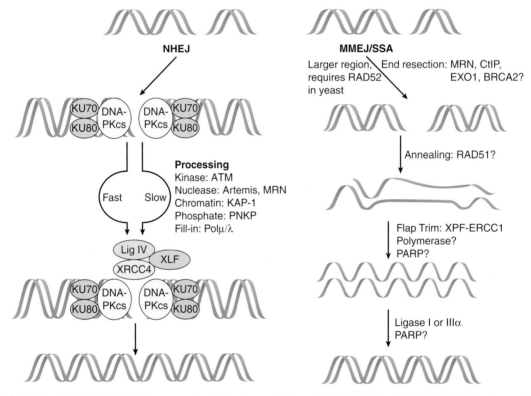

FIGURE 5–8 **NHEJ of DNA DSBs.** NHEJ is composed of subpathways that repair the DNA lesion. In the "fast" NHEJ pathway, the KU70/80 heterodimer recognizes the DNA ends and recruits the DNA-dependent protein-kinase catalytic subunit (DNA-PKcs), which autophosphorylates and forms the active DNA-PK complex. Downstream the ligase IV/XRCC4 dimer associates with the XLF/Cernuous proteins and joins the DNA ends together. In some cases, the DSB ends at the break are unligatable and require processing in the so-called slow NHEJ pathway. Repair of these ends depends at least in part on the ATM kinase and is processed by nucleases such as MRE11 or Artemis, kinases or phosphatases like PNKP, or filled in by Polμ/λ. Once competent for ligation, these ends follow the same XRCC4/ligase IV pathway above. Some lesions may require chromatin modification by KAP-1 for repair.

A less-well understood parallel pathway is microhomology-mediated end-joining (MMEJ)/single-strand annealing (SSA), which can be thought of as a hybrid pathway for DSB repair. The distinguishing features of MMEJ and SSA are poorly defined, but are differentiated primarily by the extent of the homologous regions involved and the requirement of RAD52 for SSA in yeast. The initial step includes end resection to expose homologous regions by nucleases, including MRE11, CtIP, EXO1, and BRCA2. The annealing of the homologous single-strand overhangs is facilitated by the RAD51 protein and the remaining flaps are trimmed by XPF-ERCC1. The involvement of polymerases and the PARP enzyme in this step is likely necessary but unknown. The nicks are sealed with ligase I or IIIα. Despite the disadvantage of its low fidelity, this pathway can act quickly, as required of an emergency mechanism, and, unlike HR, it does not depend on sister DNA molecules, which exist in the cells only after DNA replication. (Adapted from Dobbs et al, 2010; McVey and Lee, 2008.)

is much less understood, it is believed to contribute to deletions and chromosomal rearrangements that result in genomic instability (McVey and Lee, 2008).

The major protein complexes implicated in the NHEJ pathway are the DNA-dependent protein kinase (DNA-PK) complex and the XRCC4/ligase IV complex. Human DNA-PK consists of an approximately 460-kDa DNA-PK catalytic subunit (DNA-PKcs), and a DNA end-binding KU heterodimer (consisting of 70-kDa and 80-kDa protein subunits). The catalytic subunit shows homology to the phophatidylinositol-3 kinase (PI3K) superfamily at its C-terminus, which contains the protein kinase domain required for phosphorylating DNA-PK–associated proteins during repair. Mutations in either DNA-PKcs or in one of the KU genes result in sensitivity to ionizing radiation and reduced ability to repair radiation-induced DNA DSBs. XRCC4 forms a stable complex with DNA ligase IV and XLF, and probably links detection of the initial lesion by DNA-PK to the actual ligation reaction carried out by ligase IV (see Fig. 5–8) (Pang et al, 1997).

Much information regarding the cellular activity of the DNA-PK complex stems from research utilizing the severe combined immunodeficiency (SCID) model mouse, which has a complete lack of mature T and B cells and is radiosensitive. The DNA-PKcs protein in the SCID mouse is mutant and unstable because of a loss of the last 83 amino acids prior to the C-terminal kinase domain. Consequently, DNA-PK activity is severely reduced in tissues derived from this animal. Immunodeficiency is secondary to an inability to process and rejoin the broken DNA molecules produced endogenously during rearrangement of immunoglobulins and T-cell receptor loci (see Chap. 21, Sec. 21.3.1). These animals also show chromosomal instability in their normal cells and are susceptible to lymphoma, suggesting that these act as tumor-suppressor genes (Khanna and Jackson, 2001). Consistent with phenotypes observed in the animals, fibroblasts derived from DNA-PKcs, KU70 or KU80 deficient mice present delayed kinetics of DSB repair and overall lower DSB rejoining following ionizing radiation (see Chap. 15).

The RAD50–MRE11–NBS1 protein complex (termed MRN) acts in both HR and NHEJ pathways (see Figs. 5–7 and 5–8) and also in maintenance of telomeres (see Sec. 5.6). Mutations in the *NBS1* gene (also called the p95 or nibrin gene in humans) result in *Nijmegen breakage syndrome (NBS)*, a recessive disorder with some phenotypic similarities to ataxia telangiectasia (AT); (see Sec. 5.5), including chromosomal instability, radiosensitivity, and an increased incidence of lymphoid tumors (Featherstone and Jackson, 1998; Little, 1994). Mutations in human MRE11 have been linked to the *ataxia-telangiectasia–like disorder (ATLD)*. Cells from NBS, AT, and ATLD patients are hypersensitive to DSB-inducing agents and show radioresistant DNA synthesis (persistent DNA synthesis after irradiation that is not observed in normal cells) after exposure to ionizing radiation (Girard et al, 2000). Disruption of the mammalian RAD50 or MRE11 genes results in nonviable mice attesting to their importance in development. Biochemical studies of the yeast

and human protein complexes have shown that MRE11 has a 3' to 5' Mn^{2+}-dependent exonuclease activity on DNA substrates with blunt or 5' protruding ends and endonuclease activity on hairpin and single-stranded DNA substrates. This suggests that MRE11 may expose single-stranded regions on DNA DSB. This may promote the use of HR or may activate separate pathways related to NHEJ, called microhomology mediated end joining (MMEJ) and single-strand annealing (SSA) (see Fig. 5–8).

Although DNA DSB repair defects and increased radiosensitivity have been reported for a DNA-PKcs–deficient human glioblastoma tumor cell line, there are no human syndromes attributed to defects in DNA-PK protein function. The relative levels of DNA-PKcs protein are generally lower in rodent than in human tissues, and DNA-PKcs and KU80 protein expression varies widely among different tissue types. Evidence suggests that there is no simple relationship between tumor cell radiosensitivity and the absolute level of ATM or DNA-PK protein expression (Chan et al, 1998).

Unlike HR, NHEJ does not require homology and the NHEJ proteins simply link the ends of DNA breaks together; this usually results in the loss or gain of a few nucleotides during modification of the damaged DNA to produce ligatable ends (5'-phosphate and 3'-hydroxyl). NHEJ is therefore an error-prone pathway, but is operational throughout the cell cycle. There is evidence that RAD52 (a HR-related protein), and the KU70/80 heterodimer, a DNA end-binding protein that functions in NHEJ, compete for binding to DSBs and channel the repair of DSBs into HR or NHEJ respectively, depending on the cellular context (van Gent et al, 2001). The BRCA1 and 53BP1 proteins are also suggested to direct the choice of DNA repair pathway (Bouwman et al, 2010).

5.3.6 DNA Crosslink Repair: Fanconi Anemia Proteins

The Fanconi anemia pathway is a specialized pathway for the repair of interstrand crosslinks that can occur during S-phase. The importance of this pathway is highlighted by patients with predisposition to cancer and deficiencies in 1 of 13 Fanconi anemia complementation (FANC) proteins. In this pathway, unique FANC proteins coordinate a repair mechanism including components of translesion synthesis, HR and NER (Fig. 5–9). When a replication fork approaches an interstrand crosslink, the DNA is not able to form an open configuration for the passage of the polymerase. The FANCM protein initially recognizes the lesion, which recruits an FA-core complex and creates a large E3 ubiquitin ligase that catalyses the ubiquitylation of FANCD2 and FANCI proteins that subsequently localize to the damage site and coordinate downstream functions of nucleases (eg, FAN1), DNA polymerases, NER components, and BRCA1/2-mediated HR (Kee and D'Andrea, 2010). Together these mechanisms lead to the restart of the replication fork, thereby preventing cell death or genomic rearrangements (Moldovan and D'Andrea, 2009).

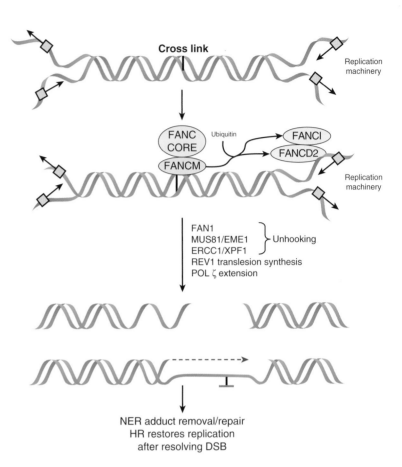

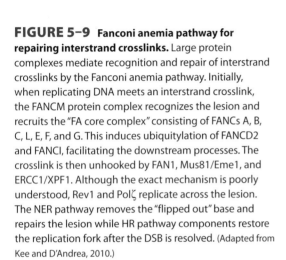

FIGURE 5–9 **Fanconi anemia pathway for repairing interstrand crosslinks.** Large protein complexes mediate recognition and repair of interstrand crosslinks by the Fanconi anemia pathway. Initially, when replicating DNA meets an interstrand crosslink, the FANCM protein complex recognizes the lesion and recruits the "FA core complex" consisting of FANCs A, B, C, L, E, F, and G. This induces ubiquitylation of FANCD2 and FANCI, facilitating the downstream processes. The crosslink is then unhooked by FAN1, Mus81/Eme1, and ERCC1/XPF1. Although the exact mechanism is poorly understood, Rev1 and Polζ replicate across the lesion. The NER pathway removes the "flipped out" base and repairs the lesion while HR pathway components restore the replication fork after the DSB is resolved. (Adapted from Kee and D'Andrea, 2010.)

5.4 DNA DAMAGE CHECKPOINTS AND DNA REPAIR

Mammalian cells have evolved complex interrelated responses to DNA damage that, as well as direct repair, induce cell-cycle checkpoints and apoptosis. Cells can halt cell-cycle progression in the G_1, S, and G_2 phases at cell-cycle checkpoints to ensure that they do not enter mitosis with damaged DNA (see Chap. 9, Sec. 9.3.1). These checkpoints are initiated by kinases and are followed by a cascade of molecular events that include posttranslational modification (ie, phosphorylation, ubiquitylation, and sumoylation) of proteins surrounding the break. There are 2 general types of cell-cycle checkpoints (Hoeijmakers, 2001; Kao et al, 2001): the mitotic spindle assembly checkpoint is responsible for ensuring that the mitotic spindle is correctly formed prior to division whereas the DNA-integrity checkpoints delay progression through the cell cycle in response to DNA damage or to defects in DNA replication (ie, G_1 to S, intra-S and G_2 to M; see also Chap. 9, Sec. 9.3) (Nelson and Kastan, 1994). Three related kinases, ATM, ATM-and RAD3-related (ATR) and DNA-PKcs, all sense DNA DSBs and function in DNA repair and also participate in blockade of the cell cycle (Perkins et al, 2002).

A concerted response to DNA DSBs includes the localization of a large number of proteins to the break site to concentrate kinase activity on substrates. Figure 5–10 outlines the DNA DSB-sensing pathways that lead to phosphorylation of downstream effector proteins. The ATM protein is held inactive in the cell as a dimer until DNA damage leads to

autophosphorylation of ATM monomers leading to its kinase activity, both of which are enhanced by the MRN complex (Bakkenist and Kastan, 2003). This activation of ATM (and simultaneous activity of DNA-PKcs) induces phosphorylation of the histone protein H2A.X at Serine-139 forming γH2AX (see Sec. 5.6), which serves as a platform for the assembly of other components, including MDC1. ATM phosphorylation of MDC1 triggers recruitment of the RNF8 E3-ubiquitin ligase, which cooperates with UBC13 to ubiquitylate H2AX and H2A histones (Huen et al, 2007; Kolas et al, 2007; Mailand et al, 2007). In turn, the RNF168-UBC13 ubiquitin ligase complex is recruited to extend ubiquitin chains (Doil et al, 2009; Stewart et al, 2009). These events are thought to modify chromatin in such a way that proteins, including 53BP1 and the RAP80-BRCA1 complex can associate along the break site. Furthermore, downstream effectors, such as p53 and CHK2, also localize to these sites, a process that appears to be mediated by protein–protein interactions of upstream components (Al-Hakim et al, 2010; Panier and Durocher, 2009). This model supposes that the local concentration of kinase activity and downstream effector proteins contributes to the initiation of cell-cycle checkpoints, and also facilitates repair mechanisms discussed above. Many of these proteins have been found to colocalize in a spatiotemporal manner at IR-induced nuclear foci as shown in Figure 5–11 for γH2AX and 53BP1.

As described above, some lesions stall replication forks during S-phase and expose ssDNA tracts. To protect them from degradation, RPA rapidly coats this DNA and leads to recruitment of ATR interacting protein (ATRIP) and ATR. ATR and

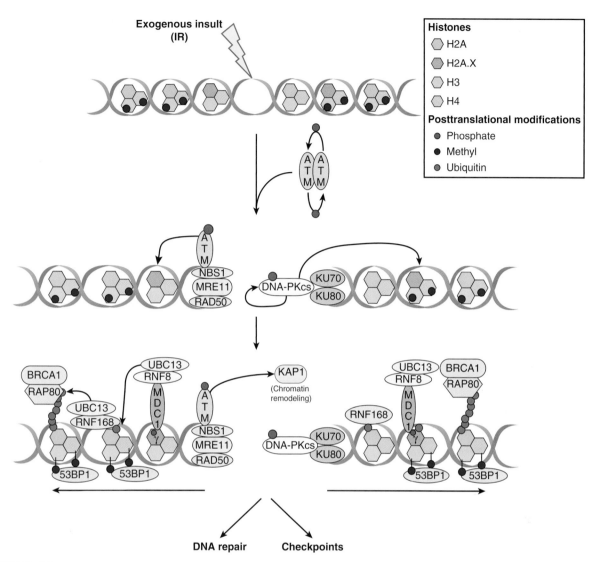

FIGURE 5–10 Signaling pathways in response to DNA DSBs induced by ionizing radiation. Signaling pathways that recognize DNA DSBs are multifaceted and likely include overlapping functions that serve to ensure checkpoints are activated even when some components do not respond properly. In addition to their role in checkpoints, these cascades also contribute to repair. When ionizing radiation (IR) creates DSBs, it leads to activation of the ATM kinase by autophosphorylation and dissociation into monomers from the inactive dimer; this process is facilitated by the MRN complex. Simultaneously, the DNA-PK complex (DNA-PKcs/KU70/KU80) (see Sec. 5.3.5) is activated, and together with ATM, phosphorylates the histone H2AX at serine-139 (forming γH2AX) in megabase domains spanning the break. This serves as a platform for the assembly of mediator of DNA damage checkpoint 1 (MDC1) which is also phosphorylated by ATM. This then recruits the E3 ubiquitin ligase RNF8, which, along with the E2-ubiquitin ligase, UBC13, ubiquitylates H2A and H2AX. This further recruits the RNF168 E3-ubiquitin ligase that, through poorly understood mechanisms, leads to the recruitment of RAP80/BRCA1 and the p53-binding protein 1 (53BP1). Multiple posttein–protein interactions, facilitated by "mediator" proteins (ie, MDC1, RNF8/168, 53BP1) surrounding the DSB are thought to concentrate the "effector" proteins (ie, p53, etc) in the vicinity of "sensor" proteins (ie, ATM, MRN) to facilitate the enactment of downstream processes, including DNA repair and checkpoints.

ATM are crosstalk partners and phosphorylate many of the same downstream substrates leading to cell-cycle checkpoints as described below and shown in Figure 5–12. Whether the DNA DSB response is mediated by ATM or ATR many of the same signaling cascades are activated to cause localization of downstream factors near the break (Bensimon et al, 2011). Importantly, the ATR-ATM pathways are likely not to be as distinct as once believed as recent evidence shows that ATR can activate ATM and vice-versa (Jazayeri et al, 2006; Stiff et al, 2006). Recent phosphoproteome experiments have shown that they share upwards of 700 protein targets, indicating that

these pathways are heavily intertwined (Matsuoka et al, 2007). These overlapping pathways increase the likelihood that sufficient checkpoint responses will take place.

The colocalization of ATM activity with effectors initiates a G_1-to-S cell-cycle checkpoint by a posttranslational stabilization of the p53 protein via direct phosphorylation of serine 15 on p53 (Canman et al, 1998). ATM also phosphorylates threonine residue 68 on the Chk2 protein, which can, in turn, phosphorylate p53. These phosphorylations lead to p53 nuclear accumulation by interfering with a nuclear export site contained within the amino terminus

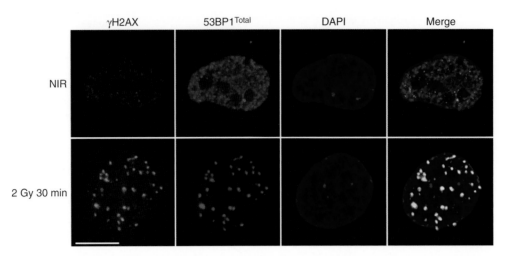

FIGURE 5–11   DNA damage-induced foci and the H2AX response. Confocal immunofluorescent images of normal human fibroblasts (GM05757) either untreated (nonirradiated [NIR]) or irradiated with 2 Gy and fixed at 30 minutes post-IR. Cells were stained for phosphorylated H2AX (γH2AX) and total 53BP1. IR induces γH2AX intranuclear foci whereas 53BP1 redistributes from a pan-nuclear nonnucleolar pattern into discrete foci that colocalize with γH2AX in the DAPI-stained nucleus (shown in blue) as shown by yellow coloration. Scale bar is 10 μm. Many DSB-responsive proteins form foci in this manner (eg, MRE11, ATM, MDC1).

of the p53 protein and by preventing degradation of p53 by MDM2 (see Chap. 7, Sec. 7.6.1; Liang and Clarke, 2001). Because p53 acts primarily as a transcription factor, current models regard its stabilization following DNA damage as a mechanism to activate the cyclin D/E-kinase complex inhibitor, p21^{WAF}, which leads to continual hypophosphorylation of the Rb protein to effect G$_1$ cell-cycle arrest. A second G$_1$ checkpoint pathway is also activated that targets the

FIGURE 5–12   Cell-cycle checkpoint activation downstream of ATM and ATR. Induction of DSBs by IR activates ATM, which phosphorylates MDM2 preventing p53 proteasomal degradation. ATM also activates, via phosphorylation, CHK2, which, in turn, phosphorylates CDC25A to inactivate its phosphatase activity and block CyclinE-CDK2-Rb–mediated S-phase entry. The stabilization of p53 is accompanied by ATM- and CHK2-phosphorylation which activate transcription of p53 target genes, such as p21. As a CDK inhibitor p21 blocks CyclinD-CDK4/5 and CyclinE-CDK2 and, therefore, S-phase entry. Activated ATM also phosphorylates SMC1 and NBS1 proteins that slow progression through S-phase by poorly defined mechanisms. DNA damage incurred during S-phase (by IR or UV) may create ssDNA. This ssDNA is coated by RPA recruiting ATR via its coactivator, ATRIP. Active ATR phosphorylates CHK1, which inactivates CDC25C. ATM activity and p53-induction of 14-3-3σ also inactivate CDC25C. Inactive CDC25C cannot remove inhibitory phosphate groups on CDK1 and therefore blocks CyclinB-mediated transition to mitosis. Crosstalk between ATM and ATR leads to simultaneous activation of many of these pathways, as described in the text.

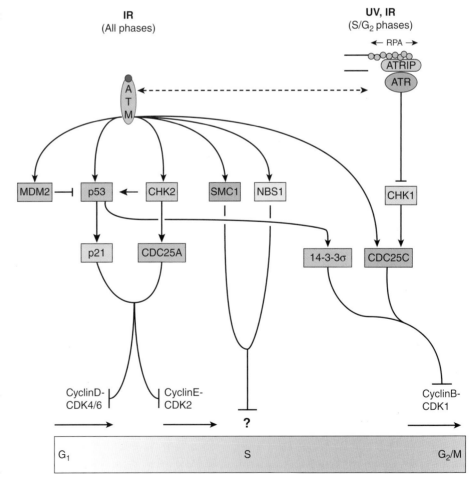

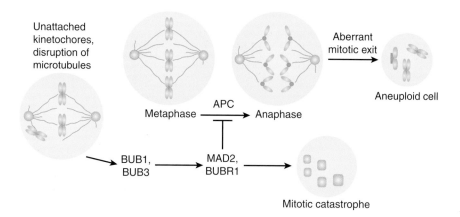

FIGURE 5–13 **Improper chromosome alignment on the mitotic spindle can activate the spindle checkpoint mediated by the BUB1, BUB3, BUBR1, and MAD2 proteins that localize to kinetochores.** An intact spindle checkpoint induces metaphase arrest through inhibition of the APC. Defective spindle-checkpoint function results from either loss of BUB1- and BUB3-dependent signaling or abrogation of MAD2, BUBR1-mediated inhibition of the APC. This leads to the absence of a functional mitotic spindle checkpoint generating aneuploid cells. (Adapted from Stewart et al, 2003.)

CDC25A phosphatase that is essential for G_1/S transition (Falck et al, 2001).

Further important targets of ATM-mediated phosphorylation are the BRCA1, NBS1, and FANCD2 proteins, which initiate both DNA repair and an S-phase DNA damage checkpoint (Cortez et al, 1999; Gatei et al, 2000; Lim et al, 2000). The ATM-mediated phosphorylation of NBS1 seems to be required for proper execution of an S-phase checkpoint as mutations in the ATM-associated serine residues (ie, Ser278, -343, or -397) of NBS1 leads to radioresistant DNA synthesis, a phenotype associated with AT cells.

Following their activation by ATM and ATR, CHK1 and CHK2 phosphorylate a conserved site (Ser216) on protein phosphatase CDC25C, which results in it being inactivated and bound by the 14-3-3σ protein. The inactive CDC25C is then incapable of removing an inhibitory phosphate group on Tyr-15 of CDC2, preventing entry into mitosis. In addition, p53-dependent transcriptional repression of the CDC2 and cyclin B promoters may contribute to the maintenance of the G_2/M checkpoint in mammalian cells, which may allow for repair of chromosomal or chromatid damage prior to cellular division. The elegant crosstalk between ATM and ATR and factors involved in DNA repair, DNA damage signaling and cell-cycle control act to maintain genomic stability and inhibit carcinogenesis (see Fig. 5–12).

Chromosome segregation is crucial for cells to maintain the integrity of their genome (Jasin, 2000). Mitotic exit occurs after ubiquitination and proteolytic degradation of cyclin B by the anaphase promoting complex (APC), which inactivates CDK1. The *mitotic spindle checkpoint* monitors the interaction between chromosomes and microtubules at highly specialized chromosomal regions called *kinetochores* (Musacchio and Hardwick, 2002). This checkpoint delays chromosome segregation during anaphase to correct any defects in the mitotic spindle apparatus; if defects persist, the cell undergoes cell death. The kinetochore-associated MAD2, BUBR1, BUB1, and BUB3 proteins are critical constituents of the spindle-checkpoint pathway: MAD2 and BUBR1 regulate mitotic progression by direct interaction and inhibition of the APC machinery and BUB1 and BUB3 also mediate mitotic arrest after disruption of microtubules as shown in Figure 5–13. Cells that lack either BUB1 or BUB3 do not undergo mitotic

arrest when treated with spindle-disrupting agents, such as the chemotherapy drugs docetaxel or vinblastine.

Genetic defects in the spindle checkpoint can lead to chromosome loss during mitosis and meiosis with links to the pathogenesis of several human tumors. For example, in human colon and breast carcinoma cells, BUB1 mutations have been identified that facilitate the transformation of cells that lack BRCA2. In other studies, MAD2 haploinsufficiency significantly elevated the rate of lung tumor development in MAD2$^{+/-}$ mice compared with age-matched controls (Stewart et al, 2003). There is potential for therapeutic intervention in cancer treatment by abrogation of cell cycle checkpoints using agents targeted at particular kinases (ie, UCN-01 for CHK1) in cells that already lack other checkpoints (ie, p53 mediated). This results in catastrophic mitotic death as a result of cell progressing into mitosis with unrepaired DNA DSBs (Lapenna and Giordano, 2009).

5.5 HUMAN DNA REPAIR DISORDERS AND FAMILIAL CANCERS

As discussed above, repair of DNA plays an important role in determining cancer predisposition. Functional analyses of DNA repair proteins and their pathways in vivo have benefited from molecular recombinant technologies whereby a specific DNA repair gene is either aberrantly expressed or rendered null (ie, gene knockout) in murine embryonic stem cells (see Chap. 2, Sec. 2.4.5). Some, but not all, DNA repair proteins are required for mammalian development as a number of the mice were embryonic lethal (ie, mice null for Rad51 and Rad50). Furthermore, repair-deficient mice are also prone to chromosomal instability and to the early onset of specific cancers (Hakem, 2008).

Several human disease syndromes are associated with pronounced cellular sensitivity to DNA-damaging agents because of hereditary deficiencies in DNA repair or in signaling pathways that are activated by DNA damage (Table 5–1). People with several of these syndromes show marked chromosomal instability and predisposition to malignancy, highlighting the importance of genetic maintenance for prevention of carcinogenesis. Some of these disorders are discussed below.

TABLE 5–1 Cancer prone human syndromes with defective DNA repair.

Syndrome	Affected Repair Pathway	Defective Protein	Main Type of Genomic Defect	Major Cancer Predisposition
Xeroderma pigmentosum (XP)	Nucleotide excision repair	XP CS	Point mutations	UV-induced skin cancer
Ataxia telangiectasia (AT)	DNA DSB response	ATM	Chromosome aberrations	Lymphomas
AT-like disorder (ATLD)	DNA DSB response	MRE11	Chromosome aberrations	Lymphomas
Nijmegen breakage syndrome (NBS)	DNA DSB response	NBS1	Chromosome aberrations	Lymphomas
BRCA1/BRCA2	Homologous recombination	BRCA1 BRCA2	Chromosome aberrations	Breast (ovarian) cancer
Werner syndrome	Homologous recombination	WRN helicase	Chromosome aberrations	Various cancers
Bloom syndrome	Homologous recombination	BLM helicase	Chromosome aberrations— sister-chromatid exchange	Leukemia, lymphoma, others
Hereditary nonpolyposis colorectal cancer (HNPCC)	Mismatch repair	MLH1 MSH2	Microsatellite instability	Colorectal cancer
Fanconi anemia	DNA crosslink repair	FANC-D2	Chromosome aberrations	Leukemia, others
Li Fraumeni	DNA DSB Response	p53, others?	Cell-cycle checkpoints	Many (eg, sarcoma) (early onset)
Riddle	DNA DSB Response	RNF168	cell-cycle checkpoints, DSB repair	Unknown

5.5.1 Ataxia Telangiectasia

The AT syndrome is an autosomal recessive disease characterized by cerebellar degeneration, immunodeficiency, chromosomal instability, cancer predisposition, radiation sensitivity (see Chap. 15, Sec. 15.4.1 and Figure 15–16), and cell-cycle abnormalities (Rotman and Shiloh, 1998; Weissberg et al, 1998). A mutation in a single gene coding for ATM is responsible for this syndrome. The ATM gene encodes a large protein that possesses a highly conserved C-terminal kinase domain related to PI3K (see Durocher and Jackson, 2001). Most mutations in ATM result in truncation and destabilization of the protein, but certain missense and splicing errors produce a less-severe phenotype. The pleiotropic clinical symptoms associated with AT may be explained partly by modification of cellular metabolism. For example, the loss of ATM function is associated with increased oxidative damage, particularly in cerebellar Purkinje cells, implicating a role for ATM in the response to reactive oxygen species and possibly explaining the cerebellar degeneration observed in AT-affected individuals. These observations support the hypothesis that ATM is associated with oxidative metabolism and the possible prevention of the DNA-damaging effects of reactive oxygen species (Rotman and Shiloh, 1998).

The association between mutation of the ATM gene and a high incidence of lymphoid malignancy in those patients with AT, together with the development of lymphoma in ATM-deficient mice, supports the hypothesis that inactivation of the ATM gene is important in the pathogenesis of sporadic lymphoid malignancy. LOH at 11q22-23 (the location of the ATM gene) is a common event in lymphoid malignancy. Frequent inactivating mutations of the ATM gene have been reported in patients with Hodgkin and non-Hodgkin lymphoma, rare sporadic T-cell prolymphocytic leukemia (T-PLL), B-cell chronic lymphocytic leukemia (B-CLL), and, most recently, mantle cell lymphoma (MCL). Furthermore, AT heterozygotes may have a slightly increased risk of breast cancer when compared to the normal population. These data suggest that ATM functions as a tumor-suppressor gene (Rotman and Shiloh, 1998).

Cells derived from AT patients and ATM$^{-/-}$ mice in culture display hypersensitivity to ionizing but not UV radiation; they exhibit chromosomal instability and a mild DNA DSB rejoining defect. ATM-deficient cells also have radioresistant DNA synthesis and further defects in the $G_1/S–$, S– and $G_2/M–$phase DNA damage checkpoints. One model suggests that ATM or ATR kinase activity requires colocalization with its substrate (ie, p53 or other proteins) at sites of DNA damage to initiate signaling within DNA repair and cell-cycle checkpoint pathways (Al Rashid et al, 2005, 2011).

A number of other diseases, including ATLD and NBS, show similar disease phenotypes to AT supporting the cooperation of their cognate molecular defects (MRE11 and NBS1, respectively) with ATM in suppression of genetic instability as discussed (see Sec. 5.4). The exact mechanism for the developmental defects in these patients is not well understood, but these syndromes have been instrumental in the understanding of the molecular pathways that control the responses to DNA damage, particularly DNA DSBs.

5.5.2 Xeroderma Pigmentosum and Related Disorders

The human XP, CS, and trichothiodystrophy (TTD) disorders exhibit cellular UV sensitivity as a consequence of deficiency in NER (see Sec. 5.3.3; Hoeijmakers, 2001). For reasons that are not understood, only XP patients are cancer-prone with a dramatic 1000-fold increase in the incidence of UV-induced skin cancer. This is caused by mutations in 1 of 7 XP genes (XPA-XPG) in their cells. CS is characterized by a TCR defect secondary to mutations in CSB and CSA genes. CS patients exhibit neurodegeneration and premature aging related to inappropriate apoptosis. TTD patients share many features of CS patients, but also have brittle hair, nails, and scaly skin, secondary to reduced expression of epidermal matrix proteins.

5.5.3 Hereditary Nonpolyposis Colon Cancer

Hereditary nonpolyposis colon cancer (HNPCC) is the most common form of hereditary colon cancer, accounting for 5% to 8% of all colon cancers. People with HNPCC also have an excess of endometrial, small bowel, and renal cancer. This familial cancer syndrome occurs secondary to genetic instability acquired through deficient MMR by virtue of mutations in 6 different MMR genes (see Sec. 5.3.1) (Harfe and Jinks-Robertson, 2000). Replication of repetitive DNA sequences, termed *microsatellites*, can result in gains or losses of these repeated units giving rise to *microsatellite instability* (MSI). The MMR system suppresses MSI. Cells from HNPCC patients (and also from sporadic colorectal tumors) can acquire runs of approximately 4 to 40 repeated mononucleotides or dinucleotides, such as TTTT or CACACA, at multiple sites within the genome as a consequence of MSI.

More than 300 different predisposing MMR genetic mutations have been documented in human cancers, mainly affecting MLH1 (approximately 50%), MSH2 (approximately 40%), and MSH6 (approximately 10%) (Friedberg, 2001). Genetically predisposed individuals with HNPCC carry a defective copy of an MMR gene in every cell and mutation rates in tumor cells with MMR deficiency are 100- to 1000-fold higher than in normal cells. Somatic inactivation of the remaining wild-type copy in a target tissue, typically colon, gives rise to a profound repair defect and increased rates of mutation in cells (ie, a "mutator" phenotype) with progressive accumulation of mutations in APC, p53, or other genes that contribute to colon cancer development (Jiricny and Nystrom-Lahti, 2000; Loeb, 1991; Peltomaki, 2001).

5.5.4 Li-Fraumeni Syndrome

One of the most frequently mutated genes in human tumors occurs in that encoding the p53 protein, which is involved at multiple points in the response to DNA damage and genetic instability, including but not limited to cell-cycle checkpoints, apoptosis, and modulating DNA repair (see Chap. 7, Sec 7.6.1). The Li-Fraumeni syndrome occurs in people with germline mutations of TP53. Originally characterized in 1969 in early onset cancers in relatives of children with rhabdomyosarcoma, p53 has since been found to be mutated in more diverse tumor types and in various families with inherited cancers (Palmero et al, 2010). In people with the Li-Fraumeni syndrome, 50% develop cancer before age 40 years, and 90% develop cancer before age 60 years. These are tumors of various histopathologies and include sarcomas and brain and breast cancers. Although mutation of other genes (eg, CHK2) have been suggested to be alternative predisposing factors for Li-Fraumeni syndrome, the evidence for such involvement is controversial (Palmero et al, 2010).

5.5.5 Fanconi Anemia

Fanconi anemia (FA) is a very rare autosomal recessive disorder with 1 in 300 people carrying mutations in 1 FANC gene; 1 to 5 in 1 million people are affected by this disorder (D'Andrea, 2010). Although rare, this syndrome has led to the identification of 13 "complementation group" proteins that are mutated or lost in FA patients and that comprise a distinct pathway in mammalian cells (see Sec. 5.3.6). The definitive test for FA is to treat lymphocytes from patients with diepoxybutane, a DNA crosslinking agent, and assess chromosome breakage. In FA patients, this leads to accumulation of breaks owing to an inability to repair interstrand crosslinks in DNA. Tumors (eg, leukemia, head and neck) develop in at least 20% of FA patients and this number would likely be much higher if bone marrow failure and other manifestations of the syndrome did not lead to early death of afflicted individuals.

5.5.6 BRCA1/2

Germline mutations in a single copy of the BRCA1 or BRCA2 tumor-suppressor gene occur in approximately 1 in 250 women and lead to early onset breast and ovarian cancer (Narod and Foulkes, 2004). The large majority of tumors from carriers display LOH such that both copies of the gene become mutated, rendering the cell BRCA1 or BRCA2 null. Mechanistic roles for BRCA1/2 have been observed in various DNA repair pathways including the FA pathway (see Sec. 5.3.6) and, HR (see Sec. 5.3.4), and in cell-cycle checkpoints and maintenance of ploidy (O'Donovan and Livingston, 2010). The defect in HR in BRCA1/2 tumors is being tested for a possible role in synthetic lethality using PARP inhibitors in ongoing clinical trials (Audeh et al, 2010; Tutt et al, 2010).

5.6 ASSAYS OF DNA DAMAGE AND REPAIR

It is important to be able to measure the DNA damage that is present in a cell, and to determine how well a cell is able to repair this damage by one of the mechanisms previously described. Table 5–2 outlines techniques that have been used to measure different types of DNA strand breaks. Modifications of these assays provide the ability to measure base damage and photoproducts that result when DNA repair pathways are defective. Techniques such as velocity sedimentation, filter elution, assays for chromosomal damage, and DNA electrophoresis have been used to study specific DNA lesions caused by radiation (Fairbairn et al, 1995; Whitaker et al, 1991). Two techniques, fluorescence in situ hybridization (FISH; see Chap. 2) and premature chromosome condensation (PCC), allow the quantification of single- or double-strand breaks following doses of IR as low as 1 Gy (Sasai et al, 1994). Other

TABLE 5–2 Assays for the detection of DNA damage following ionizing radiation.

Assay	Dose Range	Technique	Limitations
1. Sucrose velocity sedimentation	SSB > 5 Gy DSB >15 Gy	Larger DNA fragments sediment to a greater extent.	Insensitive to clinically relevant low radiation doses.
2. Filter elution	SSB > 1 Gy (alkaline elution) DSB > 5 Gy (neutral elution)	Smaller DNA fragments elute more quickly through a filter of defined pore size.	Uncertain effects of DNA conformation, cell cycle, cell number, and lysis.
3. Nucleoid sedimentation	SSB 1 to 20 Gy	Irradiated cells show altered DNA supercoiling within nucleus.	Uncertain which DNA lesion(s) are being detected.
4. Pulse-field gel electrophoresis (PFGE)	DSB > 2 Gy	Allows for resolution of DNA DSB, which can be quantified by relative migration within the gel.	Uncertain effects of DNA conformation; high number of cells in S phase may bias results of assay.
5. Comet assay	SSB > 1 Gy (alkaline lysis) DSB > 2 Gy (neutral lysis)	Following lysis, individual nuclei are subjected to agarose gel electrophoresis. The DNA that moves out of the nucleus (head) to form the "tail" of the comet is quantitated to provide a measure of DNA damage.	Requires image analysis system to quantify DNA damage; increased numbers of cells in S-phase may bias assay.
6. Fluorescence in situ hybridization (FISH)	Doses > 1 Gy	Chromosome-specific probes, which can be detected with a fluorescent ligand, are used to identify radiation-induced translocations.	May be difficult to interpret in tumor cells that contain translocations prior to irradiation.
7. Premature chromosome condensation (PCC)	Doses > 1 Gy	An irradiated interphase cell is fused to a mitotic cell. The chromosomes in the interphase cell undergo premature condensation, allowing radiation-induced chromosome damage to be scored.	May be difficult to interpret in tumor cells that contain chromosome aberrations prior to irradiation.
8. γ-H2AX intranuclear foci	Doses > 0.05 Gy	Immunofluorescence microscopy or flow cytometry using an antibody to γ-H2AX phosphoprotein.	Requires image analysis system. No standard for size of foci to count.

DSB, double-strand breaks; *SSB*, single-stranded breaks.

Source: Adapted from Whitaker et al, 1991.

techniques, such as pulsed-field gel electrophoresis (PFGE) or the Comet assay (Fairbairn et al, 1995), can facilitate the separation and quantification of large DNA fragments secondary to single- or double-strand DNA breaks following radiation, but, with exception of the comet assay, require much higher (>10 to 20 Gy) doses because of their lower sensitivity. DNA DSBs are of particular importance as they are the most lethal form of DNA damage (see Chap. 15).

IR leads to rapid phosphorylation of nucleosomal histone protein, H2AX. γH2AX is the phosphorylated form that can be quantified using a specific antibody as an intracellular marker of DNA DSBs (Rogakou et al, 1999; see Figs. 5–10 and 5–11). This early event precedes the actions of repair enzymes involved in HR and NHEJ of these breaks. Microscopically visible nuclear foci, each containing thousands of γH2AX molecules covering about 2 Mb of DNA surrounding the break, can be detected using antibody staining and fluorescence microscopy. The number of γH2AX foci has been directly correlated to the number of DNA DSBs in [125]IUdR-treated cells as each ^{125}I decay yields a DNA DSB and each DNA DSB yielded a visible γH2AX focus (Sedelnikova et al, 2002). Following IR these foci resolve with kinetics that correlate with other biochemical DSB rejoining assays (eg, PFGE) such that approximately 50% of breaks remain after 2 hours and by 24 hours following the radiation dose almost all breaks are rejoined. It is probable that increased residual nuclear foci (≥24 hours post-IR) represent non-rejoined DNA DSBs and lead to subsequent cell lethality (MacPhail et al, 2003). However, there are confounding factors that activate γH2AX, such as apoptosis and cell-cycle and oncogene signaling (Lobrich et al, 2010). This method has also been adapted to detect other types of lesions, such as 6-4PPs, to which antibodies have been generated (Vermeulen, 2011).

Using innovative microscopic and fluorescent technologies, researchers can specifically generate and visualize discrete DNA DSBs. For example, use of high fluence targeted laser microirradiation induces DNA DSBs in a spatially restricted manner within the nucleus. These can be used to monitor the recruitment of repair proteins to DNA damage, and can also be used in combination with more advanced techniques such as fluorescence recovery after photobleaching (FRAP) to determine the residence of repair proteins at the DNA damage site in live cells. Despite the utility of such methods for localization of DNA damage, there remains to be determined the exact nature of the damage created by these techniques, and conclusions drawn from such assays are typically bolstered by the more traditional techniques outlined in Table 5–2.

5.7 REGULATION OF TELOMERE LENGTH AND CANCER

Human cells have evolved a complex network of proteins that bind to chromosomal ends, called *telomeres*, to protect them from being inappropriately recognized as DNA damage. Disruption of this nucleoprotein complex, either through loss of telomere DNA or direct disruption of protein function at the telomere, signals a DNA damage response leading to cell death or cessation of cell division. Cells that retain the capacity to proliferate, such as stem cells and cancer cells, must thus find a mechanism to maintain telomere integrity. Most often, cancer cells achieve this protection through the activation of an enzyme that adds new telomere DNA onto chromosome ends, called *telomerase*. More rarely, maintenance of telomeres is achieved through recombination, exchange, or copying of existing telomere DNA tracts through mechanisms collectively referred to as "alternate lengthening of telomeres" (ALT). Together, telomerase and the nucleoprotein complex that protects telomeres ensure the maintenance of telomere integrity in dividing mammalian cells.

Pioneering genetic experiments in the fruit fly *Drosophila melanogaster* and in maize laid the foundation for our appreciation of the importance of telomeres in genome stability (reviewed in Greider, 1996). These initial experiments determined that DNA damage could result in the loss of the terminal "knob" of linear chromosomes. Loss of telomeres in maize led to fusion or loss of chromosomes and an ensuing cycle of chromosome breakage, chromosome fusion, and anaphase bridges during cell division that is referred to as the *breakage-fusion-bridge* cycle. We now appreciate that telomere integrity is critical to the viability of normal and malignant cells in many organisms, and that loss of telomere DNA is an important contributor to genomic instability.

5.7.1 Telomeres Protect Chromosomal Ends from Recognition as DNA Damage

Most linear chromosomes terminate in a long, noncoding repetitive tract of G-rich, telomeric-DNA that varies in its sequence and average length between organisms. In humans, telomeres are composed of 4 to 15 kilobase pairs (kbp) of the hexanucleotide sequence 5'-TTAGGG-3' followed by 100 to 150 nucleotides of a single-stranded TTAGGG-3' overhang. The 3' single-stranded overhang is looped back on itself in a structure termed the *t-loop* (reviewed in de Lange, 2004). Internal to the telomeric tract there are several kilobases of degenerate telomeric sequence, called *subtelomeric DNA*. The subtelomeric and telomeric regions exist in a nucleoprotein complex containing several telomere-binding proteins and chromatin-associated proteins. This nucleoprotein complex possesses a distinct nucleosomal structure that is thought to protect the chromosome ends from being perceived as damaged DNA, although in response to uncapping of telomere DNA overt chromatin remodeling is not observed (Wu and de Lange, 2008; Fig. 5–14). Telomere dysfunction, either by erosion of telomere DNA or through loss of telomere end protection, can trigger the recruitment of several DSB response factors, including γH2AX, 53BP1, MRE11/RAD50/NBS1, and phosphorylated ATM. These resultant telomere-dysfunction–induced foci (TIF) coincide with the activation of the checkpoint kinases ATR and/or ATM, which, in turn, phosphorylate Chk1 and Chk2 and lead to p53- and p21-dependent cell apoptosis and cycle arrest (reviewed in d'Adda di Fagagna, 2008). Thus, many factors that play a role in the DNA damage response elsewhere in the genome also play important roles at the telomere.

To prevent the gradual erosion of linear DNA that arises as a result of the inability of DNA polymerases to completely replicate the 5' ends of linear DNA, a special cellular mechanism must compensate for telomere loss. This mechanism entails the addition of new G-rich, single-stranded telomere DNA to chromosome ends by telomerase, which carries its own telomere-complementary RNA template (see Fig. 5–14). This enzyme employs a reverse transcriptase (*telomerase reverse transcriptase [TERT]*) and the RNA template (*telomerase RNA-TR*) to direct new telomere DNA synthesis, 1 nucleotide at a time, onto chromosome ends (reviewed in Greider and Blackburn, 1996).

Telomeric sequences added by telomerase compensate for the gradual erosion of chromosome ends to enable cells undergoing multiple divisions during cell proliferation such as stem cells and cancer cells to maintain telomere length and chromosome stability. New telomere DNA synthesis is coordinated with replication of the telomeric DNA tract by conventional DNA polymerases, and, indeed, telomerase interacts with subunits of the DNA replication machinery (reviewed in Price et al, 2010). Concomitant with or following replication, the 5' and 3' ends of telomeric DNA are processed via enzymatic pathways that have not yet been fully elaborated. During de novo telomere DNA synthesis by TERT, the telomerase RNA template is reversed transcribed into telomeric DNA (see Fig. 5–14). The assembly of active telomerase in vivo requires other components. For example, dyskerin and its protein partners NHP2, NOP10, and GAR1 bind to the 3' terminal H/ACA box on telomerase RNA to modulate telomerase assembly and stability (Egan and Collins, 2010). TCAB1 (telomerase Cajal body protein 1) interacts with dyskerin and recognizes the CAB box in the telomerase RNA, also facilitating telomerase assembly and trafficking to Cajal bodies (reviewed in Venteicher and Artandi, 2009). An excellent inventory of telomerase subunits from various organisms can be found at: http://telomerase.asu.edu/.

5.7.2 Telomere Regulation in Normal Cell Proliferation

In humans, normal cells often express low or undetectable levels of telomerase activity because of transcriptional repression of the TERT catalytic protein subunit of telomerase, and

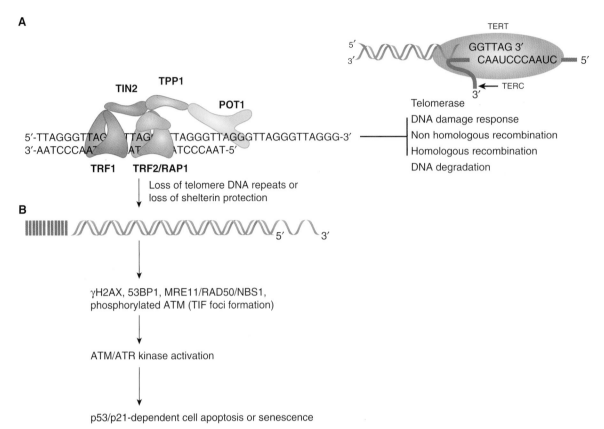

FIGURE 5–14   Telomere maintenance by telomerase and shelterin and the consequences of telomere dysfunction. A) Telomere DNA, telomerase, and shelterin (TIN2, TRF1, TRF2, POT1, RAP1, TPP1). Telomeres protect against DNA damage and degradation. The access of telomerase is limited by telomere-bound POT1 and TRF1. **B)** Dysfunctional telomeres that arise via loss of telomere DNA repeats or loss of protection of shelterin induce DNA damage foci formation in telomeres (TIF) and activate ATM or ATR kinases leading to p53/p21-dependent cell apoptosis, cell-cycle arrest, and cellular senescence. (Reproduced with permission from Lue NF, Autexier C. *Telomerases: Chemistry, Biology and Clinical Applications*. John Wiley and Sons; 2012.)

therefore undergo telomere shortening with each subsequent cell division (reviewed in Greider, 1998b). Normal cells do not replicate indefinitely in culture. The eventual loss of replicative potential is termed *cellular senescence* or the *Hayflick limit*. The time to the cessation of cell division correlates closely with a critically eroded telomere at which telomeric tracts can no longer be detected (called a telomere signal-free end [TSFE]; reviewed in Greider, 1998b). In the absence of the tumor-suppressor genes, p53 or pRb, cells can undergo additional population doublings before eventually reaching a proliferative block, called *crisis*. At crisis, cells exhibit extensive genome instability and most will undergo apoptosis. Only a small fraction of cells (approximately 1 in 10^7) survive by either activating expression of the endogenous *hTERT* gene, or via other telomerase-independent mechanisms, such as ALT. Stem cells from various human tissues express telomerase during proliferative bursts, although usually at levels sufficient only to maintain telomere integrity and insufficient to elicit overall telomere lengthening (reviewed in Blasco, 2007).

The hypothesis that cellular senescence is causally linked to "critically short" telomeres is supported by a tight correlation between them, and the finding that reintroduction of TERT into human primary cells renders them capable of indefinite proliferation; indeed reintroduction of this single gene indefinitely prolongs the life span of human cells in culture (Bodnar et al, 1998; Vaziri and Benchimol, 1998). Despite being "immortal" in a culture dish, TERT-reconstituted human cells appear to preserve their normal morphology, response to external stress, and karyotype (Vaziri et al, 1999). Thus, TERT itself does not possess the classical characteristics that define an oncogene (Greider, 1998a), although in combination with other oncogenes TERT promotes the malignant transformation of normal cells (reviewed in Hahn, 2002).

In mice, disruption of the genes encoding the telomerase RNA or TERT leads to telomere shortening in all tissues (reviewed in Liu and Harrington, 2012). For example, following several generations of breeding in the absence of the telomerase RNA, visible defects are observed in several organs and stem cell compartments in the germline, blood, and gut (Lee et al, 1998). Critically short telomeres lead to telomere-telomere fusions, which in turn activate a p53-dependent apoptotic response (Chin et al, 1999; Lee et al, 1998). Crossing telomerase-deficient mice with p53-deficient mice can extend the number of fertile generations (Chin et al, 1999), but eventually the germline cells from telomerase/p53 deficient mice also undergo apoptosis. This observation indicates that p53-independent mechanisms are involved in monitoring telomere integrity and genome instability in dividing cells (Chin et al, 1999). Tissue defects are related not to overall short telomere lengths per se, but to the inability to repair critically eroded telomeric tracts.

Telomere shortening has been linked to human syndromes with early mortality. For example, mutations in the telomerase components, TERT, TERC, DKC, NHP2, and NOP10 (and also in a shelterin component, TIN2—see below) are associated with rare human genetic disorders, including dyskeratosis congenita, aplastic anemia, and idiopathic pulmonary fibrosis (reviewed in Armanios, 2009; Calado and Young, 2009; Savage et al, 2009). In all but a few instances, these diseases are haploinsufficiency disorders, and 1 inactive allele is sufficient to confer disease. Partial loss-of-function of telomerase activity also leads to various forms of hematopoietic cancer. Similar disease phenotypes are recapitulated in murine models in which 1 or both copies of telomerase subunits or telomere-associated proteins have been deleted or mutated, alone or in combination with factors that promote genome instability (reviewed in Liu and Harrington, 2012).

Short telomeres have been observed in the peripheral blood of people with cardiovascular disease and those exposed to stress (Epel et al, 2006, 2010). Although a causal role of short telomeres has not yet been established, these observations suggest that telomere length could be a useful prognostic factor for certain lifestyle-associated diseases (Lin et al, 2011). In vitro, enforced overexpression of telomerase leads to telomere extension and can extend the life span of cells derived from people with dyskeratosis congenita harboring mutations in the telomerase RNA (Agarwal et al, 2011), and transcriptional activation of hTERT extends the replicative capacity of cells derived from HIV-infected patients (Fauce et al, 2008). Thus, telomere elongation could serve a useful therapeutic purpose in some human diseases.

5.7.3 Shelterin and Telomere Integrity

In mammals, telomeres are bound by a 6-subunit complex called shelterin, which contains the telomere-binding proteins TRF1, TRF2, and POT1, and their associated proteins RAP1, TPP1, and TIN2 (reviewed in de Lange, 2005; see Fig. 5–14). TRF1 and TRF2 bind to duplex telomeric DNA and anchor shelterin along the telomere repeats; POT1 binds to the single-stranded G-rich DNA overhang at telomeres; TIN2 is a protein scaffold for TRF1 and TRF2 and recruits POT1 to the complex via TPP1; and RAP1 associates with shelterin via binding to TRF2. Shelterin serves several regulatory roles at the telomere, including telomerase access to the telomere, telomere replication and integrity, t-loop assembly and stability, and the ability to attenuate ATM-dependent and ATR-dependent DNA damage responses (reviewed in de Lange, 2005). Shelterin function is conserved across a wide number of species, even in *Drosophila* where telomeres are maintained via a telomerase-independent mechanism of retrotransposition (Cenci et al, 2005; Longhese, 2008).

5.7.4 Telomere Maintenance and Cancer

To support long-term proliferative potential, cancer cells express telomerase activity or, more rarely, maintain telomeres via ALT. Evidence that telomerase inhibition selectively kills cancer cells was provided by studies showing that overexpression of dominant interfering variants of hTERT elicit telomere erosion and apoptosis in several cancer cell lines (Hahn et al, 1999; Herbert et al, 1999; Zhang et al, 1999). Several other lines of evidence now indicate that tumor cells must maintain minimally functional telomere reserves in order to retain proliferative potential.

In approximately 15% of cancers (across a wide variety of cancer types), cells maintain telomeres via HR between chromosome ends (reviewed in Cesare and Reddel, 2010) to employ "alternative lengthening of telomeres" (ALT). ALT cells possess promyelocytic leukemia-like nuclear bodies called APBs (ALT-associated PML bodies) that contain telomeric DNA, telomere DNA binding proteins, and DNA repair proteins and may represent sites permissive for telomere recombination. ALT cells also possess long and heterogenous telomere lengths, and carry extrachromosomal telomere DNA called t-circles (Cesare and Reddel, 2010). This latter feature may not be specific to ALT-associated cancers, as normal cells with elongated telomeres also exhibit t-circles (Pickett et al, 2011). In ALT cell lines, telomeres that are marked with a reporter construct can "jump" to new telomere locations, an observation that is consistent with direct telomere-telomere recombination (Dunham et al, 2000). Because ALT cells do not express telomerase activity, inhibition of telomerase function has no effect on their growth (Hahn et al, 1999).

As telomeres in actively dividing tumor cells are often short, and telomere lengths are longer in stem cells and other quiescent normal cells, telomerase is an attractive target for therapeutic intervention in cancer. In clinical development are several new telomere/telomerase targeting compounds including antisense oligonucleotides, G-quadruplex stabilizing substances, telomerase expression-related strategies such as telomerase promoter-driven suicide gene therapy, and telomerase immunotherapy (Harley, 2008). One such inhibitor, GRN163L is an antisense oligonucleotide directed against the RNA template of telomerase. This compound is now in Phase II clinical trials against several different types of cancer. An advantage of telomerase inhibition is that it should be efficacious against all telomerase-positive tumors, which make up more than 85% of tumor types. Compounds that disrupt telomere structure are also in development, and have the potential to treat both telomerase-positive and ALT-derived tumors (Harley, 2008). Inhibition of telomerase also holds promise for pediatric cancers but is complicated by the fact that pediatric tumors often possess longer initial telomere lengths (Tabori and Dome, 2007).

An important question is the role of critically short telomeres in the process of driving malignant transformation. For

Head and neck

(Oral cavity, larynx, oropharynx, nasopharynx)

NBS1   ATM
RAD51   CHK2
NBS1   RAD51
KU70/80   53BP1
BRCA1/2

Brain

(Glioblastoma)

FANCD2   FEN1
RAD51L   RAD51
RAD52   DNA-PKcs
DNA-PKcs   53BP1
BRCA1
NBS1

Lung

(Non-small cell, small cell)

BRCA1/2   CHK2
DNA-PKcs   RAD51
NBS1   MRE11
CHK2   KU70/80
ATM   MDC1
KU70/80   53BP1
BRCA1   BRCA1/2

Breast

BRCA1/2   *RAD51AP1*
MRE11   *ATM*
NBS1   DNA-PKcs
RAD50   KU80
CHK2   MDC1
BLM   53BP1
WRN   BRCA1/2
RAD54   RAD51
RAD51
RAD54

Gastrointestinal

(Pancreas, esophagus, colorectal)

WRN   BRCA1/2
NBS1   KU70/80
MRE11   ATM
RAD50   NBS1
CHK2   MRE11
RAD54   CHK2
BRCA2
FANCN

Genitourinary

(Ovarian, cervix, prostate, bladder)

CHK2   *BRCA1/2*
BRCA1/2   CHK2
ATM   RAD51
DNA-PKcs   MRE11
RAD17   KU70/80
NBS1   DNA-PKcs
KU70/80

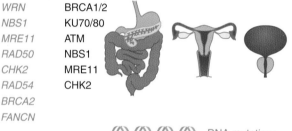
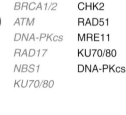
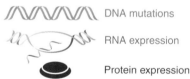

DNA mutations

RNA expression

Protein expression

FIGURE 5–15 Diagram of DNA (green; mutation, deletion, or amplification), RNA (blue; under- or overexpression), or protein (black; under- or overexpression) alterations in DNA DSB response/repair proteins that have been identified in various tumor sites as indicated.

example, BRCA2 and BRCA1 are known to participate in processes that regulate telomere integrity, and patients harboring BRCA mutations show evidence of critically short telomeres and chromosome rearrangements that are consistent with loss of telomere integrity (Bodvarsdottir et al, 2011; Bogliolo et al, 2002; McPherson et al, 2006; Wang et al, 2007). The introduction of inducible chromosome breakage sites in murine ES cells has established that chromosome breakage within telomere DNA can contribute to the breakage-fusion-bridge cycles first noted in maize (Murnane and Sabatier, 2004). In prostate cancer short telomeres are observed in precursor lesions (ie high-grade prostatic intraepithelial neoplasia, or PIN) concomitant with the onset of other chromosomal rearrangements (Vukovic et al, 2003, 2007). Experiments in mice also suggest that, in some backgrounds predisposed to cancer,

loss of telomere DNA can sometimes paradoxically lead to an increase in malignancy (Artandi and DePinho, 2010). Adjunct therapies that combine standard chemotherapeutic agents together with agents that perturb telomere function may be the best approach to achieve a rapid onset of apoptosis in telomerase-positive tumors and serve to mitigate the emergence of drug-resistant cancer.

5.8 DNA REPAIR AND CANCER TREATMENT

The PARP1 and PARP2 proteins are required for repair of DNA single-stranded breaks (SSBs) and in cells treated with small-molecule inhibitors of PARP (PARPi), unrepaired SSBs at replication forks are converted into DSBs, which require repair by HR to offset cell lethality. *Synthetic lethality* is the concept that mutation in 2 genes leads to death, whereas mutation of either alone is compatible with viability (see also Chap. 17). For example, tumor cells lacking HR function (eg, deficient in BRCA1 or BRCA2 expression) are exquisitely sensitive to PARPi because of the inability to repair replication-associated DSBs. Biomarkers that effectively predict functional losses in DNA repair activity, in addition to mutations in DNA repair genes, may therefore be useful in accurately predicting clinical PARPi efficacy (Dent and Bristow, 2011). Novel trials using PARPi may also be useful in patients who have abrogated function of the HR, FA, and *PTEN* pathways (Fraser et al, 2012). Similarly, deficiency in the MMR proteins MSH2 and MLH1 have been shown to be synthetically lethal with disruption of the DNA polymerases POLB and POLG, respectively (Martin et al, 2010), although clinically useful inhibitors of POLB or POLG are not yet available. A final example of synthetic lethality is the observation that FA defective cells are more sensitive to ATM inhibitors (Kennedy et al, 2007).

Documenting the functional loss or gain in DNA repair pathways may also be useful in sporadic tumors to individualize chemotherapy, radiotherapy, or molecular targeted therapies. Many human tumor types possess defects in DNA repair genes based on DNA, RNA, or protein analyses (Fig. 5–15), and these alterations can lead to differential sensitivity to DNA damaging agents. For example, a loss of function can lead to increased sensitivity to different chemotherapeutic agents or radiotherapy and elevated expression of the NER-associated *Ercc1* gene is a promising biomarker for the relative resistance to *cis*-platinum chemotherapy in lung cancer (Cobo et al, 2007). In another example, glioblastoma brain cancer cells that express the enzyme called *O-6-methylguanine-DNA methyltransferase (MGMT)* are better able to repair the DNA damage caused by the alkylating agent temozolomide (Hegi et al, 2005), and the presence of MGMT protein in brain tumors predicts poor response to temozolomide. Epigenetic silencing of the *MGMT/AGT* gene can prevent the synthesis of this enzyme, and as a consequence such tumors are more sensitive to killing by temozolomide. Defects in HR can also sensitize tumors to agents that are highly toxic to HR-deficient tumor cells such as mitomycin C (MMC), *cis*-platinum and IR (Chan et al, 2010).

SUMMARY

- Genetic stability is crucial to the prevention of carcinogenesis. Many proteins involved in cell-cycle checkpoint control, chromosomal stability, DNA repair, and telomerase activity act in concert with one another during cell proliferation to maintain the integrity of the genome.
- Determining the tissue specificity of the proteins involved in these responses will be important to understand the relative susceptibility of different tissues to endogenous and exogenous carcinogens.

- Multiple types of lesions occur on DNA and are repaired by concerted pathways: DNA-base mismatches (Mismatch repair), damaged bases of the DNA (Base excision repair), UV-lesions or bulky DNA-adducts (Nucleotide excision repair), Double strand breaks (homologous recombination and non-homologous end-joining) and DNA interstrand crosslinks (Fanconi Anemia pathway).
- DNA double strand breaks are the most toxic type of DNA damage. Signaling cascades respond to these lesions *in situ* to enact DNA repair mechanisms and cell cycle checkpoints to suppress mutagenesis and cell death.
- Human DNA repair-deficient, and DNA damage checkpoint-deficient syndromes and murine "genetic knockout" models provide important cellular and biochemical clues as to the temporal activity of many proteins within DNA damage signaling cascades.
- To support long-term proliferative potential, cancer cells express telomerase activity or, more rarely, maintain telomeres via ALT. Because telomeres in actively dividing tumor cells are often short, telomerase is an attractive target for therapeutic intervention in cancer. Abnormal telomere regulation can lead to genetic instability.
- Our understanding of these pathways has led to the development of molecular cancer diagnostics and therapies specific to certain proteins which normally act as gatekeepers of genomic stability. Examples include gene therapy and pharmacological means designed to inhibit DNA repair and kill cells through synthetic lethality, and telomere-specific therapies.

REFERENCES

Agarwal S, Loh YH, McLoughlin EM, et al. Telomere elongation in induced pluripotent stem cells from dyskeratosis congenita patients. *Nature* 2011;464:292-296.

Al-Hakim A, Escribano-Diaz C, Landry M-C, et al. The ubiquitous role of ubiquitin in the DNA damage response. *DNA Repair (Amst)* 2010;9:1229-1240.

Al Rashid ST, Dellaire G, Cuddihy A, et al. Evidence for the direct binding of phosphorylated p53 to sites of DNA breaks in vivo. *Cancer Res* 2005;65:10810-10821.

Al Rashid ST, Harding SM, Law C, Coackley C, Bristow RG. Protein-protein interactions occur between p53 phospho forms and ATM and 53BP1 at sites of exogenous DNA damage. *Radiat Res* 2011;175:588-598.

Ames BN, Cathcart R, Schwiers E, Hochstein P. Uric acid provides an antioxidant defense in humans against oxidant- and radical-caused aging and cancer: a hypothesis. *Proc Natl Acad Sci U S A* 1981;78:6858-6862.

Armanios M. Syndromes of telomere shortening. *Annu Rev Genomics Hum Genet* 2009;10:45-61.

Artandi SE, DePinho RA. Telomeres and telomerase in cancer. *Carcinogenesis* 2010;31:9-18.

Audeh MW, Carmichael J, Penson RT, et al. Oral poly(ADP-ribose) polymerase inhibitor olaparib in patients with BRCA1 or BRCA2 mutations and recurrent ovarian cancer: a proof-of-concept trial. *Lancet* 2010;376:245-251.

Bakkenist CJ, Kastan MB. DNA damage activates ATM through intermolecular autophosphorylation and dimer dissociation. *Nature* 2003;421:499-506.

Balajee AS, Bohr VA. Genomic heterogeneity of nucleotide excision repair. *Gene* 2000;250:15-30.

Bensimon A, Aebersold R, Shiloh Y. Beyond ATM: the protein kinase landscape of the DNA damage response. *FEBS Lett* 2011;585:1625-1639.

Besaratinia A, Pfeifer GP. Sunlight ultraviolet irradiation and BRAF V600 mutagenesis in human melanoma. *Hum Mutat* 2008;29: 983-991.

Blasco MA. Telomere length, stem cells and aging. *Nat Chem Biol* 2007;3:640-649.

Bodmer W, Bielas JH, Beckman RA. Genetic instability is not a requirement for tumor development. *Cancer Res* 2008;68: 3558-3560; discussion 3560-3561.

Bodnar AG, Ouellette M, Frolkis M, et al. Extension of life-span by introduction of telomerase into normal human cells. *Science* 1998;279:349-352.

Bodvarsdottir SK, Steinarsdottir M, Bjarnason H, Eyfjord JE. Dysfunctional telomeres in human BRCA2 mutated breast tumors and cell lines. *Mutat Res* 2011;729:90-99.

Bogliolo M, Cabre O, Callen E, et al. The Fanconi anaemia genome stability and tumour suppressor network. *Mutagenesis* 2002;17:529-538.

Bouwman P, Aly A, Escandell JM, et al. 53BP1 loss rescues BRCA1 deficiency and is associated with triple-negative and BRCA-mutated breast cancers. *Nat Struct Mol Biol* 2010;17:688-695.

Calado RT, Young NS. Telomere diseases. *N Engl J Med* 2009;361: 2353-2365.

Canman CE, Lim DS, Cimprich KA, et al. Activation of the ATM kinase by ionizing radiation and phosphorylation of p53. *Science* 1998;281:1677-1679.

Cenci G, Ciapponi L, Gatti M. The mechanism of telomere protection: a comparison between Drosophila and humans. *Chromosoma* 2005;114:135-145.

Cesare AJ, Reddel RR. Alternative lengthening of telomeres: models, mechanisms and implications. *Nat Rev Genet* 2010; 11:319-330.

Chan DW, Gately DP, Urban S, et al. Lack of correlation between ATM protein expression and tumour cell radiosensitivity. *Int J Radiat Biol* 1998;74:217-224.

Chan N, Pires IM, Bencokova Z, et al. Contextual synthetic lethality of cancer cell kill based on the tumor microenvironment. *Cancer Res* 2010;70:8045-8054.

Chin L, Artandi SE, Shen Q, et al. p53 deficiency rescues the adverse effects of telomere loss and cooperates with telomere dysfunction to accelerate carcinogenesis. *Cell* 1999;97:527-538.

Ciccia A, Elledge SJ. The DNA damage response: making it safe to play with knives. *Mol Cell* 2010;40:179-204.

Cleaver JE, Crowley E. UV damage, DNA repair and skin carcinogenesis. *Front Biosci* 2002;7:d1024-d1043.

Cobo M, Isla D, Massuti B, et al. Customizing cisplatin based on quantitative excision repair cross-complementing 1 mRNA expression: a phase III trial in non-small-cell lung cancer. *J Clin Oncol* 2007;25:2747-2754.

Cordonnier AM, Fuchs RP. Replication of damaged DNA: molecular defect in xeroderma pigmentosum variant cells. *Mutat Res* 1999;435:111-119.

Cortez D, Wang Y, Qin J, Elledge SJ. Requirement of ATM-dependent phosphorylation of brca1 in the DNA damage response to double-strand breaks. *Science* 1999;286:1162-1166.

Cox R. Molecular mechanisms of radiation oncogenesis. *Int J Radiat Biol* 1994;65:57-64.

d'Adda di Fagagna F. Living on a break: cellular senescence as a DNA-damage response. *Nat Rev Cancer* 2008;8:512-522.

D'Andrea AD. Susceptibility pathways in Fanconi's anemia and breast cancer. *N Engl J Med* 2010;362:1909-1919.

Daboussi F, Dumay A, Delacote F, Lopez BS. DNA double-strand break repair signalling: the case of RAD51 post-translational regulation. *Cell Signal* 2002;14:969-975.

Davies AA, Masson JY, McIlwraith MJ, et al. Role of BRCA2 in control of the RAD51 recombination and DNA repair protein. *Mol Cell* 2001;7:273-282.

Daya-Grosjean L, Dumaz N, Sarasin A. The specificity of p53 mutation spectra in sunlight induced human cancers. *J Photochem Photobiol B* 1995;28:115-124.

Daya-Grosjean L, Sarasin A. UV-specific mutations of the human patched gene in basal cell carcinomas from normal individuals and xeroderma pigmentosum patients. *Mutat Res* 2000;450:193-199.

de Gruijl FR, Van Kranen HJ, Mullenders LH. UV-induced DNA damage, repair, mutations and oncogenic pathways in skin cancer. *J Photochem Photobiol B* 2001;63:19-27.

de Laat WL, Jaspers NG, Hoeijmakers JH. Molecular mechanism of nucleotide excision repair. *Genes Dev* 1999;13:768-785.

de Lange T. T-loops and the origin of telomeres. *Nat Rev Mol Cell Biol* 2004;5:323-329.

de Lange T. Shelterin: the protein complex that shapes and safeguards human telomeres. *Genes Dev* 2005;19:2100-2110.

Dent RA, Bristow RG. In situ DNA repair assays as guides to personalized breast cancer chemotherapeutics: ready for prime time? *J Clin Oncol* 2011;29:2130-2132.

Dobbs TA, Tainer JA, Lees-Miller SP. A structural model for regulation of NHEJ by DNA-PKcs autophosphorylation. *DNA Repair (Amst)* 2010;9:1307-1314.

Doil C, Mailand N, Bekker-Jensen S, et al. RNF168 binds and amplifies ubiquitin conjugates on damaged chromosomes to allow accumulation of repair proteins. *Cell* 2009;136:435-446.

Dunham MA, Neumann AA, Fasching CL, Reddel RR. Telomere maintenance by recombination in human cells. *Nat Genet* 2000;26:447-450.

Durocher D, Jackson SP. DNA-PK, ATM and ATR as sensors of DNA damage: variations on a theme? *Curr Opin Cell Biol* 2001;13:225-231.

Egan ED, Collins K. Specificity and stoichiometry of subunit interactions in the human telomerase holoenzyme assembled in vivo. *Mol Cell Biol* 2010;30:2775-2786.

Epel ES, Lin J, Dhabhar FS, et al. Dynamics of telomerase activity in response to acute psychological stress. *Brain Behav Immun* 2010;24:531-539.

Epel ES, Lin J, Wilhelm FH, et al. Cell aging in relation to stress arousal and cardiovascular disease risk factors. *Psychoneuroendocrinology* 2006;31:277-287.

Essers J, Hendriks RW, Swagemakers SM, et al. Disruption of mouse RAD54 reduces ionizing radiation resistance and homologous recombination. *Cell* 1997;89:195-204.

Fairbairn DW, Olive PL, O'Neill KL. The comet assay: a comprehensive review. *Mutat Res* 1995;339:37-59.

Falck J, Lukas C, Protopopova M, Lukas J, Selivanova G, Bartek J. Functional impact of concomitant versus alternative defects in the Chk2-p53 tumour suppressor pathway. *Oncogene* 2001;20: 5503-5510.

Fauce SR, Jamieson BD, Chin AC, et al. Telomerase-based pharmacologic enhancement of antiviral function of human CD8+ T lymphocytes. *J Immunol* 2008;181:7400-7406.

Featherstone C, Jackson SP. DNA repair: the Nijmegen breakage syndrome protein. *Curr Biol* 1998;8:R622-R625.

Fraser M, Harding SM, Zhao H, Coackley C, Durocher D, Bristow RG. MRE11 promotes AKT phosphorylation in direct response to DNA double-strand breaks. *Cell Cycle* 2012;10:2218-2232.

Friedberg EC. How nucleotide excision repair protects against cancer. *Nat Rev Cancer* 2001;1:22-33.

Gatei M, Young D, Cerosaletti KM, et al. ATM-dependent phosphorylation of nibrin in response to radiation exposure. *Nat Genet* 2000;25:115-119.

Girard PM, Foray N, Stumm M, et al. Radiosensitivity in Nijmegen Breakage Syndrome cells is attributable to a repair defect and not cell cycle checkpoint defects. *Cancer Res* 2000;60:4881-4888.

Greider CW. Telomere length regulation. *Annu Rev Biochem* 1996; 65:337-365.

Greider CW. Telomerase activity, cell proliferation, and cancer. *Proc Natl Acad Sci U S A* 1998a;95:90-92.

Greider CW. Telomeres and senescence: the history, the experiment, the future. *Curr Biol* 1998b;8:R178-R181.

Greider CW, Blackburn EH. Telomeres, telomerase and cancer. *Sci Am* 1996;274:92-97.

Hahn WC. Immortalization and transformation of human cells. *Mol Cells* 2002;13:351-361.

Hahn WC, Stewart SA, Brooks MW, et al. Inhibition of telomerase limits the growth of human cancer cells. *Nat Med* 1999;5:1164-1170.

Hakem R. DNA-damage repair; the good, the bad, and the ugly. *EMBO J* 2008;27:589-605.

Hanahan D, Weinberg RA. Hallmarks of cancer: the next generation. *Cell* 2010;144:646-674.

Harfe BD, Jinks-Robertson S. DNA mismatch repair and genetic instability. *Annu Rev Genet* 2000;34:359-399.

Harley CB. Telomerase and cancer therapeutics. *Nat Rev Cancer* 2008;8:167-179.

Hegi ME, Diserens AC, Gorlia T, et al. MGMT gene silencing and benefit from temozolomide in glioblastoma. *N Engl J Med* 2005;352:997-1003.

Helleday T. Homologous recombination in cancer development, treatment and development of drug resistance. *Carcinogenesis* 2010;31:955-960.

Helleday T, Lo J, Van Gent DC, Engelward BP. DNA double-strand break repair: from mechanistic understanding to cancer treatment. *DNA Repair (Amst)* 2007;6:923-935.

Herbert B, Pitts AE, Baker SI, et al. Inhibition of human telomerase in immortal human cells leads to progressive telomere shortening and cell death. *Proc Natl Acad Sci U S A* 1999;96:14276-14281.

Heyer W-D, Ehmsen KT, Liu J. Regulation of homologous recombination in eukaryotes. *Annu Rev Genet* 2010;44:113-139.

Hiom K. Coping with DNA double strand breaks. *DNA Repair (Amst)* 2010;9:1256-1263.

Hittelman WN. Genetic instability in epithelial tissues at risk for cancer. *Ann N Y Acad Sci* 2001;952:1-12.

Hoeijmakers JH. DNA damage, aging, and cancer. *N Engl J Med* 2009;361:1475-1485.

Hoeijmakers JH. Genome maintenance mechanisms for preventing cancer. *Nature* 2001;411:366-374.

Huen MSY, Grant R, Manke I, et al. RNF8 transduces the DNA-damage signal via histone ubiquitylation and checkpoint protein assembly. *Cell* 2007;131:901-914.

Jasin M. Chromosome breaks and genomic instability. *Cancer Invest* 2000;18:78-86.

Jazayeri A, Falck J, Lukas C, et al. ATM- and cell cycle-dependent regulation of ATR in response to DNA double-strand breaks. *Nat Cell Biol* 2006;8:37-45.

Jiricny J. The multifaceted mismatch-repair system. *Nat Rev Mol Cell Biol* 2006;7:335-346.

Jiricny J, Nystrom-Lahti M. Mismatch repair defects in cancer. *Curr Opin Genet Dev* 2000;10:157-161.

Kao GD, Mckenna WG, Yen TJ. Detection of repair activity during the DNA damage-induced G2 delay in human cancer cells. *Oncogene* 2001;20:3486-3496.

Kee Y, D'Andrea AD. Expanded roles of the Fanconi anemia pathway in preserving genomic stability. *Genes Dev* 2010;24:1680-1694.

Kennedy RD, Chen CC, Stuckert P, et al. Fanconi anemia pathway-deficient tumor cells are hypersensitive to inhibition of ataxia telangiectasia mutated. *J Clin Invest* 2007;117:1440-1449.

Khanna KK, Jackson SP. DNA double-strand breaks: signaling, repair and the cancer connection. *Nat Genet* 2001;27:247-254.

Kolas NK, Chapman JR, Nakada S, et al. Orchestration of the DNA-damage response by the RNF8 ubiquitin ligase. *Science* 2007;318:1637-1640.

Kress S, Sutter C, Strickland PT, Mukhtar H, Schweizer J, Schwarz M. Carcinogen-specific mutational pattern in the p53 gene in ultraviolet B radiation-induced squamous cell carcinomas of mouse skin. *Cancer Res* 1992;52:6400-6403.

Lapenna S, Giordano A. Cell cycle kinases as therapeutic targets for cancer. *Nat Rev Drug Discov* 2009;8:547-566.

Lee HW, Blasco MA, Gottlieb GJ, Horner JW 2nd, Greider CW, Depinho RA. Essential role of mouse telomerase in highly proliferative organs. *Nature* 1998;392:569-574.

Liang SH, Clarke MF. Regulation of p53 localization. *Eur J Biochem* 2001;268:2779-2783.

Lim DS, Hasty P. A mutation in mouse rad51 results in an early embryonic lethal that is suppressed by a mutation in p53. *Mol Cell Biol* 1996;16:7133-7143.

Lim DS, Kim ST, Xu B, et al. ATM phosphorylates p95/nbs1 in an S-phase checkpoint pathway. *Nature* 2000;404:613-617.

Lin J, Epel E, Blackburn E. Telomeres and lifestyle factors: roles in cellular aging. *Mutat Res* 2011;730:85-89.

Little JB. Failla Memorial Lecture. Changing views of cellular radiosensitivity. *Radiat Res* 1994;140:299-311.

Little JB. Radiation carcinogenesis. *Carcinogenesis* 2000;21:397-404.

Liu Y, Harrington L. Murine models of dysfunctional telomeres and telomerase. In: Autexier C, Lue NF, eds. *Telomerases: Chemistry, Biology, and Clinical Applications.* 1st ed. New York, NY: John Wiley: 2012;213-242.

Lobrich M, Shibata A, Beucher A, et al. gammaH2AX foci analysis for monitoring DNA double-strand break repair: strengths, limitations and optimization. *Cell Cycle* 2010;9:662-669.

Loeb LA. Mutator phenotype may be required for multistage carcinogenesis. *Cancer Res* 1991;51:3075-3079.

Longhese MP. DNA damage response at functional and dysfunctional telomeres. *Genes Dev* 2008;22:125-140.

MacPhail SH, Banath JP, Yu TY, Chu EH, Lambur H, Olive PL. Expression of phosphorylated histone H2AX in cultured cell lines following exposure to x-rays. *Int J Radiat Biol* 2003;79: 351-358.

Mailand N, Bekker-Jensen S, Faustrup H, et al. RNF8 ubiquitylates histones at DNA double-strand breaks and promotes assembly of repair proteins. *Cell* 2007;131:887-900.

Marmorstein LY, Ouchi T, Aaronson SA. The BRCA2 gene product functionally interacts with p53 and RAD51. *Proc Natl Acad Sci U S A* 1998;95:13869-13874.

Martin SA, Lord CJ, Ashworth A. Therapeutic targeting of the DNA mismatch repair pathway. *Clin Cancer Res* 2010;16:5107-5113.

Matsuoka S, Ballif BA, Smogorzewska A, et al. ATM and ATR substrate analysis reveals extensive protein networks responsive to DNA damage. *Science* 2007;316:1160-1166.

McPherson JP, Hande MP, Poonepalli A, et al. A role for Brca1 in chromosome end maintenance. *Hum Mol Genet* 2006;15:831-838.

McVey M, Lee SE. MMEJ repair of double-strand breaks (directors cut): deleted sequences and alternative endings. *Trends Genet* 2008;24:529-538.

Moldovan GL, D'Andrea AD. How the Fanconi anemia pathway guards the genome. *Annu Rev Genet* 2009;43:223-249.

Momparler RL. Cancer epigenetics. *Oncogene* 2003;22:6479-6483.

Morgan WF, Hartmann A, Limoli CL, Nagar S, Ponnaiya B. Bystander effects in radiation-induced genomic instability. *Mutat Res* 2002;504:91-100.

Moynahan ME, Pierce AJ, Jasin M. BRCA2 is required for homology-directed repair of chromosomal breaks. *Mol Cell* 2001;7:263-272.

Murnane JP, Sabatier L. Chromosome rearrangements resulting from telomere dysfunction and their role in cancer. *Bioessays* 2004;26:1164-1174.

Musacchio A, Hardwick KG. The spindle checkpoint: structural insights into dynamic signalling. *Nat Rev Mol Cell Biol* 2002;3:731-741.

Narod SA, Foulkes WD. BRCA1 and BRCA2: 1994 and beyond. *Nat Rev Cancer* 2004;4:665-676.

Nelson WG, Kastan MB. DNA strand breaks: the DNA template alterations that trigger p53-dependent DNA damage response pathways. *Mol Cell Biol* 1994;14:1815-1823.

O'Donovan PJ, Livingston DM. BRCA1 and BRCA2: breast/ovarian cancer susceptibility gene products and participants in DNA double-strand break repair. *Carcinogenesis* 2010;31:961-967.

Offer H, Milyavsky M, Erez N, et al. Structural and functional involvement of p53 in BER in vitro and in vivo. *Oncogene* 2001;20:581-589.

Otto E, McCord S, Tlsty TD. Increased incidence of CAD gene amplification in tumorigenic rat lines as an indicator of genomic instability of neoplastic cells. *J Biol Chem* 1989;264:3390-3396.

Palmero EI, Achatz MI, Ashton-Prolla P, Olivier M, Hainaut P. Tumor protein 53 mutations and inherited cancer: beyond Li-Fraumeni syndrome. *Curr Opin Oncol* 2010;22:64-69.

Pang D, Yoo S, Dynan WS, Jung M, Dritschilo A. Ku proteins join DNA fragments as shown by atomic force microscopy. *Cancer Res* 1997;57:1412-1415.

Panier S, Durocher D. Regulatory ubiquitylation in response to DNA double-strand breaks. *DNA Repair (Amst)* 2009;8: 436-443.

Peltomaki P. Deficient DNA mismatch repair: a common etiologic factor for colon cancer. *Hum Mol Genet* 2001;10:735-740.

Perkins EJ, Nair A, Cowley DO, Van Dyke T, Chang Y, Ramsden DA. Sensing of intermediates in V(D)J recombination by ATM. *Genes Dev* 2002;16:159-164.

Pickett HA, Henson JD, Au AY, Neumann AA, Reddel RR. Normal mammalian cells negatively regulate telomere length by telomere trimming. *Hum Mol Genet* 2011;20:4684-4692.

Price CM, Boltz KA, Chaiken MF, Stewart JA, Beilstein MA, Shippen DE. Evolution of CST function in telomere maintenance. *Cell Cycle* 2010;9:3157-3165.

Richardson C, Jasin M. Coupled homologous and nonhomologous repair of a double-strand break preserves genomic integrity in mammalian cells. *Mol Cell Biol* 2000;20:9068-9075.

Rogakou EP, Boon C, Redon C, Bonner WM. Megabase chromatin domains involved in DNA double-strand breaks in vivo. *J Cell Biol* 1999;146:905-916.

Romanov SR, Kozakiewicz BK, Holst CR, Stampfer MR, Haupt LM, Tlsty TD. Normal human mammary epithelial cells spontaneously escape senescence and acquire genomic changes. *Nature* 2001;409:633-637.

Rotman G, Shiloh Y. ATM: from gene to function. *Hum Mol Genet* 1998;7:1555-1563.

Sancar A, Lindsey-Boltz LA, Unsal-Kacmaz K, Linn S. Molecular mechanisms of mammalian DNA repair and the DNA damage checkpoints. *Annu Rev Biochem* 2004;73:39-85.

Sasai K, Evans JW, Kovacs MS, Brown JM. Prediction of human cell radiosensitivity: comparison of clonogenic assay with chromosome aberrations scored using premature chromosome condensation with fluorescence in situ hybridization. *Int J Radiat Oncol Biol Phys* 1994;30:1127-1132.

Savage SA, Dokal I, Armanios M, et al. Dyskeratosis congenita: the first NIH clinical research workshop. *Pediatr Blood Cancer* 2009;53:520-523.

Sedelnikova OA, Rogakou EP, Panyutin IG, Bonner WM. Quantitative detection of (125)IdU-induced DNA double-strand breaks with gamma-H2AX antibody. *Radiat Res* 2002;158: 486-492.

Stewart GS, Panier S, Townsend K, et al. The RIDDLE syndrome protein mediates a ubiquitin-dependent signaling cascade at sites of DNA damage. *Cell* 2009;136:420-434.

Stewart ZA, Westfall MD, Pietenpol JA. Cell-cycle dysregulation and anticancer therapy. *Trends Pharmacol Sci* 2003;24:139-145.

Stiff T, Walker SA, Cerosaletti K, et al. ATR-dependent phosphorylation and activation of ATM in response to UV treatment or replication fork stalling. *EMBO J* 2006;25:5775-5782.

Svendsen JM, Harper JW. GEN1/Yen1 and the SLX4 complex: solutions to the problem of Holliday junction resolution. *Genes Dev* 2010;24:521-536.

Syljuasen RG, Krolewski B, Little JB. Molecular events in radiation transformation. *Radiat Res* 2001;155:215-221.

Tabori U, Dome JS. Telomere biology of pediatric cancer. *Cancer Invest* 2007;25:197-208.

Tlsty TD. Normal diploid human and rodent cells lack a detectable frequency of gene amplification. *Proc Natl Acad Sci U S A* 1990;87:3132-3136.

Tutt A, Robson M, Garber JE, et al. Oral poly(ADP-ribose) polymerase inhibitor olaparib in patients with BRCA1 or BRCA2 mutations and advanced breast cancer: a proof-of-concept trial. *Lancet* 2010;376:235-244.

van Gent DC, Hoeijmakers JH, Kanaar R. Chromosomal stability and the DNA double-strand break connection. *Nat Rev Genet* 2001;2:196-206.

Vaziri H, Benchimol S. Reconstitution of telomerase activity in normal human cells leads to elongation of telomeres and extended replicative life span. *Curr Biol* 1998;8:279-282.

Vaziri H, Squire JA, Pandita TK, et al. Analysis of genomic integrity and p53-dependent G1 checkpoint in telomerase-induced extended-life-span human fibroblasts. *Mol Cell Biol* 1999;19: 2373-2379.

Venteicher AS, Artandi SE. TCAB1: driving telomerase to Cajal bodies. *Cell Cycle* 2009;8:1329-1331.

Vermeulen W. Dynamics of mammalian NER proteins. *DNA Repair (Amst)* 2011;10:760-771.

Vukovic B, Beheshti B, Park P, et al. Correlating breakage-fusion-bridge events with the overall chromosomal instability and in vitro karyotype evolution in prostate cancer. *Cytogenet Genome Res* 2007;116:1-11.

Vukovic B, Park PC, Al-Maghrabi J, et al. Evidence of multifocality of telomere erosion in high-grade prostatic intraepithelial neoplasia (HPIN) and concurrent carcinoma. *Oncogene* 2003;22:1978-1987.

Wang X, Liu L, Montagna C, Ried T, Deng CX. Haploinsufficiency of Parp1 accelerates Brca1-associated centrosome amplification, telomere shortening, genetic instability, apoptosis, and embryonic lethality. *Cell Death Differ* 2007;14:924-931.

Weissberg JB, Huang DD, Swift M. Radiosensitivity of normal tissues in ataxia-telangiectasia heterozygotes. *Int J Radiat Oncol Biol Phys* 1998;42:1133-1136.

Whitaker SJ, Powell SN, Mcmillan TJ. Molecular assays of radiation-induced DNA damage. *Eur J Cancer* 1991;27:922-928.

Woodward WA, Bristow RG. Radiosensitivity of cancer-initiating cells and normal stem cells (or what the Heisenberg uncertainly principle has to do with biology). *Semin Radiat Oncol* 2009;19:87-95.

Wu P, de Lange T. No overt nucleosome eviction at deprotected telomeres. *Mol Cell Biol* 2008;28:5724-5735.

Zhang X, Mar V, Zhou W, Harrington L, Robinson MO. Telomere shortening and apoptosis in telomerase-inhibited human tumor cells. *Genes Dev* 1999;13:2388-2399.

Zhou PK, Sproston AR, Marples B, West CM, Margison GP, Hendry JH. The radiosensitivity of human fibroblast cell lines correlates with residual levels of DNA double-strand breaks. *Radiother Oncol* 1998;47:271-276.

Ziegler A, Leffell DJ, Kunala S, et al. Mutation hotspots due to sunlight in the p53 gene of nonmelanoma skin cancers. *Proc Natl Acad Sci U S A* 1993;90:4216-4220.

Oncogenic Viruses and Tumor Viruses

6

Fei-Fei Liu and Christopher D. Richardson

6.1 INTRODUCTION

Viruses are implicated in approximately 15% to 20% of all cancers (reviewed by Nevins, 2007; Ou and Yen, 2010). They can cause malignancies that include nasopharyngeal carcinoma, Burkitt lymphoma, cervical carcinoma, T-cell leukemia/lymphoma, hepatocellular carcinoma, Merkel cell carcinoma, and Kaposi sarcoma. Even more importantly, oncogenes and tumor-suppressor proteins were first identified through the study of cancer-causing viruses. For example, research with simian virus 40 led to the discovery of tumor-suppressor genes, p53 and the retinoblastoma gene (Rb). Oncogenic viruses fall into 2 groups: the DNA tumor viruses that contain either linear or circular double-stranded DNA and the RNA-containing tumor viruses (also called *retroviruses*). DNA tumor viruses usually cause malignant transformation by inhibiting the normal function (growth control) of tumor-suppressor genes (see Chap. 7, Sec. 7.6), whereas retroviruses usually deregulate signal transduction pathways (see Chap. 8).

Stehelin et al (1976) demonstrated that Rous sarcoma virus (a retrovirus that causes sarcomas in chickens) contained nucleotide sequences that were not found in similar nontransforming retroviruses. These novel retroviral sequences, however, were closely related to nucleotide sequences present in the DNA of normal chickens. This important discovery indicated that a viral transforming gene (in this case v-*src*) was derived from a normal cellular gene. Many other retroviruses have been studied since and have been shown to contain different oncogenes derived from and closely related to their cellular counterparts. The normal cellular genes from which the retroviral oncogenes (v-*onc*) are derived are referred to as *protooncogenes* (or c-*onc*). The process by which protooncogenes become integrated into the viral genome and are converted to viral oncogenes with overt transforming activity is complex; it involves recombination between the retroviral and cellular genomes following integration of a retrovirus adjacent to a cellular protooncogene. This process, known as *transduction*, is accompanied by alterations in the structure and regulation of oncogene sequences. Many of the oncogenes found in transforming retroviruses have also been identified independently in spontaneously arising tumors of nonviral origin, where they appear to be activated by other mechanisms, including point mutation, gene amplification, and chromosomal translocation.

Protooncogenes encode a wide range of protein products involved in the control of cell proliferation and differentiation, including growth factors, growth factor receptors, components of signal transduction pathways, and transcription factors that regulate the synthesis of messenger RNA (mRNA). Tumor-suppressor genes, in contrast, represent genes that are likely to play a role in negatively regulating cell growth. In this chapter, the mechanisms of cellular transformation by oncogenic viruses are described. These mechanisms provide clues to more general mechanisms of transformation caused by increases in dominantly acting oncogenes or inactivation of tumor-suppressor genes.

6.2 DNA TUMOR VIRUSES

6.2.1 Polyomaviruses

The polyomaviruses include simian virus 40 (SV40), mouse polyomavirus, and 8 human viruses, JC virus, BK virus, KI virus, WU virus, HPyV6, HPyV7, HPyV9, and Merkel cell carcinoma virus (van Ghelue et al, 2012). Presently, genome sequences of approximately 21 polyomaviruses infecting humans, nonhuman primates, birds, bats, rabbits, and rodents have been deposited in GenBank. Although the roles of this family of viruses in human cancers is still not clear, SV40 and mouse polyomavirus have yielded valuable information about the process of cellular transformation by DNA viruses (Atkin et al, 2009; Gjoerup and Chang, 2010). SV40 and mouse polyomavirus may cause tumors in newborn hamsters but have not been associated directly with human cancer. Mouse polyomavirus was found to cause tumors in the salivary glands of mice and subsequently in many other organs, leading to the name by which it is known. The SV40 virus was identified as a contaminant in poliomyelitis virus vaccines prepared in rhesus monkey cells and caused widespread concern after it was discovered that the virus yielded tumors in newborn hamsters. The virus was injected unwittingly into millions of people. Epidemiological studies of people who received the vaccine gave no evidence that it can cause cancer in humans. However, the fact that SV40 gene sequences were identified in some human tumors, including ependymomas, mesotheliomas, and osteosarcomas renewed fears that the virus might contribute to human carcinogenesis, and the presence of SV40 DNA sequences and T antigens in these tumors has been reported (reviewed in Jasani et al, 2001; Qi et al, 2011). Although it is unlikely that SV40 infection alone causes human malignancy, SV40 may act as a cofactor in the pathogenesis of these tumors. JC and BK viruses are associated with progressive multifocal leukoencephalopathy and interstitial nephritis, respectively, but are less studied. Sporadic reports also describe their presence in some primary brain tumors, osteosarcomas, lymphomas, and colon cancers (reviewed in Boothpur and Brennan, 2010). Most recently, a polyomavirus was shown to be associated with the skin cancer Merkel cell carcinoma using DNA sequencing and digital transcriptome subtraction (Feng et al, 2008). The viral genome is found in cancerous lesions derived from resident Merkel cells of the skin, which comprise the epidermal mechanoreceptors involved in touch discrimination (reviewed in Gjoerup and Chang, 2010; Schrama et al, 2012). It affects immunosuppressed individuals including the elderly, people with AIDS, and posttransplantation patients, and is normally treated with surgery and radiation. The 5-year survival rate is about 75%, 60%, and 25% for localized, regional, and lymphatic forms of this cancer, respectively.

The polyomaviruses interact with susceptible cells in 2 different ways. In permissive cells that support productive infection, the lytic cycle proceeds in 2 phases: an early phase in which nonstructural, regulatory proteins are synthesized, and a late phase during which viral DNA is replicated, coat protein is made, and progeny virions are assembled. Viral DNA is not integrated in the cellular genome during the lytic cycle. Release of mature virus particles results in lysis and cell death. Monkey cells are permissive for SV40 infection, whereas mouse cells are permissive for mouse polyoma infection. A second type of interaction leads to a small proportion of surviving transformed cells that contain viral DNA integrated randomly into host chromosomes. Transformation occurs more commonly in cells that are unable to efficiently support viral replication. In contrast to normal cells, virus-transformed cells show little or no contact inhibition and therefore grow to high cell density in culture; they give rise to multilayered and disorganized cell colonies, show anchorage-independent growth in a semisolid medium containing agar or methylcellulose, and exhibit a decreased requirement for serum. Cells transformed in culture after infection, give rise to tumors when inoculated into susceptible animals.

Polyomaviruses are small, nonenveloped icosahedral viruses that contain circular, double-stranded DNA genomes of about 5 kbp in length (Fig. 6–1). Early gene products are transcribed immediately after the virus enters the cell, followed by the transport of its genome to the nucleus of the host cell. Late genes are transcribed after viral DNA replication begins, and serve to produce viral structural proteins (VP1, VP2, VP3) and Agno-protein, in the case of SV40. The major capsid protein, VP1 interacts with the host cell receptor, which is believed to be the major histocompatability complex class I protein (MHC I) for SV40, and sialic acid for polyomavirus. Agno-protein is a small multifunctional polypeptide implicated in viral transcription, replication, assembly, and release. It can function as a viroporin, bind to other viral proteins (LT, ST, PP2A), and interacts with cellular proteins (HP1α, FEZ1, Ku70, p53, YB-1). The gene for Agno-proteins is not expressed in all polyomaviruses and its exact mechanism of action remains to be determined (Gerits and Moens, 2012). Viral DNA replication, transcription, and virion assembly occur in the nucleus. The early genes of SV40 include large T antigen, small t antigens, and 17-kDa protein (Fig. 6–1A) and the early genes of polyomavirus are large T, middle T, and small t antigens. These gene products possess transforming properties.

The large T antigens of the polyomaviruses are complex multifunctional proteins and the functional domains of SV40 T antigen are summarized in Figure 6–1B (reviewed in Cheng et al, 2009; Gjoerup and Chang, 2010). These domains are similar for the closely related large T antigens in all polyomaviruses. More than 95% of large T antigen is associated with the nucleus but a small portion is found linked to the plasma membrane. The protein is phosphorylated, O-glycosylated, adenosine diphosphate (ADP)-ribosylated, is associated with Zn^{++}, binds adenosine triphosphate (ATP), and possesses a nuclear localization signal (NLS). The large T antigen binds the viral DNA origin of replication in the form of double hexamer structures and functions as the switch between early and late transcription. This protein has DNA helicase activity, unwinds double-stranded DNA, and hydrolyzes ATP in the

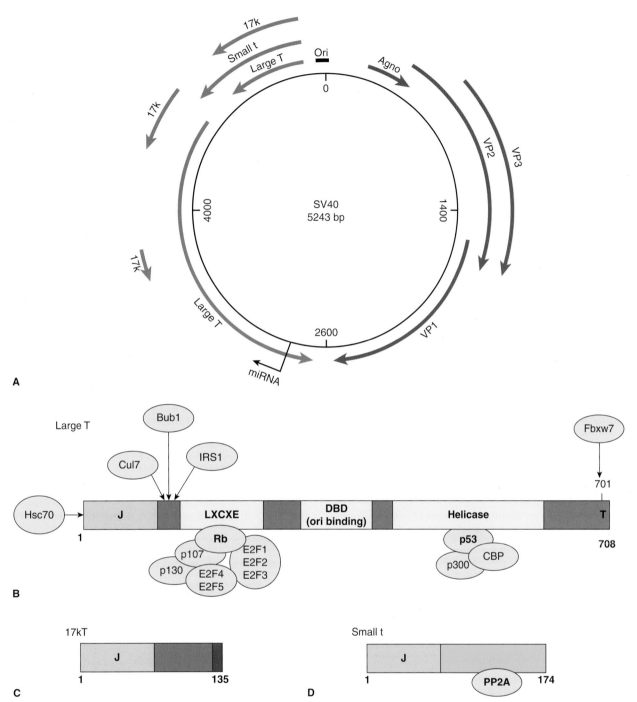

FIGURE 6-1 **Simian virus 40 (SV40) gene expression. A)** The SV40 genome consists of a circular duplex DNA molecule. Primary transcripts are expressed from opposite DNA strands that constitute early (*blue*) and late (*red*) viral mRNA. The largest of the 3 early mRNA spliced transcripts encodes large-T antigen. The shorter early transcripts encode the small t antigen and 17-kDa protein. The aminoterminal 82 residues of the small t and 17-kDa proteins are identical. The late mRNA encoding the VP1, VP2, and VP3 structural proteins and Agno-protein as indicated. **B)** Schematic representation of the functional domains of large T antigen. Both p53 and pRb, the products of 2 cellular tumor-suppressor genes, interact with large T antigen. The Rb protein binds to the LXCXE motif, which can also bind to the Rb-related proteins p107 and p130. Rb family proteins normally bind and sequester the cellular transcription factors E2F1, E2F2, E2F3, E2F4, and E2F5 inhibiting transcription. Binding of Rb to LXCXE allows the release of E2F factors resulting in transcription and cell-cycle progression into S phase (see Chap. 9, Sec. 9.2.3). The p53 and CBP/p300 proteins bind to a similar region in the helicase domain. T antigen has DNA helicase and adenosine triphosphatase (ATPase) activity for its replication function with cellular DNA polymerase and DNA binding proteins. This protein is the switch between early and late transcription, and T-antigen binds to the origin of replication through the Ori DNA binding domain (DBD). The protein is phosphorylated, binds Zn^{++}, and has a host range or species specific domain (hr/hf) at the extreme carboxyl terminus. **C)** The 17-kDa protein is a truncated version of large T antigen and contains a J region and RB binding region. It has immortalizing and transforming properties. **D)** The small t antigen is distinct in sequence and binds and inhibits the cellular phosphatase PP2A.

process. Large T antigen contains 3 domains involved in the transformation and immortalization of rodent cells (Cheng et al, 2009; Gjoerup and Chang, 2010). The N-terminal J domain stimulates both viral replication and enhances oncogenic transformation. It binds specifically to the heat shock protein Hsp70 and activates its adenosine triphosphatase (ATPase) activity during the process of chaperone-mediated protein folding. The J domain also functionally inactivates the p130 and p107 Rb proteins and promotes their degradation. Next to the J domain is another protein region, which contains the LXCXE (leu-amino acid-cysteine-amino acid-glu) motif that is found in proteins that interact with molecules in the Rb family. The Rb protein (p105) and related proteins p107 and p130 function by normally binding to and blocking the functions of E2F transcription factors. Rb preferentially binds to "activating" E2Fs (E2F4/5) whereas p107/p130 bind "repressing" E2Fs (E2F4/5). The large T antigen binds to pRb, p107, or p130, disrupting their regulator roles and activating or repressing specific genes that are associated with cell-cycle progression (reviewed in DeCaprio, 2009). Finally, another transformation domain found in the T antigen of SV40, forms complexes with p53 and led to the discovery of this tumor-suppressor gene. This interaction was originally discovered in 1979 and heralded the recognition of cellular tumor-suppressor proteins (Lane and Crawford, 1979; Linzer and Levine, 1979). T antigen binding to p53 inhibits apoptosis and favors cell-cycle progression. Transfection of the gene encoding large T antigen may alone cause the malignant transformation of normal rodent cells, although the presence of the small t antigen contributes to the full expression of an SV40-transformed phenotype. The T antigen of SV40 can also bind to other factors including cullin 7 (involved in ubiquitination), IRS1 (an insulin-like growth factor receptor), p300/CBP (histone acetylase transcription factors), Bub1 (kinase involved in mitotic checkpoint control), and Fbxw7 (ubiquitination of cyclin E, Myc, Notch, and Jun; see Chap. 8, Fig. 8–9 and Chap. 9, Fig. 9–4). These interactions are summarized in Figure 6–1B. The 3D structures of large T antigen complexed to p53 and the origin DNA was reported (Bochkareva et al, 2006; Lilyestrom et al, 2006). Expression of large T antigen alone, or in combination with small t antigen, will transform most rodent cell types. Transgenic mice that contain the SV40 large T antigen gene develop a high incidence of tumors in organs in which the gene is expressed (reviewed in Saenz Robles and Pipas, 2009).

The small t antigens of SV40 and polyomavirus also function in transformation. Small t antigen is dispensable for lytic growth of the virus but it does favor cell-cycle progression (G1-S) through activation of growth factor signal transduction pathways, via interaction with the catalytic and structural subunits of protein phosphatase 2A (PP2A). By displacing the structural subunit, small t antigen inhibits phosphatase activity and upregulates kinase activity in mitogen-activated protein kinase (MAPK), stress-activated protein kinase (SAPK), protein kinase C (PKC), phophatidylinositol-3 kinase (PI-3 kinase), protein kinase B (PKB/

AKT) and nuclear factor kappa B (NF-κB) pathways (Pallas et al, 1990). The middle T antigen of mouse polyomavirus localizes to the plasma membrane and interacts with components of signal transduction pathways including c-src and PI-3 kinase to upregulate MAPK and PKB/AKT activity (Auger et al, 1992; see Chap. 8 for details of pathways). Because middle T antigen also contains most of the sequence of small t antigen, it can also complex with and inhibit the effects of PP2A (Pallas et al, 1990). The interactions of all 3 T antigens with specific cellular components favor cell-cycle progression, cell division, activate growth factor pathways, and inhibit apoptosis. These 3 proteins account for all of the oncogenic properties of the polyomaviruses.

6.2.2 Human Adenoviruses

Adenoviruses are common and can cause acute infections of the upper respiratory tract, infantile gastroenteritis, pharyngitis, and conjunctivitis (reviewed in Berk, 2007). Most people have antibodies directed against 1 or more of these viruses. Aside from adenovirus type 12, which can cause tumors in newborn hamsters, adenoviruses have never been associated with human tumor development. Human cells infected with adenovirus undergo lytic infection, whereas rodent cells are less permissive for growth of the virus and readily survive infection to undergo transformation. The ability of human adenoviruses to induce tumors in rodents and transform cells in culture has rendered them as important tools to study malignant transformation.

Adenoviruses are icosahedral particles with "antennae-like" fibers emanating from the vertices of the icosahedron (Fig. 6–2A) that are composed of 11 structural proteins (Berk, 2007). The 35-kbp linear, double-stranded DNA genome is organized into early and late transcription units (Fig. 6–2B), containing 5 early transcription units (E1A, E1B, E2, E3, and E4), and 1 major late unit that is spliced to generate 5 families of late mRNAs (L1 to L5) that encode the structural viral proteins. Cells transformed with adenoviruses contain an incomplete viral genome that always includes the viral *E1A* (early region 1A) and *E1B* genes integrated into host DNA. This minimal region of adenovirus DNA has the capacity to transform rat embryo cells following DNA-mediated gene transfer.

Two mRNA species, 12S and 13S, are produced by differential splicing from *E1A* and encode similar proteins of 243 and 289 amino acids that function as transcription activators. These 2 proteins differ internally by an additional 46 amino acids that are unique to the 13S product. Multiple transcripts also originate from the *E1B* gene, giving rise to 2 major proteins of 19 kDa and 55 kDa, which can block apoptosis (see Chap. 9). E2 encodes the proteins E2A and E2B that function in DNA replication. E3 proteins are also multiply spliced gene products that are designated by their molecular masses and interfere with immune response. E4 proteins are a diverse family of proteins that mediate transcription, mRNA transport, modulate DNA replication, and inhibit apoptosis.

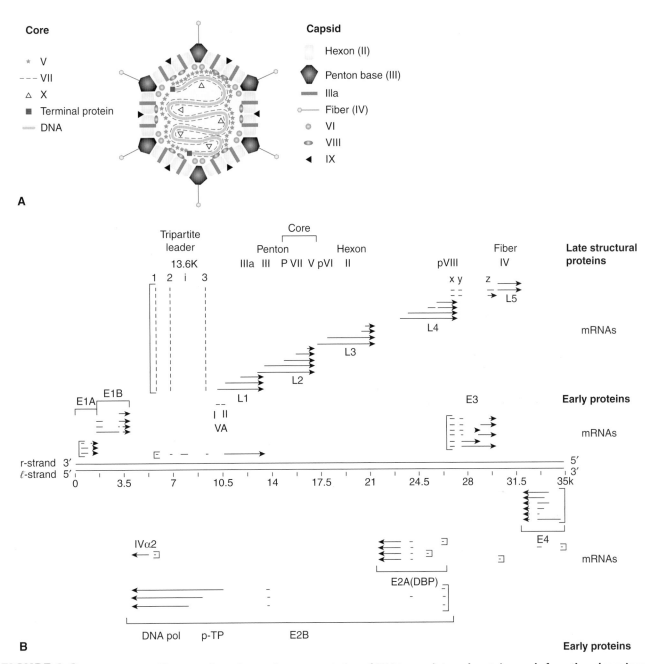

FIGURE 6-2 **The structure of human adenovirus and a representation of RNA transcripts and proteins made from the adenovirus genome. A)** The virus consists of capsid and core proteins. Core proteins include hexon, penton base, IIIa, fiber, VI, VIII, and IX proteins. The core contains the double-stranded DNA genome, major core proteins (V, VII), terminal proteins, and minor core protein (X). **B)** The genome is a template for early gene transcripts (E1A, E1B, E2, E3, E4) and late gene transcripts (L1, L2, L3, L4, L5). Early gene products cause transformation, inhibit apoptosis, regulate DNA replication, and block the immune response. Late gene products code for structural proteins (penton, core, hexon, pVIII, and fiber) and mRNA is transcribed from the major late promoter.

In gene-transfer experiments, both E1A gene products immortalize primary rodent cells and complement an activated *ras* gene to transform cells. *E1B* can replace *ras* in this type of assay to promote transformation. Additional functions attributed to E1A protein include its ability to either activate or repress transcription from cellular and viral genes dependent on enhancer sequences. Comparison of the E1A amino acid sequence among several adenovirus serotypes shows the presence of 3 conserved regions (CR1, CR2, and CR3). Mutational analysis of the E1A region has revealed that CR1 (amino acids 40 to 80) and CR2 (amino acids 121 to 139) are necessary for transformation, whereas CR3 (amino acids 140 to 188) is dispensable (Moran and Mathews, 1987). The E1A regions required for control of cell growth, blockade of differentiation, and transformation comprise the nonconserved amino terminus together with CR1 and CR2. CR2 contains the

LXCXE motif that binds to pRb and is also present in SV40 large T antigen and in the E7 protein of human papillomaviruses. E1A can activate transcription by E2F by promoting its dissociation from pRb (DeCaprio, 2009) and promotes cell-cycle progression, moving the infected cell into S phase. E1A also blocks acetylation of histones and inhibits the transcription of certain genes. Both of these processes are thought to play a role in E1A-mediated transformation.

The E1B55K protein binds p53 and inhibits its transactivation function as well as p53-dependent apoptosis (Harada and Berk, 1999). Unlike E1A, expression of the E1B55K protein alone is insufficient to stimulate resting cells to enter S phase. The E1B19K protein has many activities, all of which tend to block apoptosis and favor cell survival. It is a member of the antiapoptotic Bcl-2 family and has been shown to block both Fas and tumor necrosis factor (TNF)-mediated apoptosis by interacting with Bax (Han et al, 1996). In addition, E1B19K can upregulate SAPK (see Chap. 8, Sec. 8.2.4) to increase transcription and expression of c-jun, promoting cell survival (See and Shih, 1998).

Adenoviruses have been shown to antagonize the immune system. The E1A protein and viral-associated RNAs inhibit the protective effects of interferons α and β. E3 proteins block induction of apoptosis by cytotoxic T lymphocytes (CTLs) and macrophages, and interfere with the processing and presentation of peptide antigens (see Chap. 21, Fig. 21–2). Gene products of the E3 region can be deleted without affecting infections in culture, but these mutations dramatically reduce infections in vivo.

Adenoviruses have been evaluated extensively for cancer gene therapy with multiple reengineering strategies (Pesonen et al, 2011; reviewed in Yamamoto and Curiel, 2010). One of the earliest manipulations was Onyx-015 (or dl-1520), wherein the viruses cannot synthesize the E1B55K protein, facilitating its preferential replication in tumor cells (Bischoff et al, 1996). A similar version of the *E1B-55K*-deleted adenovirus, called H101, was developed and approved for use in China. It was administered via intratumoral injection in combination with chemotherapy for patients with head and neck squamous cell carcinoma, and demonstrated higher response rates than in patients treated with cisplatin alone (Yu and Fang, 2007). However, because of the limitations of intratumoral injections, these strategies have never evolved into broader applications or lived up to the expectations derived from animal experiments. Furthermore, an unfortunate incident resulted in a fatal outcome in one individual 4 days into a gene therapy trial (Marshall, 1999), which was likely related to a severe immune reaction directed against the adenovirus proteins in the liver. This slowed the development of adenovirus based vectors for gene therapy and oncolytic treatment. In addition the lack of specific viral receptors (CAR) in the tumor, the presence of preexisting antibodies against Ad5 serotype, and the need for more stringent replicative selectivity for cancer cells, have tempered enthusiasm for oncolytic adenovirus therapy (Yamamoto and Curiel, 2010).

6.2.3 Human Papillomaviruses

Human papillomaviruses (HPVs) are nonenveloped DNA viruses that infect epithelial cells to cause warts in the skin, condylomas in mucous membranes, and malignancies of the cervix, vulva, and anal canal, and recently, head and neck cancers (Moody and Laimins, 2010; reviewed in zur Hausen, 2002). Papillomaviruses contain a single molecule of circular double-stranded DNA that is about 8 kb in length, which encodes 8 "early" genes (*E1* to *E8*) and 2 "late" genes (*L1* and *L2*). In addition there is a noncoding regulatory region called the long control region (LCR) (Fig. 6–3A). The functions of the various proteins are as follows: L1 is the major capsid protein whereas L2 is a minor capsid protein that associates with genomic DNA. E1 directs initiation of DNA replication and E2 is a transcription activator that has an auxiliary role in replication. The function of E3 is not known, whereas E4 disrupts cytokeratins and is important for viral release. E5 is a membrane protein with transforming properties that interacts with growth factor receptors, and regulates protein trafficking. E6 is a transforming protein that targets p53 for degradation in the ubiquitin pathway. E7 is a transforming protein that binds to the Rb protein. The function of E8 remains unknown.

Papillomaviruses have been difficult to study and propagate in culture because they replicate in stratified squamous epithelium, a property that cannot be duplicated in monolayer cell cultures. The virus reaches the basal layers of the epithelium where it can replicate through a process of mechanical stress and damage to the keratinized epithelium. Virus is taken into the host cell through receptor-mediated endocytosis and is transported to the nucleus. Early gene transcription and translation of early proteins and limited replication of the viral genome occur in the basal squamous epithelial cell. The transcription and production of late capsid proteins (L1, L2), high levels of DNA replication, and virus assembly occur in the keratinized epithelium. Virus is released as the stratum corneum is sloughed from the surface of the skin or mucosa.

More than 100 different types of HPV have been identified. These viruses infect only epithelial cells and are associated mostly with benign mucosal and cutaneous lesions, such as warts in the skin and anogenital regions. Low-risk anogenital warts can be caused by several HPV types—including HPV6, -10, and -11—that infect the genital tract and are associated also with low grades of cervical intraepithelial neoplasia that regress spontaneously; they are rarely found in malignant tumors. Anogenital warts are prevalent among young sexually active adults and their incidence increased 6-fold between 1966 and 1981 during the sexual revolution.

Cervical cancer is the third most common cancer in women worldwide and is a sexually transmitted disease that is associated with high-risk HPV types including HPV16, -18, -31, -33, and -45, that are found in approximately 90% of all cervical cancers (reviewed in zur Hausen, 2002). However, these HPV types have also been detected in nonmalignant cervical tissue, and only a small proportion of women with clinically

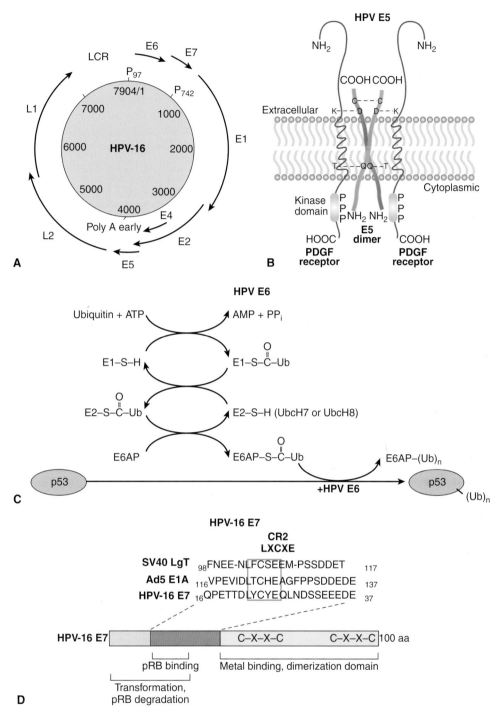

FIGURE 6–3 **A) Organization of the HPV-16 genome.** The papillomavirus genome is double-stranded circular DNA, but the genes are expressed from only 1 strand in a unidirectional manner. The coding regions for viral proteins in all 3 possible translation phases are indicated by the solid heavy lines and are based on the complete DNA sequence. *E* and *L* stand for early and late proteins, respectively. There are 6 open reading frames that code for early proteins (E1, E2, E4, E5, E6, E7) and 2 for the late structural proteins (L1, L2). P_{97} and P_{742} are the promoters used in transcription. **B)** E5 protein of papillomavirus dimerizes through an intermolecular disulfide bond linkage and interacts with platelet-derived growth factor receptor (PDGFR). Aggregation of the receptor occurs through ionic (lysine-aspartic acid, K-D) or hydrogen bond (threonine glutamine, T-Q) interactions to activate the receptor associated tyrosine kinase. **C)** E6 is a ubiquitin ligase that catalyzes the ubiquitination and subsequent degradation of p53 in the proteosomes. Ubiquitin is then transferred to a ubiquitin conjugating enzyme E2. Ubiquitin is subsequently transferred to E6-associated protein (E6AP), which binds to and ubiquitinates p53 in the presence of HPV E6. Additional ubiquitin molecules can be added to p53 and finally the polyubiquitinated p53 is degraded in the proteasome. **D)** E7 protein binds pRB through an LXCXE (leu-amino acid-cys-amino acid-glu) motif in a CR2 region along with residues in the CR1 domain. It targets the pRB protein for degradation. An adjacent domain contains metal binding and dimerization motifs that can transactivate some genes recognized by E2F. In many respects, the E7 protein is very similar in structure and function to the SV40 large T antigen and adenovirus E1A protein.

apparent high-risk HPV infection eventually develop cervical carcinoma, possibly because many of these infections may be transient. HPV infection is not sufficient for tumor development and other cofactors—such as smoking, use of oral contraceptives, recurrent infection, early pregnancy, and immunological and hormonal status—may play a role in progression to malignancy. In addition to the aforementioned malignancies, HPV has also been associated with nonmelanoma skin cancers, penile cancer, and respiratory malignant papillomas. Immunosuppressed individuals, transplant recipients, and AIDS patients are at higher risk for HPV-related malignancies.

There has been increasing recognition of HPV involvement in head and neck cancers, particularly those located in the oropharyngeal region such as the tonsils, and the base of tongue (Chung and Gillison, 2009). Approximately 60% to 70% of oropharyngeal squamous cell carcinomas diagnosed in North America are associated with HPV. There are multiple purported reasons for this increasing incidence, such as reduction in smoking, but other lifestyle issues likely contribute to this epidemic (D'Souza et al, 2007). Dissimilar to cervix cancer, greater than 90% of HPV involvement in oropharyngeal cancers is dominated by HPV16. Furthermore, HPV-associated oropharyngeal cancers overexpress the cyclin-dependent kinase (CDK) inhibitor CDKN2A or p16, such that p16 immunohistochemistry on formalin-fixed patient biopsies is a diagnostic surrogate for identifying such HPV-infected entities (Shi et al, 2009). HPV-associated oropharyngeal cancers have a superior clinical outcome, with 3-year overall survival rates of approximately 82% to 85% versus 60% to 65% between HPV-positive and HPV-negative cancers (Shi et al, 2009; Ang et al, 2010). Many possibilities have been suggested to explain this difference, including better performance status of patients (younger, more likely to be nonsmokers); increased expression of p16 hence lower proliferative potential; less deleterious *p53* mutations (Westra et al, 2008), and HPV immunological responses. Whole exome sequencing studies have documented that HPV-positive tumors harbor half the mutation rates of HPV-negative malignancies (Stransky et al, 2011). The specific mechanisms remain to be elucidated, but explain the better treatment outcomes for patients with HPV-positive tumors.

The HPV genome is maintained in benign warts as an episome (a nonintegrated, circular form). In malignant cells, HPV DNA is integrated randomly into various chromosomes, resulting in substantial deletions or disruption of the viral genome, particularly the *E2* gene, which has a negative regulatory effect on the expression of the HPV proteins E6 and E7. These latter 2 proteins are always retained and consistently expressed in cervical tumor tissue and cell lines, suggesting that 1 or both of these proteins may be required for transformation by HPV. A comparison of high-risk HPVs, such as HPV16 and HPV18, with low-risk viruses, such as HPV2, HPV4, HPV6, and HPV11, has allowed the mapping of transformation properties to *E5*, *E6*, and *E7* genes. The E5 protein can dimerize and interact with growth factor receptors, such as those for the epidermal growth factor receptor (EGFR) and platelet-derived growth factor receptor (PDGFR), leading to activation of the MAPK pathway (see Chap. 8, Sec. 8.2.4) and cell proliferation (see Fig. 6–3*B*). Gene transfer experiments with primary human fibroblasts or keratinocytes demonstrate that either the *E6* or *E7* genes from the high-risk HPV types, but not from the low-risk HPV types, extend the life span of these cells in culture (Hawley-Nelson et al, 1989; Munger et al, 1989). These cells, however, will not form tumors when injected into nude mice and enter a crisis period in culture. HPV E6 proteins interact with and inactivate the p53 tumor-suppressor protein (see Fig. 6–3*C*). E6 may have additional functions that operate in the transformation process as it can promote hyperplasia in a p53 null background. HPV E7 proteins contain domains similar to the adenovirus E1A protein and large T antigen of SV40; the transforming ability of E7 proteins depends on their binding to pRb tumor-suppressor proteins (Dyson et al, 1989) through a domain that contains the LXCXE motif (see Fig. 6–3*D*). Binding of E7 to pRb favors the degradation of the tumor suppressor and results in the release of the bound E2F transcription factor from pRb to induce cellular DNA synthesis and progression into the S phase of the cell cycle. The E7 protein from low-risk HPV types bind to pRb with at least 10-fold lower efficiency than the E7 protein of HPV16 and HPV17. The E7 protein can also interact with CDK inhibitors such as p27 and p21 (see Chap. 9, Sec. 9.2.2), which may promote the replication of papillomavirus DNA in differentiating squamous epithelial cells. Thus, related mechanisms of transformation seem to be evident for papovaviruses, adenoviruses, and papillomaviruses (see Fig. 6–3*D*).

Prophylactic vaccines directed against the high-risk papillomaviruses have been evaluated and marketed. Gardasil (Merck Pharmaceuticals) is a recombinant quadrivalent vaccine consisting of virus-like particles prepared from synthetic L1 proteins and protects against HPV6, -11, -16, and -18 after a regimen of 3 injections. This vaccine has been demonstrated to be effective for both young women and men at reducing the incidence of intraepithelia neoplastic and external genital lesions, respectively (Future II Study Group, 2007; Giuliano et al, 2011). A similar vaccine, Cervarix (GlaxoSmithKline), designed to target HPV types 16 and 18, is similarly efficacious (Paavonen et al, 2009), is also able to cross-protect against HPV31, -33, -45, and -51 (Wheeler et al, 2012). Despite success in development of these HPV vaccines, and the efficacy of primary prevention, uptake of these vaccines in developed countries ranges from 50% to 80%, indicating that there remain important challenges in these diseases (Ogilvie et al, 2010).

6.2.4 Epstein-Barr Virus

An aggressive lymphoma that affects African children was first described by Dennis Burkitt and is known as Burkitt lymphoma. Cultured cells from these lymphomas were found by Epstein and Barr to release a herpes virus that subsequently became known as *Epstein-Barr virus* (EBV). EBV is transmitted horizontally, usually via contaminated saliva, infecting more than 90% of the human population by the age of 20 years, often without any manifestation of disease (reviewed in Kieff and Rickinson, 2007; Rickinson and Kieff, 2007). EBV strains can be classified into two main types, type 1 and type 2, based on polymorphisms (genetic differences) within certain viral genes. Type 1 strains are more common in western countries, whereas both type 1 and type 2 strains are prevalent in central Africa and New Guinea. Strong epidemiological and clinical data have associated EBV infection with 3 lymphoproliferative diseases of B-cell origin—infectious mononucleosis, Burkitt lymphoma, and lymphoma of the immunocompromised host, particularly in the setting of organ transplantation and HIV infection. There is also a very strong association between EBV infection and undifferentiated nasopharyngeal carcinoma (NPC), and evidence has implicated EBV in the pathogenesis of Hodgkin disease, T-cell lymphoma, and some gastric carcinomas. Recent epidemiological studies have also implicated the virus in multiple sclerosis (Owens and Bennett, 2012). Geographic and ethnic variation has been recognized in the incidence of EBV-associated malignancies, indicating involvement of other genetic and environmental factors.

EBV contains a double-stranded DNA genome that codes for immediate-early, early, and late gene products. The B lymphocyte is the preferential target cell of EBV and the complement regulatory protein CD21, which normally protects a cell from self-destruction, and MHC II, involved in antigen presentation, are the cell receptors for this virus. CD21 binds to the viral glycoprotein gp350/220, whereas MHC II binds gp42. Two forms of infection can occur in the B cell using 2 different sets of gene products and promoters: (a) latent infection, which is accompanied by B cell proliferation, and (b) lytic infections, which are characterized by synthesis of structural proteins, generation of linear viral genomes, packaging, and the generation of mature virions.

Upon entry into the host cell, the viral genome travels to the nucleus and circularizes to establish a latent infection (Fig. 6–4A). Latency is characterized by the synthesis of 6 EBV nuclear antigens (EBNA-LP, EBNA-1, EBNA-2, EBNA-3A, EBNA-3B, and EBNA-3C). Three latent membrane proteins (LMP1, LMP2A, and LMP2B) are also synthesized during latency. EBNA-1 protein is required for DNA replication of the extrachromosomal viral plasmids in EBV-infected cells. It binds to the viral origin of replication and is essential for maintenance of multiple viral genomes in an episomal form. EBNA-1 also binds to chromosomes to enable the EBV episome to partition to progeny cells. EBNA-LP and EBNA-2 activate transcription from viral and cellular genes (including c-myc; see Chap. 7, Sec. 7.5.2). EBNA-2 protein transactivates expression of cellular and viral genes through interaction with at least 2 sequence-specific DNA-binding proteins. LMP1 has transforming effects in rodent fibroblast cell lines; it permits them to grow under low serum conditions, generate colonies in soft agar, and allows them to form tumors in nude mice (Li and Chang, 2003). In B-lymphocytes, it causes cell clumping, increased villous projections, upregulates vimentin and other

proteins, and protects cells from apoptosis through induction of Bcl-2 (see Chap. 9, Sec. 9.4.2). LMP-1 can also cause hyperplasia and lymphomas when expressed as a transgene in mice. LMP1 spans the membrane 6 times and mimics the function of TNF receptor family member, CD40. It acts as a constitutively active receptor that activates NF-κB, p38/MAPK, Jun kinase (JNK), JAK3, and PI3K (see Chap. 8, Secs. 8.2.4 and 8.2.5). The long cytoplasmic tail of LMP1 contains 3 C-terminal activating regions (CTAR1, CTAR2, and CTAR3) which interact with tumor necrosis factor receptor-associated factors (TRAFs) 1, 2, 3, and 5, TRAD1, RIP, and JAK3. Upregulation of the protein kinase pathways can stimulate the production of vascular endothelial growth factor (VEGF), interleukin (IL)-6, IL-8, CD40, fibroblast growth factor (FGF), EGFR, phosphorylation of p53, activation of Akt/PKB, and expression of DNA methyltransferase and telomerase (Soni et al, 2007; Kung et al, 2011). LMP2 proteins span the membrane of the host cell 12 times and mimic the function of the B-cell receptor (BCR; see Chap. 21, Sec. 21.3.1). LMP2A protein possesses a 119-amino acid cytoplasmic N-terminal domain that acts as a substrate for and associates with src family tyrosine kinases (Syk, Lyn). It is required to establish and maintain EBV latency and its expression in nude mice can transform epithelial cells and produce tumors. The function of LMP2A is to block activation of lytic EBV infection by sequestering the protein kinases that would mediate reactivation following crosslinking of the surface immunoglobulin that serves as the BCR (Longnecker, 2000; Dykstra et al, 2001). This association targets the kinases for ubiquitin mediated degradation. LMP2A can also activate PI3 kinase and PKB/AKT (see Chap. 8, Sec. 8.2.5) to enhance survival of the latently infected B cell. LMP2B lacks the amino terminus, involved in the interaction with protein kinases, and interacts with LMP2A to dampen its effect. The LMP2B protein is important in reactivation of the lytic phase of EBV infections.

Small RNAs are also produced by EBV during infection. The small nonpolyadenylated noncoding RNAs (Epstein-Barr early RNAs [EBERs]) are abundant viral transcripts that bind to double-stranded RNA-activated protein kinase (PKR) and inhibit its activity during the interferon-mediated antiviral response (Iwakiri and Takada, 2010). They also help block apoptosis through the induction of BCL-2 (see Chap. 9, Sec. 9.4.2). Viral micro-RNAs (miRNAs) were first discovered in EBV (Pfeffer et al, 2004; see Chap. 2, Sec. 2.4.3). They have since been found in other herpes viruses including Kaposi sarcoma herpesvirus (KSHV) and cytomegalovirus. There are more than 45 potential EBV miRNAs encoded by either the BamH1 fragment rightward open reading frame (BHRF) or BamHI RNA transcript (BART) regions of the genome. Interestingly, the BART miRNAs are predominantly expressed in cells derived from NPCs, whereas the BHRF miRNAs are expressed in B lymphocytes. These miRNAs appear to regulate viral replication, control transition between latent and lytic infections, block host innate/adaptive immunity, modulate growth of the host cell, or inhibit apoptosis (Cai et al, 2006; Grundhoff et al, 2006; Xing and Kief, 2007). Targets for the

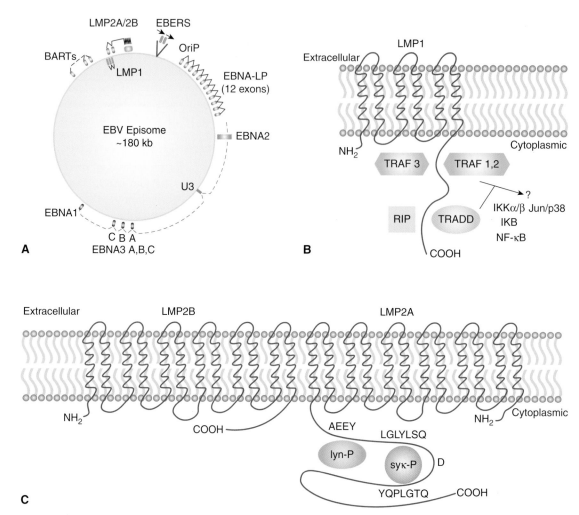

FIGURE 6–4 A) Latency-associated genes of the genome from EBV. When EBV infects a cell, the genome becomes circularized and forms an episome or plasmid. The gene products associated with latency are called Epstein-Barr nuclear antigen (EBNA); leader protein 1, 2, 3A, 3B, 3C; latent membrane protein (LMP) 1, 2A, 2B; Epstein-Barr early RNAs (EBERS); and BamHI RNA transcripts (BARTs). The transcribed gene products are multiply spliced and the exons are represented as gray rectangular boxes. The latency-associated origin of replication is OriP. **B)** LMP1 is a transforming protein that activates transcription and stimulates cell growth through interaction with TNF receptor-associated proteins (TRAF, TRADD, RIP). It stimulates cell survival pathways by activating NF-κB through phosphorylation of inhibitor of NF-κBNF-κB (IKB) and activation of c-jun. **C)** LMP2A is receptor-like protein that contains tyrosine phosphorylation domains that sequester src-like tyrosine kinases and prevent reactivation of the infected B cell from its latent state.

miRNAs include viral DNA polymerase, LMP-1, chemokines (CXCL-11), NK cell ligand (MICB), and a p53-dependent modulator of apoptosis (PUMA).

Viral latency is designed to promote the survival of the EBV episome in the face of an efficient attack by cytotoxic T-lymphocytes of the infected cell. Latency attempts to minimize the number of viral proteins and antigenic epitopes being expressed and yet retain the genetic material of EBV within the infected cell (see Chap. 21, Sec. 21.3). Initially the circularized viral genome expresses all the proteins and RNA transcripts associated with latency. This promotes a state of lymphoproliferation and replication of the viral episome. This state, referred to as latency III, is present in the rapidly proliferating B lymphocytes found in infectious mononucleosis or posttransfusion lymphoma. In latency states I and II, fewer viral proteins are expressed (they include EBNA1 and EBERs); this is the characteristic state of NPC cells, T-cell lymphomas, and gastric carcinomas. In vitro this state can be mimicked by fusing EBV-infected lymphoblastic cell lines with EBV-negative epithelial, fibroblast, or hematopoietic cells. Latency II alone is characteristic of cells in Hodgkin disease.

Reactivation of EBV from the latent state to produce structural proteins and virions can occur through a number of stimuli. These stimuli include crosslinking of BCRs with antibodies or treatment with phorbol esters, which mimic phosphatidyl inositol/diglyceride, and activate MAPK and PKC, leading to transcription of a number of genes that are involved in DNA replication. Late genes are subsequently transcribed and specify the structural proteins of EBV. In addition, an IL-10 analog (BCRF1), is transcribed in the late phase of infections and has B-cell growth properties, downregulates natural killer (NK) cells, blocks cytotoxic T-cell activity, and inhibits interferon-γ production to favor a T-helper (Th)-2 immune response by interfering with CD4+ T and NK cell functions (Hsu et al, 1990; Jochum et al, 2012; see Chap. 21, Sec. 21.3.4). Cooperation between the latent and lytic states of EBV infection is an efficient mechanism by which to propagate the viral genome and minimize the exposure of viral proteins to immune surveillance. The proteins made during latency are associated with a variety of diseases, including mononucleosis, Burkitt lymphoma, NPC, Hodgkin disease, and gastric carcinoma.

Infectious mononucleosis is a benign disease where symptoms range from mild transient fever to several weeks of pharyngitis, lymphadenopathy, swollen spleen and lymph nodes, and general malaise. Infectious mononucleosis is characterized by the proliferation of latently infected B cells coupled with the effects of reactive T cells, which eventually clear the pathogen. EBV is released from the oropharynx in localized lytic infections that appear to occur when latently infected B cells are in contact with mucosal surfaces. Linear EBV DNA, characteristic of lytic infection, is detectable in only a fraction of tonsillar lymphocytes. Epithelial cells in these local regions may become permissive to EBV infection. At the peak of an acute infection, 0.1% to 1% of the circulating B cells are positive for EBERs and the latency antigens. Expanding B-cell populations carry somatically rearranged immunoglobulin (Ig) genes that are characteristic of antigen primed polyclonal memory B cells and are capable of producing antibodies (see Chap. 21, Sec. 21.3.1). Upon resolution of infectious mononucleosis through the action of cytotoxic T-lymphocytes directed against both lytic and latent antigen epitopes, an asymptomatic carrier state is established.

Burkitt lymphoma is the most common childhood cancer in equatorial Africa and is also found in coastal New Guinea (Gromminger et al, 2012; reviewed in Molyneux et al, 2012). Climatic factors, the high incidence of *Plasmodium falciparum* malaria, as well as EBV infection, predispose children in these areas to the disease. Both type 1 and type 2 isolates of EBV have been found to be associated with Burkitt lymphoma. Tumors present at extranodal sites, most frequently in the jaw during molar tooth development, but also in the orbit of the eye, the central nervous system, and in the abdomen. It affects 3 times as many boys as girls. The tumors are monoclonal, are composed of germinal center B cells, and contain chromosome translocations between *c-myc* and the IgG heavy-chain locus (8:14) or *c-myc* and the IgG light-chain loci (8:2 or 8:22). These translocations are believed to result in deregulation of *c-myc* expression as a result of proximity to the immunoglobulin enhancer sequences, thus preventing the normal downregulation of *c-myc* expression in maturing B lymphocytes. Malaria or AIDS together with EBV may supply lymphoproliferative signals that favor translocations. High *c-myc* expression in the EBV-transformed B cell can substitute for the growth-promoting effects of

the EBV latency genes. Burkitt lymphoma is endemic in Africa, but it can also occur, although 50 to 100 times less frequently, in Europe and North America. A third form of the disease now affects patients infected with HIV; it is called AIDS-related Burkitt lymphoma. The lymphomas are "immunologically silent" and avoid surveillance by cytotoxic T lymphocytes through inhibition of proteosome-dependent antigen presentation, downregulation of MHC I, and low levels of costimulatory and cell adhesion molecules on the cell surface (see Chap. 21, Secs. 21.3.5 and 21.3.6). Normally only EBNA1 and EBERs are expressed in Burkitt lymphoma, accounting for a lack of immunogenicity against the tumors. In 30% of tumors, the p53 gene is also mutated.

Nasopharyngeal carcinoma is a relatively rare disease in Europe and North America but is almost endemic among Southeast Asian populations, particularly those of southern China. The link between NPC and EBV was first suggested by the presence of elevated antiviral antibodies in the sera of patients. DNA hybridization studies and polymerase chain reaction (PCR) amplification have subsequently confirmed that EBV is present in most tumor samples. Real-time quantitative PCR can be used to measure EBV DNA load in the plasma, and can be correlated with tumor burden and recurrence following treatment (Lin et al, 2004). The role of EBV in NPC is continuing to be elucidated; racial, genetic, and environmental cofactors all appear to be important (Lo et al, 2004). MHC I haplotype, viral LMP1 variants, dietary factors (nitrosamines in dried fish), chemical carcinogens, cytochrome P450 mutations, and physical irritants (dust and smoke) are all implicated as risk factors for NPC. Four EBV proteins, in addition to EBERs, have been detected in NPC cells, namely the nuclear antigen EBNA-1, LMP1, LMP2A, and LMP2B. The profound growth-stimulating effect of LMP1 on keratinocyte cultures suggests that LMP1 expression may exert similar effects in the nasopharyngeal epithelium. The miRNAs derived from the BART transcripts are very abundant in these tumors and probably play a significant role in carcinogenesis (Marquitz and Raab-Traub, 2012). With advances in both diagnostic and therapeutic technologies such as intensity-modulated radiation therapy (IMRT), the clinical outcome for NPC has improved over the past decade, especially for locoregional control, although challenges remain in addressing the development of distant metastases (Razak et al, 2010).

Hodgkin disease is a lymphoma characterized by a malignant population of mononuclear B and multinuclear Reed-Sternberg cells set within a background of reactive nonmalignant lymphocytes. Reed-Sternberg cells carry the genotype of a cell that has inappropriately escaped apoptotic death and have the properties of monoclonal postgerminal center (memory) B cells. They do not express conventional B- or T-cell markers. Reed-Sternberg cells express a range of cytokines that have the capacity to divert CTL recognition away from them. An association between EBV and a subset of patients with Hodgkin disease is now supported by circumstantial evidence. EBV DNA sequences and transcripts have been detected in malignant Reed-Sternberg cells and their mononuclear variants by in situ hybridization and PCR-based assays (reviewed in Kapatai and Murray, 2007). LMP1 protein has also been detected by immunohistochemical staining of lymph nodes from patients with Hodgkin disease. The association of EBV with this disease varies greatly from country to country, and Hodgkin disease in developing countries differs from that in Western countries in terms of epidemiological, pathological, and clinical characteristics. Thus, 100% of Kenyan children with Hodgkin disease were found to be EBV-positive (53 of 53 cases), whereas 51% of children from the United States and the United Kingdom (46 of 90 cases) showed evidence of EBV in the malignant cells.

Gastric carcinoma is caused by EBV in approximately 10% of all cases, and is associated with the lymphoepithelial subtype of stomach cancer (reviewed in Fukayama, 2010; Jang and Kim, 2011). It is characterized by the monoclonal growth of EBV-infected epithelial cells that express EBNA1, EBERs, BART transcripts, and small amounts of LMP2A, which is characteristic of latency state I. The LMP2A protein is believed to cause methylation of CpG motifs in the promoter region of the PTEN tumor suppressor (see Chap. 7, Sec. 7.6.2). More explicitly, LMP2A induces the phosphorylation of STAT3, which activates transcription of DNMT1 methyltransferase, and causes loss of PTEN expression through CpG island methylation of the PTEN promoter in EBV-associated gastric carcinoma. Virus-derived miRNAs are also believed to contribute to gastric carcinoma. EBV-associated gastric carcinoma affects 75,000 patients worldwide each year.

6.2.5 Hepatitis B Virus

Most individuals infected with the hepatitis B virus (HBV) develop either an acute transient illness or an asymptomatic infection that leaves them immune. However, severe liver failure associated with fulminant hepatitis can occur in approximately 1% of those infected with HBV and usually results in death. Approximately 10% of infected individuals develop chronic hepatitis, which can progress to more severe conditions, such as cirrhosis and liver cancer. There are estimated to be 500 million chronic carriers of HBV worldwide and 2 billion seropositive individuals have been exposed to the virus. There is strong epidemiological evidence indicating the importance of chronic HBV infection in the development of human hepatocellular carcinoma. Liver cancer is the fifth most common malignancy worldwide and the third leading cause of cancer death. More than 80% of individuals with liver cancer have been chronically infected by HBV. Hepatitis B is widespread throughout Asia, Africa, and regions of South America, and in some regions hepatocellular carcinoma is the leading cause of cancer death. Transmission of HBV is primarily through blood and sexual contact. In Asia, vertical transmission from mother to child during the birthing process is the main route of infection. Introduction of the recombinant vaccine derived from the membrane protein of HBV (Recombivax), which is administered as a

3-dose regimen, has limited the incidence of this virus in North America and dramatically reduced hepatitis B in the younger populations throughout Asia (Cassidy et al, 2011; Luo et al, 2012; Xiao et al, 2012).

HBV is an enveloped DNA-containing virus (reviewed in Seeger et al, 2007). The envelope contains 3 related forms of surface-exposed glycoproteins (L, M, S) that act as the major surface antigenic determinant (hepatitis B surface antigen [HBsAg]; Fig. 6–5A). The larger surface antigen (L) interacts with an unidentified HBV receptor on the plasma membranes of hepatocytes. Viral membranes surround an icosahedral nucleocapsid composed of core protein (C). This nucleocapsid contains at least 1 HBV polymerase protein (P) as well as the HBV genome. Viral DNA found in viral particles is composed of one 3.2-kb strand (minus strand) base-paired with a shorter "plus" strand of variable length. Small fragments of remnant RNA pre-genome can also be found in the virus as a consequence of replication. Because the 5' ends of both strands invariably overlap by about 300 bases, the DNA retains a circular configuration, although neither strand is itself a closed circle. The genome of HBV is organized very efficiently and its coding capacity consists of 4 overlapping reading frames that specify core protein (C), envelope surface proteins (L, M, S), polymerase (P), and the viral oncogene (X) (Fig. 6–5B). Different HBV proteins are generated by the transcription and translation of mRNAs from several start sites and in-frame initiation codons.

HBV cannot be propagated in cultured cells, and many of the steps of viral replication, such as attachment, host cell entry, and virion assembly, are poorly understood. However, several cell lines are capable of supporting HBV DNA synthesis, following transfection with viral DNA. Genome replication is complex and occurs after viral DNA is transported into the nucleus where the gap is repaired to produce covalently closed-circular DNA by using host cell enzymes (see Fig. 6–5C). Integration of HBV DNA into host chromosomes is not required for replication. Once recircularized, enhancers and promoters within the HBV DNA direct the synthesis of RNA transcripts required for viral protein synthesis (C, S, P, X) and the formation of an RNA pregenome that serves as a template for viral DNA replication. The viral polymerase (P) is actually a reverse transcriptase that first directs the synthesis of minus strand DNA from the RNA pregenome. A ribonuclease (RNase) activity associated with the polymerase subsequently degrades the RNA pregenome, and the viral polymerase uses the RNA fragments to prime synthesis of the positive-sense DNA strand. Completion of this positive strand DNA never occurs and the virus is secreted from the host cell by a process of exocytosis following virus assembly.

HBV likely causes cancer by a combination of virus-specific and host-related factors and 90% of hepatocellular carcinoma (HCC) cases develop in a cirrhotic liver (reviewed in Tsai and Chung, 2010). After 20 to 30 years of chronic infection, 20% to 30% of patients develop liver cirrhosis and liver cancer develops at an annual rate of 3% to 8% in these individuals. During

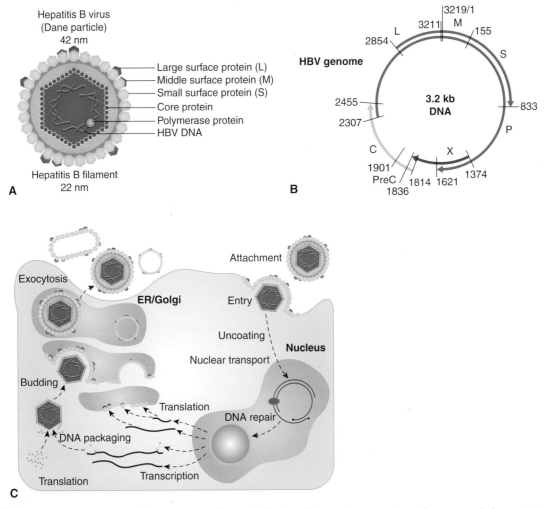

FIGURE 6-5 **A) Essential features of the structure of hepatitis B virus.** The envelope contains surface-exposed glycoproteins (L, M, S), and surrounds an icosahedral nucleocapsid composed of core protein. The nucleocapsid contains at least 1 HBV polymerase protein, as well as the HBV genome. Viral DNA in the virion is composed of one 3.2-kb strand (minus strand) base-paired with a shorter "plus" strand of variable length. **B)** The genome of HBV is compact and consists of 4 overlapping reading frames that specify core protein (C), envelope surface proteins (L, M, S), polymerase (P), and the viral oncogene (X or HBx). Different HBV proteins are generated by transcription and translation of mRNAs from several promoter start sites and in-frame initiation codons. A larger form of core protein (precore [PreC]) possesses a signal peptide, causes it to associate with the endoplasmic reticulum (ER), and allows the core antigen (hepatitis B e antigen [HBeAg]) to be secreted from the cell. The shorter form of core protein remains in the infected cell and functions as the major nucleocapsid protein. The X protein is a multifunctional polypeptide that acts as a weak oncogene in HBV infections. **C)** HBV initiates infection by binding to an unknown receptor on the hepatocyte and the membranes of the virus fuses with that of the host cell. The nucleocapsid core enters the cytoplasm and is transported to the nucleus where the viral DNA (single-stranded DNA gap) is repaired by host enzymes to form a double-stranded circle. Promoters within the HBV DNA are recognized by host cell RNA polymerase to produce RNA transcripts required for viral protein synthesis (C, S, P, X). Host RNA polymerase also directs the synthesis of an RNA pregenome that also serves as a template for the viral DNA genome. PreC is a signal sequence that allows HBeAg to be secreted.

the process of liver injury and inflammation, hepatic stellate cells become activated and transform into myofibroblast-like cells and produce liver fibrosis. Hepatocarcinogenesis is a complex multistep process involving genetic and epigenetic alteration, activation of cellular oncogenes, inactivation of tumor suppressors, and dysregulation of multiple signal transduction pathways. These include Wnt/β-catenin, p53, pRb, Ras, MAPK, Janus kinase (JAK), STAT, PI3K/Akt, Hedgehog, epidermal growth factor (EGF), transforming growth factor

(TGF)-β pathways (see Chap. 8). Viral gene products (HBx, preS2/S), random insertion of the viral genome into host chromosomal DNA, liver injury and inflammation, alcohol, and dietary carcinogens together constitute a multifactorial cause for liver cancer.

Random integration of HBV DNA fragments occurs in more than 85% of HBV-related HCC and precedes tumor formation. This process contributes to chromosomal deletions, translocation, produces fusion transcripts, causes

DNA amplification, and results in host genomic instability. Insertion of virus DNA can activate human cyclin A_2, retinoic acid receptor β, telomerase reverse transcriptase (TERT), platelet-derived growth factor (PDGF) receptor, signaling, and 60S ribosomal protein gene expression. Most integrated HBV DNA fragments contain the HBx and preS2/S genes, which can both contribute to hepatocarcinogenesis. Both these genes can upregulate signal transduction pathways and stimulate transcription of genes characteristic of growth and survival.

HBx is a multifunctional protein whose exact role in HBV infections and carcinogenesis has remained elusive (reviewed in Wei et al, 2010; Kew, 2011; Ng and Lee, 2011). It was originally called the "promiscuous transactivator" because HBx increases the synthesis of many viral and cellular gene products. The X protein is conserved in all mammalian, but not avian, hepadnaviruses, and HCC is only associated with the mammalian viruses. HBx compromises nucleotide excision repair by binding to and inactivating the UV-damaged DNA-binding protein (DDB1), which is also a component of several E3 ubiquitin ligase complexes (see Chap. 8, Fig. 8–9 and Chap. 9, Fig. 9–4). HBx could also help target the E3 ubiquitin ligase to critical cell proteins for ubiquitination and degradation. This interaction could affect STAT proteins and innate immunity, cell-cycle progression, chromosome segregation and remodeling, and produce further mutations that cause HCC. Thus, the interaction of HBx with DDB1 could impinge a number of cellular processes that could lead to HCC (Li et al, 2010; Martin-Lluesma et al, 2008). HBx affects cell signaling pathways including PKC, JAK/STAT, PI3K, SAPK, JNK, MAPK, AP-1, NF-κB, Smad, Wnt, PI3K/Akt, p53, and TGF-β (see Chap. 8). HBx can increase cytosolic calcium levels and activate calcium dependent proline rich tyrosine kinase 2, which, in turn, activates Src kinase (Yang and Bouchard, 2012). HBx decreases proteasomal degradation of β-catenin and interacts with Pin1, a Wnt signal regulator. HBx can cause transcriptional repression of the p53 gene and bind to p53 protein to inhibit its activity. TGF-β expression is upregulated by HBx in HCC tissue and shifts signaling to the oncogenic Smad3L pathway. Hepatic steatosis is also induced by HBx through transcriptional activation of the serum response factor SREBP1. HBx is a very weak oncogene, and can only lead to increased hyperplasia, malignant transformation of hepatocytes, and liver carcinoma in some strains of HBx transgenic mice. Similarly, transgenic mice containing the entire HBV genome do not spontaneously develop HCC. The only satisfactory in vivo experimental system for studying HCC caused by a hepadnavirus is the woodchuck hepatitis virus model.

HBV and hepatitis C virus (HCV, see Sec. 6.3.6) account for 90% of the approximately 6 million cases of HCC worldwide. Globally, it is the fifth most common cancer and the third leading cause of cancer death. Surgical resection and liver transplantation are the most effective treatment options, but the prognosis is usually bleak.

6.2.6 Kaposi Sarcoma-Associated Herpesvirus

KSHV, or human herpesvirus 8 (HHV-8), was identified as the pathogen responsible for a number of malignancies, including Kaposi sarcoma (KS), body cavity-based or primary effusion lymphoma, and multicentric Castleman disease (reviewed in Ganem, 2007; Mesri et al, 2010). KS is a vascular tumor of endothelial cells that affects elderly men in Mediterranean and African populations (endemic KS). However, with the onset of AIDS, a more aggressive and often lethal form of KS appeared. The virus infects the spindle cells of the skin, which are probably derived from lymphatic endothelial cells, and causes a proliferation of small red blotches over the entire body through a process of angiogenesis (Fig. 6–6). Body cavity-based or primary effusion lymphoma is a B-cell lymphoma, which occurs as malignant effusions in visceral cavities. These lymphomas are often coinfected with EBV, and in the setting of AIDS the tumors are extremely aggressive. Multicentric Castleman disease is a reactive lymphadenopathy characterized by expanded germinal centers and proliferation of endothelial vessels within involved lymph nodes. Although classified as a hyperplasia and considered nonneoplastic, it often precedes the development of non-Hodgkin lymphoma; it appears to be caused by viral secretion of IL-6. The KSHV tumors are usually found in immunosuppressed individuals and the virus is endemic in many populations without causing disease.

KSHV is a large, enveloped double-stranded DNA in the same family as the EBV. The double-stranded DNA genome is approximately 165 kbp in length and contains more than 85 open reading frames that encode virus-specific proteins. The virus can now be propagated in culture using immortalized dermal microvascular endothelial cells (Moses et al, 1999). The genome of KSHV encodes viral structural proteins, replicative enzymes, and host genes acquired through a process of "molecular piracy" that help the virus evade immune surveillance and inhibit apoptosis (see Fig. 6–6A). Many of the genes share homology with those of the EBV, and KSHV also specifies latency and lytic gene products.

The KSHV episome is maintained in the cell through use of latency-associated factors, including LANA (latency-associated nuclear antigen), which binds to viral DNA, inhibits p53-dependent transcription (Friborg et al, 1999), and binds to the retinoblastoma protein pRb (Radkov et al, 2000). It has similar properties to EBNA1 of EBV and large T antigen of SV40. LANA promotes latent replication of viral DNA, but suppresses transcription of lytic viral genes and deregulates some cellular genes. It inhibits p53 function and induces chromosomal instability (Si and Robertson, 2006) and also upregulates transcription of the proliferation gene survivin (Lu et al, 2009). LANA also induces IL-6 expression. Through its interaction with glycogen synthase kinase-3 beta (GSK-3β) it prevents the phosphorylation of β-catenin, allowing it to enter the nucleus and stimulate proliferative genes of the Wnt signal transduction pathway (see Chap. 8;

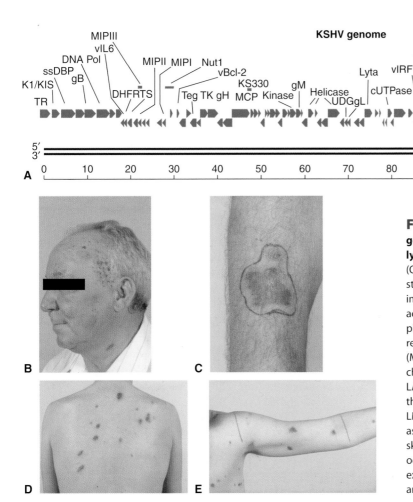

FIGURE 6–6 **A) The linearized double-stranded DNA genome of KS virus showing important genes of the lytic cycle.** The genome contains 87 open reading frames (ORFs) coding for latent proteins, reactivation proteins, and structural proteins. Host genes that help the virus evade immune surveillance and inhibit apoptosis have been acquired from chromosomes through a process of molecular piracy. These genes include vFLIP, vBcl-2, v-cyclin, interferon response factors (IRFs), and membrane cofactor protein (MCP), v-IL6, macrophage inflammatory protein (MIP) chemokines, LANA, and v-IL8R (vGCR). Genes specifying LANA, K1/KIST, and K15/LAMP maintain the viral episome in the latent state and are analogous to EBV proteins (EBNA1, LMP1, LMP2) with similar functions. **B** to **E)** Skin lesions associated with KS. Lesions present as red blotches on the skin caused by the infection of spindle cells. Angiogenesis occurs in the surrounding tissue. Panels *B* and *C* are examples of endemic or Mediterranean KS, while panels *D* and *E* illustrate epidemic or AIDS-related KS.

Fujimuro et al, 2005). LANA can also block TGF-β to inhibit normal growth arrest and apoptosis (Di Bartolo et al, 2008). Another viral protein called vFLIP (viral FLICE inhibitory protein) can interact with and block TRAF-2 association with caspase 8 (FLICE) to inhibit apoptosis (Guasparri et al, 2006). vFLIP can also activate NF-κB signaling by interacting with the IKK complex (Bagneris et al, 2008). A viral homolog to cellular D-type cyclins (v-cyclin) can associate with cyclin-dependent kinase 6 (CDK6) and phosphorylate pRB, to activate E2F-induced transcription and promote G1-S cell-cycle transition and DNA replication (see Chap. 9, Sec. 9.2.3) reviewed in Verschuren et al, 2004). The v-cyclin/CDK6 complex is resistant to the CDK inhibitors p16, p21, and p27 and phosphorylates the p27 inhibitor to trigger its degradation. Transgenic mice expressing v-cyclin on a p53(−/−) background produced lymphoma with a 100% frequency, indicating that this viral protein probably has a role in tumorigenesis (Verschuren et al, 2002). The secreted viral IL-6 cytokine has 62% sequence similarity to its host cellular homolog. It binds to host cell receptors and stimulates cell growth, VEGF production, and transformation of spindle cells and B cells. By binding to the cellular receptor (gp130), it activates transcription activators (STAT1, -3, and -5) and can stimulate genes that block apoptosis, induce

vascularization (VEGF), stimulate hematopoiesis, and prevent cell-cycle arrest caused by interferon-α (Chatterjee et al, 2002). Another viral homolog called viral G-protein–coupled receptor (v-GPCR) has sequence similarity to the cellular IL-8 receptor. Its signaling is constitutively active but also regulated by the binding of a variety of chemokines. It is known to activate MAPK, PI3K/Akt, NF-κB, and p38 pathways. It induces the expression of VEGF and cyclooxygenase-2 (COX-2) to stimulate angiogenesis and prostaglandin synthesis in endothelial cells. Transgenic mice expressing v-GPCR in hematopoietic cells developed angioproliferative lesions similar to KS in multiple organs (Yang et al, 2000; Montaner et al, 2003). Finally the kaposin family of viral proteins (A, B, C) are believed to mediate transformation (Muralidhar et al, 1998) and promote inflammation (McCormick and Ganem, 2005).

During latent infections, KSHV expresses two membrane proteins called KSHV immunoreceptor tyrosine activation motif (ITAM)-based signal transducer (K1/KIST) and latency-associated membrane protein (K15/LAMP). K1/KIST appears to have an analogous function to the LMP1 protein of EBV. It is structurally similar to the BCR and may act as a decoy molecule to prevent the reactivation of KSHV that occurs when the BCR is engaged. K1/KIST is a 46-kDa transmembrane glycoprotein that contains 2 SH2 motifs in its SH2 domain which can recruit nuclear factor of activated T cell (NFAT), syk, and vav kinases. It can also activate the PI3K/Akt/mammalian target of rapamycin (mTOR) pathway and promote cell survival (Tomlinson and Damania, 2004; Wang et al, 2006). K1/KIST can also upregulate NF-κB–dependent transcription (Samaniego et al, 2001). Like LMP1, the KIST protein has transformation properties in Rat-1 fibroblasts and primary human umbilical vein endothelial cells (Lee et al, 2005; Wang et al, 2006) Expression of K1/KIST results in secretion of VEGF (see Chap. 11, Sec. 11.4.1) and matrix metalloproteinase-9 (MMP-9) by endothelial cells. The other viral membrane protein, K15/LAMP, has similarities to both the LMP1 and LMP2A protein of EBV, and possesses up to 12 membrane-spanning domains; the cytoplasmic C terminus contains a src protein kinase-binding motif (SH2) with signal transduction properties. The constitutive phosphorylation of Y481 in the SH2 domain by Src, Lck, Yes, Hck, and Fyn protein kinases activates Ras/MAPK, NF-κB, JNK/SAPK pathways and results in the induction of IL-6, IL-8, and COX-2 (Brinkmann et al, 2003, 2007). The cytoplasmic tail of K15/LAMP also contains a TRAF binding domain that functions to upregulate NF-κB, AP-1, and ERK signaling. Overexpression of K15/LAMP seems to block the function of KIST, and prevents intracellular calcium mobilization. This protein also appears to antagonize BCR signaling and prevents reactivation of lytic infection from the latent state.

In addition to latency-associated proteins, KSHV has been shown to express up to 17 miRNA molecules from 12 genes located in the latency-associated region of the viral genome (Samols et al, 2007; reviewed in Ziegelbauer, 2011). Particular mRNAs that appear to be targeted by the viral miRNAs include osteopontin, thrombospondin-1, and plasticity-related gene 1 (Samols et al, 2007). Thrombospondin-1 has previously been reported to have tumor suppressor, antiangiogenic, and immune stimulator activities. These miRNAs probably function to maintain latency and help the virus avoid the cellular innate immune system.

As is the case with EBV, lytic replication can be triggered by chemical agents including butyrate and phorbol 12-myristate 13-acetate (PMA) that inhibit histone deacetylases and activate MAPK signaling, respectively. The viral protein Rta is a transactivator that regulates the switch from latency to a lytic infection that yields structural proteins and virus particles. It is a 691-amino acid protein that contains an N-terminal binding domain and a C-terminal transactivation domain. Rta requires interactions with cellular proteins like RBP-Jk (recombination signal binding protein Jk), AP-1, and OCT-1 in order to activate other viral transcriptional promoters. The activity of Rta can be suppressed and controlled by viral and cellular factors including interferon response factor 7 (IRF-7), KSHV Rta-binding protein (K-RBP), PARP-1, NF-κB, histone deacetylase 1 (HDAC1), KSHV bZIP, and LANA. However, Rta also has ubiquitin E3 ligase activity that can promote the degradation of these repressors (Yang et al, 2008; Yu et al, 2008). Viral infections respond to nucleotide analogs,

such as ganciclovir and acyclovir, and these agents have been shown to reduce the symptoms of KS in HIV-1 infected patients. Highly active antiretroviral therapy (HAART) has reduced the incidence of AIDS-related KS. Radiation and chemotherapy with liposomal daunorubicin or doxorubicin and rapamycin have been found to be effective in treating KS. New drug treatments that target the VEGF and angiogenesis pathways are in clinical trials for KS (see Chap. 11, Sec. 11.7; Dittmer et al, 2012; reviewed in Mesri et al, 2010). Rapamycin is probably effective because it interferes with the dependence of KS cells on the PI3K/Akt/mTOR pathway. Small molecules that inhibit mTOR include sirolimus, tacrolimus, and everolimus and are in Phase II/III trials.

A variety of DNA viruses have been implicated in human cancers. HPVs, Merkel cell carcinoma virus, EBV, and KSHV all seem to produce well-defined malignancies. The role of SV40 as a human carcinogen is still pending, but it may play a role as a cofactor in the development of mesotheliomas and some bone cancers. Recently, torque teno (TT) viruses, members of a new class of single-stranded DNA viruses (*Anelloviridae*), have been suggested to play a role in some human leukemias and colon cancer based on PCR, epidemiological evidence, and an association with red meat (zur Hausen, 2012; zur Hausen and de Villiers, 2009). Further research may confirm the role of these and other viruses in human cancer.

6.3 RNA TUMOR VIRUSES

6.3.1 Retrovirus Life Cycle

Retroviruses are enveloped viruses of approximately 120 nm in diameter (reviewed in Goff, 2007). The outer envelope is a lipid bilayer that is derived from the plasma membrane of the host cell through a "budding" process. The virus contains viral glycoproteins that are encoded by the viral *env* gene. This glycoprotein is usually cleaved during the assembly process to yield 2 subunits, SU and TM, which remain tightly associated. The envelope surrounds a nucleocapsid core composed of capsid proteins derived from the viral *gag* gene. The core includes 2 identical single strands of viral RNA that are linked together in a dimer structure through their 5′ termini and encode the capsid proteins, protease, viral polymerase, integrase, and envelope proteins (gag-pro-pol-env; Figs. 6–7A and 6–8). In addition, some classes of retroviruses (eg, HIV and human T-cell leukemia virus [HTLV]) contain accessory genes that encode proteins that assist in mRNA synthesis and viral assembly, whereas others may contain an oncogene that contributes to cellular transformation. Bound to the RNA are several copies of the enzyme reverse transcriptase (RT) encoded by the viral *pol* gene.

The life cycle of a retrovirus occurs through a sequence of discrete steps, which are illustrated in Figure 6–7B. Adsorption of the virus to a cell is mediated by an interaction between the envelope proteins of the virus and specific receptor molecules on the cell surface that leads to membrane fusion between the viral envelope and host cell plasma membrane. A fusion

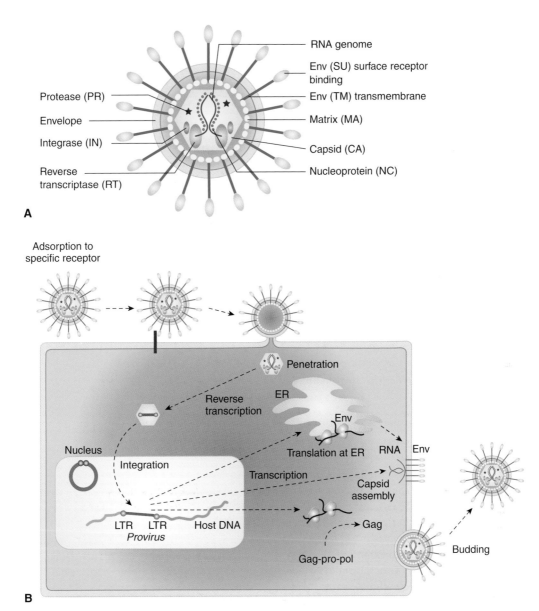

FIGURE 6-7 **The structure and life cycle of a retrovirus. A)** The virion possesses a membrane that contains an envelope protein that is cleaved into 2 subunits—surface receptor (SU) and transmembrane (TM) components. Beneath the envelope is a matrix protein (MA) that holds the membrane and the nucleocapsid together. The nucleocapsid consists of a capsid protein (CA), nucleoprotein (NC), reverse transcriptase (RT), integrase (IN), and protease (PR). The genome consists of 2 identical RNA strands. **B)** The retrovirus attaches to a specific receptor on the host cell. Its membrane subsequently fuses with that of the cell and the nucleocapsid is released into the cytoplasm. The single-stranded viral RNA genome is reverse-transcribed to a double-stranded DNA form, which has at its ends long terminal repeats (LTRs). The viral DNA migrates to the nucleus and integrates into the chromosomal DNA. The single viral transcript can form the genome for progeny viruses or can be processed and translated to generate viral structural proteins, gag or gag-pro-pol, and env. Gag and pol proteins are processed by the virus-associated protease to yield capsid (CA), and matrix (MA), polymerase (pol), and integrase (IN) proteins (see panel A). The envelope protein mRNA is translated at the rough endoplasmic reticulum and the protein precursor is cleaved to surface receptor (SU) and transmembrane (TM) subunits at the Golgi. Viral assembly occurs beneath the membrane of the host cell and the mature virus buds from the plasma membrane.

peptide found on the envelope protein mediates this event. Specificity at the level of virus adsorption accounts in large part for the restricted host and cell range of many types of viruses. HIV, for example, attaches to and enters a cell through the CD4 cell surface antigen; as a result, only CD4-positive cells are susceptible to infection by HIV. Host coreceptor molecules, such as the chemokine receptors CXCR4 and CCR5,

can add further specificity at the level of membrane fusion and entry (Berger et al, 1999). Other receptors for retroviruses include the low-density lipoprotein receptor, tv-b locus (TNF family receptor), multiple membrane spanning amino acid transporter proteins, or the sodium-dependent phosphate symporter. Retroviruses infect mice, birds, reptiles, mink, cats, cows, and monkeys, but to a lesser extent humans,

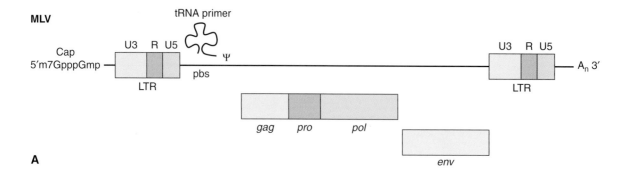

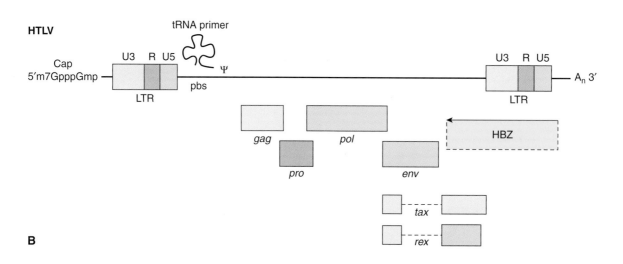

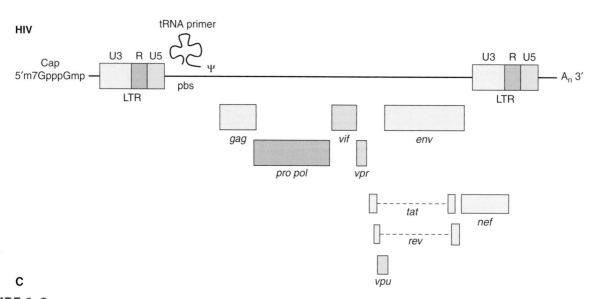

FIGURE 6–8 **Genome organization of oncogenic retroviruses. A)** Single-stranded RNA genome of Maloney leukemia virus (MLV) showing long terminal repeats (LTRs) and coding regions for gag, pol, and envelope (env) proteins. The RNA genome is 5′-capped and possesses a poly A sequence at its 3′ terminus. Ψ represents the packaging signal with which capsid protein associates. **B)** In addition to the long-terminal repeats (LTRs) and the typical *gag, pol,* and *env* genes found in other replication-competent retroviruses, a novel region exists at the 3′ end of the HTLV genome encoding 2 regulatory proteins, Tax (transactivator) and Rex (regulator of expression). Three different mRNA species have been identified for HTLV-1. The full-length genomic mRNA encodes the gag and pol proteins and is also packaged into virions. A singly spliced mRNA encodes the env protein and the doubly spliced mRNA encodes Tax and Rex. HBZ is a protein translated from an antisense transcript derived from the 3′ end of the HTLV genome. **C)** The genome of HIV also codes for structural proteins, regulatory proteins (Tat and Rev), and accessory proteins (vpr, vpu, vif, and nef).

and can cause tumors. Compared to other viruses, these agents are fragile; overcrowding, close contact, and intimate behavior facilitates their transfer from one host to another. Retroviruses cause few cancers in humans and much of what we have learned about these viruses has been derived by isolates from mice and chickens. The protooncogenes targeted by these viruses have been instrumental in the elucidation and understanding of signal transduction pathways (see Chap. 8).

Once the virus is inside the cell, loss of the viral envelope produces a core particle that is permeable to entry by deoxyribonucleotides. The RNA is then converted to double-stranded DNA through the activity of the virus-encoded RT that occurs in a large cytoplasmic complex consisting of nucleocapsid, RT, integrase, and viral RNA. The +ve sense RNA genome serves as a template in this process and a large pool of deoxyribonucleotides may trigger this process. Reverse transcription occurs through the multistep process shown in Figure 6–7B. Initially, a small nucleotide repeat sequence at both ends of the viral RNA is extended to form a long terminal repeat (LTR) that is incorporated into the double-stranded DNA. These linear DNA molecules then cross the nuclear membrane. Simple retroviruses require the breakdown of the nuclear membrane during the normal process of cellular mitosis, whereas linear DNA of HIV-related viruses can cross the nuclear membrane of a nondividing cell. One or a few molecules of viral DNA integrate randomly into the host chromosomes in association with the viral integrase molecule. The integrated form of the virus is called the *provirus*.

Once integrated, the proviral DNA acts as a template for transcription. Although both LTRs are identical and contain promoter and enhancer sequences necessary for synthesis of viral RNA, the upstream LTR acts to promote transcription whereas the downstream LTR specifies termination. Between the LTRs are coding sequences for the *gag, pro, pol,* and *env* genes (see Fig. 6–8A). In a simple retrovirus, 2 transcripts are synthesized from the proviral DNA. A full-length genomic transcript serves as the mRNA for the synthesis of both gag and gag-pro-pol fusion proteins. This transcript can also be packaged into virus particles, and therefore acts as the genome of the virus. Gag, gag-pro-pol, and genomic RNA assemble beneath the env protein at the plasma membrane of the infected cell and the complete virion buds from the cell. Maturation of the viral particle occurs during the budding process as the viral protease (Pro) cleaves the gag precursor into matrix (MA), capsid (CA), nucleocapsid (NC), protease (Pro), RT (RT), and integrase (IN) polypeptides. This maturation is crucial to produce a fully infectious virion, and this protease is the target of inhibitors (indinavir or saquinavir) currently used to treat AIDS. Retroviral infections are surprisingly benign and do not have immediate cytopathic effects on the infected host cell. However, over the long-term, disease can become apparent as a result of the acquisition of host genes or insertional mutagenesis into the host chromosome by these viruses.

A widespread role for retroviruses in human cancers has never been documented. Only HTLV-1 and -2 have been implicated in the generation of acute adult T-cell leukemia/lymphoma (ATLL). The recent report that xenotropic mouse retrovirus (XMRV) played a role in human prostate cancer and chronic fatigue syndrome has been discounted as a laboratory contamination artifact caused by genetic recombination between 2 viral genomes carried in the germline DNA of mice during prostate cancer xenograft experiments (Sfanos et al, 2012). Despite the absence of disease associated with retroviruses in human, the human genome does contain genetic material derived from endogenous retroviruses. However, these endogenous retroviruses that are incorporated into human genomic DNA are defective and carry inactivating mutations and deletions in their coding regions and LTRs are silenced through hypermethylation. The human endogenous retroviruses do not cause disease and occasionally their promoters and enhancers are used to control host gene transcription (eg, pancreatic/salivary amylase; p63 tumor suppressor). Exogenous retroviruses are inactivated by host restriction factors such as APOBEC3G (a cytidine deaminase), TRIM5α (binds a targets capsid for ubiquitination), Tetherin (prevents budding and release of the virion), and the innate immune system. Successful human retroviruses, such as HIV and HTLV, have developed accessory factors that appear to neutralize these restriction factors.

6.3.2 Acute Transforming Retroviruses

Transforming retroviruses can be separated into 2 major groups based on their different mechanisms of transformation. Some viruses contain a viral oncogene, and these have been termed *acute* or *rapidly transforming viruses*. More than 20 viral oncogenes have been identified; each of these has been found to have a counterpart in normal cells. Other viruses do not contain an oncogene and are referred to as *chronic* or *slowly transforming viruses*. Again, these cancer viruses affect mice and birds, and as yet have not been implicated in human tumorigenesis.

Acute transforming viruses are almost always replication-defective as a result of replacement of viral sequences required for replication with host-derived oncogene sequences. For example, MC29 is a defective virus containing v-myc and is missing all of the *pol* gene and parts of *gag* and *env*. As a result, these transforming viruses require the presence of replication-competent helper viruses that assist in viral replication and assembly by supplying the necessary viral gene products. Because viral oncogenes come under the control of the efficient retroviral promoter present on the LTRs and are no longer tightly regulated by cellular mechanisms that normally act on the natural promoter, these genes can be expressed at inappropriately high levels. The viral oncogenes are frequently mutated because of the poor fidelity of retroviral replication, and often contain point mutations, deletions, substitutions, and insertions when compared with the protooncogenes from which they are derived. In addition, viral oncogenes differ from protooncogenes in that they do not contain intron

TABLE 6-1   Oncogenes recovered in transducing retroviruses.

Oncogene	Retrovirus	Function of Cellular Homolog
Sis	Simian sarcoma virus	Platelet-derived growth factor
ErbB	Avian erythroblastosis virus (ES4)	Epidermal growth factor receptor
Fms	Feline sarcoma virus (McDonough)	Cerebrospinal fluid (CSF)-1 receptor
Sea	Avian erythroblastosis virus (S13)	Growth factor receptor
Kit	Feline sarcoma virus (HZ4)	Stem cell growth factor receptor
ErbA	Avian erythroblastosis virus (R)	Thyroid hormone receptor
H-ras	Murine sarcoma virus (Harvey)	G protein, guanosine triphosphatase (GTPase), signaling
K-ras	Murine sarcoma virus (Kirsten)	G protein, GTPase, signaling
Crk	Avian sarcoma virus (1, CT10)	Adaptor protein, signaling, T cell
Cbl	Casitas mouse lymphoma virus	Adaptor protein, lymphocytes, signaling
Src	Rous sarcoma virus (RSV)	Nonreceptor tyrosine kinase, signaling
Abl	Abelson murine leukemia virus	Nonreceptor tyrosine kinase, signaling
Fps	Fujinami avian sarcoma virus	Nonreceptor tyrosine kinase, signaling
Fes	Feline sarcoma virus (S-T)	Nonreceptor tyrosine kinase, signaling
Fgr	Feline sarcoma virus (G-R)	Nonreceptor tyrosine kinase, signaling
Yes	Avian sarcoma virus (Y73, Esh)	Nonreceptor tyrosine kinase, signaling
Mos	Moloney mouse sarcoma virus	Serine-threonine kinase, germ cell
Raf	Mouse sarcoma virus (3611)	Serine-threonine kinase, MAPK pathway
Mil	Avian myelocytoma virus (MH2)	Serine-threonine kinase, Raf family homolog
Akt	Avian sarcoma virus (AK-8)	Serine-threonine kinase, PKB
Jun	Avian sarcoma virus (17)	Transcription factor (AP-1 complex)
Fos	Mouse sarcoma virus (F-B-J)	Transcription factor (AP-1 complex)
Myc	Avian myelocytoma (MC29, MH2)	Transcription factor
Myb	Avian myeloblastosis virus (BAI/A)	Transcription factor
Ets	Avian myeloblastosis virus (E26)	Transcription factor, GATA-1 family homolog
Rel	Avian reticuloendotheliosis virus	Transcription factor, NF-κB family homolog
Ski	Avian retrovirus (Sloan-Kettering)	Transcription factor, muscle, MyoD family homolog
Qin	Avian retrovirus (ASV31)	Transcription factor, forkhead family homolog

(ie, noncoding) sequences. Retroviruses containing oncogenes can transform cells in culture after several days and can induce leukemias and sarcomas in infected animals relatively quickly. Expression of the v-onc gene transforms every infected cell. Consequently, polyclonal tumors develop from many different infected progenitor cells. Table 6–1 summarizes examples of oncogenes and their cellular counterparts that have been transduced by acute transforming viruses. Viral oncogenes include growth factors (v-Sis), growth factor receptors (v-erbB), intracellular tyrosine kinases (v-src, v-fps, v-fes, v-abl), serine/threonine kinases (v-Akt, v-Raf), G proteins (H-ras, Ki-ras), transcription factors (v-myc, v-erbA, v-fos, v-jun), and many other protein families (see Chap. 7).

6.3.3 Chronic Tumor Retroviruses

The replication-competent chronic tumor viruses do not contain viral oncogenes but transform infected cells through a mechanism known as *insertional mutagenesis*, in which proviral integration leads to the aberrant activation or sometimes inactivation of adjacent cellular genes. Protooncogenes may be activated by LTR promoter insertion, LTR enhancer insertion, viral poly-A site insertion that stabilizes mRNA, or viral leader insertion that increases and stabilizes mRNA. In other instances a cellular gene may be activated or inactivated by insertion of the retrovirus in the middle of a cellular gene depending upon the arrangement of exons. Several of the protooncogenes identified initially as progenitors to transducing retroviral oncogenes (c-*erb*B, c-*mos*, c-*myb*, c-*myc*, c-H-*ras*, c-K-*ras*, c-*fms*, c-*fli1*) have also been identified through insertional mutagenesis. Cytokines regulating cell growth (IL-2, IL-3, IL-10) are also activated by retroviral integration in several animal species. Usually more than 1 insertional mutation event is required to produce tumors in animals.

Avian leukemia virus (ALV) is a typical slow-acting retrovirus. In ALV-induced B-cell lymphomas, malignant clones transformed by these viruses contain proviruses integrated in the vicinity of the c-*myc* gene. In many tumors, the provirus is integrated upstream of c-*myc* and in the same transcriptional orientation. In such cases the 3′ LTR, which normally acts to terminate viral transcription, promotes transcription of c-*myc* sequences. The resulting hybrid RNA transcripts contain both viral and c-*myc* sequences and are present at levels 30- to 100-fold higher than that of c-*myc* RNA in normal tissues. Such c-*myc* transcripts appear to encode a normal c-myc protein. This mechanism is called *promoter insertion*. In other tumors, the provirus is integrated upstream of c-*myc* but oriented in the transcriptional direction opposite to that of the gene, or it is integrated downstream of the gene. The strong enhancer properties of the LTRs are then believed to be responsible for activation of c-*myc* transcription, and this mechanism of transformation is known as *enhancer insertion*. The majority of B-cell lymphomas induced by ALV contain proviral sequences adjacent to c-*myc*, but the *myc* oncogene requires the cooperative function of a second oncogene. Because integration adjacent to c-*myc* is a random, rare event and secondary genetic events are required for tumor progression, ALV-induced leukemia may arise slowly and is clonal in origin.

Other examples of transformation by chronic tumor viruses include insertion of the mouse mammary tumor virus (MMTV) next to the wnt-1/int-1 or hst/int-2 genes leading to mammary tumors in mice. The hst/int-2 protein belongs to the FGF family and can be upregulated in KS, stomach cancer, and teratocarcinomas, as well as in mouse mammary tumors. The Lck gene, normally found in T cells, NK cells, and some B cells, was found to be upregulated in lymphoma cell lines derived from thymomas of murine leukemia virus-infected mice. Other oncogenes that have been found as a result of proviral insertions include Ahi-1, Evi-1, Evi-2, Fli-1, Mlvi-1, Mlvi-3, and Pvt-1.

Proviral insertion may disrupt or alter the protein-coding sequence of resident celluiar genes. For example, in ALV-induced erythroblastosis, proviral insertions commonly map to a small region in the middle of the EGFR gene (c-*erb*B; see Chap. 7). The resulting transcripts contain viral *gag* and *env* sequences fused to c-*erb*B sequences. The amino acid sequence predicted from these hybrid transcripts contain amino acids encoded by *gag* and *env* fused to carboxy-terminal amino acid sequences encoded by c-*erb*B. Thus, expression of an altered, truncated EGFR molecule appears necessary for the development of ALV-induced erythroblastosis.

6.3.4 Human T-Cell Leukemia Virus

HTLV-1 and HTLV-2 are the only retroviruses that are known to lead directly to cancers in humans (reviewed in Lairmore and Franchini, 2007; Matsuoka and Jeang, 2011). HTLV-1 by itself can cause ATLL, a rare but virulent cancer that is endemic in southern Japan, the Caribbean, northern South America, parts of Africa, and the southeastern United States. The virus has infected approximately 20 million people worldwide and over a prolonged period of 20 to 40 years it can produce ATLL in 1% to 5% of infected individuals. Transmission of this disease may occur through blood transfusion, breast feeding, and sexual intercourse. Nucleotide sequence determination of the viral genomes has shown that the Japanese and American isolates were closely related strains of a single retrovirus now called HTLV-1.

There are 4 molecular subtypes of HTLV-1 (A to D), which reflect the geographical locations from which the virus is isolated. The virus exhibits little genetic variation and there is an approximately 98% homology between different HTLV-1 strains. HTLV-1 has since been recognized as an agent that causes ATLL. In some chronically infected patients the virus can also cause a neurodegenerative disease called HTLV-associated myelopathy (HAM) or tropical spastic paraparesis (TSP). HTLV-2 is much less common than HTLV-1 and a convincing role of this virus in human disease has not been demonstrated, although a few patients have exhibited neurological disease.

Unlike the common oncogenic retroviruses of animals, HTLV-1 does not carry a host-derived oncogene and does not activate cellular protooncogenes by insertional mutation. HTLV-1 is believed to initiate a multistep process leading to ATLL. These steps include an asymptomatic carrier state, preleukemic state, chronic/smoldering ATLL, lymphoma type, and acute ATLL. Both HTLV-1 and HTLV-2 can immortalize human peripheral blood T cells in vitro, as well as T cells from monkeys, rabbits, cats, and rats. The cellular receptor for the virus is the glucose transporter protein GLUT-1. Entry into the host cell and cell to cell fusion require the participation of coreceptors, which include cell adhesion molecules (ICAM-1, ICAM-3, V-CAM, integrins). The virus can infect either CD4+ or CD8+ T cells, but transformed cells from ATLL patients are usually CD4+ and only occasionally CD8+. Following infection of T lymphocytes by HTLV-1, surface IL-2 receptors are upregulated, and the provirus is found randomly integrated into the cellular genome. The infected cell population undergoes a transient polyclonal expansion followed by a latency period that is variable in duration; it can be as short as a few years if infection occurs in adulthood or as long as 40 years if infection occurs in infancy. Not all individuals infected by the virus develop ATLL, and the latent state may be maintained by immunological clearance of the infected cells. An infected individual will have approximately a 1% chance of developing ATLL over a lifetime. If a patient progresses to pre-ATLL, 50% of patients still have the chance of undergoing spontaneous regression. When ATLL is clinically evident, however, all the leukemic cells in a patient have a common proviral integration site in the host DNA, but no 2 patients have the same integration site. These observations suggest that HTLV-1 is derived from a single, infected, progenitor cell but that subsequent genetic events are required to induce ATLL.

Figure 6–8B illustrates the genome of HTLV-1. In addition to *gag, pol,* and *env* genes, HTLV encodes accessory proteins, Tax, Rex, p12, p13, p30, and the recently discovered HBZ, which is expressed from the antisense strand. The Tax protein is the transforming component of HTLV-1; it is critical for viral replication and functions as a transcriptional coactivator of viral and cellular gene expression (Matsuoka and Jeang, 2011). Tax protein contacts a GC-rich region in the U3 promoter region of the proviral DNA and recruits cellular transcription factors that include CREB, CREB binding protein (p300/CBP), which is a histone acetylase, the CBP-associated factor (PCAF), and transcription factors IIA, IIB, IID (Fig. 6–9A). The Tax protein is a multifunctional protein

composed of several domains (Fig. 6–9B). In addition to regulating transcription, Tax upregulates the activity of NF-κB to increase the expression of IL-2, IL-15, IL-2R, and IL-15R. Tax does this by binding to and activating the IKK complex, which targets the NF-κB inhibitor (IkB) for ubiquitination and degradation, allowing NF-κB to enter the nucleus and trigger the expression of many cytokines (Fig. 6–9C). Mutations in Tax have shown that both CREB and NF-κB activities are required for efficient transformation. Cellular genes that are responsive to transcriptional activation by Tax include *IL-2,* the α subunit of the IL-2 receptor, granulocyte-macrophage colony-stimulating factor, protooncogenes c-*sis* and c-*fos,* and proliferating cell nuclear antigen (*PCNA*). Tumor cells from ATLL patients as well as T lymphocytes transformed in culture with HTLV-1 display an activated T-cell phenotype characterized by expression of IL-2 cell surface receptors and cell adhesion molecules such as ICAM-1. Nonhuman and rodent models for HTLV-1 exhibit little disease progression. However, transgenic Tax expression under

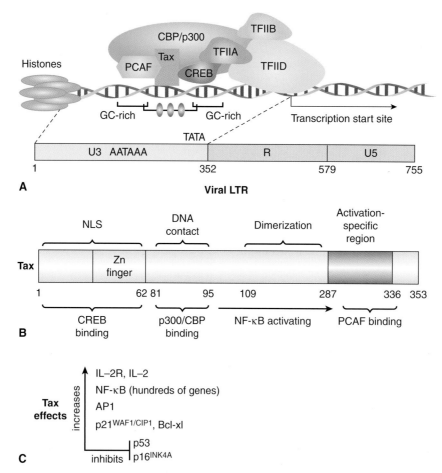

FIGURE 6–9 Molecular domains and functions of HTLV-1 Tax protein. A) Tax protein contacts a GC-rich region in the U3 promoter region of the proviral DNA LTR and recruits cellular transcription factors that include CREB, CREB binding protein (CBP/p300), which is a histone acetylase, the CBP-associated factor (PCAF), and transcription factors IIA, IIB, IID. **B)** Functional domains of Tax showing CREB binding site, nuclear localization sequence (NLS), p300/CBP binding region, NF-κB–activating domain, and PCAF binding region. **C)** Tax upregulates expression of IL-2R, AP1, p21^WAF/CIP1, and Bcl-xL, and activates NF-κB, which augments the expression of hundreds of genes, including IL-2, IL-15, IL-2R, and IL-15R. It blocks the functions of p53 and p16^INK4A.

control of the granzyme B promoter produced large granular lymphocytic leukemia in mouse T cells (Grossman et al, 1995). ATLL-like T-cell leukemia/lymphoma was produced in mice with Tax driven by the Lck promoter (Hasegawa et al, 2006; Ohsugi et al, 2007). At the molecular level, overexpression of Tax can lead to inhibition of DNA repair as a result of overexpression of the PCNA processivity factor (see Chap. 5, Sec. 5.3). Tax can also bind to PI3K and activate Akt (PKB), which both promotes cell survival and inhibits apoptosis (Sun and Yamaoka, 2005). In addition Tax can accelerate cell cycle progression by binding and stabilizing cyclin D3, cyclin D2, and Cdk4 (Marriott and Semmes, 2005; see Chap. 9, Sec. 9.2.2). It can also inactivate retinoblastoma protein (Rb) and p53 tumor suppressor (Miyazato et al, 2005). The Tax protein is also believed to be responsible for the "flower-like" polynuclear lymphocytes that characterize ATLL by interfering with mitotic spindle checkpoint control (Liu et al, 2005; Chi and Jeang, 2007). Thus, expression of the tax gene has the potential to perturb many normal cellular functions leading to malignancy.

Rex is essential for viral replication and acts post-transcriptionally to upregulate the levels of virion proteins to assure the production of infectious virus. The protein Rex binds to recognition sequence near the 3' ends of genome-length unspliced RNA and partially spliced mRNAs, allowing them to be exported from the nucleus to the cytoplasm, instead of being subjected to splicing or degradation. The Rex complex binds to the nuclear export factor exportin-1 (CRM-1) and releases the unspliced RNA in the cytoplasm for translation or packaging. This allows for production of viral structural proteins (gag, pol, pro, env) and packaging of the RNA genome. Rex is the regulatory switch between latent and productive phases of the HTLV-1 life cycle and favors the production of virus particles (Baydoun et al, 2008; reviewed in Younis and Green, 2005). Rex also stabilizes the mRNAs for IL-2, IL-2R, the kinase FynB, vascular cell adhesion molecule (VCAM)-1, and leukocyte function-associated antigen (LFA)-3. The p12 protein resides in the endoplasmic reticulum and Golgi and interacts with the chaperones calnexin and calreticulin to increase intracellular Ca^{++} levels, which results in the dephosphorylation and activation of the transcription factor NFAT that regulates proliferation and differentiation of T lymphocytes. P12 can also bind the subunits of IL-2R, the transcription factor STAT5, and the MHC-I heavy chain. P30 binds the mRNAs for Tax and Rex and tethers them inside the nucleus to inhibit their protein synthesis, thus maintaining the virus in a latent state. It also promotes cell survival and inhibits apoptosis. HBZ is a protein that is translated from an antisense transcript derived from the 3' end of the HTLV-1 genome. The protein contains a leucine zipper domain that can interact with CREB, CREB-2, CREM-Ia, ATF-I, c-Jun, JunB, JunD, and NF-κB transcription factors. It acts to suppress Tax-mediated transactivation of viral transcription at the 5'-LTR and the Hbz RNA promotes ATLL cellular proliferation. Tax is needed to initiate transformation, whereas HBZ is required for cell proliferation and maintenance of the

transformed phenotype late in ATLL when Tax expression diminishes (Satou et al, 2006; Lemasson et al, 2007).

The mean survival time for aggressive ATLL without treatment is less than 1 year. Standard treatment usually starts with cytostatic chemotherapeutic agents such as vincristine, cyclophosphamide, doxorubicin, ranimustine, vindesine, etoposide, carboplatin, and prednisone (reviewed in Goncalves et al, 2010; Matsuoka and Jeang, 2011). Alternatively, nucleoside analogs and topoisomerase inhibitors have been used, resulting in limited improvement. Chemotherapy can yield a 3-year survival rate of about 25%. The major obstacle in therapy is multidrug resistance of the ATLL cells coupled with the patients' immunodeficient state. Complications from opportunistic fungal, viral, protozoal, and bacterial infections can worsen the prognosis. Allogeneic stem cell transplantation is effective in ATLL patients, with a 3-year survival rate of about 35%. Cell-mediated immunity against HTLV-1 is augmented in 30% to 40% of the surviving patients, leading to complete remission. A humanized antibody against CCR4 that is found on T-regulatory (T-reg) cells has also been effective in treating ATLL patients. NF-κB and histone deacetylase inhibitors may offer a new direction in therapy (Rauch and Ratner, 2011). The virus-associated neurological disease, HAM/TSP, is generally untreatable and it responds poorly to treatment with corticosteroids, plasmapheresis, interferon, and antiretroviral drugs.

6.3.5 Human Immunodeficiency Virus

HIV is a member of the retrovirus family and has been classified as a lentivirus. The RNA genome of HIV encodes core (gag), polymerase (pol), and envelope (env) gene products in addition to regulatory and accessory proteins (Tat, Rev, Nef, Vif, Vpr, and Vpu) that play key roles in the pathogenesis of the viral infection (see Fig. 6–8C). Tat is a transactivating protein of the LTR promoter and Rev interacts with and directs the export of unspliced viral mRNAs to the cytoplasm and favors synthesis of viral structural proteins. Vif increases viral infectivity of certain cell types and Vpr promotes nuclear localization of proteins from the cytoplasm. Vpu enhances the release of virus from the cell. Nef is critical in maintaining high virus loads, increases circulating virions, and down-regulates surface expression of CD4 and MHC I (see Chap. 21, Fig. 21–1). The virus initiates infection by binding to the CD4 receptor on T-cells and macrophages, and penetrates into the host cell through use of chemokine coreceptors and a process of membrane fusion. Viral replication occurs as described in Figure 6–7B. HIV causes immune suppression through destruction of lymphoid tissue and depletion of CD4+ T cells. Combinations of antiretrovirus nucleotide analogs and viral protease inhibitors are used as a short-term therapy to suppress plasma viral loads. This treatment is known as HAART.

Although HIV does not cause cancer directly, it is an immunosuppressive virus that can lead to the appearance of several types of HIV associated malignancies during late-stage infections (Casper, 2011). These AIDS-related malignancies are the result of reactivation of infections with HPVs, EBV, and human herpesvirus 9 (KSHV; see Sec. 6.2.6). The cancers include smooth muscle sarcomas (leiomyosarcoma), Hodgkin disease, NPC, AIDS-related lymphomas (non-Hodgkin lymphoma, Burkitt lymphoma, primary central nervous system lymphoma), cervical cancer, anal carcinomas, HCC, lung cancer, squamous cell neoplasia, primary effusion lymphoma, and KS. HAART can be effective in treating less-aggressive cancers, but tumor-specific therapy may be indicated. With the significant improvement in morbidity, mortality, and life expectancy of AIDS patients, non-AIDS–defining malignancies have been on the rise (Deeken et al, 2012). These include cancers of the lung, breast, colon, anus, kidney, and skin, which develop over longer periods of time following successful HAART treatment. A major challenge to oncologists is how to administer chemotherapy safely and effectively to patients on retroviral therapy.

6.3.6 Hepatitis C Virus

HCV is a member of the family of viruses that includes yellow fever virus and dengue fever virus. Following the discovery of HBV in 1965, and the characterization of hepatitis A virus in 1973, it became apparent that other agents responsible for blood-borne hepatitis also existed and caused non-A, non-B hepatitis. This led to the discovery of the HCV. The HCV virion is approximately 50 nm in diameter and consists of an envelope that contains the 2 viral glycoproteins, E1 and E2. Surrounding the positive-sense, single-stranded RNA genome is the core or nucleocapsid protein. The genome encodes the structural proteins (core, E1, E2) and nonstructural proteins (p7, NS2, NS3, NS4A, NS4B, NS5A, and NS5B) which are required for viral replication (Fig. 6–10). There are 7 known genotypes of this virus that reflect their geographical distribution. HCV replication is slow and inefficient and the virus establishes persistent viral infections that are not cytotoxic. Two major barriers have hampered research in the HCV field: the virus cannot be easily propagated in cultured cells, and the previous lack of a small animal model in which to propagate and study the immunology of this pathogen and evaluate antiviral agents. Chimpanzees are the only primates besides humans that support the replication of HCV. An important breakthrough was the development of a severe combined immunodeficiency (SCID) urokinase transgenic mouse model into which human liver cells have been introduced. This murine model promises a useful tool with which to study antiviral agents and production of the virus in vivo (Mercer et al, 2001). Another major discovery was reported when a single strain of Japanese fulminant hepatitis C (JFH-1) was found to grow and produce virus particles in a hepatoma cell line (Huh 7.5) (Wakita et al, 2005). This cell line has allowed researchers to study the interaction of HCV with the innate immune system, elucidate viral receptors on the cell, and study viral RNA synthesis in association with intracellular membrane structures.

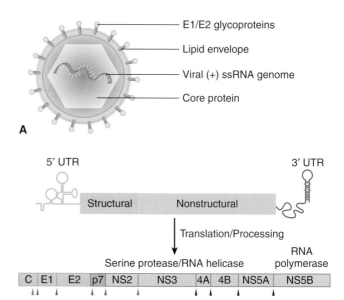

FIGURE 6–10   RNA genome and polyprotein of HCV showing structural and nonstructural viral proteins. The single open reading frame of the genome translates into a polyprotein that is processed by host and viral proteases into 10 proteins. These include structural components for capsid (C) and 2 envelope/membrane proteins (E1, E2). A viral pore protein (p7) appears to be important during virus assembly. Nonstructural proteins include a metalloprotease (NS2), protease-helicase (NS3/NS4A), RNA polymerase (NS5B), and replication factors whose functions are being defined (NS4B, NS5A). Cleavage sites for host proteases are shown in blue, the NS2 metalloprotease in red, and the NS3/NS4A serine protein in black.

HCV is blood borne and is spread through transfusions, intravenous drug use, tattoo parlors, multiple use of needles for vaccination, and sexual contact. The acute phase of hepatitis C is often mild and undiagnosed in both adults and children. Malaise, nausea, right upper quadrant pain, and dark urine may appear in about one-third of patients. Liver transaminase (alanine aminotransferase [ALT]) levels in the blood may increase and jaundice is only occasionally evident. However, HCV goes on to establish persistent viral infections and chronic disease in 60% to 80% of these patients leading to cirrhosis and HCC. Damage to the hepatocytes in the liver occurs through the effects of cytotoxic T cells and the action of Fas ligand and perforin on these target cells. The virus undergoes genetic variation in the face of a mounting humoral response and a region of the E2 proteins called the *hypervariable 2* (HVP2) region, is particularly prone to mutagenesis. Low-grade persistent viral infections appear to survive in the face of a vigorous immune response against the virus: the virus may survive immune surveillance through the generation of mutants that escape T-cell cytotoxicity (Cooper et al, 1999; Wong et al, 2001). HCV can also induce anergy in both CD4+ T-helper cells and CD8+ CTL cells (Lechner et al, 2000), which prevents clearance of virus and contributes to persistent viremia. Alcohol abuse in hepatitis C patients can accelerate the progression and severity of the disease. This could be related to alcohol induced immunosuppression or the production of proinflammatory cytokines that lead to cytotoxicity and apoptosis.

Approximately 80% of patients with HCC also have cirrhosis. The genome of HCV is not transcribed to DNA and does not integrate into the host chromosome. The HCV core protein itself has oncogenic potential based on studies with core transgenic mice. These mice can exhibit liver steatosis (lipid droplets) and develop HCC after approximately 16 months (Lerat et al, 2002). Chronic liver inflammation caused by the HCV infection is believed to be an important carcinogenic factor. Hepatocellular death as a result of chronic inflammation and subsequent regeneration of hepatocytes can yield mutagenesis in the liver. At the molecular level, core protein has been reported to activate the JNK signal transduction pathway (Tsutsumi et al, 2003), inhibit the suppressor SOCS-1 (Miyoshi et al, 2005), upregulate NF-κB activity (Tai et al, 2000), and inactivate p53 (Yin et al, 1999). Other proteins also influence host cells but whether the gene products of HCV contribute to liver cancer remains unknown.

HCV can also cause B-lymphocyte proliferative disorders, including mixed cryoglobulinemia and non-Hodgkin lymphoma (NHL) (Ferri et al, 1994). Approximately 20% to 50% NHL patients in Italy exhibit HCV infections (Ferri et al, 1997). Other studies in Japan and the United States also indicate a high prevalence of HCV in cases of NHL (Zuckerman et al, 1997). Infection of B cells with HCV can yield a mutator phenotype which is characterized by increased mutations in immunoglobulin genes, protooncogenes, and tumor-suppressor genes (Machida et al, 2004). These genes include β-catenin, BCL-6, and p53. The mutations can be induced through double-stranded DNA breaks caused by activation of error-prone DNA polymerase ζ, polymerase t, and activation-induced cytidine deaminase. This process could be induced by interaction of E2 protein of HCV with the CD81 virus coreceptor, aggregation of CD19 and CD21 and stimulation of the BCR signal transduction pathways (Weng and Levy, 2003). HCV core, NS3, and NS5A proteins have also been reported to induce reactive oxygen species, increase NO production, and cause chromosome translocations (Lai, 2002; Machida et al, 2006).

Previous treatment for hepatitis C involved the administration of pegylated interferon in combination with ribavirin over a period of 1 year and produced a sustained antiviral response in about half of infected patients, depending largely on the genotype of HCV being treated. The recent launch of NS3/4A protease inhibitors (telaprevir, boceprevir) and imminent release of NS5B polymerase inhibitors promises to cure HCV-related hepatitis for those patients that can afford treatment (Sarrazin et al, 2012). Prophylactic vaccines for hepatitis C are under development, but progress is slow and limited by the hypervariable nature of the virus (Houghton, 2011).

SUMMARY

- Viruses have proven to be important agents in promoting a diverse set of cancers. They can both cause or be important cofactors in many human malignancies.
- DNA viruses, such as SV40, adenoviruses, papillomaviruses, and gamma-herpesviruses, generally downregulate the activity of tumor suppressors such as p53 and Rb proteins, and were instrumental in the discovery and characterization of these cellular products. Histone acetylation is also modulated by these 3 viruses and favors the transcription of other genes involved in transformation.
- Transducing retroviruses can pirate cellular genes encoding growth factors, receptors, tyrosine and kinases, G-proteins, adaptors, and transcription factors, whereas chronic retroviral tumor viruses can activate similar genes through insertional mutagenesis.
- Many viruses contain genes that block apoptosis or inhibit immune recognition of the infected host cell, which favors cell survival.
- Each virus discussed in this chapter is unique in the manner in which it deregulates cell growth. However, transformation of the host cell is always achieved through viral manipulation of the cell cycle, apoptosis, and signal transduction pathways to favor growth and survival. Details between these viruses may differ, but basic principles underlie the process of cellular transformation by these agents.

REFERENCES

Ang KK, Harris J, Wheeler R, et al. Human papillomavirus and survival of patients with oropharyngeal cancer. *N Engl J Med* 2010;363:24-35.

Atkin SJL, Griffin BE, Dilworth SM. Polyoma virus and simian virus 40 as cancer models: history and perspectives. *Semin Cancer Biol* 2009;19:211-217.

Auger KR, Carpenter CL, Shoelson SE, et al. Polyoma virus middle T antigen-pp60c-src complex associates with purified phosphatidylinositol 3-kinase in vitro. *J Biol Chem* 1992;267: 5408-5416.

Bagneris C, Ageichik AV, Cronin N, et al. Crystal structure of a vFLIP-IKKγ complex: insights into viral activation of the IKK signalosome. *Mol Cell* 2008;30:620-631.

Baydoun HH, Bellon M, Nicot C. HTLV-1 yin and yang: Rex and p30 master regulators of viral mRNA trafficking. *AIDS Res* 2008;10:195-204.

Berger EA, Murphy PM, Farber JM. Chemokine receptors as HIV-1 coreceptors: roles in viral entry, tropism, and disease. *Annu Rev Immunol* 1999;17:657-700.

Berk AJ. Adenoviridae. In: Knipe DM, Howley PM, eds. *Field's Virology*. Philadelphia, PA: Lippincott, Williams, & Wilkins; 2007: 2355-2394.

Bischoff JR, Kirn DH, Williams A, et al. An adenovirus mutant that replicates selectively in p53-deficient human tumor cells. *Science* 1996;274:373-376.

Bochkareva E, Martynowski D, Seitova A, et al. Structure of the origin-binding domain of simian virus 40 large T antigen bound to DNA. *EMBO J* 2006;25:5961-5969.

Boothpur R, Brennan DC. Human polyoma viruses and disease with emphasis on clinical BK and JC. *J Clin Virol* 2010;47:306-312.

Brinkmann MM, Glenn M, Rainbow L, et al. Activation of mitogen-activated protein kinase and NF-kappaB pathways by a Kaposi's sarcoma-associated herpesvirus K15 membrane protein. *J Virol* 2003;77:9346-9358.

Brinkmann MM, Pietrek M, Dittrich-Breiholz O, et al. Modulation of host gene expression by the K15 protein of Kaposi's sarcoma-associated herpesvirus. *J Virol* 2007;81:42-58.

Cai X, Schafer A, Lu S, et al. Epstein-Barr virus microRNAs are evolutionarily conserved and differentially expressed. *PLoS Pathog* 2006;2:e0236-e0247.

Casper C. The increasing burden of HIV-associated malignancies in resource-limited regions. *Annu Rev Med* 2011;62:157-170.

Cassidy A, Mossman S, Olivieri A, et al. Hepatitis B vaccine effectiveness in the face of global HBV genotype diversity. *Expert Rev Vaccines* 2011;10:1709-1715.

Chang Y, Cesarman E, Pessin MS, et al. Identification of herpesvirus-like DNA sequences in AIDS-associated Kaposi's sarcoma. *Science* 1994;266:1865-1869.

Chang Y, Moore PS, Talbot SJ, et al. Cyclin encoded by KS herpesvirus. *Nature* 1996;382:410.

Chatterjee M, Osborne J, Bestetti G, et al. Viral IL-6-induced cell proliferation and immune evasion of interferon activity. *Science* 2002;298:1432-1435.

Cheng J, DeCaprio JA, Fluck MM, et al. Cellular transformation by simian virus 40 and polyoma virus T antigens. *Semin Cancer Biol* 2009;19:218-228.

Chi YH, Jeang KT. Aneuploidy and cancer. *J Cell Biochem* 2007;102:531-538.

Chung CH, Gillison ML. Human papillomavirus in head and neck cancer: its role in pathogenesis and clinical implications. *Clin Cancer Res* 2009;15:6758-6762.

Cooper S, Erickson AL, Adams EJ, et al. Analysis of a successful immune response against hepatitis C virus. *Immunity* 1999;10:439-449.

DeCaprio JA. How the Rb tumor suppressor structure and function was revealed by the study of adenovirus and SV40. *Virology* 2009;384:274-284.

Deeken JF, Tjen-A-Looi A, Redek MA, et al. The rising challenge of non-AIDS-defining cancers in HIV-infected patients. *Clin Infect Dis* 2012;55:1228-1235.

Di Bartolo DL, Cannon M, Liu YF, et al. KSHV LANA inhibits TGF-beta signaling through epigenetic silencing of the TGF-beta type II receptor. *Blood* 2008;111:4731-4740.

Dittmer DP, Richards KL, Damania B. Treatment of Kaposi sarcoma-associated herpesvirus-associated cancers. *Front Microbiol* 2012;3(141):1-8.

D'Souza G, Kreimer AR, Viscidi R, et al. Case-control study of human papillomavirus and oropharyngeal cancer. *N Engl J Med* 2007;356:1944-1956.

Dykstra ML, Longnecker R, Pierce SK. Epstein-Barr virus coopts lipid rafts to block the signaling and antigen transport functions of the BCR. *Immunity* 2001;14:57-67.

Dyson N, Howley PM, Munger K, et al. The human papilloma virus-16 E7 oncoprotein is able to bind to the retinoblastoma gene product. *Science* 1989;243:934-937.

Fanning E, Knippers R. Structure and function of simian virus 40 large tumor antigen. *Annu Rev Biochem* 1992;61:55-86.

Feng H, Shuda M, Chang Y, et al. Clonal integration of a polyomavirus in human Merkel cell carcinoma. *Science* 2008;319:1096-1100.

Ferri C, Caracciolo F, Zignego AL, et al. Hepatitis C infection in patients with non-Hodgkin's lymphoma. *Br J Haematol* 1994;88:392-394.

Ferri C, La Civita L, Zignego AL, et al. Viruses and cancers: possible role of hepatitis C virus. *Eur J Clin Invest* 1997;27:711-718.

Friborg J Jr, Kong W, Hottiger MO, et al. p53 inhibition by the LANA protein of KSHV protects against cell death. *Nature* 1999;402:889-894.

Fujimuro M, Liu J, Zhu J, et al. Regulation of the interaction between glycogen synthase kinase 3 and the Kaposi's sarcoma-associated herpesvirus latency-associated nuclear antigen. *J Virol* 2005;79:10429-10441.

Fukayama M. Epstein-Barr virus and gastric carcinoma. *Pathol Int* 2010;60:337-350.

Future II Study Group. Quadrivalent vaccine against human papillomavirus to prevent high-grade cervical lesions. *N Engl J Med* 2007;356:1915-1927.

Ganem D. Kaposi's sarcoma-associated herpesvirus. In: Knipe DM, Howley PM, eds. *Field's Virology*. Philadelphia, PA: Lippincott, Williams, & Wilkins; 2007:2847-2888.

Gerits N, Moens U. Agnoprotein of mammalian polyomaviruses. *Virology* 2012;432:316-326.

Giuliano AR, Palefsky JM, Goldstone S, et al. Efficacy of quadrivalent HPV vaccine against HPV infection and disease in males. *N Engl J Med* 2011;364:401-411.

Gjoerup O, Chang Y. Update on human polyomaviruses and cancer. *Adv Cancer Res* 2010;106:1-51.

Goff SP. Retroviridae: the retroviruses and their replication. In: Knipe DM, Howley PM, eds. *Field's Virology*. Philadelphia, PA: Lippincott, Williams, & Wilkins; 2007:1999-2070.

Goncalves DU, Roietti FA, Ribas JGR, et al. Epidemiology, treatment, and prevention of human T-cell leukemia virus type 1-associated diseases. *Clin Microbiol Rev* 2010;23:577-589.

Gromminger S, Mautner J, Bornkamm GW. Burkitt lymphoma: the role of Epstein-Barr virus revisited. *Br J Haematol* 2012;156:719-729.

Groom HC, Bishop KN. The tale of xenotropic murine leukemia virus-related virus. *J Gen Virol* 2012;93:915-924.

Grossman WJ, Kimata JT, Wong FH, et al. Development of leukemia in mice transgenic for the tax gene of human T-cell leukemia virus type I. *Proc Natl Acad Sci U S A* 1995;92:1057-1061.

Grundhoff A, Sullivan CS, Ganem D. A combined computational and microarray-based approach identifies novel microRNAs encoded by human gamma-herpesviruses. *RNA* 2006;12:733-750.

Guasparri I, Wu H, Cesarman E. The KSHV oncoprotein vFLIP contains a TRAF-interacting motif and requires TRAF2 and TRAF3 for signalling. *EMBO Rep* 2006;7:114-119.

Han J, Sabbatini P, Perez D, et al. The E1B 19K protein blocks apoptosis by interacting with and inhibiting the p53-inducible and death-promoting Bax protein. *Genes Dev* 1996;10:461-477.

Harada JN, Berk AJ. p53-Independent and -dependent requirements for E1B-55K in adenovirus type 5 replication. *J Virol* 1999;73:5333-5344.

Hasegawa H, Sawa H, Lewis MJ, et al. Thymus-derived leukemia-lymphoma in mice transgenic for the Tax gene of human T-lymphotropic virus type I. *Nat Med* 2006;12:466-472.

Hawley-Nelson P, Vousden KH, Hubbert NL, et al. HPV16 E6 and E7 proteins cooperate to immortalize human foreskin keratinocytes. *EMBO J* 1989;8:3905-3910.

Heise C, Sampson-Johannes A, Williams A, et al. ONYX-015, an E1B gene-attenuated adenovirus, causes tumor-specific cytolysis and antitumoral efficacy that can be augmented by standard chemotherapeutic agents. *Nat Med* 1997;3:639-646.

Higa LA, Zhang H. Stealing the spotlight. CUL4-DDB1 ubiquitin ligase docks WD40-repeat proteins to destroy. *Cell Div* 2007;2:5.

Houghton M. Prospects for prophylactic and therapeutic vaccines against the hepatitis C viruses. *Immunol Rev* 2011;239:99-108.

Hsu DH, de Waal Malefyt R, Fiorentino DF, et al. Expression of interleukin-10 activity by Epstein-Barr virus protein BCRF1. *Science* 1990;250:830-832.

Iwakiri D, Takada K. Role of EBER5 in the pathogenesis of EBV infection. *Adv Cancer Res* 2010;107:119-136.

Jang BG, Kim WH. Molecular pathology of gastric carcinoma. *Pathobiology* 2011;78:302-310.

Jasani B, Cristaudo A, Emri SA, et al. Association of SV40 with human tumours. *Semin Cancer Biol* 2001;11:49-61.

Jochum S, Moosmann A, Lang S, et al. The EBV immunoevasins vIL-10 and BNLF2a protect newly infected B cells from immune recognition and elimination. *PLoS Pathog* 2012;8:e1002704.

Kapatai G, Murray P. Contribution of the Epstein Barr virus to the molecular pathogenesis of Hodgkin lymphoma. *J Clin Pathol* 2007;60:1342-1349.

Kew MC. Hepatitis B virus x protein in the pathogenesis of hepatitis B virus-induced hepatocellular carcinoma. *J Gastroenterol Hepatol* 2011;26 Suppl 1:144-152.

Kieff ED, Rickinson AB. Epstein-Barr virus and its replication. In: Knipe DM, Howley PM, eds. *Field's Virology*. Philadelphia, PA: Lippincott, Williams, & Wilkins; 2007:2603-2654.

Kung CP, Meckes DG, Raab-Traub N. Epstein-Barr virus LMP1 activates EGFR, STAT3, and ER through effects of PKCδ. *J Virol* 2011;85:4399-4308.

Lai MM. Hepatitis C virus proteins: direct link to hepatic oxidative stress, steatosis, carcinogenesis and more. *Gastroenterology* 2002; 122:568-571.

Lairmore MD, Franchini G, Human T-cell leukemia virus types 1 and 2. In: Knipe DM, Howley PM, eds. *Field's Virology*. Philadelphia, PA: Lippincott, Williams, & Wilkins; 2007: 2071-2106.

Lane DP, Crawford LV. T antigen is bound to a host protein in SV40-transformed cells. *Nature* 1979;278:261-263.

Lechner F, Wong K, Dunbar PR, et al. Analysis of successful immune responses in persons infected with hepatitis C virus. *J Exp Med* 2000;191:1499-1512.

Lee BS, Lee SH, Feng P, et al. Characterization of the Kaposi's sarcoma-associated herpesvirus K1 signalosome. *J Virol* 2005; 79:12173-12184.

Lemasson I, Lewis MR, Polakowski N, et al. Human T-cell leukemia virus type 1 (HTLV-1) bZIP protein interacts with the cellular transcription factor CREB to inhibit HTLV-1 transcription. *J Virol* 2007;81:1543-1553.

Lerat H, Honda M, Beard MR, et al. Steatosis and liver cancer in transgenic mice expressing the structural and nonstructural proteins of hepatitis C virus. *Gastroenterology* 2002;122: 352-365.

Li HP, Chang YS. Epstein-Barr virus latent membrane protein 1: structure and functions. *J Biomed Sci* 2003;10:490-504.

Li T, Robert EI, Strubin M, et al. A promiscuous alpha-helical motif anchors viral hijackers and substitute receptors to the CUL4-DDB1 ubiquitin ligase machinery. *Nat Struct Mol Biol* 2010;17: 105-111.

Liebowitz D. Nasopharyngeal carcinoma: the Epstein-Barr virus association. *Semin Oncol* 1994;21:376-381.

Lilyestrom W, Klein MG, Zhang R, et al. Crystal structure of SV40 large T-antigen bound to p53: interplay between a viral oncoprotein and a cellular tumor suppressor. *Genes Dev* 2006;20:2373-2382.

Lin JC, Wang WY, Chen KY, et al. Quantification of plasma Epstein-Barr virus DNA in patients with advanced nasopharyngeal carcinoma. *N Engl J Med* 2004;350:2461-2470.

Linzer DI, Levine AJ. Characterization of 54K Dalton cellular SV40 tumor antigen present in SV40-transformed cells and uninfected embryonal carcinoma cells. *Cell* 1979;17:43-52.

Liu BS, Hong S, Tang Z, et al. HTLV-I Tax directly binds the Cdc20-associated anaphase-promoting complex and activates it ahead of schedule. *Proc Natl Acad Sci U S A* 2005;102:63-68.

Liu L, Eby MT, Rathore N, et al. The human herpes virus 8-encoded viral FLICE inhibitory protein physically associates with and persistently activates the Ikappa B kinase complex. *J Biol Chem* 2002;277:13745-13751.

Lo KW, To KF, Huang DP. Focus on nasopharyngeal carcinoma. *Cancer Cell* 2004;5:423-428.

Longnecker R. Epstein-Barr virus latency: LMP2, a regulator or means for Epstein-Barr virus persistence? *Adv Cancer Res* 2000; 79:175-200.

Lu J, Verma SC, Murakami M, et al. Latency-associated nuclear antigen of Kaposi's sarcoma-associated herpesvirus (KSHV) upregulates survivin expression in KSHV-Associated B-lymphoma cells and contributes to their proliferation. *J Virol* 2009;83:7129-7141.

Luo Z, Ruan B. Impact of the implementation of a vaccination strategy on hepatitis B virus infections in China over a 20-year period. *Int J Infect Dis* 2012;16:e82-e88.

Machida K, Cheng KT, Lai CK, et al. Hepatitis C virus triggers mitochondrial permeability transition with production of reactive oxygen species, leading to DNA damage and STATe activation. *J Virol* 2006;80:7199-7207.

Machida K, Cheng KT, Sung VM, et al. Hepatitis C virus induces a mutator phenotype: enhanced mutations of immunoglobulin and proto-oncogenes. *Proc Natl Acad Sci U S A* 2004;101: 4262-4267.

Marquitz AR, Raab-Traub N. The role of miRNAs and EBV BARTS in NPC. *Semin Cancer Biol* 2012;22:166-172.

Marriott SJ, Semmes OJ. Impact of HTLV-I Tax on cell cycle progression and the cellular DNA damage repair response. *Oncogene* 2005;24:5986-5995.

Marshall E. Gene therapy death prompts review of adenovirus vector. *Science* 1999;286:2244-2246.

Martin-Lluesma S, Schaeffer C, Robert EI, et al. Hepatitis B X protein affects S phase progression leading to chromosome segregation defects by binding to damaged DNA binding protein 1. *Hepatology* 2008;48:1467-1476.

Marusawa H, Hijikata M, Chiba T, et al. Hepatitis C virus core protein inhibits Fas- and tumor necrosis factor alpha-mediated apoptosis via NF-kappaB activation. *J Virol* 1999;73:4713-4720.

Matsuoka M, Jeang KT. Human T-cell leukemia virus type 1 (HTLV-1) and leukemic transformation: viral infectivity, Tax, HBZ and therapy. *Oncogene* 2011;30:1379-1389.

Matta H, Chaudhary PM. Activation of alternative NF-kappa B pathway by human herpes virus 8-encoded Fas-associated death domain-like IL-1 beta-converting enzyme inhibitory protein (vFLIP). *Proc Natl Acad Sci U S A* 2004;101:9399-9404.

McCormick C, Ganem D. The kaposin B protein of KSHV activates the p38/MK2 pathway and stabilizes cytokine mRNAs. *Science* 2005;307:739-741.

McLaughlin-Drubin ME, Munger K. Oncogenic activities of human papillomaviruses. *Virus Res* 2009;143:195-208.

Mercer DF, Schiller DE, Elliott JF, et al. Hepatitis C virus replication in mice with chimeric human livers. *Nat Med* 2001;7:927-933.

Mesri EA, Cesarman E, Boshoff C. Kaposi's sarcoma and its associated herpesvirus. *Nat Rev Cancer* 2010;10:707-719.

Miyazato AS, Sheleg S, Iha H, et al. Evidence for NF-kappaB- and CBP-independent repression of p53's transcriptional activity by human T-cell leukemia virus type 1 Tax in mouse embryo and primary human fibroblasts. *J Virol* 2005;79:9346-9350.

Miyoshi HH, Fujie H, Shintani Y, et al. Hepatitis C virus core protein exerts an inhibitory effect on suppressor of cytokine signaling (SOCS)-1 gene expression. *J Hepatol* 2005;43:757-763.

Molyneux EM, Rochford R, Griffin B, et al. Burkitt's lymphoma. *Lancet* 2012;379:1234-1244.

Montaner S, Sodhi A, Molinolo A, et al. Endothelial infection with KSHV genes in vivo reveals that vGPCR initiates Kaposi's sarcomagenesis and can promote the tumorigenic potential of viral latent genes. *Cancer Cell* 2003;3:23-36.

Moody CA, Laimins LA. Human papillomavirus oncoproteins: pathways to transformation. *Nat Rev Cancer* 2010;10:550-560.

Moran E, Mathews MB. Multiple functional domains in the adenovirus E1A gene. *Cell* 1987;48:177-178.

Moses AV, Fish KN, Ruhl R, et al. Long-term infection and transformation of dermal microvascular endothelial cells by human herpesvirus 8. *J Virol* 1999;73:6892-6902.

Munger K, Phelps WC, Bubb V, et al. The E6 and E7 genes of the human papillomavirus type 16 together are necessary and sufficient for transformation of primary human keratinocytes. *J Virol* 1989;63:4417-4421.

Muralidhar S, Pumfery AM, Hassani M, et al. Identification of kaposin (open reading frame K12) as a human herpesvirus 8 (Kaposi's sarcoma-associated herpesvirus) transforming gene. *J Virol* 1998;72:4980-4988.

Nevins JR. Cell transformation by viruses. In: Knipe DM, Howley PM, eds. *Field's Virology*. Philadelphia, PA: Lippincott, Williams, & Wilkins; 2007:209-248.

Ng SA, Lee C. Hepatitis B virus X gene and hepatocarcinogenesis. *J Gastroenterol* 2011;46:974-990.

Ogilvie G, Anderson M, Marra F, et al. A population-based evaluation of a publicly funded, school-based HPV vaccine program in British Columbia, Canada: parental factors associated with HPV vaccine receipt. *PLoS Med* 2010;7:e1000270.

Ohsugi T, Kumasaka T, Okada S, et al. The Tax protein of HTLV-1 promotes oncogenesis in not only immature T cells but also mature T cells. *Nat Med* 2007;13:527-528.

Ou JHJ, Yen TSB. *Human Oncogenic Viruses*. Hackensack, NJ: World Scientific; 2010.

Owens GP, Bennett JL. Trigger, pathogen, or bystander: the complex nexus linking Epstein-Barr virus and multiple sclerosis. *Mult Scler* 2012;18:1204-1208.

Paavonen J, Naud P, Salmeron J, et al. Efficacy of human papillomavirus (HPV)-16/18 AS04-adjuvanted vaccine against cervical infection and precancer caused by oncogenic HPV types (PATRICIA): final analysis of a double-blind, randomized study in young women. *Lancet* 2009;374:301-314.

Pallas DC, Shahrik LK, Martin BL, et al. Polyoma small and middle T antigens and SV40 small t antigen form stable complexes with protein phosphatase 2A. *Cell* 1990;60:167-176.

Pesonen S, Kangasniemi L, Hemminki A. Oncolytic adenoviruses for the treatment of human cancer: focus on translational and clinical data. *Mol Pharm* 2011;8:12-28.

Pfeffer S, Zavolan M, Grasser FA, et al. Identification of virus-encoded microRNAs. *Science* 2004;304:734-736.

Qi F, Yang H, Gaudini G. Simian virus 40 transformation, malignant mesothelioma, and brain tumors. *Expert Rev Respir Med* 2011;5:683-697.

Radkov SA, Kellam P, Boshoff C. The latent nuclear antigen of Kaposi sarcoma-associated herpesvirus targets the retinoblastoma-E2F pathway and with the oncogene Hras transforms primary rat cells. *Nat Med* 2000;6:1121-1127.

Rauch DA, Ratner L. Targeting HTLV-1 activation of NFkB in mouse models and ATLL patients. *Viruses* 2011;3: 886-900.

Razak AR, Siu LL, Liu FF, et al. Nasopharyngeal carcinoma: the next challenges. *Eur J Cancer* 2010;46:1967-1978.

Rickinson AB, Kieff E. Epstein-Barr virus. In: Knipe DM, Howley PM, eds. *Field's Virology*. Philadelphia, PA: Lippincott, Williams, & Wilkins; 2007:2655-2700.

Saenz Robles MT, Pipas JM. T antigen transgenic mouse models. *Semin Cancer Biol* 2009;19:229-235.

Samaniego F, Pati S, Karp JE, et al. Human herpesvirus 8 K1-associated nuclear factor-kappa B-dependent promoter activity: role in Kaposi's sarcoma inflammation? *J Natl Cancer Inst Monogr* 2001;28:15-23.

Samols MA, Hu J, Skalsky RL, et al. Cloning and identification of a microRNA cluster within the latency-associated region of Kaposi's sarcoma-associated herpesvirus. *J Virol* 2005;79:9301-9305.

Samols, MA, Skalsky RL, Maldonado AM, et al. Identification of cellular genes targeted by KSHV-encoded microRNAs. *PLoS Pathog* 2007;3:e65.

Sarrazin C, Hezode C, Zeuzen S, et al. Antiviral strategies in hepatitis C virus infection. *J Hepatol* 2012;56 Suppl 1: S88-S100.

Satou Y, Yasunaga J, Yoshida M, et al. HTLV-I basic leucine zipper factor gene mRNA supports proliferation of adult T cell leukemia cells. *Proc Natl Acad Sci U S A* 2006;103:720-725.

Schrama D, Ugurel S, Becker JC. Merkel cell carcinoma: recent insights and new treatment options. *Curr Opin Oncol* 2012;24: 141-149.

See RH, Shi Y. Adenovirus E1B 19,000-molecular-weight protein activates c-Jun N-terminal kinase and c-Jun-mediated transcription. *Mol Cell Biol* 1998;18:4012-4022.

Seeger, et al. Hepadnaviruses. In: Knipe DM, Howley PM, eds. *Field's Virology*. Philadelphia, PA: Lippincott, Williams, & Wilkins; 2007:2977-3030.

Sfanos KS, Aloia AL, De Marzo AM, et al. XMRV and prostate cancer—a "final" perspective. *Nat Rev Urol* 2012;10:111-118.

Shi W, Kato H, Perez-Ordonez B, et al. Comparative prognostic value of HPV16 E6 mRNA compared with in situ hybridization for human oropharyngeal squamous carcinoma. *J Clin Oncol* 2009;27:6213-6221.

Si H, Robertson ES. Kaposi's sarcoma-associated herpesvirus-encoded latency-associated nuclear antigen induces chromosomal instability through inhibition of p53 function. *J Virol* 2006;80: 697-709.

Soni V, Cahir-McFarland E, Kieff E. LMP1 trafficking activates growth and survival pathways. *Adv Exp Med Biol* 2007;597: 173-187.

Stehelin D, Varmus HE, Bishop JM, Vogt PK. DNA related to the transforming gene(s) of avian sarcoma viruses is present in normal avian DNA. *Nature* 1976;260:170-173.

Stransky N, Egloff AM, Tward AD, et al. The mutational landscape of head and neck squamous cell carcinoma. *Science* 2011;333: 157-1160.

Sun SC, Yamaoka S. Activation of NF-kappaB by HTLV-I and implications for cell transformation. *Oncogene* 2005;24:5952-5964.

Tai DI, Tsai SL, Chen YM, et al. Activation of nuclear factor kappaB in hepatitis C virus infection: implications for pathogenesis and hepatocarcinogenesis. *Hepatology* 2000;31:656-664.

Tomlinson CC, Damania B. The K1 protein of Kaposi's sarcoma-associated herpesvirus activates the Akt signaling pathway. *J Virol* 2004;78:1918-1927.

Tsai WL, Chung RT. Viral hepatocarcinogenesis. *Oncogene* 2010;29:2309-2324.

Tsutsumi T, Suzuki T, Moriya K, et al. Hepatitis C virus core protein activates ERK and p38 MAPK in cooperation with ethanol in transgenic mice. *Hepatology* 2003;38:820-828.

van Ghelue M, Khan MT, Ehlers B, Moens U. Genome analysis of the new human polyomaviruses. *Rev Med Virol* 2012; [Mar 28 Epub ahead of print].

Verschuren EW, Jones N, Evan GI. The cell cycle and how it is steered by Kaposi's sarcoma-associated herpesvirus cyclin. *J Gen Virol* 2004;85:1347-13612.

Verschuren EW, Klefstrom J, Evan GI, et al. The oncogenic potential of Kaposi's sarcoma-associated herpesvirus cyclin is exposed by p53 loss in vitro and in vivo. *Cancer Cell* 2002;2:229-241.

Wakita, T, Pietschmann, T, Kato T, et al. Production of infectious hepatitis C virus in tissue culture from a cloned viral genome. *Nat Med* 2005;11:791-796.

Wang L, Dittmer DP, CC, et al. Immortalization of primary endothelial cells by the K1 protein of Kaposi's sarcoma-associated herpesvirus. *Cancer Res* 2006;66:3658-3666.

Wang LN, Wakisaka N, Tomlinson VV, et al. The Kaposi's sarcoma-associated herpesvirus (KSHV/HHV-8) K1 protein induces expression of angiogenic and invasion factors. *Cancer Res* 2004; 64:2774-2781.

Wang WK, Levy S. Hepatitis C virus (HCV) and lymphagenesis. *Leuk Lymphoma* 2003;44:1113-1120.

Wei Y, Neuveut C, Tiollais P, et al. Molecular biology of the hepatitis B virus and role of the X gene. *Pathol Biol* 2010;58:267-272.

Weng WK, Levy S. Hepatitis C virus (HCV) and lymphomagenesis. *Leuk Lymphoma* 2003;44:1113-1120. http://www.ncbi.nlm.nih .gov/pubmed/12916862.

Westra WH, Taube JM, Poeta ML, Begum S, et al. Inverse relationship between human papillomavirus-16 infection and disruptive p53 gene mutations in squamous cell carcinoma of the head and neck. *Clin Cancer Res* 2008;14:366-369.

Wheeler CM, Castellsague X, Garland SM, et al. Cross-protective efficacy of HPV-16/18 AS04-adjuvanted vaccine against cervical infection and precancer caused by non-vaccine oncogenic HPV types: 4-year end-of-study analysis of the randomized, double-blind PATRICIA trial. *Lancet Oncol* 2012;13:100-110.

Wong DK, Dudley DD, Dohrenwend PB, et al. Detection of diverse hepatitis C virus (HCV)-specific cytotoxic T lymphocytes in peripheral blood of infected persons by screening for responses to all translated proteins of HCV. *J Virol* 2001;75:1229-1236.

Wong-Staal F, Gallo RC. The family of human T-lymphotropic leukemia viruses: HTLV-I as the cause of adult T cell leukemia and HTLV-III as the cause of acquired immunodeficiency syndrome. *Blood* 1985;65:253-263.

Xiao J, Zhang J, Wu C, et al. Impact of hepatitis B vaccination among children in Guandong Province, China. *Int J Infect Dis* 2012;16:e692-e696.

Xing L, Kieff E. Epstein-Barr virus BHRF1 micro and stable RNAs in latency III and after induction of replication. *J Virol* 2007;81: 9967-9975.

Yamamoto M, Curiel DT. Current issues and future directions of oncolytic adenoviruses. *Mol Ther* 2010;18:243-250.

Yang B, Bouchard MJ. The hepatitis B virus X protein elevates cytosolic calcium signals by modulating mitochondrial calcium uptake. *J Virol* 2012;86:313-327.

Yang TY, Chen SC, Leach MW, et al. Transgenic expression of the chemokine receptor encoded by human herpesvirus 8 induces an angioproliferative disease resembling Kaposi's sarcoma. *J Exp Med* 2000;191:445-454.

Yang Z, Yan Z, Wood C. Kaposi's sarcoma-associated herpesvirus transactivator RTA promotes degradation of the repressors to regulate viral lytic replication. *J Virol* 2008;82:3590-3603.

Yin M, Wheeler MD, Kono H, et al. Essential role of tumor necrosis factor alpha in alcohol-induced liver injury in mice. *Gastroenterology* 1999;117:942-952.

Younis I, Green PL. The human T-cell leukemia virus Rex protein. *Front Biosci* 2005;10:431-445.

Yu W, Fang H. Clinical trials with oncolytic adenovirus in China. *Curr Cancer Drug Targets* 2007;7:141-148.

Yu Y, Wang SE, Hayward GS. The KSHV immediate early transcription factor RTA incodes ubiquitin E3 ligase activity that targets IRF7 for proteosome-mediated degradation. *Immunity* 2008;22:59-70.

Ziegelbauer JM. Functions of Kaposi's sarcoma-associated herpesvirus microRNAs. *Biochim Biophys Acta* 2011;1809: 623-630.

Zuckerman E, Zuckerman T, Levine AM, et al. Hepatitis C virus infection in patients with B-cell non-Hodgkin lymphoma *Ann Intern Med* 1997;127:423-428.

zur Hausen H. Papillomaviruses and cancer: from basic studies to clinical application. *Nat Rev Cancer* 2002;2:342-350.

zur Hausen H. Red meat consumption and cancer: reasons to suspect involvement of bovine infectious factors in colorectal cancer. *Int J Cancer* 2012;130:2475-2483.

zur Hausen H, de Villiers EM. TT viruses: oncogenic or tumor-suppressive properties? *Curr Top Microbiol Immunol* 2009;331: 109-116.

Oncogenes and Tumor-Suppressor Genes

Previn Dutt and Vuk Stambolic

7.1 INTRODUCTION

Cancer is fundamentally a genetic disease. It results in expansion of a cellular population that invades and destroys surrounding organs and tissues and gains the ability to spread throughout the body. The second half of the 20th century inaugurated a steady stream of breakthroughs in the field of cancer research, largely spurred by an explosion of technologies enabling the analysis of tumors at a molecular level. Recent dramatic advancements in low-cost high-throughput sequencing of cancer genomes and the development of high-resolution genome-wide profiling of the changes in gene copy number and structure are enabling detailed mapping of the genetic events associated with cellular transformation from nonmalignant to malignant cell.

The emerging comprehensive surveys of cancer genomes are uncovering the complexity of the disease and are also beginning to guide the development of highly targeted anticancer treatments based on discrete molecular features. Importantly, these efforts are revealing the extreme genetic heterogeneity that exists amongst tumors with similar histopathology (see also Chap. 13, Sec. 13.2.2). Although a given tumor may harbor hundreds of mutations in protein coding regions, perhaps

only 10 to 15 can truly be considered to be "driver" mutations that confer a selective growth advantage to transformed cells. The remaining "passenger" mutations result from the genetic instability of cancer cells without actively contributing to oncogenesis. Distinguishing between the driver and passenger mutations is critical for the identification of therapeutic targets and the development of tailored treatment regimens with the promise of maximizing anti-cancer activity whilst minimizing side effects (Fig. 7–1) (Carter et al, 2009; Carter et al, 2010).

7.2 THE GENETIC BASIS OF CANCER

7.2.1 Historical Perspective

The earliest recorded cases of cancer were documented in ancient Egypt around 1600 BC and described 8 cases of breast cancer along with a cauterization technique used to treat the disease. The term *cancer* itself was coined by the father of medicine, Hippocrates, who also advanced the theory that the origins of the disease resided in an excess of "black bile," 1 of the 4 constituent fluids the ancient Greeks believed made up the human body. Remarkably, this humoral theory persisted as the dominant explanation for cancer for nearly 2 millennia thereafter.

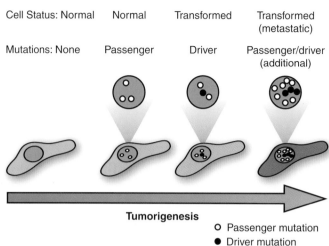

FIGURE 7–1 Passenger and driver mutations. Tumor sequencing has revealed that transformed cells acquire a genetic landscape marked by the accumulation of numerous mutations. Amongst these genetic changes, however, are a much more limited subset of driver mutations that actively impart oncogenic properties, with the remaining passenger mutations representing inert changes that are neither selected for or against during tumorigenesis. Distinguishing between driver and passenger mutations is a critical research objective as the former represent potential therapeutic targets.

The genesis of understanding cancer as a genetic disease is widely traced to experiments carried out more than a century ago, the implications of which would go largely unappreciated for decades afterward. In 1902, the German biologist Theodor Boveri manipulated the structure of sea urchin chromosomes and was able to correlate malignant cellular growth with genomic abnormalities (Balmain, 2001). Strikingly, on the basis of these findings, he presciently speculated on the existence of cell-cycle checkpoints, oncogenes, and tumor suppressors, which are now known actors in oncogenesis. However, the first correlation between chromosomal defects and cancer in humans was not reported until 1960, with the discovery of the chronic myeloid leukemia (CML)-associated Philadelphia chromosome, generated by a gene translocation (Goldman and Melo, 2008).

7.2.2 Transforming Retroviruses

Another landmark breakthrough in the field of cancer research came in 1911, when Peyton Rous demonstrated that cell-free filtrates isolated from chicken sarcomas, later determined to contain retroviruses (see Chap. 6, Sec. 6.4), were capable of inducing tumor growth when introduced into healthy birds (Rous, 1911). Rous carefully documented the various characteristics which these tumors shared with the sarcomas, such as morphological appearance and the capacity to metastasize and invade distant tissues. Although some time would pass before his work gained widespread appreciation, his experiments ultimately led to the isolation of viral oncogenes from a number of transforming tumor viruses. In 1966, Rous was awarded the Nobel Prize in Medicine or Physiology, 55 years after the publication of his seminal work.

7.2.3 The Knudson Two-Hit Hypothesis

During the 1950s and 1960s, some researchers sought to explore the genetics of cancer by employing mathematical modeling to approximate the number of mutations required to induce neoplastic transformation, based upon the frequency of cancer incidence and estimated mutation rates. In particular, these models sought to explain the synergistic increase in tumor formation observed in mice subjected to repeated exposure to carcinogens, as well as the age-dependent acceleration in the onset of human cancers. In 1953, Carl Nordling estimated that roughly 7 mutations were involved in cancer progression, based upon his analysis of the age of cancer onset in several Western countries (Nordling, 1953). Peter Armitage and Richard Doll reported a similar conclusion the following year, before revising their estimates down to 2 oncogenic mutations for tumor formation in 1957 (Armitage and Doll, 1954; Armitage and Doll, 1957). Alfred Knudson elegantly reiterated these models of multistage cancer progression in 1971, in the form of his now famous "two-hit" hypothesis (Knudson, 1971). Knudson believed that the mutational requirements of cancer progression could be delineated by comparing the incidence rates of inherited and sporadic forms of retinoblastoma. He concluded that individuals who had inherited 1 mutant allele presented the disease at a frequency consistent with a single somatic mutation, whereas individuals who had not inherited a mutant allele exhibited an age-onset pattern consistent with 2 mutations. The onset of hereditary retinoblastoma represents the archetypal example of loss of heterozygosity (LOH) at a tumor-suppressor locus, generated by the inheritance of a single mutant allele, encoding an inactive protein, along with a copy of the wild-type allele. In the heterozygous state, sufficient functional tumor suppressor is expressed from the wild-type allele to prevent the onset of tumorigenesis. Disease progression is contingent on the loss of the heterozygous state through inactivation of the wild-type allele, for example through deletion, which completely ablates expression of the tumor-suppressor activity. Subsequent research provided the molecular basis for the Knudson model, namely the necessity of homozygous inactivation of the retinoblastoma protein (Rb) on chromosome 13 for development of the disease (see Secs. 7.2.5 and 7.6.4).

7.2.4 Discovery of Oncogenes

In 1976, Michael Bishop and Harold Varmus isolated the oncogenic region of the Rous sarcoma virus, containing the *v-src* gene, by comparing the genetic content of a transformation-defective version of the virus with that of its highly transforming counterpart (Stehelin et al, 1976). Remarkably, they discovered that the normal avian DNA contained a nearly identical version of the *v-src* gene. On this basis, they advanced what was then a provocative concept, that oncogenes were altered versions of normal cellular genes, which they termed *protooncogenes*. Moreover, their findings suggested that other oncogenes might be found in the genomes of other transforming retroviruses. Indeed, many of the best known oncogenes were originally identified in viruses (see Chap. 6).

In 1982, the first somatically mutated cellular oncogenes were isolated in a number of laboratories by employing strategies that generally involved introducing DNA isolated from human cancer cell lines into mouse fibroblasts, which were then monitored for transformation. Isolation of individual genes from the transformed fibroblasts led to the identification of the activated mutant versions of the *H-RAS* and *K-RAS* oncogenes, derived from human bladder and lung carcinoma cell lines, respectively (Der et al, 1982). A year later, mutant *N-RAS* was similarly isolated from a neuroblastoma cell line (Shimizu et al, 1983).

7.2.5 Isolation of the First Tumor Suppressor

The prevailing view in the 1970s was that neoplastic transformation resulted from dominant activating mutations in oncogenes. This paradigm was challenged in the 1980s, when the retinoblastoma (*Rb1*) locus was mapped to a chromosomal region containing homozygous deletions, in both inherited and sporadic retinoblastomas (Cavenee et al, 1983). In 1986, a complementary DNA (cDNA) fragment mapping to the *Rb1* locus was isolated and found to be at least partially deleted in retinoblastomas (Friend et al, 1986). The following year, 2 groups cloned the Rb cDNA, and reported that the transcript was either expressed in a truncated form or was entirely undetectable in tumors (Fung et al, 1987; Lee et al, 1987; Kallioniemi, 2008). Collectively, these results demonstrated the existence of a recessively acting cancer gene, with the homozygous loss of the wild-type *Rb1* locus correlating with retinoblastoma development, as predicted by Knudson's theoretical work 15 years earlier (see also Sec. 7.6.4).

7.2.6 The Genomics Age and Beyond

By the beginning of the 1990s, a clearer picture of the genetic changes accompanying cancer progression had begun to emerge, leading to the realization that cancer is a disease involving a combination of either inherited or somatic mutations, resulting in the activation of oncogenes or inactivation of tumor-suppressor genes (Fig. 7–2). Since then, additional putative oncogenes and tumor suppressors have been cataloged using both classical methods, as well as novel high-throughput analyses (Table 7–1; see Chap. 2, Sec. 2.2 for techniques). Functional characterization of proteins encoded by oncogenes and tumor-suppressor

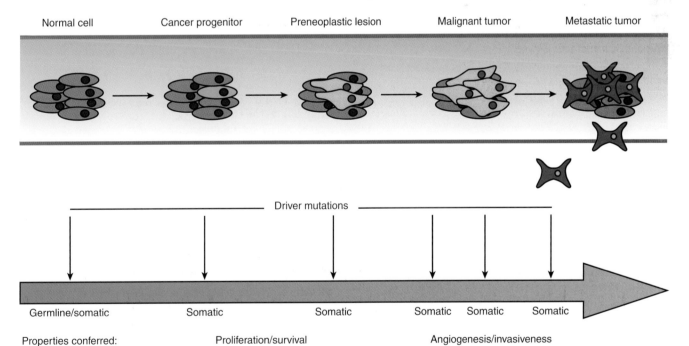

| Normal cell | Cancer progenitor | Preneoplastic lesion | Malignant tumor | Metastatic tumor |

Driver mutations

Germline/somatic   Somatic   Somatic   Somatic   Somatic   Somatic

Properties conferred: Proliferation/survival   Angiogenesis/invasiveness

FIGURE 7–2 Multistage oncogenesis. During oncogenesis, a tumor progressively acquires a set of abnormal properties that enable it to support the growing mass of cells and ultimately metastasize to distal sites. It has long been recognized that this constitutes a multistep process involving a series of oncogenic hits, potentially occurring at both the germline (inherited) or somatic level. More recently, it has been appreciated that, in addition to genetic mutations, these hits can entail changes at the epigenetic, transcriptomic, proteomic, and metabolic levels. Moreover, these tumorigenic programs can be driven by different sets of oncogenic hits and progress at different rates.

TABLE 7–1 Oncogenes and tumor-suppressor genes.

Tumor initiation, expansion, and metastasis are driven by a combination of oncogene gain-of-function and tumor-suppressor loss-of-function mutagenic events, which confer neoplastic properties on the population of cancer cells. These aberrations may occur at the genetic, epigenetic, transcriptomic, proteomic, or metabolic levels. Well-characterized oncogenes and tumor suppressors are listed, along with the tumors they are commonly associated with, as well as relevant diagnostic tests and approved targeted therapies.

Oncogene	Cancer	Diagnostic	Targeted Therapy
p110α	breast, prostate, endometrial, colorectal, cervical, head and neck, gastric, lung	PCR, sequencing	
EGFR	lung, glioma, colorectal, ovarian, breast	PCR, FISH, IHC	gefitinib, erlotinib, cetuximab
ERBB2 (HER2)	breast, gastric, ovarian, bladder	PCR, sequencing	trastuzumab, lapatinib
B-RAF	melanoma, thyroid, colorectal, ovarian	PCR, sequencing	vemurafenib
K-RAS	pancreatic, lung, colorectal, endometrial, ovarian	PCR, sequencing	
H-RAS	bladder	PCR, sequencing	
N-RAS	melanoma, AML	PCR, sequencing	
MYC	lymphomas, colorectal, breast, prostate, melanoma, neuroblastoma, ovarian	FISH, IHC	
BCR-ABL	CML, ALL, AML	FISH, PCR	imatinib, dasatinib, nilotinib
IDH1	glioblastoma, AML	PCR, sequencing	
IDH2	glioblastoma, AML	PCR, sequencing	
JAK2	CML, ALL	FISH	
KIT	gastrointestinal stromal tumors, AML, melanoma	IHC, flow cytometry	
MET	kidney, gastric, lung, head and neck, colorectal		
FLT-3	AML	PCR	
Tumor Suppressor	**Cancer**	**Diagnostic**	**Targeted Therapy**
p53	lung, colorectal, bladder, ovarian, head and neck, gastric, breast, prostate	IHC, PCR, sequencing	
PTEN	glioblastoma, melanoma, prostate, breast, endometrial, thyroid, lung, colorectal, AML, CLL	IHC, PCR, sequencing	
p16^{INK4A}	melanoma, pancreatic, lung, bladder, head and neck, colorectal, breast	IHC, PCR, sequencing	
p14^{ARF}	lung, bladder, head and neck, colorectal, breast	IHC, PCR, sequencing	
BRCA1	breast, ovarian	PCR, sequencing	
BRCA2	breast, ovarian	PCR, sequencing	
LKB1	lung, gastrointestinal, pancreatic, cervical, melanoma	PCR, sequencing	
VHL	kidney, adrenal, hemangioblastoma	PCR, sequencing	
APC	colorectal, gastric	PCR, sequencing	
FBXW7	ALL, bile duct, colorectal, gastric, endometrial, lung, pancreatic, prostate, ovarian	PCR, sequencing	
Rb	retinoblastoma, lung, bladder, esophageal, osteosarcoma, glioma, liver, CML, prostate, breast	IHC, PCR, sequencing	
NF1	neurofibroma, neuroblastoma, glioma, colorectal	PCR, sequencing	
NF2	meningioma, schwannoma, glioma	PCR, sequencing	

Abbreviations: ALL, acute lymphoblastic leukemia; *AML,* acute myelogenous leukemia; *CML,* chronic myeloid leukemia; *FISH,* fluorescent in situ hybridization; *IHC,* immunohisto-chemistry; *PCR,* polymerase chain reaction.

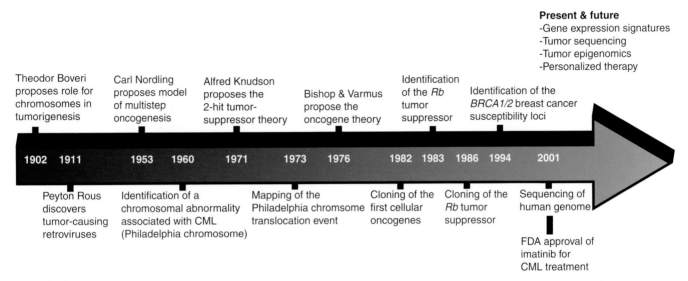

FIGURE 7–3 **Timeline of cancer discoveries.** For much of the past 2 millennia, our understanding of cancer remained relatively static. Beginning in the middle of the 19th century, technological improvements revolutionized our capacity to study the disease, and led to a number of paradigm-shifting discoveries. This process has accelerated in recent decades and we may now anticipate an era in which individual tumors can be comprehensively analyzed and personalized therapies designed to target the appropriate oncogenic mechanisms.

genes has led to an improved understanding of the processes responsible for tumorigenesis. It is now expected that a true understanding of cancer will require surveying for disease-associated changes beyond the genomic level. Of particular interest are epigenetic and microRNA factors, which influence normal cellular physiology (see Chap. 2, Sec. 2.4.3) and are often functionally altered during oncogenic progression.

Comprehensive analyses of genomic, epigenetic, transcriptomic, proteomic, and metabolic states have been rendered practical for the first time by the advent of new high-throughput technologies (see Chap. 2). Characterizations of genomic structure including single nucleotide polymorphisms (SNPs), copy number variations, insertions, deletions, and translocations can be evaluated by SNP and comparative genomic hybridization (CGH) arrays, as well as next-generation sequencing (NGS) techniques (Carter, 2007; Kallioniemi, 2008; Ansorge, 2009). Epigenetic structure is being examined using chromatin immunoprecipitation (ChIP)-based NGS and array methods, while expression profiling, of both protein- and microRNA-encoding transcripts, is undertaken with both genome-wide and more specialized array platforms (Liu et al, 2008; Laird, 2010; see Chap. 2 for more details on these technologies).

There is great anticipation for insights that may be gleaned from these inventories of oncogenic changes at various levels of cellular regulation. Basic research scientists hope to develop a clearer picture of the underlying molecular mechanisms involved in oncogenesis by delineating the precise cellular events occurring at each stage of cancer progression. The prospects for translational scientists and clinicians are no less promising, encompassing the classification of cancers into more homogeneous subtypes, the identification of novel drug targets, and the development of prognostic tools

capable of predicting metastatic propensity, therapeutic response, and survival (Fig. 7–3).

7.3 THE PROPERTIES OF NEOPLASTIC CELLS

The various tissues of the human body have evolved tightly regulated homeostatic mechanisms and lineage differentiation pathways that govern their function and regeneration if injured. Tumorigenesis is initiated when small populations of cells acquire genetic mutations that enable them to circumvent the homeostatic programs particular to their tissue microenvironment. The subsequent survival and expansion of the tumor mass is contingent on the acquisition of additional neoplastic properties, such as invasion. Ultimately, tumor cells gain metastatic potential, involving the capacity to migrate from their tissue of origin and invade distal sites to establish secondary malignancies (see Chap. 10).

Hanahan and Weinberg proposed that virtually all cancer cells exhibit certain hallmark properties: self-sufficiency in growth signals, insensitivity to antigrowth signals, evasion of apoptosis, limitless replicative potential, sustained angiogenesis, genomic instability, deregulated metabolism, the capacity for invasion and metastasis, as well as the ability to circumvent immune clearance an stimulate tumor-promoting inflammation (Hanahan and Weinberg, 2000; Hanahan and Weinberg, 2011; Fig. 7–4). Although a disproportionate number of cancer-associated mutations are found in a small group of critical regulatory proteins, each of these characteristics can be acquired through distinct sets of mutations, and the extreme genetic heterogeneity of cancer cells serves as a platform for the selection of tumor-promoting

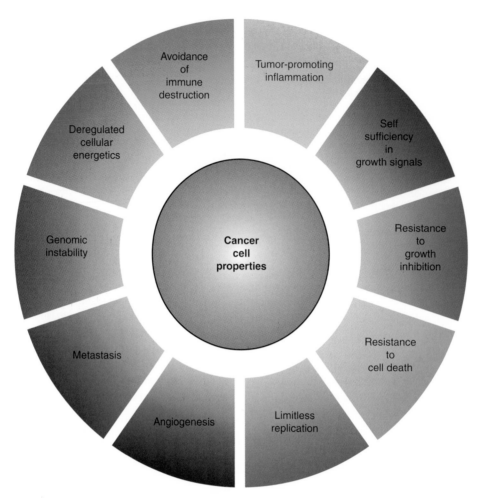

FIGURE 7–4 Properties of cancer. In 2000, Douglas Hanahan and Robert Weinberg proposed a model outlining a series of properties that distinguish cancer cells from their untransformed counterparts. In 2011, this model was updated to incorporate the findings of the ensuing decade of research. Collectively, these properties impart a capacity for tumor survival, expansion, and metastasis in circumstances in which growth would ordinarily be constrained by a variety of regulatory signals. (Adapted from Hanahan and Weinberg, 2011.)

properties. Aberrant autocrine growth signaling, as well as hyperactivation of transmembrane receptors or intracellular signal transducers can engender self-sufficiency in growth signals. Acquired insensitivity to antigrowth signals often involves inactivation of the Rb protein or inhibition of terminal differentiation. Resistance to apoptotic death is frequently associated with loss of the p53 tumor suppressor, as well as the upregulation of antiapoptotic proteins such as BCL2. The replicative potential of normal cells is limited by the progressive attrition of telomeres at chromosome ends, a tendency counteracted in malignant cells through activation of the telomerase enzyme. The nutrient requirements of expanding tumors necessitates the de novo formation of blood vessels, triggered by a combination of upregulated proangiogenic factors, such as vascular endothelial growth factor (VEGF), and downregulation of inhibitory factors like thrombospondin-1 (see Chap. 11, Sec. 11.4). The spread of tumor cells to secondary sites requires the disruption of cell–cell and cell-extracellular matrix (ECM) contacts, as well as the capacity to penetrate tissue compartments,

often through upregulation of extracellular protease activity (see Chap. 10).

Although the reductionist approach of characterizing tumors by these autonomous molecular changes in their cells can be beneficial, it is also important to conceptualize tumors within their tissue contexts. Solid tumors, in particular, are heterotypic collections of cells that include stromal compartments supporting the growth of the malignant cells. This idea was succinctly included in a model of oncogenesis advocated by Kinzler and Vogelstein, who classified cancer-associated genetic changes as gatekeeper, caretaker, and landscaper mutations (Kinzler and Vogelstein, 1996; Kinzler and Vogelstein, 1998; Fig. 7–5). The gatekeepers are generally tumor suppressors that normally constrain growth by regulating cell-cycle progression and activating apoptotic mechanisms as required. The caretakers, often DNA repair proteins, impede oncogenesis by preventing the genetic instability that favors the creation of tumorigenic mutations (see Chap. 5, Sec. 5.3). Alterations in stromal cells, which promote tumorigenesis were termed landscaper mutations.

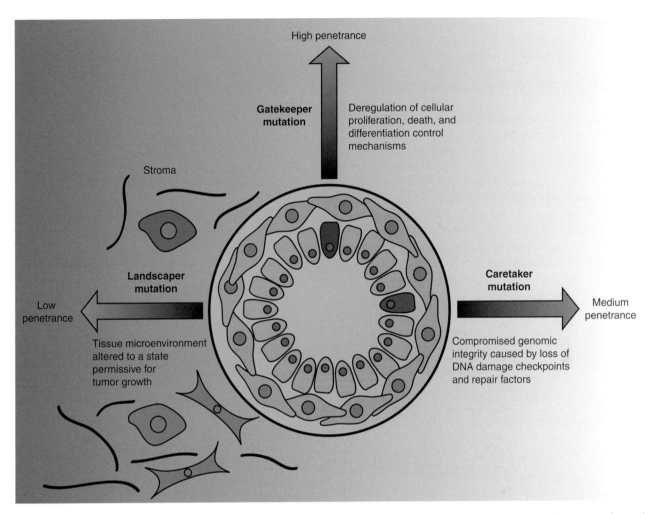

FIGURE 7-5 **Gatekeeper, caretaker, and landscaper mutations.** In the late 1990s, Kenneth Kinzler and Bert Vogelstein proposed a model of tumorigenesis based on their observations of the oncogenic mechanisms underlying hereditary colorectal cancer. Tumor-promoting genes were classified as gatekeepers, caretakers, and landscapers, according to their function. Gatekeeper genes encode proteins that regulate cell fate, be it proliferation, growth, arrest, death, or differentiation. Because deregulation of these mechanisms is likely to lead directly to abnormal growth, mutations in these genes correlate with the highest risk of cancer. Caretaker genes encode proteins that are responsible for guarding the integrity of the genome, with loss of function increasing the risk of acquiring mutations, for instance, in gatekeeper genes, that would lead to oncogenic growth. Mutations occurring in cells of the surrounding tissue stroma can create a microenvironment that is more permissive for tumorigenesis, and the associated genes were categorized as landscapers. As the functions of these genes are primarily supportive, in isolation, these mutations are much less penetrant.

Because genetic instability is a prominent feature of cancer cells (see Chap. 5, Sec. 5.2), the identification of proper therapeutic targets is dependent on determining which alterations represent causal driver mutations that promote oncogenic growth and which are neutral passenger mutations. Although many strategies are being pursued concurrently, there is as yet no clear method for distinguishing driver and passenger mutations (Carter et al, 2009; Bozic et al, 2010). Computational prediction methods have sought to identify driver mutations based on frequency of occurrence. Although it is tempting to categorize those alterations that occur at the background mutational rate as passenger mutations, rare mutations have sometimes been found to be potently oncogenic. Conversely, some genes located in mutational hot spots are disproportionately altered despite making no apparent contribution to

oncogenic progression. Moreover, variations in background mutation rates between tumors complicate such analyses. It may be that as larger datasets become available, driver mutations will be found to occur at rates and in patterns that can be distinguished from passenger mutations, although this remains speculative. The presence of clusters of mutations, both within individual genes and known signaling pathways, is strongly suggestive of driver mutation status. Other prediction strategies aim to identify genetic changes that are likely to alter the function(s) of the encoded proteins. This is most obvious in the case of frameshift and nonsense mutations that introduce stop codons, or mutations that interfere with splice sites. Anticipating the effects of missense mutations, resulting in single amino acid changes, on the activity of a given protein is more challenging, but can be facilitated by

7.4 THE BASIS OF TUMORIGENESIS

While cancer cells are defined at the cellular level by a handful of hallmark properties (see Fig. 7–4), at the molecular level, the genotypic and phenotypic changes are numerous, diverse, and complex. The genetic mutations that are responsible for cancer initiation are accompanied by additional alterations at the epigenetic, transcript, and protein levels (Fig. 7–6). Indeed, deregulation at any one of these levels may induce a cascade of additional mutagenic effects, creating the molecular basis for tumor expansion through clonal selection. In addition to point mutations, which can result in changes to amino acid sequences, other mutagenic events include gene amplifications, deletions, and insertions, as well as chromosomal translocations. The expression levels of cancer-associated genes can also be modulated epigenetically through promoter methylation, as well as the methylation, acetylation, and phosphorylation of histones (see Chap. 2, Sec. 2.3). Additional changes in the expression levels of proteins arise as a result of the modulation of transcriptional rates and messenger RNA (mRNA) stability, often involving the actions of small noncoding RNAs (see Chap. 2, Sec. 2.4.3). Much of the research effort has focused on the protein coding regions of the genome, the so-called exome, which represents only 1% to 2% of the entire human genome. The preponderance of aberrations occur in the remainder of the genome and their effects on oncogenesis, are as yet unclear. Ultimately, the deregulation of oncogenic targets, through an array of mutagenic mechanisms, is merely the means through which tumorigenesis confers the hallmark properties of cancer on transformed cells.

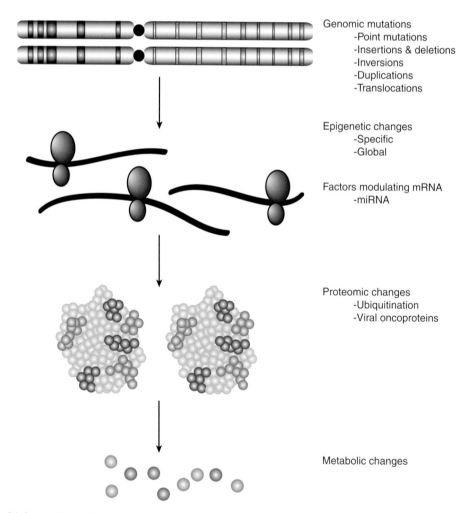

Cancer-related changes at a given regulatory level beget changes at other levels, collectively contributing to the oncogenic state

Genomic mutations
  -Point mutations
  -Insertions & deletions
  -Inversions
  -Duplications
  -Translocations

Epigenetic changes
  -Specific
  -Global

Factors modulating mRNA
  -miRNA

Proteomic changes
  -Ubiquitination
  -Viral oncoproteins

Metabolic changes

FIGURE 7–6 Cancer targets multiple regulatory levels. Cancer has long been recognized as a genetic disease, and large chromosomal abnormalities along with much smaller mutations have been cataloged since the 1960s. Previously, these were assumed to affect the function or expression of 1 or 2 proteins. More recently, broader changes affecting the epigenome, transcriptome, proteome, and the metabolic status of cells also have been associated with tumorigenesis. New oncogenic actors, such as microRNAs and oncometabolites, continue to emerge and contribute to a much more textured picture of the transformed phenotype. Moreover, oncogenic hits at any of these regulatory levels tend to engender further hits at other levels, synergistically promoting carcinogenesis. *mRNA*, Messenger RNA; *miRNA*, microRNA.

Specific oncogenes and tumor-suppressor genes are generally found to be mutated in some types of cancers but not others, and this varies among tumor subtypes that arise within the same tissue. This is puzzling when the gene in question is thought to influence fundamental cellular functions. Understanding why certain mutations or combinations of mutations occur preferentially in specific tumors is of fundamental importance, but remains speculative. The particular mutations capable of conferring neoplastic properties are dictated by the specific regulatory mechanisms that normally control these processes in the given tumor cell progenitor. Most cellular functions are regulated by multiple, partially redundant, regulatory networks. Because these networks have varying influence in different cell types, the severity of the effects caused by their disruption will also vary, and mutations in specific cancer genes will be subject to different selective pressures, depending on the cellular context in which they occur. Mutations that confer a selective advantage in one cell type may have little effect or even compromise the viability of another cell type. Factors likely to govern the effect of a particular mutation include the expression level of the gene, the existence of compensatory mechanisms, and developmental stage, as well as the modifying effects of other mutations.

7.4.1 Changes at the Genetic Level

The human genome is subject to a wide array of mutations of greatly differing sizes, ranging from point mutations affecting single nucleotides to large-scale rearrangements involving megabases of DNA (Fig. 7–7). Thousands of nucleotide variations have been cataloged in genome sequencing efforts, with many predicted to cause changes in the amino acid sequences of the encoded proteins, sometimes resulting in hyperactivation of oncoproteins or inactivation of tumor suppressors.

Although gene amplifications and deletions have long been recognized as oncogenic events, the prevalence of such cancer-associated rearrangements in the human genome has probably been underappreciated. Since the discovery of the

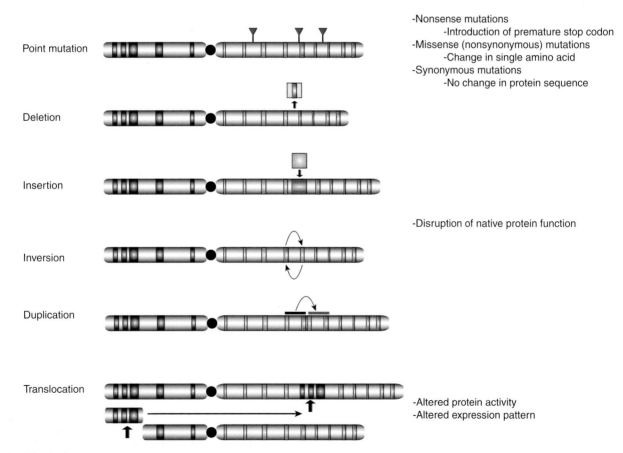

FIGURE 7–7 Classes of genetic mutations. The role of chromosome abnormalities in oncogenesis has been suspected for more than a century and specific genetic mutations have been identified since the 1960s. Whereas the available technologies once severely limited our capacity to characterize mutations, with next generation sequencing (NGS, see Chap. 2, Sec. 2.2.10), it is possible to characterize the entire set of genetic abnormalities in a given tumor cell in a relatively cost-effective manner. The number of genetic mutations in a given cancer cell is far greater than once suspected, encompassing point mutations affecting single nucleotides, deletions, insertions, inversions, and duplications, as well as intra- and interchromosomal translocations, all of varying sizes. Some mutations are functionally inert, while others can dramatically alter the activity and/or expression pattern of the affected protein(s).

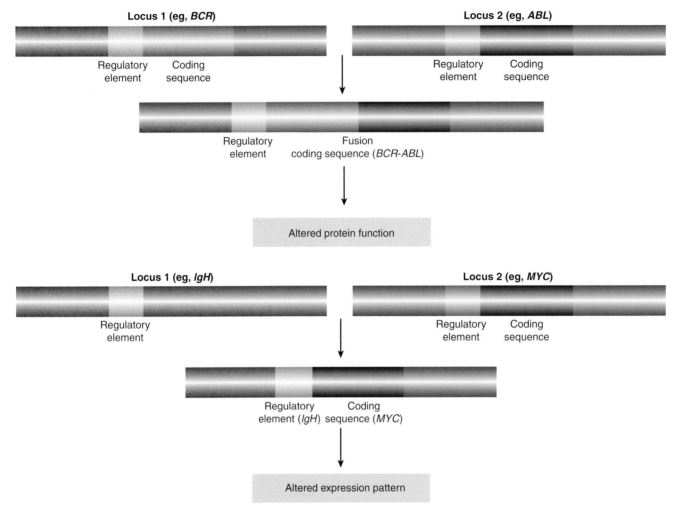

FIGURE 7–8 Effects of translocations. The first observed cancer-associated chromosomal abnormality was a reciprocal translocation between chromosomes 9 and 22, resulting in the so-called Philadelphia chromosome, identified in CML patients. The functional result of this genetic event is the creation of the BCR-ABL fusion protein, which causes the constitutive activation of the ABL kinase. This represents an example of a chromosomal translocation that alters the activity of the affected protein(s). In other translocations, it is the expression pattern of the protein that is altered, rather than its structure or direct function. One such example is the juxtaposition of the *MYC* gene with powerful transcriptional regulatory elements of the immunoglobulin heavy chain (IgH) observed, for instance, in Burkitt lymphoma, which results in a dramatic upregulation of the MYC transcription factor. Other examples are described in the text and in Table 7–2.

translocation event resulting in the generation of the onco-genic *BCR-ABL* fusion gene, additional cancer-associated gene fusions have been identified, particularly in hema-tological cancers, as well as in bone and soft-tissue sarco-mas (Nussenzweig and Nussenzweig, 2010). Increasingly, such genomic rearrangements are also being identified in epithelial-derived malignancies, including prostate, lung, and breast tumors (Table 7–2) (Kumar-Sinha et al, 2008; Edwards, 2010).

Gene fusions result from intra- or interchromosomal trans-locations, as well as deletions, inversions, and tandem dupli-cations (see Fig. 7–7). In some instances, the expression of one of the genes is altered as a result of its juxtaposition with the transcriptional regulatory elements of the second gene (see Fig. 7–8). Some follicular lymphomas feature transloca-tion events between chromosomes 14 and 18 that bring the

BCL2 gene, encoding the antiapoptotic BCL2 protein, under the control of the immunoglobulin (Ig) heavy-chain gene enhancer, rendering the cells resistant to cell death signals. Gene fusions that result in the addition or deletion of regula-tory domains can cause constitutive activation of the affected protein, as a result of forced multimerization, differential sub-cellular localization, or altered protein-protein interactions. Recombination between chromosomes 9 and 12 is found in leukemic cells of CML and acute lymphoblastic leukemia (ALL), resulting in production of the constitutively active TEL-JAK fusion tyrosine kinases that regulate cell prolifera-tion, survival, and differentiation.

On the basis of analyses of cancer genomes, it is suspected that most epithelial carcinomas also contain gene fusion events. Notably, more than half of all prostate cancers harbor a *TMPRSS2-ERG* fusion event, caused by an intrachromosomal

TABLE 7–2 Cancer-associated gene fusions.

Numerous examples of tumor-promoting gene fusions have now been identified and characterized, most frequently in hematological, bone, and soft-tissue malignancies, but also in a broad range of cancers, including prostate and lung tumors. Some of the most prominent cancer-associated fusion genes are listed. Next generation sequencing (NGS) is likely to lead to the discovery of novel gene fusions which could not be readily detected using older technologies.

Fusion Gene	Cancer
ASPSCR1-TFE3	soft tissue, kidney
BCR-ABL	CML, ALL, AML
COL1A1-PDGFB	soft tissue
EML4-ALK	lung
ETV6-NTRK3	soft tissue, kidney, breast, salivary gland
ETV6-RUNX1	ALL
EWSR1-ATF1	soft tissue
EWSR1-ERG	bone
EWSR1-FLI1	bone, soft tissue
EWSR1-WT1	soft tissue
IGH-BCL2	lymphoma
IGH-MYC	Burkitt lymphoma
MLL-ENL	AML, ALL
MLL-AF9	AML, ALL
NPM1-ALK	T-cell lymphoma
PAX3-FOXO1	soft tissue
PAX7-FOXO1	soft tissue
SS18-SSX1	soft tissue
SS18-SSX2	soft tissue
TEL-JAK	CML, ALL
TMPRSS2-ERG	prostate
TMPRSS2-ETV1	prostate
TMPRSS2-ETV4	prostate
TPM3-ALK	soft tissue, lymphoma

Abbreviations: ALL, acute lymphoblastic leukemia; *AML,* acute myelogenous leukemia; *CML,* chronic myeloid leukemia.

deletion on chromosome 21, in which the gene encoding the ERG transcription factor is brought under the control of the androgen-dependent regulatory elements of the *TMPRSS2* gene promoter, leading to its aberrant expression (Clark and Cooper, 2009). A small percentage of non–small cell lung cancers feature a fusion between the *EML4* gene and the *ALK* tyrosine kinase gene, which results in forced oligomerization and constitutive activation of the kinase (Crystal and Snow, 2011).

Gene amplification events produce regions of DNA (amplicons) containing multiple copies of oncogenes, such as the breast cancer-associated *ERBB2* (*HER2*) or *MYC*, and effectively achieve hyperactivation of oncogenic pathways by dramatically increasing oncogene dosage. The deletion of regulatory modules, such as the epidermal growth factor receptor (*EGFR*) ligand-binding domain, can also result in oncogenic deregulation of proteins. Conversely, the deletion of tumor-suppressor genes, such as *PTEN*, is also a common oncogenic event. Point mutations can affect enzymatic activity, regulatory phosphorylation sites, protein–protein interactions, protein stability, and subcellular localization. Moreover, many of the oncoproteins that are initially sensitive to a given therapeutic agent often acquire secondary mutations that render them refractory to the drug.

7.4.2 Changes at the Epigenetic Level

A number of heritable characteristics could not be solely attributed to genetics, and the field of epigenomics has sought to explore these factors (Fletcher and Houlston, 2010; see Chap. 2, Sec. 2.3). Epigenetic effects entail heritable changes in gene expression that are not the result of alterations in the primary DNA sequence and they can influence oncogenic progression. These events may also represent novel targets for therapeutic intervention (Fig. 7–9).

The preeminent epigenetic factors are DNA methylation and a pattern of acetylation, methylation, and phosphorylation of DNA-associated histone proteins that are collectively known as the *histone code.* The methylation pattern of the cellular genome, whereby DNA methyltransferases attach methyl groups to cytosines within CpG dinucleotides, specifies which genes are actively transcribed or silenced. The CpG dinucleotides are enriched within the so-called CpG islands that span the 5′ ends of some genes, typically including the promoter and first exon (Esteller, 2008). In mammals, the majority of genes have promoters containing CpG islands, and promoter methylation results in the silencing of the associated gene(s). Histone modifications alter localized chromatin structure, rendering regions either amenable or resistant to transcription. The various histone modifications do not occur independently of one another, but rather entail a complicated interplay that collectively controls gene expression.

Tumorigenesis frequently appears to coincide with both global and local epigenetic changes that are in some respects paradoxical (Chi et al, 2010; Veeck and Esteller, 2010). At a global level, the genome typically becomes hypomethylated during oncogenic progression. A sizable portion of the human genome consists of repetitive stretches of identical or similar sequences, a subset of which are transposable DNA elements that have the capacity to alter their genomic location. The methylation of these repetitive sequences is thought to block the activation and movement of transposable elements, and therefore prevent chromosomal instability. Thus, global hypomethylation of the genome may contribute to the genomic instability that is a prominent feature of transformed cells (see Chap. 5, Sec. 5.2.1).

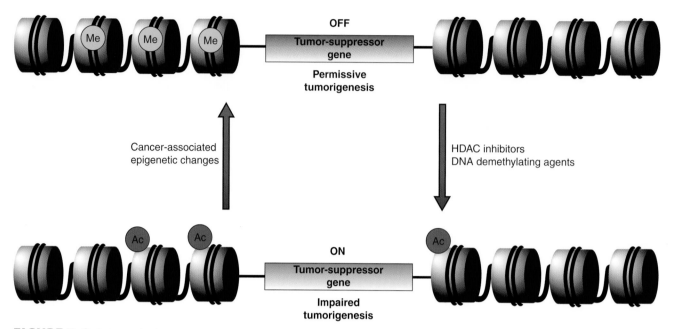

FIGURE 7–9 Epigenetic therapy. Global changes in the cellular epigenome frequently accompany transformation and the epigenetic silencing of tumor-suppressor genes or activation of oncogenes is now a recognized tumorigenic mechanism. One such example is the silencing of the p16^{INK4A} and antigen-presenting cell (APC) tumor-suppressor genes in non–small cell lung cancers. Clinical testing suggests that the tumor-suppressor genes can be reactivated through the application of DNA methyltransferase inhibitors (eg, 5′-deoxycitidine), to reduce the methylation of promoter regions, and histone deacetylase (HDAC) inhibitors (eg, entinostat) that activate gene loci through chromatin remodeling. It is anticipated that epigenetic therapies will be most effective in a combinatorial setting, enhancing the response to other anticancer agents.

Promoter methylation patterns of critical cancer-associated genes also feature prominently during tumorigenesis, with hypermethylation-associated silencing of tumor-suppressor genes and hypomethylation-mediated activation of onco-genes. Cancer-associated hypermethylation of the *Rb1* tumor-suppressor gene promoter was noted in the 1980s, and similar epigenetic targeting of other tumor suppressor promoters, including those for *BRCA1* and *PTEN*, has since been reported. A detailed understanding of the role of epigenetics in neoplastic transformation remains a work in progress. For instance, it is not clear whether the cancer-associated epigenetic modifications result from specifically targeted acts or whether they represent random epigenetic changes that are then selected for in the course of oncogenic clonal expansion.

7.4.3 Changes at the Transcript Level; microRNAs

One of the great revelations of recent biological research has been the discovery of the extensive roles of small RNAs in the control of gene expression. MicroRNAs are 20- to 30-nucleotide RNA molecules, generated by defined posttranscriptional maturation steps, that hybridize to complementary sequences in target mRNA transcripts in order to block gene expression (see Chap. 2, Sec. 2.4.3). This may be accomplished either by promoting transcript degradation or by interfering with the translation process. It is now recognized that microRNAs govern a variety of cellular processes, regulating at least

one-third of all human genes, and may have key roles in tumorigenesis. MicroRNAs that normally suppress transformation by targeting oncogenic transcripts are downregulated in some cancers, whereas those targeting tumor-suppressor transcripts are sometimes overexpressed (Croce, 2009; Garzon et al, 2009; Ryan et al, 2010).

Genes encoding microRNAs, no less than protein-encoding genes, are subject to mutations and epigenetic silencing resulting in loss of function. MicroRNA expression can also be affected by oncogenic changes occurring at any of the post-transcriptional biogenesis steps whereby the immature RNA molecule is processed into the mature microRNA form. Deletions in the 13q14 chromosomal region are common abnormalities associated with chronic lymphocytic leukemia (CLL). The underlying molecular cause was unclear as no protein-coding tumor-suppressor gene could be identified in the region. The nature of the oncogenic mechanism was only clarified when the miR-15/miR-16 microRNA gene cluster was localized to this segment and found to target the antiapoptotic BCL2 protein, which is found at elevated levels in CLL samples (Cimmino et al, 2006). The LET-7 microRNA family members, which target the *RAS* and *MYC* onco-genes, are downregulated in many cancers, including lung, breast, and colon tumors (Johnson et al, 2005; Sampson et al, 2007). Intriguingly, miRNA-29 has been shown to target the DNMT3A methyltransferase and thus could affect onco-genesis through global epigenetic effects (Fabbri et al, 2007). MicroRNAs are potentially attractive therapeutic focal points because individual molecules regulate multiple targets, theoretically affecting several oncogenic pathways simultaneously.

7.4.4 Changes at the Protein Level

Virally encoded oncoproteins often trigger tumorigenic programs by directly interacting with critical host cell regulatory proteins. The first identified human tumor virus, the Epstein-Barr herpesvirus was discovered in the 1960s when Joseph Epstein detected viral particles in Burkitt lymphoma biopsies (Caparros-Lefebvre et al, 1996; Klein et al, 2010). As most adults are Epstein-Barr virus (EBV) carriers without developing the disease, the oncogenic mechanisms are not certain, but virus-encoded proteins appear to be involved in a complex interplay with proteins of host B-cell lymphocytes, including the *p53* and *Rb* tumor suppressors (see Chap. 6; Sec. 6.2.4).

Additional human tumor viruses have since been identified, with roughly 20% of all cancers thought to have at least some viral etiology (see also Chap. 6, Sec 6.2). The hepatitis C (HCV) RNA virus constitutes a major hepatocellular carcinoma risk factor. Although a comprehensive understanding of HCV-associated hepatocarcinogenesis remains elusive, it appears that virally encoded proteins affect host cell physiology without proviral integration (Tsai and Chung, 2010). Viral proteins disrupt several signaling pathways, again including checkpoint mechanisms activated by the *p53* and *Rb* tumor suppressors. Sequences of the human papillomavirus (HPV) have been detected in human malignancies, notably cervical cancers (Munger et al, 2004) and oropharyngeal carcinomas (Miller et al, 2012). The HPV E6 gene product inactivates the p53 tumor suppressor protein and induces expression of the TERT subunit of the telomerase enzyme (see Chap. 5, Sec. 5.7). The E7 gene product destabilizes the Rb tumor suppressor, can override the inhibitory effects of the cyclin-dependent kinase (CDK) inhibitors p21[CIP1] and p27[KIP1], and interacts with a number of other host proteins, including histone deacetylases and acetyltransferases. Although there are a multitude of virus–host protein interactions, inactivating interactions between virus-encoded proteins and p53 or Rb are a recurring theme in viral–host pathogenic interactions (Levine, 2009). A detailed discussion of viruses in cancer can be found in Chapter 6.

7.5 GAIN OF FUNCTION EVENTS

7.5.1 BCR-ABL

The Philadelphia chromosome was initially described initially as a minute chromosome and assumed to be the product of a loss of genetic material from chromosome 22 (Nowell and Hungerford, 1960). Improvements in cytogenetics permitted more careful examination of chromosome defects, allowing Janet Rowley to determine that the deletion of genetic material in chromosome 22 was matched by a comparable insertion in chromosome 9 (Rowley, 1973). She speculated that the chromosomal defects observed in CML cases were the result of a translocation exchange between chromosomes 9 and 22.

By 1985, it had been determined that cells of most patients with CML feature reciprocal translocation events between the long arms of the 2 chromosomes, resulting in the creation of a *BCR-ABL* hybrid gene (see Fig 7–8). The same translocation event has been found to occur in 25% to 30% of adult and 2% to 10% of pediatric ALL, and occasionally in cases of acute myelogenous leukemia (AML) (De Klein et al, 1986).

The ABL kinase is the human homolog of the transforming sequence found in the Abelson murine leukemia virus. Whereas the protein normally shuttles between the nucleus and cytoplasm, the product of the *BCR-ABL* fusion gene is a constitutively active tyrosine kinase permanently localized in the cytoplasm. The addition of the BCR gene product appears to promote extensive multimerization of the fusion protein, facilitating self-activation by trans-autophosphorylation. During the chronic phase of CML, the BCR-ABL kinase activates a number of downstream pathways while also increasing genomic instability. In the absence of therapeutic intervention, additional genomic aberrations ultimately lead to a transition from the chronic to the advanced CML phase known as blast crisis that is more difficult to treat. At a cellular level, the blast phase is marked by increased proliferation accompanied by impaired apoptosis and differentiation, which together increase the population of blast progenitors. One noteworthy molecular change is a moderate increase in BCR-ABL levels, enhancing throughput of the relevant signaling pathways and begetting still more genetic damage.

The correlation of a disease state with a particular genetic lesion offered the possibility for targeted therapeutic intervention. The subsequent development and successful application of imatinib, which binds in the vicinity of the adenosine triphosphate (ATP)-binding site and locks BCR-ABL in an inhibited conformation, remains one of the most celebrated achievements in targeted cancer therapy.

7.5.2 MYC

MYC family members are global transcription factors (see Chap. 8, Sec. 8.2.6) that activate some target genes while repressing others, thereby affecting numerous cellular processes including proliferation, growth, apoptosis, and angiogenesis (Fig. 7–10) (Meyer and Penn, 2008; Albihn et al, 2010). Roughly 15% of all human genes are thought to be regulated by MYC proteins, so it is difficult to pinpoint the specific MYC targets that are responsible for oncogenesis. For example, MYC promotes cell-cycle progression by influencing a variety of targets, including downregulation of CDK inhibitors and upregulation of CYCLIN D1, CDK4, CDC25A, and E2F transcription factors (see Chap. 9, Sec. 9.2.2). Numerous genes, associated with the production of the constituent building blocks required for cell growth, are also controlled by the MYC proteins. Importantly, MYC deregulation appears to correlate with general chromosomal instability, although there is not yet agreement about the responsible mechanisms. Paradoxically, MYC upregulation also triggers apoptosis, and additional oncogenic mutations capable of blocking cell death are required for tumor progression. Thus, *MYC* overexpression

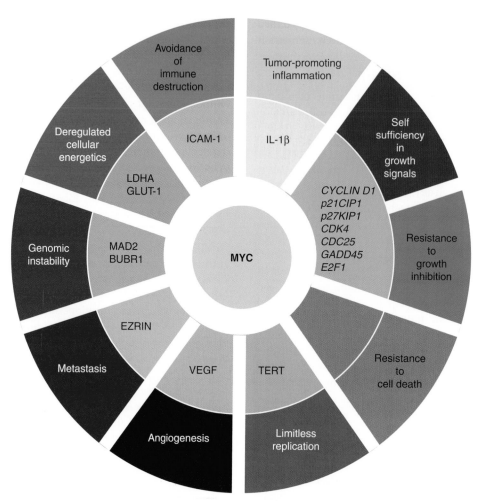

FIGURE 7-10 **MYC targets and the promotion of tumorigenesis.** The MYC transcription factor is thought to regulate the expression of roughly 15% of all human genes and is frequently upregulated in a variety of cancers. MYC upregulates the expression of some genes while repressing the expression of other targets. Unsurprisingly, given the number of genes affected by MYC, its deregulation contributes to the acquisition of many of the characteristic properties of cancer cells, as defined by Hanahan and Weinberg (2011). One notable exception is the paradoxical induction of apoptosis by MYC overexpression, necessitating the disengagement of cell death pathway(s) by additional oncogenic hits so as to foster transformation. Some of the MYC-regulated genes involved in tumorigenesis are denoted, although the particular MYC targets critical to oncogenesis will undoubtedly vary in different tumors.

results in pleiotropic downstream effects that collectively promote oncogenic transformation.

Transforming viruses can direct oncogenesis by proviral DNA integration in the proximity of protooncogenes or tumor-suppressor genes, leading to altered expression or splicing (see Chap. 6, Sec. 6.3). An interesting example is the mechanism of chicken B-cell lymphogenesis by the slowly transforming avian leukosis virus (ALV). The ability of ALV to induce lymphomas was initially puzzling because of the apparent absence of any transforming sequence in the viral genome. Nevertheless, a careful analysis of lymphomas from independently infected birds revealed proviral integration at highly specific sites, giving rise to similar viral–host hybrid RNAs (Hayward et al, 1981). The viral coding segments were often altered in ways that precluded their transcription, indicating that viral protein expression was not required for transformation. Remarkably, the hybrid RNAs were found to

include *Myc* coding sequences leading to increased expression of myc protein, suggesting that proviral integration promoted oncogenesis through upregulation of myc levels. Lymphomas in birds caused by ALV infection are slow growing as the oncogenic mechanism involves clonal selection of the rare proviral integration events in the vicinity of the *myc* protooncogene. This constituted the first observation of neoplastic transformation caused by the upregulation of a non-mutated cellular gene. Interestingly, the acutely transforming avian myelocytomatosis retrovirus (MC29), from which MYC derives its name, induces leukemia in birds through expression of v-*Gag-Myc* already encoded in the viral genome (Reddy et al, 1983).

Upregulation of *Myc* expression is observed in some mouse plasmacytomas as a result of a recombination between the *Myc* and immunoglobin (*Ig*) heavy-chain genes. Burkitt lymphomas, as well as other human B-cell lymphomas, frequently feature chromosome translocation events between chromosome 8, where the *MYC* gene is located, and chromosomes 14, 2, or 22, where the Ig heavy- and light-chain genes reside. These rearrangements have the effect of bringing the *MYC* gene under the transcriptional control of *Ig* gene enhancer elements, leading to its overexpression. Whereas genomic translocations involving *MYC* genes are common in hematopoietic cancers, heightened MYC levels are often attained in solid tumors through gene amplification. The *MYCN* gene, which is normally expressed during development, has been found amplified in neuroblastomas, and increased copy numbers of the related *MYCL1* gene have been observed in several cancers, including ovarian tumors.

7.5.3 EGFR/ERBB2

The involvement of epidermal growth factor (EGF) signaling in tumorigenesis has been recognized for 3 decades. The EGF family is comprised of 11 related ligands that stimulate intracellular signaling by binding to the EGF receptors, ERBB1 (EGFR), ERBB3, and ERBB4 (Baselga and Swain, 2009). A fourth member of the EGF receptor family, ERBB2 (HER2), cannot bind ligands itself, but is activated by dimerization with other family members (see also Chap. 8, Sec. 8.2.1). The EGF receptors are transmembrane proteins consisting of an N-terminal ligand-binding ectodomain, an intracellular kinase domain, and a C-terminal regulatory tail that contains docking sites for a number of downstream effectors. Ligand binding to the ectodomain induces receptor dimerization, transmitting conformational changes that promote kinase activation. Active receptor signaling complexes can be formed by both homodimerization and certain heterodimer combinations. The ERBB3 receptor binds ligands but has an inactive kinase domain and therefore can only transmit the EGF signal as part of a heterodimer with an active family member (Fig. 7–11).

All 3 portions of the ERBB1 receptor are subject to oncogenic mutations (Pines et al, 2010). Ligand-independent dimerization occurs as a result of point mutations or, more commonly, deletions within the ectodomain that leave the receptors in

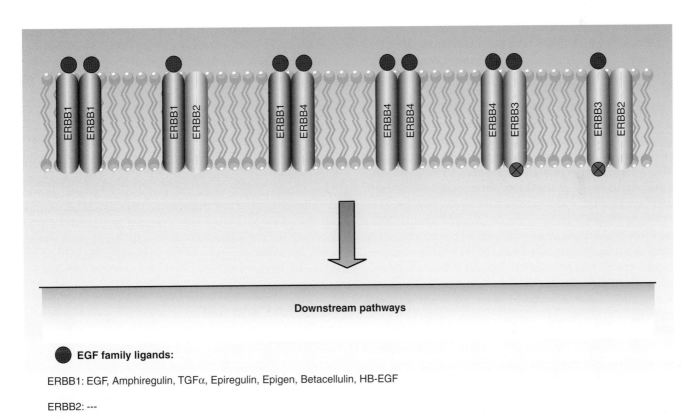

EGF family ligands:

ERBB1: EGF, Amphiregulin, TGFα, Epiregulin, Epigen, Betacellulin, HB-EGF

ERBB2: ---

ERBB3: Neuregulin 1, Neuregulin 2

ERBB4: Epiregulin, Betacellulin, HB-EGF, Neuregulin 1, Neuregulin 2, Neuregulin 3, Neuregulin 4

FIGURE 7–11 EGF receptor family. The EGF receptor family consists of 4 transmembrane proteins that couple a ligand-binding domain that responds to external stimuli with intracellular tyrosine kinase domains responsible for signal transduction. ERBB1 (EGFR), ERBB3, and ERBB4 each respond to a particular set of EGF family ligands, with some overlap, whereas ERBB2 appears to be an orphan receptor that must dimerize with ERBB1 or ERBB3 in order to engage downstream pathways. In addition, ERBB3 has an inactive kinase domain and transmits signals by dimerizing with ERBB2 or ERBB4. Collectively, these receptors regulate pathways that impact a number of cell processes, and are deregulated in a number of cancers.

a constitutively activated conformation. Many such deletion mutants have been characterized, with one notable example being the variant III mutant, lacking the exons 2 to 7 coding sequences, which is particularly common in gliomas, but also found in lung, breast, ovarian, and other cancers. Interestingly, these deletion mutants mimic the avian erythroblastosis virus v-ErbB oncoprotein, from which the EGFR family members took their names. Numerous point mutations are also found in the kinase domain, especially in non–small cell lung cancers, which promote constitutive activation, even in the absence of ligand-induced dimerization. Again, the effects of the point mutations are also closely replicated by small insertions and deletions within the kinase domain.

Activation of the EGFR receptor results in phosphorylation of tyrosine residues in the C-terminal tail, which serve as docking sites for the recruitment of downstream effectors (see Chap. 8, Sec. 8.2). Generally, activating point mutations result in the receptor tail attaining a phosphorylation status intermediate between that of unstimulated and growth factor-stimulated wild-type receptors. An important consequence of this "partial" activation is a resulting shift in the downstream signaling output from the mutant receptors. Whereas stimulated wild-type epidermal growth factor receptors (EGFRs) activate a number of downstream pathways, the mutant receptors tend to prominently activate mitogen-activated protein (MAP) kinase and phophatidylinositol-3 (PI3) kinase signaling at the expense of the other pathways. Normally, EGF signaling is attenuated by a feedback mechanism that involves the removal of the receptors from the cell membrane by endocytosis, followed by lysosomal degradation or recycling. Some point mutations have been found to disrupt this regulatory device, resulting in hyperactivation of the EGF pathway.

EGF signaling has an important physiological role in mammary development, and deregulation of downstream pathways feature prominently in many breast tumors (Schmitt, 2009). The ERBB2/ERBB3 heterodimeric receptor complex is a potent signal transducer, particularly of the PI3 kinase pathway, because the ERBB3 receptor recruits the PI3 kinase directly rather than through intermediary adaptor proteins. The *ERBB2(HER-2)* gene is amplified or overexpressed in roughly one-quarter of all human breast cancers, as well as a smaller percentage of ovarian and gastric cancers. Overexpression of the ERBB2 receptor has also been correlated with elevated ERBB3 levels. Although *ERBB2* somatic mutations have now been identified in some lung tumors, gene amplification is the most common mechanism for oncogenic upregulation of the receptor. Amplification of the *ERBB2* gene is generally an early event in breast cancer progression and is associated with poor prognosis in breast and gastric cancers.

7.5.4 PI3 Kinase

In response to specific upstream signals, the PI3 kinases phosphorylate the 3′ hydroxyl group of phosphatidylinositols, generating membrane-embedded lipid secondary messengers that activate downstream pathways (Fig. 7–12;

see also Chap. 8, Sec. 8.2.5) (Engelman et al, 2006). Although the superfamily includes a number of isoforms, the preponderance of research has focused on the Class IA PI3 kinases, which consist of p110 catalytic and p85 regulatory subunits. These preferentially convert phosphatidylinositol 4,5-bisphosphate (PIP_2) to phosphatidylinositol 3,4,5-triphosphate (PIP_3), which recruits Pleckstrin homology (PH) domain-containing proteins, such as the PKB/AKT serine/threonine kinase, to the plasma membrane for activation. The involvement of PI3 kinase signaling in oncogenesis was evident in the 1980s from the discovery of an interaction between the transforming polyoma viral middle T antigen and the p85 subunit of the kinase (Whitman et al, 1985; Otsu et al, 1991). In parallel, a constitutively active version of the p110 subunit was isolated from the genome of the ASV16 avian retrovirus, which was known to transform chicken fibroblasts (Chang et al, 1997).

More recently, activating mutations have been identified in the *PIK3CA* gene, encoding the p110 subunit, in a number of tumors, including breast, prostate, endometrial, and colon cancers (Chalhoub and Baker, 2009). These mutations result in constitutive activation of the kinase in the absence of upstream signaling, a buildup of PIP_3, and increased mobilization of downstream pathways that regulate cell processes such as growth, proliferation, survival, migration, and glucose metabolism. Remarkably, approximately 80% of all somatic PI3 kinase mutations occur at 3 hotspot residues: E542K and E545K within the helical domain, and H1047R in the kinase domain. All 3 mutations have been found to increase the in vitro activity of the kinase as well as the PI3 kinase signaling throughput in cells and tissues bearing the mutations. Amplifications of the *PIK3CA* gene are sometimes observed in cervical, head and neck, gastric, as well as lung cancers. Less frequent cancer-associated activating mutations have also been identified in the *PIK3R* gene, encoding the p85 subunit, as well as the *AKT1* gene, encoding 1 of the more prominent downstream effectors of PI3 kinase signaling.

7.5.5 RAS and RAF

The importance of MAP kinase signaling in neoplastic transformation is evident from the frequency of oncogenic mutations affecting multiple proteins in the pathway, including growth factor receptors, RAS guanosine triphosphatase (GTPase), and its immediate target, RAF (Fig. 7–13) (Karreth and Tuveson, 2009). The pathway modulates a number of cellular processes, including proliferation, growth, survival, differentiation, and migration, albeit in a tissue-dependent manner (see also Chap. 8, Sec. 8.2.3). *RAS* genes are among the most commonly mutated genes in human cancer, with a variety of aberrations detected in at least 30% of all tumors. Among the 3 *RAS* genes, the preponderance of mutations is observed in the *K-RAS* gene, especially in pancreatic, lung, colon, endometrial, and ovarian tumors. Mutations in the *H-RAS* gene are more commonly observed in bladder cancers

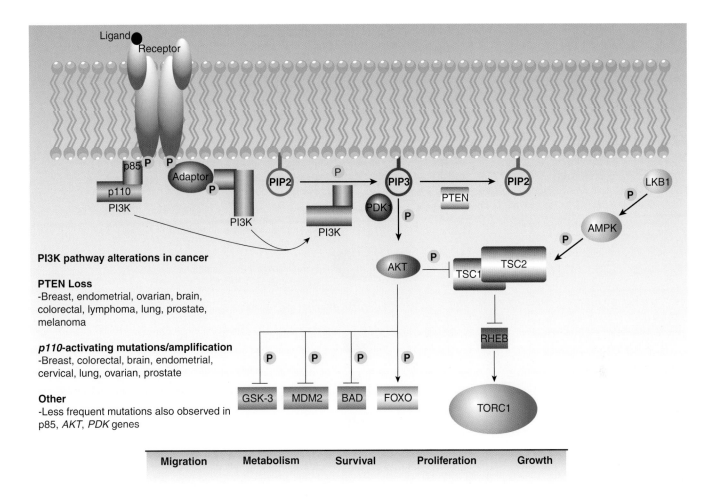

PI3K pathway alterations in cancer

PTEN Loss
-Breast, endometrial, ovarian, brain, colorectal, lymphoma, lung, prostate, melanoma

***p110*-activating mutations/amplification**
-Breast, colorectal, brain, endometrial, cervical, lung, ovarian, prostate

Other
-Less frequent mutations also observed in p85, *AKT*, *PDK* genes

FIGURE 7–12 **PI3 kinase pathway.** The PI3 kinase pathway regulates a variety of cell functions, including migration, metabolism, survival, proliferation, and growth. It is frequently deregulated in human cancers at various points. In response to external stimuli, activated receptor tyrosine kinases recruit PI3 kinase via its p85 regulatory subunit, either directly or mediated by an adaptor protein such as IRS-1. Upon recruitment, activated PI3 kinase (PI3K) converts PIP_2 (phosphatidylinositol 4,5 bisphosphate) to PIP_3 (phosphatidylinositol 3,4,5 triphosphate). This reaction is antagonized by the lipid phosphatase, PTEN, which acts as a brake on the pathway. PH-domain proteins, such as the PDK1 and AKT kinases, are recruited to the plasma membrane by PIP_3, whereupon PDK1 contributes to the activation of AKT, which then transmits the signal downstream by phosphorylating a range of targets. AKT also modulates the RHEB guanosine triphosphatase (GTPase)-TORC1 signaling axis by downregulating the TSC1–TSC2 complex, which is modulated by a number of upstream signals including activation by LKB1-AMPK in response to energy deprivation. The PI3 kinase pathway is generally overstimulated in cancers through aberrant activation of the receptors, activating mutations in the PI3 kinase catalytic subunit (p110), and through the loss of PTEN.

with *N-RAS* mutations found in neuronal, melanoma, and myeloid malignancies.

The most common mutations are gain-of-function substitutions in codons 12, 13, and 61, with many lower-frequency mutations identified throughout the protein sequence. The RAS gain-of-function mechanism is somewhat distinct in that it is the RAS GTPase enzymatic turnover that is blocked by the oncogenic mutations, effectively locking the protein into the activated guanosine triphosphate (GTP)-bound signaling state, and resulting in the upregulation of its downstream effectors.

The primary downstream effectors of RAS are the 3 RAF family serine/threonine kinases (see also Chap. 8, Sec. 8.2.3). Although a virally transduced version of C-RAF exhibits oncogenic properties, missense mutations are infrequently

observed in the *C-RAF* gene, and these rare substitutions do not generally appear to stimulate kinase activity. Similarly, mutations in the *A-RAF* gene have been detected very rarely. *B-RAF* is the most frequently mutated RAF family member with approximately 40% of malignant melanomas and 2% of all human cancers, including thyroid, colon, and ovarian cancers, exhibiting *B-RAF* mutations (Beeram et al, 2005; Maurer et al, 2011). The V600E substitution in the kinase activation loop accounts for roughly 90% of all B-RAF mutations. Development of vemurafenib, an agent that specifically targets this mutation, has led to marked improvement in outcome for patients with malignant melanoma (Chapman et al, 2011). Interestingly, mutations in the *RAS* and *B-RAF* genes are almost entirely mutually exclusive, indicative of the potency of a single oncogenic hit at either gene that evidently

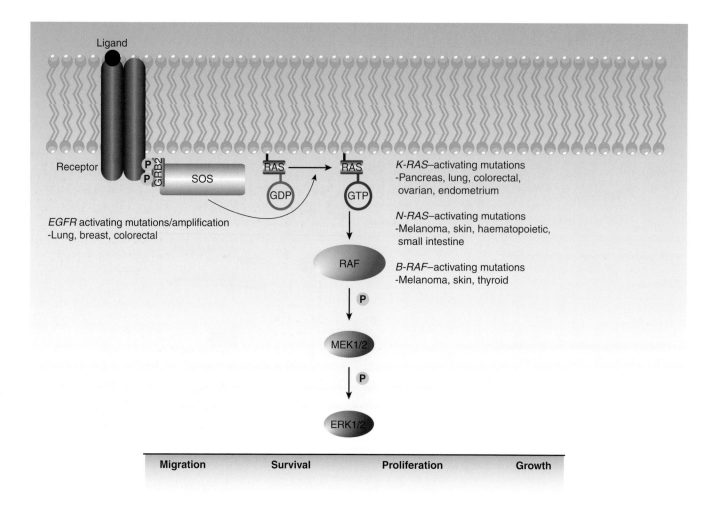

FIGURE 7-13 MAP kinase pathway. The mitogen-activated kinase (MAPK)/ERK pathway is frequently deregulated during oncogenesis. The pathway is stimulated by binding of ligands to their cognate receptors, ultimately resulting in activation of the ERK1/2 kinase. Activated receptors recruit adaptors, such as GRB2, and guanine nucleotide exchange factors (GEFs), such as SOS, which promotes the guanosine triphosphate (GTP) loading of RAS. RAF is then activated by RAS-GTP, triggering a kinase cascade resulting in the sequential activation of MEK1/2 and ERK1/2, whose downstream targets regulate a number of cell functions including migration, survival, proliferation, and growth. Overactivation of the pathway through activating mutations or amplification of receptors, as well as activating mutations in various RAS isoforms or B-RAF, is commonly observed in human cancers.

relieves virtually all the selective pressure for additional mutations in the pathway. Indeed, the B-RAF^{V600E} mutant protein is constitutively activated and essentially independent of upstream signaling from growth factor receptors or RAS. An analysis of the effects of the V600E substitution on the B-RAF structure suggested that the mutation results in the activation loop adopting an open conformation than is more accessible to substrates. Typically, this conformation change is accomplished by specific regulatory phosphorylation events particularly within the kinase activation loop.

7.5.6 IDH

Despite extensive genome-wide sequencing efforts to produce a detailed genetic map of the cancer landscape, surprisingly few novel oncogenes and tumor-suppressor genes have been identified. The *IDH1* and *IDH2* genes, encoding 2 previously unglamorous isocitrate deydrogenase metabolic enzymes,

are the most prominent examples of the worthiness of these large-scale projects. The mechanism by which these proteins contribute to tumorigenesis, though far from clear, appears to define a novel oncogenic paradigm. Now recognized as oncogenes, they were initially mistaken for tumor suppressors because the observed cancer mutations destroy their normal cellular activities.

Exon sequencing carried out on human glioblastoma multiforme, as well as other cancers, revealed somatic mutations in IDH1 and IDH2 at homologous arginine positions in some of the sampled tumors (Parsons et al, 2008; Yan et al, 2009). Functional characterization of the mutant proteins indicated that the amino acid substitutions led to a loss of function, destroying their ability to convert isocitrate into α-ketoglutarate, and suggesting that these were novel tumor suppressors. However, there was no evidence of a LOH at the *IDH* loci in human tumors, indicating that they did not conform to Knudson's 2-hit tumor-suppressor model. An alternative explanation for these findings arose from the observation that cells harboring the tumor-associated *IDH1* mutation exhibit an accumulation of a particular metabolite, 2-hydroxyglutarate (2-HG) (Dang et al, 2009). An analysis of the effects of the mutation on the IDH1 structure suggested that although the active site of the mutant enzyme failed to interact with isocitrate, its normal substrate, it was capable of interacting with α-ketoglutarate and converting it to 2-HG. Thus, the arginine substitution effectively represents both a loss-of-function and gain-of-function mutation that destroys the normal enzymatic activity while creating a novel one.

On the basis of these results, it has been proposed that 2-HG represents an oncometabolite whose ability to promote oncogenesis needs to be fully elucidated. In addition to gliomas, *IDH1* and *IDH2* mutations have also been detected in AML genomes, including a novel mutation in the *IDH2* sequence which also leads to 2-HG build up (Balss et al, 2008; Ward et al, 2010). Importantly, knockdown of *IDH1* and *IDH2* reduced

the growth of cultured AML cells, consistent with their roles as oncogenes rather than tumor-suppressor genes.

7.6 LOSS OF FUNCTION EVENTS

7.6.1 p53

The most extensively studied tumor-suppressor gene is the p53 transcription factor, which was discovered in 1979 as an interacting partner of the SV40 viral T-antigen (Brosh and Rotter, 2009). In response to cellular stresses, a variety of mechanisms converge on p53 leading to its stabilization and accumulation (Junttila and Evan, 2009). Contingent upon the extent of the stress signals, p53 then activates the expression of genes involved in DNA repair and growth arrest on the one hand, or apoptotic cell death on the other (Fig. 7–14). In the absence of p53, cells are impaired in their ability to appropriately respond to oncogenic stresses, leading to tumorigenic proliferation, growth, and genetic instability. Remarkably,

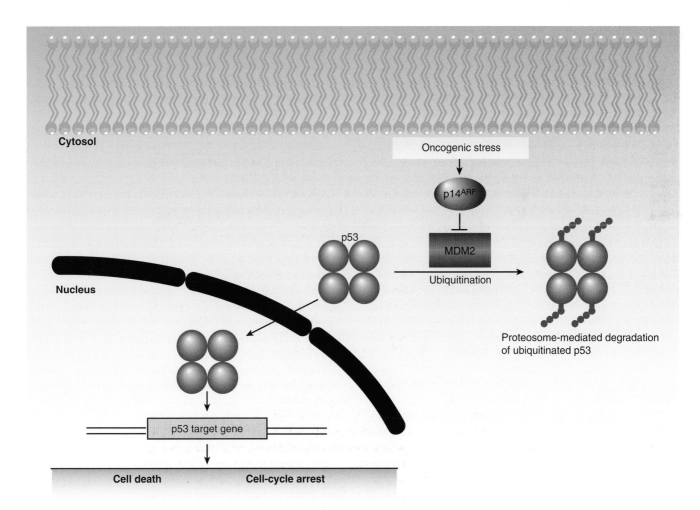

FIGURE 7–14 p53 and cell fate determination. The p53 tumor suppressor represents a critical regulatory node for cell fate determination and is the most frequently mutated gene in human cancers. The levels of p53 are normally constrained, primarily by the action of MDM2, which promotes the ubiquitination and proteasomal degradation of the protein. In response to cellular stresses, p53 is stabilized and translocates to the nucleus and regulates gene expression. Depending on the level of stress, p53 can promote different cellular outcomes, notably cell-cycle arrest, to permit the alleviation of the particular stress or, in irretrievable cases, cell death. Because oncogenic stresses can inhibit MDM2, through the activity of p14^ARF, tumorigenic progression requires either the circumvention or loss of p53 activity.

despite the vast amount of p53 research, new functions for this multitasking protein are still being discovered. Somatic mutations in the *TP53* gene, encoding the p53 protein, are found at varying frequencies in many human cancers, ranging from roughly 10% in some leukemias to more than 70% in advanced lung carcinomas. The majority of mutations in the *TP53* gene are missense substitutions, with the remainder consisting of frameshift, nonsense, and silent mutations, along with rare deletions and insertions. In addition to somatic changes, germline p53 mutations lead to Li-Fraumeni syndrome, a highly penetrant autosomal dominant disorder that causes tumor growth in a wide spectrum of tissues. For both somatic and germline mutations, oncogenic progression almost always involves LOH at the p53 locus.

Although thousands of p53 mutations have been cataloged, 6 "hotspot" residues, located in the central DNA binding domain, are mutated in a disproportionate percentage of p53-associated cancers. Two of these mutations, R248Q and R273H, affect p53 activity by interfering with its capacity to bind DNA, while the other mutations, R249S, G245S, R175H, and R282W, cause varying degrees of structural disruption. The traditional models of p53 function, in relation to oncogenesis, involve a combination of loss-of-function and dominant-negative effects, the latter mediated by dimerization of mutant p53 with wild-type p53 (thereby inhibiting normal p53 function), prior to LOH. The inability of mutant p53 to bind DNA naturally results in reduced expression of p53 targets, including the gene that encodes the MDM2 ubiquitin ligase (see Chap. 8, Fig. 8–3 and Chap. 9, Fig. 9–4), which strongly influences the turnover of p53 itself. As a consequence, mutant p53 levels are frequently, although not always, elevated in tumors, enhancing the dominant-negative effect. More recently, it has been proposed that some p53 mutations confer gain-of-function oncogenic effects, at least partly involving inactivation of the other p53 family members, p63 and p73, as well as some unrelated transcription factors. Researchers are now designing drugs (eg, PRIMA1) that selectively target cancers with mutated p53 by promoting conversion of the mutant conformation to the wild-type form, or by driving downstream effector proteins (eg, MDM2) to reengage apoptotic pathways, thereby sensitizing tumors to chemotherapy and radiotherapy (Brown et al, 2009).

7.6.2 PTEN

Initially identified during the 1990s as the major tumor suppressor at chromosome 10q23, PTEN was found to directly counter PI3 kinase signaling by acting as a lipid phosphatase for PIP_3, the product of PI3 kinase activity (see Fig. 7–12) (Chalhoub and Baker, 2009; Hollander et al, 2011). Downregulation of PTEN correlates with increased PIP_3 levels and hyperactivation of downstream PKB/AKT-mediated signaling. Although reported initially as an exclusively cytoplasmic enzyme, there is also a nuclear PTEN cohort in at least some cells. The nuclear functions of PTEN have not yet been fully documented, though, intriguingly, PTEN loss appears to correlate with genomic instability. The protein structure consists of a short N-terminal lipid-binding domain followed by the phosphatase domain, a membrane-binding C2 domain, and a C-terminal tail that influences stability and subcellular localization.

Germline *PTEN* mutations are causal in the related Cowden, Bannayan-Riley-Ruvalcaba, Proteus, and Proteus-like hamartoma syndromes, collectively known as PTHS (PTEN hamartoma tumor syndromes). These clinically distinct conditions are marked by small benign growths and, in Cowden syndrome, carry an enhanced risk for developing breast, thyroid, and endometrial cancers. Importantly, progression from benign to malignant tumor growth, in Cowden syndrome, coincides with LOH at the *PTEN* locus.

Sporadic PTEN loss-of-function, effected at the genomic, epigenomic, transcriptional, or protein levels, is found in a wide array of cancers, especially glioblastomas, melanomas, prostate, breast, and endometrial tumors. For example, genomic deletions at the *PTEN* locus have been observed in roughly 70% of glioblastomas, with biallelic inactivation occurring in roughly 25% to 40% of these malignancies. *PTEN* deletions are also observed in premalignant endometrial lesions, suggestive of a role in the initiation of endometrial carcinomas. In addition to missense substitutions, nonsense and frameshift mutations have also been observed, yielding truncated mutants that retain the phosphatase and C2 domains, but not the more C-terminal regions. These mutants lack the capacity to suppress the growth of PTEN-deficient cells, indicating a deficiency in regulation or stability. Silencing of the *PTEN* promoter by methylation has been found in some thyroid and lung cancers, as well as in melanomas and glioblastomas.

Beyond genomic and epigenomic disruptions, PTEN is also downregulated by oncogenic mechanisms operating at other regulatory levels. The miR-21 microRNA, which promotes tumorigenesis by targeting the PTEN transcript, is overexpressed in a wide array of cancers, including hematological malignancies such as AML and CLL, along with solid tumors such as glioblastomas, breast, colon, and lung cancers (Leslie and Foti, 2011). The PICT-1 protein, which stabilizes PTEN by interacting with its C-terminal tail, is lost in some neuroblastomas, and PICT-1 deficiency correlates with PTEN downregulation at the protein level. The critical role played by PTEN in suppressing tumorigenesis in many tissues is underscored by the variety of means through which its function is controlled.

7.6.3 BRCA1 and BRCA2

In 1994, linkage analysis studies correlated the *BRCA1* and *BRCA2* genes with hereditary breast cancer and hundreds of germline and somatic mutations have since been identified in both genes (Narod and Foulkes, 2004). *BRCA1* mutations associate with high-grade infiltrating ductal carcinomas, frequently exhibiting a basal, triple-negative phenotype (ie, without expression of hormone receptors or HER-2/ERBB2; see Chap. 20, Sec. 20.3), whereas *BRCA2* mutations do not appear to correlate with a particular tumor histopathology. In addition to breast cancer, *BRCA1* and *BRCA2* carriers are now also known to bear a heightened risk for developing ovarian tumors, and male carriers of *BRCA2* have an increased risk of prostate cancer.

The BRCA1/2 tumor suppressors play central roles in the maintenance of genomic integrity (Huen et al, 2010). The BRCA1 structure consists of an N-terminal RING domain, a central coiled-coil domain, and a C-terminal BRCT (BRCA1 C-terminus) domain, all of which mediate interactions critical to the functions of the protein in the realms of DNA repair, cell-cycle checkpoint control, chromatin remodeling, and ubiquitination. The RING domain, which interacts with the BARD1 protein to create an E3 ubiquitin ligase holoenzyme, is a common target for oncogenic mutations. Frequent mutations are also found in the coiled-coil and BRCT domains, which disrupt BRCA1 function by interfering with protein–protein interactions. BRCA1 is involved in the resection step of DNA double-stranded break (DSB) repair by homologous recombination, via its interaction with the MRN endonuclease complex (see Chap. 5, Sec. 5.3.4). Moreover, BRCA1 also appears to modulate DNA damage-triggered cell-cycle checkpoints by regulating activation of the Chk1 kinase (see Chap. 9, Sec. 9.3.1).

BRCA2 is a large protein containing several regions known to mediate interactions, notably 8 central BRCT repeats that bind RAD51 and C-terminal nucleic acid recognition sequences (known as OB folds) that interact with single-stranded DNA (ssDNA). Recently, 3 groups reported the successful purification of the BRCA2 protein, enabling greater mechanistic insights (Jensen et al, 2010; Liu et al, 2010; Thorslund et al, 2010). The primary function of the protein is in facilitating DNA repair by homologous recombination through the recruitment of RAD51 to the resected ssDNA stretches generated by the MRN complex at sites of DNA damage (see Chap. 5, Sec 5.3.4). BRCA1 is also involved in this phase of DNA repair via its interaction with BRCA2. Tumors which lack functional BRCA1 or BRCA2, and therefore are deficient in homologous recombination, can be selectively targeted by inhibition of poly(adenosine diphosphate-ribose) polymerase (PARP) which provides an alternative pathway for DNA repair; this is the prototype example of the use of "synthetic lethality" in the treatment of cancer (see Chap. 5, Sec. 5.8 and Chap. 17, Sec. 17.3.2).

7.6.4 Retinoblastoma Protein

The Rb protein is an important transcriptional regulator, which is inactivated in a substantial portion of human cancers, beyond the historic association alluded to in its name. In part, Rb protein acts as a cofactor interacting with and regulating the activity of transcription factors, notably those of the E2F family. In addition, Rb protein serves as an adaptor for the recruitment of epigenetic regulators, thereby impacting the chromatin status both at specific loci and at a global level. Originally, the tumor suppressor function of Rb protein

was attributed largely to its role in constraining cell-cycle progression, at the G1 to S phase transition, by influencing the expression of genes under the control of E2F transcription factors (see Chap. 9, Sec 9.2.3). In its hypophophorylated form, Rb binds E2F proteins and prevents them from activating target genes required for cell-cycle progression. In response to proliferative signals, CYCLIN/CDK complexes phosphorylate Rb protein resulting in its dissociation, thereby liberating the E2F proteins to activate the appropriate gene expression program. It is now appreciated that Rb protein also affects the expression of transcriptional targets that impact a wide array of cellular processes encompassing differentiation, cell death, genomic stability, senescence, and angiogenesis. Deregulation of any of these through Rb protein inactivation would clearly have the potential to promote various stages of tumorigenesis, although the precise Rb protein contribution likely varies in different tumors.

7.7 THERAPEUTIC STRATEGIES GUIDED BY CANCER GENETICS

The treatment of cancers with radiation and conventional chemotherapy largely entails broad-spectrum killing of both malignant and untransformed cells resulting in varying levels of toxicity. The genetic heterogeneity of cancer, although complex, presents oncologists with an opportunity for more targeted approaches. The prospect of personalized medicine is now a tangible objective, encompassing the capacity to profile the totality of aberrations in individual tumors, and then tailor treatments to maximize the targeted killing of cancer cells while reducing attendant side effects (see Table 7–1). The advent of high-throughput screening technologies has enabled the timely identification of promising targeted therapeutics from libraries of small-molecule compounds. In parallel, humanized monoclonal antibodies have been developed to interfere with oncogenic pathways at the cell surface, for example, by blocking ligand binding or tagging cancer cells for immunological clearing.

Diagnostic tests for profiling genetic changes in human tumors have become commercially available and many more are anticipated. One class of diagnostic assays scans tumor DNA for hundreds of known cancer-associated mutations. Currently, this is accomplished by high-throughput chip-based mass spectrometry platforms such as the Sequenom MassArray system, which has been used to screen panels of genes including the OncoCarta and OncoMap sets (MacConaill et al, 2009; see Chap. 2 for description of techniques). Single-nucleotide mutations, insertions, deletions, and copy number variations, as well as epigenetic changes, can all be detected with this technique. As costs are reduced by the development of next-generation DNA sequencing methods, more comprehensive probing of tumor DNA alterations will soon be available (Ansorge, 2009).

A second class of diagnostic tests is based on the profiling of tumor gene expression patterns in order to predict clinical scenarios, such as metastatic propensity, disease recurrence, and therapeutic sensitivity (Nevins and Potti, 2007). One such assay is the MammaPrint microarray test that analyzes a 70-gene signature that is predictive of metastatic spread in early stage breast tumors (van 't Veer et al, 2002). Another example, is the Oncotype DX test in which the expression levels of 21 genes are assessed by reverse-transcription polymerase chain reaction (RT-PCR) and used to predict the probability of 10-year recurrence and responsiveness to adjuvant chemotherapy in patients with early stage breast cancer (Sparano and Paik, 2008; see Chap. 20, Sec. 20.3.2). A similar test, based on a 12-gene panel, for predicting 10-year recurrence in patients with stage II colon cancer is also now available. Given the heterogeneity of genetic alterations among cancers within individual tissues, more ambitious gene expression signatures are being developed in order to distinguish tumor subtypes, thereby facilitating the design of more precise therapeutic regimens.

The discovery of the oncogenic BCR-ABL fusion protein (Sec. 7.5.1) triggered a search for compounds that could specifically inhibit the kinase. The resulting treatment of CML with the specific BCR-ABL inhibitor, imatinib, remains the benchmark for targeted cancer therapeutics. Although imatinib has proven to be highly effective in preventing the progression of CML from the chronic to blast phases, secondary mutations in the BCR-ABL kinase domain can lead to the development of therapeutic resistance. In such cases, successful management of the disease has involved countering the secondary resistance with other tyrosine kinase inhibitors, such as dasatinib. Because CML is associated with a specific genetic lesion, it is debatable whether it can truly be regarded as a paradigm for countering the progression of tumors dependent on perhaps 15 driver mutations. Such tumors are unlikely to have a single "Achilles' heel" that can be specifically targeted, and cocktails of targeted therapies will likely be required. Moreover, recent sequencing efforts have confirmed that spatially distinct regions of individual tumors are often occupied by subclonal populations of tumor cells whose genomes have acquired divergent sets of driver mutations, in addition to the common mutations present in the original clonal population. This intratumor heterogeneity also would be expected to limit any therapeutic strategy that depended on a single agent.

Several targeted therapeutics have been designed to counter hyperactivation of EGF pathways. Non–small cell lung cancers (NSCLCs), often driven by EGFR hyperactivation, have been treated with the specific EGFR inhibitors, erlotinib and gefitinib (Pines et al, 2010). Both are effective against only a subset of targeted malignancies, and this initial potency is commonly followed by the development of therapeutic resistance. Gaining an understanding of the molecular factors underlying both the initial insensitivity and acquired resistance is indispensable for guiding modifications to the therapeutic regimens.

Small-molecule EGFR inhibitors have generally proved disappointing in treating refractory colorectal cancers, although EGFR pathway activation is often observed in these tumors. Cetuximab, a humanized monoclonal antibody that binds to the EGFR ligand-binding domain promoting cytosolic internalization of the receptor, has demonstrated some clinical efficacy. Improved therapeutic response has been observed, mostly in combinatorial treatment regimens, in trial settings evaluating cetuximab as both first-line therapy, as well as in the treatment of refractory colorectal cancers. Moreover, evaluation of trial data to identify predictive biomarkers determined that tumors bearing K-ras mutations were not responsive to cetuximab, presumably because of downstream activation of the EGFR pathway.

ERBB2 (HER-2) status is an important predictive marker, in either early stage or metastatic breast cancers, for tumor sensitivity to treatment with trastuzumab, a humanized monoclonal antibody that targets the ERBB2 ectodomain (Finn and Slamon, 2003). Mammary carcinomas are screened for ERBB2 status by a combination of immunohistochemistry (IHC), to gauge receptor levels at the cell surface, and fluorescence in situ hybridization (FISH) to establish gene copy numbers. A finding of greater than 6 ERBB2 gene copies is suggestive of a tumor that may be receptive to treatment with trastuzumab. However, a substantial portion of tumors with high ERBB2 status prove to be refractory to the therapy, presumably because of additional oncogenic events, such as loss of the PTEN tumor suppressor, which obviates the requirement for upstream signals from the ERBB2 receptor for downstream pathway activation.

In light of the frequent upregulation of MAP kinase and PI3 kinase signaling in a wide array of cancers, the various actors in the pathway constitute attractive therapeutic targets. However, the clinical performance of drugs targeting these pathways has been minimal, although new compounds are being evaluated in trials. RAS hyperactivation is somewhat paradoxical in that oncogenic mutations lock the protein in an activated state by blocking enzymatic turnover. This poses a problem for drug designers who typically generate compounds designed to block the enzymatic catalysis, a conceptually simpler task for which established inhibitory strategies are known.

Deactivation of RAS requires stimulation of enzymatic turnover and, despite great effort, there is no drug capable of effectively downregulating oncogenic RAS. In addition to GTP binding, RAS activation involves membrane translocation brought about by the multistep covalent attachment of specific lipid groups near the C-terminus of the protein. Drugs, such as farnesyltransferase inhibitors (FTIs), designed to disrupt this lipidation process, have either proven ineffectual or overly toxic (Beeram et al, 2005). The prospect of interfering with the MAP kinase pathway downstream of RAS, using RAF or MEK inhibitors, is being pursued. RAF inhibitors have proven to be potent against cancers driven by the oncogenic B-RAF^{V600E} mutant, such as malignant melanoma, but, counterintuitively, have demonstrated tumorigenic properties when treating experimental cancers harboring oncogenic RAS or the wild-type RAS/RAF combination (Heidorn et al, 2010;

Chapman et al, 2011). This finding is indicative not only of the complexity of MAP kinase signaling, but also of the careful consideration which must be accorded to the full genetic context of a cancer prior to therapeutic administration. MEK inhibitors are also being assessed, although there is evidence that some RAS mutant tumors do not require MEK activation for oncogenic signaling.

Although the PI3 kinase inhibitors, Wortmannin and LY294002, have been used in research for the better part of 2 decades, a combination of poor pharmacological properties and a lack of specificity have hampered clinical applications. Despite these challenges, the prevalence of the pathway in neoplastic transformation has encouraged continued investment into the creation of drugs targeting specific PI3 kinase isoforms, and a number of compounds are at different stages of clinical development.

Many promising targets, such as RAS and MYC, may prove to be "undruggable," necessitating alternative attack strategies. Synthetic lethal studies can be exploited to uncover secondary targets, more amenable to therapeutic intervention, whose inhibition can block cancer progression driven by specific oncogenic pathways. As noted, there is interest in the use of PARP inhibitors in patients whose tumors have lost expression or function of the BRCA1 and BRCA2 DNA repair genes, and become dependent on PARP to repair DNA. Still other targets will prove promising in one genomic context, but when inhibited in the presence of other mutations may have limited effect on tumorigenesis. As noted, the targeting of upstream receptors is ineffectual when additional mutations in the *K-RAS*, *B-RAF*, *PIK3CA*, or *PTEN* genes activate the downstream pathways irrespective of receptor signaling. Granting these qualifications, the first step in dealing with a given cancer will be to define the nature of the oncogenic transformation through timely and cost-effective profiling of the tumor.

SUMMARY

- Recent years have witnessed the alleviation of many of the technological limitations that have long hampered efforts by cancer biologists to develop a comprehensive picture of the genetic events underlying tumorigenesis.
- The advent of new research platforms has created the potential for identifying virtually all oncogenic events in a given cancer in a cost-effective and high-throughput manner. For the first time, it is possible to distinguish the full mutational spectra of cancers that arise in different tissues, as well as between primary malignancies and metastasized tumors.
- One of the greatest revelations of the recent large-scale analyses is the extent of the heterogeneity afflicting cancer genomes. Moreover, it is now apparent that cancer should be viewed as a set of mutagenic alterations, occurring not only at the genomic, but also at the epigenomic, transcriptomic, proteomic, and metabolic levels.
- These changes confer a selective advantage that constitutes the transformed phenotype, encompassing properties that are particular to cancer cells. As defined by Hanahan and Weinberg, these include self-sufficiency in growth signals, insensitivity to antigrowth signals, resistance to cell death, limitless replicative potential, angiogenesis, genomic instability, deregulated metabolism, and the capacity for invasion and metastasis, as well as the ability to circumvent immune clearance and generate tumorigenic inflammation.
- The critical challenge confronting the research community is to sift among the immense list of changes occurring during transformation, so as to identify the indispensable oncogenic processes, which may then be interdicted therapeutically (see Table 7–1).
- Acquiring such an understanding requires a confluence of efforts in many fields including bioinformatics, bioengineering, and pharmacology, as well as basic biological and translational research.
- Such comprehensive efforts promise to reveal novel cancer genes, such as *IDH1* and *IDH2*, while confirming the importance of more established oncogenes, like *BCR-ABL*, *MYC*, *EGFR*, *ERbB2*, *PIK3CA*, *RAS*, and *RAF*, along with the *TP53*, *PTEN*, *BRCA1*, *BRCA2*, and *Rb* tumor-suppressor genes.
- A clearer understanding of the oncogenic processes underlying specific cancers will enable personalized therapeutic approaches, presumably leading to more effective clinical outcomes.

REFERENCES

Albihn A, Johnsen JI, Henriksson MA. MYC in oncogenesis and as a target for cancer therapies. *Adv Cancer Res* 2010;107:163-224.

Ansorge WJ. Next-generation DNA sequencing techniques. *N Biotechnol* 2009;25:195-203.

Armitage P, Doll R. The age distribution of cancer and a multistage theory of carcinogenesis. *Br J Cancer* 1954;8:1-12.

Armitage P, Doll R. A two-stage theory of carcinogenesis in relation to the age distribution of human cancer. *Br J Cancer* 1957;11: 161-169.

Balmain A. Cancer genetics: from Boveri to Mendel to microarrays. *Nat Rev Cancer* 2001;1:77-82.

Balss J, Meyer J, Mueller W, et al. Analysis of the IDH1 codon 132 mutation in brain tumors. *Acta Neuropathol* 2008;116:597-602.

Baselga J, Swain SM. Novel anticancer targets: revisiting ERBB2 and discovering ERBB3. *Nat Rev Cancer* 2009;9:463-475.

Beeram M, Patnaik A, Rowinsky EK. Raf: a strategic target for therapeutic development against cancer. *J Clin Oncol* 2005;23: 6771-6790.

Bozic I, Antal T, Ohtsuki H, et al. Accumulation of driver and passenger mutations during tumor progression. *Proc Natl Acad Sci U S A* 2010;107:18545-18550.

Brosh R, Rotter V. When mutants gain new powers: news from the mutant p53 field. *Nat Rev Cancer* 2009;9:701-713.

Brown CJ, Lain S, Verma CS, et al. Awakening guardian angels: drugging the p53 pathway. *Nat Rev Cancer* 2009;9:862-873.

Caparros-Lefebvre D, Girard-Buttaz I, Reboul S, et al. Cognitive and psychiatric impairment in herpes simplex virus encephalitis suggest involvement of the amygdalo-frontal pathways. *J Neurol* 1996;243:248-256.

Carter H, Chen S, Isik L, et al. Cancer-specific high-throughput annotation of somatic mutations: computational prediction of driver missense mutations. *Cancer Res* 2009;69:6660-6667.

Carter H, Samayoa J, Hruban RH, et al. Prioritization of driver mutations in pancreatic cancer using cancer-specific high-throughput annotation of somatic mutations (CHASM). *Cancer Biol Ther* 2010;10:582-587.

Carter N. Methods and strategies for analyzing copy number variation using DNA microarrays. *Nat Genet* 2007;39:S16-S21.

Cavenee W, Dryja T, Phillips R, et al. Expression of recessive alleles by chromosomal mechanisms in retinoblastoma. *Nature* 1983;305:779-784.

Chalhoub N, Baker SJ. PTEN and the PI3-kinase pathway in cancer. *Annu Rev Pathol* 2009;4:127-150.

Chang HW, Aoki M, Fruman D, et al. Transformation of chicken cells by the gene encoding the catalytic subunit of PI 3-kinase. *Science* 1997;276:1848-1850.

Chapman PB, Hauschild A, Robert C, et al. Improved survival with vemurafenib in melanoma with BRAF V600E mutation. *N Engl J Med* 2011;364:2507-2516.

Chi P, Allis CD, Wang GG. Covalent histone modifications—miswritten, misinterpreted and mis-erased in human cancers. *Nat Rev Cancer* 2010;10:457-469.

Cimmino A, Calin GA, Fabbri M, et al. miR-15 and miR-16 induce apoptosis by targeting BCL2. *Proc Natl Acad Sci U S A* 2006;102:13944-13949.

Clark JP, Cooper CS. ETS gene fusions in prostate cancer. *Nat Rev Urol* 2009;6:429-439.

Croce CM. Causes and consequences of microRNA dysregulation in cancer. *Nat Rev Genet* 2009;10:704-714.

Crystal AS, Snow AT. New targets in advanced NSCLC: EML4-ALK. *Clin Adv Hematol Oncol* 2011;9:207-214.

Dang L, White DW, Gross S, et al. Cancer-associated IDH1 mutations produce 2-hydroxyglutarate. *Nature* 2009;462:739-744.

De Klein A, Hagemeijer A, Bartram CR, et al. bcr rearrangement and translocation of the c-abl oncogene in Philadelphia positive acute lymphoblastic leukemia. *Blood* 1986;68:1369-1375.

Der CJ, Krontiris TG, Cooper GM. Transforming genes of human bladder and lung carcinoma cell lines are homologous to the ras genes of Harvey and Kirsten sarcoma viruses. *Proc Natl Acad Sci U S A* 1982;79:3637-3640.

Edwards PA. Fusion genes and chromosome translocations in the common epithelial cancers. *J Pathol* 2010;220:244-254.

Engelman JA, Luo J, Cantley LC. The evolution of phosphatidylinositol 3-kinases as regulators of growth and metabolism. *Nat Rev Genet* 2006;7:606-619.

Esteller M. Epigenetics in cancer. *N Engl J Med* 2008;358:1148-1159.

Fabbri M, Garzon R, Cimmino A, et al. MicroRNA-29 family reverts aberrant methylation in lung cancer by targeting DNA methyltransferases 3A and 3B. *Proc Natl Acad Sci U S A* 2007;104:15805-15810.

Finn RS, Slamon DJ. Monoclonal antibody therapy for breast cancer: herceptin. *Cancer Chemother Biol Response Modif* 2003;21:223-233.

Fletcher O, Houlston RS. Architecture of inherited susceptibility to common cancer. *Nat Rev Cancer* 2010;10:353-361.

Friend S, Bernards R, Rogelj S, et al. A human DNA segment with properties of the gene that predisposes to retinoblastoma and osteosarcoma. *Nature* 1986;323:643-646.

Fung Y, Murphree A, T'Ang A, et al. Structural evidence for the authenticity of the human retinoblastoma gene. *Science* 1987;236:1657-1661.

Garzon R, Calin GA, Croce CM. MicroRNAs in cancer. *Annu Rev Med* 2009;60:167-179.

Goldman JM, Melo JV. BCR-ABL in chronic myelogenous leukemia—how does it work? *Acta Haematol* 2008;119:212-217.

Hanahan D, Weinberg RA. The hallmarks of cancer. *Cell* 2000;100:57-70.

Hanahan D, Weinberg RA. Hallmarks of cancer: the next generation. *Cell* 2011:646-674.

Hayward WS, Neel BG, Astrin SM. Activation of a cellular onc gene by promoter insertion in ALV-induced lymphoid leukosis. *Nature* 1981;290:475-480.

Heidorn SJ, Milagre C, Whittaker S, et al. Kinase-dead BRAF and oncogenic RAS cooperate to drive tumor progression through CRAF. *Cell* 2010;140:209-221.

Hollander MC, Blumenthal GM, Dennis PA. PTEN loss in the continuum of common cancers, rare syndromes and mouse models. *Nat Rev Cancer* 2011;11:289-301.

Huen MS, Sy SM, Chen J. BRCA1 and its toolbox for the maintenance of genome integrity. *Nat Rev Mol Cell Biol* 2010;11:138-148.

Jensen RB, Carreira A, Kowalczykowski SC. Purified human BRCA2 stimulates RAD51-mediated recombination. *Nature* 2010;467:678-683.

Johnson SM, Grosshans H, Shingara J, et al. RAS is regulated by the let-7 microRNA family. *Cell* 2005;120:635-647.

Junttila MR, Evan GI. p53—a jack of all trades but master of none. *Nat Rev Cancer* 2009;9:821-829.

Kallioniemi A. CGH microarrays and cancer. *Curr Opin Biotechnol* 2008;19:36-40.

Karreth FA, Tuveson DA. Modelling oncogenic Ras/Raf signalling in the mouse. *Curr Opin Genet Dev* 2009;19:4-11.

Kinzler KW, Vogelstein B. Lessons from hereditary colorectal cancer. *Cell* 1996;87:159-170.

Kinzler KW, Vogelstein B. Landscaping the cancer terrain. *Science* 1998;280:1036-1037.

Klein G, Klein E, Kashuba E. Interaction of Epstein-Barr virus (EBV) with human B-lymphocytes. *Biochem Biophys Res Commun* 2010;396:67-73.

Knudson AG. Mutation and cancer: statistical study of retinoblastoma. *Proc Natl Acad Sci U S A* 1971;68:820-823.

Kumar-Sinha C, Tomlins SA, Chinnaiyan AM. Recurrent gene fusions in prostate cancer. *Nat Rev Cancer* 2008;8:497-511.

Laird PW. Principles and challenges of genome-wide DNA methylation analysis. *Nat Rev Genet* 2010;11:191-203.

Lee W, Bookstein R, Hong F, et al. Human retinoblastoma susceptibility gene: cloning, identification, and sequence. *Science* 1987;235:1394-1399.

Leslie NR, Foti M. Non-genomic loss of PTEN function in cancer: not in my genes. *Trends Pharmacol Sci* 2011;32:131-140.

Levine AJ. The common mechanisms of transformation by the small DNA tumor viruses: the inactivation of tumor suppressor gene products: p53. *Virology* 2009;384:285-293.

Liu CG, Calin GA, Volinia S, et al. MicroRNA expression profiling using microarrays. *Nat Protoc* 2008;3:563-578.

Liu J, Doty T, Gibson B, et al. Human BRCA2 protein promotes RAD51 filament formation on RPA-covered single-stranded DNA. *Nat Struct Mol Biol* 2010;17:1260-1262.

MacConaill LE, Campbell CD, Kehoe SM, et al. Profiling critical cancer gene mutations in clinical tumor samples. *PLoS One* 2009; 4:e7887.

Maurer G, Tarkowski B, Baccarini M. Raf kinases in cancer-roles and therapeutic opportunities. *Oncogene* 2011;30:3477-3488.

Meyer N, Penn LZ. Reflecting on 25 years with MYC. *Nat Rev Cancer* 2008;8:976-990.

Miller DL, Puricelli MD, Stack MS. Virology and molecular pathogenesis of HPV (human papillomavirus)-associated oropharyngeal squamous cell carcinoma. *Biochem J* 2012;443: 339-353.

Munger K, Baldwin A, Edwards KM, et al. Mechanisms of human papillomavirus-induced oncogenesis. *J Virol* 2004;78:11451-11460.

Narod SA, Foulkes WD. BRCA1 and BRCA2: 1994 and beyond. *Nat Rev Cancer* 2004;4:665-676.

Nevins JR, Potti A. Mining gene expression profiles: expression signatures as cancer phenotypes. *Nat Rev Genet* 2007;8:601-609.

Nordling CO. A new theory on cancer-inducing mechanism. *Br J Cancer* 1953;7:68-72.

Nowell PC, Hungerford DA. A minute chromosome in human chronic granulocytic leukemia. *Science* 1960;132:1488-1501.

Nussenzweig A, Nussenzweig MC. Origin of chromosomal translocations in lymphoid cancer. *Cell* 2010;141:27-38.

Otsu M, Hiles I, Gout I, et al. Characterization of two 85 kd proteins that associate with receptor tyrosine kinases, middle-T/pp60c-src complexes, and PI3-kinase. *Cell* 1991;65:91-104.

Parsons DW, Jones S, Zhang X, et al. An integrated genomic analysis of human glioblastoma multiforme. *Science* 2008;321: 1807-1812.

Pines G, Kostler WJ, Yarden Y. Oncogenic mutant forms of EGFR: lessons in signal transduction and targets for cancer therapy. *FEBS Lett* 2010;584:2699-2706.

Reddy EP, Reynolds RK, Watson DK, et al. Nucleotide sequence analysis of the proviral genome of avian myelocytomatosis virus (MC29). *Proc Natl Acad Sci U S A* 1983;80:2500-2504.

Rous P. Transmission of a malignant new growth by means of a cell-free filtrate. *JAMA* 1911;56:198.

Rowley JD. A new consistent chromosomal abnormality in chronic myelogenous leukaemia identified by quinacrine fluorescence and Giemsa staining. *Nature* 1973;243:290-293.

Ryan BM, Robles AI, Harris CC. Genetic variation in microRNA networks: the implications for cancer research. *Nat Rev Cancer* 2010;10:389-402.

Sampson VB, Rong NH, Han J, et al. MicroRNA let-7a down-regulates MYC and reverts MYC-induced growth in Burkitt lymphoma cells. *Cancer Res* 2007;67:9762-9770.

Schmitt F. HER2+ breast cancer: how to evaluate? *Adv Ther* 2009;26 Suppl 1:S1-S8.

Shimizu K, Goldfarb M, Suard Y, et al. Three human transforming genes are related to the viral ras oncogenes. *Proc Natl Acad Sci U S A* 1983;80:2112-2116.

Sparano JA, Paik S. Development of the 21-gene assay and its application in clinical practice and clinical trials. *J Clin Oncol* 2008;26:721-728.

Stehelin D, Varmus H, Bishop J, et al. DNA related to the transforming gene(s) of avian sarcoma viruses is present in normal avian DNA. *Nature* 1976;260:170-173.

Thorslund T, McIlwraith MJ, Compton SA, et al. The breast cancer tumor suppressor BRCA2 promotes the specific targeting of RAD51 to single-stranded DNA. *Nat Struct Mol Biol* 2010;17: 1263-1265.

Tsai WL, Chung RT. Viral hepatocarcinogenesis. *Oncogene* 2010;29: 2309-2324.

van 't Veer LJ, Dai H, van de Vijver MJ, et al. Gene expression profiling predicts clinical outcome of breast cancer. *Nature* 2002;415:530-536.

Veeck J, Esteller M. Breast cancer epigenetics: from DNA methylation to microRNAs. *J Mammary Gland Biol Neoplasia* 2010;15:5-17.

Ward PS, Patel J, Wise DR, et al. The common feature of leukemia-associated IDH1 and IDH2 mutations is a neomorphic enzyme activity converting alpha-ketoglutarate to 2-hydroxyglutarate. *Cancer Cell* 2010;17:225-234.

Whitman M, Kaplan DR, Schaffhausen B, et al. Association of phosphatidylinositol kinase activity with polyoma middle-T competent for transformation. *Nature* 1985;315:239-242.

Yan H, Parsons DW, Jin G, et al. IDH1 and IDH2 mutations in gliomas. *N Engl J Med* 2009;360:765-773.

Cellular Signaling Pathways

8

Michael Reedijk and C. Jane McGlade

8.1 INTRODUCTION

The ability of cells to receive and respond to extracellular signals is a critical process in the embryonic development of multicellular organisms as well as for the maintenance and survival of mature tissues in the adult. Changes in the physical or chemical environment of the cell can result in modifications of cell metabolism, morphology, movement, or proliferation. These responses are brought about by elaborate networks of intracellular signals transmitted by changes in protein phosphorylation and enzymatic activity, localization and the formation of protein–protein complexes. Cellular responses are triggered by the recognition of extracellular signals at the cell surface, resulting in the activation of linked cytoplasmic and nuclear biochemical cascades. These signal transduction pathways control cellular processes that range from the generalized control of cell proliferation and survival to specialized functions such as the immune response and angiogenesis. When dysregulated, signaling pathways involved in normal growth, adhesion and development contribute to malignant transformation in human cells. This knowledge has led to the development of new cancer therapeutics that specifically target aberrant signal transduction pathways. This chapter explores how signal transduction pathways are organized and highlights ongoing drug discovery efforts to target these pathways.

8.2 GROWTH FACTOR SIGNALING PATHWAYS

8.2.1 Extracellular Growth Factors and Receptor Tyrosine Kinases

In multicellular organisms, cell regulation is controlled by secreted polypeptide molecules called growth factors or cytokines, by antigen stimulation of immune cells, or by cell contact with neighboring cells and surrounding extracellular matrix. Our most detailed understanding of signal transduction pathways comes from studies of soluble growth factors and their interaction with complementary growth factor receptors expressed on responsive cells. The interaction between growth factors and receptors on the cell surface leads to the modification of intracellular biochemical signaling pathways that control cellular responses, especially cell proliferation. Cellular regulation also occurs through direct cell to cell contact or cell contact with its surrounding extracellular matrix (as discussed in Chap. 10, Sec. 10.2).

Growth factors were first identified in cell culture medium as necessary to sustain mammalian cell survival and proliferation. One of the characteristics of malignant transformation was found to be relative independence from the action of external growth factors. Many polypeptide growth factors have

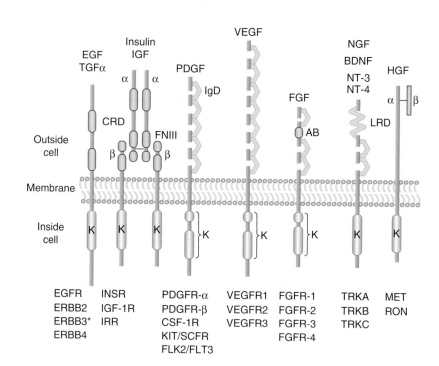

FIGURE 8–1 **The receptor protein tyrosine kinases.** Representative molecules from selected RPTK families of receptors ("R") are shown below and representative ligands above. *EGF*, epidermal growth factor; *FGF*, fibroblast growth factor; *HGF*, hepatocyte growth factor; *NGF*, nerve growth factor; *PDGF*, platelet-derived growth factor; *VEGF*, vascular endothelial growth factor. All members have a conserved intracellular kinase domain (K). Some of the common structural elements found in the extracellular ligand binding domain include the CRD (cysteine-rich domain), FNIII (fibronectin type III repeats), IgD (immunoglobulin-like domain), AB (acid-rich box), and LRD (leucine-rich domain); *TGF-α*, transforming growth factor-alpha; *IGF*, insulin-like growth factor; *BDNF*, brain derived neurotrophic factor; *NT-3*, neurotrophin 3; *NT-4*, neurotrophin 4.

been identified with diverse functions in normal embryonic development and tissue homeostasis but only a few factors are associated with the process of malignant transformation.

Polypeptide growth factors influence cell processes, such as growth, proliferation, differentiation, survival, and metabolism, via their interaction with specific transmembrane receptor protein tyrosine kinases (RPTKs). Most are small monomeric (ie, single-chain) polypeptides, such as the epidermal growth factor (EGF) and members of the fibroblast growth factor (FGF) family. There are also dimeric polypeptide growth factors (ie, those containing 2 chains of amino acids), such as platelet-derived growth factor (PDGF). In addition to being freely diffusible, growth factors can also reside in spatially restricted domains within an organism, either through binding to components in the extracellular matrix or because they are produced as membrane anchored molecules that reside on the surface of the producing cells. Figure 8–1 summarizes selected growth factors and their cognate receptors.

Receptors for growth factors are membrane spanning cell surface molecules that share the ability to phosphorylate themselves and other cytoplasmic proteins, thereby activating a signaling cascade. Most growth factor receptors are protein tyrosine kinases that specifically phosphorylate the amino acid tyrosine in protein substrates and can be subdivided into 20 different families based on distinct structural components. The main distinguishing feature amongst RPTK subgroups resides in the extracellular growth factor-binding domain at the amino terminus. Usually several hundred amino acids in length, these extracellular domains can be grouped by sequence homology, or by the presence of sequence motifs also found in other functionally unrelated molecules such as EGF repeats, immunoglobulin repeats or fibronectin type III

repeats (see Fig. 8–1). The extracellular domains of RPTKs are also commonly posttranslationally modified by glycosylation.

The extracellular domain is connected to the intracellular (cytoplasmic) domain by a short, single, hydrophobic helix transmembrane component. The cytoplasmic domain is comprised of regulatory sequences and a conserved kinase domain, which catalyzes the transfer of a phosphate group from adenosine triphosphate (ATP) onto a protein substrate. In RPTKs, the core catalytic domain is typically about 260 residues in length and is as much as 90% identical between members of this protein kinase family. The amino acids flanking the kinase domain and adjacent to the plasma membrane (juxtamembrane region) of growth factor receptors frequently contain sites of tyrosine phosphorylation and these regions often have important roles in both signal transmission and in regulation of catalytic activity. Such regulatory sequences can also reside within the catalytic domain of receptor kinases. Members of the PDGFR and vascular endothelial growth factor (VEGFR) families of receptors are distinguished by possessing a split kinase domain in which important autophosphorylation sites are present on a kinase insert within the catalytic domain (van der Geer et al, 1994).

Binding of the growth factor or ligand induces conformational changes in the extracellular domain of the receptor that facilitate dimerization (ie, joining together) or clustering of receptor tyrosine kinases (Fig. 8–2). Some ligands, such as PDGF, are themselves dimeric forms of a single subunit and naturally induce a symmetric ligand/receptor dimer. Structural studies have revealed how other ligands that exist as monomers, such as EGF, induce receptor dimerization through receptor-receptor interactions. These studies revealed that binding of EGF to the epidermal growth factor receptor (EGFR) (ERBB1) induces a conformation change that exposes

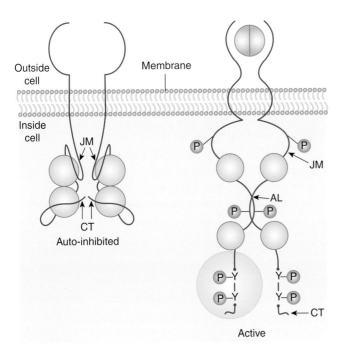

FIGURE 8-2 Growth factor receptor dimerization and activation. In the absence of ligand (eg, EGF) binding the intracellular kinase domain is inactive, held in a repressed conformation by intramolecular interactions involving the juxtamembrane region (JM), carboxyterminal tail (CT) and activation loop (AL). Ligand binding induces receptor dimerization, relief of inhibitory constraints and autophosphorylation of the intracellular domains on tyrosine residues. These autophosphorylation sites function to both enhance the catalytic activity and serve as docking sites for intracellular signaling molecules that bind to phosphotyrosine. *P*, Phosphate; *Y*, tyrosine.

a dimerization loop that mediates association of neighboring, ligand occupied receptors (Schlessinger, 2002). Similar dimerization loops are found in the other members of the EGFR family (ERBB2, ERBB3, and ERBB4) allowing the formation of heterodimers between different members of the ERBB family.

Ligand binding and receptor dimerization bring together 2 catalytic domains, resulting in intermolecular autophosphorylation (transphosphorylation) of tyrosine residues within the catalytic domain and in the noncatalytic regulatory regions of the cytoplasmic domain. Phosphorylation of key residues within the kinase activation loop induces the opening of the catalytic site and allows access to ATP and protein substrates, while phosphorylated residues in noncatalytic regions create docking sites for downstream signaling molecules that are essential for signal propagation (see Fig. 8–2) (Lemmon and Schlessinger, 2010; Pawson, 2002).

Dimerization of receptors also leads to conformational changes within the cytoplasmic domain required for full catalytic activity. RPTKs are autoinhibited through intramolecular interactions that occlude the enzyme active site and prevent access of protein substrates. The juxtamembrane region of receptors from the PDGFR family represses the activity of the kinase domain and this repression is relieved

by phosphorylation of tyrosine residues in the juxtamembrane region (Hubbard, 2004; Lemmon and Schlessinger, 2010). Similarly, the carboxyterminal tail of the angiopoietin receptor Tie2 is thought to block the active site of the kinase domain preventing substrate access (Niu et al, 2002).

Abnormal RPTKs involved in cancer are deregulated by loss of 1 or more of the regulatory mechanisms described above, making their catalytic activity ligand-independent. Identification of aberrantly activated RPTKs has led to the development of selectively targeted cancer therapeutics. For example, the ERBB2/NEU oncogene encodes a member of the EGFR family that is frequently amplified in human breast tumors (Slamon et al, 1987). Increased expression in this case is thought to increase the concentration of active dimers generating continuous and inappropriate cellular signaling. Trastuzumab, a humanized monoclonal antibody that targets the extracellular domain of ERBB2 (HER-2), is used in combination with chemotherapy to treat breast cancer and has shown improvement in survival of patients with ERBB2-positive tumors, when used as adjuvant therapy or for treatment of advanced disease (Hudis, 2007). Also, the small molecule tyrosine kinase inhibitors erlotinib and gefitinib significantly improve progression-free survival of patients with non–small cell lung cancer that harbor kinase domain-activating mutations of the EGF receptor (Cataldo et al, 2011; Lynch et al, 2004). Mutations in the juxtamembrane regulatory regions of both c-KIT and FLT3 have been implicated in gastrointestinal stromal tumors and acute myeloid leukemia, respectively, and have also been targeted with selective tyrosine kinase inhibitors (Antonescu, 2011; Kindler et al, 2010). Although RPTKs remain attractive drug targets, the development of resistance through the acquisition of second site mutations of the oncogenic kinase, argues for therapeutic strategies that combine RPTK inhibition with targeting of downstream signaling pathways (Engelman and Settleman, 2008).

8.2.2 Formation of Multiprotein Complexes and Signal Transmission

Signaling pathways downstream of activated RPTKs are activated via interactions of specific proteins that create networks of signaling molecules. These signaling networks consist of both preformed and rapidly associating protein complexes that transmit information throughout the cell. A unifying feature of cytoplasmic signaling proteins is the presence of one or more conserved noncatalytic domains that mediate sequence-specific protein–protein interactions. The modular nature of these domains allows them to be used in diverse groups of cytoplasmic signaling molecules (Pawson and Nash, 2003). Many of these domains bind specifically to short (typically less than 10 amino acids) contiguous regions of their target protein. The binding of specific domains to their target sometimes requires phosphorylation of amino acids within the sequence-specific binding motif. Proteins that contain either SH2 (Src homology 2) or PTB (phosphotyrosine binding) domains, which recognize tyrosine phosphorylated sequence

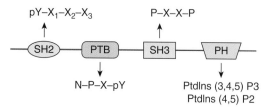

FIGURE 8–3 Examples of modular interaction domains.
Representation of the protein modules commonly found in
intracellular signaling proteins that are linked to growth factor
receptor signaling cascades. Each is shown with its consensus peptide
or phospholipid binding target. *N*, Asparagine; *P*, proline; *X*, any amino
acid; *Y*, tyrosine. The domains are represented as if linked together
on a single polypeptide to illustrate how the presence of multiple
domains within signaling molecules would facilitate the assembly of
larger signaling complexes. *SH2*, Src homology 2; *SH3*, Src homology 3;
PTB, Phosphotyrosine binding; *PH*, Pleckstrin homology.

motifs are central to the formation of signaling complexes following activation of growth factor receptor tyrosine kinases
(see Figs. 8–2 and 8–3) (Schlessinger and Lemmon, 2003).

The SH2 domain was identified as a conserved region containing approximately 100 amino acids found outside the
catalytic domain of Src family cytoplasmic tyrosine kinases.
The specificity of SH2 domain recognition is determined
both by the requirement for phosphotyrosine, common to
almost all SH2 domains and by 3 to 4 amino acids (often
termed the +1, +2, and +3 residues relative to the phosphotyrosine) on the carboxyterminal side of the tyrosine residue
(see Fig. 8–3). Individual SH2 domains bind selectively to
distinct phosphopeptide motifs, and the preferred consensus
binding sequences for most SH2 domains have been defined.
PTB domains can also specifically bind phosphotyrosine-
containing peptides but, in contrast to SH2 domains, PTB
domains recognize phosphotyrosine within a sequence motif
that includes amino acids on the aminoterminal side of the
tyrosine residue (see Fig. 8–3; Blaikie et al, 1994; Forman-Kay
and Pawson, 1999).

Activation of growth factor receptors results in the autophosphorylation of the receptor at multiple tyrosine residues
resulting in the creation of docking sites for cytoplasmic proteins that contain SH2 or PTB domains. Docking sites can also
be created by the phosphorylation of cytoplasmic molecules,
such as insulin receptor substrate-1 (IRS-1) by the insulin
receptor. As such, phosphorylated IRS-1 becomes a docking
site for SH2 domain-containing proteins (Myers et al, 1994).
In this way SH2 and PTB domains play a crucial role in linking
external signals received by a membrane receptor to cytoplasmic signaling pathways.

Since the original description of the SH2 domain, many
additional protein modules have been identified, and their
3-dimensional structures have been described and distinct target specificities defined (Seet et al, 2006). All of these interaction modules represent independently folding domains with
amino and carboxy termini in close proximity and a discrete
surface ligand-binding interface, even when incorporated into

a larger polypeptide. In addition to the tyrosine-phosphorylated
peptides described above, the specific binding partners for protein modules include phosphoserine- or phosphothreonine-
containing peptides, proline-rich peptides, and carboxyterminal
motifs, and membrane phospholipids.

Two additional protein interaction domains commonly
found in signaling molecules downstream of RPTKs are the
SH3 (Src homology 3) and PH (Pleckstrin homology) domain
(see Fig. 8–3). SH3 domains are approximately 60 amino acids
in length and are commonly found in signaling proteins in
combination with other interaction molecules. These modules often bind to proline-based motifs in target proteins
and the interaction is not dependent on changes induced by
phosphorylation (Yu et al, 1992). SH3 domains are known
to function both in the assembly of multiprotein complexes,
and also as regulatory domains in intramolecular interactions.
PH domains are protein modules of approximately 120 amino
acids in length that interact specifically with membrane phosphoinositides (phosphorylated forms of phosphatidylinositol;
PtdIns) (Harlan et al, 1994). Phosphoinositides are found at
low levels within the cell and can be rapidly modified by phosphorylation in response to signaling. Importantly, PH domains
recognize specific phosphoinositides such as PtdIns(3,4,5)P3
that are transiently produced following activation of growth
factor receptors. Thus, an important function of PH domains
is the recruitment of proteins to the membrane in the vicinity of an activated growth factor receptor (Seet et al, 2006;
Lemmon and Schlessinger, 2010).

There is an additional class of signaling proteins that have
no catalytic function (eg, NCK, CRK, and GRB2 [growth factor receptor bound-2]) and are composed entirely of SH2 and
SH3 domains. These molecules are adaptor proteins that function by interacting with signaling enzymes that do not contain
SH2 domains (or other phosphotyrosine containing modules
such as PTB domains) thereby coupling them to a tyrosine
kinase signaling complex. Each of these adaptor molecules has
a different capacity to form protein complexes as a result of
the binding specificity of its SH2 and SH3 domains, and the
result is an organized but complex network of protein-protein
interactions essential to coordinate an appropriate cellular
response (Seet et al, 2006).

Figure 8–4 illustrates two examples of how protein modules
function to activate growth factor receptor signal transduction.
The SH2 and SH3 domain-containing adaptor protein, GRB2
plays a critical role in the activation of the small guanosine
triphosphatase (GTPase) protein, RAS, a central transducer
of growth factor receptor signals. As described below, RAS
proteins are membrane-associated molecules that actively signal when bound to the guanine triphosphate nucleotide GTP.
The SH2 domain of GRB2 associates with activated growth
factor receptors while its SH3 domains are bound to proline-
based motifs in SOS (son-of-sevenless), a guanine nucleotide
exchange protein that activates RAS. Consequently, receptor
activation leads to the recruitment of the GRB2-SOS complex
close to its target, RAS, leading to its activation and downstream signaling (Lemmon and Schlessinger, 2010).

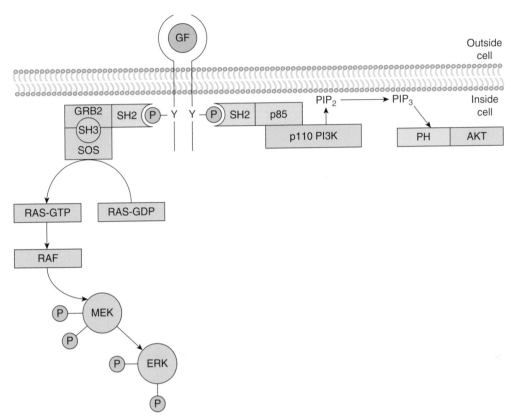

FIGURE 8–4 **Recruitment of cytoplasmic signaling molecules by receptor protein tyrosine kinases.** Binding of a receptor to a growth factor (GF) leads to phosphorylation of the intracellular domain on tyrosine (Y) residues; this interaction allows the SH2 domain-mediated association of enzymes and adaptor molecules such as GRB2 and p85. GRB2 is associated with the guanine nucleotide exchange factor SOS (son-of-sevenless). SOS recruited to activated receptor complexes then catalyzes the exchange of guanosine diphosphate (GDP) for guanosine triphosphate (GTP) on RAS. GTP-bound RAS binds the protein kinase RAF and activates a kinase cascade including MEK and ERK (see Sec. 8.2.4). The heterodimeric phosphoinositide kinase, phosphatidylinositol-3 kinase (PI3K), is comprised of a catalytic subunit, p110, and an adaptor or regulatory subunit, called p85 that contains two SH2 domains. Binding of the p85/p110 complex to activated growth factor receptors via the p85 SH2 domain activates catalytic activity of p110 which phosphorylates phosphotidylinositol 4,5 bisphosphate (PIP$_2$). The product of this reaction, phosphatidylinositol 3,4,5 triphosphate (PIP$_3$), serve as membrane anchoring site for PH domain-containing proteins such as AKT. See text for additional details.

Activation of growth factor receptors also results in the activation of phosphoinositide kinases that phosphorylate the 3′ hydroxyl group of the inositol ring. Phosphatidylinositol-3 kinase (PI3K) is a heterodimer made up of a catalytic subunit, p110, and a regulatory subunit, p85 that contains 2 SH2 domains. Following receptor activation, the PI3K is recruited to the activated receptor by the p85 SH2 domains, which binds to specific phosphotyrosine interaction motifs, leading to allosteric activation of the p110 catalytic subunit and the production of PtdIns(3,4,5)P3 (described in Sec. 8.2.5; Lemmon and Schlessinger, 2010).

8.2.3 RAS Proteins

RAS proteins control signaling pathways that regulate normal cell growth and malignant transformation. Three human RAS genes encode the proteins H-RAS, K-RAS and N-RAS and are part of a large family of low-molecular-weight GTP-binding proteins. RAS proteins have a molecular weight of 21 kDa (hence the designation p21ras) and share 85% sequence homology. The RAS proteins are GTPases that cycle between an active GTP-bound "on" and an inactive guanosine diphosphate (GDP)-bound "off" configuration in response to extracellular signals, essentially functioning as a molecular binary switch (Fig. 8–5). RAS is activated by the effects of guanine nucleotide exchange factors (GEFs), such as SOS described above, that releases RAS-bound GDP and allows GTP binding to RAS (Buday and Downward, 2008).

In the active GTP-bound form, RAS binds to a number of distinct effector proteins that, in turn, activate downstream signaling cascades. One of the best characterized effectors is the protein kinase RAF. RAS-GTP binding to RAF activates its kinase activity, and consequently activates a downstream cascade of protein kinases that include MEK and ERK (see Fig. 8–4). Additional RAS-GTP effectors include the exchange factor for another small GTPase RAL (RALGDS), and the p110 catalytic subunit of PI3K (see Fig. 8–5). Through these diverse effectors RAS proteins regulate cell-cycle progression, cell survival, and cytoskeletal organization (Reuther and Der, 2000).

Termination of RAS activity occurs through the hydrolysis of GTP, converting it to GDP by action of GTPase-activating

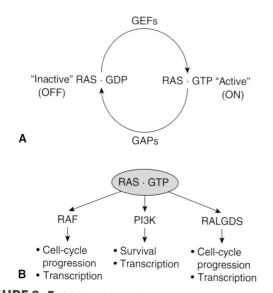

FIGURE 8–5 **RAS protein activation and downstream signaling. A)** The small GTPase RAS cycles between an inactive GDP bound state and the active GTP bound state. RAS activation is regulated by guanine nucleotide exchange factors (GEFs) that promote exchange of GDP for GTP. GTP hydrolysis requires GTPase-activating proteins (GAPs) that enhance the weak intrinsic GTPase activity of RAS proteins. **B)** Once in its active GTP bound form RAS interacts with different families of effector proteins including RAF protein kinases, PI3Ks and RAL GDS, a GEF for the RAS-related protein RAL. Activation of these downstream pathways leads to cellular responses including gene transcription, cell-cycle progression and survival.

proteins (GAPs) that promote the intrinsic GTPase activity of the RAS proteins themselves. Therefore, a balance to the activities of GEFs and GAPs determines the activity of normal RAS proteins. Both the GEFs and a number of the GAP family members, which are often represented by p120^{GAP}, are themselves regulated by receptor tyrosine kinase signaling cascades (Wittinghofer, 1998).

The normal function of RAS proteins requires posttranslational modification. Newly synthesized RAS proteins are modified by the addition of a lipid chain to a cysteine residue in the carboxy terminus of RAS proteins. This covalently linked lipid is either a farnesyl or geranylgeranyl group (collectively termed *prenylation*) and is required for RAS association with intracellular membranes. It is important for the oncogenic activity of RAS proteins. Both H-RAS and N-RAS are also subsequently modified by the addition of 2 palmitoyl long-chain fatty acids important for the correct localization of these proteins to specific parts of the membrane. RAS proteins are activated and signal from specific microdomains within the plasma membrane, as well as distinct subcellular compartments such as the Golgi and endosomes (Hancock, 2003).

Abnormalities in RAS protein activity have been identified in greater than 30% of human malignancies as a result of either mutations (most commonly in K-RAS) that render it locked in an active GTP-bound state, or activated as a result of deregulated signaling from upstream pathways (see Chap. 7, Sec. 7.5.5). RAS proteins have been targets for anticancer therapeutics. Because prenylation involves the activity of a protein farnesyl transferase

or a geranylgeranyl transferase, inhibitors of these enzymes were developed as potential inhibitors of oncogenic RAS activity (Berndt et al, 2011). Farnesyl transferase inhibitors (FTIs) were demonstrated to be potent killers of tumor cells in culture and in animal models, but results of clinical trials showed no survival advantages for most patients with solid or hematological malignancies. Inhibitors of geranylgeranyl transferase inhibitor (GTI) have shown similarly promising in vitro properties and are being evaluated in clinical trials. The efficacy of FTIs does not depend on the presence of activating RAS mutations and may be linked to the prediction that hundreds of proteins are modified by prenylation. While FTIs and GTIs were developed to inhibit RAS activity, other prenylated proteins, such as Rheb, an activator of TORC1 (described in Sec. 8.2.5), may be important targets of FTI activity in tumors. The effective use of these agents in cancer therapy will require the identification of biomarkers, perhaps the farnesyl transferase substrates themselves, of response to FTIs (Berndt et al, 2011).

8.2.4 Mitogen-Activated Protein Kinase Signaling Pathways

Mitogen-activated protein kinases (MAPKs) control highly conserved signaling pathways that regulate all eukaryotic cells. Mammalian cells contain multiple distinct MAPK pathways that respond to divergent signals including growth factors and environmental stresses such as osmotic stress and ionizing radiation. All MAPK pathways include a core 3-tiered signaling unit, in which MAPKs are activated by the sequential activation of linked serine/threonine kinases (Fig. 8–6). The MAPK pathway is activated by phosphorylation of threonine and tyrosine residues in a T-X-Y (T = threonine, X = any amino acid, Y = tyrosine) motif in the kinase activation loop. This phosphorylation is achieved by a family of dual specificity kinases referred to as MEKs or MKKs (MAPK-kinase). MEK (mitogen-activated protein [MAP]/extracellular signal-related kinase [ERK] kinase) activity is regulated by serine and threonine phosphorylation catalyzed by kinases called MAP3Ks (MAPK-kinase-kinase). A number of distinct families of MAP3Ks are activated by diverse upstream stimuli that link the activation of the MAPK signaling unit to extracellular signals. These structurally related pathways are controlled by stimuli that elicit very distinct physiological consequences (ie, mitogenesis or the stress response). Within each pathway specificity is determined by scaffold molecules that link specific core components. Similarly, although all MAPKs phosphorylate very similar consensus motifs in their target substrates, specificity of protein substrate selection is ensured by docking domains that mediate binding of specific kinases to their substrates (Sharrocks et al, 2000).

Three distinct MAPK pathways have been characterized in mammalian cells: the extracellular signal regulated kinase 1 and 2 (ERK1/2), the c-Jun N-terminal kinase or stress-activated protein kinase (JNK/SAPK), and p38. As described in Section 8.2.3, activation of RAS proteins causes the activation of RAF, a MAP3K upstream of ERK1/2. ERK kinase activation is a final signaling step that is shared amongst several pathways

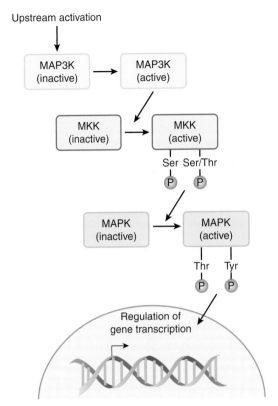

FIGURE 8–6 The MAPK core signaling module. All MAPK pathways include a core 3-tiered signaling unit, in which MAPKs are activated by the sequential activation of linked serine/threonine kinases. The MKKs are unique dual specificity kinases that phosphorylate both tyrosine (Y) and threonine (T) residues within an activation motif found in the MAPKs. P, Phosphate.

and tyrosine residues in the activation loop, which induces catalytic activation of ERK and phosphorylation of both cytoplasmic and nuclear protein substrates that regulate cell migration, proliferation, and differentiation. In the cytoplasm, activated ERK phosphorylates cytoskeletal proteins as well as the RSK family of protein kinases. Activated RSK kinases regulate translation, transcription, and survival signaling through phosphorylation of both nuclear and cytoplasmic substrates (Anjum and Blenis, 2008). Activation of ERK also induces its translocation to the nucleus where it phosphorylates and activates transcription factors (see Sec. 8.2.6), including SP1, ELK-1 and AP-1 (comprised of FOS and JUN) (Fig. 8–6).

Given the broad biological outcomes of MAPK signaling, it is not surprising that dysregulation of these pathways has been implicated in malignant transformation. Increased levels of activated ERKs are frequently found in human tumors, and often are attributable to the presence of mutations in RAS or other upstream components in growth factor signaling cascades. Activating mutations in the RAF family member BRAF, occur in 70% of malignant melanoma and at lower frequency in a wide range of other human tumors (see also Chap. 7, Sec. 7.5.5; Davies et al, 2002). The most common mutation, V600E, is a valine-to-glutamic-acid substitution in the activation loop of the kinase domain that results in constitutive activation. In Phase III clinical trials in metastatic melanoma, the selective BRAF inhibitor vemurafenib has produced tumor regression and improved survival in patients with V600E BRAF mutations (Chapman et al, 2011).

8.2.5 Phosphoinositide Signaling

Phosphoinositides are rare phospholipids of cell membranes that are dynamically regulated in response to growth factor signaling. They contribute to signal propagation by 2 main mechanisms; by serving as precursors of the second messengers diacylglycerol (DAG) and inositol triphosphate (Ins(1,4,5)P3) and Ca^{2+}, or by binding to signaling proteins that contain specific phosphoinositide binding modules. Figure 8–7 illustrates some of the important phospholipid products that function in growth factor signal transduction

stimulated by growth factor receptors, such as those for EGF, PDGF, FGF (see Chap. 7, Sec. 7.5.3), and by more diverse stimuli from cytokine receptors, and antigen receptors (Katz et al, 2007). RAF directly activates MEK-1/2 by phosphorylating it on serine residues, which enhances the availability of the catalytic site to potential substrates. Activated MEK-1/2 is a dual-specificity kinase that phosphorylates the ERK kinases. MEK-induced phosphorylation of ERK occurs on threonine

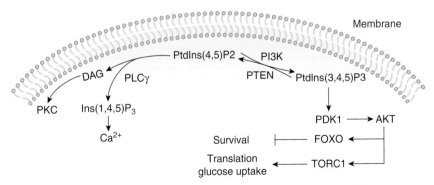

FIGURE 8–7 Phosphoinositide metabolism in growth factor signaling. The positions in the inositol ring that are modified by phosphorylation are numbered. PtdIns(4,5)P2 is hydrolyzed by phospholipase Cγ (PLCγ) to produce second messengers DAG (diacylglycerol) and inositol triphosphate (Ins(1,4,5)P3), that results in activation of Protein Kinase C (PKC) and release of calcium (Ca^{2+}) from intracellular stores. Lipid kinases (PI3K) and phosphatases (PTEN) positively or negatively regulate the phosphorylation of the inositol 3′ position and the production of PtdIns(3,4,5) P3. PtdIns(3,4,5) signals downstream to activate PDK1 and AKT and the activation of metabolic and survival pathways (see text for details).

pathways. Phosphoinositides can be phosphorylated or dephosphorylated by lipid kinases and phosphatases at distinct positions on the inositol ring in response to growth factor signaling. Activation of PI3K (described in Sec. 8.2.2), which specifically phosphorylates the 3′ position, leads to the rapid production of PtdIns(3,4,5)P3. Levels of PtdIns(3,4,5)P3 are tightly controlled by the action of inositol phosphatases. Phosphatase and tensin homolog (PTEN) is a 3′-phosphoinositide phosphatase that dephosphorylates the 3′ position of PtdIns(3,4,5)P3 and PtdIns(3,4)P2, and therefore functions as a major negative regulator of PI3K signaling (see Chap. 7, Sec. 7.6.2).

The production of PtdIns(3,4,5)P3 leads to the recruitment of the PH-domain-containing protein serine/threonine kinases PDK1 and AKT. AKT is activated by conformational changes evoked by phospholipid binding, and phosphorylation by PDK1 at threonine 308. Full activation of AKT requires phosphorylation at a second site (serine 473) by the serine kinase complex TORC2. A number of important substrates for activated AKT have been identified that fall into 2 main classes as regulators of cell survival or regulators of cell proliferation (see Chap. 9, Sec. 9.2.4). Briefly, AKT phosphorylates substrates that, in turn, lead to the activation of TORC1, the serine/threonine kinase mammalian target of rapamycin (mTOR) complex (see below) that regulates cell functions required for growth such as protein translation, glucose uptake, and glycolysis (Zoncu et al, 2011). Activated AKT also controls cell survival through the phosphorylation and nuclear exclusion of the FOXO transcription factors, preventing the expression of genes that can induce cell death (Manning and Cantley, 2007).

Mammalian target of rapamycin (mTOR) is a serine threonine kinase that interacts with additional proteins to form two distinct functional complexes, termed mTOR Complex 1 (TORC1) and 2 (TORC2). TORC1 controls a wide range of cellular processes that promote cell proliferation (see Chap. 9, Sec. 9.2.4) including protein synthesis through the phosphorylation of eukaryotic translation initiation factor binding protein (4E-BP1) and S6 kinase 1 (S6K1) that in turn promote cap-dependent protein translation. TORC1 regulates ATP production and metabolism by promoting the expression of hypoxia-inducible factor 1a (HIF1a) that regulates the expression of glycolytic genes controlling glucose metabolism (see Chap. 12, Sec. 12.2.3). TORC1 also inhibits autophagy (see Chap. 12, Sec. 12.3.6), a process required for cellular catabolism under nutrient starvation, by phosphorylation and inhibition of the activity of autophagy-related gene 13 (ATG13), which forms part of a kinase complex required to initiate autophagy. Much less is known about the functions of TORC2 but its activity also promotes cell growth through activation of protein kinases AKT (described above), serum- and glucocorticoid-induced kinase (SGK1), and protein kinase C-a (PKCa). The SGK1 kinase is activated by TORC2 and regulates ion transport and cell growth. TORC2 can also regulate actin cytoskeleton dynamics through the phosphorylation and activation of PKCa (Laplante and Sabatini, 2012).

Human malignancies are frequently associated with inactivating mutations in the PTEN gene (see Chap. 7, Sec. 7.6.2; Li et al, 1997). Loss of PTEN leads to accumulation of 3′-phosphinositides, causing deregulated AKT activity and malignant transformation (Stambolic et al, 1998). High-throughput sequencing has identified activating mutations in PI3K-CA, the p110 subunit of PI3K in a wide variety of tumors, including 25% to 40% of breast tumors, making it the most commonly mutated gene in breast cancer (Samuels and Waldman, 2010). PI3K-CA inhibitors and AKT inhibitors are being developed and tested in clinical trials, but associated toxicity has been substantial. Inhibition of mTOR (TORC1) has been more successful as a therapeutic strategy. The mTOR inhibitor, rapamycin, was originally developed as an anti-fungal agent and subsequently has been used as an immunosuppressant. Rapamycin analogs temsirolimus and everolimus have been used to treat renal cell carcinoma and other human tumors.

8.2.6 Transcriptional Response to Signaling

One important consequence of growth factor signaling is the transcription of genes that coordinate cell growth, cellular differentiation, cell death, and other biological effects. Transcription of genes is catalyzed by the enzyme RNA polymerase II and regulated by supporting molecules, collectively termed *transcription factors*. Transcription factors can activate or repress gene expression by binding to specific DNA recognition sequences, typically 6 to 8 base pairs in length, found in the promoter regions at the 5′ end of genes. The formation of RNA transcripts is influenced by the interaction of these gene-specific factors with elements of a common core of molecules regulating the activity of RNA polymerase II (Woychik and Hampsey, 2002). The activity of transcription factors can be modified, frequently by phosphorylation, through the activity of many of the signaling pathways described above, including MAPK and the PI3K pathways, which can act in the nucleus to directly modify transcription factor activity (Brivanlou and Darnell, 2002).

Transcription factors are modular, consisting of a specific DNA binding region that binds to specific DNA sequences, as described below, and an activation or repression domain, which interacts with other proteins to stimulate or repress transcription from a nearby promoter. Based on the structure of their DNA-binding domains, transcription factors can be placed into homeodomain (sometimes called *helix-turn-helix*), zinc-finger, or leucine-zipper, and helix-loop-helix (HLH), groupings (Fig. 8–8).

The homeodomain factors contain a 60-amino-acid DNA-binding domain called a *homeobox* that is similar to the helix-turn-helix domain first described in bacterial repressors. The name is derived from the *Drosophila* homeotic genes that determine body structure identity. In vertebrates, homeodomain proteins have similar properties and function as master regulators during development. The homeodomain

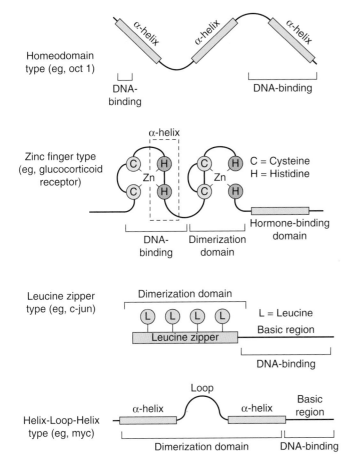

FIGURE 8–8 Transcription factor DNA-binding domain classes. The general structure of the 4 major classes of DNA-binding domains found in modular transcription factors is illustrated.

contains 3 helical regions. The third helical region, as well as amino acids at the aminoterminal end of the homeodomain, directly contact DNA.

Zinc-finger transcription factors contain a sequence of 20 to 30 amino acids with 2 paired cysteine or histidine residues that are coordinated by a zinc ion. Binding of the zinc ion folds these polypeptide sequences into compact domains with α helices that insert into the DNA (see Fig. 8–8). Members of this group of transcription factors mediate differentiation and growth signals, including those caused by binding of steroid hormones to receptors; they have been implicated in malignancy.

Leucine-zipper transcription factors contain helical regions with leucine residues occurring at every seventh amino acid, which all protrude from the same side of the α-helix. These leucines form a hydrophobic interaction surface with leucine zippers of similar proteins. Additional members of this family contain other hydrophobic amino acids in the α-helices that make up the dimerization domain. The DNA binding regions of the α-helices in either case contain basic amino acids that interact with the DNA backbone. These factors, also referred to as *basic zipper proteins*, bind to DNA as homo- or heterodimers, and include the fos/jun pair (called the AP1

transcription factor), which becomes activated by cellular stress. Members of this group also tend to become activated by proliferative and developmental stimuli.

Basic helix-loop-helix factors are similar to the basic zipper factors described above, but include a loop region that separates the 2 α-helical regions of the polypeptide. The carboxyterminal α-helix mediates formation of homo- or heterodimers that contact DNA with basic amino acids found in the aminoterminal helix.

Activation and repression domains are structurally diverse regions, ranging from the random coil conformation of acidic activation domains to the highly structured ligand-binding domains of hormone receptors. Both transcription activators and repressors exert their effects by binding to multisubunit coactivators or corepressors that act to modify chromatin structure and assembly of RNA Pol II complexes. Enzymes that regulate histone acetylation and phosphorylation are key components of transcriptional activator and repressor complexes. Histone acetylation near the promoter regions of genes facilitates the interaction of the DNA with transcription factors while deacetylation results in condensed chromatin structures that inhibit assembly of the transcription machinery at the promoter (Berger, 2007).

Alteration in transcription factor function, which can cause unregulated activation and expression of genes, or lead to inappropriate repression of others, can lead to transformation and is well documented in human cancers. Although we understand how mutation or overexpression of transcription factors such as MYC and TP53 alters their activity, we do not yet fully understand how these changes influence the gene expression or repression patterns that bring about the oncogenic state.

8.2.7 Biological Outcomes of Growth Factor Signaling

Growth factor signaling results in changes in gene expression of large numbers of genes that program the physiological responses such as cell-cycle progression, cellular differentiation, cell growth, survival, or apoptosis. Changes in gene expression downstream of growth factor signaling proceeds in 2 stages. Expression of immediate early genes, which often encode transcription factors, does not require new protein synthesis. Immediate early gene expression is followed by expression of other genes, sometimes called *delayed response genes*, which are often the products of the transcription induced by the immediate early genes (Hill and Treisman, 1999).

Cells in the G_1 phase of the cell cycle respond to external stimuli by either withdrawing from the cell cycle (Go) or advancing through the restriction point (see Chap. 9, Sec. 9.2.1) toward cell division. Progression through G_1 and entry into S phase normally requires stimulation by mitogens, such as growth factors. For example the D-type cyclins are expressed as part of the delayed early response to stimulation of growth factor signaling cascades. These D-type cyclins assemble with cyclin-dependent kinases, and the active complex phosphorylates and inactivates the retinoblastoma (Rb) protein, releasing the E2F transcription factor family that in turn activate the transcription of genes required for S-phase entry (see Chap. 9, Sec. 9.2.3). A common property of cancer cells is their ability to undergo G_1 phase progression in the absence of external mitogenic stimuli. Activating mutations in any of the growth factor signaling components upstream of G_1 checkpoint control can lead to cyclin D accumulation, which drives continuous cell cycling (Evan and Vousden, 2001; Sherr, 1996).

A second important consequence of growth factor signaling is cell survival. Normal cells require continuous exposure to survival factors, such as soluble growth factors, or cell matrix interactions, to suppress apoptosis. Tissue homeostasis is maintained through the limited supply or spatial restriction of these factors that limit cell expansion. Evasion of this control mechanism is another common feature of tumor cells. Activating mutations in survival pathways, such as activating mutations in the PI3K pathway or loss of function mutations in PTEN, can confer resistance to apoptotic signals that would normally limit deregulated cell proliferation (Evan and Vousden, 2001).

8.2.8 Suppression of Growth Factor Signaling

Signaling from activated growth factor receptors is tightly regulated both temporally and spatially. Many proteins that antagonize receptor tyrosine kinase signaling are also recruited to active receptor complexes through interactions with SH2, PTB, or TKB domains. For example, the opposing action of protein tyrosine phosphatases can eliminate docking sites for proteins containing SH2 domains or inhibit tyrosine kinase activity by dephosphorylation of regulatory phosphorylation sites in the kinase activation loop (Chernoff, 1999; Tiganis, 2002). Similarly the action of lipid phosphatases such as PTEN (described in Sec. 8.2.5) function to antagonize PI3K-AKT signaling.

Modification of proteins with ubiquitin is an important mechanism for signal termination. Ubiquitination describes the covalent attachment of 1 or more 76-amino-acid ubiquitin molecules to a target protein. Ubiquitin modification involves a multistep process in which free ubiquitin is first attached to an ubiquitin-activating enzyme (E1) and subsequently transferred to an ubiquitin-conjugating enzyme (E2), which, in partner with an ubiquitin ligase (E3), transfers ubiquitin to the specific protein substrate (Hershko and Ciechanover, 1998; Fig. 8–9). The specificity of this process is determined by the E3 ligase that selectively binds substrates (Deshaies and Joazeiro, 2009; Rotin and Kumar, 2009). The consequences of protein modification by ubiquitin can include degradation by the 26S proteasome, which is a mechanism for eliminating activated enzymes in the cytosolic compartment (see Chap. 9, Sec. 9.2.2). Ubiquitination of transmembrane proteins such as activated RPTKs is followed by their endocytosis and transfer of activated receptors to the lysosome where they are degraded. This mechanism allows

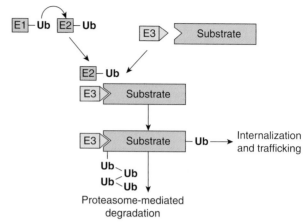

FIGURE 8–9 Ubiquitination pathway. Protein ubiquitination is a multistep process in which free ubiquitin is first attached to an ubiquitin-activating enzyme (E1) and subsequently transferred to an ubiquitin-conjugating enzyme (E2), which, in partner with an ubiquitin ligase (E3), transfers ubiquitin to the specific protein substrate. The E3 ligase provides specificity to the system by functioning as an adaptor to selectively bind substrates. Polyubiquitinated substrates are targeted for degradation by the proteasome while monoubiquitination of a substrate can serve as a signal for receptor internalization and trafficking to multivesicular bodies and the lysosome.

signal termination and return to a basal state after receiving and responding to growth factor signals.

Failure of ubiquitination of RPTKs can result in prolonged activation and oncogenic signaling (Lu and Hunter, 2009). First identified as a transforming viral oncogene, c-CBL is an E3 ligase recruited to activated RPTKs through its phosphotyrosine binding TKB domain that promotes receptor ubiquitination. Mutant forms of c-CBL that lack ubiquitin ligase activity have been identified in myeloid malignancies and lung cancer (Kales et al, 2010; Tan et al, 2010). Although the mechanisms that drive oncogenic transformation by c-CBL are not fully understood, expression of c-CBL proteins that are devoid of E3 ligase activity promotes signaling downstream of activated tyrosine kinases (Kales et al, 2010).

8.3 CYTOPLASMIC TYROSINE KINASE SIGNALING

Tyrosine kinases (TKs) also play a central role in the transmission of signals from distinct classes of cell-surface receptors that themselves do not possess intrinsic TK activity. Cytoplasmic TKs are recruited to cell-surface molecules following receptor activation, and many of the intracellular events that occur resemble those evoked by receptor TKs as described in Section 8.2. Figure 8–10 is a schematic showing selected cytoplasmic TKs. A common feature of these cytoplasmic TKs is the presence of conserved protein modules, such as SH2 and SH3 domains. These protein modules function to regulate kinase activity and also serve to couple these molecules to

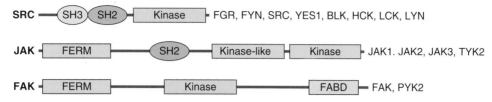

FIGURE 8-10 Cytoplasmic protein TKs. The general structure of several cytoplasmic protein TK families is illustrated. Members of each family are listed beside each diagram.

extracellular receptors. Some of the features of receptor signaling pathways that utilize cytoplasmic TKs are described below.

8.3.1 Cytokine Signaling

Cytokines regulate the proliferation, differentiation and activity of hematopoietic cell lineages through interaction with structurally and functionally related receptors of the cytokine receptor superfamily. These receptors do not contain intrinsic TK activity, but rather transmit intracellular signals through the association with the Janus kinase (JAK) family of kinases. With the exception of the receptors for granulocyte colony-stimulating factor (G-CSF) and erythropoietin (see Chap. 12, Sec. 12.1.3.1), most cytokine receptors are multisubunit complexes and contain a unique ligand binding subunit and a common or shared signaling subunit. There are 4 distinct signaling chains: the gp130 subunit (interleukin [IL]-6Rβc, where "c" denotes the chain, is common to other cytokine receptors), and the IL-3Rβc, IL-2Rβc, and IL-2Rγc chains that can transmit signals from many different ligands.

Similar to RPTK signaling, cytokine binding leads to initiation of downstream signaling events (Fig. 8–11). As the cytoplasmic domains of the common receptor subunits do not possess intrinsic TK activity, noncovalent association with the JAK family of cytoplasmic TKs is required for signal transmission (Ihle, 1995; O'Shea et al, 2002). The JAKs contain a F for 4.1 protein, E for ezrin, R for radixin and M for moesin (FERM) domain, an SH2 domain, a functional TK domain, and a kinase-like domain (or pseudokinase domain) that can exert autoinhibitory activity on the kinase domain (see Fig. 8–10). The FERM domain functions to both regulate JAK kinase activity and mediate association with receptors, while the function of the JAK SH2 domain is unclear as it does not appear to bind to tyrosine phosphorylated proteins. Upon cytokine binding, JAKs are tyrosine phosphorylated and activated, leading to phosphorylation of specific tyrosine residues on the receptor. This activated complex generates docking sites for SH2-domain containing proteins such as the STAT (signal transducers and activators of transcription) family of transcription factors (Fig. 8–11) as well as GRB2 and PI3K (described in Sec. 8.2.3). STATs are then tyrosine phosphorylated, inducing homo- or heterodimerization and subsequent transport to the nucleus where they regulate gene expression. STATs contain a conserved aminoterminal DNA binding domain that is specific to the STAT family of proteins, a conserved SH2 domain, and a carboxyterminal tyrosine residue that mediates dimerization.

In addition to tyrosine phosphorylation, STATs can be phosphorylated by serine/threonine kinases such as ERK and mTOR (see Sec. 8.2.5), and serine phosphorylation of STAT regulates its ability to activate transcription (Jatiani et al, 2010).

Both gene translocations and activating point mutations in JAK2 have been identified in myeloproliferative disorders

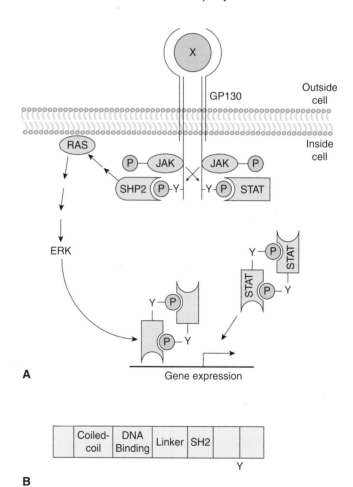

FIGURE 8–11 Cytokine receptor signaling. A) Cytokine (X) binding induces receptor dimerization resulting in JAK activation and phosphorylation of the GBP130 receptor subunit. STATs then bind the phosphorylated receptor, and are subsequently phosphorylated, inducing dimerization and transport to the nucleus where they activate downstream target genes. GBP130 phosphorylation also results in recruitment of tyrosine phosphatase SHP2, which in turn leads to RAS activation. **B)** Structure of the STATs. STATs contain a DNA binding domain, an SH2 domain, and a conserved tyrosine residue in the carboxy terminus.

and leukemia. A common feature of the translocations is a protein product that fuses the kinase domain of JAK2 with a dimerization or oligomerization domain of the fusion partner leading to constitutive kinase activation (Jatiani et al, 2010). JAK2 point mutations, such as V617F, which causes substitution of valine at amino acid 617 for phenylalanine, are found frequently in myeloproliferative diseases. Valine 617 is within the pseudokinase domain and the V617F mutation is thought to disrupt the autoinhibitory interaction between the pseudokinase and catalytic kinase domains. Several JAK2 kinase inhibitors have been developed and assessed in clinical trials. For example, ruxolitinib is a JAK2 kinase inhibitor that has shown efficacy in reducing disease burden and improving quality of life through reduction of disease-related symptoms. However, JAK2 inhibitors do not improve bone marrow pathology or reduce the number of cells with the JAK2 mutant allele or cause disease remission. As with many other targeted agents, combination therapy may be required to achieve disease remission (Jatiani et al, 2010).

8.3.2 Integrin Signaling

Mammalian cells express cell adhesion molecules that mediate their attachment to the extracellular matrix (ECM) and/or their interaction with the same or different cell types (see Chap. 10, Sec. 10.2). Most adhesion molecules are transmembrane proteins, but some are anchored in the plasma membrane by an C-terminal glycophosphatidyl-inositol moiety. Interactions between cells and the ECM are essential for cell survival and cell proliferation, and can regulate differentiation. Loss of interactions between the cell and ECM results in induction of apoptosis in both epithelial and endothelial cells. However, a common property of malignant cells is that they continue to survive and proliferate in the absence of interactions with the ECM.

Integrins are transmembrane cell-surface receptors expressed in all cell types that serve as the primary physical link between the ECM and actin cytoskeleton, and they enable direct communication across the plasma membrane. Integrins recognize and bind to specific ECM ligands (such as collagen, laminin, and fibronectin) and transduce signals leading to the activation of intracellular signaling pathways that regulate cell migration, cell polarity, cell proliferation and survival. Integrins are comprised of membrane spanning α and β subunits that associate noncovalently to form a heterodimer on the cell surface. Receptor diversity and versatility in ligand binding is determined by the extracellular domains, and through the specific pairing of 9 β subunits and 16 α subunits (see Chap. 10, Fig. 10–3). The cytoplasmic domains of both α- and β-integrin subunits are conserved among vertebrate species and *Drosophila*, and serve as a binding platform for both actin cytoskeleton binding proteins, such as α-actinin, paxillin, tensin and talin, and intracellular signaling components, such as cytoplasmic TKs, Focal Adhesion KInase (FAK) and SRC families (Fig. 8–10) (Harburger and Calderwood, 2009).

The binding of integrins to ECM ligands induces integrin clustering and subsequent recruitment of actin filaments and signaling proteins to the integrin cytoplasmic domain (see Chap. 10, Fig. 10–3). These large transmembrane adhesion complexes composed of the ECM and intracellular signaling components are called focal adhesions (FAs). The dynamic formation and remodeling of FAs assures cell adhesion to the ECM in addition to the targeted localization of actin filaments and signaling components necessary for the establishment of cell polarity, directed cell migration, and maintenance of cell proliferation and survival (Scales and Parsons, 2011). In addition to providing a physical link between the ECM and the cytoskeleton, binding of integrins to their ligands elicits a variety of intracellular signaling events (Hynes, 2002; Liu et al, 2000; Martin et al, 2002). For example, integrin signaling regulates the formation of filopodia, lamellipodia, and stress fibers through the RHO family of small GTPases CDC42, RAC, and RHO. It can also stimulate tyrosine phosphorylation and subsequent activation of cellular proteins, including the FAK and SRC cytoplasmic TKs that regulate remodeling of FAs (Fig. 8–10). Furthermore, activation of the RAS family of GTPases by integrins is important for activation of serine-threonine kinases, such as ERK, PAK, and JNK, that regulate gene expression and cell-cycle progression (Scales and Parsons, 2011).

Both up- and downregulation of integrins have been observed in tumor progression, and changes observed in integrin expression appear to be tumor- and integrin-specific (Desgrosellier and Cheresh, 2010). Loss of integrin $\alpha_2\beta_1$ is observed in some tumors while other integrins such as $\alpha_v\beta_3$, $\alpha_v\beta_6$, and $\alpha_5\beta_1$ are upregulated in epithelial tumors and associated with disease progression, metastasis, and/or tumor-induced migration of vascular endothelial cells (see Chap. 10, Sec. 10.2.3). Monoclonal antibodies and RGD peptides that block integrin ligand binding or function have been investigated as potential cancer therapeutics, and promising preclinical studies have led to a Phase III trial of the integrin-blocking peptide cilengitide in glioblastoma (Desgrosellier and Cheresh, 2010).

8.4 DEVELOPMENTAL SIGNALING PATHWAYS

Although cell–cell signaling is a fundamental aspect of early development, only a few signaling pathways are required to generate the functional and morphological diversity of cell types and patterns found in most animals. These signaling networks include WNT, Hedgehog, transforming growth factor-β (TGF-β), Notch, JAK/STAT, and nuclear hormone pathways. Depending on the cellular context, these pathways activate specific target genes and produce a spectrum of cellular signals, resulting in effects on cellular physiology and embryonic development. Predictably, abnormal activation of these crucial pathways is observed in disease states such as cancer, and understanding these pathways is central to our knowledge of cancer etiology and to the development of targeted therapy.

8.4.1 WNT Signaling

The WNT proteins are signaling molecules necessary for development of a multicellular organism. They constitute a large family of secreted glycoproteins with 19 known human members that are highly conserved throughout evolution WNT proteins bind to the Frizzled (FZ) family of transmembrane receptors of which 10 members have been identified (Fig. 8–12) Together with their coreceptors, low-density lipoprotein receptor-related proteins LRP5 and LRP6, ligand-bound FZ receptors initiate signaling to downstream intracellular targets. The affinity of FZ receptors for specific ligands determines the activation of 3 alternate intracellular pathways: (a) the canonical (ie. major) WNT pathway, which leads to regulation of gene expression through β-catenin; (b) the WNT/planar cell polarity pathway, which activates cytoskeleton reorganization through RHO and JNK; and (c) the WNT/Ca²⁺ pathway, which involves the activation of phospholipase C and protein kinase C (Gao and Chen, 2010).

The key mediator of canonical WNT signaling is β-catenin (Akiyama, 2000; Moon et al, 2002). In the absence of WNT, β-catenin is degraded through a series of phosphorylation and ubiquitination steps mediated by the "destruction complex" of proteins (Fig. 8-9; Kimelman and Xu, 2006). In the absence of β-catenin, T-cell factor (TCF) together with corepressors such as histone deacetylase (HDAC) and Groucho/transducin-like-enhancer of split (TLE) repress the transcription of WNT target genes. Upon WNT activation, the destruction complex is

inactivated, allowing β-catenin accumulation and entry into the nucleus where it interacts with the lymphoid enhanced transcription factor (LEF) and the TCF family of transcription factors to regulate transcription of specific target genes. These transcription factors bind directly to DNA but are incapable of activating gene transcription independently of β-catenin. Known target genes include *c-myc*, *cyclin D1*, and *metalloproteinase 7*.

Constitutive activation of the canonical WNT pathway has been observed in many cancers including colorectal carcinoma (CRC). Adenomatous polyposis coli (APC) is a tumor suppressor that forms part of the destruction complex and is encoded by the gene responsible for the onset of familial adenomatous polyposis (FAP), an autosomal dominant, inherited disease that predisposes patients to multiple colorectal polyps and cancers. In this disease, mutations in the APC gene result in ineffective β-catenin degradation and constitutive activation of β-catenin/TCF target genes. Consistent with this inability, in 50% of cases of sporadic CRC, mutations that protect β-catenin from degradation have been observed (Morin et al, 1997). Activating mutations in β-catenin or in other components of the canonical WNT pathway are also observed in a wide variety of human malignancies including carcinoma of the lung, breast, cervix, stomach, pancreas, ovary, prostate, hepatocellular carcinoma (HCC), and medulloblastoma (Polakis, 2007).

Targeting the WNT pathway for cancer therapy has proven successful under experimental conditions. Small molecule

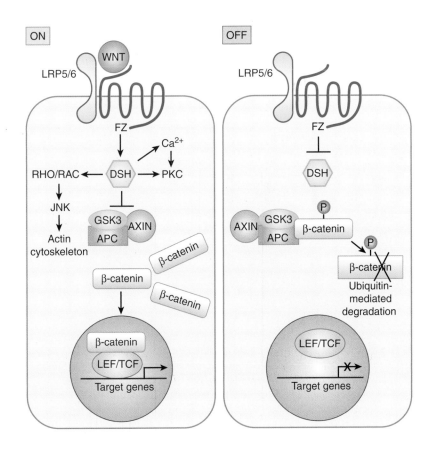

FIGURE 8–12 WNT signaling. *ON:* In the canonical WNT signaling pathway, WNT binding to Frizzled (FZ) LRP5/6 complex on the target cell results in recruitment of Dishevelled (DSH) to FZ. This interaction results in inactivation of the kinase glycogen synthase kinase 3 (GSK3), thereby stabilizing β-catenin. β-Catenin accumulates in the cytoplasm and shuttles to the nucleus where it functions as a cotranscriptional activator with LEF/TFC to regulate transcription of target genes. *OFF:* In the absence of WNT, β-catenin is phosphorylated and exists within a destruction complex (together with APC, GSK3, and AXIN) and is targeted for ubiquitin-dependent proteasomal degradation. The noncanonical WNT pathways include WNT/Ca²⁺ and WNT/Planar cell polarity pathways (see text).

antagonists of TCF/β-catenin interaction inhibit proliferation of CRC, HCC, and multiple myeloma cells (Lepourcelet et al, 2004; Sukhdeo et al, 2007; Wei et al, 2010). Furthermore, inhibition of the WNT target gene product COX-2 with nonsteroidal anti-inflammatory drug treatment of patients with FAP or a human FAP mouse model significantly reduces the number of intestinal polyps (Oshima et al, 1996; Steinbach et al, 2000).

Compounds that target the noncanonical WNT/Planar cell polarity or WNT/Ca²⁺ pathways are under development. Small molecule-mediated inhibition of RAC, a downstream effector of the WNT/PCP pathway, can suppress the growth and invasion of prostate cancer cells and leukemia cells under experimental conditions (Gao et al, 2004; Wei et al, 2008). Inhibition of PKC (protein kinase C), a WNT/Ca²⁺ pathway effector has demonstrated limited success in a number of malignancies including melanoma, non-Hodgkin lymphoma, and ovarian cancer (Swannie and Kaye, 2002). FOXY-5, an agonist of the noncanonical WNT tumor suppressor, WNT5a, can eradicate breast cancer in a mouse model (Safholm et al, 2008). In summary, both canonical and noncanonical WNT signaling pathways are potential targets for cancer therapy, but no specific modulator of WNT signaling has yet progressed into clinical trials.

8.4.2 Notch Signaling

The Notch signaling cascade is highly conserved and plays a crucial role in stem cell self-renewal (see Chap. 13, Sec. 13.4.1), cell fate determination, epithelial cell polarity/adhesion, cell division, and apoptosis (see Chap. 9, Sec. 9.4.2) in organisms from nematodes to vertebrates. Notch is a ligand-activated cell-surface receptor initially identified in *Drosophila*, and subsequently identified in *Caenorhabditis elegans* and vertebrates. Mammals possess 4 Notch proteins (NOTCH1-4) that function as receptors for 5 Notch ligands (DELTA-LIKE1, -3, -4 and JAGGED1, -2) (Fig. 8–13). Glycosylation by Fringe glycosyltransferases (LUNATIC, MANIC and RADICAL FRINGE) modifies the specificity of ligand-receptor interactions (Callahan and Egan, 2004). The Notch receptor is a large, single-pass, transmembrane protein that contains a number of conserved protein–protein interaction motifs within its 3 domains (Fig. 8–13). The large extracellular domain contains a number of EGF-like repeats involved in ligand binding, and 3 cysteine-rich Lin12/Notch repeat (LNR) regions thought to play an inhibitory role in receptor activation. This region is followed by a single transmembrane domain, and an intracellular domain composed of a RAM23 site that interacts with proteins from the CSL (CBF1/SU[H]/LAG1) family of transcription factors, 6 tandem ankyrin repeats involved in mediating protein–protein interactions with regulators of the receptor, and a proline, glutamine, serine, and threonine-rich (PEST) sequence associated with high rates of protein turnover.

Notch signaling involves complex cleavage events that occur during receptor maturation and transmission of the Notch signal. During its maturation, NOTCH is first processed into 2 distinct fragments that interact to form a heterodimer on the cell surface (see Fig. 8–13B). In this heterodimeric form, NOTCH is able to bind transmembrane ligands presented

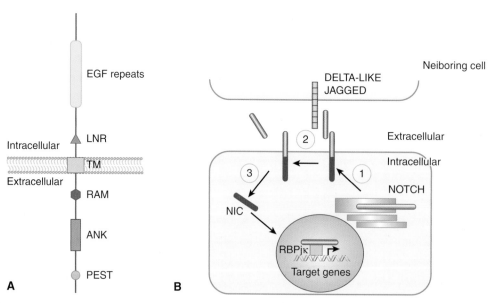

FIGURE 8–13 Notch receptor signaling. A) Schematic of the NOTCH receptor. EGF, Epidermal growth factor-like repeats; LNR, Lin12/Notch repeat region; TM, transmembrane domain; RAM, RAM23 domain; ANK, ankyrin repeats; PEST, proline, glutamate, serine, threonine-rich region. **B)** Model of Notch pathway. (1) NOTCH is first processed in the trans-Golgi network into a heterodimer which is found on the cell surface. (2) Ligand (DELTA-LIKE, JAGGED) presented on neighboring cells causes a second cleavage event that releases the extracellular domain of NOTCH. (3) This triggers a final cleavage event mediated by the γ-secretase complex, releasing the active intracellular domain of NOTCH (NIC). NIC translocates to the nucleus where it functions as a cotransactivator with the CSL family of transcription factors (such as RBPjκ) to regulate target genes.

on neighboring cells. Notch ligand-receptor interaction leads to 2 activating proteolytic cleavages of the receptor. The first cleavage event, mediated by metalloproteases of the ADAM (a disintegrin and metalloproteinase) family, releases the Notch extracellular domain. The second cleavage, executed by a presenilin-protease (γ-secretase) complex, releases the cytoplasmic domain fragment of intracellular NOTCH (NIC) from the plasma membrane (Iwatsubo, 2004; Xia and Wolfe, 2003). NIC enters the nucleus and modulates the expression of target genes predominantly by converting the CSL repressor to an activator of transcription (Honjo, 1996). Downstream targets of CBF-1 include members of the HES and HEY families, which encode basic helix-loop-helix transcriptional regulatory proteins (see Sec. 8.2.6; Iso et al, 2003).

Notch activation has been strongly linked to human cancers, most notably T-cell acute lymphoblastic leukemia (T-ALL). Here, a recurrent t(7;9)(q34;q34.3) chromosomal translocation, resulting in a dominantly active NOTCH1 receptor, was identified in a small subset of tumors (Ellisen et al, 1991). Weng et al (2004) discovered that more than 50% of T-ALLs harbored gain-of-function mutations within the NOTCH1 receptor.

Aberrant Notch signaling can also contribute to the development of solid malignancies such as breast cancer. The *Notch4* locus was identified as a common proviral integration site in MMTV-induced mammary adenocarcinomas in mice, leading to overexpression of NIC protein (Gallahan and Callahan, 1987). In human breast cancer, high-level expression of JAGGED1 and/or NOTCH1 correlates with and is an independent prognostic indicator of poor outcome (Reedijk et al, 2005). Activated Notch signaling and upregulation of genes that are required for tumor growth have been observed in breast cancer cell lines (Stylianou et al, 2006). Notch affects multiple cellular processes and aberrant Notch activity influences breast cancer progression through the maintenance of tumor-initiating cells and by promoting proliferation, motility, and survival of cancer cells. Aberrant Notch signaling has also been identified in several other solid malignancies, including prostate cancers and head and neck squamous cell carcinomas. Thus, aberrant Notch signaling contributes to the progression of a wide spectrum of human cancers.

Notch ligands or receptors may be inhibited by monoclonal antibodies, RNA interference, soluble ligands, or receptor decoys. Inhibition of enzymes involved in glycosylation or cleavage of receptors, such as γ-secretase inhibitors (GSIs) or ADAM inhibitors are also potential approaches to target Notch therapeutically. Among Notch pathway inhibitors, GSIs have the most immediate therapeutic potential. Potent GSIs have been available for over a decade and were developed originally to inhibit the γ-secretase complex that plays a role in plaque formation in Alzheimer disease. The discovery of γ-secretase-dependent NOTCH1 mutations in T-ALL accelerated the use of GSIs in preclinical studies, where induction of apoptosis and reduced cell proliferation was demonstrated in several human cancer models, including Notch-activated breast cancer cells cultured as a monolayer

(O'Neill et al, 2007) or as tumor spheres (Farnie et al, 2007). GSI treatment also blocks Notch signaling and growth of human breast cancer xenografts (Rizzo et al, 2008) and tumors in a HER-2 transgenic breast cancer mouse model (Watters et al, 2009). Several Phase I and II clinical trials with GSIs are underway.

8.4.3 Hedgehog Signaling

Hedgehog (HH) proteins act as key mediators of fundamental processes in embryonic development, and serve broad roles in the proliferation, migration, and differentiation of target cells, and in the maintenance of stem cell populations (Merchant and Matsui, 2010). HH signaling is essential to the growth, patterning, and morphogenesis of many different tissues and organs including the skin, brain, gut, lung, and bone, and HH proteins play a role in hematopoiesis (Cohen, 2003; Ingham and McMahon, 2001; Nybakken and Perrimon, 2002). The HH signaling pathway is highly conserved throughout evolution, and much of what is known about signaling in vertebrates has been inferred from studies in *Drosophila*. In humans there are 3 homologs of the *Drosophila Hh* gene; sonic hedgehog (*Shh*), desert hedgehog (*Dhh*), and Indian hedgehog (*Ihh*). The *Hh* gene products encode ligands that signal through a membrane–receptor complex including the Patched (PTC1 and PTC2) and Smoothened (SMO) receptors, which together form a molecular switch controlling activation of downstream target genes (Fig. 8–14). In the absence of ligand, PTC inhibits

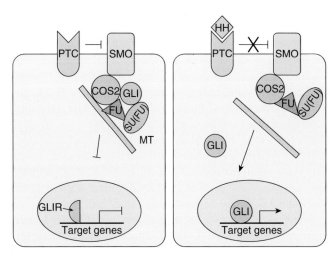

FIGURE 8–14 Hedgehog signaling. In the absence of HH, PTC silences SMO, the key signal transducer of the HH pathway. Binding of HH to PTC prevents SMO inhibition and results in nuclear translocation of activated Gli. Release of SMO inhibition results in nuclear translocation of activated GLI transcription factors and HH target gene expression. GLI is found in a complex with Fused (FU), Costal2 (COS2), and Suppressor of Fused (SU[FU]) bound to microtubules (MT). Upon activation of SMO this complex is disassembled, releasing GLI and allowing nuclear translocation and upregulation of downstream target genes. Target genes include WNT, bone morphogenetic protein (BMP), and Ptc itself.

SMO accumulation and activation (Rohatgi et al, 2007). The interaction between HH and PTC releases SMO (Corbit et al, 2005; Rohatgi et al, 2007). Activated SMO allows expression and/or proteolytic processing of 3 zinc-finger transcription factors (see Sec. 8.2.6; GLI1, -2, and -3) and ultimate transcription of HH target genes through direct interaction with the consensus binding sequence of bases in DNA 5′-tgggtggta-3′. Several regulators of HH signaling have been identified, including molecules that modify the ligand, such as Hedgehog interacting protein (HIP) and Hedgehog acyltransferase (HHAT), and proteins that function downstream of SMO, including the serine/threonine protein kinase Fused (FU) and the Suppressor of Fused (SU[FU]) (reviewed in Merchant and Matsui, 2010).

Given its critical role in development, disturbances in HH signaling can result in disease states. Inactivation of the HH signaling pathway during development results in an abnormality in which the embryonic forebrain fails to develop into 2 hemispheres, whereas abnormal activation of this pathway has been implicated in the development of malignancy. HH pathway activation in cancer may occur through different mechanisms, including activating mutations within components of the signaling pathway. For example, *Ptc1* loss-of-function or *Smo* gain-of-function mutations have been observed in sporadic basal cell carcinoma (BCC) and medulloblastoma (reviewed in Pasca di Magliano and Hebrok, 2003). Consistent with these observations, Gorlin (basal cell nevus) syndrome, which results from *Ptc1* mutation, leads to a predisposition to BCC, medulloblastoma, and rhabdomyosarcoma (Hahn et al, 1996; Johnson et al, 1996). These findings have been recapitulated in mouse models of SMO activation or PTC inactivation, where animals frequently develop BCC or medulloblastoma (Pasca di Magliano and Hebrok, 2003). Gli activation can also result in malignancy. This propensity may occur as a result of *K-ras* activating mutations that increase GLI transcriptional activity or through mutations within the *Gli* genes themselves; both mechanisms of HH activation have been observed in carcinoma of the pancreas (Ji et al, 2007; Jones et al, 2008). Mutations in *Su(Fu)*, have been identified in patients with medulloblastomas (Taylor et al, 2002). HH signaling in malignancy can also be induced by pathways that are commonly activated in human cancer, such as PI3K/AKT and MEK (see Sec. 8.2.4; Stecca et al, 2007).

Aberrant HH activation may also occur through ligand-mediated mechanisms in either autocrine or paracrine settings (reviewed in Merchant and Matsui, 2010). In multiple malignancies, including small cell lung cancer (SCLC), pancreatic adenocarcinoma, colon cancer, prostate cancer, glioblastoma, and malignant melanoma, tumor cells have been shown to synthesize HH ligand to which they also respond. In B-cell lymphoma and multiple myeloma, stromal production of HH ligand in the spleen, lymph nodes, and bone marrow supports the growth of tumor cells. Conversely, tumor production of HH ligand can stimulate HH signaling in stromal cells of the tumor microenvironment, resulting in the expression of HH target genes in those cells to increase the stromal content of tumors. Indeed, inhibition of HH signaling in tumor stroma in a mouse model of pancreatic carcinoma has been reported to improve delivery of cytotoxic chemotherapy (Olive et al, 2009).

A role for HH signaling in the maintenance of tumor initiating cells (TICs; see Chap. 13, Sec. 13.4) has been reported for multiple tumor types, including breast and pancreatic cancer, glioblastoma, multiple myeloma, and chronic myeloid leukemia (Merchant and Matsui, 2010). Analogous to normal tissue stem cells, TICs are defined by their capacity to self-renew and to regenerate tumors containing differentiated progeny identical to the original tumor.

Also suggestive of a putative role in TICs is emerging evidence that implicates HH signaling in tumor invasion and metastases (Feldmann et al, 2007). In primary colon cancer, HH signaling is upregulated in the TIC compartment and is accompanied by elevated expression of Snail, a protein involved in epithelial-to-mesenchymal transition (EMT) and metastasis (Varnat et al, 2009). Growth and metastases of primary colon cancer in a xenograft model requires active HH signaling and induction of EMT.

Numerous HH antagonists are undergoing clinical testing in a wide range of malignancies including BCC. An early encouraging report of the Smo antagonist GDC-0449, demonstrated a 55% clinical response rate, including 2 complete remissions in 33 patients with advanced BCC (Von Hoff et al, 2009). While these results are promising, results from ongoing Phase I and II clinical trials in SCLC, glioblastoma, pancreatic adenocarcinoma, colon cancer, prostate cancer, and other malignancies are pending.

8.4.4 Signal Transduction by the Transforming Growth Factor-β Superfamily

Members of the TGF-β superfamily regulate a number of developmental and homeostatic processes, such as cell proliferation, differentiation, apoptosis, cell adhesion, and migration. They constitute a highly conserved family of proteins with at least 30 vertebrate members and over a dozen structurally and functionally related proteins found in invertebrates, such as *C. elegans* and *Drosophila*. There are 2 general branches of this superfamily, including a TGF-β/activin/nodal branch and a bone morphogenic protein (BMP) branch whose members have diverse, but often complementary, effects. Some members are widely expressed during embryogenesis and in adult tissues, whereas others are expressed in only a few cell types and for restricted periods during development.

TGF-β, the prototypic member of this superfamily is a secreted growth factor synthesized as an inactive precursor and is proteolytically processed into a mature secreted ligand. Upon dimerization, TGF-β becomes biologically active and binds to a cell-surface receptor complex consisting of 2 distinct single-pass transmembrane proteins known as the type I and type II receptors, both of which contain an intracellular serine-threonine kinase domain (Fig. 8–15; Attisano and Wrana,

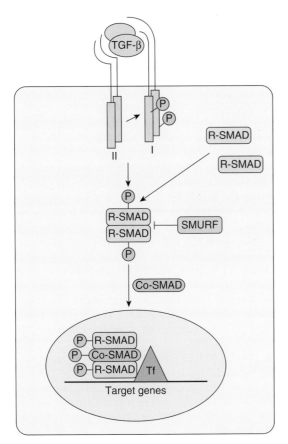

FIGURE 8–15 **TGF-β signaling.** TGF-β ligand binding induces the association of type II and type I receptor heterodimers into a heterotetrameric complex. This results in phosphorylation and subsequent activation of the type I receptor that then phosphorylates a member of the R-SMAD class of proteins (SMADs 1, 2, 3, 5, or 8). Phosphorylated R-SMADs interact with the Co-SMAD, SMAD4, and this complex then accumulates in the nucleus. SMURFs are E3 ubiquitin-protein ligases that orchestrate ubiquitin transfer to the R-SMADs causing their ubiquitination and subsequent proteasomal degradation. In the nucleus, the activated SMAD complex associates with DNA binding cofactors, coactivators and corepressors that regulate transcription of target genes. *Tf*, Transcription factors.

antagonize TGF-β signaling. An additional level of regulation of TGF-β signaling occurs with SMURF1 and SMURF2. These proteins are E3 ubiquitin-protein ligases that regulate SMAD levels. SMURFs orchestrate ubiquitin transfer to the R-SMADs causing their ubiquitination and subsequent proteasomal degradation (see Fig. 8–9).

The biological output of TGF-β signaling appears to be almost entirely determined by the type I receptor. In vertebrates there are 7 distinct type I receptors that interact with 1 of 5 type II receptors. The signal from the type I receptor is funneled through 1 of 2 groups of SMAD proteins. Specific R-SMADs recognize different DNA binding proteins and regulate distinct target genes, thereby generating diverse biological responses. For example, phosphorylation and activation of R-SMADs SMAD2 and SMAD3 transduce a TGF-β–like signal, whereas activation of R-SMADs SMAD1, SMAD5, and SMAD8 transduce signals initiated by bone morphological proteins. There is also evidence that TGF-β can signal through SMAD independent processes through the activation of RHOA, RAS, and TGF-β activated kinase I (Tak1) (Massague et al, 2000).

Mutations in the TGF-β family of ligands are responsible for a variety of human diseases, including human cancer, hereditary chondrodysplasias, and pulmonary hypertension (de Caestecker et al, 2000; Massague et al, 2000). TGF-β signaling plays an important role in cancer progression by functioning as both an antiproliferative factor and as a tumor promoter. For example, in colon cancer, TGF-β can switch from an inhibitor of primary tumor growth to a stimulator of proliferation in metastatic cells (Lampropoulos et al, 2012). Immunohistochemical staining intensity of TGF-β correlates significantly as an independent marker of colon cancer progression to metastases. Mutations in the TGF-β receptors have been identified in several human cancers with a recent meta-analysis demonstrating that the TGF-β type I 6A polymorphic allele (containing a deletion of 3 alanine residues from the N-terminus) is associated with increased cancer risk (Zhang et al, 2005). In addition, mutations in SMAD2 are found in colorectal and lung cancers, and SMAD4 mutations are found in a large number of colorectal, pancreatic, and lung cancers (Lampropoulos et al, 2012). These point mutations in the SMAD proteins lead to loss of phosphorylation of SMAD2, for example, and subsequent loss of association with SMAD4.

Agents that target TGF-β signaling are being developed, including TGF-β neutralizing antibodies, soluble TGF-βR:Fc fusion proteins, antisense oligonucleotides and inhibitors of TGF-β receptors. Some agents have reached clinical trial, including AP-12009, an antisense oligonucleotide targeting TGF-β2 messenger RNA that led to remission in some patients (Hau et al, 2007) and is in Phase III clinical trial for aggressive brain tumors. Because the TGF-β pathway has a dual role as both tumor suppressor and promoter, the clinical delivery of agents that modify TGF-β signaling must be carried out thoughtfully and their impact interpreted carefully.

2002; Dennler et al, 2002; Moustakas et al, 2001). Ligand binding induces association of the type I and type II receptors into a heterotetrameric complex. This association leads to unidirectional phosphorylation and subsequent activation of the kinase domain of the type I receptor by the type II receptor. The activated type I receptor then signals to the SMAD (for Sma and Mad proteins from *C. elegans* and *Drosophila*, respectively) family of intracellular mediators, which function to carry the signal from the cell surface directly to the nucleus. There are 3 distinct classes of SMADs: receptor-regulated or R-SMADs (SMADs 1, 2, 3, 5, and 8), common mediator or Co-SMAD4, and inhibitory SMADs 6 and 7 (Fig. 8–15). The activated type I receptor directly phosphorylates and activates the R-SMADs leading to interaction with Co-SMAD4. The inhibitory SMADs counteract the effects of R-SMADs and

SUMMARY

- A diverse array of extracellular signals activate common core signaling pathways and can, in turn, lead to very different cellular responses; seemingly small changes within individual components of a signaling pathway can have major effects on cellular function.
- Although there have been substantial advances in our knowledge of the molecular details of many signaling pathways, our understanding of how these signals integrate to bring about the phenotypic changes associated with malignancy is still limited.
- Many developments in cancer therapeutics are based upon understanding of growth factor and developmental signaling pathways and the identification of aberrantly activated signaling components.
- With a few exceptions, the development of therapeutic agents to target a single signaling pathway has led to disappointing results. This is not surprising given the redundancy of the pathways, and future strategies must include combinations that target multiple points in an oncogenic signaling network. However, since the pathways are not unique to malignant cells, toxic side effects are likely to be observed from such combined therapy.

REFERENCES

Akiyama T. Wnt/beta-catenin signaling. *Cytokine Growth Factor Rev* 2000;11:273-282.

Anjum R, Blenis J. The RSK family of kinases: emerging roles in cellular signalling. *Nat Rev Mol Cell Biol* 2008;9:747-758.

Antonescu CR. The GIST paradigm: lessons for other kinase-driven cancers. *J Pathol* 2011;223:251-261.

Attisano L, Wrana JL. Signal transduction by the TGF-beta superfamily. *Science* 2002;296:1646-1647.

Berger SL. The complex language of chromatin regulation during transcription. *Nature* 2007;447:407-412.

Berndt N, Hamilton AD, Sebti SM. Targeting protein prenylation for cancer therapy. *Nat Rev Cancer* 2011;11:775-791.

Blaikie P, Immanuel D, Wu J, Li N, Yajnik V, Margolis B. A region in Shc distinct from the SH2 domain can bind tyrosine-phosphorylated growth factor receptors. *J Biol Chem* 1994;269:32031-32034.

Brivanlou AH, Darnell JE Jr. Signal transduction and the control of gene expression. *Science* 2002;295:813-818.

Buday L, Downward J. Many faces of Ras activation. *Biochim Biophys Acta* 2008;1786:178-187.

Callahan R, Egan SE. Notch signaling in mammary development and oncogenesis. *J Mammary Gland Biol Neoplasia* 2004;9:145-163.

Cataldo VD, Gibbons DL, Perez-Soler R, Quintas-Cardama A. Treatment of non-small-cell lung cancer with erlotinib or gefitinib. *N Engl J Med* 2011;364:947-955.

Chapman PB, Hauschild A, Robert C, et al. Improved survival with vemurafenib in melanoma with BRAF V600E mutation. *N Engl J Med* 2011;364:2507-2516.

Chernoff J. Protein tyrosine phosphatases as negative regulators of mitogenic signaling. *J Cell Physiol* 1999;180:173-181.

Cohen MM Jr. The hedgehog signaling network. *Am J Med Genet A* 2003;123A:5-28.

Corbit KC, Aanstad P, Singla V, Norman AR, Stainier DY, Reiter JF. Vertebrate Smoothened functions at the primary cilium. *Nature* 2005;437:1018-1021.

Davies H, Bignell GR, Cox C, et al. Mutations of the BRAF gene in human cancer. *Nature* 2002;417:949-954.

de Caestecker MP, Piek E, Roberts AB. Role of transforming growth factor-beta signaling in cancer. *J Natl Cancer Inst* 2000;92:1388-1402.

Dennler S, Goumans MJ, ten Dijke P. Transforming growth factor beta signal transduction. *J Leukoc Biol* 2002;71:731-740.

Desgrosellier JS, Cheresh DA. Integrins in cancer: biological implications and therapeutic opportunities. *Nat Rev Cancer* 2010;10:9-22.

Deshaies RJ, Joazeiro CA. RING domain E3 ubiquitin ligases. *Annu Rev Biochem* 2009;78:399-434.

Ellisen LW, Bird J, West DC, et al. TAN-1, the human homolog of the Drosophila notch gene, is broken by chromosomal translocations in T lymphoblastic neoplasms. *Cell* 1991;66:649-661.

Engelman JA, Settleman J. Acquired resistance to tyrosine kinase inhibitors during cancer therapy. *Curr Opin Genet Dev* 2008;18:73-79.

Evan GI, Vousden KH. Proliferation, cell cycle and apoptosis in cancer. *Nature* 2001;411:342-348.

Farnie G, Clarke RB, Spence K, et al. Novel cell culture technique for primary ductal carcinoma in situ: role of Notch and epidermal growth factor receptor signaling pathways. *J Natl Cancer Inst* 2007;99:616-627.

Feldmann G, Dhara S, Fendrich V, et al. Blockade of hedgehog signaling inhibits pancreatic cancer invasion and metastases: a new paradigm for combination therapy in solid cancers. *Cancer Res* 2007;67:2187-2196.

Forman-Kay JD, Pawson T. Diversity in protein recognition by PTB domains. *Curr Opin Struct Biol* 1999;9:690-695.

Gallahan D, Callahan R. Mammary tumorigenesis in feral mice: identification of a new int locus in mouse mammary tumor virus (Czech II)-induced mammary tumors. *J Virol* 1987;61:66-74.

Gao C, Chen YG. Dishevelled: the hub of Wnt signaling. *Cell Signal* 2010;22:717-727.

Gao Y, Dickerson JB, Guo F, Zheng J, Zheng Y. Rational design and characterization of a Rac GTPase-specific small molecule inhibitor. *Proc Natl Acad Sci U S A* 2004;101:7618-7623.

Hahn H, Wicking C, Zaphiropoulous PG, et al. Mutations of the human homolog of *Drosophila* patched in the nevoid basal cell carcinoma syndrome. *Cell* 1996;85:841-851.

Hancock JF. Ras proteins: different signals from different locations. *Nat Rev Mol Cell Biol* 2003;4:373-384.

Harburger DS, Calderwood DA. Integrin signalling at a glance. *J Cell Sci* 2009;122:159-163.

Harlan JE, Hajduk PJ, Yoon HS, Fesik SW. Pleckstrin homology domains bind to phosphatidylinositol-4,5-bisphosphate. *Nature* 1994;371:168-170.

Hau P, Jachimczak P, Schlingensiepen R, et al. Inhibition of TGF-beta2 with AP 12009 in recurrent malignant gliomas: from preclinical to phase I/II studies. *Oligonucleotides* 2007;17:201-212.

Hershko A, Ciechanover A. The ubiquitin system. *Annu Rev Biochem* 1998;67:425-479.

Hill CS, Treisman R. Growth factors and gene expression: fresh insights from arrays. *Sci STKE* 1999:PE1.

Honjo T. The shortest path from the surface to the nucleus: RBP-J kappa/Su(H) transcription factor. *Genes Cells* 1996;1:1-9.

Hubbard SR. Juxtamembrane autoinhibition in receptor tyrosine kinases. *Nat Rev Mol Cell Biol* 2004;5:464-471.

Hudis CA. Trastuzumab—mechanism of action and use in clinical practice. *N Engl J Med* 2007;357:39-51.

Hynes RO. Integrins: bidirectional, allosteric signaling machines. *Cell* 2002;110:673-687.

Ihle JN. The Janus protein tyrosine kinase family and its role in cytokine signaling. *Adv Immunol* 1995;60:1-35.

Ingham PW, McMahon AP. Hedgehog signaling in animal development: paradigms and principles. *Genes Dev* 2001;15:3059-3087.

Iso T, Kedes L, Hamamori Y. HES and HERP families: multiple effectors of the Notch signaling pathway. *J Cell Physiol* 2003;194:237-255.

Iwatsubo T. The gamma-secretase complex: machinery for intramembrane proteolysis. *Curr Opin Neurobiol* 2004;14:379-383.

Jatiani SS, Baker SJ, Silverman LR, Reddy EP. Jak/STAT pathways in cytokine signaling and myeloproliferative disorders: approaches for targeted therapies. *Genes Cancer* 2010;1:979-993.

Ji Z, Mei FC, Xie J, Cheng X. Oncogenic KRAS activates hedgehog signaling pathway in pancreatic cancer cells. *J Biol Chem* 2007;282:14048-14055.

Johnson RL, Rothman AL, Xie J, et al. Human homolog of patched, a candidate gene for the basal cell nevus syndrome. *Science* 1996;272:1668-1671.

Jones S, Zhang X, Parsons DW, et al. Core signaling pathways in human pancreatic cancers revealed by global genomic analyses. *Science* 2008;321:1801-1806.

Kales SC, Ryan PE, Nau MM, Lipkowitz S. Cbl and human myeloid neoplasms: the Cbl oncogene comes of age. *Cancer Res* 2010;70:4789-4794.

Katz M, Amit I, Yarden Y. Regulation of MAPKs by growth factors and receptor tyrosine kinases. *Biochim Biophys Acta* 2007;1773:1161-1176.

Kimelman D, Xu W. Beta-catenin destruction complex: insights and questions from a structural perspective. *Oncogene* 2006;25:7482-7491.

Kindler T, Lipka DB, Fischer T. FLT3 as a therapeutic target in AML: still challenging after all these years. *Blood* 2010;116:5089-5102.

Lampropoulos P, Zizi-Sermpetzoglou A, Rizos S, Kostakis A, Nikiteas N, Papavassiliou AG. TGF-beta signalling in colon carcinogenesis. *Cancer Lett* 2012;314:1-7.

Laplante M, Sabatini DM. mTOR signaling in growth control and disease. *Cell* 2012;149:274-293.

Lemmon MA, Schlessinger J. Cell signaling by receptor tyrosine kinases. *Cell* 2010;141:1117-1134.

Lepourcelet M, Chen YN, France DS, et al. Small-molecule antagonists of the oncogenic Tcf/beta-catenin protein complex. *Cancer Cell* 2004;5:91-102.

Li J, Yen C, Liaw D, et al. PTEN, a putative protein tyrosine phosphatase gene mutated in human brain, breast, and prostate cancer. *Science* 1997;275:1943-1947.

Liu S, Calderwood DA, Ginsberg MH. Integrin cytoplasmic domain-binding proteins. *J Cell Sci* 2000;113(Pt 20):3563-3571.

Lu Z, Hunter T. Degradation of activated protein kinases by ubiquitination. *Annu Rev Biochem* 2009;78:435-475.

Lynch TJ, Bell DW, Sordella R, et al. Activating mutations in the epidermal growth factor receptor underlying responsiveness of non-small-cell lung cancer to gefitinib. *N Engl J Med* 2004;350:2129-2139.

Manning BD, Cantley LC. AKT/PKB signaling: navigating downstream. *Cell* 2007;129:1261-1274.

Martin KH, Slack JK, Boerner SA, Martin CC, Parsons JT. Integrin connections map: to infinity and beyond. *Science* 2002;296:1652-1653.

Massague J, Blain SW, Lo RS. TGFbeta signaling in growth control, cancer, and heritable disorders. *Cell* 2000;103:295-309.

Merchant AA, Matsui W. Targeting Hedgehog—a cancer stem cell pathway. *Clin Cancer Res* 2010;16:3130-3140.

Moon RT, Bowerman B, Boutros M, Perrimon N. The promise and perils of Wnt signaling through beta-catenin. *Science* 2002;296:1644-1646.

Morin PJ, Sparks AB, Korinek V, et al. Activation of beta-catenin-Tcf signaling in colon cancer by mutations in beta-catenin or APC. *Science* 1997;275:1787-1790.

Moustakas A, Souchelnytskyi S, Heldin CH. Smad regulation in TGF-beta signal transduction. *J Cell Sci* 2001;114:4359-4369.

Myers MG Jr, Sun XJ, White MF. The IRS-1 signaling system. *Trends Biochem Sci* 1994;19:289-293.

Niu XL, Peters KG, Kontos CD. Deletion of the carboxyl terminus of Tie2 enhances kinase activity, signaling, and function. Evidence for an autoinhibitory mechanism. *J Biol Chem* 2002;277:31768-31773.

Nybakken K, Perrimon N. Hedgehog signal transduction: recent findings. *Curr Opin Genet Dev* 2002;12:503-511.

O'Neill CF, Urs S, Cinelli C, et al. Notch2 signaling induces apoptosis and inhibits human MDA-MB-231 xenograft growth. *Am J Pathol* 2007;171:1023-1036.

O'Shea JJ, Gadina M, Schreiber RD. Cytokine signaling in 2002: new surprises in the Jak/Stat pathway. *Cell* 2002;109 Suppl:S121-S131.

Olive KP, Jacobetz MA, Davidson CJ, et al. Inhibition of Hedgehog signaling enhances delivery of chemotherapy in a mouse model of pancreatic cancer. *Science* 2009;324:1457-1461.

Oshima M, Dinchuk JE, Kargman SL, et al. Suppression of intestinal polyposis in Apc delta716 knockout mice by inhibition of cyclooxygenase 2 (COX-2). *Cell* 1996;87:803-809.

Pasca di Magliano M, Hebrok M. Hedgehog signalling in cancer formation and maintenance. *Nat Rev Cancer* 2003;3:903-911.

Pawson T. Regulation and targets of receptor tyrosine kinases. *Eur J Cancer* 2002;38 Suppl 5:S3-S10.

Pawson T, Nash P. Assembly of cell regulatory systems through protein interaction domains. *Science* 2003;300:445-452.

Polakis P. The many ways of Wnt in cancer. *Curr Opin Genet Dev* 2007;17:45-51.

Reedijk M, Odorcic S, Chang L, et al. High-level coexpression of JAG1 and NOTCH1 is observed in human breast cancer and is associated with poor overall survival. *Cancer Res* 2005;65:8530-8537.

Reuther GW, Der CJ. The Ras branch of small GTPases: Ras family members don't fall far from the tree. *Curr Opin Cell Biol* 2000;12:157-165.

Rizzo P, Miao H, D'Souza G, et al. Cross-talk between notch and the estrogen receptor in breast cancer suggests novel therapeutic approaches. *Cancer Res* 2008;68:5226-5235.

Rohatgi R, Milenkovic L, Scott MP. Patched1 regulates hedgehog signaling at the primary cilium. *Science* 2007;317:372-376.

Rotin D, Kumar S. Physiological functions of the HECT family of ubiquitin ligases. *Nat Rev Mol Cell Biol* 2009;10:398-409.

Safholm A, Tuomela J, Rosenkvist J, Dejmek J, Harkonen P, Andersson T. The Wnt-5a-derived hexapeptide Foxy-5 inhibits breast cancer metastasis in vivo by targeting cell motility. *Clin Cancer Res* 2008;14:6556-6563.

Samuels Y, Waldman T. Oncogenic mutations of PIK3CA in human cancers. *Curr Top Microbiol Immunol* 2010;347:21-41.

Scales TM, Parsons M. Spatial and temporal regulation of integrin signalling during cell migration. *Curr Opin Cell Biol* 2011;23: 562-568.

Schlessinger J. Ligand-induced, receptor-mediated dimerization and activation of EGF receptor. *Cell* 2002;110:669-672.

Schlessinger J, Lemmon MA. SH2 and PTB domains in tyrosine kinase signaling. *Sci STKE* 2003:RE12.

Seet BT, Dikic I, Zhou MM, Pawson T. Reading protein modifications with interaction domains. *Nat Rev Mol Cell Biol* 2006;7:473-483.

Sharrocks AD, Yang SH, Galanis A. Docking domains and substrate-specificity determination for MAP kinases. *Trends Biochem Sci* 2000;25:448-453.

Sherr CJ. Cancer cell cycles. *Science* 1996;274:1672-1677.

Slamon DJ, Clark GM, Wong SG, Levin WJ, Ullrich A, McGuire WL. Human breast cancer: correlation of relapse and survival with amplification of the HER-2/neu oncogene. *Science* 1987; 235:177-182.

Stambolic V, Suzuki A, de la Pompa JL, et al. Negative regulation of PKB/Akt-dependent cell survival by the tumor suppressor PTEN. *Cell* 1998;95:29-39.

Stecca B, Mas C, Clement V, et al. Melanomas require HEDGEHOG-GLI signaling regulated by interactions between GLI1 and the RAS-MEK/AKT pathways. *Proc Natl Acad Sci U S A* 2007;104:5895-5900.

Steinbach G, Lynch PM, Phillips RK, et al. The effect of celecoxib, a cyclooxygenase-2 inhibitor, in familial adenomatous polyposis. *N Engl J Med* 2000;342:1946-1952.

Stylianou S, Clarke RB, Brennan K. Aberrant activation of notch signaling in human breast cancer. *Cancer Res* 2006;66:1517-1525.

Sukhdeo K, Mani M, Zhang Y, et al. Targeting the beta-catenin/TCF transcriptional complex in the treatment of multiple myeloma. *Proc Natl Acad Sci U S A* 2007;104:7516-7521.

Swannie HC, Kaye SB. Protein kinase C inhibitors. *Curr Oncol Rep* 2002;4:37-46.

Tan YH, Krishnaswamy S, Nandi S, et al. CBL is frequently altered in lung cancers: its relationship to mutations in MET and EGFR tyrosine kinases. *PLoS One* 2010;5:e8972.

Taylor MD, Liu L, Raffel C, et al. Mutations in SUFU predispose to medulloblastoma. *Nat Genet* 2002;31:306-310.

Tiganis T. Protein tyrosine phosphatases: dephosphorylating the epidermal growth factor receptor. *IUBMB Life* 2002;53:3-14.

van der Geer P, Hunter T, Lindberg RA. Receptor protein-tyrosine kinases and their signal transduction pathways. *Annu Rev Cell Biol* 1994;10:251-337.

Varnat F, Duquet A, Malerba M, et al. Human colon cancer epithelial cells harbour active HEDGEHOG-GLI signalling that is essential for tumour growth, recurrence, metastasis and stem cell survival and expansion. *EMBO Mol Med* 2009;1: 338-351.

Von Hoff DD, LoRusso PM, Rudin CM, et al. Inhibition of the hedgehog pathway in advanced basal-cell carcinoma. *N Engl J Med* 2009;361:1164-7112.

Watters JW, Cheng C, Majumder PK, et al. De novo discovery of a gamma-secretase inhibitor response signature using a novel in vivo breast tumor model. *Cancer Res* 2009;69:8949-8957.

Wei J, Wunderlich M, Fox C, et al. Microenvironment determines lineage fate in a human model of MLL-AF9 leukemia. *Cancer Cell* 2008;13:483-495.

Wei W, Chua MS, Grepper S, So S. Small molecule antagonists of Tcf4/beta-catenin complex inhibit the growth of HCC cells in vitro and in vivo. *Int J Cancer* 2010;126:2426-2436.

Weng AP, Ferrando AA, Lee W, et al. Activating mutations of NOTCH1 in human T cell acute lymphoblastic leukemia. *Science* 2004;306:269-271.

Wittinghofer A. Signal transduction via Ras. *Biol Chem* 1998;379: 933-937.

Woychik NA, Hampsey M. The RNA polymerase II machinery: structure illuminates function. *Cell* 2002;108:453-463.

Xia W, Wolfe MS. Intramembrane proteolysis by presenilin and presenilin-like proteases. *J Cell Sci* 2003;116:2839-2844.

Yu H, Rosen MK, Shin TB, Seidel-Dugan C, Brugge JS, Schreiber SL. Solution structure of the SH3 domain of Src and identification of its ligand-binding site. *Science* 1992;258:1665-1668.

Zhang HT, Zhao J, Zheng SY, Chen FX. Is TGFBR1*6A really associated with increased risk of cancer? *J Clin Oncol* 2005;23: 7743-7744.

Zoncu R, Efeyan A, Sabatini DM. mTOR: from growth signal integration to cancer, diabetes and ageing. *Nat Rev Mol Cell Biol* 2011;12:21-35.

Cell Proliferation and Death

Paul Jorgensen and Razqallah Hakem

9.1 INTRODUCTION

Our cells are continuously proliferating and dying. Our development from a single-celled egg into adults with approximately 10^{14} cells requires intense cell proliferation. But our development also requires cell death; for instance, to prune excess neurons in the brain and to sculpt the fingers. As adults, most of our organs exist in a dynamic steady state, being constantly renewed by cell proliferation and death. For example, our bodies generate and destroy more than a million blood and intestinal cells *every second*. In the extreme, cells live for only a few days before dying, as is the case for neutrophils and the cells that line the small intestine. In the midst of this continual and profuse cell renewal lies the constant threat of cancer. Cancerous cells invariably contain alterations to genes encoding regulators of cell proliferation and cell death and are generally thought to arise from actively proliferating cell types.

This chapter discusses the molecular control of the cell cycle and of the processes that lead to cell death, many of which are modified in the processes of malignant transformation and tumor progression. Chapter 12 discusses the growth of tumors and the patterns of cell proliferation and cell death that influence tumor growth, together with the tumor microenvironment and metabolism with which they are closely linked. Chapter 13 discusses the properties of tumor stem cells with high proliferative potential.

9.2 MOLECULAR CONTROL OF CELL PROLIFERATION

Cell proliferation is perhaps best viewed as a combination of two distinct processes: the cell cycle, which replicates and segregates the genome, and cell growth, which doubles all the other components of the cell. The cell cycle and cell growth are intertwined in most normal and cancerous cells, but the two processes can be uncoupled, both in the laboratory and as part of normal development.

9.2.1 The Mammalian Cell Cycle

The cell cycle is partitioned into 4 phases: G_1, S, G_2, and M. This organization reflects the 2 primary goals of the cell cycle: to replicate the genome of the mother cell during DNA synthesis or S-phase, and to segregate the replicated genome into 2 daughter cells during mitosis or M-phase (Fig. 9–1). Two gap phases (G_1, G_2) separate these fundamental events. The

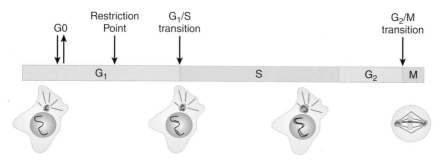

FIGURE 9–1   The key events of the cell cycle. In cells, the nucleus (orange) contains chromosomes (black). The centrosomes (green) are centred around centrioles (red). Most microtubules (blue) project from the centrosome. Chromosome and centrosome duplication begin at the start of S-phase. During mitosis, chromosomes (yellow) condense and the 2 sister chromatids become apparent, remaining joined at the centromeres, which is also the location of the kinetochores (purple) that bind the sister chromatids to bundles of microtubules from opposing poles. Cell structures are not drawn to scale.

combined G_1, S, and G_2-phases are frequently referred to as interphase. When cells cease proliferating because of insufficient nutrients, lack of growth factors, or upon differentiation, they exit the cell cycle from G_1-phase and enter a quiescent state called G_0. Most cells in the body are in the G_0 state. If cells in G_0 are instructed to start proliferating, they must transition back into G_1-phase before starting another cell cycle.

9.2.1.1 The Genome Is Duplicated During S-Phase

Replicating the genome is the first of the cell cycle's two primary objectives. Each of the more than 6 billion base pairs in the DNA of a human cell must be replicated and replicated only once. To replicate so many base pairs, DNA synthesis is initiated at thousands of replication origins scattered throughout the genome (Fig. 9–2A,B). At each replication origin, double-stranded DNA (dsDNA) is unwound into 2 single stands and large protein complexes containing DNA polymerase load onto the single-stranded DNA (ssDNA) (Fig. 9–2C). As they start to replicate the ssDNA, these protein complexes progress away from the origin, unwinding the dsDNA in front of them and leaving 2 copies of dsDNA in their wake, thereby creating a structure called a replication fork (Fig. 9–2C). When replication forks progressing away from neighboring origins of replication collide, replication stops, the DNA replication complexes are removed, and the DNA strands are ligated together (Fig. 9–2A).

Cells ensure that each stretch of interorigin DNA is replicated only once by allowing each DNA replication origin to initiate or "fire" only once per cell cycle. Origins can only initiate synthesis once each cell cycle because of a temporal separation between the formation of the prereplicative complex (pre-RC) on the origin and the initiation of replication at the origin (origin firing) (Arias and Walter, 2007). Pre-RCs are protein complexes containing DNA-binding proteins that assemble on origins at the end of the previous mitosis (see Fig. 9–2B). Once an origin is bound by a pre-RC, it is said to be "licensed" for replication, but these licensed origins remain inert throughout G_1-phase. It is only starting in S-phase that licensed replication origins "fire," when the aforementioned replication complexes containing DNA

polymerases are recruited to the pre-RC and DNA synthesis begins at the origin (see Fig. 9–2C). Pre-RC complexes cannot reassemble in S-phase, nor throughout the subsequent G_2 and early M phases. This strict separation between times during which pre-RCs can assemble and hence license the origins (G_1-phase) and during which the licensed origins can fire (S-phase), limits each origin to a single firing event and prevents rereplication of the DNA.

9.2.1.2 The Duplicated Genome Is Segregated into Two Daughter Cells During Mitosis

Segregating the replicated genomes into two daughter cells is the cell cycle's other primary objective. Chromosome segregation is powered and organized by microtubules. Microtubules and associated proteins form the mitotic spindle, a complex cellular apparatus that pulls apart the replicated chromosomes and then drags the separated sister chromatids to opposite ends of the mother cell.

Assembly of the mitotic spindle is complicated, but is facilitated by centrosomes, organelles that sit at either spindle pole and generally act to organize microtubules. Centrosomes are small (~1 µm) and consist of an electron-dense pericentriolar material of uncertain organization centered on 2 compact (200 × 500 nm), barrel-shaped cylinders of microtubules called *centrioles*. Normal cells in G_1-phase contain a single, centrally located centrosome with 2 separated centrioles (see Fig. 9–1). This single centrosome must replicate itself during the cell cycle. Centrosome replication begins in early S-phase when a daughter centriole grows orthogonally off the surface of each of the 2 original centrioles, leading to the formation of 2 proximal, but distinct, centrosomes, each centered on 2 orthogonally connected centrioles. Upon entering mitosis, the 2 centrosomes separate and move to opposite sides of the cell, with the spindle forming between them. Near the end of mitosis, the centrioles within each centrosome disengage, losing their orthogonal juxtaposition and drifting slightly apart to return to the G_1-phase configuration.

At the start of mitosis, the replicated chromosomes (46 in humans) are comprised of 2 sister chromatids that are glued together along their entire length by cohesive protein

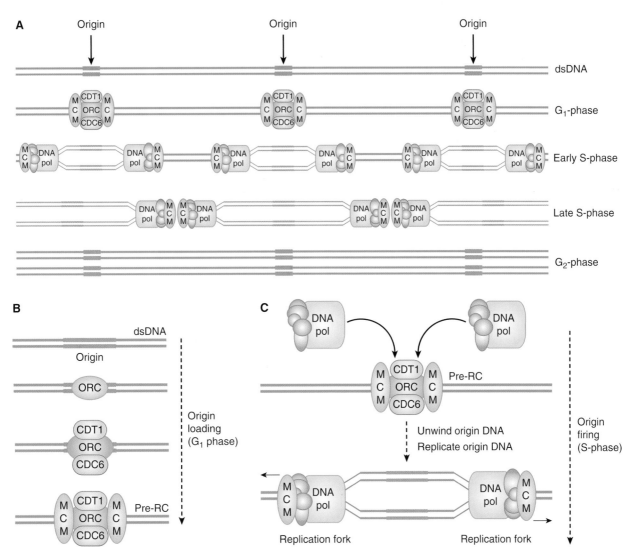

FIGURE 9–2 **The loading and firing of DNA replication origins during the cell cycle. A, B)** During G_1 phase, prereplication complexes (pre-RCs) composed of ORC, CDT1, CDC6 and MCM proteins assemble on stretches of double-stranded DNA (dsDNA) termed *replication origins* (origins). *ORC*, Origin-recognition complex; *MCM*, minichromosome maintenance complex. **A, C)** In S-phase, replication proteins, including DNA polymerase (DNA pol), are recruited by the pre-RC, leading to the unwinding of the origin DNA and the exposure of single-stranded DNA (ssDNA). The 2 exposed stands of ssDNA act as the templates for DNA replication, leading to the formation of 2 copies of dsDNA. Replication proceeds bidirectionally away from the origin, as 2 replication forks unwind DNA and then replicate the exposed ssDNA.

complexes. Although it involves multiple parallel processes that progress in a continuous fashion, mitosis continues to be described as a series of discrete phases, defined by the landmark morphological events observed under the microscope by early cell biologists (Fig. 9–3). Prophase begins with chromosome condensation in the nucleus. As long linear molecules of DNA, chromosomes must be compacted approximately 10,000-fold in order to be cleanly separated from one another and to be moved around the cell (Morgan, 2007). In the cytoplasm, the 2 centrosomes separate from one another and the microtubule spindle begins to elaborate between them, pushing the centrosomes to opposite sides of the cell. At the beginning of prometaphase, the nuclear envelope breaks down, allowing the microtubule spindle to physically interact with the chromosomes (Guttinger et al, 2009). At this point, the 2 sister

chromatids that make up each chromosome have condensed into distinct rods. During prometaphase, the sister chromatids lose most, but not all, of their length-wise cohesion but remain tightly juxtaposed at their centromeres (Peters et al, 2008). The centromere is a single, long (0.2 to 7 megabases) sequence of repetitive DNA encoded in each sister chromatid which forms a platform for the kinetochore, a large protein complex that will physically link microtubules with the sister chromatid (see Fig. 9–1). During prometaphase, each kinetochore is bound by a bundle of 20 to 25 microtubules (Walczak et al, 2010). For each sister chromatid pair, the 2 bundles emanate from opposite spindle poles. The bundles apply pulling forces on each centromere toward their respective spindle pole, but the sister chromatids remain tightly cohered at their centromeres. Under the influence of these counterbalanced pulling forces,

Interphase	Prophase	Prometaphase	Metaphase

Early anaphase	Late anaphase	Telophase

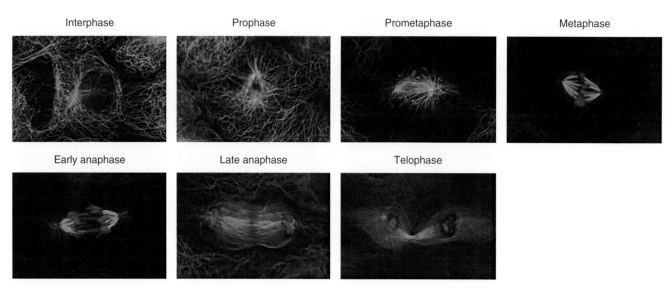

FIGURE 9–3 **The phases of mitosis.** Microtubules stained green, DNA stained blue. The events of each phase are described in the text. Note the microtubule-rich midzone between the segregated chromosomes in late anaphase. The midzone collapses into the midbody following ingression of the contractile ring during telophase. The images are of fixed and stained rat kangaroo kidney (PtK) cells, which are presented in lieu of human cells because the small numbers of chromosomes in these cells make the mitotic events clearer. (Previously unpublished images kindly provided by Jennifer Waters, Harvard Medical School.)

as well as other spindle forces, each of the 46 pairs of sister chromatids becomes bi-orientated in the center of the spindle, aligned in a plane called the metaphase plate (Dumont and Mitchison, 2009). The cell is now in metaphase, but progresses into anaphase when an abrupt and total loss of sister chromatid cohesion occurs, allowing the opposing microtubule bundles to pull the sister chromatids apart and drag them to opposite spindle poles. The spindle itself then elongates, driving the divided genomes to opposite ends of the mother cell. During the subsequent telophase, the events of early mitosis are reversed, as the chromosomes decondense, the nuclear envelopes assemble, and the spindle is taken apart. The process of cytokinesis, which splits the mother cell into 2 daughter cells, is initiated in late anaphase and is completed when both daughter cells are in early G_1-phase.

9.2.1.3 Gap Phases and Checkpoints Are Points of Decision Making

The G_1 and G_2 gap phases are decision-making periods, during which intracellular and extracellular signals determine whether the cell is prepared to enter the subsequent S-phase and M-phase. During G_2-phase, the key signal is intracellular, emanating from the newly replicated DNA. If serious DNA damage has occurred during replication, entry into mitosis is delayed. During G_1-phase, many different kinds of extracellular and intracellular information are integrated into the decision to enter S-phase. Extracellularly, the appropriate signal transduction pathways need to be activated by the binding of receptor ligands. The combination of ligands required to proliferate depends on the cell type, and so we generically refer to them in this chapter as "growth factors" (see Chap. 8, Sec. 8.2). In some cell types, G_1 arrest can also be imposed by excessive physical contact with neighboring cells.

Together, these extracellular requirements define the special niches in which cells typically proliferate in vivo. Intracellularly, serious genomic damage will block cells in G_1-phase. Cells lacking nutrients, such as essential amino acids, will also arrest in G_1-phase. Supply of nutrients is unlikely to be limiting in normal animal tissues with adequate blood supply but may be limiting within solid tumors (see Chap. 12, Secs. 12.2 and 12.3). In some mammalian cell types, a minimal cell size may also be needed to enter S-phase, a requirement that would help coordinate cell growth with the cell cycle (Jorgensen and Tyers, 2004).

When essential growth factors or nutrients are removed from cells, death by apoptosis or senescence may result (see Sec. 9.4). If the cells do not die, a transition in G_1-phase called the *restriction point* determines the cellular response (see Fig. 9–1). If growth factors or nutrients are withdrawn before the restriction point, cells will enter the quiescent G_0 state. If these factors are withdrawn after the restriction point, cells will progress through a full cell cycle before transitioning into the G_0 state early in the subsequent G_1-phase. The restriction point can occur early or late in G_1-phase, depending upon the cell type. In most cancers, control over the restriction point appears to be loosened as the cells proliferate without the appropriate combination of extracellular signals.

9.2.2 Molecular Mechanisms Central to Cell-Cycle Control

The molecular biology of the cell cycle has been explored intensively with important discoveries having been made in yeasts, frog eggs, fruit flies, cultured mammalian cells, and mice. The molecular wiring of the cell cycle has largely been conserved during eukaryotic evolution and employs the full gamut of cellular regulatory mechanisms: transcription, translation, protein degradation, protein localization, protein phosphorylation, and microRNAs. But two molecular mechanisms are particularly central to cell-cycle regulation: cyclin-dependent kinases (CDKs) and E3 ubiquitin ligases.

9.2.2.1 Cyclin-Dependent Kinase Activity Is Tightly Regulated
CDKs are the central regulators of the cell cycle.

CDK activities largely define the phases of the cell cycle, while changes in CDK activity drive transitions between these phases. CDKs exert these effects by phosphorylating hundreds of different proteins throughout the cell. But the abundance of CDKs is constant throughout the cell cycle. Multiple, overlapping, posttranslational mechanisms ensure that the catalytic activity of different CDKs is highly regulated in space and time (Fig. 9–4A).

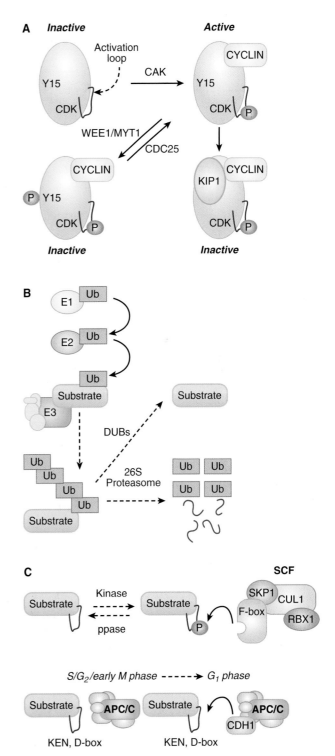

FIGURE 9–4 Molecular mechanisms central to cell cycle control. A) CDKs are the central regulators of the cell cycle. Multiple mechanisms control CDK kinase activity. To become active kinases, CDKs must bind CYCLINs, which leads to the phosphorylation (P) of their activation loop by the CDK activating kinase (CAK). CYCLIN-bound CDKs can, however, become inactivated by phosphorylation on a different residue (Y15) by WEE1/MYT1 kinases. This inhibitory phosphorylation is removed by CDC25 phosphatases. CDKs can also be inactivated upon binding CDK inhibitors (CKIs), such as KIP1. **B)** Several important cell-cycle proteins are destroyed by ubiquitin-mediated proteolysis. Ubiquitin (Ub) is activated by the E1 ubiquitin-activating protein and the covalent bond then transferred to an E2 ubiquitin-conjugating enzyme. E3 ubiquitin ligases bind to both the E2 and to the substrate protein, catalyzing the formation of a covalent bond between the ubiquitin and the substrate. Iterative rounds of ubiquitination generate a multiubiquitinated substrate, which is recognized by the 26S proteosome and degraded into peptides. If the substrate is also recognized by deubiquitinating enzymes (DUBs), the DUBs may hydrolyze the covalent bond with ubiquitin from the substrate, preempting substrate degradation. **C)** SCF complexes often recognize substrates when the F-box protein binds to a phosphorylated peptide (degron) in the substrate protein. The rate at which these substrates are degraded is set by the activity of the kinase or the phosphatase (ppase), which is often cell-cycle regulated. In contrast, anaphase promoting complex/cyclosome (APC/C) complexes recognize substrates that contain degrons called D-boxes or KEN-boxes. APC complexes are only active during late mitosis and G_1 phase when they have bound to an activating subunit, CDC20 or CDH1.

CDK activity is almost entirely dependent on the binding of a cyclin protein (see Fig. 9–4A). Once bound, a CYCLIN not only greatly stimulates the enzymatic activity of the CDK, it also influences substrate selection by the CDK. Based on sequence similarity, the human genome encodes at least 21 CDKs and 25 CYCLINs, but only a subset of the CYCLIN-CDK pairs have been shown to regulate the cell cycle (Malumbres et al, 2009). In normal cells, CDK1 forms complexes with A- and B-type CYCLINs, CDK2 forms complexes with E- and A-type CYCLINs, and CDK4 and CDK6 form complexes with D-type CYCLINs. In mice and humans, CYCLINs are expressed in small families of 2 to 3 proteins each, with the expression of different isoforms often being tissue-specific. For example, CYCLIN A1 is expressed solely in the male germline in mice, while CYCLIN A2 is expressed in all other cells (Kalaszczynska et al, 2009). CYCLINs D1, D2, and D3 are expressed in different tissues in mice, but with some overlap. CYCLINs also specify the intracellular location of CDK activity, as localized CYCLINs can focus CDK activity to the nucleus, the cytoplasm, or the Golgi apparatus. The location of some CYCLIN-CDK complexes changes dynamically during the cell cycle.

Typically, A-, B-, and E-type CYCLINs oscillate in abundance during the cell cycle, defining windows of potential CDK1 and CDK2 activity. In contrast, the abundance of D-type CYCLINs does not change appreciably during the cell cycle (see Fig. 9–5). When a CYCLIN binds a CDK, a threonine in the activation loop of the CDK is phosphorylated by the CDK-activating kinase (CAK) (see Fig. 9–4A; Merrick et al, 2008). In human cells, CAK is actually another CYCLIN-CDK complex composed of CYCLIN H-CDK7, which is constitutively active throughout the cell cycle (Harper and Elledge, 1998).

CDK activity is further shaped by repressive influences (see Fig. 9–4A). The MYT1 and WEE1 kinases inhibit CYCLIN B-CDK1 complexes by phosphorylating amino acids of CDK1. CDC25 phosphatases remove the phosphates from these amino acids. CDK activity can also be curbed by 2 families of CDK inhibitor proteins (CKIs). The INK4 family (p16^{INK4A}, p15^{INK4B}, p18^{INK4C}, p19^{INK4D}) of CKIs bind to CDK4 and CDK6 and prevent their binding to D-type CYCLINs. The CIP/KIP family (p21^{CIP1}, p27^{KIP1}, p57^{KIP2}) of CKIs are more generalized inhibitors, binding and inhibiting the activity of CYCLIN E-CDK2, CYCLIN A-CDK2, and CYCLIN B-CDK1.

9.2.2.2 Ubiquitin-Mediated Proteolysis and E3 Ligases Degrade Cell-Cycle Regulators

Critical cell-cycle events are triggered by the destruction of regulatory proteins. Protein degradation is rapid and irreversible—these properties are advantageous when regulating a dynamic and unidirectional process such as the cell cycle. The primary cellular mechanism for targeted protein degradation is ubiquitin-mediated proteolysis in which the small protein ubiquitin is covalently attached to target proteins (see Chap. 8, Sec. 8.2.8). In this process, an E1 ubiquiting-activating enzyme forms a covalent bond with free ubiquitin and then transfers this bonded ubiquitin to an E2 ubiquitin-conjugating enzyme

(see Fig. 9–4B). The ubiquitin is then transferred from the E2 enzyme to the substrate protein, a process that requires the binding of both the E2 enzyme and the substrate protein to the E3 ubiquitin-ligase. Substrate selectivity in ubiquitin-mediated proteolysis appears to be entirely conferred by the binding interaction between the substrate and the E3 ligase. The same substrate can be ubiquitinated multiple times—it is the presence of multiple ubiquitins attached to a substrate protein that result in that protein binding to and being proteolyzed by the 26S proteosome. Deubiquitinating enzymes (DUBs) can, however, hydrolyze the covalent bond between a substrate and ubiquitin, counteracting the actions of the E3 ligase. For any given ubiquitinated protein, the rate of proteolysis by the 26S proteosome is set by the relative activity of the E3 ligase and the DUB (see Fig. 9–4B; Komander et al, 2009).

SCF, CUL4-DDB1, and the anaphase promoting complex/cyclosome (APC/C) are E3 ligases with important cell-cycle roles. These 3 protein complexes are evolutionarily related to one another and share similar modular structures, with a catalytic core binding to multiple substrate binding proteins. The catalytic core of SCF complexes binds, via an adaptor protein (SKP1), to multiple substrate-binding proteins (F-box proteins) (Willems et al, 2004). As individual F-box proteins are typically able to bind many different substrates, SCF complexes catalyze the ubiquitination of a myriad of target proteins. CUL4-DDB1 complexes are similarly organized with a catalytic core which binds, via an adaptor protein (DDB1), to multiple substrate binding proteins (DWD proteins) (Jackson and Xiong, 2009). The structure of the APC/C is more complicated: its catalytic core is bound to at least 11 other proteins, and this complex then binds to substrate-binding proteins (CDC20, CDH1) in a cell-cycle–dependent manner (Hutchins et al, 2010; Peters, 2006).

Despite their structural similarities, SCF and APC/C differ in how they are activated to ubiquitinate their targets during the cell cycle (Peters, 2006; Willems et al, 2004). In both cases, short peptide sequences (degrons) in the targeted proteins are recognized by the E3 ligase complexes. In the case of SCF complexes, F-box proteins frequently recognize degrons only when they include a phosphorylated serine or threonine (see Fig. 9–4C). The SCF complexes are constitutively active, but they cannot target a substrate for degradation until that substrate is phosphorylated. Typically, SCF activity towards a given substrate is dependent on the activity of the kinase that phosphorylates that substrate. In sharp contrast, APC/C E3 ligases are only active during certain phases of the cell cycle. APC/C^{CDC20} is active during prometaphase and metaphase and APC/C^{CDH1} is active from anaphase to the end of G$_1$-phase (see Fig. 9–4C). During this time, the APC/C complexes bind to degrons that are common to their substrates, most importantly destruction (D) boxes (both APC/C complexes) and KEN boxes (APC/C^{CDH1} only) (Pfleger and Kirschner, 2000). Because these degrons are not usually phosphorylated or otherwise modified, the degradation of these substrates doesn't rely on kinases and simply occurs during the windows of APC activity.

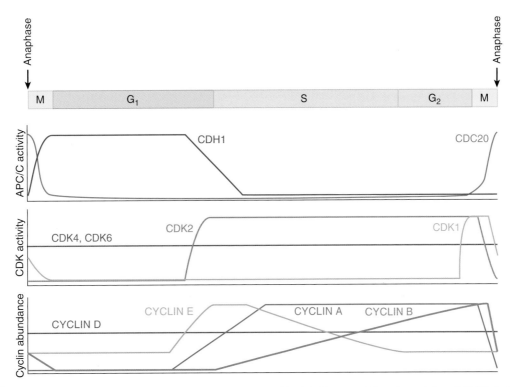

FIGURE 9–5 The pattern of CDC20- or CDH1-dependent APC/C E3 ubiquitin ligase activity, the activity of CDK1, 2, 4, and 6, and the abundance of CYCLINs A, B, D, and E during the cell cycle.

9.2.3 The Molecular Underpinnings of the Human Cell Cycle

The biochemical essence of the cell cycle is an oscillation between 2 states (Nasmyth, 1996). The first state lasts from anaphase to the end of the next G_1-phase, while the second state lasts from the beginning of S-phase to metaphase (Fig. 9–5). In the first state, CDK1 and CDK2 activity is low, APC/C^{CDH1} activity is high, and pre-RC assembly on replication origins is permitted. In the second state, CDK2 activity is high, APC/C^{CDH1} activity is low, and pre-RC assembly on replication origins is not allowed. Each biochemical state is highly stable as a result of multiple positive feedback loops that continually reinforce that state. Switching between the 2 stable states requires special mechanisms that overcome the positive feedback that maintains each state. The points at which the cell switches between the 2 states, the G_1/S transition and the metaphase-anaphase transition, are key points of cell-cycle control. The G_2/M transition is a third key point of control at which the high CYCLIN B-CDK1 activity that controls early mitosis first appears.

9.2.3.1 G_1-Phase Is a Period of Low CDK1 and CDK2 Activity and High APC/C^{CDH1} Activity
Replication origins become capable of initiating DNA replication during G_1 phase when pre-RCs assemble on them (see Fig. 9–2B; Diffley, 2004). The origin DNA is bound directly by the origin recognition complex (ORC). ORC is then bound by CDC6 and CDT1, which, in turn, recruit MCM complexes to the origin (Arias

and Walter, 2007). The absence of CDK1 and CDK2 kinase activity and the high activity of APC/C^{CDH1} during G_1 phase combine to create a biochemical environment that allows pre-RC assembly (see below).

During G_1-phase, CDK1 and CDK2 are not bound to CYCLINs and so their kinase activity is very low (see Fig. 9–4A). CYCLIN A2 and CYCLIN B protein levels are very low during G_1-phase because both proteins are substrates of APC/C^{CDH1} and because their genes are transcriptionally repressed (see Fig. 9–5). The fact that CDH1 is itself a substrate of CYCLIN A2-CDK2 and CYCLIN B-CDK1 complexes generates a self-reinforcing positive feedback loop that lasts throughout G_1 phase (Fig. 9–6A, inner loop). When phosphorylated by CYCLIN A2-CDK2 or CYCLIN B-CDK1, CDH1 dissociates from the APC/C complex, abolishing APC/C activity. Therefore, the low activity of CDK1 and CDK2 in G_1 phase prevents CDH1 from becoming phosphorylated and the activity of the APC/C^{CDH1} complex remains high, which, in turn, keeps CYCLIN A2 and CYCLIN B levels low. An additional positive feedback loop reinforces low CDK1 and CDK2 kinase activity (Fig. 9–6A, outer loop). In this loop, APC/C^{CDH1} targets the F-box protein SKP2 for degradation (Wei et al, 2004). As SCF^{SKP2} targets the CKI p27^{KIP1} for degradation (Malek et al, 2001; Wei et al, 2004), high APC/C^{CDH1} activity during G_1-phase indirectly stabilizes the CKI p27^{KIP1}. p27^{KIP1} can then bind to and inactivate any CYCLIN B-CDK1 or CYCLIN A2-CDK2 complexes that do manage to form.

Quiescence or G_0 is not simply an indefinitely prolonged G_1 period. Like G_1-phase cells, G_0-phase cells have low CDK1

A G₁ phase

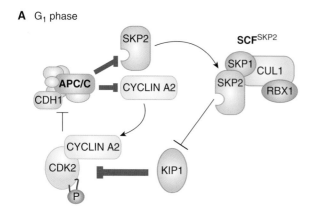

B S/G₂/early M phase

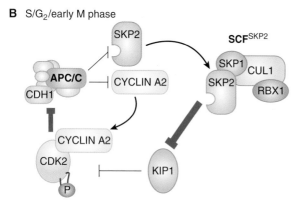

FIGURE 9–6 **Positive feedback loops between APC/C^CDH1 and CYCLIN-CDK1/2 complexes create 2 self-reinforcing states that help define the 2 primary biochemical states in the eukaryotic cell cycle. A)** In G₁-phase, APC/C and CDH1 are associated so APC/C^CDH1 activity is high. This high APC/C^CDH1 activity results in the degradation of CYCLIN A2 and SKP2. Because of the low abundance of these 2 proteins, CYCLIN A2-CDK2 and SCF^SKP2 complexes are rare. Low SCF^SKP2 activity results in relatively high p27^KIP1 abundance. p27^KIP1 helps suppress the activity of any CYCLIN A2-CDK2 complexes that do form. CYCLIN B-CDK1 has a similar place to CYCLIN A2-CDK2 in the positive feedback loops, but is not shown for simplicity. **B)** In S/G₂/early M phase, the balance of power is reversed. Now, CYCLIN A2 is abundant, so CYCLIN A2-CDK2 complexes form and suppress APC/C^CDH1 activity. Similarly, SKP2 is abundant, so SCF^SKP2 complexes form and cause the degradation of p27^KIP1.

and CDK2 activity and high APC^CDH1 activity. But in contrast to G₁-phase cells, G₀-phase cells have little to no CYCLIN D-CDK4/6 activity, as a result of sharply repressed CYCLIN D transcription. In G₀-phase cells, pre-RCs are not assembled on replication origins, apparently because the abundance of some pre-RC components is very low (Williams et al, 1998). The entry of quiescent cells into G₁-phase is a prolonged process that includes the synthesis of D-type cyclins, decreasing levels of p27^KIP1, the accumulation of CDC6, CDT1, MCM, and the assembly of pre-RCs. D-type cyclins are transcriptionally induced and *p27^KIP1* is transcriptionally repressed downstream of growth factor signaling (Sherr and Roberts, 1999; see Chap. 8).

9.2.3.2 The G₁/S Transition Marks the Rise of CDK1/2 Activity At the G₁/S transition, the positive feedback loops

that suppress CDK2 activity and keep the APC/C^CDH1 active are overturned (see Fig. 9–6B). CYCLIN D-CDK4/6 complexes are thought to have 2 key roles early in this process. First, CYCLIN D-CDK4/6 functions noncatalytically to bind p27^KIP1 protein, and prevents p27^KIP1 from inhibiting CYCLIN E-CDK2 and CYCLIN A-CDK2 (Sherr and Roberts, 1999). Second, CYCLIN D-CDK4/6 phosphorylates 3 related "pocket proteins," the Retinoblastoma (RB) protein, p107, and p130. Phosphorylation of the 3 pocket proteins leads to their release from the E2F family of transcription factors (Fig. 9–7). E2Fs complex with the DP protein and bind to sequences found in the promoters of a broad cohort of genes, many of which encode proteins important for S-phase entry or DNA synthesis. E2F4 and E2F5 bind primarily to p130 and p107, and these complexes act to repress target genes in G₀-phase and in early G₁-phase. E2F1-3 bind primarily to RB, which keeps E2F1-3 target genes inactive throughout G₁-phase (Fig. 9–7). The phosphorylation of the 3 pocket proteins by CYCLIN D-CDK4/6 decreases their affinity for E2Fs, resulting in the inhibitory E2Fs (E2F4, E2F5) leaving the nucleus and the activating E2Fs (E2F1, -2, -3) inducing a broad transcriptional program in late G₁-phase (Fig. 9–7).

The E2F transcriptional program includes the genes encoding CYCLIN E, CYCLIN A2, and EMI1. Once translated, these 3 proteins collectively overturn the G₁ state of inactive

G₀ and early G₁ phase

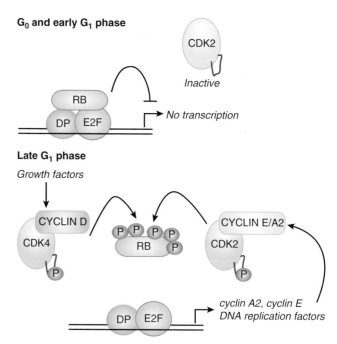

Late G₁ phase

FIGURE 9–7 **In late G₁ phase, the transcription of *cyclin E*, *cyclin A2*, and DNA replication factors is driven by the E2F1-3 transcription factors.** Five types of E2F bind to DNA-binding sites in the promoters of hundreds to thousands of genes with the assistance of the DP protein. In G₀ and early G₁ phases, these genes are repressed by either E2F4-5/p130 complexes (not shown) or E2F1-3/RB complexes. Phosphorylation of the 3 pocket proteins (RB, p130, p107) by CYCLIN D-CDK4/6 causes the pocket proteins to dissociate from the E2Fs during G₁-phase, freeing E2F1-3 to activate transcription. The onset of E2F-dependent transcription is also likely to be the molecular basis for the restriction point.

CDK1 and CDK2 and active APC/C^{CDH1}. CYCLIN E-CDK2 and CYCLIN A2-CDK2 complexes phosphorylate RB and further stimulate the expression of E2F1-3 target genes in a positive feedback loop (Fig. 9–7). CYCLIN E-CDK2 and CYCLIN A2-CDK2 also phosphorylate CDH1, causing CDH1 to dissociate from the APC/C (see Fig. 9–6A, inner loop). The assault on APC/C^{CDH1} activity is furthered by EMI1, a binding partner and direct inhibitor of APC/C^{CDH1} (Di Fiore and Pines, 2008). The loss of APC/C^{CDH1} activity leads to the accumulation of its substrate SKP2. Rising SCF^{SKP2} activity in late G$_1$ phase targets p27^{KIP1} for degradation, contributing to the rise in CYCLIN E-CDK2 and CYCLIN A2-CDK2 activity (see Fig. 9–6A, outer loop). These interlocking feedback loops, which are elaborated late in G$_1$-phase and cause the G$_1$/S transition, stabilize the new S/G$_2$/early M-phase state of high CDK2 activity and low APC/C activity (see Fig. 9–5).

The switch from low to high CDK2 activity and from high to low APC/C^{CDH1} activity is thought to be the molecular basis of the restriction point. That is, at some point in G$_1$-phase, this switching process becomes irreversible and no longer requires growth signaling pathways. As discussed above, these signaling pathways are thought to drive the G$_1$/S transition by (a) stimulating the synthesis and activity of CYCLIN D-CDK4/6 complexes, and (b) transcriptionally repressing and directly inactivating p27^{KIP1}.

9.2.3.3 The Initiation of DNA Replication and the Block to Overreplication

The rise of CYCLIN A2-CDK2 activity at the G$_1$/S transition triggers DNA replication. In at least some cell types, CYCLIN E-CDK2 also contributes to this process (Kalaszczynska et al, 2009). DNA replication also requires the CDC7 kinase, whose activity requires binding to the DBF4/ASK protein. Like CYCLIN A2, DBF4/ASK increases in abundance at the G$_1$/S transition (Jiang et al, 1999). Phosphorylation by CYCLIN A2-CDK2 and CDC7-DBF4 of the pre-RC complex assembled around a particular DNA replication origin leads to the recruitment of replication proteins to that origin. The DNA double helix at the origin is subsequently unwound by the MCM helicase (Takeda and Dutta, 2005). These events attract DNA polymerase complexes, which bind to the unwound ssDNA at the origin and initiate DNA replication (see Fig. 9–2).

The reloading of pre-RC complexes on replication origins in S-, G$_2$-, and early M-phase is prevented primarily by eliminating CDT1 activity (Fig. 9–8A; Arias and Walter, 2007). Overlapping mechanisms are likely necessary to ensure that pre-RC complexes do not reappear on any of the tens of thousands of replication origins over the many hours it takes to complete S, G$_2$, and early M phases. Two different E3 ligases target CDT1 for degradation. In S, G$_2$, and early M phases, phosphorylation of CDT1 by CYCLIN A2-CDK2 leads to CDT1 being ubiquitinated by SCF^{SKP2}. In S-phase, CDT1 also interacts with the chromatin-bound proliferating cell nuclear antigen (PCNA), which also leads to CDT1 becoming ubiquitinated. Any CDT1 that escapes ubiquitin-mediated degradation is inactivated by the Geminin protein. Geminin (GEM) binding to CDT1 prevents

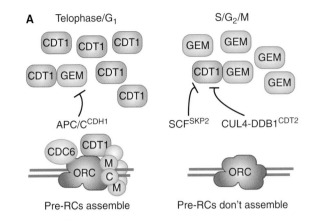

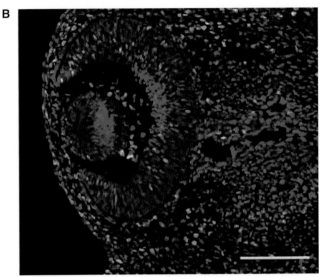

FIGURE 9–8 A) Multiple mechanisms inhibit CDT1 in S-, G$_2$-, and early M-phase, thereby preventing new pre-RCs from assembling during these cell-cycle phases. The protein stability and abundance of CDT1 and Geminin (GEM) are inversely related during the cell cycle. CDT1 is stable and abundant during telophase and G$_1$-phase, while GEM is stable and abundant during S-, G$_2$-, and early M-phase. The E3 ubiquitin ligases that target CDT1 and GEM for degradation in each phase are shown. **B)** Fluorescent proteins fused to the degron sequences of CDT1 (red) and GEM (green) localize to the nucleus and report the cell-cycle dependent instability conferred by these degrons. In the eye of a mouse that expressed both reporters in all of its cells, it is evident that cells are either red or green, depending on the cell cycle phase of that cell. (From Sakaue-Sawano et al, 2008.)

the recruitment of MCM complexes to DNA replication origins, thereby blocking a crucial step in pre-RC assembly. Geminin is itself an APC/C substrate that starts to accumulate at the G$_1$/S transition when APC/C^{CDH1} is inactivated. Therefore, CDT1 and GEM are binding partners that have reciprocal patterns of degradation and abundance during the cell cycle (Fig. 9–8B). In addition to the mechanisms that restrict CDT1 activity in S, G$_2$, and early M phases, CDC6 and components of the ORC complex may also be negatively regulated by CYCLIN A2-CDK2 and CYCLIN B-CDK1 phosphorylation during this same period (Arias and Walter, 2007; Diffley, 2004).

During DNA replication, the 2 emerging sister chromatids become connected by a protein complex called *Cohesin*. By keeping the sister chromatids tightly connected, Cohesin is critical for the segregation of the 2 chromatids into separate daughter cells during mitosis. Cohesin is also important for the repair of dsDNA breaks (DSBs) by recombination between sister chromatids (see Chap. 5, Sec. 5.3.4; Peters et al, 2008). Cohesin may link sister chromatids by simply enclosing them within the same ring of protein (Nasmyth and Haering, 2009). How Cohesin establishes sister-chromatid cohesion during S-phase remains uncertain, but it is known to require a cohort of loading and stabilization proteins (Peters et al, 2008).

9.2.3.4 G_2 and the Entrance to Mitosis

In late G_2-phase, mammalian cells experience a surge of CYCLIN B-CDK1 activity that initiates the events of early mitosis. Throughout S- and G_2-phase, the concentration of CYCLIN B rises, being induced by the FOXM1 transcription factor (see Fig. 9–5). The newly translated CYCLIN B binds to unphosphorylated CDK1. The binding of CYCLIN B allows phosphorylation of CDK1 on the activation loop, generating a momentarily active CYCLIN B-CDK1 kinase (see Fig. 9–4*A*; Deibler and Kirschner, 2010). This complex is quickly recognized in the cytoplasm by MYT1 and in the nucleus by WEE1, 2 protein kinases that phosphorylate other amino acids (particularly tyrosine 15) of CDK1 and thereby quell the kinase activity of the CYCLIN B-CDK1 complex (O'Farrell, 2001; see Fig. 9–4*A*). Throughout S- and G_2-phase, these inactive, phosphorylated CYCLIN B-CDK1 complexes accumulate in the cell.

In late G_2-phase, the stockpiled complexes are suddenly activated by a rapid loss of the inhibitory phosphorylations, a process that is driven by at least 2 positive feedback loops (O'Farrell, 2001; Lindqvist et al, 2009). In the first positive feedback loop, CYCLIN B-CDK1 phosphorylates and activates the CDC25 phosphatases, which remove the inhibitory phosphate groups. In the second positive feedback loop, CYCLIN B-CDK1 inactivates WEE1 and MYT1, thereby blocking any further phosphorylations on CDK1. As inactive CYCLIN B-CDK1 complexes accumulate for many hours during S-phase and G_2-phase, some trigger must be required to activate these positive feedback loops in late G_2-phase. A strong candidate for the late G_2-phase trigger is simply the accumulation of CYCLIN B and/or CYCLIN A2 above a threshold concentration. The time required to achieve this threshold concentration of CYCLIN B and/or CYCLIN A2 would then set the length of G_2-phase.

The elaboration of CYCLIN B-CDK1 activity in late G_2-phase is blocked by severely damaged or unreplicated DNA, a checkpoint that prevents cells from attempting to segregate damaged chromosomes (see Sec. 9.3 and Chap. 5, Sec. 5.4).

9.2.3.5 The Events of Early Mitosis Culminate in Sister Chromatid Separation

The early events of mitosis are orchestrated by 4 mitotic kinases: CYCLIN B-CDK1, Polo-like kinase 1 (PLK1), Aurora (AUR) A, and AUR B. Correspondingly, more than 1000 proteins become phosphorylated specifically during mitosis (Dephoure et al, 2008). All 4 mitotic kinases are activated at the G_2/M transition or in prophase. CYCLIN B-CDK1 activation has been discussed. Activation of PLK1, AUR A, and AUR B results from phosphorylation and from binding interactions that localize these kinases to critical locations in the mitotic cell (Fig. 9–9). At the end of mitosis, all 4 of the mitotic kinases are inactivated, in large part as a result of the resurgence of APC/C activity. CYCLIN B is targeted for degradation by APC/C^{CDC20} during metaphase, while the degradation of PLK1, AUR A, and AUR B by APC/C^{CDH1} begins in anaphase (Barr et al, 2004; Carmena et al, 2009).

The strength and location of CYCLIN B-CDK1 activity during early mitosis helps determine the sequence of early events (see Fig. 9–9; Gavet and Pines, 2010). CYCLIN B-CDK1 activity is first apparent in the cytoplasm and on the centrosomes. In early prophase, cytoplasmic CYCLIN B-CDK1 causes adherent cells to "round up" and, in collaboration with PLK1, causes the 2 centrosomes to separate and mature (Gavet and Pines, 2010). CYCLIN B-CDK1 then moves into the nucleus and by late prophase the complex is predominantly nuclear (Takizawa and Morgan, 2000). Nuclear CYCLIN B-CDK1 triggers chromosome condensation, as well as the breakdown of the nuclear envelope, in part by phosphorylating and disassembling the meshwork of intermediate filaments called *lamins* that lines the inner nuclear membrane.

Upon dissolution of the nuclear envelope, which marks the start of prometaphase, microtubules gain access to the chromatin. Microtubule interaction with the condensing chromosomes leads to the self-organization of the mitotic spindle between the 2 centrosomes (see Fig. 9–9). This process is highly complex and requires numerous proteins that move and stabilize microtubules (Gatlin and Bloom, 2010). During prometaphase, 20 to 25 microtubules bind the kinetochore of each sister chromatid (Walczak et al, 2010). By metaphase, each sister chromatid pair has formed a bipolar attachment to the mitotic spindle: one sister chromatid's kinetochore is connected by microtubules to one spindle pole, while the other sister chromatid's kinetochore is connected by microtubules to the other spindle pole (see Fig. 9–9). Each microtubule bundle exerts pulling forces on the kinetochore toward the spindle pole from which the bundle emanates. Although their kinetochores and centromeres are being pulled in opposite directions, the sister chromatids do not separate as a result of the Cohesin complexes that continue to physically connect them. The balance of these pulling and resistive forces, amongst other forces present in the mitotic spindle, cause each sister chromatid pair to align at the metaphase plate (Dumont and Mitchison, 2009). By phosphorylating multiple centrosome, spindle, and kinetochore proteins, the 4 mitotic kinases play key roles in shaping the mitotic spindle and aligning sister chromatid pairs (Carmena et al, 2009; Petronczki et al, 2008).

The loss of cohesion between the sister chromatid pairs occurs in 2 steps. During prophase and prometaphase, most of the Cohesin along the chromosomal arms dissociates, allowing the chromosomal arms to partially separate by metaphase

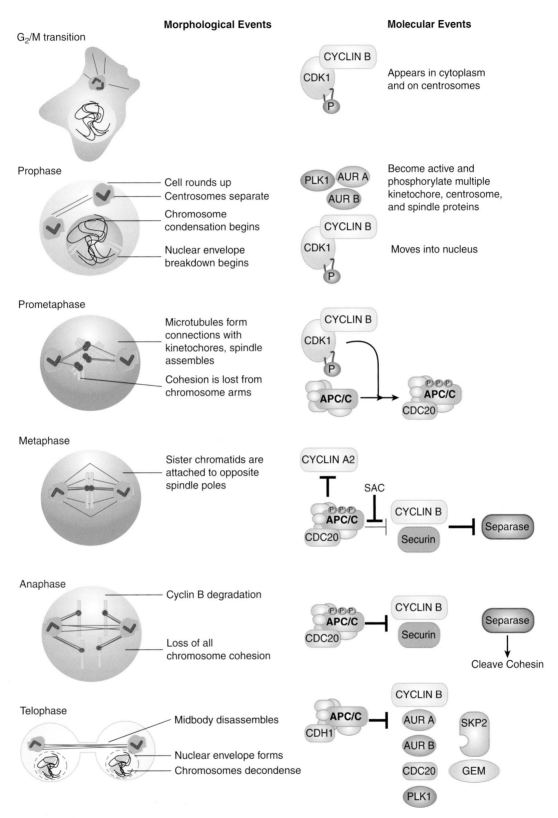

FIGURE 9–9 Major morphological and molecular events of mitosis. Schematic (left) images of cells in the primary stages of mitosis. Uncondensed DNA is in black, condensed DNA is in yellow and microtubules are in blue. Purple spheres on DNA represent kinetochores. Orthogonal red rectangles within green spheres represent centrosomes. The concentration of active CYCLIN B-CDK1 complexes is roughly indicated by the intensity of orange in the cytoplasm and nucleus. See text for details on the major molecular events. *P*, Phosphorylation; *SAC*, spindle assembly checkpoint.

(Peters et al, 2008). But, Cohesin located at the centromeres does not dissociate until the onset of anaphase. The 2-step loss of cohesion explains the X-shaped structure of chromosomes in karyotypes, which are derived from cells arrested in metaphase by spindle poisons.

The APC/C becomes active early in mitosis when CDC20 binds to the APC/C following extensive phosphorylation of the APC/C by CYCLIN B-CDK1. The bound APC/C^{CDC20} is active versus some substrates in prometaphase, including CYCLIN A2 (Geley et al, 2001), but remains inactive toward other critical substrates in prometaphase due to the inhibitory effects of the spindle assembly checkpoint (SAC; see Fig. 9–9). Once all of the kinetochores have attached to microtubules and each sister chromatid pair in under tension, cells are in metaphase, the SAC is inactivated, and the APC/C^{CDC20} becomes fully active. This fully active APC/C^{CDC20} then ubiquitinates 3 crucial substrates: securin and the 2 B-type Cyclins (B1 and B2). The proteolysis of these proteins is probably sufficient to explain the loss of sister chromatid cohesion that triggers anaphase (Oliveira et al, 2010). Securin is a binding partner and inhibitor of the protease Separase (Zou et al, 1999). In parallel to Securin, CYCLIN B-CDK1 phosphorylation of separase represses separase activity (Stemmann et al, 2001). Anaphase is initiated when the APC/C^{CDC20} simultaneously removes the 2 blocks (Securin and Cyclin Bs) to separase protease activity (Oliveira et al, 2010). Separase then cleaves the Cohesin subunit SCC1, which causes the removal of centromeric Cohesin and any Cohesin remaining on the chromosome arms. Once Cohesin is entirely removed, the sister chromatids are free to respond to the pulling forces exerted on their kinetochores and progress toward opposite spindle poles. Note that this current model of anaphase may not explain the synchrony with which the 46 pairs of sister chromatids separate.

9.2.3.6 Late Mitosis Ends with Two Genetically Identical Daughter Cells
The events of late anaphase and telophase are largely driven by the loss of protein phosphorylations that were applied earlier in mitosis by the CYCLIN B-CDK1, PLK1, and AUR B mitotic kinases (Sullivan and Morgan, 2007). Also key to late mitosis is the appearance of APC/C^{CDH1} activity (see Fig. 9–9). With the degradation of CYCLIN B during metaphase and anaphase, CYCLIN B-CDK1 kinase activity is much lower by telophase, allowing CDH1 to become dephosphorylated and bind to the APC/C (see Fig. 9–9). APC/C^{CDH1} has a much broader substrate range than APC/C^{CDC20}. As 1 of the substrates of APC/C^{CDH1} is CDC20, APC/C^{CDC20} activity is lost in late mitosis (see Fig. 9–5).

Many of the molecular details of late anaphase and telophase remain mysterious. The loss of protein phosphates applied earlier in mitosis by CYCLIN B-CDK1—most of which remain unidentified—is required to disassemble the mitotic spindle, decondense the separated chromosomes, and form nuclear envelopes around the 2 daughter genomes. One relatively well-understood event of telophase is the assembly of pre-RCs on DNA replication origins (Arias and Walter, 2007). Here the APC/C has important roles. The ubiquitin-dependent proteolysis of CYCLIN A2 in prometaphase and CYCLIN B1 and B2 in metaphase by APC/C^{CDC20} reestablishes the low-CDK1/2 activity state required for pre-RC formation (see above). In late anaphase and telophase, APC/C^{CDH1} maintains the degradation of these CYCLINs. APC/C^{CDH1} also initiates the destruction of GEM (the binding inhibitor of the pre-RC component CDT1) and SKP2 (which targets CDT1 for degradation via the SCF^{SKP2} complex) (Wei et al, 2004; Arias and Walter, 2007). As a result of APC/C^{CDH1} activity, CDT1 can accumulate in telophase, bind to ORC at DNA replication origins, and then recruit the remaining components of the pre-RC. The DNA replication origins are now prepared to initiate DNA synthesis in the next S-phase.

Separation of the daughter cells (cytokinesis) is caused by the gradual constriction of a contractile ring attached to the inner face of the plasma membrane. The contractile force appears to be provided by filaments of Myosin II motor protein interacting with filaments of Actin, although exactly how these filaments are organized to constrict the ring remains uncertain. During anaphase, the contractile ring forms on the inner plasma membrane around the center of the spindle, equidistant from each mass of chromosomes. Typically, the spindle is located in the center of the cell and so the cell divides in half, but asymmetric spindle positioning leading to asymmetric cell cleavage is common during development and in stem cell divisions. During late anaphase and telophase, the spindle's morphology changes, passing through an intermediate stage called the *midzone* before being compacted into a bundle of microtubules called the *midbody*. Ingression of the contractile ring begins in late anaphase and continues throughout telophase, with membrane vesicles fusing with the cleavage furrow to provide the increased plasma membrane required by 2 smaller cells. The midbody spans the 1 to 1.5μm diameter cytoplasmic bridge connecting the 2 future daughter cells after maximal ingression of the contractile ring (Eggert et al, 2006). Membrane vesicles are then directed by the midbody to fill the remaining hole, a process which completes the physical separation of the 2 daughter cells.

9.2.3.7 Caveats to the Current Model of the Mammalian Cell Cycle
Studies of mice carrying null alleles of core cell-cycle regulators have raised important caveats about the current model of the human cell cycle described herein. For example, mice lacking both *Cdk4* and *Cdk6* die late in development as a result of poor proliferation of hematopoietic precursor cells, but most other cell types in the embryo proliferate normally (Malumbres et al, 2009). Second, genes encoding regulatory proteins that are central to this consensus model are not always essential. SKP2, CDH1, p27^{KIP1}, CDK2, CDK4, CDK6, CYCLIN Ds, CYCLIN Es, and CYCLIN As are not required for the proliferation of many cell types in mice (eg, Geng et al, 2003; Kalaszczynska et al, 2009). Even a triple loss of CDK2, CDK4, and CDK6 still allows most cell types in the mouse embryo to proliferate (Santamaria et al, 2007). The surprising mildness of CYCLIN and CDK knockout phenotypes may be because of unusual

CYCLIN-CDK complexes (eg, CYCLIN E-CDK1) that form when the usual binding partners are missing (Santamaria et al, 2007). But these mouse knockout studies also hint that current models may be far from complete.

9.2.4 Cell Growth

Although the term *growth* is often used loosely to refer to proliferation, the term *cell growth* specifically refers to increases in cell size. Fundamentally, cell growth is a net increase in biomass, primarily proteins, RNA, and membrane lipids. For cells to proliferate and maintain their size, cell growth must, on average, double the size of the mother cell by the time of mitosis. So, in addition to doubling the amount of DNA and the number of centosomes with each cell cycle, a cell must grow sufficiently to double all its other constituent parts—ribosomes, mitochondria, lysosomes, etc.

It remains unclear how intertwined cell growth and the cell cycle are in human cells. Growth of some cells can become uncoupled from the cell cycle, arguing that they are distinct processes. For example, during the formation of the oocytes, which are giant single cells, cell growth occurs in the absence of any cell division. The uncoupling of cell growth and the cell cycle can also occur in somatic cells when the cell cycle is arrested by a DNA damage checkpoint (see Sec. 9.3). Such cell-cycle arrest usually allows cell growth to continue, resulting in oversized cells. In general, cell growth is more limiting for cell proliferation than is the cell cycle, because in animal cells the events of the cell cycle can be accomplished in far less time than it takes to double the mass of the cell. Because different amounts of time are necessary to double cell mass and to complete the cell cycle, coordination between cell growth and the cell cycle must exist at some level or else cell size would fluctuate wildly, which is not observed (Jorgensen and Tyers, 2004).

For a given human cell, cell growth, like the cell cycle, requires the appropriate combination of growth factors to bind to the cell (see Chap. 8, Sec. 8.2). Some of the molecular regulators of cell growth that lie downstream of growth factor signaling are known. c-MYC is a transcription factor encoded by the oncogene most frequently amplified in cancers. c-MYC binds to gene promoters with its binding partner MAX (see Chap. 7, Sec. 7.5.2). The widespread transcriptional program activated by c-MYC overexpression can stimulate cell growth, in part by inducing genes involved in ribosome synthesis, a process that is intrinsically related to cell growth (Eilers and Eisenman, 2008). c-MYC/MAX can also stimulate the cell cycle by activating the transcription of *cyclin D1, cyclin D2* and *cdk4*, while a c-MYC/MAX/MIZ1 complex represses the genes encoding the p21[CIP1] and p15[INK4B] proteins.

The mammalian target of rapamycin (mTOR) and phophatidylinositol-3 kinase (PI3K) signaling network (see Chap. 7, Sec. 7.5.4 and Chap. 8, Sec. 8.2.5) is a central regulator of animal cell growth and proliferation. This network integrates large amounts of extracellular and intracellular information into the decision to activate the AKT kinase and the mTORC1 kinase complex (Guertin and Sabatini, 2007). These 2 kinases then activate multiple downstream processes that drive cell growth, the cell cycle, and block cell death (Guertin and Sabatini, 2007). Genetic alterations that increase AKT and mTORC1 activity can be oncogenic. Mutations in the gene encoding PTEN (see Chap. 7, Sec. 7.6.2), a phosphatase that counteracts PI3K, can constitutively activate AKT and are common in many cancers (eg, ~40% of endometrial cancers, 30% to 40% of glioblastoma multiforme) (Liu et al, 2009; Sansal and Sellers, 2004). Amplification of the genes encoding growth factor receptors upstream of AKT and mTORC1 (eg, ERBB2 see Chap. 7, Sec. 7.5.3) are also common in cancer (Liu et al, 2009). Two rapamycin analogs (temsirolimus and everolimus, small molecular inhibitor of mTORC1) have been shown to be efficacious in the treatment of metastatic renal cell carcinoma and are in clinical trials for other types of cancer.

To grow, cells need to either import or synthesize large amounts of amino acids, nucleotides and fatty acids. In addition, large amounts of adenosine triphosphate (ATP) are required to polymerize these building blocks into proteins, RNA, and membrane lipids. Consequently, growing cells have special metabolic properties. The anabolic state is programmed by growth factor signaling pathways and transcription factors, particularly the PI3K/mTOR network and c-MYC discussed above (Jones and Thompson, 2009). The anabolic state is characterized by a number of features, particularly rapid uptake and metabolism of glucose. The rapid uptake of glucose by some cancer cells reflects their higher rate of glycolysis. Indeed, some cancer cells produce more pyruvate—the end product of glycolysis—than can be oxidized by the tricarboxylic acid (TCA) cycle in the mitochondria. The excess pyruvate is converted to lactic acid and secreted, a phenomenon commonly known as the Warburg effect (see Chap. 12, Sec. 12.3.1). Although usually thought of as an energy generating pathway, glycolysis–via the interlinked pentose phosphate pathway–also has important roles in supplying cellular building blocks, including the reducing equivalent nicotinamide adenine dinucleotide phosphate (NADPH) which is used in many anabolic reactions, the nucleotide precursor ribose-5-phosphate, the phospholipid precursor glycerol-3-phosphate, and the precursors for 4 amino acids (Jones and Thompson, 2009). The need to produce building blocks like NADPH to allow for rapid cell growth may be the molecular explanation for why some cancer cells engage in such rapid glycolysis that lactic acid must be secreted from the cell.

9.2.5 Modifications to Control of Cell Proliferation in Cancer

The first tumor suppressorgene discovered in humans was *Rb1*, whose loss was found to be the cause of familial retinoblastoma (see Chap. 7, Sec. 7.6.4). Soon after, *cyclin D1* was isolated as an oncogene in a subset of parathyroid adenomas. The *cdkn2a* locus, which contains the genes encoding the p15[INK4B] protein, the p16[INK4A] protein, and the p53 activator ARF, was then identified as a tumor suppressor in familial melanomas. These early findings anticipated a general truth about human cancers, which is that the vast majority contain genetic or epigenetic alterations that loosen control over the G_1/S transition. Typical alterations include the amplification of genes that encode proteins that drive the G_1/S transition (eg, *cyclin D1*), as well as genomic deletions, point mutations, and promoter methylations that remove G_1/S inhibitors like RB and p16^{INK4A}. In a genome-wide survey of 26 human cancer types, the tightly opposed loci encoding p15^{INK4B} and p16^{INK4A}/ARF were found to be the most frequently deleted genomic region, while the genes encoding CYCLIN D1 and CDK4 were among the 4 most frequently amplified regions (Beroukhim et al, 2010). When genetic alterations to the G_1/S machinery are considered collectively, the majority of cancers contain at least 1 such change. For example, more than 90% of liver, ovarian, testicular, and lung cancers bear alterations in the genes encoding the currently known G_1/S regulatory apparatus (Malumbres and Barbacid, 2001). Alterations to the genes encoding the G_1/S regulatory apparatus are thought to allow cancer cells to enter the cell cycle precociously, defying the extracellular signals that limit the proliferation of their normal neighbors.

A detailed understanding of the cell cycle could be important for developing better anticancer drugs. There is active preclinical development and clinical evaluation of agents designed to inhibit cell-cycle regulators. For example, clinical trials are evaluating specific inhibitors of EG5, PLK1, and the Aurora kinases as such drugs may kill mitotic cells without affecting microtubules in quiescent cells. Similarly, substantial effort has been dedicated to generating CDK inhibitors (Malumbres et al, 2008). Future generations of anticancer drugs could exploit the common alterations to the cell-cycle machinery shared by many cancers, such as defective control over the G_1/S transition, loss of the p53 response, aneuploidy, or the presence of extra centrosomes. In particular, cancers may acquire a dependence on nonessential cell-cycle components like D- and E-type CYCLIN-CDK complexes, which could be exploited by targeted therapies. Supporting such an idea, mice lacking *cyclin D1* or *cdk4* can be highly resistant to tumor formation.

9.3 GENOMIC INSTABILITY AND CHECKPOINT PATHWAYS

Nearly all cancers show evidence of genomic instability. Mutations that increase genomic instability are probably selected early in the evolution of many cancers. Consistent with this idea, many familial cancer syndromes are caused by mutations in genes encoding DNA repair proteins and checkpoint proteins (see Chap. 5, Sec. 5.5 and Chap. 7, Sec. 7.2). Genomic instability can occur through point mutations, the amplification or deletion of genomic regions, and the fusion, loss, or gain of whole chromosomes. The duplication and segregation of the genome during the cell cycle inexorably increases the risk of genomic instability. Checkpoints that arrest the cell

cycle in response to DNA damage or to difficulties in segregating the chromosomes exist to alleviate such risks.

9.3.1 The DNA Damage Checkpoints

The cell cycle is intimately associated with the detection and repair of DNA damage. (see Chap. 5) When the cell sustains genomic damage beyond a threshold level, the cell cycle arrests. Arresting the cell cycle gives time to repair this damage before entering either S-phase or mitosis, thereby preventing the replication or segregation of compromised chromosomes. Cells with severely damaged DNA can undergo malignant transformation, as demonstrated by the many hereditary cancer syndromes caused by defective DNA checkpoint and repair genes (see Chap. 5, Sec. 5.5). To protect the body from this threat, a cell's response to DNA damage can often end in that cell's death (see Sec. 9.4).

There is a 2-way flow of information between the DNA damage response and the cell cycle. Serious DNA damage arrests the cell cycle, but the cell cycle also regulates the response to DNA damage. Mechanisms that correct common chemical changes to DNA bases, such as base excision repair and nucleotide excision repair, operate constitutively. In contrast, a cell's response to DSBs, likely the most dangerous type of DNA damage, can depend on its cell-cycle phase. During G_1-phase, cells primarily repair DSBs through a nonhomologous end-joining (NHEJ) process, in which broken ends are directly ligated together, often leading to the loss of base pairs. During S- and G_2-phases, cells continue to repair DSBs by NHEJ, but also deploy homologous recombination (HR), which typically uses the replicated sister chromatid as a template for correcting damaged DNA. Unlike NHEJ, HR doesn't usually lead to any genomic instability (see Chap. 5, Sec. 5.3).

Serious DNA damage like DSBs activate DNA damage kinases that trigger cell-cycle arrest through phosphorylation of proteins that control the G_1/S and the G_2/M transitions. These phosphorylation events lead to the stabilization and activation of both the transcription factor p53 and the CKI p21^{CIP1}. p53 induces a broad transcriptional program of DNA repair proteins (Zilfou and Lowe, 2009). p21^{CIP1} suppress CYCLIN E-CDK2 and CYCLIN A2-CDK2 activity, preventing entry into S-phase. For cells in S- and G_2-phase, DNA damage kinases inactivate all 3 CDC25 phosphatases and activate the WEE1 kinase. These actions arrest cells before the G_2/M transition point by preventing the surge of CYCLIN B-CDK1 activity that drives cells into mitosis (Reinhardt and Yaffe, 2009).

9.3.2 The Spindle Assembly Checkpoint

The SAC is essential for the human cell cycle, serving to delay anaphase until all the replicated chromosomes are bi-orientated and under tension (Musacchio and Salmon, 2007). The primary defect detected by the SAC is kinetochores that are not attached to microtubules. A single unattached kinetochore can prevent anaphase in mammalian cells (Rieder et al, 1995). Properly bi-orientated pairs of sister chromatids will also experience tension between their cohered centromeres, as the 2 microtubule bundles pull the 2 kinetochores in opposite directions. Insufficient levels of tension between centromeres can also lead to activation of the SAC, although the exact mechanism is unresolved (Musacchio and Salmon, 2007).

The SAC blocks anaphase by preventing the full activation of APC/C^{CDC20}. The result is stabilized Securin and CYCLIN B, which can suppress Separase and maintain the metaphase state for a long, though not indefinite, period of time (Brito and Rieder, 2006).

9.3.3 Mitotic Errors, Aneuploidy, and Oncogenesis

In the multihit genetic model of oncogenesis, it is evident that genomic instability that arises during S-phase can contribute to cancer formation. For instance, errors by DNA polymerases can introduce point mutations into genes encoding tumor suppressors, while DSBs can cause chromosomal translocations that lead to the misexpression of oncogenes. But cancers are marked not just by such discrete genetic changes, but also by wholesale changes in the number of chromosomes (aneuploidy), which presumably arise from errors in mitosis. More than 90% of clinically detected solid tumors are aneuploid. Although they typically have less bizarre karyotypes than solid tumors, hematopoietic cancers also frequently show loss or gain of one or more chromosomes (Weaver and Cleveland, 2006).

Despite the strong connection between aneuploidy and solid tumors, it is not clear that aneuploidy is a cause, as opposed to a consequence, of cancer. Aneuploidy is generally detrimental to the proliferation of normal cells, presumably because it creates subtle imbalances in the expression levels of the hundreds or thousands of genes present on a supernumery chromosome. But as a general rule, molecular mechanisms proposed to cause cancer are thought to increase—not decrease—the rate of cell proliferation. How then could aneuploidy be a cause of cancer? First, in contrast to the general presumption that drivers of cancer must increase the rate of cell proliferation, cell proliferation in solid tumors is often considerably slower than in normal renewing tissues (see Chap. 12, Sec. 12.1). Second, populations of aneuploid cells will have greater genetic variability and presumably greater phenotypic variability. In some circumstances, the altered expression of multiple genes resulting from certain combinations of chromosome numbers may generate advantageous phenotypes. Such phenotypic diversity could allow aneuploid populations of cancer cells to rapidly evolve in response to physiological stresses, such as hypoxia or immune responses, or to medical interventions, such as chemotherapy.

When misregulated, several proteins involved in mitosis have been shown to induce tumors in mice. These results suggest that the aneuploidy that results from mitotic errors can be a cause of cancer. Misregulation of mitotic proteins can cause aneuploidy by at least three interconnected mechanisms: chromosomal instability, extra centrosomes, and tetraploidy (Weaver and Cleveland, 2006).

Chromosome instability is the failure to properly segregate 1 copy of the sister chromatid pairs to each of the 2 daughter cells, a failure that results in 2 aneuploid daughter cells. In normal cells, missegregation of a chromosome—leading to 1 daughter cell inheriting both sister chromatids—is a rare event, occurring once every 50 to 100 cell cycles. But in some cancer cell lines, chromosomes can be missegregated nearly every cell cycle (Thompson and Compton, 2008).

Extra centrosomes are a common feature of cancers. In normal cells, centrosomes are similar to chromosomes in that they are replicated during S-phase and then segregated during mitosis. In fact, cells appear to use a similar strategy to ensure that both chromosomes and centrosomes replicate only once per cell cycle: there are distinct windows of time for becoming competent for replication and for actually undergoing replication. The 2 centrioles in a centrosome become competent for replication in telophase when they disengage from each other. Upon entering S-phase, each of the disengaged centrioles initiates construction of a new orthogonal centriole, thereby generating two pairs of centrioles and hence 2 centrosomes. But, once cells have entered S-phase, the pairs of centrioles cannot become competent for another round of replication until they disengage in the subsequent telophase. Therefore, in normal cells, centrosomes are only duplicated once per cell cycle. But, cell-cycle defects that weaken the blocks against centriole rereplication appear to arise during the evolution of many cancers (Nigg, 2002). At the start of mitosis, the presence of extra centrosomes results in a spindle with more than 2 poles being formed. If such a multipolar spindle is stable, the resulting anaphase typically generates 3 or more daughter cells. In such cases, the daughter cells usually die as a consequence of profound aneuploidy. Frequently, however, multipolar spindles collapse into bipolar spindles prior to anaphase, with the extra centrosome clustered around 1 of the 2 spindle poles (Ganem et al, 2009). Such divisions generate only 2 daughter cells but often result in chromosome missegregation as a result of additional attachments being made to kinetochores by the extra centrosome.

Tetraploid cells can arise when anaphase or cytokinesis fail. Some tissues, such as the liver, intentionally give rise to tetraploid cells. But in most cell types, tetraploidy usually results from errors. Because centrosomes are not segregated when tetraploid cells form, tetraploid cells almost always have excessive centrosomes, which may help explain the high rates of chromosomal instability in tetraploid cells (Ganem et al, 2007).

9.4 CELL DEATH

The balance between cell viability and cell death is critical for all organisms, and involves a network of proteins and communication amongst several signaling pathways. Impaired cell death is associated with various human pathologies, including immunodeficiency, autoimmunity, neurodegenerative diseases and cancer. Similar to proliferation, cell death is also essential for embryonic and postnatal development and for tissue homeostasis.

Different types of cell death occur in mammalian cells, including apoptosis (or programmed cell death) and necrosis. Autophagic cell death has been also reported, but current evidence supports a more prominent role of autophagy in cell survival rather than cell death (see Chap. 12, Sec. 12.3.7; Kroemer and Levine, 2008). While initially most of the focus has been placed on apoptosis, which is a highly regulated mechanism involving interplay among a large number of pro- and antiapoptotic proteins, mounting evidence has emerged to support the genetic regulation of necrosis. Although many proteins have been shown to play critical roles in the different types of mammalian cell death mechanisms, recent studies have unraveled additional functions for a number of these proteins in other important cellular processes.

9.4.1 Morphological Changes Associated with Different Types of Cell Death

Morphological changes within dying cells provide important criteria to distinguish between apoptosis and necrotic cell death. Changes associated with apoptosis include rounding up of the cell, plasma membrane blebbing, cytoplasm shrinkage, alteration of membrane asymmetry, and condensation and fragmentation of the nucleus (Fig. 9–10A). Cells at late stages of apoptosis become fragmented into apoptotic bodies that are eliminated by phagocytic cells without triggering inflammation.

Necrosis-associated cellular changes are manifested by swelling of the cell, mitochondria and cytoplasmic organelles, followed by focal rupture of the plasma membrane. Moderate chromatin condensation is also displayed by necrotic cells. More advanced stages of necrosis are associated with disintegration of all cellular components and inflammation (see Fig. 9–10B).

Transcriptional changes, protein levels and posttranslational modifications can also help differentiate among the different types of cell death.

9.4.2 Mechanisms of Apoptosis

The first evidence that apoptosis is genetically regulated arose from studies of the nematode *Caenorhabditis elegans* (Kinchen and Hengartner, 2005). During the development of this invertebrate, 131 of the 1090 somatic cells died by apoptosis, and genetic screens identified several genes required for this process. Loss-of-function mutations of *C. elegans egl-1*, *ced-3* or *ced-4*, or gain-of-function mutations of *ced-9* result in survival of the 131 cells programmed to die. The Ced-4 proapoptotic protein binds to Ced-3 and Ced-9, and genetic studies demonstrated that Ced-4 functions downstream of Ced-9 but upstream to Ced-3 (Fig. 9–11). These genetic studies of apoptosis in *C. elegans* have contributed remarkably to our knowledge of the mechanisms of apoptosis in mammalian cells. In 2002, Sydney Brenner, Robert Horvitz, and John Sulston were

Apoptotic cell

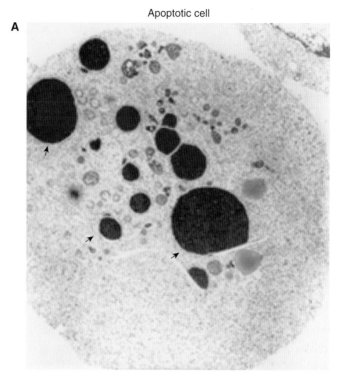

Necrotic cell

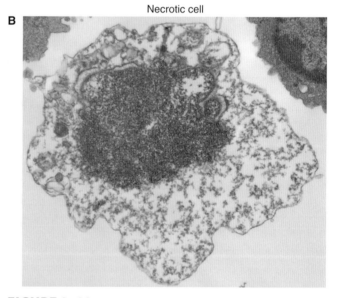

FIGURE 9–10 **Morphological changes within dying cells.** Transmission electron microscopy images of apoptotic (**A**) and necrotic (**B**) cells. Arrows indicate fragmented and condensed nuclear chromatin.

awarded the Nobel Prize in Medicine or Physiology for their elucidation of the genetic regulation of organ development and programmed cell death in *C. elegans*.

Apoptosis is triggered in mammalian cells in response to endogenous stimuli (eg, growth factor deprivation) or exogenous stimuli (eg, irradiation or genotoxic chemotherapeutic drugs). Apoptosis is also induced in response to inadequate cell–matrix interactions and this specific type of apoptosis is

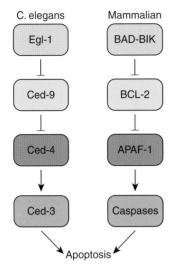

C. elegans   Mammalian

Egl-1   BAD-BIK

Ced-9   BCL-2

Ced-4   APAF-1

Ced-3   Caspases

Apoptosis

FIGURE 9–11 **Major regulators of apoptosis in *C. elegans* and their mammalian orthologs.** Schematic of the major components of the apoptotic pathway in *C. elegans* (left). Mammalian cells have evolved several orthologs to the pro- and antiapoptotic proteins of *C. elegans* (right; see text).

known as *anoikis*. In addition, programmed cell death is also critical for embryonic development, and for the elimination of autoreactive T and B cells (Conradt, 2009).

Biochemical and genetic studies have demonstrated the existence of multiple orthologs of the *C. elegans* apoptotic proteins Ced-9, Ced-4, and Ced-3. These studies also demonstrated the existence of 2 major apoptotic pathways in mammalian cells; the death receptor (also known as extrinsic) apoptotic pathway and the mitochondrial (also known as intrinsic) apoptotic pathway (Fig. 9–12). Mammalian apoptotic pathways are highly controlled and their regulation involves various proteins including anti-apoptotic (eg, BCL-2 and BCL-X$_L$) and proapoptotic (eg, caspases "CASP," FAS, BIM, and BAX) proteins (Fig. 9–13).

Biochemical studies have proven instrumental for the identification and characterization of the components involved in the initiation, propagation, or inhibition of the mammalian apoptotic signaling pathways. Genetic studies in mice possessing a disruption within, or overexpression of, specific pro- or antiapoptotic genes have been critical to demonstrate the in vivo apoptotic functions of these proteins, and have helped to identify developmental defects and diseases associated with impaired apoptosis.

9.4.2.1 BCL-2 Family Members and Their Roles in Apoptosis
The mammalian *Bcl-2* gene, a homolog of the *C. elegans Ced-9*, is a prototypical member of the BCL-2 family that includes antiapoptotic proteins such as BCL-2, BCL-X$_L$, BCL-W, A1, and MCL-1, and proapoptotic proteins, such as BAX, BCL-X$_S$, BAK, BAD, BIK, BIM, BID, and PUMA (see Fig. 9–13; Tait and Green, 2010). Proteins of the BCL-2 family are essential for the initiation and regulation of mammalian apoptosis. These proteins share several conserved domains

known as "BCL-2 homology" (BH) regions including BH1, BH2, BH3, and BH4. These domains allow the formation of homo- and heterodimers between BCL-2 family members and are essential for the function of these proteins. BCL-2 family members play important roles in the regulation of apoptosis. For example, overexpression of BCL-2 in mammalian cells inhibits the release of Cytochrome *C* as well as other factors important for apoptosis (eg, apoptosis-inducing factor [AIF], SMAC, and OMI) from the mitochondrial intermembrane space into the cytosol. Overexpression of BCL-2 also prolongs the survival of cells and increases their resistance to a variety of apoptotic stimuli, including glucocorticoids, phorbol esters, ionomycin, anti-CD3 monoclonal antibodies, irradiation, and chemotherapeutic agents.

9.4.2.2 Role of Caspases in Apoptosis
Mammalian caspases, "cysteine-dependent aspartate specific proteases," are the orthologs of the *C. elegans* protein Ced-3. The first caspase (ICE or CASP1) was identified in 1993 on the basis of its similarity to Ced-3. More than 14 mammalian caspases have since been cloned (Fig. 9–14; Li and Yuan, 2008). Caspases are present in the cytosol in their inactive forms (procaspases or zymogens). To be activated, they require proteolytic cleavage at specific aspartate residues. Active caspases are heterotetrameric complexes composed of 2 large subunits (~20 kDa) and 2 small subunits (~10 kDa) (see Fig. 9–14). All caspases contain an active site pentapeptide (QACXG; X is R, Q, or G). Although caspases are primarily known for their apoptotic function, caspases such as CASP1 and CASP11 play important roles in inflammation. Mounting evidence supports that CASP8 also possesses nonapoptotic functions (see below).

Caspases possess a wide range of expression patterns throughout mammalian tissues. The finding that caspases are able to sequentially process and activate other caspases, together with the structural studies of these proteins, has allowed the classification of caspases into "initiators" (eg, CASP8, CASP9 and CASP10) or "executioners" of apoptosis (eg, CASP3, CASP6, and CASP7). Initiator procaspases contain large prodomains, whereas executioner procaspases contain small prodomains.

Hundreds of caspase substrates have been identified, including cytoskeleton proteins (eg, Actin and Gelsolin), nuclear proteins (eg, Lamin A and B), proteins involved in DNA damage repair (eg, PARP, RAD51, and DNA-PKcs), cell-cycle proteins (eg, p21, p27, CDC27, and RB), cytokines (eg, IL-1β and IL-18) and apoptotic proteins (eg, Caspases, BCL-2, BCL-X$_L$, BID, BAX, and ICAD) (Luthi and Martin, 2007). The caspase-activated DNase (CAD) is inactive when associated with its inhibitor ICAD (also known as DNA fragmentation factor [DFF]). In response to apoptotic stimuli, ICAD is cleaved by caspases allowing the release of the active endonuclease CAD to cleave DNA of apoptotic cells to produce internucleosomal DNA cleavage, a characteristic of apoptosis.

A number of caspases also have proinflammatory functions. These caspases include CASP1, -4, -5, -11, and -12 (Li and

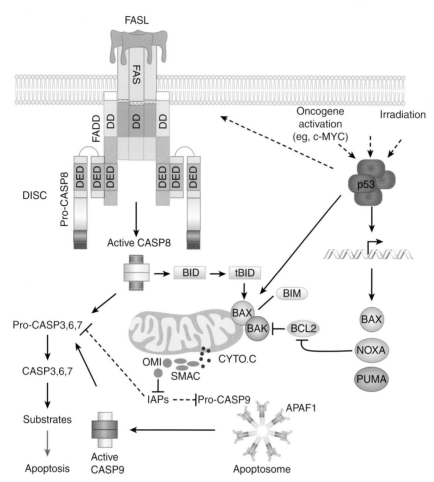

FIGURE 9–12 Schematic of the 2 major apoptotic pathways in mammalian cells. The death receptor pathway is exemplified by the events that occur following engagement of FAS (CD95) by its ligand FASL (CD95L). FAS/FASL interaction leads to the trimerization of the FAS receptor and the recruitment of the adaptor protein FADD to the cytoplasmic tail of FAS. The interaction FAS/FADD is mediated by their respective death domains (DD). This interaction allows the recruitment of CASP8 (and CASP10 in human cells) and the formation of the death-inducing signaling complex (DISC). The presence of these caspases in the DISC results in their oligomerization, autoactivation and subsequent processing of downstream effector caspases (CASP3, -6, and -7). Once activated, effector caspases cleave various cellular proteins leading to apoptotic cell death. The mitochondrial apoptotic pathway is triggered in response to various stimuli including oncogenic activation and DNA damage. Activation of the tumor suppressor and transcriptional factor p53 in response to cellular stresses leads to the transcriptional activation of several proapoptotic genes (eg, BAX, PUMA, NOXA, and FAS). Activation of BAX and BAK leads to outer membrane permeabilization and the release to the cytosol of of a number of mitochondrial proteins including Cytochrome C (CYTO.C). CYTO.C clusters with APAF-1 and the pro-CASP9, forming the apoptosome. The oligomerization of pro-CASP9 within the apoptosome leads to its activation and the subsequent processing of downstream caspases and cell death. In certain cell types, the cleavage of BID by CASP8 generates tBID, a truncated form of BID that translocates to the mitochondria and cooperates with BAX-BAK in inducing the mitochondrial apoptotic pathway.

Yuan, 2008). CASP8 is important in other cellular functions, including blood vessel formation during embryogenesis and mitogen- or antigen-induced proliferation of T and B cells (Su and Lenardo, 2008).

The hierarchical involvement of caspases in the extrinsic and intrinsic apoptotic pathways, impaired apoptosis in their absence, and the nonapoptotic functions ascribed for the caspases all highlight the importance of this family of proteins.

9.4.2.3 Cytochrome *c*, APAF-1, and Apoptosis The apoptosis protease activating factor-1 (APAF-1) is the first identified mammalian ortholog of Ced-4. Studies of APAF-1

have demonstrated its critical role for the intrinsic apoptotic pathway (Tait and Green, 2010). APAF-1 is a 130-kDa protein composed of 3 functional domains: a short N-terminal CARD, a central Ced-4 homology domain, and a long C-terminal "WD-40" repeat domain. Following the release of Cytochrome *C* from mitochondrial intermembrane space, it binds to APAF-1, and induces its conformational change and oligomerization, thus leading to the formation of the apoptosome (see Fig. 9–12). Similar to the death-inducing signaling complex (DISC) and CASP8, the apoptosome recruits, dimerizes, and activates the initiator CASP9, thus leading to apoptosis. A number of studies have demonstrated that Cytochrome *C*, APAF-1, and CASP9 are all required for the activation of the

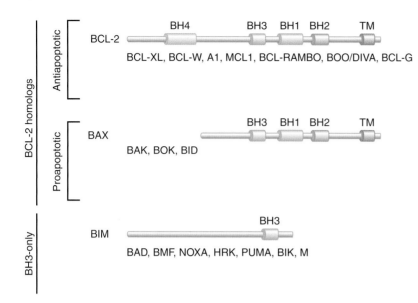

FIGURE 9–13 **BCL-2 family members include both anti- and proapoptotic proteins and are classified into different groups.** The antiapoptotic group of BCL-2 homologs (eg, BCL-2, BCL-XL, and MCL1) contain 4 BCL-2 homology (BH) domains (BH1 to BH4), and a transmembrane domain (TM). Members of the proapoptotic group of BCL-2 homologs (eg, BAX, BAK, and BID) contain TM, BH1, BH2, and BH3, but lack BH4. Finally, the BH3-only proteins (eg, BIM, NOXA, and PUMA) lack all the domains of the BCL-2 family members with the exception of BH3.

downstream effectors CASP3, -6, and -7. Transcriptional regulation of APAF-1 has been reported to be mediated by E2F1 and p53, suggesting its possible contribution to E2F1- and p53-mediated apoptosis. The BCL-2 family member and

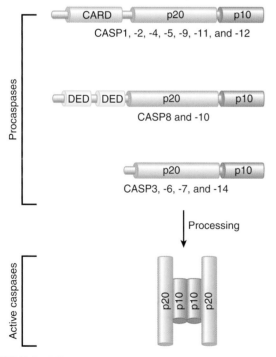

FIGURE 9–14 **Mammalian caspases.** Caspases exist in an inactive form (procaspases) that require autoprocessing or proteolytic cleavage by upstream caspases in order to be activated. The first group of caspases (CASP1, -2, -4, -5, -9, -11, and -12) contain caspases that contain caspase recruitment domain (CARD) and the subunits p20 and p10. The second group include CASP8 and CASP10, which possess 2 N-terminal death effector domains (DEDs) and the subunits p20 and p10. The third group contains CASP3, -6, -7, and -14. These caspases contain only the 2 subunits, p20 and p10. The processing of procaspases allows the formation of active caspases that consist of heterotetrameric complexes composed of 2 p20 and 2 p10 subunits.

antiapoptotic protein BCL-X$_L$ interacts with APAF-1 and CASP9, and forms a ternary complex. Through this interaction, BCL-X$_L$ negatively regulates CASP9 activation.

By mediating apoptosome formation, Cytochrome C and APAF-1 play essential roles in the mitochondrial apoptotic pathway.

9.4.3 The Mitochondrial Apoptotic Pathway

Apoptotic stimuli, which trigger the mitochondrial or intrinsic apoptotic pathway, activate BAX and BAK and lead to mitochondrial outer membrane permeabilization and the release of a number of proteins important for apoptosis (eg, Cytochrome C, SMAC, and OMI) from the mitochondrial intermembrane space into the cytosol (see Fig. 9–12; Tait and Green, 2010). Mitochondrial membrane permeabilization is suppressed by the antiapoptotic BCL-2 family members (eg, BCL-2 and BCL-X$_L$), as they bind and inhibit activated BAX or BAK as well as other BH3-only proteins. Once in the cytosol, Cytochrome C forms the apoptosome with APAF-1 and CASP9, thus leading to activation of CASP9, which, in turn, processes and activates downstream effector caspases. This leads to cleavage of various cellular substrates, and cell death.

Caspase activity is modulated by various members of the family of inhibitors of apoptosis (IAPs). IAPs were originally discovered in baculoviruses and shown to suppress the host cell death response to viral infection (Altieri, 2010). Currently, 8 human IAPs have been identified, including the X-linked IAP (XIAP), Survivin, and cellular IAP1 and -2 (c-IAP1 and c-IAP2). Several IAPs bind directly to caspases such as CASP3, -7, and -9 and inhibit their functions. This IAPs-mediated inhibition of caspases can be antagonized by the proteins SMAC and OMI (see Fig. 9–12). When SMAC and OMI are released from the mitochondrial intermembrane space into the cytosol, they bind directly to XIAP and suppress its inhibition of caspases. In addition to their roles in apoptosis, IAPs are also involved in other processes including nuclear factor kappa B (NF-κB) signaling, cell division, and cellular stress responses.

The mitochondrial apoptotic pathway is essential for the response to DNA damage and oncogenic activation. The tumor suppressor p53 plays a critical role in this apoptotic pathway as it controls the transactivation of a number of essential pro-apoptotic BCL-2 family members including PUMA, BAX, and NOXA. In addition to controlling different cellular processes, including proliferation (see Sec. 9.4.1), the activated oncogene c-MYC (see Chap. 7, Sec. 7.5.2) also induces apoptosis (Meyer and Penn, 2008). c-MYC induced apoptosis is p53 dependent (see Fig. 9–12). Deregulated c-MYC also promotes the accumulation of the tumor suppressor ARF that sequesters MDM2 in the nucleolus, thus releasing p53 from MDM2-mediated inhibition. Thus the ARF-MDM2-p53 pathway is important for c-MYC–induced apoptosis.

Posttranslational modifications play important roles in the regulation of the mitochondrial apoptotic pathway (Newton and Vucic, 2007). For example, MCL-1 is ubiquitinated by ARF-BP1, targeting it for proteasomal degradation (Fig. 9–4B). Evidence exists that IAPs ubiquitinate mammalian caspases and the *Drosophila* IAP (DIAP1) polyubiquitinates the caspase orthologs Dronc, Dcp-1, and drICE leading to their nondegradative inactivation. Polyubiquitination of BCL-2, BAX, BIK, NOXA, BID, and BIM has also been reported to lead to their proteasomal degradation, thus controlling their levels of expression.

Deregulation of this apoptotic pathway has been associated with a number of diseases, including cancer.

9.4.4 The Death Receptor Apoptotic Pathway

The death receptor or extrinsic apoptotic pathway is initiated by the interaction of the death receptors, members of the tumor necrosis factor (TNF) receptor superfamily, with their ligands (Wilson et al, 2009). The death receptors share the presence of an approximately 80-amino-acid motif known as the death domain (DD) in their cytoplasmic tails. Six human death receptors have been identified and include FAS (also known as CD95 or APO-1), TNFR-1, death receptor (DR) 3, DR4 (also known as TRAILR1), DR5 (also known as TRAILR2), and DR6. Several ligands for these death receptors have been identified and include TNF and LTα (TNFR1), FASL (FAS), TL1A (DR3), and APO2L/TRAIL (DR4 and DR5). The ligand for DR6 remains unknown.

The death receptor apoptotic pathway is exemplified by the FAS-induced apoptotic signaling pathway (see Fig. 9–12; Strasser et al, 2009). Following FAS/FASL interaction, the FAS receptor proteins aggregate to form a trimer and recruit the adaptor protein FADD (FAS-associated death domain) that contains 2 protein interaction domains, a death domain, and a death effector domain (DED). FAS/FADD interaction allows the recruitment of the DED-containing initiator pro-CASP8 (and also pro-CASP10 in human) and the formation of the DISC. Dimerization of pro-CASP8 within the DISC allows its autoprocessing, activation and the formation and release of its

active tetrameric form into the cytosol. Active CASP8 in the cytosol processes its substrates including the effector CASP3, CASP6 and CASP7, and the BH3-only protein BID. Cellular FLICE-like inhibitory protein (cFLIP), a pseudo-CASP8 protein with a nonfunctional catalytic domain, inhibits the death receptor apoptotic pathway by precluding the recruitment of CASP8 to the DISC.

p53 also affects the death receptor apoptotic pathway as demonstrated by p53 transactivation of FAS and DR5 in response to DNA damage (see Figs. 9–12 and 9–15). Posttranslational modifications, including ubiquitination, also play important roles in the death receptor apoptotic pathway (Wertz and Dixit, 2010). In response to stimulation of DR4 or DR5, the E3 ligase CULLIN-3 polyubiquitinates CASP8 present at the DISC. This ubiquitination event recruits the ubiquitin-binding polypeptide p62 that mediates CASP8 aggregation, thus increasing its activation and processing (Jin et al, 2009). c-FLIP, an inhibitor of CASP8 and CASP10, is transcriptionally upregulated by NF-κB and is also regulated by ubiquitylation. The E3 ligase ITCH has been shown to mediate the polyubiquitylation of c-FLIP, leading to its proteasomal degradation (Chang et al, 2006).

Communication between the death receptor and mitochondrial apoptotic pathways is best demonstrated by CASP8 cleavage of BID. This cleavage generates a truncated form of BID (tBID) that cooperates with BAX to form openings in the outer mitochondrial membrane, leading to release of proteins including Cytochrome C from the mitochondrial intermembrane space (see Fig. 9–12). This CASP8 processing of BID amplifies the death receptor apoptotic pathway. In addition, stimulation of the mitochondrial pathway leads to the

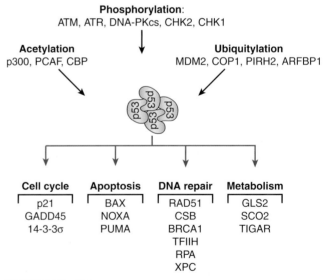

FIGURE 9–15 The tumor suppressor p53 is a mutlifunctional protein highly regulated by posttranslational modifications. Examples of proteins involved in p53 posttranslational modifications (eg, acetylation, phosphorylation, and ubiquitylation) are indicated. Activated p53 plays major roles in a number of cellular processes including cell cycle, apoptosis, DNA repair, and metabolism. Examples of p53 transcriptional targets involved in these cellular processes are indicated (see also Chap. 7, Sec. 7.6.1).

activation of the effector caspases, such as CASP3 and CASP6, that can subsequently process and activate CASP8.

Impaired apoptosis owing to mutations in the components of the death receptor apoptotic pathway has been observed in human and mouse cells. For example, resistance to stimuli that activate this pathway was observed in cells deficient for CASP8, FADD, FAS, FASL, or in cells overexpressing c-FLIP (Strasser et al, 2009). Similar to the mitochondrial apoptotic pathway, the death receptor apoptotic pathway also plays critical roles in development and tissue homeostasis, and is dysregulated in a number of diseases including cancer.

9.4.5 Apoptosis, Developmental Defects, and Disease

Deregulation of apoptosis is associated with human diseases, including immunodeficiency, neurodegeneration, and autoimmunity. Similarly, studies of genetically modified mice deficient in or overexpressing anti- or proapoptotic proteins demonstrate an essential role of apoptosis in the prevention of embryonic and postnatal developmental defects, and to restrain the development of various diseases, including autoimmunity.

9.4.5.1 Antiapoptotic BCL-2 Family Members and Disease

BCL-2 inhibits apoptosis in response to a wide range of stimuli that target the mitochondrial apoptotic pathway. In addition to cancer, overexpression of the prosurvival BCL-2 family members also promotes the development of other diseases, including autoimmunity. Transgenic mice expressing the human BCL-2 in T and B cells develop an autoimmune disorder characterized by antinuclear antibodies and glomerulonephritis (Strasser et al, 1991).

Deficiency of the prosurvival BCL-2 family members (eg, BCL-2, BCL-X$_L$ or MCL-1) results in increased cell death and promotes the development of a number of pathologies (Youle and Strasser, 2008). Mice deficient for BCL-2 display polycystic kidney disease and loss of mature B and T cells as a consequence of increased apoptosis. Bcl-$2^{-/-}$ mice die by 6 weeks of age. Inactivation of Bcl-X$_L$ in mice results in embryonic lethality by day 14 of gestation, which underscores the important role of BCL-X$_L$ in the regulation of programmed cell death during the development of embryonic nervous system and lymphoid organs. Similarly, analysis of mice deficient for MCL-1 demonstrated the importance of this antiapoptotic protein for the survival and implantation of the zygote, while conditional gene targeting of Mcl-1 results in the premature death of immature and mature B and T cells and hematopoietic stem cells (Opferman et al, 2003).

9.4.5.2 Proapoptotic BCL-2 Family Members and Disease

The proapoptotic members of the BCL-2 family also play critical roles in apoptosis and their deregulation has been associated with various pathologies (Youle and Strasser, 2008). While $Bax^{-/-}$ mice display male sterility and mild lymphoid hyperplasia, $Bak^{-/-}$ mice display no such abnormalities.

However, perinatal lethality was observed in $Bax^{-/-}Bak^{-/-}$ mice. The small subset of double mutant mice that survive to adulthood accumulate lymphoid and myeloid cells and typically develop lymphoadenopathy and splenomegaly. The surviving $Bax^{-/-}Bak^{-/-}$ mice also accumulate cells of the central nervous system and fail to remove their interdigital webs.

Other mouse models deficient for 1 or more BH3-only proteins have been generated (Youle and Strasser, 2008). For example, $Bid^{-/-}$ mice display hepatocyte resistance to FAS-induced apoptosis and suffer fatal hepatitis. Mice deficient for either BIM or PUMA display resistance to various apoptotic stimuli that target the intrinsic apoptotic pathway. Similar to $Bax^{-/-}Bak^{-/-}$ mice, mice lacking both BIM and PUMA displayed higher resistance to apoptosis compared to single mutants, thus indicating cooperation between these 2 proteins. $Puma^{-/-}$ mice possess a normal life span and show no increased predisposition to diseases. In contrast, because of its important roles in the deletion of autoreactive T and B cells and its requirement for the downregulation of immune responses, $Bim^{-/-}$ mice display splenomegaly and lymphadenopathy, and in a C57BL/6x129SV genetic background they develop a fatal systemic lupus erythematosus (SLE)-like autoimmune disease. Recent studies demonstrate that the autoimmunity of $Bim^{-/-}$ mice is further exacerbated in a Fas mutant background (Strasser et al, 2009). These studies demonstrate the collaboration of the mitochondrial and the death receptor apoptotic pathways in the elimination of autoreactive cells and the prevention of autoimmune disorders.

Collectively, the data strongly support that both the anti- and the pro-apoptotic BCL-2 family members are important for in vivo apoptosis, and that deregulation of a number of proteins in this family leads to developmental defects and immune disorders.

9.4.5.3 Caspases and Disease

Mice deficient for specific caspases demonstrate the crucial role for apoptosis in development (Li and Yuan, 2008). $Casp3^{-/-}$ and $casp9^{-/-}$ mice exhibit a similar brain defect characterized by ectopic masses of supernumerary cells that escape apoptosis during brain development (Fig. 9–16; Hakem et al, 1998; Woo et al, 1998). $Casp12^{-/-}$ mice are resistant to apoptosis induced in response to stress to the endoplasmic reticulum, but undergo apoptosis in response to other stimuli (eg, FAS or dexamethasone). $Casp2^{-/-}$ mice are viable, and although most of $casp2^{-/-}$ cells fail to show any significant defect in apoptosis, $casp2^{-/-}$ B lymphoblasts display defective cytolysis mediated by Perforin and Granzyme B. $Casp2^{-/-}$ females display excess ovarian germ cells and resistance of oocytes to antineoplastic drug-induced apoptosis.

The autoimmune lymphoproliferative syndrome (ALPS), a rare inherited human disorder, is characterized by lymphoproliferation, accumulation of CD4$^-$CD8$^-$ (double-negative) T lymphocytes and autoantibody production (Su and Lenardo, 2008). This syndrome is associated with heterozygous mutations of FAS or $FASL$. ALPS patients are at an increased risk to develop lymphomas. Mice that carry homozygous mutations of FAS or FASL also develop an ALPS-like

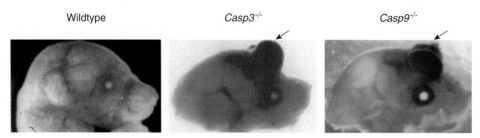

Wildtype   Casp3⁻/⁻   Casp9⁻/⁻

FIGURE 9–16 Developmental defects associated with deficiency of caspases. Postnatal day 1 wild-type, Caspase 3 deficient (*casp3⁻/⁻*), and Caspase 9 deficient (*casp9⁻/⁻*) mice are shown. Arrows point to the characteristic perturbation of brain (cortex and forebrain) structures observed in both *casp3⁻/⁻* and *casp9⁻/⁻* mutants.

syndrome characterized by splenomegaly, lymphadenopathy, hypergammaglobulinemia, autoantibody production, and glomerulonephritis. Homozygous mutations of *CASP8* are associated with an ALPS-like syndrome. Patients with this rare syndrome are immunodeficient and display lymphadenopathy, splenomegaly, and impaired lymphocyte activation. *Casp8⁻/⁻* mice display defects in the heart and neural tube, accumulate erythrocytes, and die by embryonic day 12 (Li and Yuan, 2008). Remarkably, similar to the ALPS-like syndrome of CASP8 mutant patients, mice with specific inactivation of *casp8* in T-cell lineage are also immunodeficient, exhibit impaired T-cell homeostasis characterized by T-cell lymphopenia, and have impaired responses to viral infection (Salmena et al, 2003). These mice also have short lifespans as they develop an age-dependent and fatal lymphoproliferative disorder (Salmena and Hakem, 2005). In addition, CASP8 deficiency in the B-cell lineage promoted development of lymphomas in mouse models (Hakem et al., 2012).

Caspases are therefore important for in vivo apoptosis. Impairment of their functions can lead to defective embryonic and postnatal development, and promote the development of diseases including immunodeficiency and lymphoproliferation.

9.4.6 Mechanisms Leading to Necrosis

Although necrosis was thought initially to be a nonregulated process, recent studies demonstrate that necroptosis, a programmed type of necrosis, is highly regulated by a network of proteins (Christofferson and Yuan, 2010). Ligands binding to death receptors upon the plasma membrane of normal cells leads to CASP8-dependent cleavage and inactivation of the receptor-interacting protein RIPK1 and RIPK3 (also known as RIP1 and RIP3, respectively) (Fig. 9–17). Activated CASP8 also cleaves downstream targets including the executioner Caspases 3, 6, and 7, and thus promotes cell death by apoptosis. However, together with the presence of defective death receptor signaling, cells lacking CASP8 activity fail to induce cleavage of RIPK1 and RIPK3. These kinases are therefore normally active in CASP8 deficient cells and can trigger cell death by necroptosis. T cells deficient for CASP8 die by necroptosis and inhibitors of necroptosis (eg, necrostatin 1) rescue the survival of these T cells. A genome wide short-interference RNA screen for regulators of necrosis has identified 432 genes

that regulate this type of necrotic cell death (Hitomi et al, 2008). BMF, a BH3-only BCL2 family member was found to be important for death receptor-induced necrosis. Recent data demonstrated that genetic inactivation of *Ripk3* rescues embryonic lethality of *casp8⁻/⁻* mice and restores survival of their T cells (Peter, 2011). Similarly, the absence of *Ripk1* rescued the embryonic lethality of *Fadd⁻/⁻* mice and the proliferative defects of their T cells.

These genetic data demonstrate the strong interactions between the mechanisms that control apoptotic and necrotic cell death.

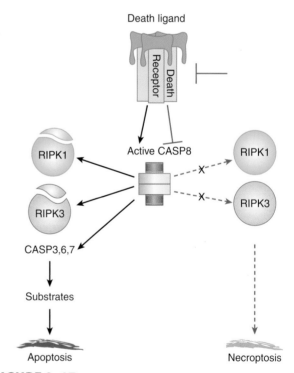

FIGURE 9–17 Representation of the crosstalk between apoptosis and necroptosis. In response to the binding of ligands to death receptors (eg, TNFR1) on the plasma membrane, active CASP8 inactivates RIPK1 and RIPK3 by proteolytic cleavage and also processes downstream caspases to promote apoptosis. In the case where death receptor signaling is impaired or CASP8 is lost or inhibited, the executioner caspases are not activated and RIPK1 and RIPK3 are not cleaved and thus remain active. Active RIPK1 and RIPK3 trigger necroptosis, a programmed necrotic cell death.

9.4.7 Modifications to Control of Cell Death in Cancer

Resisting programmed cell death has been proposed as 1 of 6 hallmarks of cancer (Hanahan and Weinberg, 2000). A number of tumor suppressors (eg, p53) and oncogenes (eg, c-MYC, BCL-2; see Chap. 7, Sec. 7.5.2) important for human cancer are involved in the regulation of apoptosis. The *p53* gene, important for promoting apoptosis and suppressing proliferation, is mutated in more than 50% of human tumors. Consistent with the critical role p53 plays in suppressing human cancer, mouse models for p53 deficiency have increased predisposition for various types of tumors (Lozano, 2010).

p53 is required for the apoptotic response to various stimuli, including DNA damage, oncogenic activation, hypoxia, and ribosomal stress. As a transcription factor, p53 controls the expression of genes involved in different cellular processes such as apoptosis, proliferation, metabolism, and DNA repair (see Fig. 9–15). Apoptotic genes that are transcriptionally activated by p53 include *Bax*, *Noxa* and *Puma*.

The *Bcl-2* gene, was identified initially in studies of human follicular B-cell lymphoma carrying the translocation t(14-18). This chromosomal translocation results in the overexpression of BCL-2 and inhibition of apoptosis. The antiapoptotic protein MCL-1 is also overexpressed in a number of human malignancies including B-cell lymphoma, and myeloma (Warr and Shore, 2008). Mutations of the proapoptotic proteins are also observed in human cancers. Thus, human *Bax* was reported to be mutated in colon cancer and hematopoietic malignancies (Meijerink et al, 1998; Rampino et al, 1997). Loss of CASP8 expression because of hypermethylation of its promoter has been observed in human neuroblastomas with N-MYC amplification, small cell lung carcinoma, and in relapsed glioblastoma multiforme. Inactivation of human *Casp8* by somatic mutations is observed in hepatocellular carcinomas and advanced gastric cancer (Fulda, 2009). In addition to cancer development, loss of CASP8 is also reported to promote metastasis of neuroblastoma.

Studies of mouse models have confirmed the important role apoptosis plays in suppressing cancer. Transgenic mice overexpressing BCL-2 in lymphocytes develop lymphomas (McDonnell and Korsmeyer, 1991) and risk for lymphoma was also increased in transgenic mice overexpressing MCL-1 in hematopoietic and lymphoid tissues (Zhou et al, 2001). BCL-2 inhibits c-MYC–induced apoptosis and, consequently, transgenic mice overexpressing both BCL-2 and c-MYC in B-cell lineages (Strasser et al, 1990) or mammary glands (Jager et al, 1997) display elevated cancer risk compared to *c-Myc* transgenic mice. c-MYC–induced tumorigenesis is also promoted by the overexpression of the antiapoptotic proteins BCL-X$_L$ and MCL-1 (Campbell et al, 2010; Cheung et al, 2004).

Radiation and most chemotherapeutic agents (eg, platinum derivatives) used in the clinic trigger the death of tumors. There is a continous effort to generate novel compounds to modulate cell death, particularly apoptosis, and improve the response of cancer patients to therapies (Ashkenazi, 2008 #991; Davids, 2012 #990). Some of these compounds are currently in clinical trials as single agents or in combination with other chemotherapeutic drugs. Compounds that activate the death receptor pathway include agonists and human monoclonal antibodies to proapoptotic receptors DR4 and DR5 and their ligand APO2L/TRAIL. Radiation and most chemotherapeutic agents kill through activation of the mitochondrial apoptotic pathway; therefore, significant efforts have been made to identify compounds to activate this pathway. Approaches have been designed to inhibit the prosurvival members of BCL-2 family or activate its pro-apoptotic members. This is exemplified by the small molecule BH3 mimetic ABT-737, and the closely related and orally bioavailable ABT-263. These compounds bind to BCL-2, BCL-X, and BCL-W and kill tumors by displacing pro-apoptotic proteins from BCL-2. Promising results have been obtained with ABT-263, and several clinical trials are underway to assess therapeutic benefit of its combination with standard anti-cancer agents.

In addition to promoting development of a number of diseases, including neurodegenerative diseases and immune disorders, defective apoptosis also promotes cancer development. Mechanisms that lead to cell death or survival can be targeted to improve cancer therapy.

SUMMARY

- The entry of resting cells into cycle, and the orderly progression of cells to synthesize DNA and subsequently to divide at mitosis is tightly regulated by the synthesis, activation and subsequent degradation of proteins.
- Different CDKs are activated by phosphorylation after binding to corresponding CYCLINs, and allow progression around the cell cycle. Other families of proteins inhibit CDKs, so that both positive and negative effectors contribute to regulation of cell-cycle progression.
- Expression of molecules that regulate the cell cycle may become disturbed in malignant cells with a resulting loss of control of cell proliferation.
- Various checkpoints arrest the cell cycle in response to DNA damage or to difficulties in segregating the chromosomes, but these may also be modified in the development of malignancy.
- Different cell death mechanisms, including the programmed apoptosis and necroptosis, exist in mammalian cells. Communication between these cell death mechanisms has been identified and is thought to balance prosurvival and prodeath signals.
- Deregulation of cell death processes leads to multiple developmental defects and disease in several tissue types.
- Deregulation of apoptosis (eg, overexpression of BCL-2 or downregulation of CASP8) has been associated with human cancer.
- Specific inhibitors of apoptosis or necroptosis have been developed. Based on the importance of cell death processes in diseases, these inhibitors might have great potentials for therapeutic intervention.

ACKNOWLEDGMENTS

PJ thanks Rick Deibler, Amit Tzur, James Orth, Kevin Haigis, Jennifer Waters, and Matthew Vander Heiden for sharing their expertise. PJ thanks Marc Kirschner and Jason Moffat for support.

REFERENCES

Altieri DC. Survivin and IAP proteins in cell-death mechanisms. *Biochem J* 2010;430:199-205.

Arias EE, Walter JC. Strength in numbers: preventing rereplication via multiple mechanisms in eukaryotic cells. *Genes Dev* 2007;21: 497-518.

Ashkenazi A. Directing cancer cells to self-destruct with pro-apoptotic receptor agonists. *Nat Rev Drug Discov* 2008;7: 1001-1012.

Barr FA, Sillje HH, Nigg EA. Polo-like kinases and the orchestration of cell division. *Nat Rev Mol Cell Biol* 2004;5:429-440.

Beroukhim R, Mermel CH, Porter D, et al. The landscape of somatic copy-number alteration across human cancers. *Nature* 2010;463: 899-905.

Brito DA, Rieder CL. Mitotic checkpoint slippage in humans occurs via cyclin B destruction in the presence of an active checkpoint. *Curr Biol* 2006;16:1194-1200.

Campbell KJ, Bath ML, Turner ML, et al. Elevated Mcl-1 perturbs lymphopoiesis, promotes transformation of hematopoietic stem/progenitor cells, and enhances drug resistance. *Blood* 2010;116: 3197-3207.

Carmena M, Ruchaud S, Earnshaw WC. Making the Auroras glow: regulation of Aurora A and B kinase function by interacting proteins. *Curr Opin Cell Biol* 2009;21:796-805.

Chang L, Kamata H, Solinas G, et al. The E3 ubiquitin ligase itch couples JNK activation to TNFalpha-induced cell death by inducing c-FLIP(L) turnover. *Cell* 2006;124:601-613.

Cheung WC, Kim JS, Linden M, et al. Novel targeted deregulation of c-Myc cooperates with Bcl-X(L) to cause plasma cell neoplasms in mice. *J Clin Invest* 2004;113:1763-1773.

Christofferson DE, Yuan J. Necroptosis as an alternative form of programmed cell death. *Curr Opin Cell Biol* 2010;22:263-268.

Conradt B. Genetic control of programmed cell death during animal development. *Annu Rev Genet* 2009;43:493-523.

Davids MS, Letai A. Targeting the B-cell lymphoma/leukemia 2 family in cancer. *J Clin Oncol* 2012;30:3127-3135.

Deibler RW, Kirschner MW. Quantitative reconstitution of mitotic CDK1 activation in somatic cell extracts. *Mol Cell* 2010;37: 753-767.

Dephoure N, Zhou C, Villen J, et al. A quantitative atlas of mitotic phosphorylation. *Proc Natl Acad Sci U S A* 2008;105:10762-10767.

Di Fiore B, Pines J. Defining the role of Emi1 in the DNA replication-segregation cycle. *Chromosoma* 2008;117:333-338.

Diffley JF. Regulation of early events in chromosome replication. *Curr Biol* 2004;14:R778-86.

Dumont S, Mitchison TJ. Force and length in the mitotic spindle. *Curr Biol* 2009;19:R749-61.

Eggert US, Mitchison TJ, Field CM. Animal cytokinesis: from parts list to mechanisms. *Annu Rev Biochem* 2006;75:543-566.

Eilers M, Eisenman RN. Myc's broad reach. *Genes Dev* 2008;22: 2755-2766.

Fulda S. Caspase-8 in cancer biology and therapy. *Cancer Lett* 2009; 281:128-133.

Ganem NJ, Godinho SA, Pellman D. A mechanism linking extra centrosomes to chromosomal instability. *Nature* 2009;460: 278-282.

Ganem NJ, Storchova Z, Pellman D. Tetraploidy, aneuploidy and cancer. *Curr Opin Genet Dev* 2007;17:157-162.

Gatlin JC, Bloom K. Microtubule motors in eukaryotic spindle assembly and maintenance. *Semin Cell Dev Biol* 2010;21: 248-254.

Gavet O, Pines J. Progressive activation of cyclinB1-Cdk1 coordinates entry to mitosis. *Dev Cell* 2010;18:533-543.

Geley S, Kramer E, Gieffers C, et al. Anaphase-promoting complex/cyclosome-dependent proteolysis of human cyclin A starts at the beginning of mitosis and is not subject to the spindle assembly checkpoint. *J Cell Biol* 2001;153:137-148.

Geng Y, Yu Q, Sicinska E, et al. Cyclin E ablation in the mouse. *Cell* 2003;114:431-443.

Guertin DA, Sabatini DM. Defining the role of mTOR in cancer. *Cancer Cell* 2007;12:9-22.

Guttinger S, Laurell E, Kutay U. Orchestrating nuclear envelope disassembly and reassembly during mitosis. *Nat Rev Mol Cell Biol* 2009;10:178-191.

Hakem A, El Ghamrasni S, Maire G, et al. Caspase-8 is essential for maintaining chromosomal stability and suppressing B-cell lymphomagenesis. *Blood* 2012;119:3495-3502.

Hakem R, Hakem A, Duncan GS, et al. Differential requirement for caspase 9 in apoptotic pathways in vivo. *Cell* 1998;94:339-352.

Hanahan D, Weinberg RA. The hallmarks of cancer. *Cell* 2000;100: 57-70.

Harper JW, Elledge SJ. The role of Cdk7 in CAK function, a retro-retrospective. *Genes Dev* 1998;12:285-289.

Hitomi J, Christofferson DE, Ng A, et al. Identification of a molecular signaling network that regulates a cellular necrotic cell death pathway. *Cell* 2008;135:1311-1323.

Hutchins JR, Toyoda Y, Hegemann B, et al. Systematic analysis of human protein complexes identifies chromosome segregation proteins. *Science* 2010;328:593-599.

Jackson S, Xiong Y. CRL4s: the CUL4-RING E3 ubiquitin ligases. *Trends Biochem Sci* 2009;34:562-570.

Jager R, Herzer U, Schenkel J, Weiher H. Overexpression of Bcl-2 inhibits alveolar cell apoptosis during involution and accelerates c-myc-induced tumorigenesis of the mammary gland in transgenic mice. *Oncogene* 1997;15:1787-1795.

Jiang W, McDonald D, Hope TJ, Hunter T. Mammalian Cdc7-Dbf4 protein kinase complex is essential for initiation of DNA replication. *EMBO J* 1999;18:5703-5713.

Jin Z, Li Y, Pitti R, et al. Cullin3-based polyubiquitination and p62-dependent aggregation of caspase-8 mediate extrinsic apoptosis signaling. *Cell* 2009;137:721-735.

Jones RG, Thompson CB. Tumor suppressors and cell metabolism: a recipe for cancer growth. *Genes Dev* 2009;23:537-548.

Jorgensen P, Tyers M. How cells coordinate growth and division. *Curr Biol* 2004;14:R1014-R1027.

Kalaszczynska I, Geng Y, Iino T, et al. Cyclin A is redundant in fibroblasts but essential in hematopoietic and embryonic stem cells. *Cell* 2009;138:352-365.

Kinchen JM, Hengartner MO. Tales of cannibalism, suicide, and murder: Programmed cell death in C. elegans. *Curr Top Dev Biol* 2005;65:1-45.

Komander D, Clague MJ, Urbé S. Breaking the chains: structure and function of the deubiquitinases. *Nat Rev Mol Cell Biol* 2009;10:550-563.

Kroemer G, Levine B. Autophagic cell death: the story of a misnomer. *Nat Rev Mol Cell Biol* 2008;9:1004-1010.

Li J, Yuan J. Caspases in apoptosis and beyond. *Oncogene* 2008;27:6194-6206.

Lindqvist A, Rodriguez-Bravo V, Medema RH. The decision to enter mitosis: feedback and redundancy in the mitotic entry network. *J Cell Biol* 2009;185:193-202.

Liu P, Cheng H, Roberts TM, Zhao JJ. Targeting the phosphoinositide 3-kinase pathway in cancer. *Nat Rev Drug Discov* 2009;8:627-644.

Lozano G. Mouse models of p53 functions. *Cold Spring Harb Perspect Biol* 2010;2:a001115.

Luthi AU, Martin SJ. The CASBAH: a searchable database of caspase substrates. *Cell Death Differ* 2007;14:641-650.

Malek NP, Sundberg H, McGrew S, et al. A mouse knock-in model exposes sequential proteolytic pathways that regulate p27Kip1 in G1 and S phase. *Nature* 2001;413:323-327.

Malumbres M, Barbacid M. To cycle or not to cycle: a critical decision in cancer. *Nat Rev Cancer* 2001;1:222-231.

Malumbres M, Harlow E, Hunt T, et al. Cyclin-dependent kinases: a family portrait. *Nat Cell Biol* 2009;11:1275-1276.

Malumbres M, Pevarello P, Barbacid M, Bischoff JR. CDK inhibitors in cancer therapy: what is next? *Trends Pharmacol Sci* 2008;29:16-21.

McDonnell TJ, Korsmeyer SJ. Progression from lymphoid hyperplasia to high-grade malignant lymphoma in mice transgenic for the t(14; 18). *Nature* 1991;349:254-256.

Meijerink JP, Mensink EJ, Wang K, et al. Hematopoietic malignancies demonstrate loss-of-function mutations of BAX. *Blood* 1998;91:2991-2997.

Merrick KA, Larochelle S, Zhang C, et al. Distinct activation pathways confer cyclin-binding specificity on Cdk1 and Cdk2 in human cells. *Mol Cell* 2008;32:662-672.

Meyer N, Penn LZ. Reflecting on 25 years with MYC. *Nat Rev Cancer* 2008;8:976-990.

Morgan DO. *The Cell Cycle: Principles of Control.* London, UK: New Science Press; 2007.

Musacchio A, Salmon ED. The spindle-assembly checkpoint in space and time. *Nat Rev Mol Cell Biol* 2007;8:379-393.

Nasmyth K. At the heart of the budding yeast cell cycle. *Trends Genet* 1996;12:405-412.

Nasmyth K, Haering CH. Cohesin: its roles and mechanisms. *Annu Rev Genet* 2009;43:525-558.

Newton K, Vucic D. Ubiquitin ligases in cancer: ushers for degradation. *Cancer Invest* 2007;25:502-513.

Nigg EA. Centrosome aberrations: cause or consequence of cancer progression? *Nat Rev Cancer* 2002;2:815-825.

O'Farrell PH. Triggering the all-or-nothing switch into mitosis. *Trends Cell Biol* 2001;11:512-519.

Oliveira RA, Hamilton RS, Pauli A, et al. Cohesin cleavage and Cdk inhibition trigger formation of daughter nuclei. *Nat Cell Biol* 2010;12:185-192.

Opferman JT, Letai A, Beard C, et al. Development and maintenance of B and T lymphocytes requires antiapoptotic MCL-1. *Nature* 2003;426:671-676.

Peter ME. Programmed cell death: Apoptosis meets necrosis. *Nature* 2011;471:310-312.

Peters JM. The anaphase promoting complex/cyclosome: a machine designed to destroy. *Nat Rev Mol Cell Biol* 2006;7:644-656.

Peters JM, Tedeschi A, Schmitz J. The cohesin complex and its roles in chromosome biology. *Genes Dev* 2008;22:3089-3114.

Petronczki M, Lenart P, Peters JM. Polo on the Rise-from Mitotic Entry to Cytokinesis with Plk1. *Dev Cell* 2008;14:646-659.

Pfleger CM, Kirschner MW. The KEN box: an APC recognition signal distinct from the D box targeted by Cdh1. *Genes Dev* 2000;14:655-665.

Rampino N, Yamamoto H, Ionov Y, et al. Somatic frameshift mutations in the BAX gene in colon cancers of the microsatellite mutator phenotype. *Science* 1997;275:967-969.

Reinhardt HC, Yaffe MB. Kinases that control the cell cycle in response to DNA damage: Chk1, Chk2, and MK2. *Curr Opin Cell Biol* 2009;21:245-255.

Rieder CL, Cole RW, Khodjakov A, Sluder G. The checkpoint delaying anaphase in response to chromosome monoorientation is mediated by an inhibitory signal produced by unattached kinetochores. *J Cell Biol* 1995;130:941-948.

Sakaue-Sawano A, Kurokawa H, Morimura T, et al. Visualizing spatiotemporal dynamics of multicellular cell-cycle progression. *Cell* 2008;132:487-498.

Salmena L, Hakem R. Caspase-8 deficiency in T cells leads to a lethal lymphoinfiltrative immune disorder. *J Exp Med* 2005;202:727-732.

Salmena L, Lemmers B, Hakem A, et al. Essential role for caspase 8 in T-cell homeostasis and T-cell-mediated immunity. *Genes Dev* 2003;17:883-895.

Sansal I, Sellers WR. The biology and clinical relevance of the PTEN tumor suppressor pathway. *J Clin Oncol* 2004;22:2954-2963.

Santamaria D, Barriere C, Cerqueira A, et al. Cdk1 is sufficient to drive the mammalian cell cycle. *Nature* 2007;448:811-815.

Sherr CJ, Roberts JM. CDK inhibitors: positive and negative regulators of G1-phase progression. *Genes Dev* 1999;13:1501-1512.

Stemmann O, Zou H, Gerber SA, et al. Dual inhibition of sister chromatid separation at metaphase. *Cell* 2001;107:715-726.

Strasser A, Harris AW, Bath ML, Cory S. Novel primitive lymphoid tumours induced in transgenic mice by cooperation between myc and bcl-2. *Nature* 1990;348:331-333.

Strasser A, Jost PJ, Nagata S. The many roles of FAS receptor signaling in the immune system. *Immunity* 2009;30:180-192.

Strasser A, Whittingham S, Vaux DL, et al. Enforced BCL2 expression in B-lymphoid cells prolongs antibody responses and elicits autoimmune disease. *Proc Natl Acad Sci U S A* 1991;88:8661-8665.

Su HC, Lenardo MJ. Genetic defects of apoptosis and primary immunodeficiency. *Immunol Allergy Clin North Am* 2008;28:329-351, ix.

Sullivan M, Morgan DO. Finishing mitosis, one step at a time. *Nat Rev Mol Cell Biol* 2007;8:894-903.

Tait SW, Green DR. Mitochondria and cell death: outer membrane permeabilization and beyond. *Nat Rev Mol Cell Biol* 2010;11:621-632.

Takeda DY, Dutta A. DNA replication and progression through S phase. *Oncogene* 2005;24:2827-2843.

Takizawa CG, Morgan DO. Control of mitosis by changes in the subcellular location of cyclin-B1-Cdk1 and Cdc25C. *Curr Opin Cell Biol* 2000;12:658-665.

Thompson SL, Compton DA. Examining the link between chromosomal instability and aneuploidy in human cells. *J Cell Biol* 2008;180:665-672.

Tsujimoto Y, Finger LR, Yunis J, et al. Cloning of the chromosome breakpoint of neoplastic B cells with the t(14;18) chromosome translocation. *Science* 1984;226:1097-1099.

Walczak CE, Cai S, Khodjakov A. Mechanisms of chromosome behaviour during mitosis. *Nat Rev Mol Cell Biol* 2010;11:91-102.

Warr MR, Shore GC. Unique biology of Mcl-1: therapeutic opportunities in cancer. *Curr Mol Med* 2008;8:138-147.

Weaver BA, Cleveland DW. Does aneuploidy cause cancer? *Curr Opin Cell Biol* 2006;18:658-667.

Wei W, Ayad NG, Wan Y, et al. Degradation of the SCF component Skp2 in cell-cycle phase G1 by the anaphase-promoting complex. *Nature* 2004;428:194-198.

Wertz IE, Dixit VM. Regulation of death receptor signaling by the ubiquitin system. *Cell Death Differ* 2010;17:14-24.

Willems AR, Schwab M, Tyers M. A hitchhiker's guide to the cullin ubiquitin ligases: SCF and its kin. *Biochim Biophys Acta* 2004; 1695:133-170.

Williams GH, Romanowski P, Morris L, et al. Improved cervical smear assessment using antibodies against proteins that regulate DNA replication. *Proc Natl Acad Sci U S A* 1998;95:14932-14937.

Wilson NS, Dixit V, Ashkenazi A. Death receptor signal transducers: nodes of coordination in immune signaling networks. *Nat Immunol* 2009;10:348-355.

Woo M, Hakem R, Soengas MS, et al. Essential contribution of caspase 3/CPP32 to apoptosis and its associated nuclear changes. *Genes Dev* 1998;12:806-819.

Youle RJ, Strasser A. The BCL-2 protein family: opposing activities that mediate cell death. *Nat Rev Mol Cell Biol* 2008;9:47-59.

Zhou P, Levy NB, Xie H, et al. MCL1 transgenic mice exhibit a high incidence of B-cell lymphoma manifested as a spectrum of histologic subtypes. *Blood* 2001;97:3902-3909.

Zilfou JT, Lowe SW. Tumor suppressive functions of p53. *Cold Spring Harb Perspect Biol* 2009;1:a001883.

Zou H, McGarry TJ, Bernal T, Kirschner MW. Identification of a vertebrate sister-chromatid separation inhibitor involved in transformation and tumorigenesis. *Science* 1999;285: 418-422.

Tumor Progression and Metastasis

10

Yang W. Shao, Rama Khokha, and Richard P. Hill

10.1 TUMOR PROGRESSION

10.1.1 Cellular Aspects of Tumor Progression

Cancer is not a static disease. In many tumors (eg, colon, breast, cervical, pancreatic, melanoma), there appears to be an orderly progression from benign tissue to premalignant lesion to frank malignancy. In other tumors, premalignant lesions may not have been identified, but it is likely the tumor has passed through less-malignant stages before detection. The pathological and clinical criteria for tumor progression are often specific to a given type of tumor, but include local spread along tissue planes and into various tissue spaces and cavities. Tumors also have the capacity to invade and spread from their origins to other organs in the body; This process is referred to as *metastasis*. Increasing numbers and types of genetic abnormalities accompany tumor progression and metastasis.

More than 50 years ago, Foulds defined tumor progression as "the acquisition of permanent, irreversible qualitative changes in one or more characteristics of a neoplasm" that cause the tumor to become more autonomous and malignant. In 1986, Nowell proposed that such changes arise because cancer cells tend to be genetically unstable and described a conceptual model to explain the process of tumor progression (Fig. 10–1). The key features of this model are the generation of mutant cells within a tumor and the selection and outgrowth of more autonomous cells to become dominant subclones in the population, leading to progression of the tumor and increasing malignancy. Many studies have confirmed the genetic instability of malignant cells (see Chap. 5, Sec. 5.2 and Chap. 7, Sec. 7.4), and have identified somatic DNA copy number changes and mutations using genome-wide analyses (see Chap. 2, Sec. 2.7) that are becoming routine in cancer research and in the clinic. Consistent with this model, recent studies have identified different clonal populations within tumors, raising the possibility for a minor (resistant) subpopulation to cause tumor recurrence following therapy (Navin et al, 2011). The growth and development of various cells within a tumor is largely subject to constraints associated

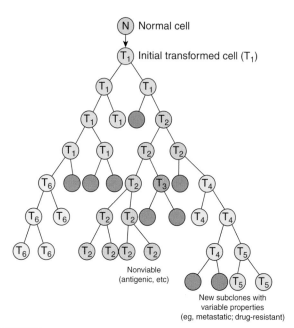

FIGURE 10–1   Schematic showing the clonal evolution of tumors. New subclones arise by mutation. Many of these may become extinct (indicated by dark shading) but others may have a growth advantage and become dominant. All of the subclones (indicated by T_2 to T_6) may share common clonal markers, but many of them have new properties leading to heterogeneity.

with interactions among the tumor cells, the stromal cells, and the extracellular environment. Thus the normal homeostatic mechanisms that control cell proliferation in the body (see Chap. 9, Sec. 9.2) are not completely lost in tumor cells, but rather the cells may become increasingly less responsive to them. In addition, tumor cells acquire autonomous means to grow, becoming less dependent on extraneous growth factors (Kopfstein and Christofori, 2006). These findings are consistent with the original concepts of Foulds that there are many different paths to malignancy. Tumors are thus evolving cell communities with properties that continue to change as they grow. The role of the stromal cell populations and the extracellular microenvironment is increasingly recognized as a critical element in tumor development and progression (Hanahan and Weinberg, 2011).

10.1.2 Molecular Genetics of Tumor Progression

Genetic instability of tumor cells may arise as a result of genetic and/or epigenetic changes. Epigenetic changes such as methylation of cytosine bases in DNA or modifications to chromatin structure (eg, by methylation, acetylation, sumoylation, or phosphorylation) can modify the expression of genes and are an important mechanism for "silencing" genes during normal differentiation (see Chap. 2, Sec. 2.3). Genetic changes may occur by point mutation, deletion, gene amplification, chromosomal translocation or other mechanisms (see Chap. 5, Sec. 5.2). A cell is continually exposed to both external and internal stresses, such as reactive oxygen species, which may cause DNA damage. Moreover, there are inherent errors made by DNA polymerases whenever DNA is being replicated. Normally such damage is either repaired by the various DNA repair mechanisms in the cell (see Chap. 5, Sec. 5.3) or damaged cells undergo apoptosis (see Chap. 9, Sec. 9.4). However, these mechanisms are not perfect, leading to a natural frequency of mutation in cells.

Many cancer cells appear to have an increased frequency of mutation because of deficiencies in their ability to repair lesions in DNA and/or decreased activation of apoptosis, so that mutated cells may survive and proliferate. For example, the breast cancer-related genes, BRCA1/2, are linked with DNA double-strand break repair. Oxidative lesions and deficiencies of mismatch repair have been demonstrated in tumor cells, particularly those from patients with certain types of colon cancer. A deficiency in mismatch repair can result in up to a 1000-fold increase in the mutation frequency. Failures in DNA damage repair may result in mutations or alterations in the expression of the many oncogenes and tumor-suppressor genes that are associated with different human cancers (see Chap. 7). Mutations in these genes are not necessarily more frequent than in other genes; rather the mutations are selected for in the process of cancer development, and thus are the ones that are most frequently detected. However, because of their genetic instability, cancer cells may also carry many "passenger" mutations that play little or no known role in their cancer phenotype.

The multiple changes that must occur in cells during tumor development and progression are illustrated by the model established by Vogelstein and colleagues describing the progression of colon cancer (Fearon and Vogelstein, 1990; Fig. 10–2). This model provides a paradigm for multistep carcinogenesis that has been applied to many other cancers (eg, breast, pancreatic, bladder, and lung), although recent studies have emphasized that the steps do not always occur in a specific order. These concepts have been reinforced by studies involving genetic manipulation of normal human primary cells that have demonstrated that sequential modifications involving activation of oncogenes or inactivation of tumor suppressors can result in their transformation (Hahn et al, 1999). Thus a molecular description of tumor progression envisages that cancers progress as a result of a series of (selected) genetic and epigenetic changes. Some of these changes are shared between different cancers, but changes unique to specific types of cancer also occur and the sequence of the multisteps may not always follow the same time line in different individual cancers of the same type.

As a result of their genetic and epigenetic changes, cells within animal and human tumors demonstrate considerable heterogeneity in their phenotypes. This heterogeneity includes morphology, karyotype, surface markers, biochemical pathways, cell proliferation, metastatic ability, and sensitivity to therapeutic agents. The ability of tumor cells to disseminate and form metastases represents the most malignant characteristic of a cancer. Therefore, it is important to understand

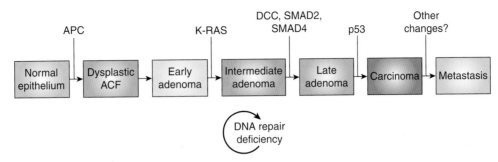

FIGURE 10-2 Genetic changes associated with colorectal tumorigenesis. Anaphase promoting complex (APC) mutations initiate the neoplastic process, and tumor progression results from mutations in the other genes indicated. Patients with familial adenomatous polyposis (FAP) inherit APC mutations and develop numerous dysplastic aberrant crypt foci (ACF), some of which progress as they acquire the other mutations indicated in the figure. The tumors from patients with hereditary nonpolyposis colorectal carcinoma (HNPCC) go through a similar although not identical series of mutations; DNA repair deficiency speeds up this process. K-*ras* is an oncogene that requires only 1 genetic event for its activation. The other specific genes indicated are tumor-suppressor genes that require 2 genetic events (1 in each allele) for their inactivation. Chromosome 18q21 may contain several different tumor-suppressor genes involved in colorectal neoplasia, with DCC (deleted in colon cancer), SMAD2 and SMAD4 genes proposed as candidates. A variety of other genetic alterations have each been described in a small fraction of advanced colorectal cancers. These may be responsible for the heterogeneity of biological and clinical properties observed among different cases.

how cancer cells metastasize and to determine the underlying genetic and molecular causes of metastasis. As described in Sections 10.4 and 10.5, metastases probably arise from a small subset of cells within a primary tumor that have undergone genetic or epigenetic changes that enhance their ability to metastasize. This feature of tumors has made it difficult to determine the cellular and molecular properties critical for metastatic spread, as the bulk of the tumor cell population may not reflect the specific properties of the individual cells responsible for the metastases.

10.2 TUMOR MICROENVIRONMENT

10.2.1 Extracellular Matrix

Most mammalian cells are in contact with an extracellular matrix (ECM). The composition and structure of the ECM is specific to location and developmental stage. For example, epithelial cells have specialized lateral, apical, and basal borders. The latter's interactions with the basement membrane are instrumental for the formation, maintenance, and polarized differentiated state of the epithelial cell sheet. The basement membrane, a specialized form of ECM, is composed of laminin, type IV (and VII) collagen, entactin/nidogen, and heparan sulfate proteoglycan (HSPG), as well as smaller amounts of fibronectin, vitronectin, and chondroitin sulfate proteoglycans. To exert tissue-specific control, basement membranes vary in composition while maintaining a common set of structural and mechanical properties (Rowe and Weiss, 2009). There are at least 7 forms of laminin and 6 type IV collagen chains that interact with other ECM proteins to generate a 3-dimensional (3D) interlocking structural network. In contrast to epithelial cells, mesenchymal cells are not attached to each other or to a basement membrane, but are surrounded by an ECM that contains the interstitial collagens types I to III, elastin, proteoglycans, fibronectin, and vitronectin. Other

specialized tissue-specific ECM molecules include tenascin, thrombospondin, and osteopontin. The highly organized 3D matrix provides an adhesive environment for cells and other molecules, such as growth factors. Interaction of cells with the ECM is essential for growth and survival, and the ECM can also regulate the differentiation of a variety of cell types. Depriving normal cells of such interactions results in the induction of apoptosis (anoikis) in epithelial and endothelial cells (Boudreau et al, 1995), or cell-cycle arrest in fibroblasts (Fang et al, 1996). Transformed cells are often defective in secreting fibronectin and in laying down an organized matrix and a common property of malignant cells is their ability to survive and proliferate with a lower dependence on interactions with an ECM than normal cells. Many studies report disruption of basement membrane continuity and collagen degradation at sites of tumor cell invasion, and breakdown of ECM integrity is considered a rate-limiting step in tumor progression and metastasis.

The ECM provides structural elements that can interact with various molecules expressed on the cell surface (cell adhesion molecules; see Sec. 10.2.3). These latter molecules also interact with specific signal transduction pathways in the cell. Growth factors can be soluble, or embedded within the matrix, or anchored to the cell surface in close proximity to their cell surface receptors that are also directly linked to cell signaling (see Chap. 8). Within this complex milieu are also extracellular, plasma membrane-bound, and ECM-bound proteinases. Normally, a balance exists in the biochemical activities of these various molecular entities, which is often disrupted within the tumor cell microenvironment. Aberrant proteolysis is an important means of offsetting the balance and can exert a "ripple" effect on multiple classes of molecules during tumor progression and metastasis. It is one hallmark of tumor cells that underlies their metastatic dissemination. Proteolysis is influenced by and localized via cell adhesion molecules, and it, in turn, acts on an array of substrates, including the ECM, cell adhesion molecules, growth factors, and cytokines, and their receptors and binding proteins. For example, increased matrix metalloproteinase (MMP)-mediated activity brings about remodeling of the ECM and basement membranes and influences cell adhesion by cadherins. As discussed in Section 10.5.6, loss of E-cadherin can promote epithelial-to-mesenchymal transition (EMT) in cells, potentially creating a phenotype leading to more aggressive cancers.

10.2.2 Cellular Proteinases and Their Inhibitors

As indicated above (and in Secs. 10.4 and 10.5), a series of tissue barriers (eg, basement membrane, interstitial connective tissue) are traversed by tumor cells during invasion and metastasis by processes involving proteolytic breakdown of the ECM. Mammalian proteinases fall into 4 major classes (serine-, cysteine-, aspartic-, and metalloproteinases), and many of these are associated with increased aggressiveness of tumor cells, and are functionally implicated during metastasis (Table 10–1). These diverse proteases have distinct structures and most have endogenous inhibitors that maintain a balance to keep proteolysis under strict control in normal tissues. Both the enzymes and their inhibitors may be aberrantly expressed by cancer cells and multiple other cell types within the tumor microenvironment.

Metalloproteinases comprise the biggest family of proteases in the human genome with a total of 186 members. MMPs, including membrane type (MT)-MMPs, and are the major enzymes responsible for degradation of ECM proteins. Extracellular MMPs are often secreted in a latent form (pro-MMP), and subsequently activated. The MMPs chelate 2 zinc ions: 1 is present in the active site and the other associates with the pro-MMP to stabilize the inactive state (Egeblad and Werb, 2002). These enzymes can be autocatalyzed, activated by other MMPs, or activated by a serine proteinase. Cell-surface anchored proteases, such as MT-MMPs, are activated by proprotein convertases, some of which are also critical for the localization and cell-surface activation of soluble pro-MMPs. For example MT1-MMP is essential for the activation of pro-MMP2 at the cell surface. Interactions among different classes of proteases also generate complex proteolytic cascades which can amplify their activity. Within the metalloproteinase family, the ADAMs (a disintegrin and metalloproteinase)

are unique in that they possess both adhesion and proteolytic domains (Werb, 1997). These transmembrane proteases act as "sheddases" to release cell surface anchored growth factors and cytokines in a process called *ectodomain shedding*; in addition, they are critical for the activation of receptor-mediated pathways such as NOTCH and epidermal growth factor receptor (EGFR) (Murphy, 2009).

Plasminogen activators (urokinase type [uPA] and tissue type [tPA]) are serine proteinases that act on circulating plasminogen to release plasmin and have long been associated with malignant cells. The activity of plasminogen and plasmin is localized to the cell surface by the uPA receptor (uPAR), which also associates with integrins and can bind to vitronectin in the ECM (Laufs et al, 2006). Increased expression of uPA has been correlated with metastasis in a number of cancers including human epidermal growth receptor 2 (HER2)-positive breast cancer (see Chap. 20, Sec. 20.3.3). The level of expression of plasminogen activator inhibitor (PAI)-1 also provides an independent unfavorable prognostic factor for the development of metastases for a population of hormone receptor- and lymph node-positive breast cancer patients (Schmitt et al, 2011). Among serine proteases, kallikreins are coded by a contiguous cluster of protease genes in the human genome and have been studied extensively for their utility as serum cancer biomarkers. For example, prostate-specific antigen (PSA) is the most commonly used kallikrein for routine evaluation of prostate cancer progression.

Cathepsins are cysteine proteases generally present on intracellular cell membranes localized to endosomal or lysosomal vesicles. Their proteolytic activity was presumed to be restricted to the intracellular compartment, but it was later discovered that cathepsins can also be found outside the cell during pathological conditions and their presence in body fluids is a prognostic indicator for several cancers. Slight structural differences between the eleven cathepsins are responsible for differences in substrate specificity and inhibition by their endogenous inhibitors. Cathepsins B, H, and L are particularly associated with tumor progression. An imbalance between the cathepsins and their inhibitors can occur during tumor progression and may be responsible for direct digestion of the ECM or activation of other proteolytic enzymes, such as uPA.

Proteinase inhibitors are produced by both malignant and normal cells. Examples of these inhibitors are PAI-1 and PAI-2, the cathepsin inhibitors, cystatins, kininogens and stefins, and

TABLE 10–1 Proteinases in specific catalytic classes.

Catalytic Type	Numbers (Human/Mouse)	Associated with Malignancy	Specific Inhibitors	Substrates
Cysteine	143/153	Cathepsins B, L, H	Kinogens, cystatins, stefins	ECM
Aspartic	21/27	Cathespins D	Not known	ECM
Metallo	186/197	MMPs 2, 3, 7, 9, 11, 13, 14	TIMPs	ECM, GFs/cytokines
Serine	176/227	uPA, tPA	PAIs	Plasminogen, latent MMPs

ECM, Extracellular matrix; *GF*, growth factor; *MMP*, matrix metalloproteinase; *PAI*, plasminogen activator inhibitor; *TIMP*, tissue inhibitor of metalloproteinase; *tPA*, tissue plasminogen activator; *uPA*, urokinase plasminogen activator.

Adapted from Puente et al, 2003.

tissue inhibitors of metalloproteinases (TIMPs). Under physiological conditions a balance between activated proteinases and their inhibitors keeps proteolysis under strict control; but when this balance is disrupted, (malignant) cells can invade tissues. Downregulation of TIMP-1 activity in immortalized murine fibroblasts, using transfected antisense RNA (see Chap. 2, Sec. 2.4.3), was found to confer invasive capacity and ability to form metastatic tumors in nude mice (Khokha et al, 1989). Increased levels of TIMP-1, TIMP-2, or TIMP-3 reduce the invasive and metastatic ability of malignant cells, and TIMP-1 provides increased resistance to metastatic colonization of organs. Gain- and loss-of-function studies have addressed the causal role of specific TIMPs and cystatins with various processes underlying tumorigenesis (Egeblad and Werb, 2002), and some studies suggest that TIMPs can function in a manner independent of their MMP-inhibitory function. However, the relationship between advanced malignancy and increased proteolytic activity (such as that arising from increased MMP or decreased TIMP expression) is not always clear. For example, increased MMP activity during cancer progression can be associated with a favorable prognosis, as is the case of MMP-12 in colon cancer, and increased TIMP expression has been identified to be a poor prognostic indicator in many studies (Egeblad and Werb, 2002). The recognition that proteolysis influences basic cellular processes, including cell division, differentiation, dissociation, and death (Hojilla et al, 2003) highlights the complexity of the proteolytic balance and the difficulty of predicting how changes in this balance may affect cancer progression.

10.2.3 Cell Adhesion Molecules

The cell–cell and cell–ECM interactions during invasion and metastasis depend upon several classes of molecules expressed on the cell surface, including integrins and cadherins, as well as the ligands that bind to these molecules. Cell adhesion molecules (CAMs) are transmembrane proteins with extracellular and intracellular domains, the intracellular domains are usually connected to the cytoskeleton or to signaling molecules. Although originally named for cell adhesion, CAMs have multiple functions, including a major role in signaling from outside to inside a cell and vice versa. The formation and breaking of adhesive bonds between tumor cells and their environment provides information to the cell about its environment and may lead to changes in the expression of specific genes that determine cell proliferation, invasion, or other processes.

Integrins are expressed in all cell types and are involved in the regulation of cellular functions during embryonic development, wound healing, inflammation, homeostasis, bone resorption, apoptosis, cell proliferation, tumor cell growth, and metastasis. They make up a family of widely expressed transmembrane receptors for proteins of the ECM, such as fibronectin, laminin, vitronectin, and collagens. These adhesion molecules are obligate heterodimers, comprising noncovalently associated α and β subunits, each of which spans the plasma membrane and typically possess a short cytoplasmic domain. Receptor diversity and versatility in ligand binding is determined by the extracellular domains through the specific pairing of 18 α and 8 β subunits, to form a family of 24 recognized heterodimers (Hynes, 2002). The cytoplasmic domain of the β subunit interacts directly with components of the actin cytoskeleton, such as α-actinin and talin, allowing its localization to focal adhesion plaques (FAPs) that form at points of contact between integrins and the ECM. FAPs represent the submembranous termini of actin stress fibers, indicating that integrins provide a structural bridge between the ECM and the actin cytoskeleton (Fig. 10–3). FAPs also contain a number

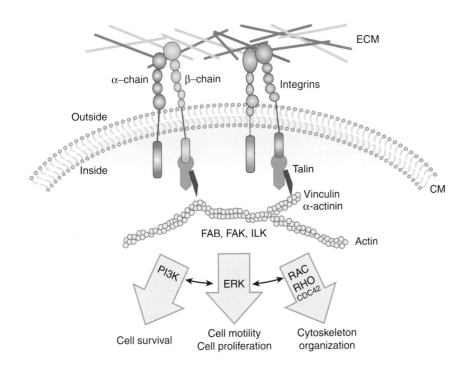

FIGURE 10–3 Schematic of integrin receptors with linkage to their major downstream signal transduction pathways. An integrin receptor contains 2 subunits (α and β); different combinations of α and β subunits lead to the structural and functional variety of the integrin receptors. Integrin receptors are important players in the "outside-in" signaling system, they can sense the changes in the environment, and transduce the signals into the cell through the signal transduction pathways shown.

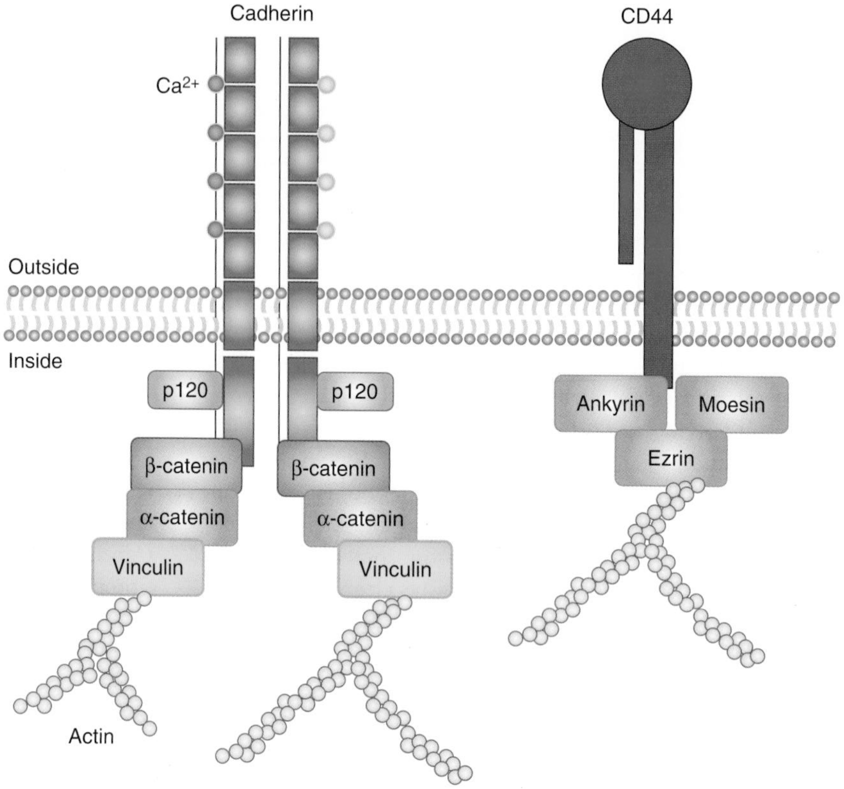

FIGURE 10–4 Schematic of the structures of cadherins and CD44. Cadherins are defined by their signature calcium binding domains. Different cadherins can have various number of repeats of calcium binding domains. Cadherins can also activate important signaling pathways, such as Wnt signaling, through their intracellular association with (p120, α and β) catenins. CD44 has many isoforms; the standard isoform is designated CD44s, while the splice variants are designated CD44v. The intracellular domain of CD44 can associated with ezrin, which is also an important player in metastasis. The function of CD44 is largely controlled by its posttranslational modifications.

of protein tyrosine kinases, such as the focal adhesion kinase (FAK), p125, and the integrin-linked kinase (ILK). It is well established that integrins act as part of signal-transduction complexes that allow cells to "sense" (and respond to) their extracellular environment (Desgrosellier and Cheresh, 2010). Integrin activation may act to prolong and intensify signaling from growth factor receptors and can be a positive mediator of angiogenesis (see Chap. 11, Sec. 11.4.7). In a recent study done with in vitro ECM gels, metastatic cells lost their proliferation capability when the $\alpha_3\beta_1$ integrin was knocked down, resulting in defective FAK signaling. This suggests that the $\alpha_3\beta_1$–FAK interaction might play a role in ECM signaling in primary tumor cells when they first migrate to other organs and thus promote metastasis (Shibue and Weinberg, 2009). The expression of integrin receptors is altered in malignant cells as compared with their normal counterparts, but the loss or gain of expression of a particular integrin has not been linked directly to malignant transformation.

Cadherins are intercellular adhesion receptors that play important roles in assembling adherens junctions and desmosomes. Distinct members of the cadherin family are principal constituents of each type of junction, mediating calcium-dependent adhesion between similar cells. There are more than 20 recognized cadherins and protocadherins. E-cadherin (*CDH1*), the major epithelial cadherin, contains 4 conserved extracellular domains, a fifth extracellular domain possessing conserved cysteine residues, a transmembrane domain, and a cytoplasmic domain. Calcium binding sites lie between adjacent extracellular domains. The cytoplasmic domain

associates with cellular proteins such as catenins, which act to link cadherins to the actin cytoskeleton and to signal-transduction components (Cavallaro et al, 2002; Fig. 10–4). An important connection between cadherins, catenins, and tumor progression was made with the observation that the APC (adenoma polyposis coli) tumor-suppressor protein (see Fig. 10–2) and β-catenin form physiological complexes with axin and glycogen synthase kinase (GSK)-3β, in which β-catenin can be phosphorylated by GSK-3β and targeted for ubiquitin-mediated degradation. This complex thereby acts to control the level of β-catenin in the cell. Besides binding APC and cadherins, β-catenin can also enter the nucleus and associate with LEF/TCP transcription factors, upregulating genes involved with cell growth such as c-Myc and cyclin D1. Mutations in APC, which are associated with the formation of adenomas, cluster within the β-catenin binding region, yielding truncated APC peptides that are unable to bind to β-catenin. This reduces its degradation and increases its availability to diffuse to the nucleus and activate cell growth. Degradation of β-catenin is also disrupted if the activity of GSK-3β is blocked by activation of the Wnt-signaling pathway (see Chap. 8, Sec. 8.4.1 and Fig. 8–12). Loss of E-cadherin and increased levels of N-cadherin (CDH2) are correlated with cellular invasiveness and, as discussed in Section 10.5.6, are associated with the so-called EMT. Disruption of cadherin-catenin complexes leads to disruption of the cytoskeleton, which, in turn, may affect signal transduction, as there is evidence that cytoskeletal proteins can act as a scaffold for the components of signal transduction pathways.

CD44 is a cell-surface glycoprotein identified as the major receptor mediating cellular interactions with hyaluronate, a glycosaminoglycan component of the ECM. Its principal physiological functions include aggregation, migration, and activation of cell functions. CD44 is widely expressed and exists in multiple forms with variable glycosylation. All CD44 isoforms contain a cytoplasmic domain, which may link CD44 to actin filaments through interactions with ankyrin, ezrin, and moesin (see Fig. 10–4). Alternative splicing of the messenger RNA (mRNA) to produce these variable isoforms (CD44v) is regulated in a tissue-specific manner or by antigen activation in lymphocytes. CD44 isoforms are overexpressed by many tumors, and their expression has been correlated with clinical outcome in several human malignancies (Jothy, 2003). Recent studies suggest that CD44 is a surface protein that is expressed preferentially on subpopulations of cells that are able to induce high frequencies of tumor growth in xenograft models (tumor initiating or cancer stem cells; see Chap. 13, Sec. 13.4.5). The potential role of the different isoforms of CD44 has not been well defined in such cells. CD44 has been reported to be expressed at the invading edges of murine carcinoma cells and is required in melanoma cells for migration on type IV collagen and for invasion of the basement membrane. Osteopontin, a secreted glycoprotein widely implicated in invasion and metastasis, binds to CD44, inducing a variety of signaling cascades associated with adhesion, migration and invasion, suggesting its interactions with CD44 may play a role in its malignancy-promoting potential (Anborgh et al, 2010).

The ERM proteins (containing ezrin, radixin, and moesin motifs) serve an important role linking the actin network cytoskeleton and the cell membrane. They provide a means by which a cell can sense environmental changes and respond to growth factors. ERM proteins normally form aggregates with each other and assume an inactive conformation. Upon tyrosine and threonine phosphorylation, ezrin becomes activated and switches into an active conformation, which allows for its translocation from the cytoplasm to the plasma membrane, bringing F-actin to the cell surface. The ERM proteins are especially abundant at cell protrusions such as membrane ruffles and microvilli. Ezrin is also reported to bind to CAMs such as CD43, CD44, and intercellular adhesion molecules (ICAMs). Many of these CAMs affect cell migration and invasiveness, and have been implicated in metastasis. Recently, ezrin was identified as a metastasis-associated gene that is related to prognosis of a number of cancers (Bruce et al, 2007). A high level of ezrin expression has been linked with poor prognosis in pediatric and adult osteosarcoma (Khanna et al, 2004). In a mouse model of osteosarcoma, it was shown that ezrin is required for metastasis, and possibly functions to provide a survival advantage to tumor cells when they reach a secondary site.

10.2.4 The Pathophysiological Microenvironment

As a solid tumor grows, the rate of cancer cell proliferation surpasses the ability of the existing vasculature to supply growth factors, nutrients, and oxygen, and to remove the catabolites produced by the cells. The result of this imbalance between supply and demand is a microenvironment containing regions of hypoxia (low oxygen concentration), low glucose levels, low pH, and elevated interstitial fluid pressure (IFP). There is spatial and temporal heterogeneity in the tumor microenvironment, both between different tumors and within an individual tumor. Furthermore, the tumor microenvironment has been linked to a more aggressive phenotype, playing multiple roles in tumor progression and metastasis (Finger and Giaccia, 2010; Lunt et al, 2009). Multiple clinical studies have demonstrated a connection between tumor hypoxia and disease progression in a variety of human tumors, including carcinomas of the cervix, prostate, and the head and neck, and soft-tissue sarcomas (see Chap. 12, Sec. 12.2.2). Furthermore, studies in animal models have shown that hypoxia in tumors increases metastatic dissemination to the lungs or lymph nodes. The mechanisms by which tumor hypoxia might increase metastatic potential are discussed in more detail in Section 10.5.7.

10.3 METASTASIS

10.3.1 The Spread of Cancer

The 2 major routes of metastatic spread are via lymphatic vessels and/or blood vessels (Fig. 10–5). Metastases are subdivided into 2 groups: those in regional lymph nodes, which are usually regarded as having disseminated via the lymphatic circulation, and those that arise at distant organs, which are spread via the blood circulation system. Metastasis is an ominous feature in cancer progression and most deaths caused by cancer are caused by metastases. The T (= Tumor) N (= Nodes) M (= Metastasis) system of cancer staging is now used widely in clinical management. In this system, cancers are divided into stages based on tumor size, presence of involved lymph

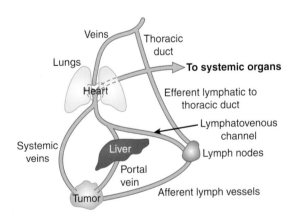

FIGURE 10–5 **The major routes by which cancer cells can spread from a primary tumor are through the lymphatic or blood vessels.** These 2 systems are interconnected as illustrated. The vascular drainage for tumors of the gastrointestinal tract is usually via the portal circulation, whereas for tumors at other sites in the body, drainage is via the systemic veins. (Adapted with permission from Sugarbaker, 1980.)

nodes, and presence of distant metastases. Prognosis is closely correlated with the stage of the disease at diagnosis and treatment decisions depend on it. Local treatment is of limited effectiveness in the presence of metastatic disease and systemic therapies may be used to a greater extent.

The kinetics of tumor spread varies between individuals, and it does not always correlate with primary tumor size. This suggests that the ability to establish metastases is not present in all primary tumor cells. In addition to properties such as avoidance of cell-cycle arrest and apoptosis, cells that leave primary tumors and establish metastases require additional abilities (see Sec. 10.4). Tumor cells are generally very inefficient at forming metastases (see Sec. 10.3.3) and often are detected in the blood circulation of patients without evidence of metastatic disease. Oncogene-driven tumors in mouse models do not necessarily develop distant metastases (Klein, 2003). A recurring theme is that tumor cells often gain metastatic abilities by turning on endogenous gene programs that are involved in normal tissue development and homeostasis. An example is provided by epithelial tumor cells that undergo EMT, a process normally involved in embryonic development and wound healing, to gain motility and survival advantages for metastasis (see Sec. 10.5.6). Furthermore, the invasive and migratory functions that are responsible for normal epithelial cell branching (eg, in the mammary gland) can be hijacked by tumor cells to expand into surrounding tissue (Ewald et al, 2008). Tumor cells in hypoxic regions can express hypoxia-inducible factors (HIFs) to initiate the angiogenesis process to compensate for lower nutrient and oxygen supplies.

10.3.2 Organ Preference

Distant metastases from different types of tumors tend to occur in specific target organs (Table 10–2). Paget's soil-and-seed hypothesis postulated that tumor cell–host organ interactions can favor or hinder metastatic development. The structure and organization of capillaries and adjacent parenchyma and tissue function vary widely in different organs; therefore, organ-specific adhesive interaction between endothelial cells

TABLE 10–2 Typical sites of metastasis of the common tumors.

Tumor Type	Principle Sites of Metastasis
Lung	Brain, bone, adrenal gland, and liver
Breast	Bone, lung, liver, and brain
Prostate	Bone
Colon	Liver and lung
Pancreas	Liver and lung
Skin	Lung, brain, skin, and liver
Sarcoma	Lung
Uveal	Liver

and tumor cells or between tumor cells and available growth factors in the organ can influence successful establishment of metastatic growth. This concept is supported by studies that show tumor cells expressing certain surface molecules have enhanced abilities to arrest, extravasate into, and grow in specific target organs (see Sec. 10.5). In addition, other factors, such as the dynamics of blood flow, are also likely to explain organ preference. In colon cancer, the mesenteric circulation delivers tumor cells from the bowels to the liver, a common site of metastasis, while blood flow carries osteosarcoma cells from the bone to lung capillaries, and osteosarcoma metastases to the lung are common.

Organ specificity also occurs in animal models. Tumor cells that form large numbers of metastatic deposits in 1 organ (eg, the lung following intravenous injection) are not necessarily capable of doing so in another organ (eg, the liver following intraportal injection). Furthermore populations of tumor cells that have enhanced ability to form metastases in specific organs can be isolated by serially selecting cells from metastases in these organs. Cells forming metastases preferentially in the lung will "home" to a lung lobe even when it is transplanted ectopically into a subcutaneous site; such cells do not form metastases in other organs that are transplanted ectopically. The classic example of serial selection is the isolation of the B16F10 cell population from B16 mouse melanoma cells (Fidler, 1973). The procedure (Fig. 10–6) involved serial intravenous injection of the cells into isogenic animals, with selection at each stage for cells that had formed lung metastases. The cells forming lung metastases were grown in culture to expand their number before being reinjected into animals. After 10 such passages, a population of cells was obtained (termed *B16F10 cells*) that was approximately 10 times as efficient at forming *experimental* lung metastases after intravenous injection as the starting B16F1 cell population. Interestingly, these cells were not more capable of forming *spontaneous* metastasis when implanted at a local site, suggesting that selecting for increased ability to grow in lung does not affect the invasive properties necessary for initial escape from the primary tumor. However, selection for B16 melanoma cells with increased spontaneous metastatic ability (B16BL6) was achieved by selecting for cells that could invade through the wall of the mouse bladder in vitro, and then expanding these cells in culture and selecting again for invasion through the mouse bladder over multiple cycles. Other investigators have also been successful, using similar approaches, in selecting cell populations from a number of rodent tumors that have enhanced experimental metastatic ability in a variety of organs including lung, liver, ovary, and brain. However, such selection procedures do not always yield cells with increased metastatic ability (Ling et al, 1985; Stackpole et al, 1991), leading to the suggestion that some properties that contribute to metastatic ability may not be stably maintained within the tumor cell population during the selection procedures and may function only transiently to promote metastasis.

The organ specificity of metastatic human tumor cells has been tested in immune-deficient hosts (eg, athymic

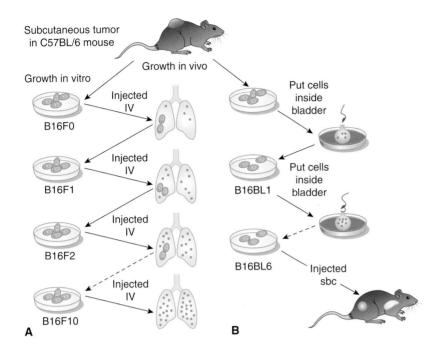

FIGURE 10–6 Procedures used for selecting highly metastatic cell populations from B16 melanoma cells. A) The B16F10 cells were selected by passing the cells 10 times through the lungs of mice, while (**B**) the B16BL6 cells were selected by requiring them to invade 6 times through the walls of mouse bladders. *sbc*, subcutaneous IV, intravenously.

nude mice or SCID [severe combined immune deficient] mice). These studies have demonstrated that the local site of growth of an implanted tumor may influence its capacity to seed spontaneous metastases and that tumors transplanted in orthotopic sites (tissue of the same pathological type as the tumor) are more likely to seed metastases (locally to lymph nodes or distantly to other organs) than tumors grown in ectopic sites (Fujihara et al, 1998). A refinement to these models is the transplantation of human tissue (eg, fetal bone) into SCID mice to generate (so-called) SCID-hu models. When human tumor cells are implanted locally or injected intravascularly into such mice, they show similar organ preference for metastasis to that seen in clinical practice and the metastases occur preferentially in the human tissue rather than the same murine tissue (Namikawa and Shtivelman, 1999).

Chemokines (molecules used by leukocytes to home to specific organs) may play an important role in organ specificity of metastasis. It has been reported that human breast cancer cells have high expression of the chemokine receptors CXCR4 and CCR7, while their respective ligands (CXCL12 and CCL21) are highly expressed in organs in which breast cancer cells have a high propensity to form metastases (lung, liver, regional lymph nodes, and bone marrow). Blocking of CXCL12/CXCR4 interaction significantly impaired formation of metastasis by a human breast cancer cell line in lung and lymph nodes in an experimental system, and this pathway is being targeted for cancer therapy. In a similar context, organ specificity may also occur as a result of specific molecular signatures that are expressed in the microvasculature in individual normal tissues (and tumors). The technique of phage display, which allows the identification and purification of small peptides that will specifically recognize and bind to the molecules involved is providing opportunities for imaging and directed therapy of cancer and other diseases (Mueller et al, 2009; Ruoslahti, 2002; Whitney et al, 2010).

10.3.3 Metastatic Inefficiency

The establishment of metastases by tumor cells appears to be an inefficient process. Blood samples taken from the renal vein in patients just prior to surgery for renal cell carcinoma allowed estimates that tumor cells were being released at rates of 10^7 to 10^9 cells per day (Glaves et al, 1988). Two of the 11 patients had no evidence of metastatic disease 30 and 55 months after the surgery. Similarly, patients with peritoneovenous shunts for malignant ascites have shown no evidence that release of large numbers of tumor cells into the blood increases the number of metastases observed. Studies in animals also support this concept, as only a few circulating cells are able to form metastases. In experimental metastasis (or colonization) assays, tumor cells are injected directly into the arterial or venous blood circulation and allowed to disseminate and arrest at various sites. It is rare that even 1% of such cells form tumor nodules and it is usually orders of magnitude lower.

The inefficiency of the metastatic process leads naturally to the question of whether metastasis is a random or a specific process. A small subpopulation of the cells in a tumor might express properties that confer a higher probability of being able to form metastases, but it is also possible that all tumor cells might have an equal (low) probability of forming metastases, but only a few manage to survive through the various stages of the process (see Sec. 10.4). Support for the random nature of the metastatic process derives from studies that have failed to demonstrate that cells obtained from metastases are consistently more metastatic than cells from the parent tumor (Weiss and Ward, 1990), which is not consistent with what

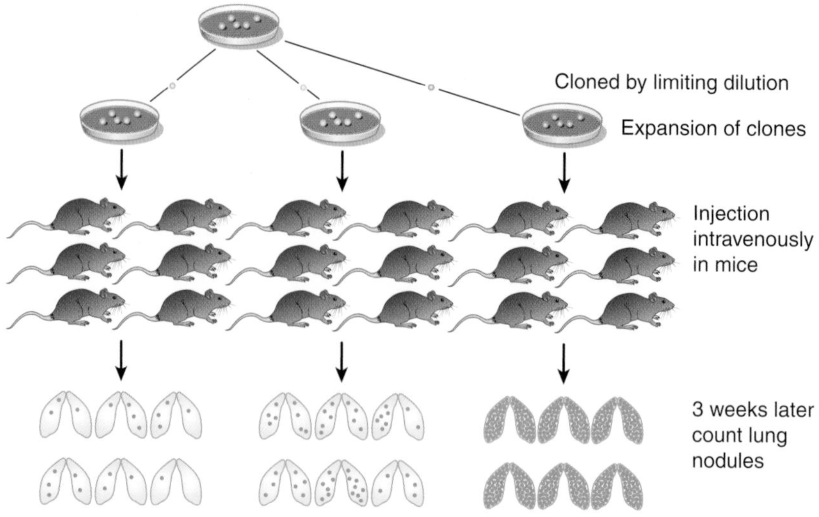

FIGURE 10-7 **Clonal heterogeneity is demonstrated by establishing a series of clones from a tumor cell population and, after expansion, testing them for metastatic ability.** Although there is some variability in the number of nodules observed in different animals injected with cells from the same clone, there is much greater variability between the clones.

would be expected if cells from metastases were expressing a stable phenotype that predisposed them to form metastases. Support for the specific nature of metastasis derives from experimental studies. When clones of B16 melanoma cells were isolated, expanded in culture and the cells tested for their ability to form experimental metastases, the variability in metastases for cells from a single clone was found to be much less than that observed when different clones were compared (Fidler and Kripke, 1977). These results indicated wide heterogeneity in metastatic ability between the different clones (Fig. 10–7) and were replicated in a number of cells lines. They suggest the presence of preexisting metastatic variants within a cell population. However, the finding that metastatic properties can be unstable cast doubt on this interpretation and gave rise to the clonal heterogeneity model of metastasis formation (Hill et al, 1984). This model proposes that, although some of the multiple properties necessary for a cell to metastasize may be relatively stably expressed, others are expressed only transiently, giving rise to unstable clonal heterogeneity. However, the wide variety of properties that have been demonstrated to promote metastasis makes it unlikely that any 1 model will adequate depict the whole picture. To better understand the process, metastasis is often divided into a few sequenced steps: invasion, intravasation and survival in the circulation, extravasation, and, finally, establishment of a new growth (Fig. 10–8). These steps provide a simplified view of the complex set of biological events involved in the process. In each step, expression of specific molecular factors may help the tumor cells to survive and proceed to the next step in the process (see Sec. 10.4).

10.3.4 Circulating Tumor Cells

Distant metastases usually arise through the distribution of tumor cells into the circulating blood system. Tumor cell dissemination can be an early event and may persist throughout the growth of the primary tumor, although it is likely that the survival time of such cells in the circulation is quite short

(hours). It is now possible to detect (small numbers) of circulating tumor cells (CTCs) in the blood of many patients, and the numbers of such cells have been associated with overall survival in some patient groups. However, their isolation and characterization remains a significant challenge partly because of their low frequency (<1000 CTCs/mL of blood vs. millions of blood cells) (Pantel et al, 2008). The 2 main approaches for detecting these CTCs are immunological assays employing antibodies against cell-surface proteins specifically expressed on the cancer cells, and polymerase chain reaction (PCR)-based molecular assays detecting cancer cell-specific transcripts. The most common surface protein used in CTC detection is epithelial cell adhesion molecule (EpCAM), because many tumors are of epithelial origin, but other markers, such as various cytokeratins, have also been used. Identifying appropriate CTC markers is an ongoing research process and far from perfect (Wicha and Hayes, 2011). New sensitive methods such as in vivo multiphoton intravital flow cytometry may help to advance the detection of CTC in the blood of cancer patients.

Whole-genome copy number analysis and gene expression profiling have been used to analyze CTCs and have indicated that most CTC are dormant and in a nonproliferative state, possibly as a result of mechanisms of adaptive immunity (Koebel et al, 2007). However, CTCs can proliferate in cell culture systems if given appropriate growth factors, such as epidermal growth factor (EGF) and fibroblast growth factor 2 (FGF2). If the growth of CTCs is susceptible to reactivation in the patient this could clearly influence the overall outcome of treatment and the molecular nature of CTCs is being intensively investigated in this context. In breast cancer, ERBB2 expression on CTCs is associated with poor prognosis, and in gastric cancer, uPAR expression on CTCs is associated with metastatic relapse. This suggests ERBB2 and uPAR might play roles affecting the reactivation process of CTCs in their respective cancer types. CTCs that express angiogenesis and hypoxia-associated markers such as vascular endothelial growth factor (VEGF), VEGFR-2, FAK, and HIF-1, are also

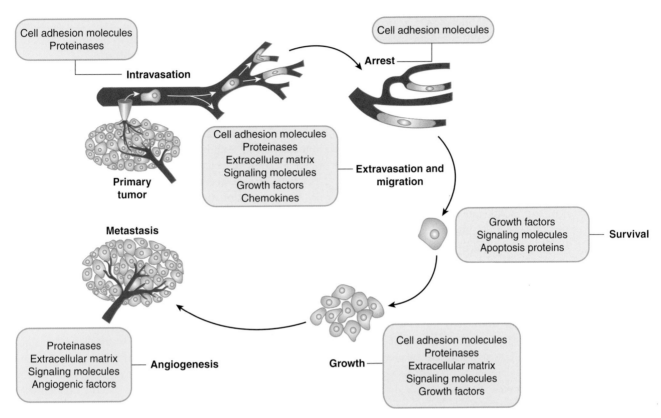

FIGURE 10-8 **Schematic of the sequential steps in the metastatic process.** Various types of molecules that are thought to be involved at each stage are listed.

thought to be associated with aggressive disease and poor prognosis (Bednarz-Knoll et al, 2011). Some CTCs have been shown to exhibit EMT (see Sec. 10.5.6), which may enhance their ability to form metastases.

Because the detection of CTCs can have prognostic value in early stages of the disease, their presence is being included in international tumor staging systems. It is hoped that CTC detection might allow monitoring of the disease and potentially treatments could be customized based on the molecular profiling of these cells.

10.4 STEPS IN THE METASTATIC PROCESS

10.4.1 Detachment from the Primary Tumor, Local Invasion, and Intravasation

Detachment or shedding of cells into blood or lymphatic vessels (intravasation) may occur as a result of prior invasion of the tumor mass into vessels or because the abnormal vasculature of tumors permits passage of cells into the circulation. Angiogenic factors such as VEGFs and FGFs can induce vascular remodeling (see Chap. 11) and thereby facilitate intravasation. Tumor blood vessels are less well-organized and leaky in comparison to their normal counterparts, providing

additional opportunities for cell penetration. The poor alignment of endothelial cells in tumor vessels has been reported to allow CTCs to home back to the original tumor, as has been observed in a mouse model of breast cancer (Kim et al. 2009). This phenomenon of cross-seeding is enhanced by tumor-derived chemoattractive cytokines such as interleukin (IL)-6 and IL-8. Tumor cells may also fine-tune surface molecules to interact with endothelial cells so as to increase their survival. For example, tumor cells can downregulate KAI1/CD82, a surface molecule that interacts with the Duffy antigen receptor for chemokine (DARC) on the endothelial cell to induce senescence of tumor cells (Bandyopadhyay et al, 2006). Loss of CD82 is correlated with metastatic progression in patients, and the knockout of DARC abrogates the suppressive effect of CD82. Studies with certain human tumor (eg, melanoma and glioblastoma) cells have shown that these tumor cells can form vascular channels and endothelial cells, and may in this way gain ready access to the vascular space (Hendrix et al, 2002). Detachment of cancer cells from the primary tumor mass may involve decreased expression of adhesion molecules involved in the "homotypic" adhesion of cells to one another or may depend on the expression of motility factors (eg, hepatocyte growth factor [HGF], autotoxin, or autocrine motility factor), which are glycoproteins found to promote cell movement through interaction with cell-surface molecules linked to the Rho/Rac/Cdc42 guanosine triphosphatase (GTPase) intracellular signaling system. Disruption of

E-cadherin expression in a mouse model of pancreatic cancer was found to enhance invasive properties and metastasis (Perl et al, 1998). Tumor cells may gain motility by overexpressing RhoC, a small calcium-dependent GTPase, that is normally responsible for sensing extracellular signals and controlling cytoskeletal actin organization. RhoC-deficient mice have normal primary tumor formation but reduced cancer cell mobility and drastically reduced metastases (Narumiya et al, 2009). The EMT process, in which a polarized epithelial cell assumes a mesenchymal cell phenotype, is also now considered to be coincident with the process of cancer cell migration (see Sec. 10.5.6). Local invasion and intravasation may also involve breakdown of the ECMs and basement membrane. Various proteases, including MMPs, play a major role in this process (see Secs. 10.2.2 and 10.5.1).

10.4.2 Survival in the Blood Stream

Once tumor cells break free of constraints at the primary site, they can gain access to the blood (or lymphatic) vessels (see Fig. 10–8). While in the blood vessels, tumor cells may travel with platelets to evade immune surveillance, ensuring their survival. Platelets are small, terminally differentiated anuclear cells shed from megakaryocytes. The basic biological function of platelets, such as blood clotting, is also exploited by tumor cells to their advantage. With the help of a number of other coagulation factors, activated platelets assemble and can form tumor cell–platelet aggregates. This aggregation, in combination with the adhesive properties of platelets, effectively arrests tumor cells in the capillaries of target organs. In addition, many platelet-surface molecules and platelet-derived factors enhance metastasis. For example, mice deficient in the platelet-specific receptor glycoprotein Ib-alpha (GPIb-α) have a 15-fold reduction of lung metastatic foci formation in an experimental metastasis model (Jain et al, 2007). In addition, α-granules released by platelets contain many growth-promoting factors, such as EGF, VEGF, HGF, and transforming growth factor (TGF)-β (Gay and Felding-Habermann, 2011).

Although CTCs can be detected in many patients, as discussed in Section 10.3.4, it appears that most tumor cells that reach the circulation are arrested in the first capillary bed that they encounter (first-pass capillary bed). Early experimental studies in which radiolabeled tumor cells were injected into the systemic or portal veins indicated that the majority of cells are arrested initially in the lung or liver capillaries, respectively. More recent work has used genes encoding markers, such as green fluorescent protein (GFP) or luciferase to provide direct visualization of tumor cell arrest following intravenous injection, or the growth of the tumor and its metastases in situ (Hoffman, 2002). Combined with such labels, the technique of intravital videomicroscopy (IVVM) has confirmed the early arrest of tumor cells in "first-pass" capillary beds and permitted dynamic study of events in the process of experimental metastasis as discussed below (MacDonald et al, 2002). It is this effect that probably accounts for the high level of

metastases in lung and liver, but some tumor cells succeed in passing through the first-pass organ to become CTCs or to establish metastases in other (preferred) sites.

10.4.3 Extravasation

After tumor cells arrive at the distant organ, they may extravasate into the new tissue (see Fig. 10–8). As discussed in Sections 10.2.2 and 10.5.1, this process involves the activity of a variety of proteases, of which MMPs are believed to play a major role. Several groups have reported in vivo studies of extravasation using IVVM. Chambers and colleagues observed that the majority of arrested cells were able to extravasate, even cells with reduced proteolytic capability or nonmalignant fibroblasts, suggesting that this process may not be a major barrier to the metastatic process (MacDonald et al, 2002). Other IVVM studies, however, found that extravasation was a formidable barrier to metastasis, and tumor cells were observed to proliferate intravascularly. Yet others observed that tumor cell extravasation was dependent on CAMs and could occur in precapillary vessels upon stimulation of the endothelial cells by inflammatory growth factors. Because the structural organization of capillary walls varies in different organs, tumor cells may need specific capabilities for infiltration at different sites. Recent studies of gene expression in patients with advanced metastatic disease have indicated that tumor cells trapped in the lung capillaries produce factors such as epiregulin (EREG), cyclooxygenase-2 (COX-2), MMP-1, and cytokine angiopoietin-like 4 (ANGPTL4) to remodel the pulmonary vasculature. These factors modify the integrity of lung endothelia and provide entry points into the lung parenchyma. Genetic and pharmaceutical inhibition of these factors significantly reduced metastatic extravasation (Gupta et al, 2007). Some of these genes seem to be general metastasis-promoting factors; for example, COX-2 is also a potent mediator of metastasis to the brain, and RNA interference-mediated knockdown of COX-2 expression decreases brain metastatic activity of certain breast cancer cell lines (Bos et al, 2009). Genes such as $\alpha_{2,6}$-sialyltransferase can facilitate passage through the blood–brain barrier by enhancing adhesion to brain endothelial cells and can act as a specific promoter of brain metastasis. Various other cell-surface molecules, such as chemokine receptors (eg, CXCR4) and growth factor receptors (eg, c-MET), have also been reported to augment metastasis. Conceivably, they accomplish this by recruiting tumor cells to target organs and enhancing their survival and growth.

10.4.4 Initiation of a New Growth (Colonization)

Following infiltration, the majority of tumor cells die as a result of selective pressure from the foreign environment, but a few (rare) tumor cells may successfully initiate growth inside the target organ. This may be accomplished by their incorporation into sites in the organ that are receptive to tumor growth (metastatic niches; see Sec. 10.5.8). There is also evidence that tumor cells that initiate metastatic growth can modify the target organ to make the environment more favorable for their outgrowth. For example, tumor cells in the bone achieve this by disrupting normal bone homeostasis. Through the secretion of parathyroid hormone-related peptide (PTHrP), IL-6, tumor necrosis factor α (TNF-α), and other factors, tumor cells stimulate the release of receptor activator of nuclear factor-κB ligand (RANKL) by osteoblasts. RANKL, in turn, stimulates myeloid progenitor cells to differentiate into osteoclasts. Osteoclasts can digest bone structures and create space for establishment of metastasis. Moreover, the lytic action of osteoclasts releases TGF-β, insulin-like growth factor I (IGF-I), and bone morphogenetic proteins (BMPs). These factors then further enhance tumor cell survival, thus creating a vicious cycle. To further increase the efficiency of the cycle, tumor cells also suppress the production of the RANKL antagonist osteoprotegerin (OPG), increasing the efficacy of RANKL (Chen et al, 2010). Denosumab, a monoclonal antibody targeting RANKL that breaks this vicious cycle, was recently approved for treating patients with bone metastasis. In the lung, inhibitor of differentiation-1 (Id1) has been implicated in bypassing senescence and promoting tumor outgrowth by desensitizing the cells to p21-dependent cell-cycle arrest (Swarbrick et al, 2008). In a mouse cancer model driven by Ras and Id1, inactivation of Id1 caused widespread senescence in established tumors within 10 days.

10.4.5 Metastatic Latency and Dormancy

After entering the target organ a few cells may survive but enter dormancy (Goss and Chambers, 2010). The dormant cells can remain in target organs for years before resulting in a metastatic growth. This has been particularly observed in breast cancer. Immunosurveillance has been suggested as being responsible for limiting the metastatic growth of the dormant cells. Because dormant tumor cells are not actively dividing, they are often harder to treat, as most drug treatments preferentially target dividing cells (see Chap. 17, Sec. 17.4). Doxorubicin was shown to reduce macrometastases but was ineffective against dormant tumor cells in a mouse model of mammary cancer. A number of factors, such as VEGF and Id1, have been implicated in reactivating dormant tumor cells but more research is needed to understand this critical event, and target these cells therapeutically (Sleeman et al, 2011).

10.5 MOLECULAR MECHANISMS OF METASTASIS

10.5.1 Protease Activity at the Invasive Front

Proteolysis must function at the tumor cell surface to facilitate invasion and degradation of the basement membrane. Extracellular proteinases, transmembrane proteinases, cell-surface molecules, and intracellular factors all contribute to generating pericellular zones of proteolysis. Mechanisms known to underlie the proteolytic activation at the cell membrane include the activation of plasmin by uPA and its receptor uPAR, and the activation of pro-MMP-2 within a trimolecular complex generated by MT1-MMP, MMP-2, and TIMP-2 (Hernandez-Barrantes et al, 2000; Overall et al, 2000). MT1-MMP activity associated with tumor progression has been observed at the leading edge of migrating cells. For the cell surface activation of pro-MMP-2 in the trimolecular complex, MT1-MMP must itself be activated by a proprotein convertase called *furin*. Mature furin can cycle between the Golgi and the cell surface, and activate MT1-MMP at both locations. The association of pro-MMP-2 with $\alpha_2\beta_1$ integrin-bound collagen was found to provide a reserve of the enzyme for subsequent activation of the trimolecular complex. By comprehensively comparing multiple MMPs in experimental systems that utilize 3D matrix composites, Weiss and colleagues found that MT1-, MT2-, or MT3-MMPs constitute the minimal requirement for basement membrane transmigration, and that MT1-MMP is the dominant protease mobilized for cancer cell trafficking through 3D interstitial ECM barriers (Rowe and Weiss, 2009). Several secreted MMPs, especially MMP-2 and MMP-9, have also been extensively studied in human cancer and experimental systems and have been shown to facilitate tumor cell invasion and motility, although their primary function in vivo may be to facilitate bulk ECM turnover during tissue remodeling (Kessenbrock et al, 2010).

The integrin $\alpha_v\beta_3$ may also localize active MMP-2 to the cell surface. Their colocalization was observed on newly developing blood vessels and on the tumor invasive front, and inhibition of their binding reduced tumor growth and angiogenesis (Silletti et al, 2001). Recently, it was shown that MT1-MMP catalyzes shedding of the α_3 integrin ectodomain in ovarian carcinoma cells, and this associates with formation of multicellular aggregates, an important step in ovarian cancer metastasis (Moss et al, 2009). Shedding of MMP-9–dependent E-cadherin may also play a role in the dissemination of ovarian cancer cells. CD44 provides a means of anchoring active MMP-9 to the cell surface of invadopodia in breast cancer and melanoma cells, and was found to be critical for MMP-9–mediated cell migration (Dufour et al, 2010). The association of CD44 with hyaluronic acid also has been shown to increase MMP-2 secretion and CD44 has been found to recruit MMP-7 and direct localization of MT1-MMP to the cell membrane. These findings highlight the complex spatial coordination between adhesion molecules and enzymatic activity, which bring about controlled activation of metalloproteinases and, ultimately, the digestion of ECM at the leading edge of invasive tumor cells.

10.5.2 Protease Activity in the Tumor Microenvironment

Beyond ECM degradation, studies using transgenic and knockout mouse models of MMPs and TIMPs have documented that proteolysis affects the early, as well as the late, stages of cancer progression. Protease activity impacts directly on cell growth, cell survival, angiogenesis, and inflammation (Fig. 10–9). Metalloproteinases and TIMPs alter the release of potent growth factors such as VEGF, TGF-β, and IGF-II, which are either sequestered in the ECM or exist in complexes with their binding proteins. Proteolytic cleavage of already synthesized factors results in altered bioavailability of growth signals to cancer cells and impact the process of cell proliferation.

Activation of EGFR (see Chap. 8, Sec. 8.2), which is overexpressed in many human cancers, follows ADAM-mediated release of members of the EGF family of growth factors, including amphiregulin, TGF-α, and HB-EGF. Similarly, processing of Notch (see Chap. 8, Sec. 8.2.4), a master regulator of cell differentiation, requires a 3-step proteolytic activation with ADAMs performing the second cleavage of the receptor. MMPs and TIMPs also influence apoptosis signals, such as

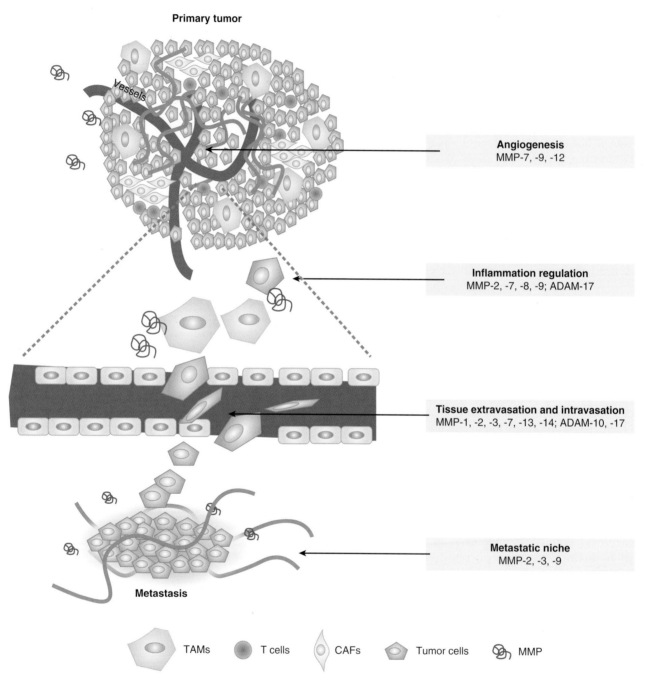

Primary tumor

Vessels

Angiogenesis
MMP-7, -9, -12

Inflammation regulation
MMP-2, -7, -8, -9; ADAM-17

Tissue extravasation and intravasation
MMP-1, -2, -3, -7, -13, -14; ADAM-10, -17

Metastatic niche
MMP-2, -3, -9

Metastasis

TAMs   T cells   CAFs   Tumor cells   MMP

FIGURE 10–9 **Metalloproteinases (MMPs) play multiple roles in tumor progression and metastasis.** These enzymes are contributed by both stromal cells and tumor cells. Different MMPs are implicated in the various processes. Specific MMPs that promote each of the listed processes during metastatic dissemination are shown as examples. The figure shows vertically an expansion of intravasation and extravasation events in the vasculature of the tumor and metastatic organ, respectively. *TAM*, Tumor-associated macrophage. *CAF*, Cancer-associated fibroblast. (Adapted from Nguyen et al., 2009).

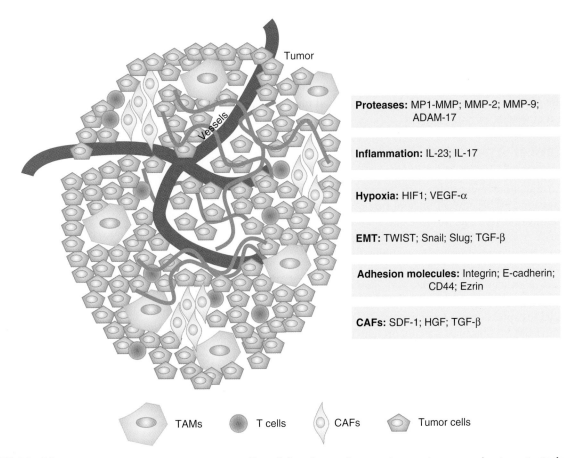

TAMs   T cells   CAFs   Tumor cells

Proteases: MP1-MMP; MMP-2; MMP-9; ADAM-17

Inflammation: IL-23; IL-17

Hypoxia: HIF1; VEGF-α

EMT: TWIST; Snail; Slug; TGF-β

Adhesion molecules: Integrin; E-cadherin; CD44; Ezrin

CAFs: SDF-1; HGF; TGF-β

FIGURE 10–10 **Mutual interactions between tumor cells and the microenvironment promote progression to metastasis.** Tumor cells can express some of the factors listed above, such as Snail or Slug, to promote progression. Futhermore, tumor cells can influence their microenvionment and induce the production of tumor-promoting factors from neighboring or incorporated "normal" cells (CAFs and TAMs). Many of the critical factors for tumor survival and motility, such as TNF-α and TGF-β, are provided by the tumor microenvironment. *CAF,* Cancer-associatrd fibroblast; *TAM,* tumor-associated macrophage.

those feeding into Fas-mediated death receptor signaling (see Chap. 9, Sec. 9.4.4). In addition, proteolytic activity regulates capillary ingrowth, vascular stability and access of tumor cells to vascular and lymphatic networks. Overall, manipulation of the expression of TIMPs reveals that they universally inhibit angiogenesis, invasion, and metastasis, but their effects on cell proliferation and apoptosis are both tissue-specific and context-dependent (Cruz-Munoz and Khokha, 2008).

Several nonneoplastic host cells, including fibroblasts, endothelial cells, leukocytes, and bone marrow-derived cell populations, are recruited during tumor development, and the composite of these stromal and cancer cells creates a complex microenvironment (Fig. 10–10). Metalloproteinase activity contributes to generating this microenvironment and can further facilitate tumor progression. For example, metalloproteinase activity, as regulated by the TIMP3-ADAM17 interactions, is important for the systemic release of molecules such as cell-surface-bound TNF-α. This pleiotropic cytokine is situated at the apex of cytokine cascades and NF-κB signaling that underlies immune cell crosstalk with cancer cells. Chemokines that influence immune cell motility are similarly processed by proteases. MMP cleavage of members of the

monocyte chemoattractant protein (MCP) family of chemokines renders them receptor antagonists with inflammation-dampening effects (McQuibban et al, 2002). MMP-1 and MMP-3 process CCL8/MCP-2, which has antitumor activity in a melanoma model. MMP-8 is mainly produced by neutrophils, and was shown to exert a tumor-suppressive effect in a model of carcinogen-induced skin cancer (Balbin et al, 2003). Other chemokines, including CXCL1/KC (neutrophil-attracting) and CXCL11 (Th1-lymphocyte-attracting), are also substrates of MMPs and thus, proteolysis can affect neutrophil content or T-cell response (see Chap. 21, Sec. 21.4). Metalloproteinases can also cleave RANKL, which can subsequently promote metastasis to bone.

10.5.3 Ameboid Movement and Cell Motility

The idea that cell penetration of ECM-imposed structural barriers depends exclusively on proteolysis has been challenged by studies in collagen gels showing that tumor cells can acquire rounded, amoeboid-like shape and perform mechanical displacement of intact ECM fibrils by relying on increased cell deformation and reduced cell-ECM adhesion. This protease-independent amoeboid tumor cell migration is likened to that of leukocytes (Croft and Olson, 2008). The importance of this alternate mechanism of migration in the metastatic process is currently uncertain, partially because of concerns about whether these gels truly mimic the 3D ECM barriers found in vivo (Sabeh et al, 2009).

10.5.4 Cancer-Associated Fibroblasts

Mesenchymal cell types, including cancer-associated fibroblasts (CAFs) and pericytes, coevolve with cancer cells during tumor progression and become an integral part of the paracrine communication (see Fig. 10–10). CAFs were thought initially to arise from local fibroblasts by acquiring a modified "activated" phenotype. However, later studies linked their origin to bone marrow-derived cells or transdifferentiation from epithelial or even endothelial cells. TGF-β is considered a critical activating factor for CAFs, which are typically identified through the expression of a set of markers (ie, α-smooth muscle actin [α-SMA]; fibroblast specific protein-1 [FSP-1]/S100A4; FAP; neuron-glial antigen-2 [NG-2]; platelet-derived growth factor-β receptor [PDGFR-β]), whereas pericytes are more loosely defined but are thought to depend on PDGF and TGF-β signaling. These stromal cell types can contribute to cancer promotion by the delivery of key growth signals (HGF, FGF) and survival signals (insulin-like growth factors [IGFs]) that can counter death signals and activate downstream oncogenic signaling. They inherently provide ECM components for interaction with integrins resulting in the activation of specific signal transduction pathways. CAFs also overexpress metalloproteinases, chemokines (SDF-1 or CXCL12, IL-6, CXCL8) and angiogenic factors (VEGFs, FGFs) that can lead to the generation of a proangiogenic and proinflammatory microenvironment. Consistent with this, when they are coinjected with tumor cells CAFs promote xenograft growth. They have been observed at the sites of metastases, and SDF-1 is known to promote the recruitment of endothelial progenitors, whereas activated pericytes can affect vessel permeability, both of which are critical mechanisms in angiogenesis. The gene expression profiles of CAFs have demonstrated their heterogeneity in individual tumors and resulted in identification of CAF subsets, which may have prognostic value. The importance of understanding these cells, originally considered to be bystanders, is emphasized by the observation that mice deficient in specific CAF markers show decreased metastasis, and that CAFs may alter the drug-sensitivity of cancer cells (Ostman and Augsten, 2009).

10.5.5 Tumor-Associated Macrophages

Tumor-associated macrophages (TAMs) are important players in promoting cancer progression (see Fig. 10–10) and high TAM content in the tumor mass correlates with poor prognosis of patients (Qian and Pollard, 2010). In the local microenvironment, tumor cells can direct the differentiation of TAMs, which exhibit several protumorigenic and prometastatic

functions, including induction of inflammation, secretion of growth factors and MMPs, promotion of angiogenesis, and suppression of cytotoxic effects (Sica et al, 2008). The inflammatory state of TAMs is controlled by the transcription factor NF-κB, which, in turn, is activated through toll-like receptors (TLRs; see Chap. 21, Sec. 21.2.2). TAMs exert most of their inflammatory effects through cytokines. Cytokines such as IL-6 cause the endothelial lining of the tumor vessels to become leaky, resulting in the recruitment of more inflammatory cells and providing escape routes into the bloodstream for tumor cells. TNF-α produced by TAMs can activate NF-κB and AP-1 family of transcription factors in the tumor cells, stimulating their cell proliferation and survival. Specific inhibition of NF-κB activity in myeloid cells through ablation of IkB kinase (IKK)-α resulted in a reduction of inflammation and inhibition of tumor progression. In contrast, inactivation of STAT3 (a transcription factor that functions to suppress inflammation—see Chap. 8, Sec. 8.3.1) in myeloid cells is associated with abundant expression of inflammatory cytokines such as TNF-α and IL-6 that have been shown to promote chronic colitis and invasive colorectal cancer in animal models (Grivennikov et al, 2009). Another crucial cytokine produced by TAMs is IL-23. IL-23 acts by enhancing the activity of Th17 cells and inhibiting the activity of T-regulatory cells. The Th17 cell is a T-helper cell subclass with strong inflammatory effects, and they are generally associated with tumor progression.

10.5.6 Epithelial-to-Mesenchymal Transition

Epithelium is a highly polarized structure composed of polygonal-shaped cells with abundant cell–cell tight junctions. It lines the outer surface, as well as the inner organ surface, of the body. Epithelial cells make contact with a basal membrane, and both cell–cell and cell–matrix adhesions are necessary for their survival. Different epithelial cell populations are heterogeneous, depending on the tissue/organ involved. In contrast, mesenchymal cells are spindle-shaped and highly migratory, which is essential for their role in supporting tissue/organ development. EMT (Fig. 10–11) is a process during which an epithelial cell loses its apical–basal polarity and becomes a mesenchymal-like cell with increased migratory ability, resistance to apoptosis, and increased production of ECM components (Kalluri and Neilson, 2003). During this process, epithelial cells often lose the expression of cell-surface and cytoskeletal proteins mediating adhesion, such as E-cadherin, cytokeratin, zona occludens 1 (ZO-1), and laminin. Instead, they gain proteins that are often seen on mesenchymal cell surface such as N-cadherin, vimentin, fibronectin, and α-SMA. The resulting mesenchymal-like cell eventually detaches from the basal membrane and migrates away from the epithelial layer. This process occurs extensively in the embryo at different stages of maturation and development of organs, and in wound healing (Hay, 1995). In tumors it is hypothesized that

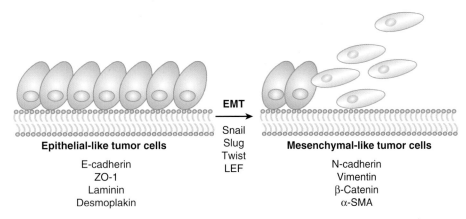

FIGURE 10–11 During tumor progression, epithelial tumor cells often undergo EMT to gain anchorage-independent survival and motility. Epithelial cells usually express markers such as E-cadherin, ZO-1, laminin, and desmoplakin. Through the aberrant expression of transcription factors such as Snail and Slug, these epithelial cells lose their epithelial markers and start to express mesenchymal markers, such as N-cadherin, vimentin, β-catenin, and α-SMA. Many of these markers are also functionally associated with the epithelial or mesenchymal characteristics. For example, E-cadherin and N-cadherin activate different intracellular programs that give rise to the epithelial-like or mesenchymal-like properties.

this embryonic program may be reactivated to drive an initial important step in metastasis, but may then be reversed mesenchymal to epithelial transition (MET) when the cell establishes a new growth (Kalluri and Weinberg, 2009). This latter (MET) step may help to explain why it has been difficult to observe evidence of the EMT process in human tumor specimens (Tarin et al, 2005).

Various studies link loss of E-cadherin to EMT. Treatment with a monoclonal anti–E-cadherin antibody disrupted cell–cell junctions in MDCK cells, activation of a fusion protein that abolishes E-cadherin expression induced EMT in mouse mammary epithelial cells, while expression of E-cadherin induced a MET-like process with reestablishment of cell junctions and decreased proliferation in cells that had already undergone EMT. Cancer cell lines with loss of E-cadherin expression show higher tumorigenicity as xenografts in nude mice, and, in some cancers, E-cadherin levels relate inversely to prognosis. Mutations in the E-cadherin gene causing either loss or truncation of the protein have been identified in human breast and gastric cancers, possibly rendering these tumors more prone to EMT and metastasis. Similarly, epigenetic mechanisms such as transcriptional repression and promoter silencing by hypermethylation also contribute to E-cadherin downregulation in various carcinomas. Transcription factors that play roles in EMT such as TWIST, Snail (Snai1), and Slug (Snai2), also repress E-cadherin expression (Medici et al, 2008).

TGF-β, normally a negative regulator of epithelial cell growth, is another key player in EMT. In various in vitro studies, TGF-β has been shown to induce EMT-like changes in epithelial cell lines. Two pathways downstream of TGF-β are at least partially responsible for its transforming effect, Smad and p38/RhoA (see Chap. 8, Sec. 8.4.4). Studies using in vitro cell lines suggest that activation of p38 is indispensable. Other signals that induce EMT include HGF, which activates the receptor tyrosine kinase c-Met, as well as EGF and PDGF, activating

their respective receptors. Multiple recent studies have linked noncoding microRNAs (see Chap. 2, Sec. 2.4.3) as regulators of EMT, both positively and negatively. MicroRNA family members, miR-200 and miR-205, prevent EMT by inhibiting Zeb-1 and Zeb-2, known repressors of E-cadherin expression. In contrast, miR-21 expression is elevated in many carcinomas and supports TGF-β-dependent EMT (Shi et al, 2010).

10.5.7 Role of Hypoxia

Hypoxia drives the expression of a large number of metastasis-related genes through the specific HIF1/2 transcription factors and has been found to relate to metastatic disease in many experimental models and in some clinical studies (Finger and Giaccia, 2010; Lunt et al, 2009). As discussed in Chapter 12, Section 12.2, cells in tumors may be exposed to hypoxia as a consequence of diffusion limitations (prolonged or chronic hypoxia) or of perfusion limitations (acute or cyclic hypoxia). Both types of exposure are reported to modify gene expression, and in experimental studies in vitro, both were found to affect metastatic properties of cells. In animal models or patients, it is currently not possible to determine directly whether cells which form metastases derive from areas of chronic or acute hypoxia, but studies that have deliberately induced increased levels of acute (cyclic) hypoxia in tumors in animal models have demonstrated increase development of metastases, suggesting that exposure to acute (cyclic) hypoxia can play an important role in the metastatic process (Lunt et al, 2009). Many specific mechanisms of metastasis are reported to be affected by hypoxia, as discussed below, but the specific genes involved may be different in different cell types.

EMT-promoting genes, such as TWIST and Snai1/2, can be upregulated by hypoxia in multiple cell lines, including ovarian, renal cell, pancreatic, and colon cancer lines, causing loss of E-cadherin. Other important adhesion molecules that can be mediated by hypoxia are the β_1 integrins that have been found to correlate with invasive capacity in pancreatic cancer cell lines. Hypoxia also can induce the expression of uPA, uPAR, MMP-2, and MMP-9 in a variety of cell lines, leading to an increase in metastatic invasion both in vitro and in vivo. Blocking uPAR activity with a monoclonal antibody was reported to almost abolish metastatic disease in mice bearing human melanoma xenografts. Similarly, hypoxic exposure of a human breast carcinoma line in vitro resulted in the downregulation of TIMP and concomitant upregulation of MMP-9, causing increased invasive capacity, an effect that could be blocked by using an inhibitor of MMPs. Other studies demonstrated hypoxia-mediated upregulation of MMP-2 activity and a positive correlation with metastatic ability in lung and melanoma tumor models. Hypoxia has been shown to increase transcription of c-MET thereby sensitizing the cells to HGF, significantly increasing the invasive capacity of tumor cells.

The SDF-1/CXCR4 signaling complex plays a key role in tumor cell motility and homing. In vivo studies using a human breast cancer line showed that the formation of both spontaneous and experimental lung metastases could be significantly reduced using a monoclonal antibody against CXCR4, demonstrating its importance in the metastatic process. CXCR4 and SDF1 have been shown to be upregulated by tumor hypoxia, facilitating the development of metastatic disease. The presence of SDF-1 at secondary sites, such as lung, lymph nodes, and bone, concomitant with the expression of its receptor on CTCs may enable cell adhesion and extravasation at the secondary site. The ECM protein, lysyl oxidase (LOX), has also been identified as a hypoxia-regulated gene involved in metastatic disease (Erler et al, 2006). LOX was found to be positively correlated with tumor hypoxia in breast cancer patients, and there was a significant relationship between LOX expression and distant metastases. In vitro studies demonstrated a role for LOX in invasion and migration through regulation of FAK activity, suggesting multiple roles for hypoxia-induced LOX in the formation of metastatic disease. Another important ECM protein that is hypoxia-regulated is the secreted glycophosphoprotein osteopontin (OPN), which is expressed by multiple different cell types (osteoclasts, osteoblasts, epithelial cells, and endothelial cells). OPN has roles in cell adhesion, angiogenesis, prevention of apoptosis, and the anchorage-independent proliferation of tumor cells. Its expression has been found to correlate with increased metastatic potential in breast, prostate, colon, and head and neck cancers, and in soft-tissue sarcoma (Anborgh et al, 2010).

VEGF-A is a potent inducer of tumor angiogenesis (see Chap. 11, Sec. 11.4.1) that is upregulated in response to hypoxia by both HIF-1 dependent and independent mechanisms. Its receptors, VEGFR-1 and -2, are also induced under hypoxic conditions. The role of this protein in metastatic disease has been examined extensively, with some studies suggesting a link between VEGF-A expression and metastatic disease, and others not, consistent with the concept that angiogenesis is a result of multiple factors of varying importance in different tumor types. However, in driving the development of neovasculature, VEGF-A may provide a mechanism of transport for the tumor cells, as well as enhancing the intravasation and extravasation stages of the metastatic process because of increased vascular permeability. VEGF-A also plays a role in macrophage migration, and TAMs are reported to localize in hypoxic regions in tumors.

Using expression microarray, OPN was identified to be the most consistently upregulated gene in relation to tumor progression (Agrawal et al, 2002). High levels of OPN in the serum also have been reported to correlate with increased levels of hypoxia and poorer treatment outcome in head and neck and non–small cell lung tumors (Le et al, 2003; Mack et al, 2008).

10.5.8 Metastatic Niches and Microvesicles

A recent addition to the metastatic process is the concept that a "premetastatic niche" can be created in distant organs to which CTCs can "home" (Carlini et al, 2011). Although tumor cells are the driving force of metastasis, these new findings suggest that the host cells within the tumor microenvironment play a key role in influencing metastatic behavior. Specifically, bone marrow-derived hematopoietic progenitor cells expressing VEGFR-1 have been shown to precede the arrival of even single metastatic cells at distant sites. They are postulated to build a microenvironment suitable for tumor cell growth, although blockade of VEGFR-1 was insufficient to prevent metastasis in the widely used B16 melanoma and Lewis lung tumor metastasis models (Dawson et al, 2009). Molecular processes that have been identified in niche creation include the upregulation of specific integrins and their ECM ligands or increased expression of inflammatory chemoattractants. For example, $\alpha_4\beta_1$ integrin expression on progenitor cells can allow their interaction with fibronectin-expressing metastatic cells. Secreted soluble factors are key players in bone marrow cell mobilization during metastasis, and S100A8 or S100A9 expressed in the niche can attract macrophages. Metalloproteinases are also likely candidates for promoting the formation of a metastatic niche, as this involves altered matrix proteins, VEGF, TGF-β, and TNF-α bioavailability, chemokine activity, and immune cell interaction. In addition hypoxia-induced LOX was recently associated with the development of metastatic niches (Erler et al, 2009). Mechanisms for how such niches are initiated, the extent of the role they play in the overall metastatic process, and whether factors secreted from the primary tumor are required for their initiation are currently unclear and require further investigation.

Membrane vesicles (exosomes) derived from both tumor and host cells have also been recognized to promote tumor growth and metastasis, possible through promotion of metastatic niches (Peinado et al, 2011). Microvesicles are generated by the outward budding and fission of membrane vesicles from the cell surface. They are released from cells upon activation, malignant transformation, stress, or death, and can be found in various biological fluids, including blood and urine. These structures contain "cargo" including proteins (receptors, antigens), lipids, and nucleic acids (DNA, mRNA, microRNA), and can be endocytosed by other cells or interact with their cell surface receptors through fusion. This process occurs frequently in platelets and tumor cells, and such exosomes can provide a means for horizontal transfer of bioactive molecules to stimulate tumor progression, immune response, invasion, angiogenesis, and metastasis. For example, microvesicles from platelets were found to induce angiogenesis and metastasis in lung and breast cancers, and those released from tumor cells contained tetraspanins that could recruit endothelial cells. Molecular information harbored in the circulating microvesicles is being explored for its prognostic and predictive significance (Pap, 2011).

10.5.9 Metastasis-Suppressor Genes

A small number of genes are reported as metastasis-suppressor genes. These genes are defined strictly as those whose products reduce the metastatic behavior of tumor cells without affecting their tumorigenic capacity. The detailed mechanisms by which these genes act are diverse and involve every step in the metastatic cascade. However, only a few genes have been investigated in enough detail to be certain about their mechanism(s) of action or even that they truly conform to the second part of the definition. The nm-23 (NME-1) gene was the first metastasis-suppressor gene isolated and it has several isoforms (Lee et al, 2009). Inverse correlations between expression levels and metastatic potential have been observed in a number of different cancers including breast cancer and melanoma. NME-1 has nucleoside diphosphate kinase (NDPK) activity as well as exonuclease and histidine kinase activity. It also appears to play a role in maintenance of genomic stability. Mutations in both NDPK and exonuclease activity still allow suppression of metastasis and the activities associated with them vary by cell type. It is unclear which of the various activities plays the critical role in suppressing cancer metastasis. The KAI-1/ CD82 gene is a member of the Tetraspanin (TM4SP) family of adhesion molecules that play a role in lymphocyte differentiation and function. It has been reported to have a p53 binding site in its promotor, and the loss of KAI-1 correlated with loss of p53. Loss of expression is implicated in metastases in cancers of the prostate, breast and colon and in melanoma. KiSS-1 appears to be involved in cell signaling, as a posttranslationally-modified version of this protein, called metastatin, has been reported to bind to a G-protein–coupled receptor (Axor12) and preliminary evidence suggests that activation of this receptor can alter signaling through FAK. MKK4 is also a molecule associated with signaling, through the stress-activated protein kinase (SAPK) pathway (see Chap. 8, Sec. 8.2.4), and both these molecules may act to increase the likelihood that a tumor cell will be able to initiate growth at a new (metastatic) site. Breast metastasis suppressor-1 (BrMS-1), which is frequently altered in late-stage breast cancers, is a transcriptional repressor and causes downregulation of phosphatidylinositol

(4,5) bisphosphate (PtdIns(4,5)P2). In vivo experiments have demonstrated that BrMS-1 inhibits several steps of metastasis, including the ultimate step, colonization at the secondary site. To date, however, whether gene regulation effects are direct versus indirect has not been clearly demonstrated. Hurst and Welch (2011) have reviewed clinical and experimental information about these and other possible metastasis-suppressor genes.

10.5.10 Genome-Wide Analyses and Metastatic Signatures

Recent advances in sequencing and microarray technologies (see Chap. 2) have enabled genome-wide analyses of primary tumors and researchers are increasingly using -omic approaches (eg, genome, transcriptome, proteome, or methylome) to study metastasis. One of the most common approaches is the gene expression profiling of tumors (transcriptome), and this approach has been applied to examining metastatic propensity of tumors. A seminal paper identified a group of 70 genes expressed in the primary tumors of breast cancer patients, which formed a profile that was capable of predicting survival and the likelihood of developing distant disease (van de Vijver et al, 2002). In a retrospective analysis, this profile was claimed to outperform the best predictions based on histological and clinical criteria, thus providing a capability to select early stage patients who needed adjuvant chemotherapy, and thereby avoiding exposing those who did not need such treatment to the toxicity involved (Knauer et al, 2010). Another study identified an expression profile involving 128 genes that distinguished between primary tumors and metastases of a range of different types of adenocarcinomas (Ramaswamy et al, 2003). This gene set was subsequently refined down to a group of 17 genes that retained a broad diagnostic ability to predict outcome in a range of tumor types (lung, breast and prostate adenocarcinomas and medulloblastoma but not lymphoma). Interestingly, predictive gene signatures from various studies often do not overlap with each other. This has been explained by the heterogeneity of the various patient pools from which the signatures are derived.

These technologies have been extensively applied to breast cancer, allowing specific subgroups with prognostic differences to be identified. Various tests using molecular profiling are currently commercially available to assist treatment decisions for patients with early stage breast cancer (Eroles et al, 2012). Clinical studies have demonstrated benefit in such tests for choice of drug treatment in patients with node-negative breast cancer, who may have undetected distant metastases, but there remain questions about which patient populations are most appropriate for these tests and whether they are applicable to other cancers (Oakman et al, 2010).

In addition to global RNA expression profiles, changes in genome-wide DNA copy number have been examined in cancers. Hu et al (2009) found consistent copy number gains on chromosome 8q22 in breast cancer patients with poor prognosis. Through computational analyses of this region, they were able to identify metadherin (MTDH) as a metastasis-promoter gene. Knocking down MTDH in several cell lines resulted in significant reduction of lung metastases in an experimental model of metastasis in mice. Hu et al (2009) also showed that gain of MTDH was associated with poor prognosis in an independent patient cohort. In another study on colorectal cancer, comparison of DNA copy number profiles from metastasis-free patients and patients harboring liver or peritoneal metastases identified copy number gains on chromosome 20q that preferentially associated with liver metastasis (Bruin et al, 2010).

Whole-genome sequencing is another powerful tool for understanding the metastatic process. In pancreatic cancer, comparison of mutations between primary malignancies and their corresponding metastases led to the identification of single-nucleotide changes that only existed in the metastases (Campbell et al, 2010). Furthermore, relying on extensive analyses of the sequencing data, an evolutionary path of the tumor cells was constructed and sequential mutations acquired by tumor cells that eventually led to metastases were identified (as illustrated by Fig. 10–2). Whole-genome methylation profiling is also being applied to metastasis research. Fang et al (2011) identified a methylation signature associated with low metastatic risk and high survival rate in breast cancer. The methylation status was able to account for many of the transcriptional differences between the poor- and good-prognosis patients, and was independent of other breast cancer markers. Its predictive potential is shared by other malignancies, such as glioma and colon cancer. As these new sequencing technologies become more affordable and more widely available, it is expected that they will lead to deeper insights in metastatic dissemination of each cancer type to specific distant organs.

10.6 TREATMENT OF METASTASES

Current cancer therapeutics largely focus on the primary tumor and it is generally assumed that the sensitivity of the cells in metastases is similar to that of the primary tumor. Specific treatment of identified solitary metastases may occur with focused radiotherapy or surgery, but there has been limited success in the development and clinical use of drugs specifically targeted against the metastatic process (Perret and Crepin, 2008). As described above, this process can be broken down into various stages and studies in preclinical models have demonstrated the potential to block metastasis formation by blocking essentially all the stages. However, clinical applications of some of these approaches have not shown much benefit to date. For example, an important step in the process is the arrest of CTCs, and many anticoagulant drugs have been assessed for their ability to inhibit metastases (Hejna et al, 1999). There have been consistent reports of reduced metastases in animal systems by treatment with heparin, warfarin, and inhibitors of platelet aggregation (prostacyclin and

dipyridamole), but there is only limited information from clinical trials. One large trial of the use of warfarin in patients with lung, colon, head and neck, and prostate cancer led to little or no improvement in survival (Zacharski et al, 1984). Similarly, the use of peptides, blocking the integrin motif RGD, which is involved in binding of cells to fibronectin, were also largely ineffective in clinical studies, although they showed considerable promise in preclinical studies. New integrin antagonists not based on the RGD motif are currently in early clinical development.

Other stages of the metastatic process are intravasation and extravasation of the tumor cells into the circulation and from the circulation into a secondary site. Despite the important roles that MMPs appear to play in these processes, the development of synthetic inhibitors against metalloproteinases as cancer therapeutics has thus far not been very successful, although the clinical studies were largely in late stage patients and not specifically designed to study effects on formation of metastases (Zucker et al, 2000). The tremendous heterogeneity of metalloproteinase expression with respect to particular members and the cell type responsible for its expression and overlapping substrate profiles of metalloproteinases may be the reason for the lack of effect observed and more specific inhibitors are under development. The plasminogen activator system is also being investigated, particularly as uPAR and PAI-1 have been found to be strong predictors of treatment outcome in breast cancer in various tests and genetic screens. Clinical studies are in progress with inhibitors of this proteolytic system (Schmitt et al, 2011).

Agents targeted at the angiogenic process, which also is critical for the development of macrometastases, have also not proved very successful in clinical studies, although, again, many of these agents are tested in patients with advanced disease. Studies of the compound, razoxane, which "normalizes" the structure of tumor blood vessels and was found to be effective as an antimetastatic agent in animal models, did suggest improved outcome in patients with soft-tissue sarcoma when combined with vindesine and radiation and surgery (Rhomberg et al, 2008). Unfortunately, razoxane development was halted because of a possible link to leukemia.

One limitation to the successful development of clinical therapies to prevent metastasis formation is that microscopic metastases are often present prior to detection and treatment of the primary tumor. Prevention of secondary metastases (ie, metastases from metastases) might be useful in palliation, but the potential for increased cure through the use of antimetastatic agents is limited to patients in whom metastases are seeded after diagnosis and prior to eradication of the primary tumor or in cases where tumor cells have seeded to other sites in the body but are in a dormant state. Tumor cells are known to enter the circulation at the time of surgery, but seeding at the time of surgery is probably the sole source of metastases for only a small proportion of patients. The recent discovery of the development of "premetastatic niches" (see Sec. 10.5.8), may provide an opportunity for early (preventative) treatment for the development of metastases using inhibitors of components of this process such as LOX.

SUMMARY

- Cancer is a multistep process that progresses through benign and premalignant changes to frank malignancy. It involves a number of genetic or epigenetic changes that may be very extensive in late-stage cancer.
- The development of metastatic potential is one of the late stages of the process of tumor progression and is the major cause of death in cancer patients.
- Several major steps are involved in the process of metastasis, including the ability to invade into and out of blood vessels, to survive in the circulation, and to arrest and grow at a new site.
- A range of properties (particularly those relating to cell adhesion, secretion of proteolytic enzymes, and initiation of a new growth) are involved in this process.
- Metastasis is an inefficient process and may depend partially on random survival factors associated with traversing the various stages of the metastatic process. Some types of primary tumors demonstrate organ-site specificity in the development of metastases.
- Cellular interactions with the ECM play an important role in development of metastasis and are mediated through CAMs, such as integrins and cadherins. The formation and breakdown of adhesive bonds between tumor cells and their environment during metastasis provides information to the cell via signaling about its environment. This can lead to changes in gene expression and determine cell proliferation, invasion, and other processes.
- Proteolytic enzymes, such as the families of serine proteases and metalloproteinases, play important functions in the breakdown of ECM components to enhance the invasive properties of tumor cells, and can release and/or activate growth factors that assist the growth of tumor cells at a new metastatic site.
- Infiltrating stromal cells, particularly CAFs and TAMs, play an important role in tumor growth and metastasis.
- Specific changes in cellular phenotype from epithelial to mesenchymal may play a role in the ability of cancer cells of epithelial origin (carcinoma cells) to metastasize.
- The identification of specific cellular or genetic properties that characterize all metastatic cells has proven elusive. Rather, many different cellular changes are capable of producing phenotypes that increase the ability of tumor cells to form metastases and these may be specific to different cancer subtypes.
- A number of metastasis-associated gene signatures have been identified that have prognostic significance particularly in breast cancer. The role that these different genes play in metastasis from individual tumors remains to be determined.

REFERENCES

Agrawal D, Chen T, Irby R, et al. Osteopontin identified as lead marker of colon cancer progression, using pooled sample expression profiling. *J Natl Cancer Inst* 2002;94: 513-521.

Anborgh PH, Mutrie JC, Tuck AB, Chambers AF. Role of the metastasis-promoting protein osteopontin in the tumour microenvironment. *J Cell Mol Med* 2010;14:2037-2044.

Balbin M, Fueyo A, Tester AM, et al. Loss of collagenase-2 confers increased skin tumor susceptibility to male mice. *Nat Genet* 2003; 35:252-257.

Bandyopadhyay S, Zhan R, Chaudhuri A, et al. Interaction of KAI1 on tumor cells with DARC on vascular endothelium leads to metastasis suppression. *Nat Med* 2006;12:933-938.

Bednarz-Knoll N, Alix-Panabieres C, Pantel K. Clinical relevance and biology of circulating tumor cells. *Breast Cancer Res* 2011;13:228.

Bos PD, Zhang XH, Nadal C, et al. Genes that mediate breast cancer metastasis to the brain. *Nature* 2009;459:1005-1009.

Boudreau N, Sympson CJ, Werb Z, Bissell MJ. Suppression of ICE and apoptosis in mammary epithelial cells by extracellular matrix. *Science* 1995;267:891-893.

Bruce B, Khanna G, Ren L, et al. Expression of the cytoskeleton linker protein ezrin in human cancers. *Clin Exp Metastasis* 2007; 24:69-78.

Bruin SC, Klijn C, Liefers GJ, et al. Specific genomic aberrations in primary colorectal cancer are associated with liver metastases. *BMC Cancer* 2010;10:662.

Campbell PJ, Yachida S, Mudie LJ, et al. The patterns and dynamics of genomic instability in metastatic pancreatic cancer. *Nature* 2010;467:1109-1113.

Carlini MJ, De Lorenzo MS, Puricelli L. Cross-talk between tumor cells and the microenvironment at the metastatic niche. *Curr Pharm Biotechnol* 2011;12:1900-1908.

Cavallaro U, Schaffhauser B, Christofori G. Cadherins and the tumour progression: is it all in a switch? *Cancer Lett* 2002;176: 123-128.

Chen YC, Sosnoski DM, Mastro AM. Breast cancer metastasis to the bone: mechanisms of bone loss. *Breast Cancer Res* 2010;12:215.

Croft DR, Olson MF. Regulating the conversion between rounded and elongated modes of cancer cell movement. *Cancer Cell* 2008; 14:349-351.

Cruz-Munoz W, Khokha R. The role of tissue inhibitors of metalloproteinases in tumorigenesis and metastasis. *Crit Rev Clin Lab Sci* 2008;45:291-338.

Dawson MR, Duda DG, Fukumura D, Jain RK. VEGFR1-activity-independent metastasis formation. *Nature* 2009;461:E4, discussion E5.

Desgrosellier JS, Cheresh DA. Integrins in cancer: biological implications and therapeutic opportunities. *Nat Rev Cancer* 2010;10:9-22.

Dufour A, Zucker S, Sampson NS, Kuscu C, Cao J. Role of matrix metalloproteinase-9 dimers in cell migration: design of inhibitory peptides. *J Biol Chem* 2010;285:35944-35956.

Egeblad M, Werb Z. New functions for the matrix metalloproteinases in cancer progression. *Nat Rev Cancer* 2002;2:161-174.

Erler JT, Bennewith KL, Cox TR, et al. Hypoxia-induced lysyl oxidase is a critical mediator of bone marrow cell recruitment to form the premetastatic niche. *Cancer Cell* 2009;15:35-44.

Erler JT, Bennewith KL, Nicolau M, et al. Lysyl oxidase is essential for hypoxia-induced metastasis. *Nature* 2006;440:1222-1226.

Eroles P, Bosch A, Perez-Fidalgo JA, Lluch A. Molecular biology in breast cancer: Intrinsic subtypes and signaling pathways. *Cancer Treat Rev* 2012;38:698-707.

Ewald AJ, Brenot A, Duong M, Chan BS, Werb Z. Collective epithelial migration and cell rearrangements drive mammary branching morphogenesis. *Dev Cell* 2008;14:570-581.

Fang F, Orend G, Watanabe N, Hunter T, Ruoslahti E. Dependence of cyclin E-CDK2 kinase activity on cell anchorage. *Science* 1996; 271:499-502.

Fang F, Turcan S, Rimner A, et al. Breast cancer methylomes establish an epigenomic foundation for metastasis. *Sci Transl Med* 2011;3:75ra25.

Fearon ER, Vogelstein B. A genetic model for colorectal tumorigenesis. *Cell* 1990;61:759-767.

Fidler IJ. Selection of successive tumour lines for metastasis. *Nat New Biol* 1973;242:148-149.

Fidler IJ, Kripke ML. Metastasis results from preexisting variant cells within a malignant tumor. *Science* 1977;197:893-895.

Finger EC, Giaccia AJ. Hypoxia, inflammation, and the tumor microenvironment in metastatic disease. *Cancer Metastasis Rev* 2010;29:285-293.

Fujihara T, Sawada T, Hirakawa K, et al. Establishment of lymph node metastatic model for human gastric cancer in nude mice and analysis of factors associated with metastasis. *Clin Exp Metastasis* 1998;16:389-398.

Gay LJ, Felding-Habermann B. Contribution of platelets to tumour metastasis. *Nat Rev Cancer* 2011;11:123-134.

Glaves D, Huben RP, Weiss L. Haematogenous dissemination of cells from human renal adenocarcinomas. *Br J Cancer* 1988; 57:32-35.

Goss PE, Chambers AF. Does tumour dormancy offer a therapeutic target? *Nat Rev Cancer* 2010;10:871-877.

Grivennikov S, Karin E, Terzic J, et al. IL-6 and Stat3 are required for survival of intestinal epithelial cells and development of colitis-associated cancer. *Cancer Cell* 2009;15:103-113.

Gupta GP, Nguyen DX, Chiang AC, et al. Mediators of vascular remodelling co-opted for sequential steps in lung metastasis. *Nature* 2007;446:765-770.

Hahn WC, Counter CM, Lundberg AS, Beijersbergen RL, Brooks MW, Weinberg RA. Creation of human tumour cells with defined genetic elements. *Nature* 1999;400:464-468.

Hanahan D, Weinberg RA. Hallmarks of cancer: the next generation. *Cell* 2011;144:646-674.

Hay ED. An overview of epithelio-mesenchymal transformation. *Acta Anat (Basel)* 1995;154:8-20.

Hejna M, Raderer M, Zielinski CC. Inhibition of metastases by anticoagulants. *J Natl Cancer Inst* 1999;91:22-36.

Hendrix MJ, Seftor RE, Seftor EA, et al. Transendothelial function of human metastatic melanoma cells: role of the microenvironment in cell-fate determination. *Cancer Res* 2002;62:665-668.

Hernandez-Barrantes S, Toth M, Bernardo MM, et al. Binding of active (57 kDa) membrane type 1-matrix metalloproteinase (MT1-MMP) to tissue inhibitor of metalloproteinase (TIMP)-2 regulates MT1-MMP processing and pro-MMP-2 activation. *J Biol Chem* 2000;275:12080-12089.

Hill RP, Chambers AF, Ling V, Harris JF. Dynamic heterogeneity: rapid generation of metastatic variants in mouse B16 melanoma cells. *Science* 1984;224:998-1001.

Hoffman RM. Green fluorescent protein imaging of tumor cells in mice. *Lab Anim (NY)* 2002;31:34-41.

Hojilla CV, Mohammed FF, Khokha R. Matrix metalloproteinases and their tissue inhibitors direct cell fate during cancer development. *Br J Cancer* 2003;89:1817-1821.

Hu G, Chong RA, Yang Q, et al. MTDH activation by 8q22 genomic gain promotes chemoresistance and metastasis of poor-prognosis breast cancer. *Cancer Cell* 2009;15:9-20.

Hurst DR, Welch DR. Metastasis suppressor genes at the interface between the environment and tumor cell growth. *Int Rev Cell Mol Biol* 2011;286:107-180.

Hynes RO. Integrins: bidirectional, allosteric signaling machines. *Cell* 2002;110:673-687.

Jain S, Zuka M, Liu J, et al. Platelet glycoprotein Ib alpha supports experimental lung metastasis. *Proc Natl Acad Sci U S A* 2007; 104:9024-9028.

Jothy S. CD44 and its partners in metastasis. *Clin Exp Metastasis* 2003;20:195-201.

Kalluri R, Neilson EG. Epithelial-mesenchymal transition and its implications for fibrosis. *J Clin Invest* 2003;112:1776-1784.

Kalluri R, Weinberg RA. The basics of epithelial-mesenchymal transition. *J Clin Invest* 2009;119:1420-1428.

Kessenbrock K, Plaks V, Werb Z. Matrix metalloproteinases: regulators of the tumor microenvironment. *Cell* 2010;141: 52-67.

Khanna C, Wan X, Bose S, et al. The membrane-cytoskeleton linker ezrin is necessary for osteosarcoma metastasis. *Nat Med* 2004;10: 182-186.

Khokha R, Waterhouse P, Yagel S, et al. Antisense RNA-induced reduction in murine TIMP levels confers oncogenicity on Swiss 3T3 cells. *Science* 1989;243:947-950.

Kim MY, Oskarsson T, Acharyya S, et al. Tumor self-seeding by circulating cancer cells. *Cell* 2009;139:1315-1326.

Klein CA. The systemic progression of human cancer: a focus on the individual disseminated cancer cell—the unit of selection. *Adv Cancer Res* 2003;89:35-67.

Knauer M, Cardoso F, Wesseling J, et al. Identification of a low-risk subgroup of HER-2-positive breast cancer by the 70-gene prognosis signature. *Br J Cancer* 2010;103:1788-1793.

Koebel CM, Vermi W, Swann JB, et al. Adaptive immunity maintains occult cancer in an equilibrium state. *Nature* 2007; 450:903-907.

Kopfstein L, Christofori G. Metastasis: cell-autonomous mechanisms versus contributions by the tumor microenvironment. *Cell Mol Life Sci* 2006;63:449-468.

Laufs S, Schumacher J, Allgayer H. Urokinase-receptor (u-PAR): an essential player in multiple games of cancer: a review on its role in tumor progression, invasion, metastasis, proliferation/dormancy, clinical outcome and minimal residual disease. *Cell Cycle* 2006;5: 1760-1771.

Le QT, Sutphin PD, Raychaudhuri S, et al. Identification of osteopontin as a prognostic plasma marker for head and neck squamous cell carcinomas. *Clin Cancer Res* 2003;9: 59-67.

Lee JH, Marshall JC, Steeg PS, Horak CE. Altered gene and protein expression by Nm23-H1 in metastasis suppression. *Mol Cell Biochem* 2009;329:141-148.

Ling V, Chambers AF, Harris JF, Hill RP. Quantitative genetic analysis of tumor progression. *Cancer Metastasis Rev* 1985; 4(2):173-192.

Lunt SJ, Chaudary N, Hill RP. The tumor microenvironment and metastatic disease. *Clin Exp Metastasis* 2009;26:19-34.

MacDonald IC, Groom AC, Chambers AF. Cancer spread and micrometastasis development: quantitative approaches for in vivo models. *Bioessays* 2002 Oct;24(10):885-893.

Mack PC, Redman MW, Chansky K, et al. Lower osteopontin plasma levels are associated with superior outcomes in advanced non-small-cell lung cancer patients receiving platinum-based chemotherapy: SWOG Study S0003. *J Clin Oncol* 2008;26:4771-4776.

McQuibban GA, Gong JH, Wong JP, Wallace JL, Clark-Lewis I, Overall CM. Matrix metalloproteinase processing of monocyte chemoattractant proteins generates CC chemokine receptor antagonists with anti-inflammatory properties in vivo. *Blood* 2002;100:1160-1167.

Medici D, Hay ED, Olsen BR. Snail and slug promote epithelial-mesenchymal transition through beta-catenin-T-cell factor-4-dependent expression of transforming growth factor-beta3. *Mol Biol Cell* 2008;19:4875-4887.

Moss NM, Liu Y, Johnson JJ, et al. Epidermal growth factor receptor-mediated membrane type 1 matrix metalloproteinase endocytosis regulates the transition between invasive versus expansive growth of ovarian carcinoma cells in three-dimensional collagen. *Mol Cancer Res* 2009;7:809-820.

Mueller J, Gaertner FC, Blechert B, Janssen KP, Essler M. Targeting of tumor blood vessels: a phage-displayed tumor-homing peptide specifically binds to matrix metalloproteinase-2-processed collagen IV and blocks angiogenesis in vivo. *Mol Cancer Res* 2009;7:1078-1085.

Murphy G. Regulation of the proteolytic disintegrin metalloproteinases, the "Sheddases". *Semin Cell Dev Biol* 2009;20:138-145.

Namikawa R, Shtivelman E. SCID-hu mice for the study of human cancer metastasis. *Cancer Chemother Pharmacol* 1999;43 Suppl: S37-S41.

Narumiya S, Tanji M, Ishizaki T. Rho signaling, ROCK and mDia1, in transformation, metastasis and invasion. *Cancer Metastasis Rev* 2009;28:65-76.

Navin N, Kendall J, Troge J, et al. Tumour evolution inferred by single-cell sequencing. *Nature* 2011;472:90-94.

Nguyen DX, Bos PD, Massague J. Metastasis: from dissemination to organ-specific colonization. *Nat Rev Cancer* 2009;9:274-284.

Nowell PC. Mechanisms of tumor progression. *Cancer Res* 1986;46: 2203-2207.

Oakman C, Santarpia L, Di Leo A. Breast cancer assessment tools and optimizing adjuvant therapy. *Nat Rev Clin Oncol* 2010;7: 725-732.

Ostman A, Augsten M. Cancer-associated fibroblasts and tumor growth—bystanders turning into key players. *Curr Opin Genet Dev* 2009;19:67-73.

Overall CM, Tam E, McQuibban GA, et al. Domain interactions in the gelatinase A.TIMP-2.MT1-MMP activation complex. The ectodomain of the 44-kDa form of membrane type-1 matrix metalloproteinase does not modulate gelatinase A activation. *J Biol Chem* 2000;275:39497-39506.

Pantel K, Brakenhoff RH, Brandt B. Detection, clinical relevance and specific biological properties of disseminating tumour cells. *Nat Rev Cancer* 2008;8:329-340.

Pap E. The role of microvesicles in malignancies. *Adv Exp Med Biol* 2011;714:183-199.

Peinado H, Lavotshkin S, Lyden D. The secreted factors responsible for pre-metastatic niche formation: old sayings and new thoughts. *Semin Cancer Biol* 2011;21:139-146.

Perl AK, Wilgenbus P, Dahl U, Semb H, Christofori G. A causal role for E-cadherin in the transition from adenoma to carcinoma. *Nature* 1998;392:190-193.

Perret GY, Crepin M. New pharmacological strategies against metastatic spread. *Fundam Clin Pharmacol* 2008;22:465-492.

Puente XS, Sanchez LM, Overall CM, et al. Human and mouse proteases: a comparative genomic approach. *Nat Rev Genet* 2003;4(7):544-558.

Qian BZ, Pollard JW. Macrophage diversity enhances tumor progression and metastasis. *Cell* 2010;141:39-51.

Ramaswamy S, Ross KN, Lander ES, Golub TR. A molecular signature of metastasis in primary solid tumors. *Nat Genet* 2003;33:49-54.

Rhomberg W, Eiter H, Schmid F, Saely CH. Combined vindesine and razoxane shows antimetastatic activity in advanced soft tissue sarcomas. *Clin Exp Metastasis* 2008;25:75-80.

Rowe RG, Weiss SJ. Navigating ECM barriers at the invasive front: the cancer cell-stroma interface. *Annu Rev Cell Dev Biol* 2009;25: 567-595.

Ruoslahti E. Specialization of tumour vasculature. *Nat Rev Cancer* 2002;2:83-90.

Sabeh F, Shimizu-Hirota R, Weiss SJ. Protease-dependent versus -independent cancer cell invasion programs: three-dimensional amoeboid movement revisited. *J Cell Biol* 2009; 185:11-19.

Schmitt M, Harbeck N, Brunner N, et al. Cancer therapy trials employing level-of-evidence-1 disease forecast cancer biomarkers uPA and its inhibitor PAI-1. *Expert Rev Mol Diagn* 2011;11: 617-634.

Shi M, Liu D, Duan H, Shen B, Guo N. Metastasis-related miRNAs, active players in breast cancer invasion, and metastasis. *Cancer Metastasis Rev* 2010;29:785-799.

Shibue T, Weinberg RA. Integrin beta1-focal adhesion kinase signaling directs the proliferation of metastatic cancer cells disseminated in the lungs. *Proc Natl Acad Sci U S A* 2009;106:10290-10295.

Sica A, Allavena P, Mantovani A. Cancer related inflammation: the macrophage connection. *Cancer Lett* 2008;267:204-215.

Silletti S, Kessler T, Goldberg J, Boger DL, Cheresh DA. Disruption of matrix metalloproteinase 2 binding to integrin alpha v beta 3 by an organic molecule inhibits angiogenesis and tumor growth in vivo. *Proc Natl Acad Sci U S A* 2001;98:119-124.

Sleeman JP, Nazarenko I, Thiele W. Do all roads lead to Rome? Routes to metastasis development. *Int J Cancer* 2011;128:2511-2526.

Stackpole CW, Alterman AL, Valle EF. B16 melanoma variants selected by one or more cycles of spontaneous metastasis to the same organ fail to exhibit organ specificity. *Clin Exp Metastasis* 1991;9:319-332.

Sugarbaker EV. Patterns of metastasis in human malignancies. In: Marchalonis JJ, Hanna MD, Fidler IJ, eds. *Cancer Biology Reviews* Vol 2. New York: Marcel-Dekker; 1980.

Swarbrick A, Roy E, Allen T, Bishop JM. Id1 cooperates with oncogenic Ras to induce metastatic mammary carcinoma by subversion of the cellular senescence response. *Proc Natl Acad Sci U S A* 2008;105:5402-5407.

Tarin D, Thompson EW, Newgreen DF. The fallacy of epithelial mesenchymal transition in neoplasia. *Cancer Res* 2005;65: 5996-6000; discussion 6000-6001.

van de Vijver MJ, He YD, van't Veer LJ, et al. A gene-expression signature as a predictor of survival in breast cancer. *N Engl J Med* 2002;347:1999-2009.

Weiss L, Ward PM. Contributions of vascularized lymph-node metastases to hematogenous metastasis in a rat mammary carcinoma. *Int J Cancer* 1990;46:452-455.

Werb Z. ECM and cell surface proteolysis: regulating cellular ecology. *Cell* 1997;91:439-442.

Whitney M, Crisp JL, Olson ES, et al. Parallel in vivo and in vitro selection using phage display identifies protease-dependent tumor-targeting peptides. *J Biol Chem* 2010;285:22532-22541.

Wicha MS, Hayes DF. Circulating tumor cells: not all detected cells are bad and not all bad cells are detected. *J Clin Oncol* 2011;29: 1508-1511.

Zacharski LR, Henderson WG, Rickles FR, et al. Effect of warfarin anticoagulation on survival in carcinoma of the lung, colon, head and neck, and prostate. Final report of VA Cooperative Study #75. *Cancer* 1984;53:2046-2052.

Zucker S, Cao J, Chen WT. Critical appraisal of the use of matrix metalloproteinase inhibitors in cancer treatment. *Oncogene* 2000;19:6642-6650.

Angiogenesis

Janusz Rak

11.1 INTRODUCTION: THE TUMOR–VASCULAR INTERFACE

An important feature of malignancies is the associated emergence of new and abnormal contact points between cancer cells and the various facets of the host vascular system (Folkman and Kalluri, 2003; Kerbel, 2008). Prior to transformation many normal epithelial tissues (eg, in the gut, skin, and exocrine glands) are functionally linked to, but often anatomically separated from, the vasculature, for instance, by basement membranes and connective tissue layers (Rak, 2009). These barriers are compromised during the course of the malignant process, resulting in abnormal, often direct and reciprocal interactions between vascular components (endothelial cells, blood cells, plasma, or lymph) and cancer cells at this new *tumor–vascular interface.*

Tumor–vascular interactions are important for disease progression, because of several "outside-in" effects, such as supply of oxygen, nutrients, growth factors, metabolites, paracrine and adhesive tumor–vascular interactions, recruitment/retention of the host immune, inflammatory, and bone marrow-derived progenitor cells, as well as delivery of drugs, hormones, and regulatory molecules. The vascular interface also mediates important "inside-out" processes, notably, intravasation of metastatic cancer cells, emission of angiogenesis-regulating, proinflammatory, procoagulant, hormonal, and metabolic (eg, cachexia-inducing) signals, as well as shedding of tumor-related microvesicles (exosomes) containing biologically active molecules (Rak, 2009). The nature of the tumor–vascular interface is influenced by a succession of genetic and epigenetic alterations in cancer cells, microenvironmental influences (hypoxia, inflammation), as well as host genetic background, accompanying diseases (comorbidities), ageing, and other factors (Kerbel, 2008).

The term *angiogenesis* and its evolving meaning have a long history. The term was first used by John Hunter in 1787, and later reintroduced in 1935 by Artur Tremain Hertig, to describe non-cancer-related blood vessel growth processes (Roy-Chowdhury and Brown, 2007). Works of Lewis (1927), Sandison (1928), Ide (1939), and Algire (1945), as well as Greenblatt and Shubik (1968) gradually led to a description of vascular expansion associated with a developing cancer, along with some of the first experimental approaches to study the related processes. It was not until the early 1970s that the concept of targeting angiogenesis for therapeutic purposes (antiangiogenesis) was proposed by Judah Folkman (Folkman, 1971). This form of therapy is now a part of the clinical management in several malignancies. Further development of these approaches depends on improving our understanding of mechanisms governing the response of the vascular system to an emerging malignancy, and the relationships, both local and systemic, between cancer cells and the vascular and nonvascular host tissues (Folkman, 2007).

11.2 CONSTITUENTS OF THE VASCULAR SYSTEM

11.2.1 Blood Vessel and Lymphatic Networks

Blood circulation ensures the delivery of oxygen, nutrients, macromolecules, hormones, and cells (eg, immune, inflammatory, or stem cells), to the vicinity of every living cell, while removing catabolites and waste products. To remain viable, each mammalian cell must be located no further than 100 to 180 μm from the nearest functional (perfused) blood vessel capillary. Directionality, efficiency, and organ-specificity of the blood flow are developmentally preprogrammed by the geometry, physical properties, and hierarchical architecture (arborization) of the vascular system. Thus, cardiac output is directed through the tree of arteries of decreasing caliber and changing wall structure, including elastic, muscular-type, and contractile arteries, as well as smaller and precapillary arterioles, which eventually branch into capillary blood vessels. Capillaries converge to form the postcapillary venules, followed by small, midsize, and large veins that differ from their corresponding arteries by lower pressure, velocity, and

content of blood (eg, low oxygen levels), as well as by thinner wall structure and (in some segments) the presence of intraluminal valves to maintain flow directionality.

Each blood vessel is composed of a crucial inner lining (endothelium) made of endothelial cells, which are surrounded by 1 or more supportive layers containing cells with contractile characteristics of smooth muscle (mural) cells, sheaths (laminae) of extracellular matrix (ECM) and other components (eg, innervation). Collectively, these structures (Fig. 11–1) provide an inner surface that is resistant to coagulation, serve as a source of intercellular and biomechanical signals required for endothelial cell survival, and afford physical support and contractility of mural cells, as appropriate for the vessel caliber and site-dependent function (Carmeliet and Jain, 2011).

Capillary blood vessels (Fig. 11–1) constitute the main point of molecular exchange between tissues and the circulating blood. Capillaries are thin walled tubes of blood endothelial cells (ECs), with lumen 8 to 20 μm in diameter, and exterior wrapped in collagen type IV-rich basement membranes, which also envelope discontinuous layers of smooth muscle-like cells (SMCs), which at the capillary level are known as pericytes (PCs). The permeability of EC layers for molecules is tightly regulated. Thus, while capillaries in most of the vascular beds are permeable to fluids and certain micromolecules (oxygen, certain ions), but highly restrictive to macromolecules, in the brain such passage is controlled even more tightly, a property known as the blood–brain barrier (BBB), while being less restrictive in endocrine organs (Carmeliet and Jain, 2011).

Fluid released (extravasated) through the capillary walls into the intercellular tissue space (interstitium) is collected by lymphatic capillaries (lymphatics) (Tammela and Alitalo, 2010). Lymphatic vascular networks are present in almost all organs, except for the central nervous system (CNS), bone marrow (BM), and avascular tissues, such as cartilage, cornea and epidermis. Lymphatic endothelial cells (LECs) are connected to the surrounding ECM by specialized fibrillin-containing anchoring filaments (Alitalo et al, 2005). Capillary lymphatics are open ended and thin walled, have discontinuous or absent basement membrane, and lack PCs, all of which predisposes them to efficiently "collect" interstitial fluid, macromolecules, and cells (see Fig. 11–1). Lymphatics drain their content (lymph) to the regional lymph nodes, while the larger lymphatic channels subsequently converge, forming a common central duct (thoracic duct), which carries the lymph to the left subclavian vein (Tammela and Alitalo, 2010). Thus, in adults 1 to 2 L of interstitial fluid containing molecules and cells enter the lymphatic system per day, and eventually reach the general circulation. In this manner also, metastatic cancer cells may reach lymph nodes and the blood circulation (Tammela and Alitalo, 2010).

11.2.2 Properties of Cells Involved in Vascular Structures

Several populations of cells contribute to the maintenance, growth, and remodeling of vascular structures (Fig. 11–2);

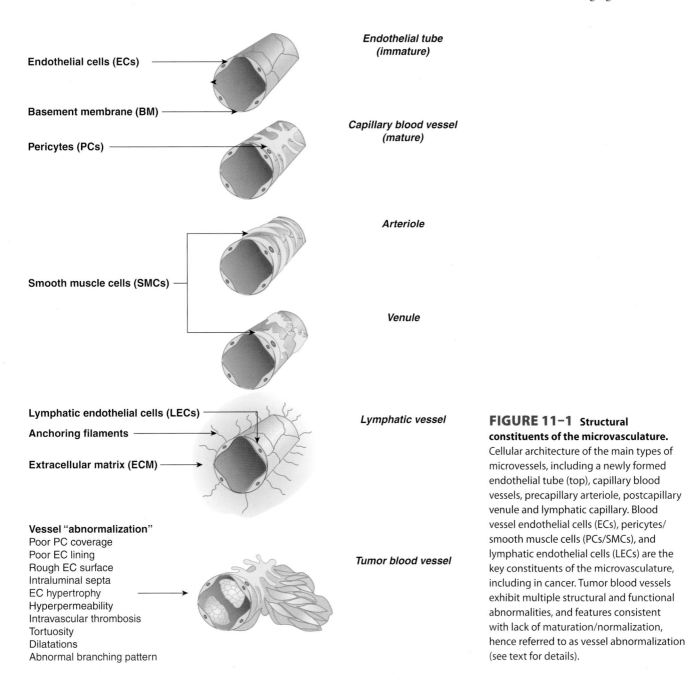

Endothelial cells (ECs)

Basement membrane (BM)

Pericytes (PCs)

Endothelial tube (immature)

Capillary blood vessel (mature)

Arteriole

Smooth muscle cells (SMCs)

Venule

Lymphatic endothelial cells (LECs)

Anchoring filaments

Extracellular matrix (ECM)

Lymphatic vessel

Vessel "abnormalization"
Poor PC coverage
Poor EC lining
Rough EC surface
Intraluminal septa
EC hypertrophy
Hyperpermeability
Intravascular thrombosis
Tortuosity
Dilatations
Abnormal branching pattern

Tumor blood vessel

FIGURE 11–1 **Structural constituents of the microvasculature.** Cellular architecture of the main types of microvessels, including a newly formed endothelial tube (top), capillary blood vessels, precapillary arteriole, postcapillary venule and lymphatic capillary. Blood vessel endothelial cells (ECs), pericytes/smooth muscle cells (PCs/SMCs), and lymphatic endothelial cells (LECs) are the key constituents of the microvasculature, including in cancer. Tumor blood vessels exhibit multiple structural and functional abnormalities, and features consistent with lack of maturation/normalization, hence referred to as vessel abnormalization (see text for details).

they include resident endothelial (ECs, LECs) and mural cells. The latter include SMCs in larger vessels, and PCs in capillaries, permanently incorporated into the vascular wall. Bone marrow-derived cells (BMDCs) may also take transient residence within (around) the vascular wall, as is the case for several subsets of progenitor and regulatory cells of myeloid and endothelial origin (De Palma and Naldini, 2006).

Endothelial cells line the entire inner surface of the circulatory system. In this fashion, they control the properties of blood and those of perivascular tissues. In the adult, endothelial cells are usually quiescent (more than 99.9%), with a cell turnover time ranging between 6 weeks and many years, and somewhat faster at vascular branching points; exceptions include wound healing and cyclical changes in female reproductive organs. Endothelial cells exhibit several common properties, such as flat morphology, anticoagulant luminal surfaces, and the expression of certain specific molecules (pan-endothelial markers), which include CD31 (PECAM), CD144 (VE-cadherin), von Willebrand factor (vWF), CD202b (TIE2), CD34 (sialomucin), CD146 (P1H12 antigen/MUC18), and CD105 (endoglin). However, endothelial cells may also display regional differences dependent on vessel type, caliber, and organ site (Folkman and Kalluri, 2003).

Mural cells enforce the integrity of the endothelial tube. These elongated and contractile cells provide blood vessels with mechanical resistance, functional stability and vasoconstrictive properties (Carmeliet and Jain, 2011). In capillaries, PCs form processes that extend along the vessel axis making

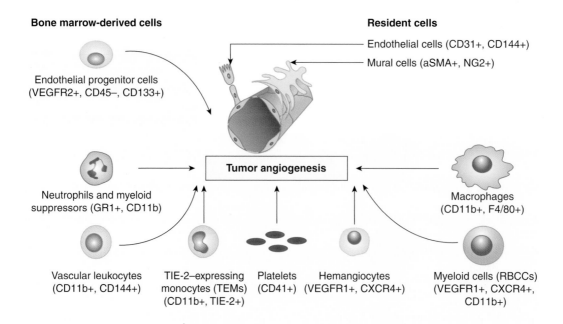

FIGURE 11–2 **Cell populations involved in tumor angiogenesis.** Vascular growth is coordinated by structural resident cells in the preexisting blood vessels, as well as by several populations of circulating cells (shaded area), mostly of bone marrow origin. Although the structural contribution of endothelial progenitor cells (EPCs) in tumor neovascularization remains controversial, the regulatory function of these cells and that of several types of myeloid cells is increasingly well established, for example, as sources of vascular endothelial growth factor (VEGF), alternative angiogenic factors, guidance signals, proteolytic activity, and other effects. Angiogenic fibroblasts, cancer cells, and immune effectors are not included in this diagram for simplicity (see text for details).

contacts with several endothelial cells. In this manner endothelial cells receive survival signals and become less dependent on soluble mediators. Mural cell-specific antigens (markers) include α smooth muscle actin (αSMA), desmin, CD13, 3G5 ganglioside, CD248 (endosialin), NG2 chondroitin sulphate proteoglycan, RGS5, and platelet-derived growth factor receptor beta (PDGFRβ). PCs are actively recruited to, and retained at, the developing vessel wall through signaling mechanisms involving angiopoietin 1 (ANG1) and its endothelial receptor (TIE2/TEK), as well as through action of multiple other factors (Yancopoulos et al, 2000; Jones et al, 2001).

Bone marrow-derived regulatory and progenitor cells maintain vascular homeostasis at the systemic level (see Fig. 11–2). Local cytokine release leads to the recruitment and retention of various populations of BMDCs. These include endothelial progenitor cells (EPCs), also known as circulating endothelial progenitors (CEPs), to distinguish them from more differentiated circulating endothelial cells (CECs) that may slough off the vessel wall as a result of damage, or cell death (Bertolini et al, 2010). EPCs/CEPs have been implicated in formation of new blood vessels, vascular regrowth, and metastasis, but their ability to differentiate into mature ECs and contribute to the vessel wall still remains controversial. They may, however, play a role in maintenance of the existing endothelial layers (Xu, 2006). Tumor-associated endothelial cells were recently found to contain a subset of cells with multipotential (stem-like) properties and the capability to differentiate into chondrocytes and bone cells, and to trigger calcification (Dudley et al, 2008).

In addition to EPCs, several types of myeloid cells play regulatory roles during remodeling and maintenance of the vasculature, including changes occurring in the course of cancer. The best-described subpopulations of these cells encompass: (a) tumor-associated M2-type macrophages, characterized by the expression of F4/80 and CD11b antigens (F4/80+/CD11b+); (b) monocytes expressing TIE2 receptor (TIE2+/CD11b+); (c) recruited bone marrow circulating cells (VEGFR1+/CXCR4+/CD11b+); (d) hemangiocytes (VEGFR1+/CXCR4+); (e) vascular leukocytes (CD11b+/VE-cadherin+); and (f) angiogenic neutrophils (GR1+/CD11b+). Proangiogenic properties have also been ascribed to other myeloid cells, such as mast cells (MCs), dendritic cells (DCs), and hemopoietic stem cells (HSCs) (De Palma and Naldini, 2006; Ahn and Brown, 2009). Several of these cell types not only produce angiogenic factors (eg, vascular endothelial growth factor [VEGF]-A or Bv8 [*Bombina variegata*-secreted protein 8]), but also express overlapping markers with endothelial cells (Bertolini et al, 2010).

11.3 PROCESSES LEADING TO BLOOD VESSEL FORMATION

11.3.1 Vasculogenesis

Vasculature is the first organ system to develop during embryogenesis, around midgestation in mice (Ema and Rossant, 2003). The process (Figs. 11–3 and 11–4) consists of

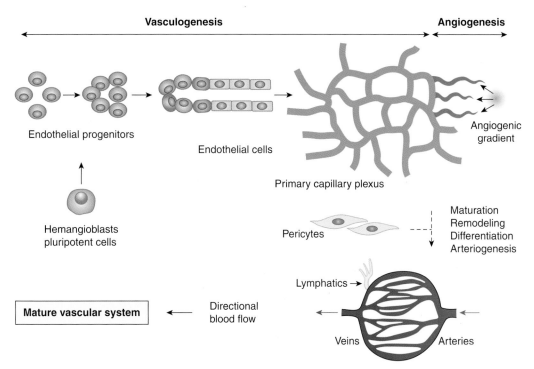

FIGURE 11–3 **Development of the vascular system.** A spectrum of blood vessel-forming processes is activated during development, and partially reactivated during postnatal vascular growth (wound healing, pregnancy, vascular diseases, and cancer). Endothelial cells, the key organizing element of the vascular system emerge from their precursors, which are a product of the lineage commitment of earlier precursors (hemangioblasts) in the embryonic mesenchyme, or may potentially arise through transdifferentiation of other cells. Vasculogenesis entails coalescence of endothelial progenitors, their differentiation to endothelial cells and formation of primitive vascular tubes, which organize themselves into a homogenous, directionless, and largely nonperfused network (primary capillary plexus). Angiogenesis is a process of outgrowth of vascular structures from the preexisting primary plexus, or mature vasculature. During development, angiogenesis is accompanied by the antithetical process leading to removal of superfluous vessels (pruning), both of which are essential for the establishment of the proper hierarchy (arborization) of the vascular network and for directional blood flow from arterial to the venous side of the circulation. The integrity of the emerging capillary blood vessels is ensured by arrival of PCs (vessel maturation). The arterial vessels that supply blood to the expanding microcirculation undergo a remodeling and circumferential growth processes, often referred to as *arteriogenesis*; see the text and references for further details. (Carmeliet and Jain, 2011; Ema and Rossant, 2003.)

at least 4 distinct phases (Carmeliet and Jain, 2011), including (a) the emergence of endothelial progenitors (angioblasts); (b) coalescence and differentiation of angioblasts to form the primitive network of endothelial tubes (vasculogenesis), a structure known as the *primary capillary plexus*; (c) branching of new vascular projections (sprouts) from the preformed endothelial tubes (angiogenesis); and (d) remodeling, expansion, and diversification of the vascular network to form the arterial and the venous side of the circulation, a process which defines the directionality of the blood flow.

As the vascular system matures, the ingress of mural cells (vascular maturation) stabilizes the endothelial channels. Some of these channels may be superfluous, or nonfunctional, which leads to their regulated regression (pruning). At the same time, branching and angiogenesis lead to the establishment of a vascular hierarchy where some vessels become supply lines for smaller capillaries. To meet the volumetric and mechanical requirements, these supplying vessels undergo circumferential expansion and wall remodeling, a process termed *arteriogenesis* (Carmeliet and Jain, 2011). Remodeling and diversification of various segments of the vascular tree serves to meet the unique

metabolic, structural and mechanical requirements of different organs and tissues. Thus, the vascular architecture of the heart muscle differs from that of the liver or kidney, as well as between other organ sites (Folkman and Kalluri, 2003). Conversely, tissue growth and geometry may be influenced by the vasculature, which, for example, controls mechanisms of liver regeneration and influences organ size (Folkman and Kalluri, 2003).

11.3.2 Endothelial Repair

EPCs can be recruited to sites of pathological losses in endothelial lining (denudation). EPC-dependent endothelial repair is thought to contribute to attenuation of the vascular damage in the course of inflammatory diseases such as atherosclerosis (Xu, 2006). These cells may also home to intravascular clots and facilitate formation of inner vascular channels within them (recanalization).

11.3.3 Angiogenesis

Angiogenesis is a process whereby new vascular structures emerge from ones that have already been established in the

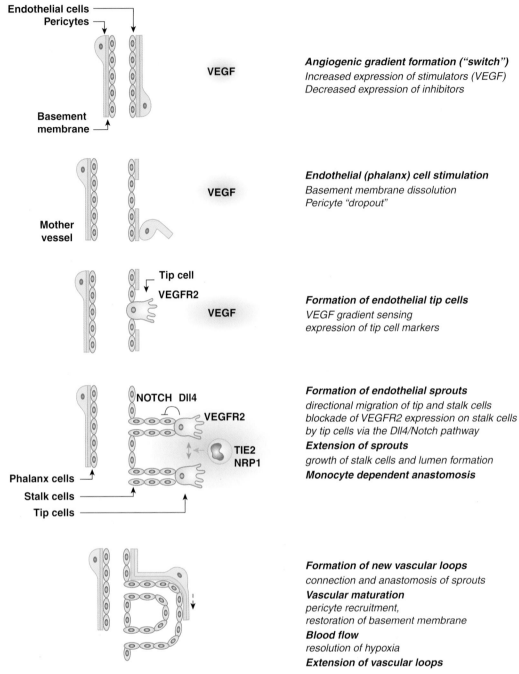

Angiogenic gradient formation ("switch")
Increased expression of stimulators (VEGF)
Decreased expression of inhibitors

Endothelial (phalanx) cell stimulation
Basement membrane dissolution
Pericyte "dropout"

Formation of endothelial tip cells
VEGF gradient sensing
expression of tip cell markers

Formation of endothelial sprouts
directional migration of tip and stalk cells
blockade of VEGFR2 expression on stalk cells
by tip cells via the Dll4/Notch pathway
Extension of sprouts
growth of stalk cells and lumen formation
Monocyte dependent anastomosis

Formation of new vascular loops
connection and anastomosis of sprouts
Vascular maturation
pericyte recruitment,
restoration of basement membrane
Blood flow
resolution of hypoxia
Extension of vascular loops

FIGURE 11–4 Sprouting angiogenesis. The change in balance between angiogenesis stimulators and inhibitors (angiogenic switch) and especially local upregulation of VEGF and formation of the VEGF gradient leads to stimulation of vascular responses known as sprouting angiogenesis. Stimulated blood vessels undergo a series of structural changes that consist of localized dissociation of pericytes ("dropout") from the endothelial tube, dissolution of the basement membrane and recruitment of the angiogenesis-directing cells (tip cells) from the endothelial monolayer (phalanx cells). Capillaries enlarge (to form mother vessels) and deploy cohorts of endothelial cells (stalk cells) led by VEGF gradient-seeking tip cells expressing high levels of VEGFR2 and DLL4. Interaction of tip cell-related DLL4 with NOTCH on following stalk cells suppresses VEGFR2 expression on the latter cell subset and ensures that they don't become superfluous tip cells. Vascular sprouts extend and undergo lumen formation. TIE2–expressing monocytic cells orchestrate the encounter and connection (anastomosis) of nearby sprouts to complete the formation of a functional vascular loop. Capillary loops can extend further to promote an increased tissue perfusion, a process known as looping angiogenesis, and operative during granulation tissue formation.

surrounding tissues or within the tumor mass (see Fig. 11–3). In cancer, this process is viewed as the key source of vascular growth associated with tumor formation and metastasis, and one that occurs via at last 3 different mechanisms:

(a) intussusception; (b) vascular splitting; and (c) sprouting angiogenesis (Carmeliet and Jain, 2011). Intussusception leads to division of a larger or dilated capillary vessel into smaller channels, as a result of external pressure exerted by extravascular tissue. Similarly, separation of the vascular lumen into several branches can be achieved by formation of intraluminal septa (splitting). Both of these processes lead to formation of additional capillary loops that could enlarge and make contacts with a greater volume of the adjacent tissue (Carmeliet and Jain, 2011).

Sprouting angiogenesis constitutes the main mechanism leading to the expansion of cancer-related microvascular networks (see Fig. 11–4). The exposure of a precapillary vessel to the gradient of proangiogenic activity (eg, VEGF expression induced by hypoxia [see Sec. 11.5.3 and Chap. 12, Sec. 12.2]) leads to several orchestrated responses, which begin with vessel dilatation giving rise to formation of a thin-walled, regionally distended structure known as a "mother vessel" (Pettersson et al, 2000). This transition reflects the activation state of the still intact monolayers of endothelial cells, here referred to as phalanx cells (Carmeliet and Jain, 2011). Formation of mother vessels is often followed by responses of mural cells (PCs), leading to their focal detachment from the endothelial tube (PC dropout), which thereby becomes liberated from the structural constraints, more exposed to extravascular stimuli, and capable of deployment of endothelial cells (Carmeliet and Jain, 2011). The centerpiece of these complex endothelial-PC interactions is the upregulation of angiopoietin 2 (ANG2) in endothelial cells, exposed to high levels of VEGF. In endothelial cells, ANG2 acts as an autocrine antagonist of the TIE2 receptor tyrosine kinase expressed on the surface of these cells (Fig. 11–5). In this context, ANG2 binding relieves phosphorylation of TIE2, as a result of displacement of its natural PC-derived agonist, angiopoietin 1 (ANG1). Inactivation of the ANG1/TIE2 interaction disrupts the pathway that normally mediates the stable PC-endothelial contact, and as a consequence liberates endothelial cells that may now form new outgrowths (Yancopoulos et al, 2000). An important step required for endothelial liberation is the focal dissolution of the capillary basement membrane by matrix metalloproteinases (MMPs; Fig. 11–6), which also release additional angiogenic factors from the ECM stores (Carmeliet and Jain, 2011).

The exposure of endothelial phalanx cells to extravascular angiogenic gradients triggers the process of coordinated formation, movement, and extension of angiogenic sprouts (see Fig. 11–4). Each sprout is composed of a single specialized tip cell equipped with hair-like, ligand-sensing projections (filopodia), containing high concentrations of VEGF receptors (especially VEGFR2) (Gerhardt et al, 2003). Tip cells also express other molecules (eg, platelet-derived growth factor B [PDGF-B]), as well as high levels of a transmembrane protein known as Delta-like ligand 4 (DLL4), the expression of which is induced by VEGF (Noguera-Troise et al, 2006). DLL4 acts as the key ligand for the NOTCH receptor present on endothelial stalk cells that follow each migrating tip cell (see Chap. 8, Sec. 8.4.2). This interaction involving the activation of the Notch pathway suppresses VEGFR2 expression in stalk cells adjacent to a tip cell, which prevents them from producing DLL4, and thereby becoming tip cells themselves. In this manner, the Notch pathway enforces the unique identity ("leadership") of the tip cell within the cellular hierarchy of each vascular sprout (Noguera-Troise et al, 2006). Indeed, when the DLL4/NOTCH interaction is inhibited, multiple tip cells and sprouts emerge, leading to hyperdense, nonperfused and dysfunctional capillary networks, a phenomenon known as *nonproductive angiogenesis* (Noguera-Troise et al, 2006). The vascular branching through formation of new sprouts may be fine-tuned with the contribution of another NOTCH ligand, Jagged 1. Jagged 1 blocks the effects of DLL4 on stalk cells leading to a controlled stimulation of processes leading to formation of additional tip cells and sprouts (Carmeliet and Jain, 2011).

Tip cells serve as guidance devices for endothelial sprouts, the numbers and directions of which they control, as they move along the path of angiogenic (VEGF) gradients (Gerhardt et al, 2003). Cohorts of stalk cells follow each tip cell and contribute to the sprout extension by directional collective migration and cell division, the latter occurring mainly at the sprout base (Gerhardt et al, 2003). Eventually neighboring sprouts connect (anastomose), a process regulated by a subset of tissue macrophages expressing TIE2 and Neuropilin 1 (NRP1) receptors (Fantin et al, 2010). Formation of endothelial sprouts is accompanied by generation of the vascular lumen. This may occur either through the merger of intracellular vacuoles within endothelial cells, or by formation of intercellular spaces between them, as they form cohorts of cells aligned in parallel (Carmeliet and Jain, 2011). Collectively, these processes of growth, lumen generation, and sprout anastomosis result in formation and extension of functional endothelial capillary loops, which may take up their roles in perfusion of new regions of the tissue or tumor mass (see Fig. 11–4).

11.3.4 Vascular Maturation

Maturation of vessels involves assembly of the mural cell layer around the newly formed endothelial tube (Carmeliet and Jain, 2011). Tumor-associated capillaries were traditionally thought to be devoid of PCs, but more recent studies confirmed the presence of these cells and their impact on the properties of the tumor microcirculation (McDonald and Choyke, 2003). Indeed, angiogenic endothelial cells, including tip cells, secrete PDGF-B, which is deposited onto the heparin sulphate proteoglycan chains and serves as a chemoattractant for regional PCs expressing PDGFRβ (Gaengel et al, 2009). PCs also secrete ANG1, which orchestrates their interactions with endothelial cells and acts as an endothelial survival factor by activating the TIE2 receptor (Hanahan, 1997; Jones et al, 2001). Vascular maturation is also critically dependent on sphingolipid signaling, notably generation of the Sphingosine 1 phosphate (S1P), which regulates N-cadherin, an adhesion molecule that links endothelial cells and PCs (Gaengel et al, 2009). Upon their attachment to the endothelial tube (see Fig. 11–1), PCs differentiate and assume a more mature phenotype, a process that is thought to be regulated by transforming growth factor beta 1 (TGFβ1) (Gaengel et al, 2009). PC coverage of endothelial structures and the vascular

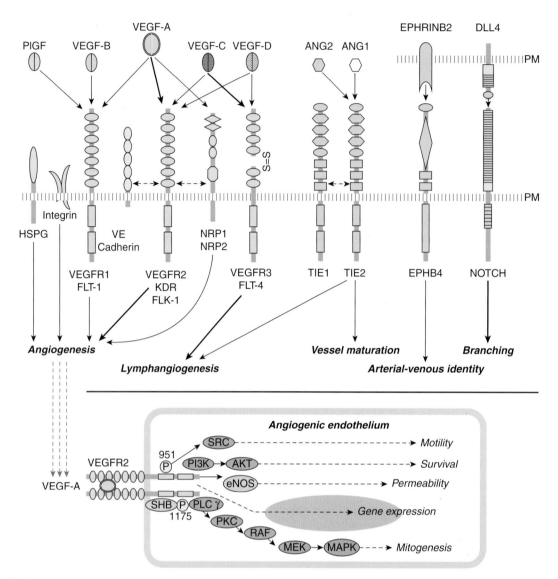

FIGURE 11–5 **Some of the key elements of the signaling circuitry involved in blood vessel formation and tumor angiogenesis.** Top panel: Ligands, receptors and co-receptors involved in angiogenic signaling. Note that EphrinB2 and DLL4 are transmembrane ligands. Domain structure, signaling properties, targets, and crosstalk are detailed in the related references. Bottom panel: Outline of signaling pathways and their effector mechanisms downstream of VEGF-A/VEGFR2. Numbers indicate phosphorylated tyrosines. *PM*, cellular plasma membrane.

maturation (stabilization) processes are profoundly affected by endothelial oxygen sensor Prolyl hydroxylase 2 (PHD2) (Carmeliet and Jain, 2011), and a number of other mechanisms responsible for cellular integrity, hypoxia response, and survival (see Chap. 12, Sec. 12.2). Overall, vascular maturation provides newly formed capillaries with structural support and mechanical resistance, and reduces endothelial cell demand for soluble survival factors, such as VEGF (Carmeliet and Jain, 2011).

11.3.5 Lymphangiogenesis

Formation of new lymphatics from preexisting lymphatic vessels is called *lymphangiogenesis* (Tammela and Alitalo, 2010). There are only small differences in the spectrum of proteins

synthesized in lymphatic endothelial cells (LECs) and vascular ECs. However, the properties of these cells, their function, and their responses to stimuli are markedly different (Alitalo et al, 2005). Studies of LECs and lymphangiogenesis have been advanced by a recent description of their distinct markers, such as the Prospero homeobox transcription factor (PROX-1), Podoplanin, and Lymphatic vessel hyaluronan receptor-1 (LYVE-1) (Alitalo et al, 2005). Lymphatics are also dependent on the activity of the forkhead transcription factor FOX2c. However, the centerpiece of the unique pathway governing lymphangiogenesis consists of two VEGF-related growth factors, VEGF-C and VEGF-D. These factors interact with a distinct receptor expressed preferentially on LECs (and on ECs in certain tumors), known as VEGFR-3/FLT-4 (Alitalo et al, 2005; see Fig. 11–5).

Proteases involved in angiogenesis

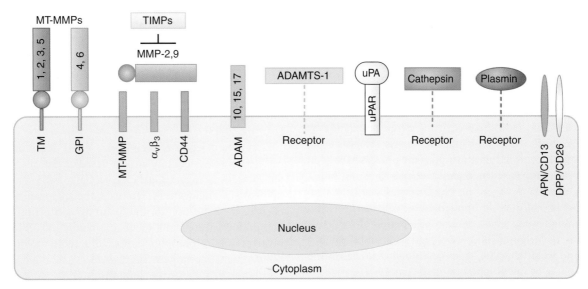

FIGURE 11–6 **Proteolytic mechanisms involved in angiogenesis and endothelial cell function.** Families of cellular and pericellular proteases involved in angiogenesis: *ADAM*, disintegrin and metalloproteinase domain-containing protein; *ADAMTS*, disintegrin and metalloproteinase domain-containing protein with thrombospondin motif; *APN*, aminopeptidase; *DPP*, diaminopeptidase; *GPI*, glycosyl-phosphatidylinositol anchor; *MT-MMP*, membrane-type matrix metalloproteinase; *TIMPs*, tissue inhibitors of metalloproteinases; *TM*, transmembrane region; *uPA*, urokinase plasminogen activator; *uPAR*, uPA receptor. (Adapted from van Hinsbergh et al, 2006.)

The essential roles of these mediators in lymphangiogenesis is evident from studies on disruption of the respective genes in mice (eg, Vegf-C or Fox2c), which halts lymphatic system development. However, important clues have also been derived from expression studies. For example, the transmembrane guidance molecule, EPHRIN-B2 is coexpressed on the surface of LECs with its receptor EPHB4. This pathway was found to control lymphatic sprouting, as well as interaction of LECs and smooth muscle cells, and to play an essential role in remodeling of the lymphatic vasculature. Moreover, in the context of LECs (unlike in vascular ECs) ANG2 acts as an agonist of the TIE2 receptor, similarly to ANG1, a pathway crucial for lymphangiogenesis. Indeed, a germline *ANG2* deletion in mice leads to lymphatic defects, which can be rescued by the expression of ANG1 (Augustin et al, 2009).

Proliferation, migration, and survival of LECs are regulated by a complex network of growth factors that straddle the processes of lymphangiogenesis and angiogenesis. Thus, VEGF-related factors, VEGF-C, and to some extent also VEGF-D stimulate lymphangiogenesis by interacting with VEGFR3/FLT-4. This interaction stimulates responses of LECs, but mainly when VEGF-C/D are present in their immature, proteolytically unprocessed forms. When proteolytically processed, these factors bind not only to VEGFR3 on LECs, but also to VEGFR2 on ECs, whereby they also stimulate angiogenesis. Moreover, VEGFR3 is also expressed on certain ECs under pathological conditions. Therefore, VEGF-C may stimulate angiogenesis also through this route (Tammela and Alitalo, 2010). Conversely, VEGF-A (often refered to simply as VEGF) may contribute to lymphangiogenesis through its interaction with VEGFR3 expressed on some LECs. VEGF-C also binds to Neuropilin-2 (NRP2), a semaphorin receptor, which interacts with VEGFR3 in a manner that is required for efficient lymphangiogenesis. VEGFR3 activation and lymphangiogenesis regulation also involve β_1 and α_9 integrins along with several other factors, such as Hepatocyte growth factor (HGF), Insulin-like growth factors 1 and 2 (IGF-1 and IGF-2), PDGF-B, and Fibroblast growth factors (FGFs). These interactions trigger formation of new lymphatic capillaries in a manner reminiscent of angiogenesis (Tammela and Alitalo, 2010).

11.3.6 Vasculogenic Mimicry

In some contexts nonendothelial cells may adopt endothelial-like phenotypes and line vascular channels (Hendrix et al, 2003). This process occurs in the normal placenta, where trophoblast epithelium enters the myometrium at sites of spiral arteries. This causes epithelial-to-endothelial transformation of trophoblastic cells, including the expression of several markers normally associated with ECs (CD31, CD144, Integrin $\alpha_v\beta_3$). Aberrant differentiation also occurs after subcutaneous injection of pluripotent embryonic stem (ES) cells into mice, and results in formation of aggressive teratomas, which contain blood vessels partially derived from ES cells (Li et al, 2009), albeit not always in high proportions (Rak, 2009). Similar transdifferentiation events were described in the bone marrow of patients with chronic myelogenous leukemia (CML), also in lymphoma, uveal melanoma, and glioblastoma (Hendrix et al, 2003; Ricci-Vitiani et al, 2010).

The extent, significance, a nd molecular mechanisms of these processes are not fully understood, but several regulators have been implicated, including: tissue factor (TF), TF pathway inhibitor 2 (TFPI-2), phosphatidyl inositol 3 kinase (PI3K), focal adhesion kinase (FAK), MMPs, Ephrins, and Laminin chains (Dome et al, 2007).

11.3.7 Vascular Cooption

Cancer cells can exploit the preexisting tissue vasculature by growing around, and enveloping, the vessels (Holash et al, 1999). Various forms of this nonangiogenic process have been observed in highly vascular organs, such as lung and brain, as well as in melanoma and in liver metastases of colorectal cancer (Dome et al, 2007). Although cancer cells can grow and migrate along blood vessels, at least for a period of time, this interaction may trigger blood vessel regression and thrombosis (Brat and Van Meir, 2004), and is eventually followed by the onset of an angiogenic reaction (Holash et al, 1999).

11.4 MOLECULAR REGULATORS OF VASCULAR GROWTH

Formation of new vascular networks, whether in health or disease, is based on the ability of the constituent cells to participate in the web of intercellular communications. The mediators of these interactions can be broadly divided into several categories, including (a) specialized ("professional") signaling effectors required for vascular homeostasis, (b) pleiotropic effectors endowed with angiogenesis-regulating activities (stimulators and inhibitors), along with other functions, and (c) other regulators that link angiogenesis to processes, such as hemostasis, bone marrow stimulation, neuronal growth, or immunity (Carmeliet and Jain, 2011). Although this molecular network contains redundancies, feedbacks and complex response patterns, at the heart of it are individual key molecules that can serve as potential targets for the anti-angiogenic therapy (Table 11–1 and Figs. 11–5 to 11–10). Key elements of this molecular circuitry are shown in Figure 11–5 and are discussed below.

11.4.1 Vascular Endothelial Growth Factor Family

VEGF-A, also known as vascular permeability factor (VPF), is the key member of a larger family of related polypeptides, which also includes VEGF-B, VEGF-C, VEGF-D, VEGF-E, VEGF-F, and placenta growth factor (PlGF), all related to platelet-derived growth factor (PDGF) (Dvorak et al, 1995; Ferrara, 2005). These ligands form functional homo- and heterodimers and interact with at least 4 different receptors (VEGFRs), of which VEGFR1/FLT-1, VEGFR2/KDR/FLK-1), and VEGFR3/FLT-4 are signaling tyrosine kinases (RTKs), while Neuropilin 1 (NRP1) is a coreceptor (Ferrara, 2005). The relatively selective (albeit not exclusive) expression of

VEGFRs by ECs (of blood vessels, lymphatics, and in tumors) allows VEGFs to control vascular processes in a potent and combinatorial manner (see Fig. 11–5). Thus, VEGFR1 binds VEGF-A, VEGF-B and PlGF, while VEGFR2 interacts mainly with VEGF-A (and VEGF-E), and VEGFR3 interacts preferentially with VEGF-C and VEGF-D. NRP1, the semaphorin receptor involved in neuronal guidance, is also expressed by ECs, where it acts as a coreceptor for VEGFR2. NRP1 binds only certain VEGF-A splice isoforms (eg, VEGF165) (Ferrara, 2005).

Germline deletion of each of the VEGF receptors leads to early embryonic lethality amidst vascular defects (Carmeliet and Jain, 2011), suggesting their essential role in vascular development and angiogenesis. However, the angiogenic responses elicited by exposure to the naturally occurring VEGF-A homodimers are mainly mediated mainly by VEGFR2. This involves robust phosphorylation and recruitment of intracellular signaling targets (see Fig. 11–5). Although VEGFR1 also binds VEGF-A with high affinity (10-fold greater than VEGFR2), the phosphorylation of this receptor in ECs is weak, and deletion of its kinase domain is relatively inconsequential for vascular development (Carmeliet and Jain, 2011). Indeed, VEGFR1 is often expressed as a splice variant composed of the soluble extracellular domain (sFlt-1), which acts as a natural VEGF antagonist (VEGF "sink") (Carmeliet and Jain, 2011). However, VEGFR1 does possess an important regulatory function for macrophages, and certain cancer cells, in which it mediates migratory responses in response to VEGF (Carmeliet and Jain, 2011).

The crucial role of VEGF/VEGF-A is underscored by the unprecedented embryonic lethality and profound vascular defects in mouse embryos lacking even a single *vegf* allele (haploinsufficiency) (Carmeliet and Jain, 2011; Ferrara, 2005). Indeed, VEGF-A acts as a potent mitogen, motility, and survival factor for ECs, and a chemoattractant for their progenitors (Ferrara, 2005). These powerful influences are regulated by the organ- and context-specific alternative splicing of the VEGF-A transcript resulting in several protein isoforms. The main species generated during this process are designated according to the number of their constituent amino acids and include VEGF121 (121 amino acids), VEGF145, VEGF165, VEGF189, and VEGF206 (Ferrara, 2005). This splicing removes various sequences from within the region encoded by exons 6 and 7, while leaving the sequences corresponding to exons 1 to 5 and 8 intact.

Consequently, VEGF-A splice isoforms exhibit reduced heparin binding, increased solubility and diminished association with both cellular membranes and the ECM, depending on their size. Thus, the shortest VEGF121 isoform is highly soluble, while VEGF189 is mostly cell bound, and VEGF165 expresses intermediate properties, and the greatest angiogenic activity. The latter is a function of the more stable angiogenic gradient that VEGF165 (VEGF164 in the mouse) can form within the interstitial space in tissues. This gradient favors directional responses of tip cells and robust sprouting. In addition, unlike VEGF121, VEGF165 interacts with both VEGFR2 and NRP1, which is thought to contribute to more pronounced endothelial responses (Ferrara, 2005). Notably, the VEGF-A splicing process also results in expression of alternative ligands endowed with antagonistic (antiangiogenic) activities. For instance, one such variant, VEGF165b, interferes with angiogenesis, and exerts a modulating influence on responses of blood vessels to angiogenic growth factors involved in tissue remodeling and inflammation (Nowak et al, 2008).

The remaining members of the VEGF family play more restricted roles in vascular processes, and germline deletions of the respective genes do not have haploinsufficient consequences. VEGF-C/D control lymphangiogenesis, while VEGF-B provides additional survival protection to ECs. VEGF-E is a VEGF-like gene found in the genome of the *Orf* virus (Ferrara, 2005). In some instances, the effects of these factors become prominent only under pathological conditions (eg, in the case of PLGF). Finally, although VEGF-related factors were originally viewed as having mainly paracrine effects, VEGF-A was recently shown to be expressed at low, but functionally meaningful, levels by ECs themselves, which contributes to vascular homeostasis (Lee et al, 2007).

11.4.2 Platelet-Derived Growth Factor Family

This family of VEGF-related growth factors consists of 4 members: PDGF-A, PDGF-B, PDGF-C, and PDGF-D, the homo- or heterodimers of which interact preferentially with 1 of 2 main cellular receptor tyrosine kinases, namely, PDGFRα and PDGFRβ, (Andrae et al, 2008). While PDGFs play multiple roles in development, disease, and cancer, they are also central to vascular growth, especially blood vessel maturation. Thus, PDGF-BB homodimers are produced at high levels in endothelial tip cells and in phalanx cells of arteriogenic vessels, whereby they attract mural cells harboring PDGFRβ (Andrae et al, 2008). Other members of this family may also contribute to various angiogenic events indirectly, for example, by influencing the expression of angiogenesis-related genes (eg, VEGF) in cancer cells and fibroblasts (Dong et al, 2004). Indeed, recent studies suggest that these mechanisms may bypass the requirement for VEGF and contribute to tumor resistance to VEGF-directed therapies (Shojaei et al, 2009).

11.4.3 Prokineticins

This family of VEGF-unrelated growth factors has been found to induce VEGF-like effects in ECs, especially in endocrine organs. This includes growth, migration, permeability, fenestration (formation of trans-endothelial openings), and angiogenesis (LeCouter et al, 2002). These mediators consist of the endocrine gland VEGF/prokineticin 1 (EG-VEGF/PK1) and *Bombina variegata*-secreted protein 8/prokineticin 2 (Bv8/PK2), which both interact with their respective G-protein–coupled receptors (PK-R1 and PK-R2) (Ferrara, 2010). Although prokineticins appear to have a role in homeostasis of the microcirculation in endocrine glands, they are also

found in cancer, where they may be produced by myeloid cells and contribute to VEGF-independent angiogenesis (Shojaei et al, 2009).

11.4.4 Angiopoietins and TIE Receptors

At least 3 related ligands known as angiopoietins (ANG1, -2, and -4) play diverse roles in endothelial cell survival, vascular development and maturation, as well as angiogenesis and lymphangiogenesis in humans (Ang3 is a mouse ortholog of ANG4) (Yancopoulos et al, 2000; Jones et al, 2001). Angiopoietins interact with TIE2/TEK receptor tyrosine kinase expressed preferentially (but not exclusively) on ECs, which also harbor a related orphan receptor known as TIE1 with poorly understood function. Nonetheless, both TIE1 and TIE2 receptors are essential for vascular development (Augustin et al, 2009). Their activity is controlled by the vascular endothelial receptor tyrosine phosphatase (VE-PTP) (Li et al, 2009). As mentioned earlier, the best understood function of the angiopoietin/TIE2 circuitry is in the regulation of EC survival, vascular permeability, and recruitment of mural cells. In this setting, ANG1 emanates from perivascular tissues and acts as the TIE2 agonist. In contrast, ANG2 is produced largely by ECs exposed to VEGF, and it blocks ANG1/TIE2 interaction, thereby destabilizing endothelial-PC contacts (see Fig. 11–5). Thus, in the presence of VEGF, the exposure to ANG2 promotes vascular sprouting, but when VEGF levels are low, ANG2 promotes vascular regression (Augustin et al, 2009 for review).

11.4.5 Notch Pathway

Cell-cell contact-dependent regulatory interactions often involve Notch receptors (NOTCH 1 to 4) and their 5 cell-associated ligands, including Jagged (JAG) 1, JAG 2, Delta-like 1, 3, and 4 (DLL1, DLL3, and DLL4) (Dufraine et al, 2008). NOTCH 1 and 4 are expressed in ECs (NOTCH 4 preferentially) and, along with DLL4, are required for proper vascular development. DLL4 is expressed in angiogenic tip cells and plays a role in maintaining their identity, whereas JAG 1 may be involved in modulating these effects and recruitment of additional tip cells. JAG 1 may also mediate direct interactions between endothelial and mural cells, or between tumor cells and the vasculature (Dufraine et al, 2008). Another Notch ligand, DLL1, is involved in vascular remodeling and arteriogenesis. Interactions with these ligands trigger proteolytic release of the intracellular domain of NOTCH (ICN), which is responsible for modulation of gene expression and cellular effects (Dufraine et al, 2008).

11.4.6 Ephrins and EPH Receptors

The definition of arterial and venous identity in the developing vascular system is largely attributed to the unique bidirectional signaling mechanism mediated by transmembrane ligands of the ephrin family, notably Ephrin B2 (on the arterial side) and their EPHB4 receptors (on the venous side;

see Fig. 11–5). The expression of other Ephrins (eg, A1, A2, B1 and B3) and additional EPH receptors (EPHB2, EPHB3) is also observed in ECs, including in tumors. These Ephrins are implicated in various angiogenesis-related processes, such as endothelial–PC interactions, interactions of blood vessels with tumor cells, and cooperation with other angiogenic factors. The latter is exemplified by Ephrin B2-dependent regulation of VEGFR2 endocytosis and signaling (Wang et al, 2010).

11.4.7 Vascular Integrins, Cadherins, and Adhesion Molecules

Adhesion molecules connect ECs with their extraluminal, intercellular, and intraluminal surroundings (see Fig. 11–7). Thus, direct interaction between the abluminal surfaces of ECs and the extravascular ECM (basement membrane) is essential for survival, homeostasis, and angiogenic activity of these cells. Quiescent ECs are anchored to the permanent basement membrane, which is composed of laminin and collagen type IV. In contrast, angiogenic ECs are surrounded by provisional ECM containing fibrin, vitronectin, fibronectin, and partially proteolyzed collagens. These various interactions are mediated by a family of heterodimeric, transmembrane ECM receptors, known as *integrins* (each composed of α and β subunits), which recognize specific motifs within their target ECM proteins (eg, RGD peptides).

Integrins are viewed as functional hubs that localize and regulate the activities of other angiogenic effectors, including VEGFR2, other receptors, MMPs, angiopoietins, and

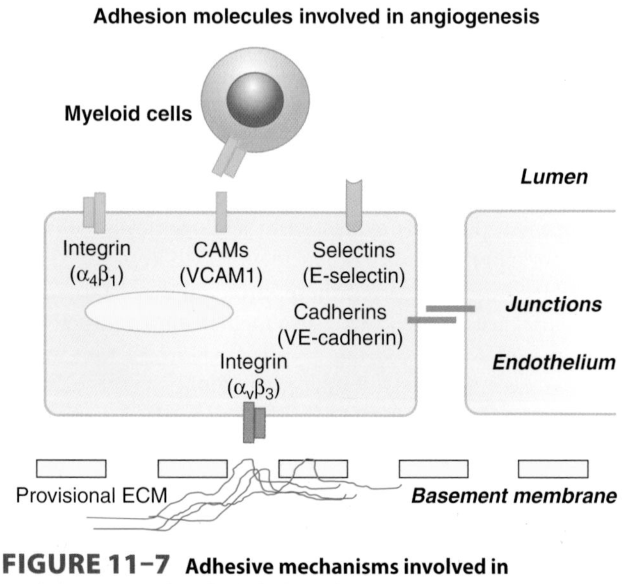

FIGURE 11–7 Adhesive mechanisms involved in angiogenesis and endothelial cell function. Endothelial cells interact homotypically through gap and tight junctional mechanisms, the latter involving lineage specific VE-Cadherin (CD144). Interactions with provisional ECM composed of proteolyzed collagen, fibrin, and vitronectin are mediated by $\alpha_v\beta_3/\beta_5$ integrins. Cell adhesion molecules (CAMs), selectins, and integrins mediate interactions with circulating cells and platelets, play a role in mechanosensing, inflammation and permeability; see text.

intracellular signal transducing kinases (PKB/AKT, FAK, ILK, SRC). Growth factors upregulate the expression of several Integrins on the surface of ECs in blood vessels ($\alpha_v\beta_3$, $\alpha_v\beta_5$, $\alpha_1\beta_1$, $\alpha_2\beta_1$, $\alpha_4\beta_1$, $\alpha_5\beta_1$) and lymphatics ($\alpha_1\beta_1$, $\alpha_2\beta_1$, $\alpha_4\beta_1$, $\alpha_9\beta_1$) (Avraamides et al, 2008). Although acute pharmacological disruption of the adhesive function of certain integrins ($\alpha_v\beta_3$) resulted in antiangiogenic effects (Cheresh and Stupack, 2002), the corresponding gene targeting studies suggested a more complex involvement. This is illustrated by the enhanced, rather than reduced, tumor angiogenesis in β_3/β_5-deficient mice (Reynolds et al, 2002). Indeed, other mutations of vascular integrins may either reduce (β_3 mutant, $\alpha_1\beta_1$), or increase ($\alpha_2\beta_1$) adult angiogenesis (Avraamides et al, 2008).

In contrast to the outward-oriented adhesion that is mediated by endothelial integrins, vascular endothelial cadherin (VE-cadherin/CD144) mediates formation of intercellular junctions between ECs within the vascular tube. This contact contributes to the unique properties of the endothelial lining (barrier function, restricted permeability, homotypic adhesion) (Nyqvist et al, 2008). VE-cadherin is selectively expressed by the cells of endothelial lineage and serves as their genetic marker. Importantly, gene targeting studies revealed that VE-cadherin is essential for vascular development, and for the functionality of some of its key regulators, such as VEGFR2 (Carmeliet and Jain, 2011). N-cadherin is also expressed by ECs, albeit not as selectively, and is required for vascular integrity and developmental angiogenesis. Cadherins bind to other cadherins on the adjacent cells and orchestrate formation of physical contacts, referred to as adherens junctions. These structures along with tight junctions (involving claudins) influence the functional integration of the endothelial lining.

Interactions between the endothelium and circulating immune, myeloid, inflammatory, and progenitor cells, and platelets are mediated by a diverse class of intraluminal adhesion molecules, including selectins (eg, E-selectin), integrins ($\alpha_4\beta_1$/VLA4), and members of the immunoglobulin family of cell adhesion molecules (CAMs, eg, ICAM-1/2 and VCAM1), all of which play different roles in angiogenesis (Francavilla et al, 2009).

11.4.8 Angiogenesis-Regulating Proteases

During blood vessel formation, the dissolution of the endothelial basement membrane, liberation of progenitor cells from the bone marrow, release of VEGF and other growth factors from their ECM stores, and the activation/modulation of the coagulation system, all involve various classes of proteases and their endogenous inhibitors (Kalluri and Zeisberg, 2006; van Hinsbergh et al, 2006). Of particular note are matrix metalloproteinases (MMPs) and their tissue inhibitors (TIMPs 1 to 4), often expressed in the tumor microenvironment (see Fig. 11–6). These molecules participate in ECM breakdown, generation of angiogenesis-regulating protein fragments, regulation of tumor and endothelial cell invasion, and may also act as ligands of cellular receptors (Kessenbrock et al, 2010). The main MMPs involved in tumor angiogenesis are MMP-1, MMP-2, MMP-9, and MMP-14. Their role is illustrated by the impairment of tumor neovascularization in mice with disrupted *MMP9* gene expression (Kessenbrock et al, 2010). Other proteases involved in angiogenesis include cathepsins, coagulation factor VIIa, thrombin (IIa), urokinase-type plasminogen activator (uPA), as well as members of the disintegrin and metalloproteinase domain (ADAM) and thrombospondin motif-containing (ADAMTS) families of proteases (van Hinsbergh et al, 2006).

11.4.9 Angiogenesis Stimulators and Inhibitors

The mechanisms described above are required for the execution of one or more of the angiogenic programs, but they are not necessarily the only or initial triggers of tumor angiogenesis. In cancer and other angiogenesis-dependent diseases, vascular growth may be initiated by a global shift in expression of several molecules, and the related cumulative change in the regulatory environment, the constituents of which are broadly classified as angiogenesis stimulators and inhibitors (see Table 11–1). It is believed that the onset of angiogenesis ("angiogenic switch," see Fig. 11–8) is triggered when the balance between these opposing influences is tilted beyond a certain discrete threshold, and in favor of stimulators (Folkman and Kalluri, 2003). Although this transition may appear as a binary event, the biological mechanisms involved can be complex, discontinuous, incremental, or oscillatory. The angiogenic threshold and the magnitude of endothelial cell responses may also differ depending on the genetic background and several other factors (Rohan et al, 2000). Furthermore, the composition of angiogenic factors may change over time during tumor progression (see Fig. 11–8), leading to a series of transitions rather than a single switch (Folkman and Kalluri, 2003).

Stimulators of angiogenesis include factors acting directly on ECs, such as VEGF, PlGF, FGF1/2, HGF, or interleukin 8 (IL-8). Similar effects can also result from indirect actions of their potent inducers, for example, transforming growth factors alpha or beta (TGFα, TGFβ) and several other cytokines and chemokines (eg, pleiotrophin). Some of these factors may act by recruitment of inflammatory cells (eg, IL-6), or bone marrow progenitor cells (eg, VEGF or stromal derived factor 1 [SDF1]), or through concomitant stimulation of both endothelial and inflammatory cells (eg, IL-8) (Kerbel, 2008).

The endogenous angiogenesis inhibitors are thought to maintain blood vessels in their quiescent state, or limit the magnitude of angiogenic responses, both locally and systemically (Folkman and Kalluri, 2003). Angiogenesis inhibitors belong to different classes of molecules, including certain ECM proteins (thrombospondins 1 and 2) (Bouck et al, 1996), or their proteolytic fragments (endostatin, tumstatin, arresten), fragments of enzymes and zymogens (angiostatin, PEX domain), fragments of coagulation-related chemokines (platelet factor 4 [PF4]), and of hormones (prolactin 16-kDa fragment), along with certain cytokines (interferons α, β, and γ) (Folkman and Kalluri, 2003; see Table 11–1).

11.4.10 Coagulation System and Platelets as Regulators of Tumor Angiogenesis

The discovery of VEGF in 1983 (Senger et al, 1983), and its role as a vascular permeability factor (VPF), originally linked angiogenesis to the coagulation system, especially through the observation of the associated extravascular leakage of plasma and formation of proangiogenic fibrin matrix (Dvorak et al, 1995). Although tumor angiogenesis was found to occur also in the absence of fibrinogen and fibrin, proangiogenic activities can be ascribed to several effectors of the coagulation system, such as TF/thromboplastin, thrombin and several others (Rickles et al, 2003). These factors may act directly on ECs, or stimulate the expression of VEGF, IL-8, and other angiogenic proteins by cancer cells and stroma. An important role is attributed to circulating blood platelets (Pinedo et al, 1998), which may serve as reservoirs and carriers of angiogenic factors (eg, plasma VEGF) and inhibitors (PF4, TSP-1). Indeed, platelets appear to take up, accumulate and segregate such factors in their granules and may selectively release them at sites of angiogenesis (Klement et al, 2009).

In addition to simple molecular signals (eg, soluble VEGF), ECs and other elements of the tumor microenvironment may receive and emit more complex (multimolecular) messages, encapsulated in cell membrane-derived structures known as *microvesicles*, *microparticles*, or *exosomes*. Microvesicles may deliver angiogenic growth factors (VEGF, FGF), inflammatory cytokines (IL-1), enzymes (MMPs), enzyme inducers (EMMPRIN), and other mediators, including messenger RNA (mRNA), microRNA, and DNA. Interestingly, microvesicles derived from cancer cells may also contain active and phosphorylated oncoproteins that may enter and reprogram ECs (eg, trigger autocrine production of VEGF) thereby possibly contributing to tumor angiogenesis (Al-Nedawi et al, 2009).

11.5 TUMOR ANGIOGENESIS

11.5.1 The Onset and Progression of Angiogenesis in Cancer

Cancer cells are dependent on their proximity to vascular networks for their growth, survival, and metastatic dissemination (Folkman and Kalluri, 2003). Sometimes these requirements are satisfied by vascular cooption, invasion of the preexisting vessels, postnatal vasculogenesis, or vascular mimicry as described earlier. However, in most human cancers the vascular dependence of tumor cells is met through the onset of angiogenesis, that is, tumor formation and progression can be regarded as *angiogenesis dependent* (Folkman and Kalluri, 2003). In some cases VEGF expression can be rate limiting for these events, which therefore can be viewed as VEGF dependent. Because of the central role of VEGF in developmental angiogenesis, this concept has undergone considerable (excessive) generalization, and has influenced design of antiangiogenic agents and

TABLE 11–1   Key molecular regulators of tumor angiogenesis.

Examples of angiogenic effectors required for endothelial and mural cell function		
Regulator	**Main Receptor(s)**	**Biological Activity**
VEGF-A/VEGF	VEGFR2 (VEGFR3, VEGF1), NRP1	Stimulator of angiogenic functions, migration and survival of ECs, including formation of tip cells
VEGF-C	VEGFR3 (VEGFR2)	Stimulator of angiogenesis (ECs) and lymphangiogenesis (LECs)
ANG 1	TIE2	Positive regulator of endothelial–mural interactions, EC survival, and vessel maturation
ANG 2	TIE2	Negative regulation of endothelial–mural interactions, stimulator of lymphangiogenesis
DLL4	NOTCH	Inhibitor of tip cells formation
JAG1	NOTCH	Stimulator of tip cell formation
EPHRINB2	EPHB4	VEGFR internalization/signaling, arterial identity, tube formation
PDGF-B	PDGFRβ	Recruitment of mural cells, vessel maturation
TGFβ1	TGFβRII	Differentiation of mural cells, ECM formation
Integrins (α_v, β_1, β_5)	ECM proteins	EC survival, migration morphogenesis

Examples of stimulators involved in tumor angiogenesis		
PlGF	VEGFR1	Stimulates angiogenesis by interaction with ECs and BMDCs
Acidic FGF (FGF-1)	FGFRs 1 to 4	Stimulator of EC mitogenesis, survival, and angiogenesis
Basic FGF (FGF-2)	FGFRs 1 to 4	Stimulator of EC mitogenesis, survival, and angiogenesis
FGF-3	FGFRs 1 to 4	Stimulator of EC mitogenesis, survival, and angiogenesis
FGF-4	FGFRs 1 to 4	Stimulator of EC mitogenesis, survival, and angiogenesis
IL-8	CXCR1	Stimulator of ECs and inflammatory cells
IL-6	IL-6R	Stimulator of inflammatory angiogenesis
TNFα	TNFR1 (55)	EC stimulator and VEGF inducer
Bv8	GPCR	Stimulator of endocrine and tumor ECs
PD-ECGF/TP	Unclear	Stimulator of angiogenesis
Angiogenin	170-kDa receptor	Stimulator of angiogenesis and RNAse
MMP9	ECM proteins	Matrix metalloproteinase that breaks down ECM and releases angiogenic growth factors

Examples of endogenous angiogenesis inhibitors	
Inhibitor	**Biological Activity**
TSP-1	Interacts with CD36 receptor, Integrins, and other proteins causing growth inhibition and apoptosis of angiogenic ECs
Endostatin	Proteolytic fragment of collagen XVIII with antiangiogenic activity
Angiostatin	Proteolytic fragment of plasminogen with antiangiogenic activity
Tumstatin	Proteolytic fragment of collagen IV α_3 chain
sFlt-1/sVEGFR1	Soluble splice variant of VEGFR1 with the ability to neutralize VEGF and block VEGFR2 signaling
VEGF165b	Splice variant of VEGF with antiangiogenic activity
PEX	Inhibitor of EC invasion and MMP activity
INFα(β)	Inhibits release of angiogenic growth factors

Abbreviations: ANG (1, 2), angiopoietin; *BMDC*, bone marrow-derived cells; *Bv8, Bombina variegata* protein; *DLL4*, delta-like 4; *EC*, endothelial cell; *ECM*, extracellular matrix; EPH, Ephrin; *FGF*, fibroblast growth factor; *GPCR*, G-protein–coupled receptor; *IFN*, interferon; *IL-6*, interleukin 6; *IL-8*, interleukin 8; *JAG1*, jagged 1; *LEC*, lymphatic endothelial cell; *MMP9*, matrix metalloproteinase 9; *PD-ECGF/TP*, platelet-derived endothelial cell growth factor/thymidine phosphorylase; *PDGF*, platelet derived growth factor; *PlGF*, placenta growth factor; *TNFα*, tumor necrosis factor alpha; *TSP-1*, thrombospondin 1; *VEGF*, vascular endothelial growth factor. See text for more details.

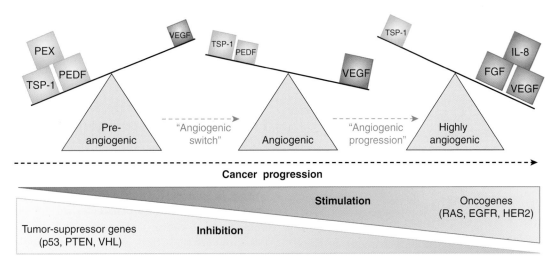

FIGURE 11–8 Angiogenic switch and progression during tumor development. Preangiogenic state in early tumor development is marked by the preponderance of angiogenesis inhibitors (TSP-1, PEDF, PEX), which override the effects of angiogenesis stimulators (VEGF) expressed at low levels. Aggressive tumor growth is triggered by the change in balance between these factors, leading to the increase in the net stimulatory activity and the onset of angiogenesis ("angiogenic switch"). The underlying qualitative and quantitative changes in levels of angiogenesis stimulators and inhibitors are driven by tumor microenvironment (hypoxia, inflammation) and genetic progression of cancer cells (mutations in oncogenes and tumor suppressors). Continued escalation of these molecular changes with progressive disease may result in exuberant proangiogenic microenvironment with increasingly active and redundant stimulatory networks (angiogenesis progression), but excessive amounts of VEGF may be incompatible with robust angiogenesis. Abbreviations: PEDF, pigment epithelium derived factor (angiogenesis inhibitor); TSP-1, thrombospondin 1; PEX, non-catalytic fragment of MMP (all angiogenesis inhibitors); FGF, fibroblast growth factor; IL-8, interleukin 8; VEGF, vascular endothelial growth factor/VEGF-A (angiogenesis stimulators); see text.

clinical trials to evaluate them. Thus, the majority of clinically used antiangiogenic drugs are presently directed at VEGF or VEGFRs (Table 11–2) (Ferrara, 2005).

The processes of vascular maturation are also disorganized in the context of cancer, which results in an incomplete and heterogeneous PC coverage (McDonald and Choyke, 2003). These defects may impact the susceptibility of tumor blood vessels to VEGF-directed therapies, as ECs devoid of PC contacts are more dependent on VEGF for survival (Ferrara, 2005). When such therapies exhaust their antiangiogenic impact a preponderance of more mature (resistant) and well-perfused tumor blood vessels is often observed. Incomplete blood vessel suppression combined with a shift toward better perfused and more mature microcirculation is often referred to as *vessel normalization* (Jain, 2001). Although this process may diminish the impact of VEGF inhibitors, it might also be exploited therapeutically, for example, by taking advantage of the increased delivery of anticancer chemotherapy agents to cancer cells that are better supplied with blood due to a more functional ("normalized") vascular network (Jain, 2001). Moreover, PCs themselves may serve as therapeutic targets in cancer, especially in situations where they support a significant proportion of tumor blood vessels (Carmeliet and Jain, 2011).

11.5.2 Mechanisms Triggering Tumor Neovascularization

The onset of tumor angiogenesis is often viewed as an early event in the course of disease progression, and one that permits the emerging tumor mass to expand beyond the size of 1 to 2 mm in diameter. The "preangiogenic" phase of tumor growth is defined by the limits of oxygen and macromolecule diffusion from the preexisting host vasculature (see Fig. 11–8). Other factors that influence the limits of preangiogenic tumor growth include the ability of cancer cells to tolerate hypoxia and metabolic deprivation (Folkman and Kalluri, 2003; see Chap. 12, Sec. 12.3), as well as the degree to which such cells can utilize vascular cooption and other alternative, nonangiogenic mechanisms of gaining an access to vascular networks (Holash et al, 1999). Beyond the boundaries of perivascular diffusion, cancer cells either undergo growth arrest, or enter a state of dynamic dormancy, defined by a balance between growth and cell death, without a net increase in the tumor mass (Folkman and Kalluri, 2003). Such exposure may eventually drive the onset of angiogenesis due to secondary changes in phenotype.

As mentioned earlier, the onset of angiogenesis ("angiogenic switch"; see Fig. 11–8) is often attributed to the net increase in the activity of angiogenesis-stimulating influences over those of inhibitors (Folkman and Kalluri, 2003). Cancer cells play a central and causative role in these events, and their role may be either direct (as producers of angiogenic factors), or more indirect, for example related to their ability to cause a hypoxic shift in the tissue microenvironment, recruitment/activation of proangiogenic stromal cells, and/or induction of inflammatory responses (Rak, 2009). Even within the same lesion the various subsets of cancer cells may differ in their proangiogenic activity. In some instances, this capacity appears to be particularly pronounced in the case of tumor-initiating cells (TICs), or cancer stem cells (CSCs), a notion particularly well studied in the case of brain tumors (Gilbertson and Rich, 2007). The major underlying trigger of a cancer cell-related angiogenic phenotype lies with the interplay between the effects of intracellular oncogenic pathways and responses to the extracellular tumor microenvironment, especially hypoxia and inflammation (see Chap. 12).

11.5.3 Hypoxia as a Trigger of Tumor Angiogenesis

Hypoxia acts as the primary physiological trigger of blood vessel formation, for example, during development, ischemia, and wound healing. Hypoxia is usually defined as tissue oxygen level below 10 to 15 mm Hg (see Chap. 12, Sec. 12.2), and may originate from several changes, such as increased oxygen consumption, low capillary density, poor blood perfusion, and the presence of vascular occlusion. Hypoxic regions (and areas of necrosis) are relatively common in advanced solid tumors, and their presence is usually associated with poor prognosis. Poor oxygenation evokes cellular responses involving the expression of genes that control intrinsic coping mechanisms, such as glycolytic metabolism, cellular quiescence, cell survival, and DNA repair, as well as those responsible for extracellular effects such as erythropoiesis and angiogenesis (Bristow and Hill, 2008).

The best described amongst the hypoxia response pathways is the activation of hypoxia-inducible transcription factors 1 and 2 (HIF1/2; see Chap. 12, Sec. 12.2.3). Several angiogenesis-related genes are targets of the HIF pathway, including VEGF, SDF1, ANG2, PlGF, PDGF-B, stem cell factor (SCF), and endothelial VEGFR1 (Rey and Semenza, 2010). Hypoxia also leads to downregulation of some angiogenesis inhibitors, notably thrombospondin 1 (TSP1) (Laderoute et al, 2000). HIF-mediated transcription is also involved in angiogenic responses of ECs themselves and contributes to vascular permeability and vessel 'abnormalization' (Fig. 11–9), followed by increased shedding of metastatic cancer cells into the blood stream (Carmeliet and Jain, 2011). Hypoxia provokes tumor cell invasiveness (Rey and Semenza, 2010) and HIF has been proposed as a factor that maintains the cancer stem cell population (Hill et al, 2009). Several other transcription factors may contribute to proangiogenic responses under hypoxia, including: nuclear factor kappa B (NF-κB), NF-IL6, MTF-1, and EGR-1.

Hypoxia triggers both angiogenesis (locally) and arteriogenesis (remotely), but the nature of these two events is fundamentally different (Carmeliet and Jain, 2011). Hypoxia serves as a potent inducer of local VEGF production (along with other factors), which in normal tissues acts as a self-limiting growth stimulus for capillaries. Angiogenesis causes an increase in blood vessel numbers, improves perfusion and tissue reoxygenation, which causes cessation of the hypoxic stimulus. Arteriogenesis occurs upstream of these events and outside of the boundaries of the hypoxic tissue, and ensures the parallel enlargement of feeding vessels through the effects of monocytes and nitric oxide (NO) (Carmeliet and Jain, 2011).

11.5.4 Tumor Vasculogenesis

Vasculogenesis involves incorporation of circulating EPCs into the capillary wall of the emerging tumor vasculature (Rafii et al, 2002). Although the nature and extent of this process is somewhat controversial, the presence of circulating cells with EPC-like characteristics in tumor-bearing animals and in cancer patients is well established, as is the ability of such cells to populate certain vascular structures (Asahara et al, 1997; Bertolini et al, 2010). Moreover, experiments involving chimeric animals harboring genetically tagged bone marrow suggest that EPCs may contribute to as much as 50%, or (more frequently) to as little as 0.01% of tumor blood vessels (Ahn and Brown, 2009). Similarly, in cancer patients who have previously undergone a gender-incompatible bone marrow transplant, donor-related EPCs (containing chromosomes or genes that distinguish them from the recipient) were found to contribute to only a minor fraction (approximately 5%) of the tumor vasculature (Peters et al, 2005).

The incorporation of EPC-like cells into tumor blood vessels may be stimulated by cancer therapy. For example, when acute administration of cytoreductive, or antivascular agents provokes emission of bone marrow activating cytokines, EPC-like cells are found to emerge within the circulation and home to the tumor mass in relatively large numbers (Shaked et al, 2006). It is proposed that this is a result of the combined action of circulating VEGF, granulocyte colony-stimulating factor (G-CSF), SDF1, and adhesion mediated by α_4 integrin. In this manner EPC-like cells may contribute to tumor revascularization and diminished antitumor effect of antivascular agents (Shaked et al, 2006). An important role in orchestrating the EPC recruitment is attributed to the ID1 transcriptional repressor (Rafii et al, 2002).

11.5.5 Proangiogenic Effects of Oncogenic Pathways

Cancer cells often express strongly proangiogenic properties (eg, overproduction of VEGF), even without exposure to hypoxia (Rak, 2009). This intrinsic and constitutive proangiogenic phenotype is triggered by the expression of several dominant oncogenes, examples of which include *H-Ras, K-Ras, Src, Myc, EGFR,* and *HER2* (Rak, 2009). In addition, the loss-of-function mutations affecting tumor-suppressor genes, such as *p53, PTEN, p16^{INK4a},* and *VHL,* also exert potent angiogenic effects, often in a cumulative manner (Bouck et al, 1996; Rak, 2009). These changes are executed through the pleiotropic impact these genetic events have on the cellular angiogenic transcriptome and proteome

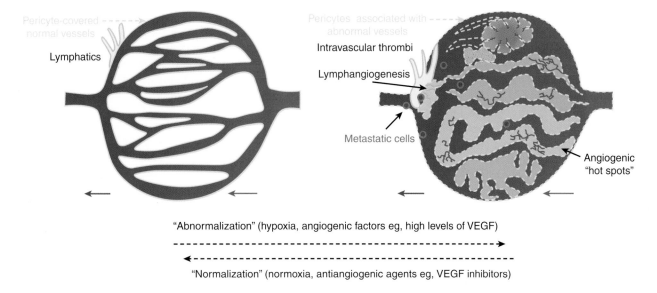

"Abnormalization" (hypoxia, angiogenic factors eg, high levels of VEGF)

-->

<--

"Normalization" (normoxia, antiangiogenic agents eg, VEGF inhibitors)

Normal microcirculation	Tumor (abnormal) microcirculation
(i) Structural characteristics	**(i) Structural characteristics**
• Continuous endothelium	• Discontinuous endothelium
• Intact basement membrane	• Incomplete basement membrane
• Complete and close pericyte coverage	• Loose and incomplete pericyte coverage
• Innervation	• No innervation
• Proper arborization and quasifractal branching	• Abnormal and chaotic branching
• Gradual changes in lumen diameter	• Paradoxical changes in lumen diameter
• No shunts or corkscrew structures	• Shunts and corkscrew structures
• No blunt ends or tortuosities	• Blunt ends and tortuosities
• Organ-specific architecture	• Heterogenous vascular density ("hot spots")
(ii) Functional characteristics	**(ii) Functional characteristics**
• Quiescent endothelial cells	• Proliferating, activated endothelial cells
• Intact junctional structures	• Abnormal/absent junctional structures
• Patent and perfused vascular branches	• Sluggish flow, poorly perfused vascular branches
• Proper tissue oxygenation and viability	• Tissue hypoxia and necrosis
• Nonleaky nonhemorrhagic capillaries	• Leaky and hemorrhagic capillaries (blood lakes)
• Intact barrier function	• Penetrable for metastatic cells
• Properly organized fenestrations and transport	• Abnormal fenestrations and transport
• Intact anticoagulant luminal surfaces	• Intravascular thrombi
• Proper lymphatic drainage (normal interstitial pressure)	• Poor lymphatic drainage (high interstitial pressure)
(iii) Molecular characteristics	**(iii) Molecular characteristics**
• Expression of pan-endothelial markers	• Expression of pan-endothelial markers
• Low VEGF/VEGFR pathway activity	• High VEGF/VEGFR pathway activity
• High ANG1/TIE2 pathway activity	• High ANG2/TIE2 pathway activity
• Absence tumor endothelial markers (eg, TEM8)	• Expression of tumor endothelial markers (eg, TEM8)

FIGURE 11–9 Tumor-related changes in vascular characteristics. Disorganized regulatory network in the tumor microenvironment leads to formation of blood vessels that are structurally, functionally, and molecularly abnormal (vessel "abnormalization"). Some of these abnormalities provide targets for antiangiogenic therapy that can selectively obliterate tumor blood vessels. Blood vessel-directed agents may either destroy blood vessels or restore, at least partially, some of their normal characteristics (vessel normalization); see text for details.

(angiome), via activation of kinase cascades, transcription factors and microRNA networks, such as the miR-17-92 cluster (Dews et al, 2006).

The most studied angiogenic effects of oncogenic mutations include upregulation of the key vascular stimulators—VEGF, FGF, IL-6, IL-8, or ANG1—coupled with downregulation of angiogenesis inhibitors, especially TSP-1, endostatin, tumstatin, and pigment epithelium-derived factor (PEDF) (Bouck et al, 1996; Rak, 2009). However, oncogene-regulated mediators of angiogenesis also include phospholipids, proteolytic enzymes, and microvesicles containing multiple angiogenic proteins (Al-Nedawi et al, 2009).

Activated oncogenic pathways often mimic or exacerbate cellular responses to hypoxia. For example, the extremely high levels of VEGF, florid angiogenesis, and hypervascularity observed in sporadic clear cell renal cell carcinoma (CCRCC) are largely attributed to the high frequency (70%) of the loss-of-function mutations affecting the *VHL* gene (Kaelin Jr, 2008). The resulting activation of HIF-dependent responses (see Chap. 12) drives transcription of VEGF and other vascular changes, even in the absence of overt oxygen deprivation. Similarly, while VEGF expression is upregulated by hypoxia in numerous types of nontransformed cells, the expression of *RAS* and other oncogenes in cancer cells can cause a marked amplification of these responses, leading to more exuberant production of VEGF (Mazure et al, 1996).

11.5.6 Inflammation

Tumor angiogenesis is profoundly affected by inflammatory cells and their soluble mediators. The sources of inflammatory reaction in cancer can be either extrinsic (infection), intrinsic (oncogenic mutations), immunological, or microenvironmental (Mantovani et al, 2008). These processes trigger recruitment of different subsets of inflammatory cells, especially M2-polarized (tumor-promoting) macrophages and other types of myeloid cells (see Fig. 11–2). There is also a growing interest in TIE2-expressing macrophages, mast cells (MCs), and granulocytes, many of which produce proteolytic enzymes, proangiogenic growth factors, cytokines, and chemokines (VEGF-A, Bv8, IL-8) (Schmid and Varner, 2010). VEGF-A exerts promigratory effects on macrophages, but inhibits antitumor immune responses, thereby tilting the regulatory balance toward tumor-promoting processes. Both tumor cells and stroma may contribute to these events through the activation of abnormal cellular "defense" mechanisms orchestrated by transcription factors (eg, NF-κB, HIF, and STAT [signal transducers and activators of transcription]), in response to the hostile tumor microenvironment (Mantovani et al, 2008).

11.5.7 Angiogenic Activation of Tumor Stroma

The presence of host cells (stroma) within the tumor mass is central to the onset of angiogenesis. Stromal cells likely contribute to endothelial cell quiescence in normal tissues by producing architectural constraints and angiogenesis inhibitors. In cancer, stromal cells may undergo functional changes described as "activation," or may even sustain genetic mutations (Hill et al, 2005). The sources of cancer-associated fibroblasts are likely diverse, ranging from cooption of resident connective tissue cells, their phenotypic reprogramming, changes in ECs, eg, endothelial-to-mesenchymal transition (EnMT), or analogous processes involving cancer cells, that is, epithelial-to-mesenchymal transition (EMT) (Kalluri and Zeisberg, 2006). Cancer-associated fibroblasts have long been known to exhibit elevated production of VEGF-A, and may also produce other angiogenic factors. For example,

production of PDGF-C by these cells was found to contribute to the resistance of tumors to therapies directed at VEGF-A. Hypoxia, paracrine interactions, activation of the coagulation system, inflammation, and oncogenic lesions may all contribute to the recruitment and stimulation of the angiogenic tumor stroma (Dvorak, 1986).

11.6 MODIFIERS OF TUMOR ANGIOGENESIS

Although most tumors express various elements of the angiogenic phenotype, the dynamics of the related vascular responses is often context dependent. This is defined by the tumor type (grade/molecular profile), or by host-dependent influences. The latter may be a function of individual characteristics of cancer patients, for example, their genetic background, age, metabolic conditions (eg, obesity, diabetes, atherosclerosis), and other comorbidities, such as thrombosis, postsurgical responses, constitutive levels of circulating growth factors, hormones, and other regulators. These host-related factors may impact various aspects of angiogenesis, such as microvessel density, endothelial cell proliferation, vascular branching patterns, and the numbers of recruited bone marrow cells at the tumor site.

11.6.1 The Impact of Genetic Background on Tumor Angiogenesis

A similar angiogenic stimulus may evoke angiogenic responses of differential nature and magnitude because of relatively subtle changes in the host genetic background. For example, different strains of mice exhibit inherently differential angiogenic reactions in response to stimulation with the same recombinant angiogenic growth factors (Rohan et al, 2000). Tumor angiogenesis was found to be constitutively altered in mice deficient for ID1 transcriptional repressor, β_1 Integrins, β_3/β_5 Integrins, and other factors (Lyden et al, 1999; Reynolds et al, 2002). Similarly, mice expressing different levels of VEGF-A (eg, due to introduction of a hypomorphic VEGF allele) exhibit alterations in angiogenesis, including in association with cancer (Sung et al, 2010). Polymorphisms of the VEGF gene in humans regulate both the angiogenic activity and responses to antiangiogenic agents, for example, in breast cancer patients administered bevacizumab (see Sec. 11.7.1.3; Schneider et al, 2009). Supernumerary chromosome 21, which is associated with Down's syndrome, impedes VEGF production and angiogenesis through the action of DSCR1 and DYRK1a genes (Reynolds et al, 2010). Moreover, otherwise silent heterozygosity of host cells for certain tumor-suppressor genes may influence regulation of angiogenesis and tumor progression. For example, in the murine model of neurofibromatosis where host tissues have the $NF1^{+/-}$ genotype, the related increase in proangiogenic mast cell recruitment is required for the efficient growth of $NF1^{-/-}$ tumors (Yang et al, 2008). Similar influences may also exist in cancer patients.

11.6.2 Modulation of Tumor Angiogenesis by Vascular Ageing and Comorbidities

Although cancers are more prevalent in adults and the elderly then in children, they may occur at any age, and the age of onset can influence tumor angiogenesis (Reed and Edelberg, 2004). This is exemplified not only by the uniqueness of malignancies affecting children, adolescents, and young adults (including some of their vascular phenotypes), but also by the age-related differences in more common cancers. For example, the age of patients affected by CCRCC may vary by up to 5 decades. During this time, the vascular system undergoes profound changes, including alterations in the state of endothelial, bone marrow, inflammatory, and other cellular compartments. Ageing impacts responses to hypoxia, impedes production of angiogenic growth factors and efficiency of vascular repair, it increases procoagulant tendencies and leads to cardiovascular decline. Age-related alterations in the vasculature may influence the responses to antiangiogenic therapies, and can be further compounded by age-related comorbidities affecting the macro- and microvasculature, eg, atherosclerosis (Rak, 2009).

11.6.3 Properties of the Tumor Microcirculation

Tumor blood vessels exhibit high levels of architectural, cellular, and molecular heterogeneity, in comparison to normal tissues (Jain, 2001). These anomalies include loss of proper arborization (hierarchy), unusual patterns of branching (trifurcation), paradoxical lumen dilatations, formation of corkscrew and blind ended structures, and abnormal vascular connections (shunts). Tumor blood vessels may contain capillaries with either incomplete or hypertrophic endothelial cell lining (eg, in brain tumors), which may fold into intraluminal projections and septa, and interact poorly with the surrounding PCs (McDonald and Choyke, 2003). Perivascular microhemorrhages and spaces filled with blood (blood lakes) are common in tumors along with vascular occlusion and regression (Holash et al, 1999). Regional abnormalities of the vessel wall often result in the leakage of plasma, macromolecules, and clotting factors into the extravascular space. This leads to extravascular activation of the coagulation system and deposition of crosslinked fibrin, as well as formation of intravascular occlusive thrombi (Brat and Van Meir, 2004). A combined effect of these changes amounts to sluggish, intermittent, often bidirectional and inefficient blood flow, poor tissue perfusion, hypoxia, and necrosis (Folkman and Kalluri, 2003).

Structural abnormalities of tumor blood vessels are associated with a shift in the EC phenotype. Thus, tumor-associated ECs may exhibit elevated mitotic indices (Denekamp, 1982), changes in cell shape, and regional heterogeneity in the expression of molecular markers. They express abnormal levels of various proteins and phospholipids (eg, exposed phosphatidylserine) (Neri and Bicknell, 2005). Some tumor ECs

overexpress proangiogenic receptors (eg, VEGFR2 or TIE2), that stimulate angiogenic activity. Molecular profiling of ECs isolated from blood vessels of certain human and murine tumors has also revealed the expression of molecules normally absent in the vasculature, and often referred to as *tumor endothelial markers* (TEMs) (Seaman et al, 2007).

Tumor ECs may also exhibit genetic changes, for example, abnormal ploidy (Hida et al, 2004), marker chromosomes, or expression of mutant oncogenes, suggesting that some tumor cells (especially CSCs) may contribute to the endothelial lining (Ricci-Vitiani et al, 2010). The unique molecular make up of tumor ECs can be used to guide the development of blood vessel-directed anticancer therapies (Neri and Bicknell, 2005).

11.6.4 Tumor Lymphangiogenesis

Solid tumors often exhibit high interstitial fluid pressure indicative of poor lymphatic drainage (see also Chap. 12, Sec. 12.2.4). This property was long regarded as an indication that lymphatics are absent in growing tumor masses, but more recent studies provided evidence to the contrary. For instance, lymphangiogenesis and expression of lymphangiogenic growth factors (VEGF-C/D) and their receptors (VEGFR3) were detected both within and around tumors, and their contribution to lymph node metastasis is well documented. Indeed, expression of VEGF-C/D in cancer cells increases their metastatic capacity in animal models. Lymph nodes are also the major and early sites of metastasis a property of considerable prognostic significance in human cancers (eg, in breast, gastrointestinal, renal, colorectal, and other malignancies). These observations suggest that agents that block lymphangiogenesis may possess anticancer and antimetastatic activity (Tammela and Alitalo, 2010).

11.6.5 Tumor Initiating Cells and Blood Vessels

The ability to initiate clonal neoplastic growth, disease recurrence, and metastasis is often attributed to a subset of cancer cells known as CSCs, or TICs (see Chap. 13). There is an emerging relationship between CSCs and angiogenesis, of which two major scenarios are being considered. First, because the expression of stem cell properties and marker molecules (eg, Oct4) is, in some cases, induced by hypoxia, some CSCs may reside in poorly perfused tumor regions, possibly distant from the vasculature (Hill et al, 2009). In contrast, normal neuroectodermal stem cells and their malignant counterparts (CSCs) appear to be located in areas adjacent to blood vessels, and in regions referred to as *perivascular niches* (Gilbertson and Rich, 2007). In glioblastoma, brain TICs expressing CD133 antigen are found to exhibit elevated production of VEGF and an increased proangiogenic activity, largely as a result of the constitutive activation of the hypoxia response pathway mediated by HIF2 (Gilbertson and Rich, 2007). TICs may also exhibit altered procoagulant properties (Rak, 2009), and their abundance may be depleted following antiangiogenic therapies. Although the links between angiogenesis and CSCs are rather complex, their tumor initiating activity implicitly involves the vasculature (eg, during metastasis) (Gilbertson and Rich, 2007). CSCs have also been proposed to transdifferentiate to form tumor endothelium (Ricci-Vitiani et al, 2010), but this notion remains controversial.

11.7 BLOOD VESSEL-DIRECTED ANTICANCER THERAPIES

The concept of targeting blood vessels to achieve anticancer effects was initially developed by Judah Folkman (Folkman, 1971, 2007). After nearly 4 decades of experimental and clinical exploration, this modality is now a part of clinical management in several human cancers (see Table 11–2), with at least 6 different agents approved for human use by the Food and Drug Administration (FDA) in the United States. Targeting tumor blood vessels in cancer is based on functional and molecular differences that separate properties of the tumor microcirculation from the corresponding segments of the normal vasculature. Agents and techniques that target tumor blood vessels may act on ECs, or on mural cells directly (direct inhibitors). Alternatively, therapeutics may interfere with events and cells stimulating or supporting tumor vasculature (indirect inhibitors).

11.7.1 Antiangiogenic Therapies

Antiangiogenic agents are designed to block formation of new tumor blood vessels through several approaches ranging from targeting the specific signaling circuitry of ECs (eg, by blocking VEGF or VEGFR2), to exploiting naturally occurring angiogenesis inhibitory pathways (see Table 11–2). Whether a particular agent possesses an antiangiogenic activity can be determined using several functional angiogenesis assays conducted either on cultured ECs or in animals (Jain et al, 1997). Those tests analyze survival, proliferation, migration, and formation of tube-like structures by cultured ECs, ingrowth of capillaries into the chick chorioallantoic membrane, sprouting in avascular sites in animals (corneal micropocket assays), or in pellets of ECM (Matrigel) implanted subcutaneously into mice (Jain et al, 1997). In animal models and in the clinic antiangiogenic activity may also be deduced from tumor responses, as measured by functional imaging (see Chap. 14), for example, Doppler ultrasound, magnetic resonance (MRI), or positron emission tomography (PET), that allow the assessment of several relevant parameters, such as tissue metabolism, oxygenation, vascular permeability, or blood flow (Jain et al, 2009). Also changes in the density of blood vessels within the tumor mass (microvascular density [MVD] counts), shifts in circulating angiogenic cytokines (VEGF, IL-8), the presence of apoptotic ECs in peripheral blood, or changes in levels of CECs (EPCs) can be used in support of the antiangiogenic mechanism of a particular anticancer drug (Kerbel, 2008).

In spite of the growing understanding of biological events surrounding the antiangiogenic activity of various agents, the establishment of clinically useful predictive biomarkers for therapeutic antiangiogenesis has been challenging (Hanrahan et al, 2010). Nevertheless, hundreds of antiangiogenic agents have been evaluated thus far, and they can be broadly assigned into several main categories as summarized in Table 11–2 and Figure 11–10.

11.7.1.1 First-Generation, Exogenous Antiangiogenic Agents In early studies, several natural compounds or their derivatives were empirically found to possess activities against ECs. Examples of such agents include the fungal product fumagillin (and its derivative TNP470), penicillamine (copper chelator), carboxyaminotriazole, suramin, and 2-methoxyestradiol (2ME2) (Folkman and Kalluri, 2003). The mechanisms of action of many of these agents remain unclear. Thalidomide is an agent whose antiangiogenic activity is at least partially linked to the teratogenic effects of this drug and its grim earlier legacy (D'Amato et al, 1994). Thalidomide's pleiotropic immunomodulating and antiangiogenic effects and those of the related agent, lenalidomide, are the basis of their recent use in the treatment of multiple myeloma and other malignancies (Cook and Figg, 2010).

11.7.1.2 Agents Based on the Activity of Endogenous Angiogenesis Inhibitors The ability of tissues to elaborate endogenous angiogenesis inhibitors inspired drug development aimed at therapeutic antiangiogenesis (Folkman, 2007). Several agents in this category have been evaluated, including antiangiogenic cytokines, such as interferon-α (IFNα), antiangiogenic fragments of ECM proteins (endostatin), fragments of plasminogen (angiostatin, K5), peptides related to TSP1 (ABT-510), and several other agents (Folkman and Kalluri, 2003). With few exceptions, the mechanisms of antiangiogenic activity of these agents are either complex, or have not been fully elucidated. In clinical settings, the therapeutic efficacy of these agents in cancer has been relatively modest, and only 1 drug in this category (YH-16-recombinant endostatin [Endostar]) is currently (2012) approved for human use, outside of North America (Cook and Figg, 2010).

11.7.1.3 Molecularly Targeted Antiangiogenic Agents Understanding of molecular pathways involved in angiogenesis has led to the development of several classes of targeted antiangiogenic agents. These can be broadly divided into 3 major categories: (a) neutralizing antibodies against angiogenic ligands, or their receptors, usually designated by generic names ending with "-mab" (eg, bevacizumab); (b) traps, which are agents designed to neutralize angiogenic factors by virtue of containing high affinity sites (ectodomains) derived from the corresponding cognate cellular receptors (eg, VEGF-trap/Aflibercept); and (c) small molecule inhibitors of angiogenic receptors, with generic names ending with "-nib" (eg, sunitinib).

TABLE 11-2 Examples of blood vessel-targeting agents developed to treat cancer.

Antiangiogenic agents (AAs)
(i) Molecularly targeted agents designed to obliterate key angiogenic pathways

Drug	Type	Target	Stage of Development (2012)
Bevacizumab	Neutralizing huMoAb	VEGF	Approved for human use
Sunitinib	TKI	VEGFR1-3, PDGFRα/β, KIT, FLT3, RET, CSF1R	Approved for human use
Sorafenib	TKI	VEGFR2-3, C-RAF, B-RAF, VEGF-C, FLT3, FGFR1, PDGFβ, KIT, p38	Approved for human use
Pazopanib	TKI	VEGFR1 to 3, PDGFRα/β, KIT, FGFR1, -3, -4, FMS	Approved for human use
Vandetanib (ZD6474)	TKI	VEGFR2, EGFR, RET	Approved for human use
Axitinib	TKI	VEGFR1 to 3, PDGFR, KIT	Approved for human use
Cabozantinib (XL184)	TKI	VEGFR2, MET, RET, KIT, FLT3, TIE2	In clinical development
VEGF-trap	Soluble VEGF "receptor-body"	VEGF-A, -B, PlGF	In clinical development
Cilengitide	Cyclic peptide	$\alpha_v\beta_3/\beta_5$ Integrin	In advanced clinical trials

(ii) Agents with direct but not fully elucidated antiangiogenic activity

Drug	Type	Target	Stage of Development (2012)
Endostar	Protein fragment	Unclear	In human use (China)
ABT510	Peptide	Endothelial CD36	In clinical development
2-Methoxyestradiol (2ME2)	Sterol	HIF-1α, Tubulin	Investigational agent
TNP470 (Lodamin)	Small molecule (slow release)	Complex activity	Investigational agent

(iii) Indirect-acting antiangiogenic agents designed to block oncogenic pathways

Drug	Type	Target	Stage of Development (2012)
Trastuzumab	Neutralizing huMoAb	HER-2	Approved for human use
Cetuximab	Neutralizing huMoAb	EGFR	Approved for human use
Gefitinib	TKI	EGFR	Approved for human use
Erlotinib	TKI	EGFR	Approved for human use
Lapatinib	TKI	EGFR, HER-2	Approved for human use
Imatinib	TKI	ABL, PDGFRβ, KIT	Approved for human use
Dacomitinib (PF00299804)	TKI	Irreversible pan-ERB inhibitor	In development
Tipifarnib	FTI	Ras, farnesylated proteins	In clinical development

(iv) Agents with antiangiogenic activity developed for non-antiangiogenic indications

Drug	Type	Target	Stage of Development (2012)
Chemotherapy (metronomic)	Various agents (CTX, VBL, TMZ, TAX)	Stress-response pathways, DNA, cytoskeleton	Under clinical exploration
Celecoxib	Small molecule	COX-2	Under clinical exploration
Thalidomide and analogs (Lenalidomide)	Small molecule	Inflammatory pathways	Approved in multiple myeloma, under investigation

(v) Antivascular agents/vascular disrupting agents

Drug	Type	Target	Stage of Development (2012)
Vadimezan (ASA404)	Flavonoid	EC survival	Advanced clinical trials
Combretastatin A-4 disodium phosphate (CA4P)	Tubulin binding	Tubulin assembly	Advanced clinical trials
Ombrabulin (AVE8062)	Tubulin binding	Tubulin assembly	Advanced clinical trials
ABT-751	Tubulin binding	Tubulin assembly	Advanced clinical trials
OXi4503	Tubulin binding	Tubulin assembly	Early clinical trials

Abbreviations: CTX, Cyclophosphamide; *EGFR*, epidermal growth factor receptor, *FTI*, protein farnesyltransferase inhibitor; *huMoAb*, humanized monoclonal antibody; *TAX*, paclitaxel; *TKI*, tyrosine kinase inhibitor; *TMZ*, temozolomide; *VBL*, vinblastin; *VEGFR*, vascular endothelial growth factor receptor; see text for more details.

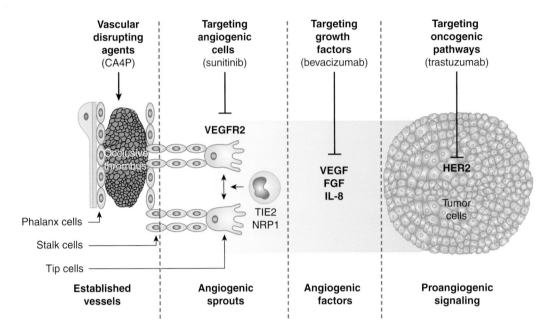

Examples of assays designed to detect blood vessel-directed effects:

- *Flow measurements in tumor models (Doppler)*

- *Tumor models—microvascular imaging, and density count*

- *Skinfold window—vascular imaging and pattern analysis*

- *Matrigel implant—imaging vascular ingrowth and perfusion*

- *CAM—chick chorioallantoic membrane assay, vessel imaging, and quantification*

- *Cornea micropocket assay— measurement of vessel growth toward angiogenic stimulus*

- *Endothelial tube formation in vitro (collagen, matrigel, fibrin)*

- *Endothelial growth and invasion assays in vitro*

- *Measurements of angiogenic growth factor levels (ELISA, microarrays)*

- *Measurements of tumor vascularity and perfusion*

- *Bioassays for angiogenic activity in the presence of vascular cells*

FIGURE 11–10 Some of the main strategies to target tumor vasculature. Development of the tumor microcirculation can be therapeutically opposed in several ways, including blocking mechanisms of the "angiogenic switch" through the use of antagonists of oncogenic pathways, such as trastuzumab, a neutralizing antibody that binds to HER-2 oncoprotein. Angiogenic factors, such as VEGF, can also be obliterated using neutralizing antibodies (eg, bevacizumab). Cells involved in angiogenic responses, namely, endothelial cells, PCs, and myeloid cells, can be prevented from responding to angiogenic growth factors by agents blocking their receptors, such as VEGFR2-directed drugs (eg, sunitinib or pazopanib). These cells can also be targeted using direct angiogenesis inhibitors (thrombospondin, tumstatin, integrin inhibitors, metronomic chemotherapy, and other agents). While these strategies generally prevent formation of new blood vessels, vascular disrupting agents (VDAs) obliterate the already established tumor vasculature by causing endothelial damage and thrombosis. Several assays have been developed to detect and measure the responses of the microcirculation to these respective insults (bottom panel); see text for details.

Targeted antiangiogenic therapeutics in clinical use (and multiple experimental agents) are largely directed against the VEGF/VEGFR pathway. In 2004, the humanized monoclonal antibody directed against VEGF-A (bevacizumab) became the first antiangiogenic agent to be approved for treatment of metastatic colorectal cancer (Hurwitz et al, 2004). Subsequently, at least 5 additional small-molecule oral agents, targeting VEGF receptors and other RTKs (multikinase inhibitors), have entered medical practice in oncology (Table 11–2). Currently, VEGF/VEGFR antagonists are being used to treat several human cancers, even though limited long term activity and toxicity continue to present challenges. These key indications include metastatic renal cell carcinoma (MRCC), hepatocellular carcinoma (HCC), metastatic colorectal cancer

(MCRC), non–small cell lung cancer (NSCLC), and glioblastoma (GBM). Antiangiogenics often provide a considerable, albeit mostly transient, benefit to at least a subset of patients (Kerbel, 2008). It is unclear why in other cancers (eg, in pancreatic adenocarcinoma or malignant melanoma) these agents are ineffective.

Additional angiogenic pathways, including PDGF/PDGFR (sunitinib, imatinib), FGF/FGFR (brivanib), Angiopoietin/TIE2 (AMG-386), HGF/Met (foretinib), EPHRINB2/EPH4 (JI-101), and DLL4/NOTCH (REGN421), are under investigation (see Table 11–2) (Cook and Figg, 2010). Targeted agents have also been developed against other molecular effectors of angiogenesis, with a more complex role, such as $\alpha_v\beta_3/\alpha_v\beta_5$ Integrins (cilengitide), EGFL7 endothelial-binding ECM protein (MEGF0444A), and protein kinase (PK) C-β (enzastaurin) (Cook and Figg, 2010). Agents that are expected to have greater selectivity against cancer-related pathological angiogenesis and lymphangiogenesis, outside of common vascular pathways are also under development. Examples of such agents include inhibitors of PlGF (anti-PlGF antibody/TB-403), Bv8 (anti-Bv8 antibody), VEGF-C (VEGFR3-trap), VEGFR3 (anti-VEGFR3 antibody), PDGF-C (anti–PDGF-C antibody), and NRP1 and NRP2 (antibodies), as well as inhibitors of PHD2 (DMOG) and HIF (EZN-2968), the effects of which are not always restricted to ECs, and may involve mural, stromal and other cells (Carmeliet and Jain, 2011).

The exposure to antiangiogenic agents, especially those targeting VEGF, may trigger vascular remodeling. It is believed that downregulation, or blockade of VEGF acutely exposes ECs to the residual excess of ANG2. In the absence of VEGF-dependent survival/stimulating signals, ANG2 blocks the remaining TIE2 survival pathway and leads to endothelial cell apoptosis, resulting in vessel thrombosis, collapse, and regression (Hanahan, 1997). However, regression of capillaries does not obliterate the tissue "memory" of the prior capillary network. Instead, upon the disappearance of ECs tissue still contains the networks of their related basement membranes (capillary "sleeves"), which may serve as a scaffold for rapid endothelial regrowth upon restoration of VEGF supply, for example, once the antiangiogenic therapy has been discontinued (reviewed in Carmeliet and Jain, 2011).

11.7.2 Antiangiogenic Effects of Agents Targeting Oncogenic Pathways

The angiogenic switch in cancer cells represents another attractive therapeutic target. Examples are inhibitors of the protein farnesyltransferase, which block not only the transforming activity of mutant *H-ras*, but also VEGF upregulation driven by this oncogene in cultured cancer cells (Rak, 2009). Recent studies demonstrate similar effects of other oncogene-directed agents, including trastuzumab (HER2), cetuximab (EGFR), imatinib (BCR-ABL), and several others, an activity coupled with overt antiangiogenic mechanism demonstrable in vitro and in vivo (Rak, 2009). Moreover such agents may possess a dual activity against proangiogenic mechanisms operative in both cancer cells and in the endothelium. For example, farnesyltransferase inhibitors (tipifarnib, lonafarnib), or epidermal growth factor receptor (EGFR) inhibitors (gefitinib, erlotinib) may exert their effects by blocking farnesylation or EGFR signaling, respectively, in both cancer cell and endothelial compartments. Several anticancer agents under development inhibit 2 or more molecular targets (multikinase or "dirty" inhibitors). For example, by combining the inhibitory effects against VEGF and epidermal growth factor (EGF) receptors certain agents (vandetanib, AEE788) can act on both tumor cell and EC populations, including tumor-associated ECs that express abnormally high levels of EGFR. Indeed, combinatorial action of the multikinase inhibitors (eg, sunitinib or sorafenib) may explain some aspects of their clinical activity (Rak, 2009; Cook and Figg, 2010).

11.7.3 Antiangiogenic Effects of Other Therapeutics

The proangiogenic circuitry activated in endothelial, stromal, and cancer cells involves pleiotropic signaling pathways whose functions have often been studied outside of angiogenesis (see Chap. 8). Drugs that interfere with such pathways have been found to possess unsuspected antiangiogenic activities (Kerbel et al, 2000). Thus cyclooxygenase 2 (COX-2) regulates the expression of several angiogenic stimulators in cancer cells and the nonsteroidal antiinflammatory drugs (eg, celecoxib), which block this pathway, also possess antiangiogenic activity (Tsujii et al, 1998). Other pathways (agents) that are being studied in this context include mammalian target of rapamycin (mTOR; temsirolimus, everolimus), proteasome complexes (bortezomib), coagulation factors (heparin), steroid receptors, and antiangiogenic effects of anticancer chemotherapeutics.

The increased mitogenic activity of tumor-associated ECs may make them susceptible to traditional cytotoxic anticancer agents and radiation (Denekamp, 1982). These effects may be present in the context of the usual chemotherapy protocols, but they rapidly dissipate posttreatment because of vascular regrowth and mobilization of BMDCs. This occurs during "drug holidays" taken to allow for hemopoietic recovery (Kerbel, 2008). However, when chemotherapy drugs are given continuously at lower doses, their is reduced, drug holidays are no longer needed, and the antiangiogenic effects may be amplified, even in the presence of tumor cell resistance to the same agent. This approach is known as *metronomic chemotherapy*, and exhibits considerable antiangiogenic activity, especially when combined with VEGF inhibitors and other endothelial-targeting agents (Browder et al, 2000; Klement et al, 2000).

11.7.4 Vascular Disrupting Agents

While antiangiogenesis mainly targets new vascular growth, the already preformed tumor blood vessels are targets of another class of therapeutics, referred to as vascular disrupting agents (VDAs) (Tozer et al, 2005; McKeage and Baguley, 2010). The goal of this therapy is to provoke a selective vascular shutdown, or "infarction," within the tumor vasculature, mainly by compromising the viability, continuity, and antithrombotic properties of the endothelial lining. Unlike antiangiogenesis, the effects of VDAs are rapid (begin within less than an hour), and result in acute intravascular thrombosis, vascular shutdown, ischemia, and tumor necrosis. Although these effects are dramatic in the center of the tumor mass, they dissipate in the periphery, leaving a viable rim of cancer cells supplied by the intact extratumoral vasculature, which is not susceptible to VDA treatment (Tozer et al, 2005). The residual disease and local vascular regrowth involving mobilization of cells from the bone marrow may lead to rapid tumor regrowth post-VDA treatment; this could be mitigated by combining VDAs with other agents, including inhibitors of angiogenesis and proper timing of these sequential treatments (Shaked et al, 2006).

The small-molecule VDAs are directed against vulnerable points of the tumor associated vasculature, especially tubulin and EC survival mechanisms (McKeage and Baguley, 2010). Two classes of these agents are under investigation (see Table 11–2), namely, (a) flavonoids (ASA404), which act mainly in a tubulin-independent manner, and (b) tubulin-binding agents. Some of the most studied compounds in this group include combretastatin A-4 phosphate (CA4P), AVE 8062, ABT-751, and OXi4503 (McKeage and Baguley, 2010).

11.7.5 Challenges Associated with Targeting Tumor Blood Vessels

11.7.5.1 Tumor-Specific Efficacy of Antiangiogenic Agents
The distinct nature of tumor blood vessels, the quiescence of normal ECs, and their initially presumed absence of genetic instability were originally taken as an indication that, unlike conventional anticancer agents, therapies directed against blood vessels should be selective, nontoxic, universally applicable, and devoid of the risk of drug resistance. However, clinical experience with the approved agents indicated that their effects may vary considerably between different cancers and individual patients. Thus, inhibitors of the VEGF pathway (bevacizumab, sunitinib, sorafenib) have shown efficacy only in a narrow spectrum of specific diseases. Even if antiangiogenic therapy elicits initial response, relapse eventually occurs in most cases and in spite of continued treatment, a pattern reminiscent of the acquired resistance to other anticancer agents.

11.7.5.2 Mechanisms of Resistance to Blood Vessel-Directed Agents
Acquired resistance to antiangiogenic agents can be a function of changes affecting ECs and their angiogenic mechanisms, or result from properties and abundance of host stromal cells. Such resistance can also be brought about by altered tumor microenvironment or genetic drift (or selection) of cancer cells. For example, progressive acquisition of oncogenic mutations may shift the expression of angiogenesis regulators leading to their increasing redundancy, and the failure of pathway-specific antiangiogenic agents (eg, VEGF inhibitors) (Rak, 2009). In addition, the expression of oncogenes and loss of tumor suppressors (eg, p53) may render cancer cells more capable of withstanding ischemic effects of antiangiogenesis (Yu et al, 2002). Examples of stromal cell-dependent resistance mechanisms that can circumvent VEGF inhibition include production of PDGF-C by fibroblasts, or Bv8 by tumor-associated granulocytes (Shojaei et al, 2009). Alternative mechanisms of angiogenesis (cooption, vasculogenic mimicry), increased vessel maturation (normalization), endothelial cell aneuploidy, autocrine reprogramming, rapid regrowth of blood vessels post-therapy, or influx of endothelial progenitors may all contribute to diminished therapeutic responses (Bergers and Hanahan, 2008). Hypoxic stress or production of cytokines may sometimes provoke more invasive behavior (or selection) amongst residual cancer cells, including increased metastasis. A better understanding of processes underlying resistance and invasiveness in this context is required to develop new more effective agents. Combinations between different antiangiogenic drugs and with other therapies may further improve the outcomes of this relatively new anticancer treatment modality.

11.7.5.3 Side Effects of Blood Vessel-Directed Agents
Antiangiogenic agents are not absolutely selective and may block normal functions of angiogenic factors, or cause off-target effects that lead to toxicity. One common toxicity is the impairment of wound healing and the related risk of bleeding. In addition, VEGF pathway inhibitors may sometimes cause thrombosis, hypertension, and proteinuria as a consequence of their systemic impact on vascular homeostasis, vascular tone, or kidney function (Eremina et al, 2007). Other side effects may include fatigue, skin rash, hypothyroidism, and other poorly understood toxicities (Verheul and Pinedo, 2007).

11.7.5.4 Biomarkers of Therapeutic Response to Antiangiogenic Agents
The chronic nature of therapeutic responses to antiangiogenic agents and their biological complexity make the effective monitoring of their anticancer effects challenging (Bertolini et al, 2010). Consequent therapeutic impact, individual responsiveness of a cancer patient, or early signs of drug resistance can sometimes be captured by using vascular imaging techniques and blood assays (Jain et al, 2009). The latter include measuring the levels of circulating endothelial-like cells, interleukins (eg, IL-6 or IL-8), TSP1, and other molecules (SDF1a, VEGF), and in some cases multiplex platforms that detect and profile several factors simultaneously (Jain et al, 2009). Still, new technologies are needed to improve the robustness and accuracy of antiangiogenic biomarkers for the expedited clinical development of new agents, and their more individualized use in cancer patients.

SUMMARY

Angiogenesis is perhaps the most critical host tissue response to an emerging malignancy. It creates a tumor–vascular interface, which signifies the transition from a local cellular defect to the systemic disease that most cancers eventually become. Because of these considerations angiogenesis has become a validated therapeutic target in cancer.

The key features of tumor angiogenesis covered in this chapter are:

- Tumor growth and metastasis are dependent on the interaction (interface) between cancer (stem) cells and the vascular system.
- Endothelial cells (ECs) are the central drivers of blood vessel formation.
- In growing vessels, ECs form specialized structures (sprouts), and in so doing differentiate into distinct subsets of tip, stalk, and phalanx cells.
- Endothelial homeostasis is regulated by their surrounding mural cells, systemically acting BMDCs and their products (growth factors, enzymes, and ECM). Vascular growth is triggered by the excess of angiogenesis-stimulating factors relative to inhibitors.
- VEGF and its receptors are the key molecular regulators of vascular development, homeostasis, and growth, but in cancer, this pathway may become dispensable.
- Tumor blood vessels exhibit several structural, cellular, and molecular anomalies, which can be exploited as therapeutic targets.
- Several hundred agents targeting tumor blood vessels are in preclinical and clinical development, of which at least 6 have been approved to treat cancer (by 2012).
- Agents targeting blood vessels are broadly divided into drugs blocking blood vessel growth (antiangiogenics) and drugs able to selectively destroy established tumor vessels (VDAs).
- Although effective, antiangiogenic agents can trigger tumor resistance and exhibit side effects.

REFERENCES

Ahn GO, Brown JM. Role of endothelial progenitors and other bone marrow-derived cells in the development of the tumor vasculature. *Angiogenesis* 2009;12:159-164.

Al-Nedawi K, Meehan B, Rak J. Microvesicles: messengers and mediators of tumor progression. *Cell Cycle* 2009;8:2014-2018.

Alitalo K, Tammela T, Petrova TV. Lymphangiogenesis in development and human disease. *Nature* 2005;438:946-953.

Andrae J, Gallini R, Betsholtz C. Role of platelet-derived growth factors in physiology and medicine. *Genes Dev* 2008;22:1276-1312.

Asahara T, Murohara T, Sullivan A, et al. Isolation of putative progenitor endothelial cells for angiogenesis. *Science* 1997; 275:964-967.

Augustin HG, Koh GY, Thurston G, et al. Control of vascular morphogenesis and homeostasis through the angiopoietin-Tie system. *Nat Rev Mol Cell Biol* 2009;10:165-177.

Avraamides CJ, Garmy-Susini B, Varner JA. Integrins in angiogenesis and lymphangiogenesis. *Nat Rev Cancer* 2008;8: 604-617.

Bergers G, Hanahan D. Modes of resistance to anti-angiogenic therapy. *Nat Rev Cancer* 2008;8:592-603.

Bertolini F, Marighetti P, Shaked Y. Cellular and soluble markers of tumor angiogenesis: From patient selection to the identification of the most appropriate postresistance therapy. *Biochim Biophys Acta* 2010;1806:131-137.

Bouck N, Stellmach V, Hsu SC. How tumors become angiogenic. *Adv Cancer Res* 1996;69:135-174.

Brat DJ, Van Meir EG. Vaso-occlusive and prothrombotic mechanisms associated with tumor hypoxia, necrosis, and accelerated growth in glioblastoma. *Lab Invest* 2004;84: 397-405.

Bristow RG, Hill RP. Hypoxia and metabolism. Hypoxia, DNA repair and genetic instability. *Nat Rev Cancer* 2008;8:180-192.

Browder T, Butterfield CE, Kraling BM, et al. Antiangiogenic scheduling of chemotherapy improves efficacy against experimental drug-resistant cancer. *Cancer Res* 2000;60: 1878-1886.

Carmeliet P, Jain RK. Molecular mechanisms and clinical applications of angiogenesis. *Nature* 2011;473:298-307.

Cheresh DA, Stupack DG. Integrin-mediated death: an explanation of the integrin-knockout phenotype? *Nat Med* 2002;8:193-194.

Cook KM, Figg WD. Angiogenesis inhibitors: current strategies and future prospects. *CA Cancer J Clin* 2010;60:222-243.

D'Amato RJ, Loughnan MS, Flynn E, et al. Thalidomide is an inhibitor of angiogenesis. *Proc Natl Acad Sci U S A* 1994;91: 4082-4085.

De Palma M, Naldini L. Role of haematopoietic cells and endothelial progenitors in tumour angiogenesis. *Biochim Biophys Acta* 2006; 1766;1:159-166.

Denekamp J. Endothelial cell proliferation as a novel approach to targeting tumor therapy. *Br J Cancer* 1982;45:136-139.

Dews M, Homayouni A, Yu D, et al. Augmentation of tumor angiogenesis by a Myc-activated microRNA cluster. *Nat Genet* 2006;38:1060-1065.

Dome B, Hendrix MJ, Paku S, et al. Alternative vascularization mechanisms in cancer: Pathology and therapeutic implications. *Am J Pathol* 2007;170:1-15.

Dong J, Grunstein J, Tejada M, et al. VEGF-null cells require PDGFR alpha signaling-mediated stromal fibroblast recruitment for tumorigenesis. *EMBO J* 2004;23:2800-2810.

Dudley AC, Khan ZA, Shih SC, et al. Calcification of multipotent prostate tumor endothelium. *Cancer Cell* 2008;14:201-211.

Dufraine J, Funahashi Y, Kitajewski J. Notch signaling regulates tumor angiogenesis by diverse mechanisms. *Oncogene* 2008;27: 5132-5137.

Dvorak HF. Tumors: wounds that do not heal. *N Engl J Med* 1986;315:1650-1659.

Dvorak HF, Brown LF, Detmar M, et al. Vascular permeability factor/vascular endothelial growth factor, microvascular hyperpermeability, and angiogenesis. *Am J Pathol* 1995;146: 1029-1039.

Ema M, Rossant J. Cell fate decisions in early blood vessel formation. *Trends Cardiovasc Med* 2003;13:254-259.

Eremina V, Baelde HJ, Quaggin SE. Role of the VEGF—a signaling pathway in the glomerulus: evidence for crosstalk between components of the glomerular filtration barrier. *Nephron Physiol* 2007;106:32-37.

Fantin A, Vieira JM, Gestri G, et al. Tissue macrophages act as cellular chaperones for vascular anastomosis downstream of VEGF-mediated endothelial tip cell induction. *Blood* 2010;116:829-840.

Ferrara N. Role of myeloid cells in vascular endothelial growth factor-independent tumor angiogenesis. *Curr Opin Hematol* 2010;17:219-224.

Ferrara N. VEGF as a therapeutic target in cancer. *Oncology* 2005;69 (Suppl 3):11-16.

Folkman J. Angiogenesis: an organizing principle for drug discovery? *Nat Rev Drug Discov* 2007;6:273-286.

Folkman J. Tumor angiogenesis: therapeutic implications. *N Engl J Med* 1971;285:1182-1186.

Folkman J, Kalluri R. Tumor angiogenesis. In: Kufe DW, Pollock RE, Weichselbaum RR, et al, eds. *Cancer Medicine*. Hamilton, Ontario: BC Decker, 2003:161-194.

Francavilla C, Maddaluno L, Cavallaro U. The functional role of cell adhesion molecules in tumor angiogenesis. *Semin Cancer Biol* 2009;19:298-309.

Gaengel K, Genove G, Armulik A, Betsholtz C. Endothelial-mural cell signaling in vascular development and angiogenesis. *Arterioscler Thromb Vasc Biol* 2009;29:630-638.

Gerhardt H, Golding M, Fruttiger M, et al. VEGF guides angiogenic sprouting utilizing endothelial tip cell filopodia. *J Cell Biol* 2003; 161:1163-1177.

Gilbertson RJ, Rich JN. Making a tumour's bed: glioblastoma stem cells and the vascular niche. *Nat Rev Cancer* 2007;7:733-736.

Hanahan D. Signaling vascular morphogenesis and maintenance. *Science* 1997;277:48-50.

Hanrahan EO, Lin HY, Kim ES, et al. Distinct patterns of cytokine and angiogenic factor modulation and markers of benefit for vandetanib and/or chemotherapy in patients with non-small-cell lung cancer. *J Clin Oncol* 2010;28:193-201.

Hendrix MJ, Seftor EA, Hess AR, et al. Vasculogenic mimicry and tumour-cell plasticity: lessons from melanoma. *Nat Rev Cancer* 2003;3:411-421.

Hida K, Hida Y, Amin DN, et al. Tumor-associated endothelial cells with cytogenetic abnormalities. *Cancer Res* 2004;64:8249-8255.

Hill R, Song Y, Cardiff RD, et al. Selective evolution of stromal mesenchyme with p53 loss in response to epithelial tumorigenesis. *Cell* 2005;123:1001-1011.

Hill RP, Marie-Egyptienne DT, Hedley DW. Cancer stem cells, hypoxia and metastasis. *Semin Radiat Oncol* 2009;19:106-111.

Holash J, Maisonpierre PC, Compton D, et al. Vessel cooption, regression, and growth in tumors mediated by angiopoietins and VEGF. *Science* 1999;284:1994-1998.

Hurwitz H, Fehrenbacher L, Novotny W, et al. Bevacizumab plus irinotecan, fluorouracil, and leucovorin for metastatic colorectal cancer. *N Engl J Med* 2004;350:2335-2342.

Jain RK. Normalizing tumor vaculature with anti-angiogenic therapy: A new paradigm for combination therapy. *Nat Med* 2001;7:987-989.

Jain RK, Duda DG, Willett CG, et al. Biomarkers of response and resistance to antiangiogenic therapy. *Nat Rev Clin Oncol* 2009;6: 327-338.

Jain RK, Schlenger K, Hockel M, et al. Quantitative angiogenesis assays: progress and problems. *Nat Med* 1997;3:1203-1208.

Jones N, Iljin K, Dumont DJ, et al. Tie receptors: new modulators of angiogenic and lymphangiogenic responses. *Nat Rev Mol Cell Biol* 2001;2:257-267.

Kaelin WG Jr. The von Hippel-Lindau tumour suppressor protein: O_2 sensing and cancer. *Nat Rev Cancer* 2008;8:865-873.

Kalluri R, Zeisberg M. Fibroblasts in cancer. *Nat Rev Cancer* 2006;6: 392-401.

Kerbel RS. Tumor angiogenesis. *N Engl J Med* 2008;358:2039-2049.

Kerbel RS, Viloria-Petit A, Klement G, et al. "Accidental" anti-angiogenic drugs. anti-oncogene directed signal transduction inhibitors and conventional chemotherapeutic agents as examples. *Eur J Cancer* 2000;36:1248-1257.

Kessenbrock K, Plaks V, Werb Z. Matrix metalloproteinases: regulators of the tumor microenvironment. *Cell* 2010;141:52-67.

Klement G, Baruchel S, Rak J, et al. Continuous low-dose therapy with vinblastine and VEGF receptor-2 antibody induces sustained tumor regression without overt toxicity. *J Clin Invest* 2000;105: R15-R24.

Klement GL, Yip TT, Cassiola F, et al. Platelets actively sequester angiogenesis regulators. *Blood* 2009;113:2835-2842.

Laderoute KR, Alarcon RM, Brody MD, et al. Opposing effects of hypoxia on expression of the angiogenic inhibitor thrombospondin 1 and the angiogenic inducer vascular endothelial growth factor. *Clin Cancer Res* 2000;6:2941-2950.

LeCouter J, Lin R, Ferrara N. Endocrine gland-derived VEGF and the emerging hypothesis of organ-specific regulation of angiogenesis. *Nat Med* 2002;8:913-917.

Lee S, Chen TT, Barber CL, et al. Autocrine VEGF signaling is required for vascular homeostasis. *Cell* 2007;130:691-703.

Li Z, Huang H, Boland P, et al. Embryonic stem cell tumor model reveals role of vascular endothelial receptor tyrosine phosphatase in regulating Tie2 pathway in tumor angiogenesis. *Proc Natl Acad Sci U S A* 2009;106:22399-22404.

Lyden D, Young AZ, Zagzag D, et al. Id1 and Id3 are required for neurogenesis, angiogenesis and vascularization of tumour xenografts. *Nature* 1999;401:670-677.

Mantovani A, Allavena P, Sica A, et al. Cancer-related inflammation. *Nature* 2008;454:436-444.

Mazure NM, Chen EY, Yeh P, et al. Oncogenic transformation and hypoxia synergistically act to modulate vascular endothelial growth factor expression. *Cancer Res* 1996;56:3436-3440.

McDonald DM, Choyke PL. Imaging of angiogenesis: from microscope to clinic. *Nat Med* 2003;9:713-725.

McKeage MJ, Baguley BC. Disrupting established tumor blood vessels: an emerging therapeutic strategy for cancer. *Cancer* 2010; 116:1859-1871.

Neri D, Bicknell R. Tumour vascular targeting. *Nat Rev Cancer* 2005; 5:436-446.

Noguera-Troise I, Daly C, Papadopoulos NJ, et al. Blockade of Dll4 inhibits tumour growth by promoting non-productive angiogenesis. *Nature* 2006;444:1032-1037.

Nowak DG, Woolard J, Amin EM, et al. Expression of pro- and anti-angiogenic isoforms of VEGF is differentially regulated by splicing and growth factors. *J Cell Sci* 2008;121:3487-3495.

Nyqvist D, Giampietro C, Dejana E. Deciphering the functional role of endothelial junctions by using in vivo models. *EMBO Rep* 2008;9:742-747.

Peters BA, Diaz LA, Polyak K, et al. Contribution of bone marrow-derived endothelial cells to human tumor vasculature. *Nat Med* 2005;11:261-262.

Pettersson A, Nagy JA, Brown LF, et al. Heterogeneity of the angiogenic response induced in different normal adult tissues by vascular permeability factor/vascular endothelial growth factor. *Lab Invest* 2000;80:99-115.

Pinedo HM, Verheul HM, D'Amato RJ, et al. Involvement of platelets in tumour angiogenesis? *Lancet* 1998;352:1775-1777.

Rafii S, Lyden D, Benezra R, et al. Vascular and haematopoietic stem cells: novel targets for anti-angiogenesis therapy? *Nat Rev Cancer* 2002;2:826-835.

Rak J. Ras oncogenes and tumour vascular interface. In: Thomas-Tikhonenko A, ed. *Cancer Genome and Tumor Microenvironment.* New York, NY: Springer; 2009:133-165.

Reed MJ, Edelberg JM. Impaired angiogenesis in the aged. *Sci Aging Knowledge Environ* 2004;2004:pe7.

Rey S, Semenza GL. Hypoxia-inducible factor-1-dependent mechanisms of vascularization and vascular remodelling. *Cardiovasc Res* 2010;86:236-242.

Reynolds LE, Watson AR, Baker M, et al. Tumour angiogenesis is reduced in the Tc1 mouse model of Down's syndrome. *Nature* 2010;465:813-817.

Reynolds LE, Wyder L, Lively JC, et al. Enhanced pathological angiogenesis in mice lacking beta3 integrin or beta3 and beta5 integrins. *Nat Med* 2002;8:27-34.

Ricci-Vitiani L, Pallini R, Biffoni M, et al. Tumour vascularization via endothelial differentiation of glioblastoma stem-like cells. *Nature* 2010;468:824-828.

Rickles FR, Patierno S, Fernandez PM. Tissue factor, thrombin, and cancer. *Chest* 2003;124:58S-68S.

Rohan RM, Fernandez A, Udagawa T, et al. Genetic heterogeneity of angiogenesis in mice. *FASEB J* 2000;14:871-876.

Roy-Chowdhury S, Brown CK. Cytokines and tumor angiogenesis. In: Caligiuri MA, Lotze MT, eds. *Cancer Drug Discovery and Development.* Totowa, NJ: Humana Press; 2007:245-266.

Schmid MC, Varner JA. Myeloid cells in the tumor microenvironment: modulation of tumor angiogenesis and tumor inflammation. *J Oncol* 2010;2010:201026.

Schneider BP, Radovich M, Miller KD. The role of vascular endothelial growth factor genetic variability in cancer. *Clin Cancer Res* 2009;15:5297-5302.

Seaman S, Stevens J, Yang MY, et al. Genes that distinguish physiological and pathological angiogenesis. *Cancer Cell* 2007;11:539-554.

Senger DR, Galli S, Dvorak AM, et al. Tumor cells secrete a vascular permeability factor that promotes accumulation of ascites fluid. *Science* 1983;219:983-985.

Shaked Y, Ciarrocchi A, Franco M, et al. Therapy-induced acute recruitment of circulating endothelial progenitor cells to tumors. *Science* 2006;313:1785-1787.

Shojaei F, Wu X, Qu X, et al. G-CSF-initiated myeloid cell mobilization and angiogenesis mediate tumor refractoriness to anti-VEGF therapy in mouse models. *Proc Natl Acad Sci U S A* 2009;106:6742-6747.

Sung HK, Michael IP, Nagy A. Multifaceted role of vascular endothelial growth factor signaling in adult tissue physiology: an emerging concept with clinical implications. *Curr Opin Hematol* 2010;17:206-212.

Tammela T, Alitalo K. Lymphangiogenesis: molecular mechanisms and future promise. *Cell* 2010;140:460-476.

Tozer GM, Kanthou C, Baguley BC. Disrupting tumour blood vessels. *Nat Rev Cancer* 2005;5:423-435.

Tsujii M, Kawano S, Tsuji S, Sawaoka H, Hori M, DuBois RN. Cyclooxygenase regulates angiogenesis induced by colon cancer cells. *Cell* 1998;93:705-716.

van Hinsbergh V, Engelse MA, Quax PH. Pericellular proteases in angiogenesis and vasculogenesis. *Arterioscler Thromb Vasc Biol* 2006;26:716-728.

Verheul HM, Pinedo HM. Possible molecular mechanisms involved in the toxicity of angiogenesis inhibition. *Nat Rev Cancer* 2007;7:475-485.

Wang Y, Nakayama M, Pitulescu ME, et al. Ephrin-B2 controls VEGF-induced angiogenesis and lymphangiogenesis. *Nature* 2010;465:483-486.

Xu Q. The impact of progenitor cells in atherosclerosis. *Nat Clin Pract Cardiovasc Med* 2006;3:94-101.

Yancopoulos GD, Davis S, Gale NW, et al. Vascular-specific growth factors and blood vessel formation. *Nature* 2000;407:242-248.

Yang FC, Ingram DA, Chen S, et al. Nf1-dependent tumors require a microenvironment containing Nf1+/− and c-kit-dependent bone marrow. *Cell* 2008;135:437-448.

Yu JL, Rak JW, Coomber BL, et al. Effect of p53 status on tumor response to antiangiogenic therapy. *Science* 2002;295:1526-1528.

Tumor Growth, Microenvironment, and Metabolism

12

Rob A. Cairns, Ian F. Tannock, and Bradly Wouters

12.1 TUMOR GROWTH AND CELL KINETICS

Tumors grow because the homeostatic mechanisms that maintain the appropriate number of cells in normal tissues are defective, leading to an imbalance between cell proliferation and cell death and to expansion of the cell population. The use of autoradiography with tritiated thymidine in the 1950s and 1960s, and the subsequent application of flow cytometry, have allowed a detailed analysis of tumor growth in terms of the kinetics of proliferation of the constituent cells. The proliferative rate of tumor cells varies widely between tumors; slowly proliferating or nonproliferating cells are common, and there is often a high rate of cell death. Several normal tissues, including bone marrow and intestine, contain cells with high rates of proliferation, and damage to these cells is often dose-limiting for chemotherapy. The rate of cell proliferation in tumors may be an important factor in determining prognosis and response to therapy.

12.1.1 Growth of Human Tumors

Because tumors are generally treated rather than observed, most of the data on growth rates of untreated human cancers are from studies that were undertaken prior to the development of more effective therapies. Accurate measurements could be made only on tumors from selected sites, and most studies have examined lung metastases using serial chest radiographs. There have been only a few reported measurements of the growth of untreated primary tumors (which generally were removed by operation or irradiated). Because there is a limited observation period between the time of tumor detection and either death of the host or initiation of therapy, such measurements represent only a small fraction of the history of the tumor's growth (see Fig. 12–1). Despite these limitations, Steel (1977) was able to review measurements of the rate of growth of more than 600 human tumors, and a few general conclusions may be stated:

1. There is wide variation in growth rate, even among tumors of the same histological type and site of origin.
2. Childhood tumors and adult tumors that are known to be responsive to chemotherapy (eg, lymphoma, cancer of the testis) tend to grow more rapidly than less-responsive tumors.
3. Lung metastases tend to grow more rapidly than the primary tumor in the same patient.
4. Over the period of observation, the time for the tumor volume to double was often constant, implying exponential growth. Doubling times for lung metastases of common tumors in humans were in the range of 2 to 3 months; Table 12–1 summarizes the doubling times for various types of cancer.

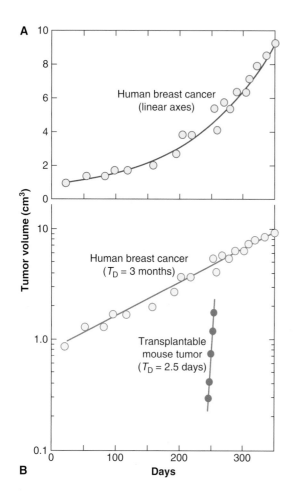

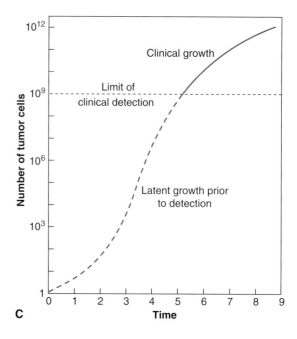

FIGURE 12–1 **A) Growth rate of a human breast cancer using linear axes. B)** Growth of the same tumor using a logarithmic scale for tumor volume. **C)** Hypothetical growth curve indicating initial latency and later slowing of tumor growth.

Exponential growth of tumors will occur if the rates of cell production and of cell loss or death are proportional to the number of cells present in the population. Exponential growth often leads to the false impression that tumor growth is accelerating with time (see Fig. 12–1). Increase in the diameter of a human tumor from 0.5 to 1.0 cm may escape detection, whereas an increase from 5 to 10 cm is dramatic and is likely to cause new clinical symptoms. Both require 3 volume doublings; during exponential growth they will occur over the same period of time.

Many internal tumors are unlikely to be detected until they grow to approximately 0.5 to 1.0 g (~10 to 13 mm in diameter), and tumors of this size will contain approximately 500 to 1000 million (0.5 to 1.0×10^9) cells. There is indirect evidence that many tumors arise from a single cell (see Sec. 12.1.3), and a tumor containing approximately 10^9 cells will have undergone approximately 30 doublings in volume prior to clinical detection (because of cell loss, this will involve more than 30 consecutive divisions of the initial cell). After 10 further doublings in volume, the tumor would weigh approximately 1 kg (10^{12} cells), a size that may be lethal to the host. Thus, the range of size over which a tumor is detectable clinically represents a rather short and late part of its total growth history (Fig. 12–2). There is evidence (eg, for breast cancer) that the probability of seeding

of metastases increases with the size of the primary tumor, but the long preclinical history of the tumor may allow cells to metastasize prior to detection. Thus "early" clinical detection may be expected to reduce, but not to prevent, the subsequent appearance of metastases.

The growth rate of a human tumor in its preclinical phase can only be estimated indirectly or inferred from observations of spontaneous or induced tumors in animals. Tumor growth may be slow at very early stages of development when tumor cells may have to overcome immunological and other host defense mechanisms, and induce proliferation of blood vessels to support them (see Chap. 11, Sec. 11.5). Deceleration of growth of large tumors is also observed, probably as a result of increasing cell death and decreasing cell proliferation as tumor nutrition deteriorates (see Sec. 12.1.4). Also, tumors often contain a high proportion of nonmalignant cells, such as macrophages, lymphocytes, and fibroblasts, and the proliferation and migration of these cells will influence changes in tumor volume.

12.1.2 Cell-Cycle Analysis

As discussed in Chapter 9, Section 9.2.1, the cell cycle is divided into a short mitotic (M) phase that can be recognized morphologically, a subsequent variable G_1 (G = Gap) phase, a

TABLE 12–1 Volume doubling time (T_D) for representative human tumors.

Tumor Type	Number of Tumors	Volume Doubling Time* (weeks)
Primary lung cancer		
Adenocarcinoma	64	21
Squamous cell carcinoma	85	12
Anaplastic carcinoma	55	11
Breast cancer		
Primary	17	14
Lung metastases	44	11
Soft-tissues metastases	66	3
Colon/rectum		
Primary	19	90
Lung metastases	56	14
Lymphoma		
Lymph node lesions	27	4
Lung metastases of		
Carcinoma of testis	80	4
Childhood tumors	47	4
Adult sarcomas	58	7

*Geometric mean values (to account for skewed distribution).

Source: Data from Steel, 1977.

the S-phase of the cell cycle, although these methods have now been supplanted by automated techniques based on flow cytometry. The proportion of thymidine-labeled cells at a short interval after administration of tritiated (^{3}H) thymidine (the *labeling index*) is a measure of the proportion of cells that were in S-phase (^{3}H-thymidine has a short half-life in the circulation). In the *percent-labeled-mitoses* (PLM) method, serial biopsies (or serial specimens from identical animals) are taken at intervals after a single injection of ^{3}H-thymidine, and the proportion of mitotic cells that are radiolabeled is estimated from autoradiographs prepared from these biopsies. Time-dependent changes in this proportion can provide estimates of the duration of phases of the cell cycle (see Steel, 1977, for details). Although this method is labor intensive, it has provided most of the available estimates of the duration of the different cell-cycle phases in human tumors and normal tissues. The PLM method and other techniques for estimating duration of cell-cycle phases, which are described below, tend to give information about the faster proliferating cells in the population, and are insensitive to the presence of more slowly proliferating cells.

Flow cytometry is a method that separates and sorts cells based on cellular fluorescence. Cells can be tagged with fluorescent markers (eg, monoclonal antibodies) to a wide range of molecules, including cell-surface receptors, molecules involved in signaling pathways, and proteins that are expressed in different phases of the cell cycle. Several fluorescent dyes (eg, propidium iodide, ethidium bromide, mithramycin, and Hoechst 33342) bind to DNA in proportion to DNA content. Cells are then directed in single file through a laser beam to excite the dye, and the fluorescence emission is collected and displayed as a DNA distribution (Fig. 12–3A); cells can also be sorted on the basis of their fluorescence intensity. Minimally toxic agents, such as 5-bromodeoxyuridine (BrdUrd) or 5-ethynyl-2′-deoxyuridine (EdU), can be incorporated into newly synthesized DNA (like tritiated thymidine) and recognized by

discrete period of DNA synthesis (or S-phase), and a G_2-phase that precedes mitosis. Much of the information about the duration of phases of the cell cycle in tumors and normal tissues was derived by using autoradiography to detect the selective uptake of radioactive (^{3}H or ^{14}C) thymidine during

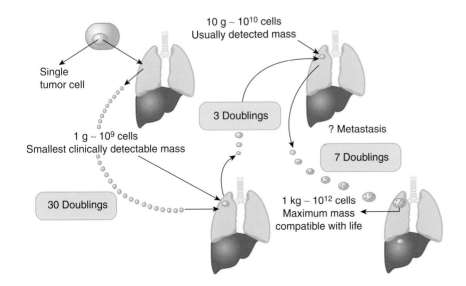

FIGURE 12–2 A human solid tumor must undergo approximately 30 to 33 doublings in volume from a single cell before it achieves a detectable size at a weight of 1 to 10 g. Metastases may have been established prior to detection of the primary tumor. Only a few further doublings of volume lead to a tumor whose size is incompatible with life. (Adapted from Tannock, 1983.)

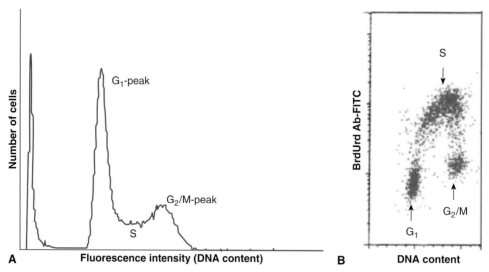

FIGURE 12–3 **A) DNA distribution for a human bladder cancer cell line produced by flow cytometry.** Cells were stained with acridine orange. The peak at the origin represents cellular debris. **B)** Use of flow cytometry to sort HL-60 cells on the basis of their uptake of bromodeoxyuridine (BrdUrd) (recognized by an antibody tagged to fluorescein isothiocyanate [FITC]) in relation to DNA content; cells in different cell-cycle phases are indicated. (Adapted from Darzynkiewicz et al, 2011.)

fluorescent-tagged antibodies. Analysis of the distribution of uptake of these precursors in relation to DNA content (Fig. 12–3B) can then provide estimates of the proportion of cells with 2N DNA content (ie, G_1 and most nonproliferating cells), 4N DNA content (G_2 and mitotic cells), and intermediate DNA content (S-phase cells), while time-dependent changes in these distributions can provide estimates of cell cycle phase duration (Darzynkiewicz et al, 2011). Many tumors are aneuploid (ie, the content of DNA in G_1-phase tumor cells differs from that of normal cells) allowing separation of tumor cells and normal cells within the tumor. Some proteins (eg, the nuclear protein Ki-67) appear to be expressed uniquely in cycling cells and can be recognized by fluorescent-labeled antibodies. Fluorescent-tagged monoclonal antibodies that recognize cyclins and other molecules involved in cell-cycle regulation can also be used to determine their expression at different times during the mitotic cycle (see Chap. 9, Sec. 9.2.3), and expression of cell cycle-dependent molecules in human tumor cells can be related to prognosis (see Sec. 12.1.5).

In most normal tissues of the adult, only a small proportion of the cells are actively proliferating. The remaining cells have either lost their capacity for proliferation through differentiation, or are G_0 cells that can proliferate in response to an appropriate stimulus. Examples of the latter include stem cells in the bone marrow (see Sec. 12.1.4) and cells in skin that participate in wound healing. Most tumors also contain slowly proliferating or nonproliferating cells, and the term *growth fraction* describes the proportion of cells in the tumor population that is proliferating—or, more accurately, those that are rapidly proliferating—as available techniques do not separate truly nonproliferating cells from those that are cycling at a rate slower than the mean. Proliferating cells in tumors can be

recognized using cytometry with an antibody against Ki-67, as described above. Most anticancer drugs are more toxic to rapidly proliferating cells (see Chap. 17, Sec. 17.5) and the growth fraction (Ki-67–positive cells) therefore indicates the proportion of tumor cells that might be sensitive to cycle-dependent chemotherapy.

The overall rate of cell production can be estimated from the growth fraction and the median length of the cell cycle (T_c), but since the value of T_c is often unknown, it is easier to estimate this from the proportion of S-phase cells (obtained by flow cytometry or from the labeling index) and the length of S-phase (T_s) with an added constant (λ) to account for the relative position of S-phase in the cell cycle. This parameter is usually called the *potential doubling time of the tumor* ($T_{pot} = \lambda T_s/LI$) and is the expected doubling time of the tumor in the absence of cell loss. However, the frequent occurrence of necrosis and of apoptotic cells in tumors and the ability of tumor cells to metastasize from a primary tumor indicates that there is considerable cell death or loss from many tumors. Thus the value of T_{pot} is usually much shorter than the measured volume doubling time (V_D) because of this cell loss (Steel, 1977). The fractional rate of cell loss from tumors can be estimated by comparing T_{pot} with the V_D (Fractional cell loss = $1 - T_{pot}/V_D$).

12.1.3 Cell Proliferation in Normal Tissues

Thymidine labeling and flow cytometry have been used to compare the overall rate of cell proliferation in a variety of normal tissues (Table 12–2). The side effects of chemotherapy that are common to many drugs (eg, myelosuppression, mucositis, hair loss, and sterility) are observed in

TABLE 12–2 Proliferative rates of selected normal tissues in adults.

Rapid	Slow	None
Bone marrow	Lung	Muscle
GI mucosa	Liver	Bone
Ovary	Kidney	Cartilage
Testis	Endocrine glands	Nerve
Hair follicles	Vascular endothelium	

Note: Acute side effects of chemotherapy occur commonly in rapidly proliferating tissue.

rapidly proliferating tissues, reflecting the greater activity of most anticancer drugs against rapidly proliferating cells (see Chap. 17, Sec. 17.5). Acute effects of radiation injury are also observed in these tissues, because irradiated cells often die when they attempt mitosis (see Chap. 16, Sec. 16.5). The proliferation and differentiation of hemopoietic cells in the bone marrow and epithelial cells in the intestine are described below as examples of renewal tissues in which the pattern of cell proliferation is an important determinant of anticancer therapy.

12.1.3.1 Bone Marrow

Morphologically recognizable cells in bone marrow and blood have an orderly progression of differentiation from myeloblasts to polymorphonuclear granulocytes, from pronormoblasts to red blood cells, and from megakaryocytes to platelets (see Chap. 17, Fig. 17–10). The earlier bone marrow precursor cells cannot be recognized morphologically, but can be enriched by flow cytometry using fluorescent markers to antigens that are expressed selectively on their surface such as CD34 (Doulatov et al, 2010). The hematopoietic stem cell may undergo self-renewal or may produce progeny that are early precursor cells, which proliferate and differentiate to produce cells of the granulocyte (G), erythroid (E), megakaryocyte (Meg), monocyte (M), and lymphoid (L) lineages (see Chap. 17, Fig. 17–10). Older thymidine-labeling studies demonstrated a very high rate of cell proliferation among recognizable precursors of granulocytes and red cells; these are among the most rapidly proliferating cells in the human body, with a mean duration of T_s and T_c of approximately 12 and 24 hours, respectively. The more mature cells in each series undergo differentiation without proliferation. Stem cells and other early precursor cells proliferate quite slowly under resting conditions, but may proliferate rapidly to restore the bone marrow population following depletion of more mature functional cells (eg, by cancer chemotherapy) or after bone marrow ablation and transplantation.

The pattern of proliferation and differentiation in the bone marrow provides an explanation for the decrease in mature granulocytes at 10 to 14 days after cycle-active chemotherapy and their recovery by 21 to 28 days (see Chap. 17, Fig. 17–10).

The rapidly proliferating intermediate precursor cells are most likely to be killed by chemotherapy. Effects on granulocytes and other normal cells in the peripheral blood are not seen immediately because the later maturing cells are nonproliferating. Recovery of the bone marrow occurs when earlier precursors are stimulated to proliferate, following release of growth factors that follows loss of the mature functional cells.

The growth factors that stimulate hemopoietic precursor cells to proliferate and differentiate into lineage-specific cells have been characterized, and several of them are now produced by recombinant techniques for clinical use. Granulocyte colony-stimulating factor (G-CSF) stimulates early cells in the granulocyte series and is used widely to decrease the duration and extent of myelosuppression after chemotherapy, and hence to lower the incidence of infection and hospitalization. Erythropoietin is produced by the kidney to stimulate erythroid cell precursors; recombinant erythropoietin and molecules derived from it (erythroid-stimulating factors) are used to treat anemia and accompanying fatigue, and to decrease the need for blood transfusion, but can be associated with increased blood clotting. Thrombopoietin stimulates the maturation of megakaryocytes and production of platelets to guard against bleeding. Clinical trials have been undertaken with recombinant thrombopoietin and derived agents in attempts to treat primary thrombocytopenia and to prevent thrombocytopenia (ie, a low platelet count and consequent bleeding) following chemotherapy, but the presence of neutralizing antibodies and other problems have limited their clinical utility (Vadhan-Raj, 2010).

12.1.3.2 Intestine

The functional part of the small intestine consists of numerous villi that project into the lumen and provide a large absorptive surface (Fig. 12–4). The villi are lined by a single layer of differentiated epithelial cells that do not proliferate, and apoptotic cell death (see Chap. 9, Sec. 9.4) and shedding of cells into the lumen occur at the top of the villi. These cells are replaced by upward migration of cells lining crypts, which lie between and at the base of the villi. There is a high rate of cell proliferation in the crypts of the intestine, but proliferation of cells at the base of the crypts occurs more slowly (Fig. 12–4) and some of these cells act as progenitors or intestinal stem cells for the entire crypt and surrounding villi. Analogous to bone marrow, proliferation of stem cells in the crypts is influenced by paracrine and autocrine signaling factors (Walters, 2005). Some cycle-dependent drugs and radiation may cause severe mucosal damage to the intestine, resulting in diarrhea and/or intestinal bleeding, although this toxicity is less often dose-limiting for anticancer drugs than toxicity to the bone marrow.

12.1.4 Cell Proliferation in Tumors

Typical values for the percent of S-phase cells (labeling index) are in the range of 3% to 15% for many types of human solid tumors, but higher values are evident in faster-growing malignancies, including acute leukemia and some lymphomas.

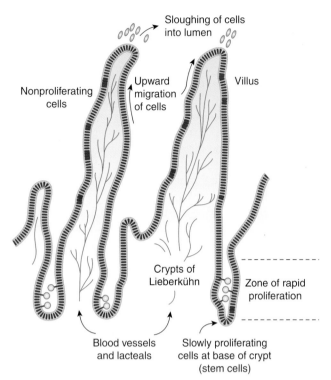

Sloughing of cells
into lumen

Nonproliferating
cells

Upward
migration
of cells

Villus

Crypts of
Lieberkühn

Zone of rapid
proliferation

Blood vessels
and lacteals

Slowly proliferating
cells at base of crypt
(stem cells)

FIGURE 12–4 Model for cell proliferation and migration in the small intestine. Slowly proliferating cells in the bases of the crypts probably act as stem cells for the entire cell population. Other cells in the lower two-thirds of the crypts proliferate rapidly, with nuclei of mitotic cells visible in the lumens of the crypts. Cells migrate up the villi to replace those sloughed into the lumen.

However, the rate of cell proliferation is usually less than that of some cells in normal renewing tissues such as the intestine or bone marrow. Thus, growth of tumors is not simply the result of an increased rate of cell proliferation as compared to the normal tissue of origin. Rather, there is defective maturation and the population of malignant cells increases because the rate of cell production exceeds the rate of cell death or removal (loss) from the population.

Information about the duration of the cell cycle and of its constituent phases in human tumors is available from a few early studies in which ^{3}H-thymidine was injected into patients and where serial biopsies allowed the generation of a PLM curve. A larger number of estimates of the duration of T_s and of T_{pot} have been derived after injection of BrdUrd, followed by a tumor biopsy and analysis by flow cytometry. The distributions of these estimates tend to be lognormally distributed but mrsn values for T_s tend to be in the range of 12 to 24 hours. Typical values of mean T_c are in the range of 2 to 3 days, but this estimate is subject to uncertainty because the distribution of cell-cycle times is broad, and the techniques used to measure it tend to give information about the faster proliferating cells in the population. Estimates of the T_{pot} range from approximately 4.5 to approximately 20 days, and are much longer than estimates of mean T_c, implying that many human tumors have a low growth fraction. If some of the slowly proliferating or nonproliferating cells in

human tumors retain the properties of a tumor stem cell (ie, they can repopulate the tumor if stimulated to divide; see Chap. 13, Sec. 13.4), a low growth fraction may be a factor that contributes to the relative resistance of human tumors to cycle-active chemotherapy. Estimates of mean values of T_{pot} are, in turn, much lower than estimates of V_D for common human tumors (typically 2 to 3 months; see Table 12–1). It follows that the rate of cell loss in many human tumors is in the range of 75% to 90% of the rate of cell production.

Studies of human and animal tumors demonstrate considerable heterogeneity in labeling and mitotic indices within different parts of the same tumor or its metastases. Factors that may contributes to this heterogeneity include differentiation, as there is often an inverse relationship between differentiation and proliferative rate, the presence of genetically distinct clones of cells in a mature tumor (Marusyk et al, 2012), and variability in nutrient availability within the tumor microenvironment (see Sec. 12.2; see also Chap. 13, Sec. 13.2). Necrosis occurs commonly in solid tumors, and orderly structures ("tumor cords") can sometimes be observed in which a tumor blood vessel and tumor necrosis are separated by a distance that in humans is commonly about 150 to 200 μm. This is estimated to be the approximate distance oxygen can diffuse in tissue before being completely metabolized by the cells in the tissue (Figs. 12–5 and 12–6; Thomlinson and Gray, 1955). The presence of such structures facilitated older studies of cell proliferation in relation to the blood supply. This relationship can now be evaluated by quantifying the proportion of Ki-67– or BrdUrd-labeled–positive cells in relation to blood vessels, recognized by an antibody to CD31, which is expressed on endothelial cells, using computer techniques and immunohistochemistry (Huxham et al, 2004). Not surprisingly, well-nourished tumor cells close to blood vessels have higher levels of rapidly proliferating cells than poorly nourished cells close to a region of necrosis (see Figs. 12–5 and 12–6; eg, Tannock, 1970; Huxham et al, 2004). The presence of slowly proliferating cells at a distance from functional blood vessels has implications for tumor therapy: Such cells may be resistant to radiation because of hypoxia (see Sec. 12.2.1 and Chap. 16, Sec. 16.4), and to anticancer drugs because of their low proliferative rate (see Chap. 17, Sec. 17.5) and limited drug access (see Chap. 19, Sec. 19.3.3). This is a major concern if such cells are also more likely to be tumor stem cells (see Chap. 13, Sec. 13.4).

Because cell proliferation and cell death in tumors depend on a supply of nutrients through the vasculature, the rate of tumor growth is likely to depend on the rate of expansion of functional tumor blood vessels by angiogenesis (see Chap. 11, Sec. 11.5). In experimental animals, the proliferation rate of capillary endothelial cells appears to be slower than that of surrounding tumor cells (Denekamp and Hobson, 1982), which may lead to decreasing tumor vasculature and slowing of growth in larger tumors.

Renewal tissues such as bone marrow and intestinal mucosa represent a hierarchy of cells produced by cell division and differentiation from a small number of stem cells (see

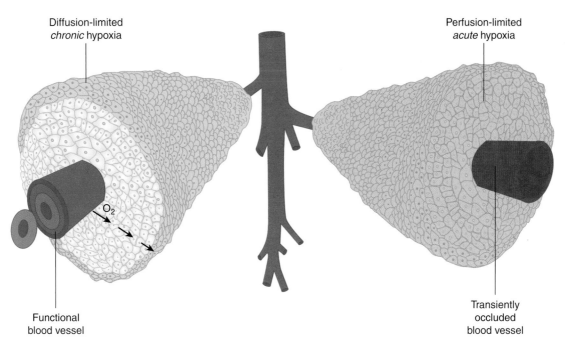

Diffusion-limited
chronic hypoxia

Perfusion-limited
acute hypoxia

O₂

Functional
blood vessel

Transiently
occluded
blood vessel

FIGURE 12–5 **Mechanisms leading to hypoxia in solid tumors.** *Left:* Oxygen metabolism (consumption) results in the establishment of oxygen gradients around isolated perfused vessels. Oxygenation values range from 4% to 5% near the vessel wall to complete anoxia. *Right:* Changes in blood perfusion, including complete vessel occlusion, result in acute changes in oxygenation in large numbers of tumor cells.

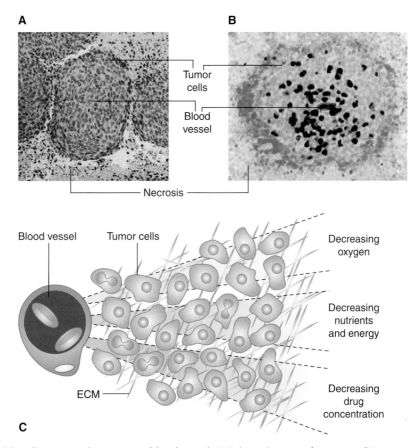

A

B

Tumor
cells

Blood
vessel

Necrosis

Blood vessel   Tumor cells

Decreasing
oxygen

Decreasing
nutrients
and energy

ECM

Decreasing
drug
concentration

C

FIGURE 12–6 **A) Viable cells surrounding a tumor blood vessel. B)** Relation between frequency of Ki-67–positive (black) proliferating cells and distance from tumor blood vessels recognized by an antibody to CD31 in an experimental tumor. **C)** Diffusion gradients of oxygen and other metabolites in solid tumors. (Reproduced from Minchinton and Tannock, 2006, with permission.)

Sec. 12.1.3). Most tumors arise in renewal tissues, and there is substantial evidence that many tumors are (a) clonal, in that all of the tumor cells express a common genetic marker (Fearon et al, 1987; Fialkow, 1974), and (b) contain a limited population of stem cells with the capacity to regenerate the tumor after treatment (see Chap. 13, Sec. 13.4). Other cells in the tumor population may have lost the capacity for cell proliferation (eg, through differentiation) or have only limited potential for cell proliferation (analogous to morphologically recognizable precursor cells in bone marrow, such as myelocytes). Proliferative potential and proliferative rate are quite different, and tumor cells with stem cell properties might be proliferating rather slowly, similar to stem cells in bone marrow or at the base of the intestinal crypts (see Sec. 12.1.3).

12.1.5 Cell Proliferation and Prognosis

The relationship between proliferative parameters and response to treatment with chemotherapy is complex. There may be a higher chance of response to chemotherapy in malignancies with a high proportion of proliferating cells, although intrinsic drug sensitivity of the cells is likely to be the major determinant of response. In contrast, malignancies with a high proportion of proliferating cells grow more rapidly both in the absence of effective treatment and during regrowth after partially effective therapy. A further confounding factor arises because analysis of DNA distributions does not provide information about the proliferative status of the cells that are able to regenerate the tumor, the putative tumor stem cells.

A technique for dissolving paraffin, followed by dispersion and staining of the cells, has allowed flow cytometry to be applied to the study of fixed tissue that is stored in paraffin blocks. Provided that attention is paid to quality control, this technique can provide a useful retrospective analysis of the relationship between kinetic parameters of human tumors and the subsequent outcome of the patients (Hedley et al, 1993).

Multiple studies of the relationship between cell-cycle parameters and outcome for several types of tumor have been done. In many studies, both DNA index (ie, the DNA content of G_1 tumor cells relative to that of normal cells) and S-phase fraction give prognostic information that is additional to the traditional prognostic factors of tumor stage and grade. In general, aneuploid tumors have a poorer prognosis than diploid tumors, and tumors with a higher proportion of proliferating cells have a poorer prognosis than tumors with a lower proportion of proliferating cells (eg, Hedley et al, 1993). The expression within tumors of cyclins, cyclin-dependent kinases (CDKs) and their inhibitors (see Chap. 9, Sec. 9.2.3) have also been reported to influence outcome, with the general, but not universal, finding that upregulation of positive regulators of the cell cycle (ie, cyclins and CDKs) are associated with poorer outcome, whereas upregulation of inhibitors is associated with better outcome (eg, Tsilhias et al, 1999; Keyomarsi et al, 2002).

12.2 TUMOR MICROENVIRONMENT

The microenvironment of solid human tumors is unlike that of normal tissues, as it is characterized by extreme heterogeneity in availability of oxygen and other nutrients, in patterns of metabolism, and in pH. The loss of normal homeostatic mechanisms uncouples cellular proliferation from growth signals and as a consequence, areas within the tumor become deficient in oxygen and other nutrients.

12.2.1 Hypoxia and Its Biological and Therapeutic Relevance

Oxygen is particularly important in solid tumors given its ability to influence metabolism, gene expression, and response to therapy. Oxygen is supplied through the vasculature, and is metabolized in the mitochondria by respiring cells, where it serves as a terminal electron acceptor during oxidative phosphorylation. The consumption of oxygen in this process establishes the oxygen demand of a given tissue, and in most tissues this demand is adequately met by the supply of oxygen through the local vasculature. The oxygen concentration of most normal tissues is maintained at around 50 to 70 μM, which is the equivalent of exposure to 5% to 7% O_2 in the gas phase or a partial pressure (pO_2) of 40 to 50 mm Hg. Note that even for normal tissues, this level of oxygenation is considerably lower than that in the normal atmosphere (~21% O_2). In various physiological and pathological situations, the oxygen concentration can fall, and when it drops to levels equivalent to 3% or below, cells within the tissue will activate oxygen-sensitive signaling pathways to allow adaptation of the cell and the tissue to oxygen deprivation. In tumors, the vasculature is often insufficient to meet the oxygen demand of rapidly proliferating cells, giving rise to oxygen gradients surrounding isolated tumor vessels. Estimates of the oxygen diffusion distance from an individual vessel range from 75 to 200 μm depending on the respiration rate (oxygen consumption rate) of the cells within the tissue in question and the equivalent pO_2 of the blood.

Hypoxia occurs when the oxygen demand exceeds oxygen supply. In tumors, this situation arises through 2 mechanisms, both of which are linked to the abnormal vasculature that characterizes many tumors. In the first mechanism, the rapid proliferation of tumor cells coupled with their reduced ability to suppress proliferation when nutrients are limiting leads to a situation of nonequilibrium in which the developing vasculature is unable to keep pace with the requirements of the expanding tumor. The lack of sufficient blood vessels creates gradients of oxygen around vessels, and at distances greater than approximately 100 μm gives rise to diffusion limited or "chronic" hypoxia (see Fig. 12–5). Similar gradients in other vascular-supplied molecules that are metabolized as they diffuse through tissue, including chemotherapeutic agents, will also occur. Chronic hypoxia can also arise in nonvascularized tumor nodules, again at distances dictated by the oxygen consumption rate. Chronic hypoxia was hypothesized to exist in tumors as early as 1955 by Thomlinson and Gray (1955) based on histological examination of human tumors. These authors noted that tissue necrosis was often observed at distances from vasculature consistent with the oxygen diffusion distance.

A second mechanism for development of tumor hypoxia occurs through transient changes in blood perfusion within tumor vasculature (see Figs. 12–5 and 12–6). Tumor vessels are often immature, leaky, lack smooth muscle cells, and have structural abnormalities, including blind ends and arterial–venous shunts that together result in unstable blood flow (see Chap. 11, Sec. 11.5 and Fig. 11–9); this can lead to "acute" or "perfusion-limited" hypoxia (Dewhirst et al, 2008; Pries et al, 2010). Regional tumor oxygenation can vary because of transient changes in blood flow that occur over periods ranging from 15 minutes to several hours. Complete vessel occlusion can result in rapid induction of hypoxia in all of the tumor cells that depend on that particular vessel for oxygen supply. As discussed below, the consequences of these 2 different mechanisms for generation of hypoxic cells in tumors can be very different from the perspective of both biology and therapy.

There is substantial heterogeneity of oxygenation and other microenvironmental factors in human cancer. This heterogeneity, although expected given the known causes of hypoxia, was only fully recognized when techniques became available to measure oxygenation in human tumors with needle electrodes and with exogenously administered markers of hypoxia that could be detected by immunohistochemistry (see also Chap. 16, Sec. 16.4.3). The spatial patterns of oxygen depend on both the distribution and functionality of the tumor blood vessels. A common misconception is that hypoxia is found primarily at the "core" of large solid tumors. Immunohistochemical studies from both animal and human tumors have confirmed that hypoxia can exist around any perfused vessel in a tumor (Fig. 12–7) (Kaanders et al, 2002). Also, there is at most a weak correlation between the degree of hypoxia and tumor size. Rather, regional variations in the levels of hypoxia are observed within tumors, reflecting regional differences in microvessel density and/or function. Because of the steep gradients in oxygen around perfused vessels, the equivalent oxygen concentration can fall from perivascular levels of approximately 5% to complete anoxia over only about 150 μm or about 10 cell diameters.

The spatial heterogeneity in oxygen levels has implications for its assessment in patients. Immunohistochemistry is the only method that provides an assessment of oxygenation at the cellular level. Single biopsies will not necessarily reflect the overall oxygenation of the tumor, and multiple samples from various parts of the tumor will be necessary to estimate the overall level of hypoxia and its variation. Other techniques, including oxygen needle electrodes and imaging of hypoxia with positron emission tomography (PET) tracers (see Chap. 14, Sec. 14.3.3), may provide a more global view of hypoxia, but measurements are regional averages of oxygenation over a defined volume within which the cellular oxygen concentration can vary from normal to complete anoxia. Needle electrodes are inserted and measurements taken as the

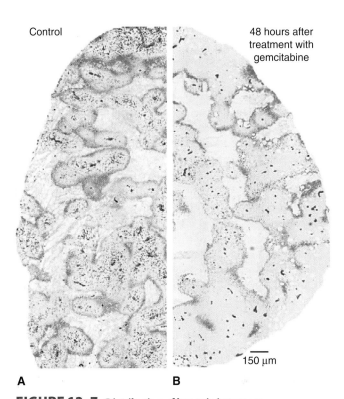

FIGURE 12–7 Distribution of hypoxia in tumors.
The heterogeneous distribution of hypoxia is revealed in tumor xenografts using pimonidazole immunohistochemistry. These figures illustrate the concept that hypoxia is heterogeneously distributed throughout the tumor and can potentially be found around any vessel. (Reproduced from Minchinton and Tannock, 2006, with permission.)

needle moves along a track through the tumor. Multiple tracks provide a frequency histogram of oxygen values (see Chap. 16, Fig. 16–12) that can reflect the overall distribution of oxygen values, but each measurement represents an average oxygen concentration over the sampling volume.

Spatial heterogeneity impacts on the biological and therapeutic consequences associated with hypoxia. For example, as discussed below, hypoxia is associated with an increased likelihood of distant metastasis. The ability of hypoxic cells to enter the circulation is likely to be much higher in regions of acute hypoxia, which can occur near blood vessels, than for chronic hypoxia. Indeed, laboratory data indicate that exposure to transient hypoxia promotes distant metastasis (see Chap. 10, Sec. 10.5.7; Chaudary and Hill, 2007). For chemotherapy, hypoxic cells are often found in regions where it is difficult to deliver therapeutic drugs effectively (see Chap. 19, Sec. 19.3.3).

Gradients surrounding isolated vessels result in oxygen concentrations that range from normal to complete anoxia. Complete anoxia is also expected to arise quickly in tumor cells surrounding temporarily occluded vessels, whereas partial vessel occlusion or a reduction in blood flow will result in a reduced oxygen concentration around the affected vessel and thus an acute drop in concentration across the entire gradient. Direct oxygen electrode and immunohistochemical studies in both animal and human tumors confirm the presence of cells at all possible oxygen concentrations. Hypoxic cells are resistant to radiation therapy (see Chap. 16, Sec. 16.4.1), but the oxygen sensitivity for this effect is significantly different from that for activation of hypoxia-inducible factor (HIF) transcription factors (discussed below) and for induction of changes in metabolism and angiogenesis. Therefore, the level of hypoxia and the fraction of hypoxic cells that is relevant depend upon the end point being considered.

The oxygen concentration in tumors also changes with time. Even when oxygen gradients around perfused vessels are stable, cellular proliferation results in movement of cells through this gradient. In rapidly proliferating mouse tumors, it has been estimated that a cell could be displaced by newly formed cells from a well-oxygenated region near the vessel to an anoxic region on the border of necrosis within 100 hours (4 to 5 doubling times). In human tumor xenografts, hypoxic cells can remain viable for up to 10 days (Durand and Sham, 1998), although this is likely to vary amongst different tumors. Thus, in addition to proliferation rates, the proportion of viable cells at low oxygenation concentration is influenced by the tolerance of the tumor cells to hypoxia. A rapid rate of proliferation coupled with high tolerance to hypoxia would be expected to produce tumors with large regions of chronic hypoxia, a feature that has been correlated with poor prognosis in patients. The contribution of changes in blood perfusion to overall levels of hypoxia also varies amongst different tumors and in some tumors accounts for a large proportion of the hypoxic cells at any given time (Durand and Aquino-Parsons, 2001). Fluctuations in regional blood flow and oxygen concentration occur over periods of approximately 30 minutes to 2 hours (Cardenas-Navia et al, 2004), and can result in periodic cycling between different oxygen concentrations. The rapid changes in oxygenation associated with perfusion-limited hypoxia present an additional challenge associated with attempts to measure oxygenation in patient tumors.

Tumor biology and response to treatment are strongly influenced by the duration of exposure to hypoxia. Transient exposures to anoxia may be better tolerated than more prolonged exposures arising at the ends of oxygen gradients at the border with necrosis. Adaptive mechanisms occur during the slow transition to longer periods of chronic hypoxia within oxygen gradients and these may have a stronger effect on gene expression and create different biological effects than the transient stress induced by acute hypoxia. Changes in oxygenation over time are also thought to be important mechanisms that can improve therapeutic outcome when treatment is delivered over longer periods of time. For example, hypoxic cells are resistant to radiotherapy (see Chap. 16, Sec. 16.4.1) and may also be resistant to many forms of chemotherapy because of poor drug distribution and through secondary effects that reduce their proliferation (see Chap. 19, Sec. 19.3.2). Thus, after a single dose of either treatment, the hypoxic cells have a selective survival advantage and the overall proportion of viable hypoxic cells in the tumor will increase. However, when treatment is fractionated over time, reoxygenation of previously hypoxic cells between treatments may result in the

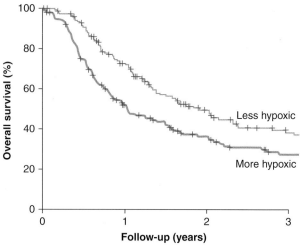

FIGURE 12–8 Hypoxia and patient outcome. A metaanalysis of oxygen electrode measurements made in head and neck cancer across several centers demonstrates an independent prognostic role for hypoxia and poor response to radiotherapy (from Nordsmark et al, 2006). This may be a result of the intrinsic resistance of hypoxic cells to radiation (the "oxygen effect"), and/or as a consequence of biological changes that occur as a result of hypoxia that promote malignancy.

proportion of viable hypoxic cells being reduced to levels more typical of that before treatment. Although reoxygenation may allow the tumor to be more responsive to fractionated treatments (see Chap. 16, Sec. 16.6.4), this process may paradoxically also "rescue" previously hypoxic tumor cells that would have died in the absence of treatment.

Given the heterogeneity in space, time, and severity of levels of hypoxia, it is difficult to ascribe a single value to characterize the hypoxic status of a given tumor. For clinical studies with oxygen electrodes, investigators have defined the level of hypoxia as the proportion of readings below a defined pO_2 value—typically 2.5, 5, or 10 mm Hg. Defined in this way, the hypoxic fraction of individual tumors can range from 0% to 100%. For immunohistochemical studies with hypoxic markers, the hypoxic fraction is usually determined as the proportion of cells (or tissue area) with a staining intensity above an arbitrary threshold. Even when defined in this suboptimal way, these approaches have provided insights into the impact of hypoxia on patient outcome. Figure 12-8 demonstrates results from the meta-analysis of 397 head and neck patients from 7 institutions who had oxygen measurements taken prior to treatment with radiotherapy (Nordsmark et al, 2006; see also Chap. 16, Fig. 16–12). This analysis indicates that pretreatment tumor oxygenation status is a significant determinant of outcome, with high levels of hypoxia predicting poor prognosis.

12.2.2 Hypoxia and the Malignant Phenotype

The association of hypoxia with poor clinical outcome is not limited to treatment with radiotherapy; measurements of hypoxia can provide prognostic value independent of treatment modality, even for patients treated with surgery alone where there is no "intrinsic" resistance of hypoxic cells (Hockel et al, 1996). Numerous laboratory and clinical observations suggest that the prognostic value of hypoxia is associated not only with its ability to mediate resistance to therapy, but also with increased malignancy. For example, several clinical studies have found an association between hypoxia and metastases (Hockel et al, 1996; Airley et al, 2001) and hypoxia is prognostic of overall survival in cervix cancer (Fyles et al, 2006). Several independent animal model systems have demonstrated that exposure to transient acute hypoxia can promote metastasis (see Chap. 10, Sec. 10.5.7; Chaudary and Hill, 2007). Together, these findings suggest that the biological changes associated with hypoxia in human tumors are associated with a more aggressive phenotype (Harris, 2002).

At least 3 mechanisms may contribute to the association of hypoxia and increased malignancy. The first is through hypoxia-mediated selection of cells with mutations that confer both tolerance to hypoxia and increased aggressiveness. For example, p53 promotes hypoxia-induced cell death, and loss or mutation of p53 can lead to both increased levels of viable hypoxic cells, along with other aggressive phenotypes linked to loss of this tumor-suppressor protein (see Chap. 7, Sec. 7.6.2). Secondly, there are links between hypoxia and genomic instability (Bristow and Hill, 2008). Hypoxia can suppress the expression of genes involved in several DNA repair pathways including base excision repair (BER), mismatch repair (MMR), and double-stranded break (DSB) repair (see Chap. 5, Sec. 5.3). As a result, tumor hypoxia provides an environment to not only select cells with specific mutations, but one that may also directly promote mutation. Development of mutations may be further exacerbated in cells exposed to transient hypoxia, since reoxygenation is associated with the production of reactive oxygen species (ROS) that create DNA damage. A third proposed mechanism stems from changes in oxygen-sensitive signaling pathways, including those designed specifically for adaptation to hypoxic stress. These pathways constitute important physiological mechanisms mediating response to stress, but in tumors can promote adverse changes that affect cellular metabolism, angiogenesis, cell survival, and metastasis.

12.2.3 Sensing and Responding to Hypoxia

12.2.3.1 Hypoxia-Inducible Factor
HIF is an essential transcription factor that regulates numerous cellular and tissue adaptive responses during hypoxia (Fig. 12–9A). It is a heterodimer composed of an oxygen-labile α-subunit (HIF-1α, HIF-2α), and a constitutively expressed HIF-1β subunit. In the presence of oxygen, the α-subunit is ubiquitinated by the von Hippel-Lindau (VHL) protein and targeted for degradation (see Chap. 8, Fig. 8–9 and Chap. 9, Fig. 9–4; Ivan et al, 2001; Jaakkola et al, 2001). Degradation requires hydroxylation of 2 proline residues (P402 and P564 in

HIF-1α), which is carried out by 1 of 3 known HIF prolyl hydroxylases (PHD1 to -3). These enzymes require oxygen as a cofactor, and thus function as oxygen-sensing molecules (Epstein et al, 2001). During hypoxia, the PHD enzymes are unable to hydroxylate HIF-1α, resulting in its stabilization and formation of an active HIF heterodimer that is capable of inducing up to 200 different genes (Harris, 2002; Semenza, 2003). In addition to destabilizing HIF-1α, oxygen concentration also regulates its transcriptional activity. In the presence of oxygen, the factor inhibiting HIF (FIH) promotes hydroxylation of an asparagine residue in the transcription activation domain, which prevents its association with other proteins important for transcriptional activity. Genes regulated by HIF include those that promote metabolic adaptation at the cellular level through regulation of glucose uptake, glycolysis, and oxidative phosphorylation (Table 12–3). HIF also stimulates tumor angiogenesis through its ability to regulate genes such as vascular endothelial growth factor (VEGF; see Chap. 11, Sec. 11.4.1). HIF activation may also account for a component of the increased metastatic capacity of hypoxic cells through induction of genes such as *LOX*, VEGF-C, *Met*, and *CXCR4* (see Chap. 10, Sec. 10.5.7; Pennacchietti et al, 2003; Staller et al, 2003; Erler et al, 2006; Chaudary et al, 2011).

HIF activation occurs during normal physiological processes and is sensitive to relatively mild tissue hypoxia, below approximately 2% oxygen, levels much higher than needed to cause substantial resistance to radiation. Thus, the proportion of HIF-expressing cells in tumors is expected to be greater than the fraction of radiation-resistant cells. This difference also influences comparisons of direct measurements of tumor hypoxia with those inferred from so-called endogenous markers of hypoxia. HIF-target genes such as carbonic anhydrase 9 (CA9) and glucose transporter 1 (GLUT-1) have been used as markers in immunohistochemical studies to evaluate tumor hypoxia, but have limited correlation with other direct measures of oxygenation. This is further complicated because HIF is also regulated by oxygen-independent mechanisms. The most extreme example occurs in renal cell carcinoma, where loss of the VHL protein leads to constitutive activation of HIF. Oncogene activation can also lead to increased synthesis and activity of HIF independent of hypoxia.

Laboratory experiments with cells and animal tumor models have suggested that targeting HIF might be an effective therapeutic strategy. However, despite numerous attempts it has been difficult to develop drugs that are specific inhibitors of HIF. Most drug development has focused on targeting pathways downstream of HIF, such as VEGF, or enzymes such as CA9, which regulate tumor pH in response to hypoxia.

12.2.3.2 Unfolded Protein Response
The endoplasmic reticulum (ER) is a specialized organelle where membrane-based and secreted proteins are folded and glycosylated. A disruption in ER homeostasis or an increase in protein flux through the ER can lead to the accumulation of unfolded proteins and activation of the unfolded protein response (UPR;

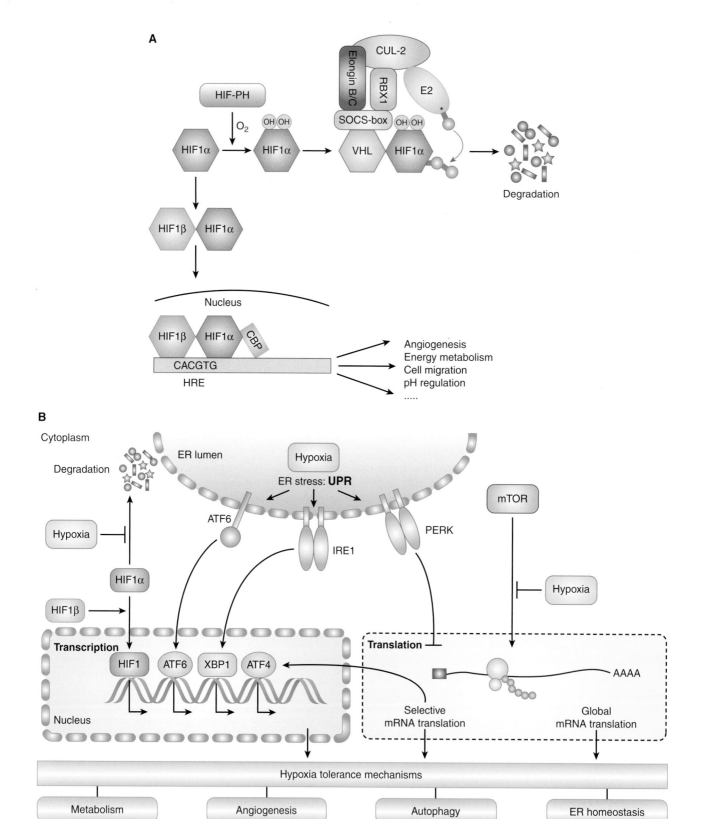

FIGURE 12–9 **A) HIF activity is regulated by oxygen.** HIF1α is hydroxylated on 2 proline residues in an oxygen-dependent reaction by 1 of the 3 HIF prolyl hydroxylases (HIF-PH enzymes). Hydroxylation leads to its recognition by the von Hippel-Lindau (VHL) protein, which subsequently mediates its ubiquitination by the Elongin B/C-CUL2-RBX1 complex and an E2 ubiquitin ligase. Ubiquitinated HIF-1α is then degraded in the proteasome. In the absence of oxygen, HIF-1α forms a heterodimer with HIF1β, which then moves into the nucleus and activates genes (together with CBP) that contain a HIF consensus-binding sequence in their promoter. These genes promote numerous biological changes that promote change in metabolism and angiogenesis. **B) Cell signaling in response to hypoxia.** Hypoxia results in the activation of HIF and the unfolded protein response (UPR), as well as inhibition of mammalian target of rapamycin (mTOR). These distinct oxygen-sensitive signaling pathways promote adaption to hypoxic stress through a multitude of downstream effectors that influence cellular metabolism, autophagy, endoplasmic reticulum (ER) stress, and angiogenesis. The UPR consists of 3 signaling arms initiated by PERK, IRE1 and ATF6. Each of these arms results in the activation of a different transcription factor (ATF4, XBP1, and ATF6), which collectively function to prevent and mitigate the consequences of ER stress. These 3 pathways can also influence cellular phenotypes in ways that promote malignancy through increased invasion and metastasis.

TABLE 12–3 Important pathways and genes controlled by HIF.

Pathway	Examples of HIF Target Genes
Metabolism	*Glut-1, Gapdh, PDK1, CA9, Mt-4, Ldh-A*
Angiogenesis	*Vegf, Pdgf, Flt-1*
Metastasis	*CXCL12(Sdf-1), Lox-1, Cxcr-4, c-Met*

see Fig. 12–9*B*). The UPR is mediated by 3 distinct ER stress sensors: PERK (PKR-like ER kinase), inositol-requiring protein-1 (IRE-1), and activating transcription factor-6(ATF6). All 3 of these sensors are activated rapidly during severe hypoxia (<0.2% equivalent) as a consequence of an unexplained disruption in protein folding. During hypoxia, PERK phosphorylates and inactivates eIF2α, leading to a block in new protein synthesis (Koumenis et al, 2002). PERK activation also leads to selected synthesis of the ATF4 transcription factor and downstream activation of genes involved in adaptation to ER stress. IRE-1 and ATF6 activation result in additional transcriptional responses that support both adaptation and recovery from ER stress. The activation of the UPR occurs within minutes of hypoxic exposure and is important for adaptation and cell survival. Defects in the PERK and IRE-1 signaling pathways result in increased cell death during hypoxia and prevent or slow tumor growth in animal models, indicating their importance for cellular adaptation to hypoxia (Wouters and Koritzinsky, 2008).

UPR activation has been observed in human tumors and is associated with poor disease-free survival, possibly reflecting the presence of hypoxia (Davies et al, 2008). UPR-dependent genes, such as *ATF4,* are also known to be overexpressed in cancer, primarily in hypoxic perinecrotic regions of human tumors (Ameri et al, 2004). Several downstream pathways are likely to contribute to the importance of the UPR in hypoxic cells. Because protein synthesis is a large consumer of cellular energy, its suppression via PERK may assist in maintaining energy homeostasis (Kraggerud et al, 1995). PERK activation also has been shown to promote survival by promoting transcriptional changes in CA9 that regulates tumor pH and by promoting autophagy, a process in which cells capture and degrade components of their own cytoplasm to sustain survival during times of starvation (see Sec. 12.3.7; Rouschop et al, 2010).

12.2.3.3 Mammalian Target of Rapamycin The mammalian target of rapamycin (mTOR) kinase acts as a central regulator of cellular metabolism by integrating upstream signaling pathways that monitor growth factors, energy, and nutrients, and coupling them to regulation of protein synthesis, ribosomal biogenesis, autophagy, and metabolism (Guertin and Sabatini, 2007; see Figs. 12–9*B* and 12–10). Many oncogenes and tumor suppressors function in pathways whose activation in cancer results in hyperactive mTOR signaling.

Hypoxia, in contrast, inhibits mTOR signaling through multiple pathways both upstream and downstream of the kinase, particularly in concert with other stresses or when hypoxic conditions are chronic (Wouters and Koritzinsky, 2008). Cells that are genetically engineered to be unable to inhibit mTOR during hypoxia show reduced tolerance to hypoxia, and produce tumors with a smaller proportion of radioresistant hypoxic cells (Dubois et al, 2009).

Tumor cells exposed to severe hypoxic stress may inhibit mTOR as a means to reduce protein synthesis and energy expenditure, and thus promote cell survival. Inhibition of mTOR also promotes tolerance to hypoxia through mechanisms that involve changes in apoptosis and/or autophagy (Erler et al, 2004). Inhibition of mTOR stimulates autophagy, which can assist in maintaining essential metabolism in nutrient- and oxygen-deprived cells (see Sec. 12.3.7). Consistent with this, autophagy has been observed in poorly vascularized xenografts (Degenhardt et al, 2006), as well as in animal models of the ischemic brain (Adhami et al, 2006) and myocardium (Yan et al, 2005). Finally, although inhibition of mTOR leads to an overall reduction in protein synthesis, certain classes of genes are able to bypass this inhibition and become selectively translated. This so-called cap-independent translation affects several important genes, including both HIF-1α and VEGF (Richter and Sonenberg, 2005). This effect has also been shown to facilitate tumor growth in locally advanced breast cancers (Braunstein et al, 2007).

New drugs that inhibit mTOR (eg, temsirolimus and everolimus) have been approved for specific anticancer indications. These agents are able to slow proliferation by reducing mTOR activity and inhibit overall metabolic activity. However, given that inhibition of mTOR also promotes tolerance to hypoxia, these agents could result in an increase in the proportion of viable hypoxic cells and as a consequence reduce the effectiveness of other therapies (Weppler et al, 2007).

12.2.4 Heterogeneity in Tumor pH and Interstitial Fluid Pressure

12.2.4.1 Tumor pH The abnormal structure and function of the vasculature causes abnormal and highly heterogeneous biochemical conditions in the tumor microenvironment in addition to affecting tumor oxygenation. As a result of an imbalance in the production and elimination of metabolic acids such as lactic and carbonic acid, extracellular pH levels in solid tumors are often acidic relative to normal tissues (Yamagata et al, 1998). However, adaptive responses mediated by membrane transport proteins and carbonic anhydrase enzymes allow maintenance of normal or even elevated intracellular pH (Parks et al, 2011). Experimental models suggest that like hypoxia, acidic extracellular conditions contribute to the malignant phenotype by increasing tumor invasiveness and metastasis. Although there is not yet a complete understanding of the mechanisms responsible for pH regulation in tumor cells, strategies to target the adaptive response to acidic conditions are under

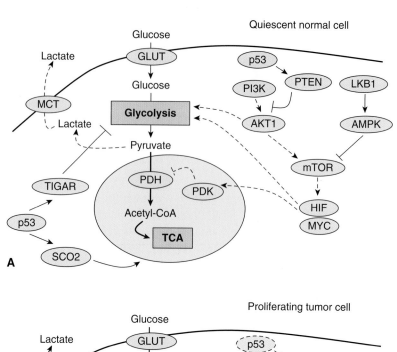

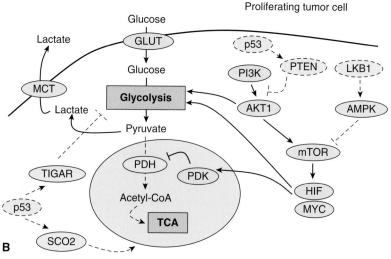

FIGURE 12-10 Molecular regulation of aerobic glycolysis. The shift to aerobic glycolysis in tumor cells (**B**) relative to normal cells (**A**) is driven by multiple oncogenic signaling pathways. Phosphatidylinositol-3 kinase (PI3K) activates the oncogenic kinase AKT, which stimulates glycolysis by directly regulating glycolytic enzymes and by activating the mammalian target of rapamycin (mTOR) kinase. The liver kinase B1 (LKB1) tumor suppressor, through adenosine monophosphate-activated protein kinase (AMPK) activation, opposes the glycolytic phenotype by inhibiting mTOR. mTOR alters metabolism in a variety of ways, but it has an effect on the glycolytic phenotype by enhancing HIF-1 activity, which engages a hypoxia adaptive transcriptional program. HIF-1 increases the expression of glucose transporters, glycolytic enzymes, and pyruvate dehydrogenase kinase, isozyme 1 (PDK1), which blocks entry of pyruvate into the tricarboxylic acid cycle (TCA) cycle. MYC cooperates with HIF in activating several glycolytic genes, but also increases mitochondrial metabolism. The tumor-suppressor p53 opposes the glycolytic phenotype by suppressing glycolysis via TP53-induced glycolysis and apoptosis regulator (TIGAR), increasing mitochondrial metabolism via cytochrome c oxidase assembly protein 2 (SCO2) and supporting expression of the phosphatase and tensin homolog (PTEN) tumor supressor. Solid lines represent more active pathways; dashed lines represent less active pathways. Pink protein labels indicate proteins whose function is commonly impaired in tumor cells.

investigation. The concentrations of critical nutrients are also altered in solid tumors. Measurements of glucose, glutamine and other metabolites reveal that spatial and temporal heterogeneity exists, as well as large intertumor variation. These conditions also require tumor cells to appropriately respond and adapt in order to continue to survive and proliferate.

12.2.4.2 Interstitial Fluid Pressure

A further abnormality encountered in the tumor microenvironment is elevated interstitial fluid pressure (IFP) (Fukumura and Jain, 2007). Tumors lack functional lymphatics, which results in a buildup of fluid in the extracellular space and increased IFP, especially when combined with an abnormal and leaky vasculature. This phenomenon has been measured in a variety of solid tumors, and predicts for poor outcome in some circumstances (Fyles et al, 2006). Impaired delivery of chemotherapeutic agents and altered levels of cytokines and growth factors are thought to be responsible for the reduced effects of treatment.

12.3 TUMOR METABOLISM

The abnormal conditions present in the tumor microenvironment play a major role in determining the metabolic phenotype of tumor cell (Lunt et al, 2009). The relationship between the tumor microenvironment and cellular metabolism is not one of simple cause-and-effect in which biochemical conditions in the tumor influence cellular metabolism. Because metabolite concentrations are governed by both supply via the vasculature and demand by the tissue (or vice versa), changes in metabolism of both the tumor and normal stromal cell have a profound effect on local microenvironmental conditions. Because of the dynamic nature of the tumor microenvironment, it is likely that the metabolic phenotype of tumor cells can change to adapt to the prevailing local conditions.

Critical phenotypes characteristic of tumor cells are caused by a series of mutational events that combine to alter multiple cellular signaling pathways affecting proliferation and survival. Thousands of point mutations, translocations, amplifications,

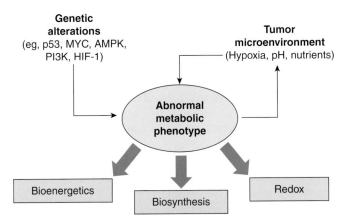

FIGURE 12–11 Determinants of the tumor metabolic phenotype. The metabolic phenotype of tumor cells is controlled by intrinsic genetic mutations and external responses to the tumor microenvironment. Oncogenic signaling pathways controlling growth and survival are often activated by loss of tumor suppressors (such as p53) or activation of oncogenes (such as PI3K). The resulting altered signaling modifies cellular metabolism to match the requirements of cell division. Abnormal microenvironmental conditions such as hypoxia, low pH, and/or nutrient deprivation elicit responses from tumor cells that further affect metabolic activity. These adaptations serve to optimize tumor cell metabolism for proliferation by providing appropriate levels of energy in the form of adenosine triphosphate (ATP), biosynthetic capacity, and maintenance of balanced reduction-oxidation (redox) status.

and deletions have been detected in cancer cells and the mutational spectrum can differ even among seemingly identical tumors. Bioinformatic analyses of large data sets have suggested that cancer-related driver mutations affect a dozen or more core signaling pathways and processes responsible for tumorigenesis, many of which are described in other chapters. Multiple molecular mechanisms, both intrinsic and extrinsic, converge to alter cellular metabolism to support growth and survival of the cancer cells. Furthermore, some of these metabolic alterations appear to be absolutely required for malignant transformation.

Genetic alterations to oncogenes and tumor suppressors (see Chap. 7) and the cellular response to extracellular microenvironmental conditions both contribute to the development of an abnormal metabolic phenotype. These metabolic alterations provide support for 3 of the most basic needs of dividing cells (Fig. 12–11):

- Rapid generation of energy in the form of adenosine triphosphate (ATP);
- Biosynthesis of the macromolecular building blocks required to generate daughter cells; and
- Maintenance of appropriate cellular reduction-oxidation (redox) status required to prevent excessive oxidative damage and to provide reducing power for anabolic enzymatic reactions.

To meet these needs, cancer cells acquire alterations to the metabolism of all 4 major classes of macromolecules:

carbohydrates, proteins, lipids, and nucleic acids. Many similar metabolic alterations are also observed in rapidly proliferating normal cells, where they represent appropriate responses to physiological growth signals (Newsholme et al, 1985; Vander Heiden et al, 2009). However, for cancer cells, these adaptations represent responses to the inappropriate growth and survival signals generated by acquired genetic mutations. Furthermore, these metabolic alterations must be implemented in a stressful and dynamic tumor microenvironment, where concentrations of critical nutrients and waste products, such as glucose, glutamine, oxygen, and lactate, are spatially and temporally heterogeneous (see Sec. 12.2).

12.3.1 Aerobic Glycolysis (The Warburg Effect)

In addition to the ATP required to maintain normal cellular homeostasis, proliferating tumor cells must also generate the energy required to support cell division. Furthermore, tumor cells must evade the checkpoint controls that would normally block proliferation under the stressful metabolic conditions characteristic of the abnormal tumor microenvironment. During the course of transformation and progression, these selective pressures result in a reprogramming of core metabolic pathways. The best characterized, and most universal metabolic phenotype observed in tumor cells is an increase in glycolysis. In this process, glucose is converted to lactate and secreted from the cell, rather than being completely oxidized to CO_2 via oxidative phosphorylation in the mitochondria (see Fig. 12–10). This is referred to as the Warburg effect, after Otto Warburg, who first described the phenomena (Warburg, 1956). This mode of glucose utilization and ATP production is similar to the Pasteur effect, which is the normal shift toward glycolytic ATP production that occurs during periods of oxygen limitation. However, the Warburg effect is observed in tumor cells even under normal oxygen concentrations (Warburg, 1956). As a result, unlike most normal cells, many transformed cells derive a substantial amount of their energy from aerobic glycolysis, converting the majority of incoming glucose into lactate rather than metabolizing it in the mitochondria via oxidative phosphorylation. Although ATP production by glycolysis can be more rapid than by oxidative phosphorylation, it is far less efficient in terms of ATP generated per molecule of glucose consumed. This shift therefore demands that tumor cells increase their rate of glucose uptake so as to meet their energy requirements.

Aerobic glycolysis is a common feature of many tumors, but there remains debate about the selective advantage that glycolytic metabolism provides to proliferating tumor cells. Initial work by Warburg and others focused on the concept that tumor cells develop defects in mitochondrial function, and that aerobic glycolysis was a necessary adaptation to cope with a decrease in ATP generation by oxidative phosphorylation. However, functional mitochondrial defects in tumors are relatively rare (Frezza and Gottlieb, 2009), and most tumor cells retain the capacity for oxidative phosphorylation and continue to consume oxygen at rates similar to those observed in normal tissues (Weinhouse, 1976). In fact, mitochondrial function is critical for transformation in some model tumor systems (Funes et al, 2007). Other explanations for the shift toward aerobic glycolysis include the concept that glycolysis has the capacity to generate ATP at a higher rate compared to oxidative phosphorylation, so it could be advantageous as long as glucose supplies are not limited. Alternatively, it has been proposed that glycolytic metabolism arises as an adaptation to the hypoxic conditions that develop during the early avascular phase of tumor growth, as it allows for ATP production and maintenance of bioenergetic homeostasis in the absence of oxygen. Adaptation to the resulting acidic microenvironment caused by excess lactate and carbonic acid production may further drive the evolution of the glycolytic phenotype (Gillies et al, 2008).

Another explanation for increased aerobic glycolysis in tumors is that this pathway serves to balance the need of proliferating cells for energy with the equally important need for macromolecular building blocks and maintenance of redox homeostasis (see Sec. 12.3.4). Several important subsidiary biosynthetic metabolic pathways rely on glycolytic intermediates, including the hexosamine pathway, uridine diphosphate (UDP)-glucose synthesis, glycerol synthesis, and the pentose phosphate pathway. The pentose phosphate pathway is also a key means of producing nicotinamide adenine dinucleotide phosphate (NADPH), which provides reducing power for many biosynthetic reactions and maintenance of antioxidant systems. In addition, by removing the burden of energy production from the mitochondria, high rates of aerobic glycolysis allow the tricarboxylic acid (TCA) cycle to act as a hub for biosynthesis of fatty acids and amino acids rather than as a site of energy generation.

The reliance of cancer cells on increased glucose uptake has proven useful for tumor detection and monitoring. The glycolytic phenotype of tumor cells serves as the basis for clinical [18F] fluorodeoxyglucose positron emission tomography (FDG-PET) imaging (see Chap. 14, Sec. 14.3.3). FDG-PET employs a radioactive glucose analog that is taken up by cells along with glucose, but cannot be further metabolized and is trapped intracellularly. Imaging of fluorodeoxyglucose (FDG) detects regions of high glucose uptake, and allows identification and monitoring of many tumor types, as well as generating data regarding the importance of glucose as a fuel for malignancies (Jadvar et al, 2009). Attempts to exploit the glycolytic phenotype of tumor cells for therapy have been less successful: There have been attempts to block aerobic glycolysis, using compounds such as 2-deoxyglucose, but effective therapeutic strategies have yet to be devised. Several novel therapeutic approaches targeting the glycolytic process are undergoing evaluation, including the inhibition of lactate dehydrogenase, and the inactivation of the monocarboxylate transporters (MCT) responsible for conveying lactate across the plasma membrane (see Fig. 12–10) (Le et al, 2010).

Although aerobic glycolysis is the most well documented metabolic phenotype of tumor cells, it is not a universal

feature of human cancers (Moreno-Sanchez et al, 2007). Moreover, even in relatively glycolytic tumors, oxidative phosphorylation is not completely shut down. Clinical FDG-PET data, as well as in vitro and in vivo experimental studies show that tumor cells are capable of using alternative fuel sources. It is estimated that up to 30% of human tumors are considered FDG-PET–negative depending on the tumor type (Jadvar et al, 2009). Amino acids, fatty acids, and even lactate have been shown to act as fuels for tumor cells in certain genetic and microenvironmental contexts.

Much of the work on cancer metabolism has focused on rapidly proliferating tumor models and cells grown in vitro. Because the rate of cell division can alter the metabolism of normal cells and tissues, some of the metabolic properties associated with malignancy may simply relate to rapid cell proliferation. It is unclear to what extent the metabolic phenotypes of tumor cells, including the Warburg effect, will prove to be important in low-grade slow-growing tumors, where metabolic demands may not be as extreme. Future clinical data describing the metabolic profiles of human tumors will be required to determine which metabolic alterations are most prevalent in specific tumor types and how they relate to changes in common oncogenic signaling pathways.

12.3.2 Regulation of Aerobic Glycolysis

12.3.2.1 The PI3K pathway   The PI3K (phophatidylinositol-3 kinase) pathway is one of the most commonly altered signaling pathways in human cancers (see Chap. 7, Sec. 7.5.4 and Chap. 8, Sec. 8.2.5). This pathway is activated by mutations in tumor-suppressor genes such as *PTEN*, mutations in components of the PI3K complex itself, or by aberrant signaling from receptor tyrosine kinases (Wong et al, 2010). Once activated, the PI3K pathway not only provides strong growth and survival signals to tumor cells but also has profound effects on their metabolism.

The best-studied effector molecule downstream of PI3K is AKT1, also known as protein kinase B (PKB). Upon activation, AKT1 exerts its effects by phosphorylating key signaling substrates involved in proliferation, survival and metabolism. AKT1 is an important driver of the tumor glycolytic phenotype and stimulates ATP generation via multiple mechanisms, ensuring that cells have the bioenergetic capacity required to respond to parallel growth signals. AKT1 stimulates glycolysis by increasing the expression and membrane translocation of glucose transporters, and by phosphorylating key glycolytic enzymes such as hexokinase and phosphofructokinase-2 (Robey and Hay, 2009). The elevated and prolonged AKT1 signaling that is associated with transformation inhibits the forkhead box subfamily O (FOXO) transcription factors, resulting in a host of complex transcriptional changes that also increase glycolytic capacity (Khatri et al, 2010). Finally, AKT1 strongly activates mTOR kinase by phosphorylating and inhibiting its negative regulator, tuberous sclerosis 2 (TSC2) (Robey and Hay, 2009). The mTOR protein functions as a key metabolic integration point, coupling growth signals to nutrient availability (see Sec. 12.2.3). Normally, activated mTOR stimulates protein and lipid biosynthesis and cell growth in response to sufficient nutrient and energy conditions and growth signals, but it is often constitutively activated in tumors (Guertin and Sabatini, 2007). At the molecular level, mTOR directly stimulates messenger RNA (mRNA) translation and ribosome biogenesis, and indirectly causes other metabolic changes by activating transcription factors such as HIF-1 (see Sec. 12.2.3). The subsequent HIF-1–dependent metabolic changes are a major determinant of the glycolytic phenotype downstream of PI3K, AKT1, and mTOR (see Fig. 12–10).

12.3.2.2 HIF-1 and MYC

The HIF-1 and HIF-2 complexes are the major transcription factors responsible for changes in gene expression during the cellular response to hypoxia (see Sec. 12.2.3). Although these 2 transcription factors transactivate an overlapping set of genes, the effects on central metabolism have been better characterized for HIF-1. In addition to its stabilization under hypoxic conditions, HIF-1 can be activated under normoxic conditions by oncogenic signaling pathways, including PI3K, and by mutations in tumor-suppressor proteins such as VHL (Kaelin, 2008), succinate dehydrogenase (SDH), and fumarate hydratase (FH) (King et al, 2006), which cause defects in its normal degradation. HIF-1 amplifies the transcription of genes encoding glucose transporters and most of the glycolytic enzymes, increasing the capacity of the cell to perform glycolysis (Semenza, 2010). In addition, HIF-1 activates the pyruvate dehydrogenase kinases (PDKs), which phosphorylate and inactivate the mitochondrial pyruvate dehydrogenase complex, thereby reducing the flow of glucose-derived pyruvate into the TCA cycle (Papandreau et al, 2006; see Fig. 12–10). This reduction in pyruvate flux into the TCA cycle decreases the rate of oxidative phosphorylation and oxygen consumption, reinforcing the glycolytic phenotype and sparing oxygen under hypoxic conditions. Inhibitors of HIF-1 or the PDKs might reverse some of the metabolic effects of tumorigenic HIF-1 signaling, and several such candidates, including the PDK inhibitor dichloroacetic acid (DCA), are under evaluation for their therapeutic utility.

The oncogenic transcription factor MYC also has a number of important effects on cell metabolism (see Chap. 7, Sec. 7.5.2). MYC can collaborate with HIF in the activation of a number of glucose transporters, glycolytic enzymes, lactate dehydrogenase A, and PDK1 (Dang et al, 2008). However, unlike HIF, MYC also activates the transcription of targets that increase mitochondrial function, especially the metabolism of glutamine, which is discussed below.

12.3.2.3 Adenosine Monophosphate-Activated Protein Kinase

Adenosine monophosphate (AMP)-activated protein kinase (AMPK) is a critical sensor of energy status and plays an important role in cellular responses to metabolic stress, coupling energy status to growth signals. AMPK opposes the effects of AKT1 by acting as a potent inhibitor of mTOR (see Fig. 12–10). The AMPK complex thus functions as a metabolic checkpoint, regulating the cellular response to available metabolic energy. AMPK becomes activated in response to an increased AMP:ATP ratio, and is responsible for shifting cells to an oxidative metabolic phenotype and inhibiting cell proliferation (Shackelford and Shaw, 2009). Tumor cells must overcome this checkpoint in order to proliferate in response to activated growth signaling pathways, especially in a nutrient deficient microenvironment. A number of oncogenic mutations and signaling pathways can suppress AMPK signaling (Shackelford and Shaw, 2009), effectively uncoupling fuel signals from growth signals, and allowing tumor cells to continue to divide under abnormal nutrient conditions. This uncoupling permits tumor cells to respond to inappropriate growth signaling pathways activated by oncogenes and the loss of tumor suppressors. Accordingly, many cancer cells exhibit a loss of appropriate AMPK signaling, which may also contribute to their glycolytic phenotype.

Given the role of AMPK, it is not surprising that the gene which encodes liver kinase B1 (LKB1), the upstream kinase necessary for AMPK activation, has been identified as a tumor-suppressor gene (see Fig. 12–10). Inherited mutations in *LKB1* are responsible for Peutz-Jeghers syndrome (Jenne et al, 1998). This syndrome is characterized by the development of benign gastrointestinal and oral lesions, and an increased risk of developing a broad spectrum of malignancies. *LKB1* is also frequently mutated in sporadic cases of non–small cell lung cancer and cervical carcinoma. Recent evidence suggests that *LKB1* mutations are tumorigenic as a consequence of the resulting decrease in AMPK signaling and loss of mTOR inhibition (Shackelford and Shaw, 2009). The loss of AMPK signaling permits the activation of mTOR and HIF-1, and therefore may also support the shift toward glycolytic metabolism. Clinically, there is interest in evaluating whether AMPK agonists can be used to recouple fuel and growth signals in tumor cells and shut down cell growth. Two such agonists are the commonly used antidiabetic drugs metformin and phenformin.

12.3.2.4 p53

Although the transcription factor and tumor-suppressor p53 is best known for its functions in the DNA damage response (DDR) and apoptosis pathways (see Chap. 5, Sec. 5.4 and Chap. 7, Fig. 7–12), it is also an important regulator of metabolism (Vousden and Ryan, 2009). p53 activates the expression of hexokinase II, which converts glucose to glucose-6-phosphate (G6P). G6P then either enters the glycolytic pathway to produce ATP, or enters the pentose phosphate pathway (PPP), which supports macromolecular biosynthesis by producing reducing potential in the form of reduced NADPH and/or ribose building blocks for nucleotide synthesis. p53 inhibits the glycolytic pathway by upregulating the expression of p53-induced glycolysis and apoptosis regulator (TIGAR), an enzyme that decreases levels of the glycolytic activator fructose-2,6-bisphosphate (see Fig. 12–10) (Vousden and Ryan, 2009). Wild-type p53 also acts to support the expression of PTEN, which inhibits the PI3K pathway, thereby suppressing glycolysis (Stambolic et al, 2001). Furthermore, p53 promotes oxidative phosphorylation by activating the expression of SCO2, which is required for assembly of the cytochrome c oxidase complex of the electron transport chain (Matoba et al, 2006). Thus, the loss of p53 may also be a major force behind the acquisition of the glycolytic phenotype.

12.3.2.5 Pyruvate Kinase

Pyruvate kinase (PK) catalyzes the final, and ATP-generating step of glycolysis, in which phosphoenolpyruvate (PEP) is converted to pyruvate (Mazurek et al, 2005). Multiple isoenzymes of PK exist in mammals: type L, found in the liver and kidneys; type R, expressed in erythrocytes; type M1, found in muscle and brain; and type M2, present in self-renewing cells such as embryonic and adult stem cells (Mazurek et al, 2005). PKM2 is also overexpressed by many tumor cells, and PKM2 expression by lung cancer cells was found to confer a tumorigenic advantage over cells expressing the PKM1 isoform (Christofk et al, 2008). While PKM1 is highly active, and would be expected to efficiently promote glycolysis and rapid energy generation, the tumor associated PKM2 is characteristically found in a less active state (Mazurek et al, 2005; Christofk et al, 2008). Initially, this observation seemed paradoxical: PKM2 represented a tumor-specific glycolytic enzyme that slowed ATP generation and antagonized the Warburg effect. However, the switch to PKM2 provides an advantage to tumor cells, because by slowing the last step of glycolysis, it allows glucose-derived carbohydrate metabolites to be diverted to other metabolic pathways. Interestingly, the oncoprotein MYC has been found to promote the expression of PKM2 over PKM1 by modulating exon splicing (David et al, 2010). MYC upregulates the expression of heterogeneous nuclear ribonucleoproteins (hnRNPs), which bind to PK mRNA, leading to preferential production of PKM2.

12.3.3 Glutamine Metabolism

Although glutamine is not an essential amino acid, cell culture medium must be supplemented with high concentrations of glutamine in order to support robust cell proliferation, and some cultured tumor cell lines derive the majority of their ATP from glutamine catabolism (Reitzer et al, 1979). More recently, it was found that oncogenic transformation can stimulate glutamine uptake and catabolism (glutaminolysis) and that many tumor cells are critically dependent on this amino acid (Wise et al, 2008). After glutamine enters the cell via specific plasma membrane transporters, glutaminase enzymes remove an ammonium ion, converting it to glutamate, which has several fates (Fig. 12–12). Glutamate can be converted directly into glutathione (GSH) by the enzyme glutathione cysteine ligase (GCL). Reduced GSH is one of the most abundant antioxidants found in mammalian cells, and is vital to controlling the redox state of all subcellular compartments. Glutamate can also be converted to α-ketoglutarate (α-KG) and enter the TCA cycle. This process, termed *anaplerosis*, supplies the alternative carbon input required for the TCA cycle to act as a biosynthetic hub and permits

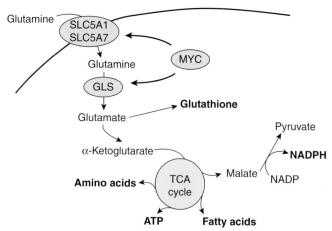

FIGURE 12–12 Glutamine metabolism. Glutamine enters cells via specific transporters (SLC5A1 and SLC5A7) and is converted to glutamate by the enzyme glutaminase (GLS). Glutamate can be converted to glutathione so as to combat oxidative stress or enter the TCA cycle as α-ketoglutarate so as to provide ATP and macromolecular building blocks for cell growth and division. Key products of glutamine metabolism are shown in bold. Oncogenic proteins, including MYC, can enhance this process at several levels and render tumor cells highly dependent on exogenous glutamine.

the production of other amino acids and fatty acids. Some glutamine-derived carbon can exit the TCA cycle as malate and serve as a substrate for malic enzyme 1 (ME1) which produces NADPH (DeBerardinis et al, 2007). The mechanisms regulating the fate of glutamine in tumor cells are not completely understood, and it is likely that genetic background and microenvironmental factors play a role.

One factor that plays a major role in regulating glutaminolysis is the oncogene MYC (see Chap. 7, Sec. 7.5.2). Thus MYC promotes not only proliferation but also the production of the macromolecules and reducing power required for cell growth and division. MYC increases glutamine uptake by directly increasing the expression of the glutamine transporters SLC5A1 and SLC7A1 (Gao et al, 2009). Furthermore, MYC indirectly increases the level of glutaminase 1 (GLS1), the key first enzyme of glutaminolysis, by repressing the expression of microRNAs-23a/b, which function to inhibit GLS1 (see Chap. 2, Sec. 2.4.3) (Gao et al, 2009). It is now clear that MYC supports antioxidant capacity by driving the production of NADPH via the PPP, by promoting the PKM2 isoform as described above, and also by increasing the synthesis of GSH through glutaminolysis. New techniques for measuring glutamine and its metabolites should soon permit the detailed examination of glutamine metabolism and MYC expression in tumors in patients.

12.3.4 Metabolic Alterations Support Balanced Redox Status

Redox status refers to the balance of the reduced versus the oxidized state of a biochemical system. In biological systems, this balance is influenced by the level of reactive oxygen species (ROS) relative to the capacity of antioxidant systems to eliminate ROS, as well as the relative concentrations of key substrates involved in oxidation reduction reactions. ROS are a diverse class of molecules produced in all cells as a normal byproduct of metabolic processes. ROS are heterogeneous in their chemical properties and cause a number of effects, depending on their concentrations. At low levels, ROS can act as signaling molecules to increase cell proliferation and survival through post-translational modification of kinases and phosphatases (Lee et al, 2002). Production of these low levels of ROS is required for homeostatic signaling events. At moderate levels, ROS induce the expression of stress-responsive genes downstream of transcription factors such as HIF-1α and NRF2, which trigger the expression of proteins providing pro-survival signals and antioxidant defense mechanisms (Gao et al, 2007). However, at high levels, ROS can overwhelm antioxidant systems, and damage macromolecules, including DNA, proteins, and lipids. Cells counteract the detrimental effects of ROS by producing antioxidant molecules such as reduced GSH and thioredoxin (TRX), along with enzymes such as superoxide dismutase and catalase. These molecules act to reduce excessive ROS so as to prevent irreversible cellular damage. Several of these antioxidant systems, including GSH and TRX, rely on the reducing power of NADPH to maintain their activities. In highly proliferative tumor cells, ROS regulation is critical because of the presence of oncogenic mutations that promote aberrant metabolism and protein translation, resulting in elevated rates of ROS production. Transformed cells counteract the accumulation of ROS by further upregulating antioxidant systems, creating a dynamic equilibrium between high levels of ROS production and high levels of antioxidant molecules (Trachootham et al, 2009; Fig. 12–13).

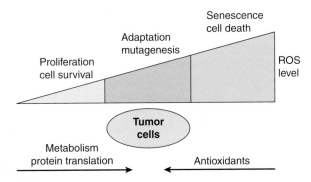

FIGURE 12–13 **Relationship between ROS level and cancer.** The impact of ROS on cell fate depends on ROS levels. Low levels of ROS provide a beneficial effect, supporting cell proliferation and survival pathways. However, once ROS levels become excessively high, they cause detrimental oxidative stress that can lead to cell death. To counter such oxidative stress, cells employ antioxidant systems that prevent ROS from accumulating to high levels. In cancer cells, aberrant metabolism, protein translation, and microenvironmental conditions generate abnormally high ROS levels. Through additional mutations and adaptations, cancer cells exert tight regulation of ROS and antioxidants in such a way that the cells survive and ROS are reduced to moderate levels.

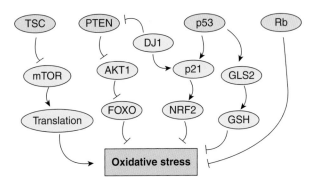

FIGURE 12–14 **Tumor suppressors influence oxidative stress.** Loss of the tumor supressors tuberous sclerosis 1 (TSC), phosphatase and tensin homolog (PTEN), p53, and retinoblastoma 1 (Rb), shaded in gray, leads to increased oxidative stress by increasing ROS production or by preventing the induction and maintenance of appropriate antioxidant defense mechanisms. TSC inhibits the mammalian target of rapamycin (mTOR), reducing the oxidative stress resulting from metabolism associated with protein translation. PTEN inhibits the ability of AKT1 to inhibit the FOXO transcription factor, which also increases oxidative stress. p53 can bolster antioxidant defenses by increasing the activity of the NRF2 antioxidant trascription factor via the p21 protein, and by stimulating glutathione production by upregulating glutaminase 2 (GLS2). The oncogenic DJ1 protein can contribute to both of these pathways by inhibiting PTEN, and by helping to stabilize NRF2. The Rb tumor suppressor enhances antioxidant defenses via a number of downstream mechanisms.

12.3.4.1 Rb, PTEN, and p53 Contribute to Redox Maintenance Fully transformed tumor cells alter their metabolic pathways and regulatory mechanisms so that ROS and antioxidants are tightly controlled and maintained at elevated levels compared to normal cells. However, during the process of tumorigenesis, the initial loss of tumor suppressors may cause cells to become overloaded with the products of aberrant metabolism and lose control of redox balance. Several mechanisms downstream of commonly mutated tumor suppressors may contribute to increased oxidative stress (Fig. 12–14). For example, when the tumor-suppressor *TSC2* is deleted, mTOR becomes hyperactive. This mTOR activity leads to an upregulation of protein translation and increased ROS production (Ozcan et al, 2008). Data from experimental systems indicates that cells lacking retinoblastoma (Rb) tumor-suppressor function, which normally participates in the antioxidant response, are more sensitive to apoptosis as a consequence of this cellular stress (Li et al, 2010). Similar results have been seen with loss of PTEN, where increased activation of AKT leads to FOXO transcription factor inactivation and increased oxidative stress because of a reduction in the antioxidant defense molecules normally maintained by FOXO (Nogueira et al, 2008).

The tumor-suppressor p53 may promote oxidative stress during the induction of apoptosis (see Chap. 9, Sec. 9.4.3 and Fig. 9–12), yet it also plays a significant role in reducing oxidative stress as a defense mechanism. Glutaminase 2 (GLS2) is upregulated by p53 and drives de novo GSH synthesis

(Suzuki et al, 2010). Furthermore, via the p53 target gene CDK inhibitor 1A (*CDKN1A*), which encodes p21 (see Chap. 9, Sec. 9.2.2), p53 promotes the stabilization of the NRF2 transcription factor (see Fig. 12–14) (Chen et al, 2009). NRF2 is an important antioxidant transcription factor that upregulates the expression of several antioxidant and detoxifying molecules. Loss of p53 in a cancer cell inactivates this redox maintenance mechanism. Thus it might be possible to exploit clinically loss-of-function p53 mutations or other tumor-suppressor genes by applying additional oxidative stress, since malignant cells might be selectively killed.

12.3.4.2 DJ1

Much of our understanding of ROS and oxidative stress has emerged from the field of neurodegenerative disease. Similar mechanisms maintain appropriate redox status in both neurons and cancer cells. One protein involved in preventing neurodegeneration that has been investigated in the context of cancer is DJ1 (also known as PARK7). Similar to p21, DJ1 acts to stabilize NRF2 and thereby promotes antioxidant responses (Clements et al, 2006). DJ1 is mutated and inactive in several neurodegenerative disorders, most notably Parkinson disease (Gasser et al, 1997). In these disorders, it is believed that loss of DJ1 function leads to elevated oxidative stress in the brain, and increased neuronal cell death (see Fig. 12–14). *DJ1* has also been described as an oncogene, and in patients with lung, ovarian, and esophageal cancers, high DJ1 expression in the tumor predicts a poor outcome (Kim et al, 2005). DJ1 stimulates AKT activity both in vitro and in vivo by regulating the function of the tumor-suppressor PTEN (see Fig. 12–14) (Kim et al, 2005). Although this function appears to be a logical candidate for the mechanism underlying a tumorigenic role of DJ1, high DJ1 expression may also promote tumor progression by reducing the oxidative stress caused by aberrant cell proliferation and thereby preventing ROS-induced cell death.

Supporting the notion that loss of DJ1 prevents appropriate redox control in cancers, an inverse correlation has been reported between cancer risk and Parkinson disease. A recent metaanalysis of patients with Parkinson disease determined that they have an approximately 30% lower risk of developing cancers compared with controls (Bajaj et al, 2010). The lower risk was associated with several different cancer types, including lung, prostate, and colorectal cancers. Additional investigation of the cancer risk of patients with other neurodegenerative disorders may provide key insights into potential therapeutic exploitation of the heightened need to maintain redox balance in a cancer cell.

12.3.5 Metabolic Oncogenes and Tumor Suppressors

Although many signaling pathways commonly altered in tumors have profound effects on cellular metabolism, few key metabolic enzymes themselves are consistently mutated. However, several metabolic enzymes have been shown to be important oncogenes and tumor suppressors.

12.3.5.1 Fumarate Hydratase and Succinate Dehydrogenase

The TCA cycle enzymes FH and SDH have been identified as classical tumor suppressors (see Chap. 7, Sec. 7.6). Loss-of-function mutations in these enzymes cause disruption of the TCA cycle and lead to hereditary cancer syndromes, predisposing patients to paraganglioma and pheochromocytoma in the case of SDH, and to leiomyoma and renal cell carcinoma in the case of FH (Selak et al, 2005). The biochemical mechanisms responsible for driving tumorigenesis in these situations are still being clarified, but they appear to involve the induction of a pseudohypoxic phenotype, caused by inhibition of the PHD enzymes responsible for causing the degradation of HIF (Selak et al, 2005). However, other mechanisms, including an increase in ROS production and alterations to other PHD substrates, may be involved. The restricted tumor spectrum observed in these syndromes indicates that the capacity of these mutations to cause cancer may be dependent on cellular context.

12.3.5.2 Isocitrate Dehydrogenases

Isocitrate dehydrogenase 1 and 2 (*IDH1/2*) have been identified as genes commonly mutated in glioma and acute myeloid leukemia (AML) (Mardis, 2009; Parsons et al, 2008). These genes normally function to regulate cellular redox status by producing NADPH during the conversion of isocitrate to α-KG in the cytoplasm and mitochondria, respectively. IDH1 and IDH2 are homologous, and structurally and functionally distinct from the nicotinamide adenine dinucleotide (NAD)-dependent enzyme IDH3, which functions in the TCA cycle to produce the reduced form of nicotinamide adenine dinucleotide (NADH) required for oxidative phosphorylation.

The *IDH1* and *IDH2* mutations associated with the development of glioma and AML are restricted to critical arginine residues required for isocitrate binding in the active site of the protein (R132 in IDH1 and R172 or R140 in IDH2) (Dang et al, 2009). Affected patients are heterozygous for these mutations, suggesting that these alterations cause an oncogenic gain-of-function. The spectrum of mutation differs in the 2 diseases, with the *IDH1 R132H* mutation predominating in gliomas (>90%), whereas a more diverse collection of mutations in both *IDH1* and *IDH2* are found in AML.

The specific mutations cause the IDH1 and IDH2 proteins to acquire a novel enzymatic activity that converts α-KG to 2-hydroxyglutarate (2-HG) in an NADPH-dependent manner (Dang et al, 2009; Gross et al, 2010). This change causes the mutated IDH1 and IDH2 enzymes to switch from NADPH production to NADPH consumption, with consequences for cellular redox balance. The product of the novel reaction, 2-HG, is a poorly understood metabolite normally present at low concentrations in cells and tissues. However, in patients bearing somatic *IDH1* or *IDH2* mutations, 2-HG builds up to high levels in glioma tissues, and in the leukemic cells and sera of AML patients and may be directly oncogenic (Dang et al, 2009; Gross et al, 2010).

Studies of IDH1 and IDH2 have established a new paradigm in oncogenesis: a driver mutation that confers a new metabolic enzymatic activity that produces a potential oncometabolite. The molecular mechanisms by which *IDH1* and *IDH2* mutations contribute to tumorigenesis are under investigation, as is the possibility that these mutant enzymes may be useful targets for therapy. Although *IDH1* and *IDH2* mutations are clearly powerful drivers of glioma and AML, they appear to be rare or absent in other tumor types, illustrating the importance of specific cellular context in understanding metabolic perturbations in cancer cells.

12.3.6 Autophagy

Autophagy has emerged as an important link between cellular metabolism and hypoxia in the microenvironment of solid tumors. Autophagy literally means "self-eating" and is a process that is responsible for the basal turnover (degradation) of long-lived cellular proteins. It occurs through generation of a double-membrane vesicle referred to as an *autophagosome* that captures cytoplasmic contents destined for degradation. The outer membrane of the autophagosome fuses with a lysosome to form an autolysosome, resulting in the degradation of the inner membrane and its contents by enzymes present within the lysosome. The degradation products (amino acids, lipids) are delivered back to the cytoplasm and can be used in essential metabolic processes. Autophagy occurs at a low basal rate in all cells, but can be strongly induced by particular forms of cell stress, including those often present in the microenvironment of tumors.

Autophagy serves at least 2 critical cellular functions that are relevant in cancer. First, it is important for the removal and degradation of damaged organelles and misfolded protein aggregates. This includes removal of damaged mitochondria that would otherwise "leak" electrons and produce ROS through a selective form of autophagy sometimes referred to as mitophagy. The ability to remove and degrade these otherwise toxic cellular components is thought to provide a tumor-suppressor function in some instances during early tumorigenesis. Indeed, mutations in genes, such as *Beclin1*, that regulate the initiation of autophagy have been observed in some types of cancer. Second, and perhaps more important, autophagy plays an essential metabolic function and is required to maintain cell survival during conditions of extreme metabolic stress. Autophagy is activated as part of a "starvation" response when cells are unable to import nutrients to sustain essential metabolic pathways. In this role, autophagy functions to degrade cytoplasmic components to provide essential products for sustaining cellular metabolism and energy homeostasis. This function is particularly important within hypoxic regions of solid tumors where maintaining energy homeostasis becomes critical for cell survival, and each of the HIF, UPR, and mTOR pathways described above are capable of stimulating rates of autophagy during hypoxia (Fig. 12–15). In some tumors, activation of growth-promoting oncogenes including *K-ras* is sufficient to render cells constitutively dependent on autophagy for their continued survival. Thus, in most advanced cancers, autophagy rates are markedly induced and function to

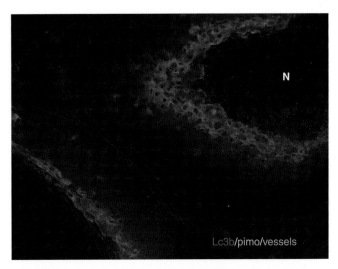

FIGURE 12–15 Hypoxia and autophagy. Immunostaining of a head and neck cancer xenograft reveals colocalization of hypoxia (green; pimonidazole immunohistochemistry) and autophagy (red; LC3 immunohistochemistry). Blood vessels are shown in blue; N = necrosis. Activation of autophagy can protect hypoxic and other tumor cells experiencing metabolic stress by promoting energy homeostasis. (From Rouschop et al, 2010.)

promote cell survival. Consequently, autophagy and the genes/pathways that regulate it, have emerged as new therapeutic targets. Current clinical strategies for inhibiting autophagy include the use of agents such as hydroxychloroquine that disrupt lysosomal pH regulation and thus prevent autolysosome formation and degradation of captured cytoplasmic content.

SUMMARY

- The growth of tumors is dependent on the rate of proliferation and of death of the cells within them. In many human tumors, the rate of cell production is only slightly higher than the rate of cell death and many cells may not be actively cycling, so that the median doubling time of tumors (typically about 2 months for common human solid tumors) is much longer than the cell cycle time of the proliferating tumor cells (typically about 2 to 3 days).

- Factors that influence the rates of proliferation and cell death in tumors include nutrient molecules in the microenvironment, which, in turn, depend on angiogenesis and the expansion of the vascular network of the tumor, and the molecular signals that are influenced by endogenous and exogenous factors.

- Tumor cells grow within a unique microenvironment characterized by deficiencies in vasculature and vascular function. This results in the generation of highly heterogeneous regions where tumor cells are exposed to elevated levels of waste products (lactate), low pH, high IFP, and hypoxia. Each of these features can influence tumor biology and tumor response to treatment in adverse ways.

- Mutations in oncogenes and tumor-suppressor genes affect the core metabolism of tumor cells, reengineering it to support cell growth and division. Such metabolic alterations help to balance 3 critical requirements of proliferating cells: supply of energy in the form of ATP; supply of macromolecular building blocks for cell growth and division; and maintenance of redox homeostasis. The unique and stressful microenvironmental conditions in solid tumors further distort the metabolic phenotype, affecting progression, treatment response, and patient outcome.
- Tumor hypoxia, in particular, leads to a series of biological changes that can promote enhanced malignancy primarily through the action of HIF transcription factors driving several oxygen-sensitive signaling pathways. In addition, very low levels of oxygen induce the unfolded protein response to reduce metabolic demand under conditions of severe energy "starvation."
- Autophagy is a further important mechanism of cell survival in the adverse microenvironment of solid tumors. It is activated as part of the "starvation" response when cells are unable to obtain nutrients to sustain essential metabolic pathways. Autophagy functions to degrade cytoplasmic components to provide essential products for sustaining cellular metabolism and energy homeostasis. This function is particularly important within hypoxic regions of solid tumors where maintaining energy homeostasis becomes critical for cell survival.
- A more complete understanding of the unique aspects of tumor metabolism may reveal opportunities for novel diagnostic and therapeutic strategies.

REFERENCES

Adhami F, Liao G, Morozov YM, et al. Cerebral ischemia-hypoxia induces intravascular coagulation and autophagy. *Am J Pathol* 2006;169:566-583.

Airley R, Loncaster J, Davidson S, et al. Glucose transporter glut-1 expression correlates with tumor hypoxia and predicts metastasis-free survival in advanced carcinoma of the cervix. *Clin Cancer Res* 2001;7:928-934.

Ameri K, Lewis CE, Raida M, et al. Anoxic induction of ATF-4 through HIF-1-independent pathways of protein stabilization in human cancer cells. *Blood* 2004;103:1876-1882.

Bajaj A, Driver JA, Schernhammer ES. Parkinson's disease and cancer risk: a systematic review and meta-analysis. *Cancer Causes Control* 2010;21:697-707.

Braunstein S, Karpisheva K, Pola C, et al. A hypoxia-controlled cap-dependent to cap-independent translation switch in breast cancer. *Mol Cell* 2007;28:501-512.

Bristow R, Hill GRP. Hypoxia and metabolism. Hypoxia, DNA repair and genetic instability. *Nat Rev Cancer* 2008;8:180-192.

Cardenas-Navia LI, Yu D, Braun RD, et al. Tumor-dependent kinetics of partial pressure of oxygen fluctuations during air and oxygen breathing. *Cancer Res* 2004;64:6010-6017.

Chaudary N, Hill RP. Hypoxia and metastasis. *Clin Cancer Res* 2007; 13:1947-1949.

Chaudary N, Milosevic M, Hill RP. Suppression of vascular endothelial growth factor receptor 3 (VEGFR3) and vascular endothelial growth factor C (VEGFC) inhibits hypoxia-induced lymph node metastases in cervix cancer. *Gynecol Oncol* 2011; 123:393-400.

Chen W, Sun Z, Wang XJ, et al. Direct interaction between Nrf2 and p21(Cip1/WAF1) upregulates the Nrf2-mediated antioxidant response. *Mol Cell* 2009;34:663-673.

Christofk HR, Vander Heiden MG, Harris MH, et al. The M2 splice isoform of pyruvate kinase is important for cancer metabolism and tumour growth. *Nature* 2008;452:230-233.

Clements CM, McNally RS, Conti BJ, et al. DJ-1, a cancer- and Parkinson's disease-associated protein, stabilizes the antioxidant transcriptional master regulator Nrf2. *Proc Natl Acad Sci U S A* 2006;103:15091-15096.

Dang CV, Kim JW, Gao P, et al. The interplay between MYC and in cancer HIF. *Nat Rev Cancer* 2008;8:51-56.

Dang L, White DW, Gross S, et al. Cancer-associated IDH1 mutations produce 2-hydroxyglutarate. *Nature* 2009;462: 739-744.

Darzynkiewicz Z, Traganos F, Zhao H, Halicka HD, Li J. Cytometry of DNA replication and RNA synthesis: historical perspective and recent advances based on "click chemistry". *Cytometry A* 2011;79: 328-337.

David CJ, Chen M, Assanah M, et al. HnRNP proteins controlled by c-Myc deregulate pyruvate kinase mRNA splicing in cancer. *Nature* 2010;463:364-368.

Davies MP, Barraclough DL, Stewart C, et al. Expression and splicing of the unfolded protein response gene XBP-1 are significantly associated with clinical outcome of endocrine-treated breast cancer. *Int J Cancer* 2008;123:85-88.

DeBerardinis RJ, Mancuso A, Daikhin E, et al. Beyond aerobic glycolysis: transformed cells can engage in glutamine metabolism that exceeds the requirement for protein and nucleotide synthesis. *Proc Natl Acad Sci U S A* 2007;104:19345-19350.

Degenhardt K, Mathew R, Beaudoin B, et al. Autophagy promotes tumor cell survival and restricts necrosis, inflammation, and tumorigenesis. *Cancer Cell* 2006;10:51-64.

Denekamp J, Hobson B. Endothelial-cell proliferation in experimental tumours. *Br J Cancer* 1982;46:711-720.

Dewhirst MW, Cao Y, Moeller B. Cycling hypoxia and free radicals regulate angiogenesis and radiotherapy response. *Nat Rev Cancer* 2008;8:425-437.

Doulatov S, Notta F, Eppert K, Nguyen LT, Ohashi PS, Dick JE. Revised map of the human progenitor heirarchy shows the origin of macrophages and dendritic cells in early lymphoid development. *Nat Immunol* 2010;11:585-593.

Dubois L, Magagnin MG, Cleven AH, et al. Inhibition of 4E-BP1 sensitizes U87 glioblastoma xenograft tumors to irradiation by decreasing hypoxia tolerance. *Int J Radiat Oncol Biol Phys* 2009; 73:1219-1227.

Durand RE, Aquino-Parsons C. Clinical relevance of intermittent tumour blood flow. *Acta Oncol* 2001;40:929-936.

Durand RE, Sham E. The lifetime of hypoxic human tumor cells. *Int J Radiat Oncol Biol Phys* 1998;42:711-715.

Epstein AC, Gleadle JM, McNeill LA, et al. *C. elegans* EGL-9 and mammalian homologs define a family of dioxygenases that regulate HIF by prolyl hydroxylation. *Cell* 2001;107:43-54.

Erler JT, Bennewith KL, Nicolau M, et al. Lysyl oxidase is essential for hypoxia-induced metastasis. *Nature* 2006;440: 1222-1226.

Erler JT, Cawthorne CJ, Williams KJ, et al. Hypoxia-mediated down-regulation of Bid and Bax in tumors occurs via hypoxia-inducible factor 1-dependent and -independent mechanisms and contributes to drug resistance. *Mol Cell Biol* 2004;24:2875-2889.

Fearon ER, Hamilton SR, Vogelstein B. Clonal analysis of human colorectal tumors. *Science* 1987;238:193-197.

Fialkow PJ. The origin and development of human tumors studied with cell markers. *N Engl J Med* 1974;291:26-35.

Frezza C, Gottlieb E. Mitochondria in cancer: not just innocent bystanders. *Semin Cancer Biol* 2009;19:4-11.

Fukumura D, Jain RK. Tumor microenvironment abnormalities: causes, consequences, and strategies to normalize. *J Cell Biochem* 2007;101:937-949.

Funes JM, Quintero M, Henderson S, et al. Transformation of human mesenchymal stem cells increases their dependency on oxidative phosphorylation for energy production. *Proc Natl Acad Sci U S A* 2007;104:6223-6228.

Fyles A, Milosevic M, Pintilie M, et al. Long-term performance of interstitial fluid pressure and hypoxia as prognostic factors in cervix cancer. *Radiother Oncol* 2006;80:132-137.

Gao P, Tchernyshyov I, Chang TC, et al. c-Myc suppression of miR-23a/b enhances mitochondrial glutaminase expression and glutamine metabolism. *Nature* 2009;458:762-765.

Gao P, Zhang H, Dinavahi R, et al. HIF-dependent antitumorigenic effect of antioxidants in vivo. *Cancer Cell* 2007;12:230-238.

Gasser T, Müller-Myhsok B, Wszolek ZK, et al. Genetic complexity and Parkinson's disease. *Science* 1997;277:388-389.

Gillies RJ, Robey I, Gatenby RA. Causes and consequences of increased glucose metabolism of cancers. *J Nucl Med* 2008;49 Suppl 2:24S-42S.

Gross S, Cairns RA, Minden MD, et al. Cancer-associated metabolite 2-hydroxyglutarate accumulates in acute myelogenous leukemia with isocitrate dehydrogenase 1 and 2 mutations. *J Exp Med* 2010;207:339-344.

Guertin DA, Sabatini DM. Defining the role of min cancer TOR. *Cancer Cell* 2007;12:9-22.

Harris AL. Hypoxia—a key regulatory factor in tumour growth. *Nat Rev Cancer* 2002;2:38-47.

Hedley DW, Shankey VT, Wheeless LL. DNA cytometry consensus conference. *Cytometry* 1993;14:471-500.

Hockel M, Schlenger K, Aral B, et al. Association between tumor hypoxia and malignant progression in advanced cancer of the uterine cervix. *Cancer Res* 1996;56:4509-4515.

Huxham LA, Kyle AH, Baker JH, et al. Microregional effects of gemcitabine in HCT-116 xenografts. *Cancer Res* 2004;64:6537-6541.

Ivan M, Kondo K, Yang H, et al. HIFalpha targeted for VHL-mediated destruction by proline hydroxylation: implications for O2 sensing. *Science* 2001;292:464-468.

Jaakkola P, Mole DR, Tian YM, et al. Targeting of HIF-alpha to the von Hippel-Lindau ubiquitylation complex by O2-regulated prolyl hydroxylation. *Science* 2001;292:468-472.

Jadvar H, Alavi A, Gambhir SS. 18F-FDG uptake in lung, breast, and colon cancers: molecular biology correlates and disease characterization. *J Nucl Med* 2009;50:1820-1827.

Jenne DE, Reimann H, Nezu J, et al. Peutz-Jeghers syndrome is caused by mutations in a novel serine threonine kinase. *Nat Genet* 1998;18:38-43.

Kaanders JH, Wijffels KI, Marres HA, et al. Pimonidazole binding and tumor vascularity predict for treatment outcome in head and neck cancer. *Cancer Res* 2002;62:7066-7074.

Kaelin WG Jr. The von Hippel-Lindau tumour suppressor protein: O2 sensing and cancer. *Nat Rev Cancer* 2008;8:865-873.

Keyomarsi K, Tucker SL, Buchholz TA, et al. Cyclin E and survival in patients with breast cancer. *N Engl J Med* 2002;347:1566-1575.

Khatri S, Yepiskoposyan H, Gallo CA, et al. FOXO3a regulates glycolysis via transcriptional control of tumor suppressor TSC1. *J Biol Chem* 2010;285:15960-15965.

Kim RH, Peters M, Jang Y, et al. DJ-1, a novel regulator of the tumor suppressor PTEN. *Cancer Cell* 2005;7:263-273.

King A, Selak MA, Gottlieb E. Succinate dehydrogenase and fumarate hydratase: linking mitochondrial dysfunction and cancer. *Oncogene* 2006;25:4675-4682.

Koumenis C, Naczki C, Koritzinsky M, et al. Regulation of protein synthesis by hypoxia via activation of the endoplasmic reticulum kinase PERK and phosphorylation of the translation initiation factor eIF2alpha. *Mol Cell Biol* 2002;22:7405-7416.

Kraggerud SM, Sandvik JA, Pettersen EO. Regulation of protein synthesis in human cells exposed to extreme hypoxia. *Anticancer Res* 1995;15:683-686.

Le A, Cooper CR, Gouw AM, et al. Inhibition of lactate dehydrogenase A induces oxidative stress and inhibits tumor progression. *Proc Natl Acad Sci U S A* 2010;107:2037-2042.

Lee K, Esselman WJ. Inhibition of PTPs by H(2)O(2) regulates the activation of distinct pathways APK M. *Free Radic Biol Med* 2002;33:1121-1132.

Li B, Gordon GM, Du CH, et al. Specific killing of Rb mutant cancer cells by inactivating TSC2. *Cancer Cell* 2010;17:469-480.

Lunt SJ, Chaudary N, Hill RP. The tumor microenvironment and metastatic disease. *Clin Exp Metastasis* 2009;26:19-34.

Mardis ER, Ding L, Dooling DJ, et al. Recurring mutations found by sequencing an acute myeloid leukemia genome. *N Engl J Med* 2009;361:1058-1066.

Marusyk A, Almendro V, Polyak K. Intra-tumor heterogeneity: a looking glass for cancer? *Nat Rev Cancer* 2012;12:323-334.

Matoba S, Kang JG, Patino WD, et al. p53 regulates mitochondrial respiration. *Science* 2006;312:1650-1653.

Mazurek S, Boschek CB, Hugo F, et al. Pyruvate kinase type M2 and its role in tumor growth and spreading. *Semin Cancer Biol* 2005;15:300-308.

Messner HA. Assessment and characterization of hemopoietic stem cells. *Stem Cells* 1995;13(suppl 3):13-18.

Minchinton AI, Tannock IF. Drug penetration in solid tumours. *Nat Rev Cancer* 2006;6:583-592.

Moreno-Sánchez R, Rodríguez-Enríquez S, Marín-Hernández A, et al. Energy metabolism in tumor cells. *FEBS J* 2007;274:1393-1418.

Newsholme EA, Crabtree B, Ardawi MS. The role of high rates of glycolysis and glutamine utilization in rapidly dividing cells. *Biosci Rep* 1985;5:393-400.

Nogueira V, Park Y, Chen CC, et al. Akt determines replicative senescence and oxidative or oncogenic premature senescence and sensitizes cells to oxidative apoptosis. *Cancer Cell* 2008;14:458-470.

Nordsmark M, Loncaster J, Aquino-Parsons C, et al. The prognostic value of pimonidazole and tumour pO2 in human cervix carcinomas after radiation therapy: a prospective international multi-center study. *Radiother Oncol* 2006;80:123-131.

Ozcan U, Ozcan L, Yilmaz E, et al. Loss of the tuberous sclerosis complex tumor suppressors triggers the unfolded protein response to regulate insulin signaling and apoptosis. *Mol Cell* 2008;29:541-551.

Papandreou I, Cairns RA, Fontana L, et al. HIF-1 mediates adaptation to hypoxia by actively downregulating mitochondrial oxygen consumption. *Cell Metab* 2006;3:187-197.

Parks SK, Chiche J, Pouyssegur J. pH control mechanisms of tumor survival and growth. *J Cell Physiol* 2011;226:299-308.

Parsons DW, Jones S, Zhang X, et al. An integrated genomic analysis of human glioblastoma multiforme. *Science* 2008;321:1807-1812.

Pennacchietti S, Michieli P, Galluzzo M, et al. Hypoxia promotes invasive growth by transcriptional activation of the met protooncogene. *Cancer Cell* 2003;3:347-361.

Pries AR, Hopfner M, le Noble F, et al. The shunt problem: control of functional shunting in normal and tumour vasculature. *Nat Rev Cancer* 2010;10:587-593.

Reitzer LJ, Wice BM, Kennell D. Evidence that glutamine, not sugar, is the major energy source for cultured HeLa cells. *J Biol Chem* 1979;254:2669-2676.

Richter JD, Sonenberg N. Regulation of cap-dependent translation by eIF4inhibitory proteins E. *Nature* 2005;433:477-480.

Robey RB, Hay N. Is Akt the "Warburg kinase"?-Akt-energy metabolism interactions and oncogenesis. *Semin Cancer Biol* 2009;19:25-31.

Rouschop KM, van den Beucken T, Dubois L, et al. The unfolded protein response protects human tumor cells during hypoxia through regulation of the autophagy genes MAP1LC3B and ATG5. *J Clin Invest* 2010;120:127-141.

Selak MA, Armour SM, MacKenzie ED, et al. Succinate links TCA cycle dysfunction to oncogenesis by inhibiting HIF-alpha prolyl hydroxylase. *Cancer Cell* 2005;7:77-85.

Semenza GL. Targeting HIF-1 for cancer therapy. *Nat Rev Cancer* 2003;3:721-732.

Semenza GL. HIF-1: upstream and downstream of cancer metabolism. *Curr Opin Genet Dev* 2010;20:51-56.

Shackelford DB, Shaw RJ. The LKB1-AMPK pathway: metabolism and growth control in tumour suppression. *Nat Rev Cancer* 2009; 9:563-575.

Stambolic V, MacPherson D, Sas D, et al. Regulation of PTEN transcription by p53. *Mol Cell* 2001;8:317-325.

Staller P, Sulitkova J, Lisztwan J, et al. Chemokine receptor CXCR4 downregulated by von Hippel-Lindau tumour suppressor pVHL. *Nature* 2003;425:307-311.

Steel GG. *Growth Kinetics of Tumours: Cell Population Kinetics in Relation to the Growth and Treatment of Cancer*. Oxford, England: Clarendon Press; 1977.

Suzuki S, Tanaka T, Poyurovsky MV, et al. Phosphate-activated glutaminase (GLS2), a p53-inducible regulator of glutamine metabolism and reactive oxygen species. *Proc Natl Acad Sci U S A* 2010;107:7461-7466.

Tannock IF. Biology of tumor growth. *Hosp Pract* 1983;18:81-93.

Tannock IF. Population kinetics of carcinoma cells, capillary endothelial cells, and fibroblasts in a transplanted mouse mammary tumor. *Cancer Res* 1970;30:2470-2476.

Thomlinson RH, Gray LH. The histological structure of some human lung cancers and the possible implications for radiotherapy. *Br J Cancer* 1955;9:539-549.

Trachootham D, Alexandre J, Huang P. Targeting cancer cells by ROS-mediated mechanisms: a radical therapeutic approach? *Nat Rev Drug Discov* 2009;8:579-591.

Tsihlias J, Kapusta L, Slingerland J. The prognostic significance of altered cyclin-dependent kinase inhibitors in human cancer. *Annu Rev Med* 1999;50:401-423.

Vadhan-Raj S. Clinical findings with the first generation of thrombopoietic agents. *Semin Hematol* 2010;47:249-257.

Vander Heiden MG, Cantley LC, Thompson CB. Understanding the Warburg effect: the metabolic requirements of cell proliferation. *Science* 2009;324:1029-1033.

Vousden KH, Ryan KM. p53 and metabolism. *Nat Rev Cancer* 2009; 9:691-700.

Walters JR. Recent findings in the cell and molecular biology of the small intestine. *Curr Opin Gastroenterol* 2005;21:135-140.

Warburg O. On the origin of cancer cells. *Science* 1956;123: 309-314.

Weinhouse S. The Warburg hypothesis fifty years later. *Z Krebsforsch Klin Onkol Cancer Res Clin Oncol* 1976;87:115-126.

Weppler SA, Krause M, Zyromska A, et al. Response of U87 glioma xenografts treated with concurrent rapamycin and fractionated radiotherapy: possible role for thrombosis. *Radiother Oncol* 2007; 82:96-104.

Wise DR, DeBerardinis RJ, Mancuso A, et al. Myc regulates a transcriptional program that stimulates mitochondrial glutaminolysis and leads to glutamine addiction. *Proc Natl Acad Sci U S A* 2008;105:18782-18787.

Wong KK, Engelman JA, Cantley LC. Targeting the PI3K signaling pathway in cancer. *Curr Opin Genet Dev* 2010;20:87-90.

Wouters Koritzinsky BGM. Hypoxia signalling through mTOR and the unfolded protein response in cancer. *Nat Rev Cancer* 2008;8:851-864.

Wouters BG, Koritzinsky M. Hypoxia signalling through mTOR and the unfolded protein response in cancer. *Nature reviews. Cancer* 2008;8:851-864.

Yamagata M, Hasuda K, Stamato T, et al. The contribution of lactic acid to acidification of tumours: studies of variant cells lacking lactate dehydrogenase. *Br J Cancer* 1998;77:1726-1731.

Yan L, Vatner DE, Kim SJ, et al. Autophagy in chronically ischemic myocardium. *Proc Natl Acad Sci U S A* 2005;102:13807-13812.

CHAPTER 13

Heterogeneity in Cancer: The "Cancer Stem Cell" Hypothesis

Craig Gedye

13.1 INTRODUCTION: CAN WE IDENTIFY THE CANCER CELLS THAT KILL PATIENTS?

Every patient's cancer is different. Cancers arising from the same organ have different histology and metastatic proclivity, are more or less aggressive, and have different responses to therapy. There are many interdependent mechanisms and dimensions of heterogeneity that account for this variability between cancers. There is also heterogeneity within individual cancers, between stromal cells with a normal genome and mutated malignant cells, between differently mutated malignant clones, between epigenetically different subpopulations within clonal populations, and between cells within different microenvironments within the tumor (Fig. 13–1; see Chap. 12, Sec. 12.2). Recognition of this heterogeneity gives rise to the intriguing possibility that a subset of cancer cells are resistant to treatment, may cause primary tumor recurrence or seed distant metastasis, and may be identifiable a priori. A surgeon's concern in ensuring complete resection of primary tumors ("negative margins") where more invasive cancer cells may reside, the prognostic relevance of circulating tumor cells (see Chap. 10, Sec. 10.3.4), and the resistance of disseminated micrometastases to adjuvant chemotherapy are phenomena that might be explained by "special" cells within a cancer, so-called cancer stem cells, cells that must be targeted to achieve long-term remission or cure. The cancer stem cell (CSC) hypothesis states that only a minority of cancer cells has the potential to (a) self-renew, (b) proliferate indefinitely, and (c) differentiate to give rise to more differentiated tumor cells (Reya et al, 2001). This chapter addresses the competing models that attempt to account for this epigenetic heterogeneity, led by the CSC hypothesis, but first describes the stromal and genetic heterogeneity of human cancers.

13.2 HETEROGENEITY IN CANCER

13.2.1 Stromal Heterogeneity in Cancer

Every seed needs appropriate soil to germinate and grow, and all cancers have a stromal component that supports, and often protects, malignant cells. Cancer cells recruit, manipulate, and nurture this microenvironment to establish and maintain their nutrition and survival. Stromal cells include endothelial cells that line tumor blood vessels and lymphatics; pericytes to support mature endothelium in larger vessels; cancer-associated fibroblasts that both provide physical scaffolding and interact with and influence malignant cells; and tumor-associated macrophages, lymphocytes, and other leucocytes. Cancer-associated fibroblasts produce

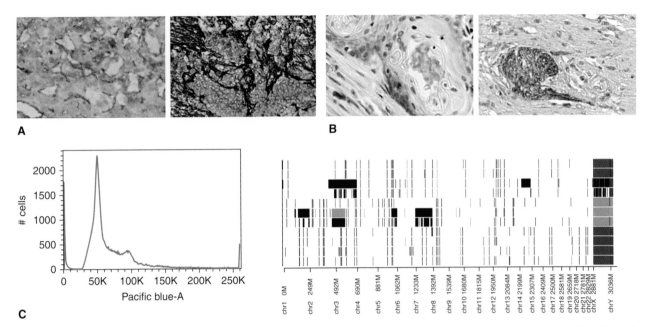

FIGURE 13–1 **Cancers are heterogeneous.** This heterogeneity must be represented and considered in many interdependent dimensions. For example, (**A**) cancers show stromal heterogeneity as many cells within cancers are nonmalignant (*left*, CD31+ endothelial cells (brown) in renal carcinoma; *right*, collagen-positive fibroblasts (brown) in ovarian carcinoma), (**B**) epigenetic heterogeneity, where malignant cells have different phenotypes that can be associated with different functional behaviors (*left*, CD44+ cells (brown) in head and neck carcinoma; *right*, N-cadherin–positive cells (brown) in colorectal carcinoma), and (**C**) genetic heterogeneity, where different clonal populations within cancer have different genomic mutations (*left*, distribution of cells with different DNA content analyzed by flow cytometry (Pacific blue-A staining is proportional to DNA content); *right*, DNA microarray showing gains (blue, green) and losses (orange, red) of DNA across different chromosomes (X-axis), which shows the "copy-number variation" against the normal human genome (background white).

an extracellular matrix (ECM) consisting of collagen and various other molecules (see Chap. 10, Sec. 10.2.1). The stromal component of a tumor can be sparse, for example, in melanoma or large cell lymphomas where the malignant population dominates, or profuse, such as in pancreatic adenocarcinoma, which is typically dominated by a thick fibrous stroma. At the extreme is Hodgkin lymphoma, where rare malignant Reed-Sternberg cells sit isolated in a sea of reactive inflammatory cells (Fig. 13–2). This variability in the tumor microenvironment influences the effectiveness of cancer treatments and may itself be a legitimate target of cancer treatment (see Chap. 19, Sec. 19.3). It also raises the prospect that CSCs may be treatable by influencing their interaction with the stromal niche (see Sec. 13.5.3).

13.2.2 Genetic Heterogeneity in Cancer

Most cancers contain multiple identifiable mutations in their cells. Genetic heterogeneity between different patients' cancers is believed to be a major determinant of variable histology and of clinical behavior. For example, patients with microsatellite instability in colorectal carcinoma may have a better prognosis, but conversely, their tumors may be more unresponsive to chemotherapy. This may occur because microsatellite unstable tumors tend to have more mutations than other colorectal cancers (Kucherlapati et al, 2012), and this greater genetic complexity may allow for a more adaptable genetic evolution when exposed to the selection pressure of

chemotherapy. The different driver mutations in individual patients' cancers are becoming important in selecting treatment—examples include the selective use of hormonal agents and human epidermal growth receptor (HER)-2–targeted therapies in subgroups of women with breast cancer, and the use of BRAF and c-KIT inhibitors in different subsets of melanoma (see Chap. 7, Sec. 7.5).

Individual cancers are thought to arise from the sequential acquisition of multiple mutations, each, in turn, conferring a survival advantage to a clonal population of cells, an evolutionary process first proposed by Nowell (1976) (see Chap. 10, Sec. 10.1.1). This process has perhaps best been documented in colorectal cancer where the transition from adenoma to dysplastic adenoma to carcinoma to invasive and metastatic carcinoma has been shown to parallel the acquisition of mutations in genes such as *APC, K-RAS, PI3KCA,* and *TP53* (Jones et al, 2008). This progression is almost certainly a stochastic process as many different genetic clones can be identified in the premalignant lesions associated with various cancers, for example, in melanoma, renal cell carcinoma, colorectal carcinoma, and pancreatic carcinoma (Campbell et al, 2010). The evolution of intratumoral cancer clones may not be sequential; for example, multiple genetically distinct leukemia-initiating cell subclones have been demonstrated in children with acute lymphoblastic leukemia. These diverse clones have differing abilities to generate xenografts, and if the dominant subclone is capable of growth in the mouse microenvironment, this portends a

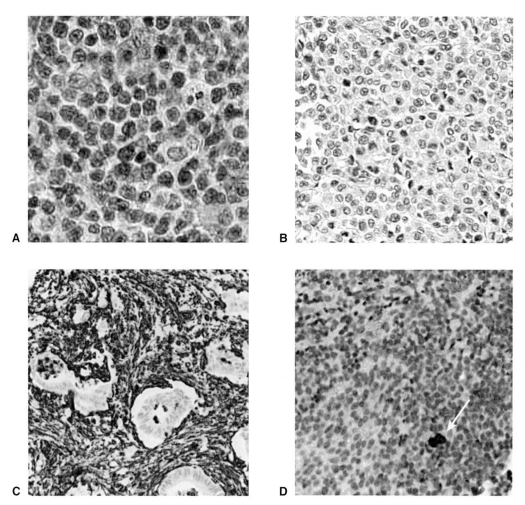

FIGURE 13–2 Different cancers have different stromal microenvironment. For example, in large cell lymphoma (**A**) and melanoma (**B**) the cancer exists as sheets of tumor cells, with few stromal cells present. In contrast, some cancers have a dense infiltrate of genomically normal fibroblasts or leucocytes (**C**), pancreatic adenocarcinoma with stroma stained brown) and Hodgkin lymphoma (**D**), with rare malignant Reed-Sternberg cell stained for the cell surface marker CD15 [arrow]).

poor clinical outcome (Notta et al, 2011). With the advent of faster, cheaper, and more detailed DNA sequencing (see Chap. 2, Sec. 2.2.10), rarer clonal populations can be identified in many cancers (Fig. 13–3). Rapid sequencing of thousands of single cancer cells has identified various clonal patterns in breast carcinoma, including very small clonal populations with highly aberrant genomes (Navin and Hicks, 2011). There is also evidence that as cancers progress to an advanced stage that a dominant clone usually predominates within the primary tumor and in metastases, presumably as a result of a process of genetic selection. In men with metastatic hormone-refractory prostate cancer, for example, examination of the cancer genome performed by single-nucleotide polymorphisms in DNA microarrays of the in situ primary and multiple bone metastases showed that most cancers were monoclonal across all sites (Liu et al, 2009). Whether cancer progression, treatment resistance, and clinical failure are caused by properties inherent in the dominant clone or by outgrowth and rapid selection of rarer subclones, is likely to be variable but of critical importance to each cancer patient's management.

13.2.3 Intratumoral Epigenetic Heterogeneity

Although mature cancers often contain a dominant clone of malignant cells, the properties of individual malignant cells in this clone may be variable. These properties are governed by epigenetic changes that influence the expression of genes within the common genome (see Chap. 2, Sec. 2.3) and by microenvironmental influences (see Chap. 12, Sec. 12.2).

Well-established, clinically apparent cancers represent a relatively late stage in the development of a malignancy. Each gram of cancer may contain half a billion cancer cells, and may shed large numbers of cancer cells into the blood circulation each day. Evidence that only a small proportion of these mobilized tumor cells leads to clinical metastases (see Chap. 10, Sec. 10.3.3) begs the question whether all cancer cells have equivalent potential to form metastases given the appropriate microenvironment (a stochastic process), or whether different cancer cells have intrinsically different self-renewal and differentiation potentials (ie, whether there is an intratumoral hierarchy (Fig. 13–4). Many theories have been

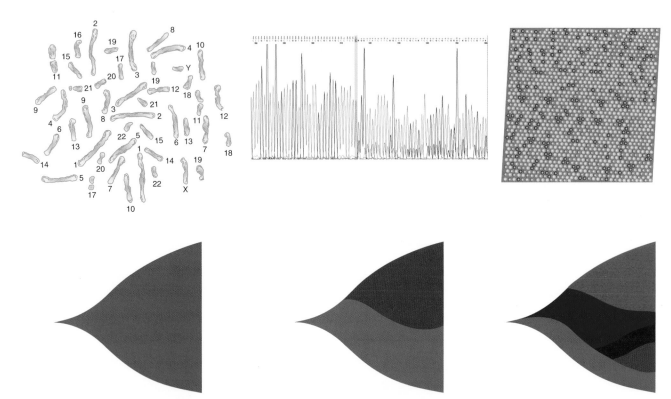

FIGURE 13–3 **Increasingly detailed genomic data from successive generations of DNA sequencing technology reveal the clonal structure of cancer cell populations.** Early techniques, such as karyotyping, allowed recognition of large chromosomal changes, while single base pair sequencing showed the primary sequence of these and other mutations. Second- and third-generation technologies, such as pyrosequencing and bridge amplification ("next-gen sequencing" where every nucleotide base-pair is individually digitally counted by changes in red, blue or green fluorescence), allow "deep" sequencing to detect rare clones (represented in different colors here to show their outgrowth and evolution from previous clones) within tumor cell populations, and even parallel sequencing of single cancer cell clones.

proposed to account for this epigenetic heterogeneity but 2 are dominant: (a) stochastic production of tumor cells with different properties, often linked with evidence of epithelial-to-mesenchymal transition (EMT) and (b) the hierarchical CSC hypothesis. The main focus of this chapter is on the CSC hypothesis, but it first discusses EMT.

13.3 EPITHELIAL-TO-MESENCHYMAL TRANSITION

EMT is a process that is described in a variety of biological scenarios to account for the ability of cells to transdifferentiate from one morphology and function to another, specifically

FIGURE 13–4 **Two mutually exclusive theories can be proposed to account for epigenetic tumor heterogeneity.** **A)** Every cancer cell might have the potential to self-renew (circular arrow) to maintain the primary tumor or form a new metastasis, if it receives appropriate microenvironmental signals. Tumor maintenance or dissemination is therefore a random or stochastic process, and variation between different behaviors may involve transition to and from epithelial to mesenchymal phenotypes. **B)** Conversely, cancers may be organized hierarchically in a disordered parody of normal stem cell hierarchies, where only a subpopulation of CSCs has the potential to self-renew, proliferate extensively, and differentiate to form the bulk of the tumor consisting of non–stem cancer cells with a terminally differentiated phenotype. By definition, non–stem cells cannot dedifferentiate to CSC.

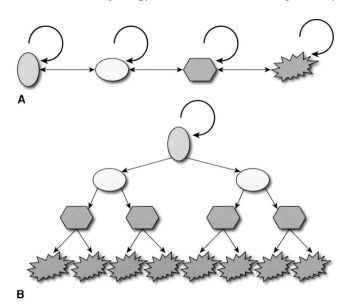

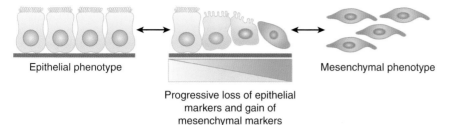

FIGURE 13–5 **The EMT describes the process of transformation of cells with a polarized, epithelial phenotype to cells with a motile, mesenchymal phenotype.** This process is thought to occur during normal development and wound healing, and there is increasing evidence that similar processes occur in cancer. (Adapted from Kalluri and Weinberg, 2009.)

to transform from a polarized epithelial phenotype to a motile, mesenchymal cell phenotype (Kalluri and Weinberg, 2009) (Fig. 13–5; see also Chap. 10, Sec. 10.5.6). The reverse of this process is termed mesenchymal-to-epithelial transition (MET), and both processes occur in embryogenesis and wound healing and are proposed to occur in cancer.

EMT has been studied in many in vitro and model systems and involves molecular events that give rise to morphological and functional alterations of cell behavior. Through the influence of extracellular signals from molecules such as transforming growth factor (TGF)-β, Wnt, and platelet-derived growth factor (PDGF) (see Chap. 8, Sec. 8.4), cells with a polarized epithelial phenotype upregulate the expression of proteins and molecules that drive the cell to reorganize its cytoskeleton (eg, desmin), disconnect from underlying ECM (eg, metalloproteinases), and migrate through the local environment or more distally via vascular channels (eg, vimentin; see Chap. 10, Sec. 10.5).

EMT is thought to occur in at least 3 situations: embryogenesis, wound healing, and malignancy. EMT might occur in cancer because mutated cancer cells may be more easily influenced by microenvironmental signals, as receptors for these molecules may be overexpressed, and downstream signaling pathways may be constitutively activated by the acquisition of further mutations. Many aspects of EMT have been translated from development and wound healing to cancer biology, but there is criticism of the EMT concept as it applies to malignancy, because much of the evidence is based on mouse models, in vitro experiments, and correlative pathological studies (Tarin, 2005).

Evidence for EMT in cancer includes the observation that cultured human epithelial cancer cells can express markers of EMT, such as loss of E-cadherin expression, and upregulation of expression of N-cadherin, smooth muscle actin, vimentin, TWIST, SNAIL, and S100A4. Cancer cells expressing these markers can be found at the "leading edge" of patients' tumors during histopathology, and are thus hypothesized to account for the population of cancer cells that can be shed into the circulation and become metastatic (Brabletz et al, 2001; see also Chap. 10, Sec. 10.5), and this phenomenon has been directly observed in xenograft models (Stoletov et al, 2010). There is also clinical evidence for the relevance of EMT in cancer. For example, markers of EMT are associated with poor prognosis in gastric carcinoma (Ryu et al, 2012), renal cell carcinoma (Mikami et al, 2011), breast carcinoma (Nes et al, 2012), and non–small cell lung carcinoma

(Hung et al, 2009). Expression of EMT markers in cancer cells is also associated with resistance to treatment, including cytotoxic chemotherapy, hormonal agents, and drugs targeting growth factor signaling pathways such as epidermal growth factor (EGF) and HER2. It is unclear if EMT can be targeted to improve cancer management, but several studies suggest that targeting microRNAs (see Chap. 2, Sec. 2.4.3) associated with EMT (such as the miR-200 family) may assist in differentiating mesenchymal-phenotype cancer cells to epithelial-phenotype cells, which may then be more susceptible to chemotherapy (Wang, Li et al, 2010).

13.4 CANCER STEM CELLS

13.4.1 The Cancer Stem Cell Hypothesis

The CSC model posits that a hierarchy exists within each individual patient's cancer, such that only a subset of malignant cells has the potential to self-renew, proliferate extensively, and differentiate to recapitulate the primary tumor's morphological and antigenic heterogeneity (Ailles and Weissman, 2007). Conversely cancer "non–stem cells" may retain some limited proliferative potential but do not to have the ability to propagate the primary tumor or seed distant metastases. The CSC model essentially represents tumors as caricatures of renewing tissues, such as the bone marrow, intestine, and skin, where it is well established that a limited number of stem cells has the capacity to self-renew and to produce progeny that differentiate and carry out the normal function of that tissue (see Chap. 12, Sec. 12.1.3). When applied to cancer, the CSC hypothesis has important implications: If only a subset of cells within a tumor is able to repopulate or seed fresh cancers, then these cells are the true targets for therapy, and if current therapies fail to eliminate these cells, then even apparent complete clinical responses will be noncurative. Instead of a cancer being compared to an infection such as an abscess, where all bacteria must be eliminated to cure an infection, cancer may be viewed rather like the organizational hierarchy of a beehive, with a queen bee, workers, and drones; only survival of the queen bee will allow reestablishment of the colony. Not every CSC is fated to form a new metastasis (Shackleton et al, 2009). CSC remain subject to the influence of the stromal microenvironment, for example to the degree of vascularization or local hypoxia, to the ambient pH and composition of the ECM. For example, although the murine melanoma cell line B16 is an aggressive cancer model where almost every cell is functionally a CSC, only 1 in 100 cells can survive to form metastases in an intravenous metastasis model (Luzzi et al, 1998).

There is controversy regarding the CSC hypothesis, in part because of misconceptions about the model. First, the CSC hypothesis does not imply that somatic stem cells in the corresponding normal tissue are necessarily the cells-of-origin for cancer. Somatic stem and progenitor cells are likely to be the cell-of-origin in some (perhaps most) cancers (eg, medulloblastoma, germ cell tumors), but some terminally differentiated cells, which can be much longer-lived than previously assumed (Rawlins and Hogan, 2008), may have sufficient time to acquire oncogenic mutations in a stepwise fashion, allowing them to evade apoptosis and senescence, proliferate independently of microenvironmental signals, and reactivate their self-renewal potential. The variation in histology, differentiation, and phenotype in cancers arising from a single tissue may be partly a result of different cells of origin. Second, the expression in cancer of genes and pathways that are expressed and active in embryonic stem cells and normal somatic stem cells, such as OCT4 (octamer-binding transcription factor 4, also known as POU5F1), NANOG, BMI1 (BMI1 polycomb ring finger oncogene), and the Hedgehog, NOTCH, and WNT signaling pathways (see Chap. 8, Sec. 8.4) is not proof of the existence of "cancer stem cells." Their reexpression in cancer most likely reflects the parsimonious use of molecular programs useful for self-renewal, asymmetric cell division, dormancy, migration/metastasis, proliferation,

and differentiation, which are properties of both somatic stem cells and cancer cells (Table 13–1). Expression of these "stemness" genes has been invoked in other models of epigenetic heterogeneity in cancer, such as BMI1 in EMT (Yang et al, 2010), and their presence does not imply a hierarchical organization in cancer.

The CSC hypothesis and other models based on epigenetic mechanisms of heterogeneity are not mutually exclusive. As much of the experimental data to support the existence of CSCs is based on samples taken from "late" clinical human cancers, it is difficult to determine whether the CSC hypothesis can account for events within early carcinogenesis. Stromal, epigenetic, and genetic mechanisms of tumor heterogeneity are likely to be involved in every clinical cancer. Unraveling the interconnections between these different mechanisms is an important challenge in cancer research.

13.4.2 Historical Perspective of the CSC Hypothesis

Paget's recognition that metastases "seed" into organs that provide a fertile "soil" provided the conceptual framework that tumor cells must interact with their microenvironment, and that some tumor cells may be more fit than others for this process (Paget, 1889). Pierce and his colleagues demonstrated that teratocarcinomas and mouse squamous cell carcinomas contained highly tumorigenic cells that could differentiate into morphologically differentiated cell types that were unable to form tumors when transplanted in

TABLE 13–1 Shared signaling pathways in stem cells, cancer, and cancer stem cells.

Pathway	Stem Cell	Cancer	Cancer Stem Cell
BMI1	Self-renewal of HSC and neural stem cells	Upregulated in AML and overexpressed in medulloblastoma	Overexpressed in, and induces self-renewal of leukemic stem cells (Lessard and Sauvageau, 2003)
Hedgehog pathway	Maintenance of HSC, development of skin, postnatal and adult brain	Implicated in basal cell carcinoma and medulloblastoma	Regulates self-renewal and tumorigenicity in glioma and myeloma (Peacock et al, 2007)
WNT signaling pathway	Maintenance of HSC and normal intestinal epithelial cells	WNT overexpressed in many human cancers	β-CATENIN loss reduces self-renewal of normal and CML stem cells (Zhao et al, 2007)
NOTCH signaling pathway	Self-renewal of HSC and neural stem cells	Mutation or aberrant activation of NOTCH1 cause T-ALL in humans	NOTCH pathway inhibition depletes stem-like cells in glioblastoma (Fan et al, 2010)
HOX gene family	Self-renewal, proliferation and differentiation of HSC	Prognostic marker in AML, described in T-ALL and drives leukemogenesis in a murine model	MEIS1 regulates MLL leukemia stem cell potential and hierarchy (Somervaille et al, 2009)
SOX gene family	Pivotal regulators of developmental programs such as fate determination and differentiation	Expressed in many cancers	Controls growth and metastasis in lung cancer stem cells (Xiang et al, 2011)
NANOG	Regulator of self-renewal in embryonic stem cells	Expressed in many cancers	Promotes stem-like behavior in androgen-resistant prostate cancer stem cells (Jeter et al, 2009)
TGF-β	Activin and Nodal necessary for pluripotency	Accelerator to break cell-cycle regulation; pivotal to EMT and metastasis	Inhibition of differentiation and tumorigenesis (Piccirillo et al, 2006) by glioma stem cells

Abbreviations: AML, acute myeloid leukemia; CML, chronic myeloid leukemia; EMT, epithelial-to-mesenchymal transition; HSC, hematopoietic stem cell; T-ALL, T-cell lymphocytic leukemia. Genes: BMI1, BMI1 polycomb ring finger oncogene; HOX, homeobox genes; TGF-β, transforming growth factor beta.

mice (Pierce and Wallace, 1971). He described cancers as a "caricature" of normal tissue renewal, whereby tumor stem cells divide and differentiate giving rise to terminal post-mitotic differentiated cells (Pierce and Speers, 1988). Till and McCulloch provided the first experimental evidence of normal tissue stem cells (Till and McCulloch, 1961), when they injected lethally irradiated mice with donor mouse bone marrow to determine the minimum number of cells required to repopulate the marrow of the recipient mouse. Colonies of cells from all 3 blood lineages were seen to form in the spleen and bone marrow of recipient mice. When these single-cell-derived colonies were subsequently transplanted into secondary recipient mice, some clones could again give rise to blood cells from multiple lineages. A frankly unethical experiment from the 1950s provided the first clinical evidence that tumor formation is limited to a subpopulation of human cancer cells. Cancer cells from patients with ovarian, cervical, and uterine cancer were cultured in vitro following palliative surgery and reinjected into the same patient subcutaneously (Brunschwig et al, 1965). Even when a million cancer cells were implanted, only approximately 50% of these injections developed into a palpable nodule. Hamburger and Salmon (1977) demonstrated in clonogenic assays that only a fraction of cells from freshly excised human tumors could form colonies in tissue culture (including myeloma, lymphoma, neuroblastoma, ovarian carcinoma, chronic lymphocytic leukemia, small cell lung cancer, and melanoma). This result led the authors to speculate that these rare clonogenic cells had been tumor stem cells in vivo, although their results might have been caused by an inadequate environment to support growth in tissue culture. Other scientists demonstrated that only a fraction of mouse lymphoma cells were capable of forming colonies in an irradiated mouse (Bruce and Van Der Gaag, 1963). Hewitt (1979) also demonstrated that large numbers of cells were needed to transplant spontaneously arising murine tumors into syngeneic mice, again implying that the putative CSC was rare.

13.4.3 Methods Used to Study Cancer Stem Cells

CSCs are defined both by their ability to generate tumors upon serial transplantation in immune-deficient animals (ie, high reproductive capacity) and by their ability to recapitulate the genetic and phenotypic heterogeneity of the original tumor (Fig. 13–6). The proposed CSC subpopulation should demonstrate potent tumor initiation by regenerating the tumor when a limited number of cancer cells are injected. Evidence for CSC self-renewal is obtained by observing xenograft formation after serially transplanting reisolated CSC into secondary and tertiary recipient mice. At each stage, larger doses of marker-negative, cancer "non–stem cells" (eg, CD133$^-$ or CD44$^-$; see below) should fail to engraft in mice. The second criterion is that the injected CSC must differentiate and recapitulate the phenotype of the tumor from which they were derived, although multilineage differentiation as seen in normal somatic stem cells is not a requirement for transplanted cells to be labeled as CSC. Based on the above properties, CSC are defined functionally as tumor-initiating cells (TICs), xenograft-initiating cells, or cancer-initiating cells.

CSCs must be identifiable a priori, and a variety of markers can be used to separate cancer and normal cells, many of which are cell-surface proteins. CSC markers have been discovered by trial and error, but have frequently been translated from normal stem cell biology to the cancer setting. For example CD133 (prominin-1 [PROM1]) is a marker for neural stem cells and has been applied to neuroectodermal tumors such as glioblastoma (Lenkiewicz et al, 2009). Cancer cells are usually obtained from solid human tumors donated by patients immediately after their surgical removal. Tumors are usually mechanically disaggregated, then digested to a single cell suspension by use of enzymes such as collagenase, hyaluronidase and DNase (Ailles et al, 2009). The resulting single-cell suspension can be examined by flow cytometry, cultured briefly in vitro, or injected into

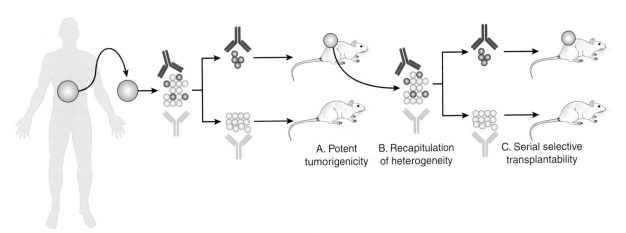

FIGURE 13–6 The CSC hypothesis is tested experimentally using the serial xenotransplantation assay. CSCs are functionally defined by their ability to **(A)** potently initiate xenograft tumors in immunocompromised mice, which **(B)** recapitulate the heterogeneity and phenotype of the original patient tumor, and upon reisolation from the xenograft **(C)** retain this selective tumorigenicity in serial xenograft experiments.

A. Potent tumorigenicity   B. Recapitulation of heterogeneity   C. Serial selective transplantability

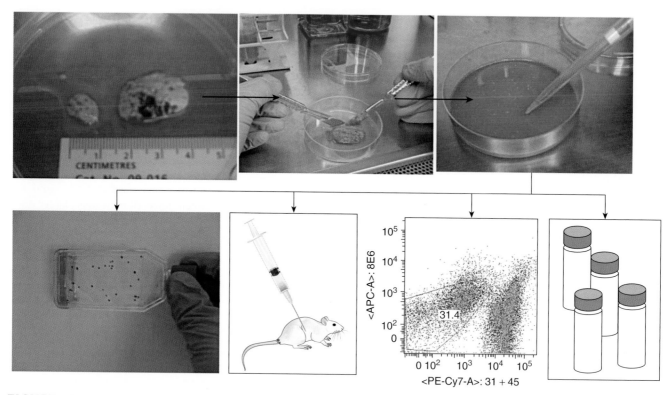

FIGURE 13–7 **Methods to study the CSC hypothesis in solid tumors.** Cancer samples are mechanically dissociated and then enzymatically digested and filtered to generate a suspension of single cells. This single cell suspension can be used for a variety of experiments, for example, to establish new cancer cell lines, to measure the tumor-forming ability of these cancer cells by injection into immunocompromised mice, or analysis by flow cytometry (in this example ~30% of cells are cancer cells, while ~70% of cells express hematopoietic, endothelial or fibroblast markers). Finally, cells can be saved for later use by cryogenic freezing.

immunocompromised mice (Fig. 13–7). Flow cytometry uses fluorescently labeled antibodies to measure semiquantitatively proteins and antigens on intact cells. Viable cells can also be sorted (fluorescence-activated cell sorting [FACS]) into different subpopulations (Alexander et al, 2009). For example stromal cells in tumors can be obtained by sorting CD45+ hematopoietic cells or CD31+ endothelial cells. From the remaining cancer cells one may then identify a population of cells suspected of being CSCs, for example, by selecting CD133+ cells (Fig. 13–8). Magnetic cell separation uses antibodies conjugated to tiny paramagnetic beads, which allow cells to be physically separated in a high magnetic field (Palmon et al, 2012). Cell function and behavior can also be used to identify CSC. For example, the "side-population" method takes advantage of the ability of normal stem cells and CSC to efflux water -soluble fluorescent dyes such as Hoechst 33342. More dormant, slow-cycling, infrequently dividing cells can be identified by staining a cell population with lipophilic fluorescent dyes, such as PKH26, then selecting fluorescent cells after a period of time in culture; CSC are thought to be less likely to divide and are therefore brighter. Finally, CSC can be isolated using a fluorescent dye that is only liberated inside cancer cells expressing aldehyde dehydrogenases (ALDHs), enzymes that are preferentially expressed in normal and CSCs.

Once cancer cells have been processed, characterized, and segregated, they can then be used for in vivo and in vitro experiments. These experiments can evaluate their ability to form xenografts in mice by limiting dilution assay, and can assess the smallest number of cells injected that are capable of forming a tumor.

Early experiments in stem cell biology used lethally irradiated mice (Till and McCulloch, 1961) to investigate repopulation of normal hematopoietic stem cells of the same inbred strain of mice, but investigation of human cancer cell biology requires immunocompromised mice. Athymic nude mice have been employed as recipients of xenografts since the 1960s, but these mice have residual antitumor immunity because of natural killer (NK) cell activity, and better engraftment is observed using the severe combined immunodeficiency (SCID) mouse that lacks T and B lymphocytes. Improved engraftment was seen when the SCID mouse was crossed with the nonobese diabetic (NOD) mouse model, yielding NOD/SCID mice. These immunocompromised mouse models have been refined further, using mice that have mutation in the Rag2 or interleukin-2 receptor γ chain (IL2Rγ$^{-/-}$) genes or similar mice crossed with the NOD/SCID mouse forming the NOD/SCID/IL2Rγ$^{-/-}$ or NSG mouse, which lack NK-cell activity as well as B- and T-cell activity.

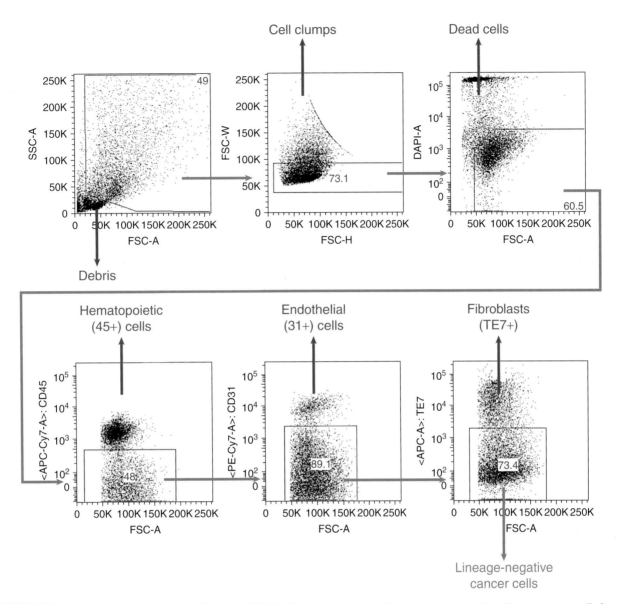

FIGURE 13–8 **Fluorescence-activated cell sorting (FACS) allows the selection of normal stromal and malignant cancer cells from solid tumors and leukemias.** After separating off debris (ie, cells that have clumped together, or cells that are dead), antibodies to cell surface markers, such as CD45 and CD31, can be used to separate hematopoietic and endothelial cells, respectively. Each blue "gate" is a subset of cells from the previous plot. For example, just over half of cells in this sample (bottom left panel) are white blood cells, and of the remaining 48% of cells, ~10% are endothelial cells. Remaining cells that do not express a lineage marker, so-called lineage-negative cells are the remaining cancer cells, from which proposed CSC populations can be selected by markers such as CD133 and CD44. FSC and SSC represent forward scatter and side scatter, optical properties of the cells that help discriminate their size and complexity. DAPI, APC-Cy7, APC, and PE-Cy7 are all fluorescent dyes used to identify different cell populations. Percent of cells in the boxed areas are indicated.

Injections into NOD/SCID or NSG mice are often performed in conjunction with Matrigel, a heterogeneous mixture of basement membrane proteins secreted by mouse sarcoma cells, which enhances tumor transplantability. Whether this enhancement is a result of tumor cell aggregation within a gel or a result of growth factors embedded in the matrix remains unclear, but it does not appear to be caused by collagen or laminin components of the matrix alone. Finally, mouse xenograft experiments can be further refined using various forms of "humanization," either via incorporation of human tissue,

such as fetal bone or adult skin, or the addition of human growth factors.

Although the functional definition of a CSC is assessed via in vivo tumor-forming experiments, surrogate in vitro assays may allow for rapid screening of drug activity and interrogation of signaling pathways in CSCs. There are criticisms of these cell-culture models, particularly as the microenvironment for cancer cells growing in a culture dish is very different to that within the primary tumor. For example, glioblastoma cells grown in bovine serum acquire in vitro mutations that transform them into cell lines with geno-types and phenotypes that do not represent the genotype and phenotype of the patients' tumor (Lee et al, 2006). This property may contribute to the often quite large differences between the phenotypes and genotypes of cell lines derived from human cancers and the ex vivo tumors themselves (van Staveren et al, 2009).

Improvements to these models are evolving. For example, human tumor cells cultured de novo as "tumor spheres" in defined serum-free media (Brewer et al, 1993) can generate cell lines with morphological heterogeneity that express markers of a primitive stem-like phenotype and form xenografts that are invasive and maintain the genotype of the original tumor. Cell lines grown in defined media have been employed to demonstrate the efficacy of targeting glioblastoma stem cells by various stem-cell-signaling pathways, but most of these in vitro models are not well validated in representing properties of CSC (Pollard et al, 2009). Once tumors or cell lines have formed, their genotype, phenotype, and differentiation status must be studied to see that it remains constant with each subsequent passage, and that it represents an accurate reproduction of the original patient's tumor. Flow cytometry, immunohistochemistry, messenger RNA (mRNA) expression by polymerase chain reaction (PCR) or gene expression microarray and genotype by karyotype or copy-number variation microarray are all methods in common use (see Chap. 2).

Finally, techniques to study the epigenetic regulation of CSCs are improving rapidly and should provide further mechanistic data on the validity of the CSC hypothesis (and EMT). Whole-genome methylation arrays, whole-genome histone modification arrays, microRNA, and noncoding RNA arrays are becoming increasingly comprehensive (see Chap. 2, Sec. 2.6.2), and suitable for small samples that are typically available when studying CSCs obtained directly from a patient's tumors.

13.4.4 Cancer Stem Cells in Hematological Malignancies

The renaissance of the CSC hypothesis followed the isolation of leukemia-initiating cells in acute myeloid leukemia (AML) (Lapidot et al, 1994; Fig. 13–9). Leukemic cells from the bone marrow and peripheral blood of patients with AML could be engrafted in SCID mice supplemented with human stem cell factor (SCF) and a human granulocyte-macrophage colony-stimulating factor (GM-CSF) interleukin-3 (IL-3) fusion protein. Some mice developed a morphologically and histochemically identical disease to the original patient. Large doses of AML cells were required for engraftment. In vitro clonogenic assays showed similar rare frequencies (0.3% to 0.9%) of AML colony-forming units (CFUs) in primary patient samples or from AML cells extracted in bone marrow aspirates from transplanted mice, suggesting that the potential to engraft leukemia into SCID mice remained a rare property. The authors then examined the cell-surface phenotype of AML cells using flow cytometry, and discovered that AML cells expressing a phenotype similar to normal human hematopoietic stem cells (CD34++/CD38−) were much more likely to engraft in SCID mice than CD34+/CD38+ or CD34− cells. In more immunocompromised NOD/SCID mice, which have far fewer NK lymphocytes, AML cells could engraft at much lower doses (10- to 20-fold). Using established statistical methods, the SCID leukemia-initiating cell (SL-IC) assay was shown to be reproducible, although there was a wide variation in the SL-IC frequency from different patients, suggesting underlying differences between their leukemias. Subsets of AML cells were again isolated by flow cytometry and injected into

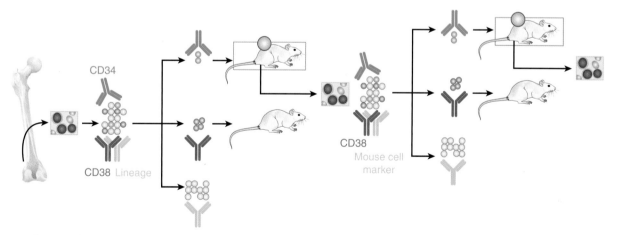

FIGURE 13–9 CSC in hematological cancers. Using cell-surface markers established from normal hematopoietic stem cell biology, leukemic stem cells were discovered in a series of elegant experiments; these leukemic cells were negative for the progenitor cell marker CD38, but expressed the normal stem cell marker CD34. To accurately measure the "stem" and "non-stem" cancer cells, other antibodies (in blue) are used to identify and segregate non-cancerous cells (eg, lymphocytes and macrophages) from the human sample (the "lineage" cells) and mouse cells from the xenografted leukemia sample. Mice that engraft the leukemia are represented here with a purple circle. Cells could be serially passaged through several generations of mice, and maintained the same phenotype and morphology as the leukemia from the original patient.

NOD/SCID mice. CD34[+] cells were able to engraft whereas CD34[-] cells did not, and the CD34[++]/CD38[-] AML subset were highly enriched for SL-IC. As few as 5000 CD34[++]/CD38[-] cells could engraft a NOD/SCID mouse, whereas 5×10^5 CD34[+]/CD38[+] could not. AML cells isolated from mice injected with CD34[++]/CD38[-] leukemia stem cells showed a similar pattern of cell-surface markers (immunophenotype) and similar morphology compared to the original cancer, implying in vivo differentiation of engrafted SL-IC. Finally, evidence of in vivo self-renewal of SL-IC was obtained, showing that CD34[++]/CD38[-] cells could be isolated from primary xenografted animals and transplanted into secondary recipients with similar efficiencies of engraftment and recapitulation of ex vivo phenotype (Lapidot et al, 1994).

Bonnet and Dick (1997) extended these findings by demonstrating that similar to the hierarchy within normal hematopoietic stem cells, that there is a "hierarchy within the hierarchy" of human AML leukemic stem cells (LSCs). Donor AML populations were transfected with a lentivirus encoding green fluorescent protein (GFP). The lentivirus stably incorporates into the genome of individual cells at a random location, and Southern blotting can be used to track this insertion site, thus allowing tracking of each clone in each mouse. This genetically engineered protein was used as a fluorescent marker to separate human AML cells from unmarked mouse cells, and also provided a means of tracking clonal progeny of an individual AML cell through serial xenografts in recipient mice. From serial transplantation of samples from multiple patients into mice, it became apparent that there were several different populations of LSCs, which the authors termed short-term, long-term, and quiescent long-term SL-ICs. In some cases, quiescent SL-IC did not contribute to leukemogenesis until transplanted into a third serial mouse, and after 6 months ex vivo. Clonal tracking demonstrated that long-term SL-IC gave rise to short-term SL-IC, and that quiescent long-term SL-IC gave rise to both short-term and long-term SL-IC, demonstrating a "hierarchy within the hierarchy" and conclusive evidence of CSC within AML. The similarity of this hierarchy to normal hematopoiesis suggests that the cell-of-origin for AML may be a normal hematopoietic stem cell (Hope et al, 2004).

Chronic myeloid leukemia (CML) provides a compelling example of the CSC model in clinical practice. Since the discovery of the oncogenic BCR-ABL translocation (see Chap. 7, Sec. 7.5.1), and the development of small-molecule tyrosine kinase inhibitors such as imatinib (see Chap. 7, Sec 7.7 and Chap. 17, Sec. 17.3.1), survival in this disease has increased substantially. However, despite the rapid disappearance of malignant cells from the blood of patients treated with these agents, there is evidence that CML stem cells remain dormant within the bone marrow, and that a fraction of these CML stem cells are resistant to BCR-ABL inhibition and can undergo further clonal evolution to give rise to blast crisis (Chu et al, 2011).

CSCs have proven more challenging to study in other hematological malignancies, such as lymphomas and myeloma. This may be related to the broad heterogeneity in genetic,

histochemical, and clinical subtypes in lymphoma, and perhaps also because of the fastidiousness of these cancers for their microenvironment. For example, addition of a humanized microenvironment improves engraftment and growth of human myeloma in immunocompromised mouse models, perhaps by providing an appropriate niche or bone marrow stromal cells that can secrete supportive human cytokines (Tassone et al, 2005).

13.4.5 Cancer Stem Cells in Solid Tumors

CSCs have been identified in many solid cancers, including squamous cell carcinoma of the head and neck (Prince et al, 2007), colorectal cancer (Dalerba et al, 2007; O'Brien et al, 2007; Ricci-Vitiani et al, 2007), pancreatic carcinoma (Hermann et al, 2007; Li et al, 2007), hepatocellular carcinoma (Ma et al, 2007; Yang et al, 2008), ovarian carcinoma (Zhang et al, 2008; Stewart et al, 2011), and prostate carcinoma (Collins et al, 2005; Patrawala et al, 2006), as well as cancers of the breast, brain, and melanoma that are discussed in detail below (Fig. 13–10).

13.4.5.1 Breast Cancer Breast CSCs were the first to be identified in a solid malignancy (Al-Hajj et al, 2003). Cells from 8 patients with metastatic pleural effusions and from 1 primary breast cancer were either FACS sorted or passaged through mice and sorted from xenografts. These sorted cell populations were orthotopically implanted in the mammary fat pad of female, estrogen-supplemented NOD/SCID mice that had been further immunocompromised by treatment with etoposide. The authors describe 3 series of experiments, refining the selected cell population at each step. Initially, the authors separated cells on the basis of CD44, CD24, and epithelial cell adhesion molecule (EpCAM), showing that CD44[+], EpCAM[+], and CD24[-] cell populations were all more tumorigenic than CD44[-], EpCAM[-], and CD24[+] populations at cell doses of 2 to 8×10^5 cells. Dead cells were excluded with a fluorescent-soluble viability dye. Mouse cells in xenografted tumors were depleted by using anti-H2K[d] (mouse major histocompatibility class) antibody, and the populations were enriched for tumor cells by sorting and discarding cells expressing "lineage" markers such as CD2, CD3, CD10, CD16, CD18, CD31, CD64, and CD140b, which are expressed on lymphocytes, NK cells, monocytes, B cells, endothelial cells, and fibroblasts. Within the remaining "lineage-negative" cells a CD44[+]/CD24[-] population was found in all tumors, ranging from 11% to 35% of cells (median: 15%) that was highly enriched (10- to 50-fold) for tumor-forming ability versus CD44[+]/CD24[+/-] cells (Fig. 13–10A). In a final round of purification in 3 tumors, the EpCAM[+]/CD44[+]/CD24[-]/Lineage[-] cell population (0.5% to 2.5% of all cancer cells) was found to be enriched more than 50-fold for tumor-forming cells, and as few as 200 cells could form a tumor when injected into the immunocompromised mice.

The authors demonstrated that tumor-forming potential was not related to cell cycle (ruling out brisker proliferation),

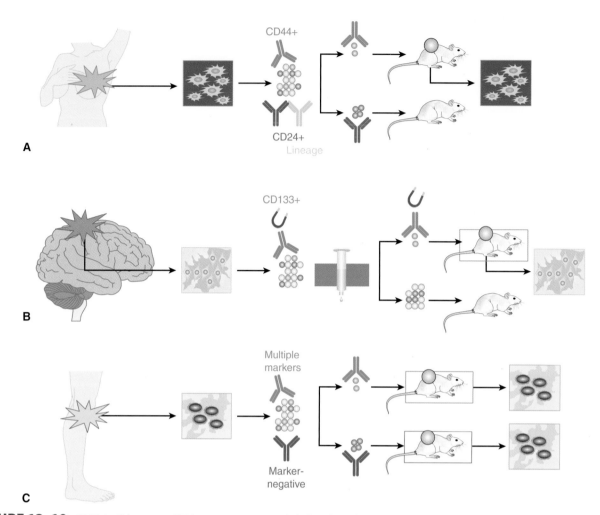

FIGURE 13–10 CSC in solid tumors. **A)** Lineage-negative, epithelial marker-positive, CD44⁺, and CD24⁻ breast cancer stem cells can form xenografts in the mouse mammary fat pad. **B)** Magnetically separated CD133⁺ glioma stem cells orthotopically implanted into mouse brain can recapitulate human glioma xenograft complexity; CD133⁻ cells cannot. **C)** Although several CSC markers had been proposed in melanoma, a systematic examination of 22 heterogenously expressed markers in melanoma failed to discover a marker that could enrich the already very frequent tumorigenic cells in melanoma; almost all malignant cells in melanoma appear to be CSCs.

and showed that tumors derived from this highly selected sub-population gave rise to a heterogeneous xenograft with similar characteristics and cellular markers to the primary human tumor. Finally, the authors demonstrated in vivo self-renewal of CD44⁺/CD24⁻/Lineage⁻ tumor-forming cells from 3 tumors that were able to be serially transplanted through multiple mice, yielding similar heterogeneous xenografts at each passage with no evidence of decreased ability to generate tumors.

13.4.5.2 Brain Tumors CSCs were next characterized in the brain tumors, glioblastoma and medulloblastoma (Singh et al, 2003; Singh et al, 2004). Freshly excised tumors from adults and children were cultured in chemically defined serum-free neural stem cell (NSC) media (Reynolds and Weiss, 1992); all tumors grew nonadherently as neurosphere-like clusters, and the rate of sphere formation and subsequent proliferation was proportional to the grade of the tumor. In vitro self-renewal was measured by assessing the rate of secondary sphere

formation in a limiting dilution assay; clonogenicity, the ability to form a new colony, again matched tumor grade. Karyotyping revealed that sphere-forming cells had an abnormal phenotype, thus excluding contaminating NSCs. CD133 was selected as a putative marker for brain CSCs as it had been used as a marker to select normal brain stem cells (Uchida et al, 2000). CD133⁺ cells were isolated from glioblastoma serum-free nonadherent cell cultures using magnetic bead separation (Fig. 13–10B). CD133⁺ cells were highly clonogenic compared to CD133⁻ cells, and showed higher proliferation and sphere formation at limiting dilutions of cells. In primary tumor specimens, CD133⁺ cells accounted for between 6% and 45% of all cells. Sphere-forming cells were exposed briefly to fetal calf serum to induce differentiation, and the phenotype of each cell line roughly matched the differentiation profile of the primary tumor, suggesting that the CD133⁺ stem-like cells within these glioblastoma and medulloblastoma serum-free cell lines could differentiate to recapitulate the phenotype of the original patient's tumor.

In subsequent work CD133+ (5.7% to 28.8%) and CD133− cells isolated directly from freshly excised human medulloblastomas and glioblastomas were injected orthotopically into the brains of NOD/SCID mice at decreasing doses of cells (ie, at limiting dilution). Tumors developed in 16 of 19 mice injected with CD133+ cells, some from injection of as few as 100 CD133+ cells. Injections of up to 100,000 CD133− cells did not form tumors. Viable CD133− cells could be detected at the injection sites by species-specific pan-centromeric probes, showing that CD133− cancer cells could survive but not form tumors. The tumors arising from the CD133+ cell injections were excised and examined by immunohistochemistry, showing close resemblance to the primary patient's tumor on the basis of immunophenotype and percentage of CD133 expression. These resected xenografts also showed reproducible karyotypes that were similar to the primary tumors. Taken together these data indicate that these xenografts were derived from the injected human CD133+ cells and had undergone differentiation in vivo to recapitulate the original tumor phenotype. Finally, self-renewal of CD133+ cells was demonstrated in vivo by excision of the tumors derived from CD133+ cells, sorting CD133+ and CD133− cells and injecting these into secondary NOD/SCID-recipient mice. As few as 100 CD133+ cells could regenerate a tumor similar to the primary tumor, whereas CD133− cells could not.

Other studies have indicated that CD133 may not mark a CSC population within every glioblastoma. Two groups reported on glioma cell lines established in serum-free stem cell media showing that some glioma lines contained CD133+ cells, while other lines were completely negative for CD133 expression (Beier et al, 2007; Gunther et al, 2008). CD133− glioma lines tended to grow more slowly in vitro and in vivo and had a different gene expression profile compared to CD133+ glioma lines. Thus the absence of a putative CSC marker in some cancers does not immediately invalidate the CSC hypothesis, but rather suggests that just as different patients' tumors show different genotypes, they can also demonstrate different patterns of epigenetic heterogeneity. In mouse models of lung cancer, it appears that genetic and epigenetic heterogeneity are intimately linked, where the mouse stem cell marker Sca-1 marked tumor-propagating cells in *K-ras/p53* mutant mouse tumors, but not in *K-ras* mutant tumors, while in EGFR mutant tumors, only the Sca-1-negative cells could form new tumors (Curtis et al, 2010). Finally, there is recent evidence that reexpression of "stemness" programs by reexpression of genes promoting self-renewal such as *MYC*, *OCT4*, and *SOX2*, may induce a degree of reprogramming stress that can lead to increased mutation rates in vitro (Ji et al, 2012). Mathematical modeling also suggests that the presence of a "CSC" population within human tumors allows them to evolve more rapidly, lending them a competitive advantage (Naugler, 2010). These observations hint at the interrelatedness of genetic and epigenetic heterogeneities in human cancers.

13.4.5.3 Melanoma The first isolation of CSCs from patient samples of melanoma was performed using the CD133 and ABCB5 cell-surface markers (Schatton et al, 2008). Melanomas were found to express more ABCB5 than benign melanocytic nevi, thick primary melanomas expressed more than thin primary melanomas, and melanomas metastatic to lymph nodes expressed more ABCB5 than primary lesions, thus suggesting that ABCB5 is a molecular marker of melanoma progression (Kim et al, 2006). ABCB5 staining was found in all 7 fresh melanoma biopsies that were transplanted to form xenografts, and ABCB5 tended to stain areas of xenografts with less melanin. In a limited number of melanoma samples, malignant melanoma-initiating cells (MMICs) marked by ABCB5 expression were demonstrated to be a rare subpopulation in NOD/SCID mice (CSC frequency of ~1/111,000, compared to a tumor-forming frequency of 1 in ~1,000,000 unsorted melanoma cells).

In contrast to the above work, studies by Morrison and colleagues have challenged the existence of melanoma CSCs and the overall relevance of the CSC hypothesis. This group performed similar xenograft experiments in melanoma with 2 additional refinements: they injected melanoma cells mixed with high-concentration Matrigel into more severely immunocompromised mice, the NSG strain that entirely lacks NK cell activity (compared to the NOD/SCID strain in which low NK cell activity is present) (Quintana et al, 2008). The rationale was that these conditions would be most permissive for melanoma xenograft formation. This group found that tumor-forming cells in melanoma were common, such that around 1 in 4 unselected melanoma cells implanted subcutaneously could form a xenograft, and some xenografts were generated after injecting a single melanoma cell per mouse. In further experiments, they demonstrated that melanoma cells sorted for a large panel of markers, such as ABCB5 and CD133, showed equivalent ability to grow into heterogeneous xenografts, expressing both marker-positive and marker-negative cells (Fig. 3–10C; Quintana et al, 2010). Thus no selection by a particular marker, no hierarchy, and thus no "CSC" could be demonstrated in melanoma. Initial experiments used cells from multiply passaged xenografts or from advanced stages III and IV melanoma patients, but this pattern of high tumor-forming ability (the frequency of TICs was ~30%) was maintained even when using single unselected cells isolated from patients with stage II melanomas (Quintana et al, 2010). Thus with sufficient optimization of the xenotransplant model, tumor-forming cells in melanoma were found to be common.

13.4.6 Criticisms of the Cancer Stem Cell Hypothesis

The observation that a xenograft could grow from almost any single unselected melanoma cell led to controversy regarding the validity of the CSC hypothesis, but, in turn, this has focused experimental design and helped drive the field forward. Criticisms of the CSC hypothesis have been discussed in detail elsewhere (Gedye et al, 2011), and can be divided into conceptual, technical, and analytical arguments. First,

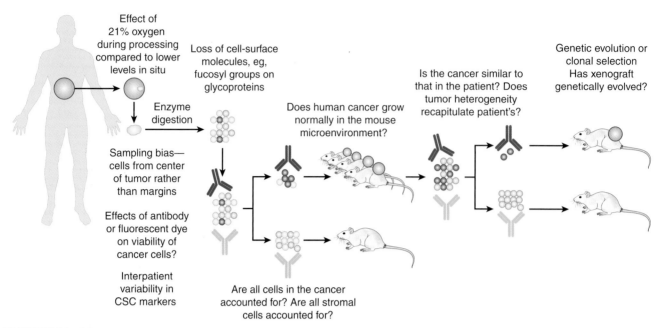

FIGURE 13–11 Technical criticisms of the CSC hypothesis. The "gold-standard" CSC assay of serial xenotransplantation has a number of technical challenges that may introduce bias into observations. Some of these challenges are unavoidable (eg, sampling at the tumor margin may not be clinically appropriate), but many are testable (eg, identifying novel markers for stromal cells, humanizing the murine microenvironment). Addressing these challenges will advance our understanding of tumor heterogeneity, and may or may not support the CSC hypothesis.

the concept of a normal stem cell hierarchy, and by extension a CSC hierarchy, has been challenged by Lander (2009), who pointed out that complex, seemingly hierarchical phenomena can arise from simple rules. The flocking of birds is an excellent example, where only 3 rules specifying separation, direction, and speed are needed to model this complex behavior. Observers also suffer from the cognitive bias of tending to see ordered patterns in random data. Second, there are technical criticisms of the experiments that support the CSC hypothesis, although addressing them is helping to advance the field (Fig. 13–11). For example, after the use of Matrigel and NSG mice in melanoma, many groups reevaluated their models by transplanting tumor cells into NSG mice and found that TICs remain rare in epithelial cancers (Ishizawa et al, 2010) and leukemia (Vargaftig et al, 2012). Other technical objections include the loss of CSC marker expression during tumor dissociation, failure to account for stromal cells such as fibroblasts, and the interspecies difference in tumor microenvironment between mice and humans. Finally, the analysis of CSC experiments has been criticized because mathematical analysis shows that the absolute number of CSCs appears to vary depending upon the context; for example, in some datasets, the absolute number of CSCs in the "negative" cell population outweighs the number in the selected "CSC marker-positive" fraction (Hill 2006; Stewart et al, 2011).

An alternative model for epigenetic heterogeneity is the concept of phenotypic plasticity (Scheel and Weinberg, 2011), where cancer cell populations are in a dynamic equilibrium controlled by epigenetic mechanisms that allow the cells to switch between different cell phenotypes in response to microenvironmental stimuli. For example, in 2 recent

publications studying melanoma and non–small cell lung cancer cell lines, the histone demethylases JARID1A and JARID1B were found to be expressed in a small proportion of cells at any one time (Roesch et al, 2010; Sharma et al, 2010). In melanoma cell lines, KDM5B (also known as JARID1B) was expressed in slow cycling cells lacking expression of the proliferation marker Ki-67, but that showed evidence of stem cell-like properties, such as dye exclusion, label retention, and self-renewal. Knockdown of JARID1B was initially associated with an increase in proliferation, followed by eventual exhaustion of cell growth, suggesting that JARID1B+ cells were necessary for maintenance of the cell line. The expression of JARID1B was not hierarchal; JARID1B+ cells could be derived from JARID1B-negative cells suggesting a dynamic plasticity between cell phenotypes rather than a CSC structure.

In parallel, Sharma et al (2010) found that in cancer cell lines exposed to an EGFR tyrosine kinase inhibitor, gefitinib (see Chap. 17; Sec. 17.3.1), that although most cancer cells rapidly died, a tiny (~0.3%) quiescent subpopulation of "drug-tolerant persister" (DTP) cells survived and gradually began to proliferate. Importantly, cell lines could become drug-sensitive again after growth in the absence of drug, suggesting plasticity in the drug-tolerant phenotype. DTP cells expressed high levels of the histone demethylase KDM5A (also known as JARID1A) and in some cell lines also expressed the CSC marker CD133. Knockdown of KDM5A in these cell lines prevented the epigenetic mechanism of chromatin remodeling and modification, and completely abrogated the survival of the DTP cells. Inhibition of chromatin remodeling by inhibition of histone deacetylation (by the histone deacetylase inhibitor SAHA (suberoylanilide

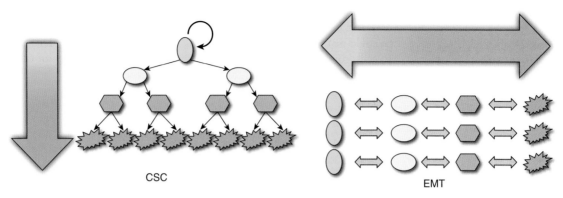

FIGURE 13–12 **CSC and EMT may be 2 sides of the same coin.** Increasing experimental evidence suggests considerable overlap in the cell-surface markers and biological pathways involved. The main difference remains the irreversibility of the hierarchical CSC hypothesis, where stem-like cells proliferate to terminally differentiated postmitotic progeny, whereas there is reversibility implied in the EMT model; cells with a migratory mesenchymal phenotype may take on an epithelial phenotype under the appropriate environmental stimuli.

hydroxamic acid), or by upstream inhibition of insulin-like growth factor signaling) prevent DTP cells from surviving.

Finally, a recent examination of cell phenotypes in genomically normal embryonic stem cell cultures showed the presence of embryonic stem (ES) cells in a so-called super state, where a small (~0.2% to 1.5%) fraction of cells were "totipotent" rather than simply pluripotent (Macfarlan et al, 2012). By fluorescent cell tracking, it could be seen that all cells within the culture had the potential to express this phenotype. Modification of histones, for example, by methylation of histone 3 lysine 4 (H3K4) and acetylation of H3 and H4, was shown to partially control this process, again demonstrating an epigenetic basis for this phenotypic plasticity.

There are, therefore, several competing models to account for epigenetic heterogeneity in normal and malignant tissues. Most biological models have uncertainties and exceptions, and rather than one model being "right" or "wrong," perhaps the CSC hypothesis and EMT models may be interrelated, though the evidence for each model has been approached from different experimental directions. This interrelationship can be exemplified by studies examining CD44+/CD24− cells in breast cancer. CD44+/CD24− breast cancer cells were described initially as breast CSCs (Al-Hajj et al, 2003). Conversely breast cancer cells that were found to be resistant to hormonal therapy (Creighton et al, 2009), chemotherapy (Li et al, 2008), or radiation (Lagadec et al, 2010), that were immunoevasive (Reim et al, 2009) or had undergone EMT (Mani et al, 2008) were found subsequently to express this same cell surface CD44+/CD24− phenotype. EMT and CSC may thus be 2 sides of the same coin (Fig. 13–12), and the mechanisms of histone modification identified in models of phenotypic plasticity might provide a mechanistic model underpinning epigenetic heterogeneity.

13.4.7 Clinical Evidence Supporting the Cancer Stem Cell Hypothesis

Although both the EMT (see Sec. 13.3 and Chap. 10; Sec. 10.5.6) and CSC models can be critiqued at many levels, the true relevance of a biological model lies in its ability to improve understanding of cancer biology and clinical management. A growing body of clinical evidence supports the CSC hypothesis, including the association of CSC phenotypes with clinical outcome and with mechanisms of resistance to therapy. The novel insights afforded by a better understanding of epigenetic heterogeneity are leading to innovations in cancer therapy that are being tested in the clinic.

The CSC phenotype correlates with markers of patient outcome such as progression, survival, and distant metastasis. This has been documented from examination of the expression of single markers and from multiplex datasets.

For example, increased expression of the glioblastoma stem cell marker CD133 predicted poor patient survival (Kong et al, 2008). Multiple studies also show an association between higher CD133 expression and increased risk of progression, poorer survival and poorer response to therapy in colorectal carcinoma (Sanders and Majumdar, 2011).

Liu et al (2007) compared the gene-expression profile of CD44+/CD24− breast CSCs with that of normal breast epithelium, deriving a 186-gene "invasiveness" gene signature (IGS) that was independently and significantly associated with both overall and metastasis-free survival in women with breast cancer. Intriguingly the IGS was also associated with prognosis in medulloblastoma, lung cancer, and prostate cancer, suggesting that this signature is relevant to other cancers. Gene expression profiling of functionally validated leukemic stem cell populations yielded a signature of "stemness" associated with poor prognosis (Eppert et al, 2011). In this study, multiple patients' samples were engrafted in mice, but showed different phenotypes of leukemic stem cell subsets (eg, CD34+, CD34+/CD38−). Despite these differences in marker expression, a core gene expression signature was present in the engrafting leukemic stem cell subset.

Pece et al (2010) isolated slow-cycling mammary gland stem cells in mammosphere culture from normal human breast biopsies, using a fluorescent dye that is retained by nondividing cells. Gene expression array analysis compared dividing (nonfluorescent) versus nondividing (fluorescent) cells, identifying a putative signature of human mammary stem cells.

This gene signature of slow-cycling cells identified cell markers such as CD49f, Delta and Notch-like EGF-related receptor (DNER), and delta-like-1 (DLL1), which could be used to isolate prospectively normal mammary stem cells from mammosphere cultures. The gene signature was also able to predict tumor grade in breast carcinoma; high grade 3 tumors highly expressed the mammary stem cell signature compared with low grade 1 tumors.

Additionally cancer cells expressing markers such as CD49f, DNER and DLL1 were much more frequent in grade 3 tumors. A gene expression signature of normal intestinal stem cells in mice, defined by ephrin-B2+ cells, was shown to be predictive of poor clinical outcome in human colorectal carcinoma (Merlos-Suarez et al, 2011). Also, in a recent study using single-cell PCR (see Chap. 2, Sec. 2.2.5) from individual colonic cells, gene expression signatures could be defined for different normal tissue compartments, such as enterocytes, goblet cells, and cells from the top (cells that are proliferating and differentiating) and bottom (where cells are more quiescent and "stem-like") of the crypt (Dalerba et al, 2011). The gene signature of these terminally differentiated top-of-crypt cells was associated with improved prognosis in patients with colorectal carcinoma. In addition, colorectal cancer xenografts were generated from decreasing numbers of injected EpCAM$^+$/CD44$^+$ colorectal CSC, including 1 xenograft derived from a single EpCAM$^+$/CD44$^+$ colorectal CSC. This clonally derived tumor recapitulated almost perfectly the heterogeneity observed in the patient's tumor, providing further evidence in support of the CSC hierarchy within colorectal carcinoma.

Patterns of failure of cancer therapy are also consistent with the CSC hypothesis. Surgery is important in the treatment of most solid malignancies, and surgical margin status is correlated with local control of disease and long-term survival in many tumor types, including head and neck cancer. Some tumors recur at the site of resection despite apparently adequate margins; Prince et al (2007) demonstrated that the CD44$^+$/BMI1$^+$ CSCs detected in head and neck squamous carcinoma are most often positioned in a peristromal location at the leading edge of the tumor, abutting connective tissue, and may be the cause of recurrence. Calabrese et al (2007) showed that glioblastoma stem cells are located in a perivascular location, perhaps accounting for the propensity of glioma to extend beyond the apparent tumor margin, leading to frequent disease relapse following attempted curative surgery.

Some types of resistance to chemotherapy can be accounted for by the CSC hypothesis (see Chap. 19, Sec. 19.3.5). Liu et al (2006) showed that CD133$^+$ CSC in de novo glioblastoma cell lines are intrinsically more chemoresistant than more differentiated cells; Li et al (2008) showed intrinsically resistant breast CSC; and Dylla et al (2008) showed that colorectal CSCs are more likely to survive treatment with oxaliplatin chemotherapy. Finally, in del(5q) myelodysplasia, a subpopulation of quiescent, CD34$^+$, CD38$^{-/low}$, and CD90$^+$ myelodysplastic stem cells was found to persist and eventually cause treatment failure in patients who had clinical complete remissions after treatment with lenalidomide (Tehranchi et al, 2010).

Resistance to radiation treatment has also been shown to be an intrinsic property of human glioblastoma CSC (Bao, Wu, McLendon et al, 2006) and breast CSC (Diehn and Clarke, 2006). The mechanism of radioresistance of CSCs may be a result of lower levels of reactive oxygen species compared to more differentiated cancer cells, which allows CSCs to mitigate DNA damage caused by radiotherapy (Diehn et al, 2009; Brunner et al, 2012).

13.5 TARGETING CANCER STEM CELLS

The CSC hypothesis is informing advances in cancer therapy, although it is unlikely that cancer would be adequately treated by attempting to eliminate CSCs alone, as more differentiated cancer cells, such as "progenitor" or "transit-amplifying" cells, are likely to retain sufficient proliferative potential to cause patient death. Rather, targeting CSCs is likely to be useful as an adjunct to standard therapies that debulk the tumor, such as surgery, radiotherapy, and chemotherapy. CSC-focused therapies may be most useful in the neoadjuvant and adjuvant settings, in conjunction with attempted curative treatment of primary disease (Table 13–2).

13.5.1 Differentiation Therapy

One implication of the CSC hypothesis is that cotreatment with agents that cause differentiation of quiescent stem-like cancer cells to cycling progenitor/transit-amplifying cells might make them more susceptible to therapy. A clinical example of this phenomenon is the use of all-*trans*-retinoic acid (ATRA) and arsenic trioxide in the treatment of M3 acute promyelocytic leukemia (APML). ATRA and arsenic trioxide act by different mechanisms to destabilize the *PML-RARα* fusion translocation oncogene which is the driver event in most cases of APML. These agents cause differentiation and loss of self-renewal in the leukemic promyelocytes, and are so effective when combined that clinical trials have shown durable complete remissions in patients without the need for cytotoxic chemotherapy (Park and Tallman, 2011).

Efforts to overcome resistance to chemotherapy associated with CSCs in other cancers are being tested in preclinical models and entering early phase clinical trials (see Chap. 19, Sec. 19.3.5). For example, parthenolide, a natural product derived from the traditional medicinal herb feverfew that inhibits the nuclear factor kappa B (NF-κB) pathway, has been shown to induce apoptosis in LSCs while sparing normal hematopoiesis in xenograft models of AML (Guzman et al, 2007). NOTCH4 has been shown to regulate breast CSCs and γ-secretase inhibitors of the NOTCH pathway (see Chap. 8, Sec. 8.4.2), are in early phase clinical trials in breast cancer (McDermott and Wicha, 2010). In another preclinical example, Gupta et al (2009) used high-throughput drug screening to identify salinomycin as a selective inhibitor of CD44$^+$/CD24$^-$ breast cancer stem-like cells in breast cancer cell lines.

TABLE 13–2 Targeting cancer stem cells.

Cancer	Target	Intervention	Mechanism	Outcome
Acute myeloid leukemia	mTOR	Rapamycin	Inhibition of self-renewal	LSC depletion and HSC renewal (Yilmaz et al, 2006)
	CD44	Anti-CD44 antibody	Immunotherapy	LSC depletion and loss of self-renewal and niche (Jin et al, 2006)
	CD47	Anti-CD47 antibody	Immunotherapy	Blocking CD47 enables phagocytosis of LSC (Majeti et al, 2009)
Breast carcinoma	NF-κB pathway	Parthenolide, thiocarbamates	Differentiation	Reduced tumor growth (Zhou et al, 2008)
	NOTCH pathway	Gamma-secretase inhibitor	Inhibition of self-renewal	Reduced mammosphere formation (Grudzien et al, 2010)
	AKT	Perifosine	Inhibition of self-renewal	Reduced tumorigenicity (Korkaya et al, 2009)
Glioblastoma multiforme	VEGF	Bevacizumab	Niche targeting	Loss of CSC niche (Calabrese et al, 2007)
	Hedgehog pathway	Cyclopamine	Inhibition of self-renewal	Neurosphere depletion and loss of tumorigenicity (Bar et al, 2007)
	BMPR2	BMP4	Differentiation	Loss of tumorigenicity (Piccirillo et al, 2006)
Colorectal carcinoma	MHC and NK ligands	δγT-lymphocytes	Immunotherapy	CSC targeted killing (Todaro et al, 2009)
	IL4	IL-4Rα antagonist or anti–IL-4 neutralizing antibody	Reversal of chemoresistance	Efficient xenograft control with chemotherapy (Todaro et al, 2007)

Abbreviations and gene names: BMP4, bone morphogenetic protein 4; BMPR2, bone morphogenetic protein receptor type II; CD44, hyaluronic acid receptor; HSC, hematopoietic stem cell; IL4, interleukin-4; LSC, leukemic stem cell; MHC, major histocompatibility complex; mTOR, mammalian target of rapamycin; NF-κB, nuclear factor kappa-light-chain-enhancer of activated B cells; NK, natural killer; VEGF, vascular endothelial growth factor.

The combination of cyclopamine, rapamycin, and gemcitabine was shown to be effective against primary human pancreatic carcinoma xenografts, whereas any combination of 2 agents was no more effective than gemcitabine alone (Mueller et al, 2009). Cyclopamine is a natural product derived from the corn lily that inhibits the Hedgehog pathway (see Chap. 8, Sec. 8.4.3), and in pancreatic carcinoma, this signaling pathway was shown to be critical to CSC self-renewal, migration, and proliferation. Cyclopamine has proven toxic in humans, but a number of synthetic inhibitors of the Hedgehog pathway are in clinical trials in basal cell carcinoma, pancreatic carcinoma, medulloblastoma, head and neck squamous carcinoma, and non–small cell lung cancer (Clayton and Mousa, 2011).

13.5.2 Immunological Targeting of Cancer Stem Cells

Attempts to improve or induce immunological surveillance, recognition, and destruction of residual CSC after debulking with chemotherapy, radiation, or surgery provide a rational approach to try to improve outcome for patients (see Chap. 21, Sec. 21.5). For example, Cioffi et al (2012) demonstrated the potential of a bispecific antibody in targeting pancreatic CSCs, showing that cytotoxic CD8+ T lymphocytes could be "redirected" against primary human pancreatic xenografts. The bispecific antibody, MT110, is synthesized to recognize 2 different antigens; one F(ab) region recognizes CD3, a pan-lymphocyte marker, and the other recognizes EpCAM, a molecule highly expressed on CSCs in pancreatic cancer. The CSC subpopulation within these tumors was not resistant to this treatment, and an improvement in survival was seen in a mouse xenograft model. Phase I clinical trials suggest evidence of activity, but also led to dose-limiting diarrhea and raised liver enzymes in humans. Cellular immune responses to CSCs have also been investigated, for example, through a γδT-cell response to colorectal CSCs (Todaro et al, 2009). Recognition and killing of colorectal CSCs was augmented by pretreatment with zoledronate to upregulate isoprenoids on the surface of CSCs. Finally, vaccination against antigens expressed on stem cells or CSCs shows some preclinical evidence of activity in targeting CSCs. Vaccination of immunocompetent mice with murine ES cells generated a robust immune response that rendered these mice strongly resistant to subsequent engraftment with a murine lung cancer cell line. This was not a result of an allogeneic immune response, as vaccination with syngeneic embryonic fibroblasts failed to generate similar protection (Yaddanapudi et al, 2012). Ning et al (2012) employed an analogous experimental plan, but vaccinated immunocompetent mice with stem-like cancer cells from murine cancer cell lines. Mice were immunized with ALDH+ stem-like cells isolated from cell lines prior to inoculation with the cancer cell line itself (Ma and Allan,

2011). Immunized mice showed in vivo and in vitro immune responses that also slowed tumor progression. There are many complexities and challenges in active cancer immunotherapy (Cebon et al, 2007) but human studies of active vaccination against CSC have commenced.

13.5.3 Targeting the Cancer Stem Cell Niche

Somatic and ES cells can only exist in a tightly regulated stem cell niche, with bidirectional signaling to maintain their phenotype, which, in turn, maintains the cells required for their niche support (Moore and Lemischka, 2006). Evolving evidence suggests that CSCs may also exist within, and signal to maintain, a functional niche, providing another potential target for cancer treatment. Bao, Wu, Sathornsumetee et al (2006) found that vascular endothelial growth factor (VEGF) was highly expressed by CD133$^+$-derived glioma stem cell cultures and xenografts compared with matched CD133$^-$ cells. This secretion was further enhanced under hypoxic culture conditions. When CD133$^+$ glioma stem cell-conditioned media was applied to endothelial cell (EC) cultures, it significantly enhanced EC migration and tube formation. The anti-VEGF antibody bevacizumab abrogated these proangiogenic effects and also suppressed tumor xenograft formation.

Calabrese et al (2007) demonstrated that primary brain cancers exist within and exert control over vascular niches that allow them to maintain the CSC subpopulation. Using multiphoton laser-scanning immunofluorescence microscopy to digitally reconstruct tumor sections, nestin-positive cells were found to colocate with capillaries in 4 glioma biopsies. In vitro experiments showed that CD133$^+$ brain CSC interact with ECs in coculture, and, in turn, these ECs were able to maintain and propagate the CD133$^+$ fraction of tumors. Finally, the authors demonstrated that ECs promoted tumor formation of CD133$^+$ brain CSCs in orthotopic xenografts, and that disruption of the vascular niche by erlotinib and the antiangiogenic agent bevacizumab directly ablated the self-renewing CSC population and inhibited xenograft growth (Calabrese et al, 2007).

Several recent publications suggest that glioblastoma stem cells can contribute directly to the tumor microenvironment by differentiating into tumor ECs. In human tumors (Ricci-Vitiani et al, 2010; Wang, Chadalavada et al, 2010) and in lentiviral lineage-restricted Cre-Lox mouse models (Soda et al, 2011), which permit the introduction of oncogenes in limited numbers of cells in vivo, glioblastoma cells differentiated into CD31$^+$CD144$^+$ ECs, which contribute to functional blood vessels. Some of these vessels lacked VEGF receptors and were insensitive to VEGF-targeted therapies. A similar process was also described in ABCB5$^+$ VEGFR2+ melanoma cells. This finding illustrates an additional level of complexity in the biology of CSCs in the context of their microenvironment and in the challenge faced in advancing cancer therapy.

SUMMARY

- Cancers are heterogeneous.
- Cancer heterogeneity is multidimensional; some cells in a cancer are malignant cells while others are host stromal cells; there is almost always clonal heterogeneity within the malignant cell population; there is phenotypic heterogeneity within the dominant malignant clone.
- Epigenetic heterogeneity may be stochastic, with every cell having the potential to self-renew and recapitulate the tumor; the EMT and phenotypic plasticity models may explain this stochastic model.
- Epigenetic heterogeneity may be hierarchal; only a subset of "CSCs" have the potential to self-renew, proliferate indefinitely, and differentiate to non–stem cancer cells.
- These models of tumor heterogeneity may not be mutually exclusive; experimental evidence supporting EMT and the CSC hypothesis can identify similar markers associated with similar behaviors.
- CSCs have been best demonstrated in AML, but have also been demonstrated in solid tumors, such as breast carcinoma, colorectal carcinoma, and head and neck squamous carcinoma.
- Tumor-initiating cells are common in some cancers such as melanoma, leading to criticisms of the relevance of the CSC hypothesis.
- Cell-surface glycoproteins, such as CD133/prominin-1 and CD44 can be used as markers to identify CSCs.
- The clinical relevance of the CSC hypothesis is supported by prognostic, mechanistic and therapeutic evidence.
- Gene expression signatures of CSCs are predictive of poor patient prognosis.
- Identification of "stemness" signaling pathways is leading to new therapeutic modalities, such as inhibiting the Hedgehog pathway.
- The CSC hypothesis is a leading candidate to account for epigenetic heterogeneity in human cancers.

REFERENCES

Ailles L, Prince M, Yu JS. Cancer stem cells. In: Walker JM, ed. *Head and Neck Squamous Cell Carcinoma*. Totowa, NJ: Humana Press; 2009:568:175-193.

Ailles LE, Weissman IL. Cancer stem cells in solid tumors. *Curr Opin Biotechnol* 2007;18:460-466.

Al-Hajj M, Wicha MS, Benito-Hernandez A, Morrison SJ, Clarke MF. Prospective identification of tumorigenic breast cancer cells. *Proc Natl Acad Sci U S A* 2003;100:3983-3988.

Alexander CM, Puchalski J, Klos KS, et al. Separating stem cells by flow cytometry: reducing variability for solid tissues. *Cell Stem Cell* 2009;5:579-583.

Bao S, Wu Q, McLendon RE, et al. Glioma stem cells promote radioresistance by preferential activation of the DNA damage response. *Nature* 2006;444:756-760.

Bao S, Wu Q, Sathornsumetee S, et al. Stem cell-like glioma cells promote tumor angiogenesis through vascular endothelial growth factor. *Cancer Res* 2006;66:7843-7848.

Bar EE, Chaudhry A, Lin A, et al. Cyclopamine-mediated hedgehog pathway inhibition depletes stem-like cancer cells in glioblastoma. *Stem Cells* 2007;25:2524-2533.

Beier D, Hau P, Proescholdt M, et al. CD133(+) and CD133(−) glioblastoma-derived cancer stem cells show differential growth characteristics and molecular profiles. *Cancer Res* 2007;67: 4010-4015.

Bonnet D, Dick JE. Human acute myeloid leukemia is organized as a hierarchy that originates from a primitive hematopoietic cell. *Nat Med* 1997;3:730-737.

Brabletz T, Jung A, Reu S, et al. Variable beta-catenin expression in colorectal cancers indicates tumor progression driven by the tumor environment. *Proc Natl Acad Sci U S A* 2001;98: 10356-10361.

Brewer GJ, Torricelli JR, Evege EK, Price PJ. Optimized survival of hippocampal neurons in B27-supplemented Neurobasal, a new serum-free medium combination. *J Neurosci Res* 1993;35: 567-576.

Bruce WR, Van Der Gaag H. A quantitative assay for the number of murine lymphoma cells capable of proliferation in vivo. *Nature* 1963;199:79-80.

Brunner TB, Kunz-Schughart LA, Grosse-Gehling P, Baumann M. Cancer stem cells as a predictive factor in radiotherapy. *Semin Radiat Oncol* 2012;22:151-174.

Brunschwig A, Southam CM, Levin AG. Host resistance to cancer. Clinical experiments by homotransplants, autotransplants and admixture of autologous leucocytes. *Ann Surg* 1965;162:416-425.

Calabrese C, Poppleton H, Kocak M, et al. A perivascular niche for brain tumor stem cells. *Cancer Cell* 2007;11:69-82.

Campbell PJ, Yachida S, Mudie LJ, et al. The patterns and dynamics of genomic instability in metastatic pancreatic cancer. *Nature* 2010;467:1109-1113.

Cebon J, Gedye C, John T, Davis ID. Immunotherapy of advanced or metastatic melanoma. *Clin Adv Hematol Oncol* 2007;5:994-1006.

Chu S, McDonald T, Lin A, et al. Persistence of leukemia stem cells in chronic myelogenous leukemia patients in prolonged remission with imatinib treatment. *Blood* 2011;118:5565-5572.

Cioffi M, Dorado J, Baeuerle P, et al. EpCAM/CD3-bispecific T-cell engaging antibody MT110 eliminates primary human pancreatic cancer stem sells. *Clin Cancer Res* 2012;18:465-474.

Clayton S, Mousa SA. Therapeutics formulated to target cancer stem cells: Is it in our future? *Cancer Cell Int* 2011;11:7.

Collins AT, Berry PA, Hyde C, Stower MJ, Maitland NJ. Prospective identification of tumorigenic prostate cancer stem cells. *Cancer Res* 2005;65:10946-10951.

Creighton CJ, Li X, Landis M, et al. Residual breast cancers after conventional therapy display mesenchymal as well as tumor-initiating features. *Proc Natl Acad Sci U S A* 2009;106: 13820-13825.

Curtis SJ, Sinkevicius KW, Li D, et al. Primary tumor genotype is an important determinant in identification of lung cancer propagating cells. *Cell Stem Cell* 2010;7:127-133.

Dalerba P, Dylla SJ, Park IK, et al. Phenotypic characterization of human colorectal cancer stem cells. *Proc Natl Acad Sci U S A* 2007;104:10158-10163.

Dalerba P, Kalisky T, Sahoo D, et al. Single-cell dissection of transcriptional heterogeneity in human colon tumors. *Nat Biotechnol* 2011;29:1120-1127.

Diehn M, Cho RW, Lobo NA, et al. Association of reactive oxygen species levels and radioresistance in cancer stem cells. *Nature* 2009;458:780-783.

Diehn M, Clarke MF. Cancer stem cells and radiotherapy: new insights into tumor radioresistance. *J Natl Cancer Inst* 2006;98: 1755-1757.

Dylla S, Beviglia L, Park I, et al. Colorectal cancer stem cells are enriched in xenogeneic tumors following chemotherapy. *PLoS ONE* 2008;3:e2428.

Eppert K, Takenaka K, Lechman ER, et al. Stem cell gene expression programs influence clinical outcome in human leukemia. *Nat Med* 2011;17:1086-1093.

Fan X, Khaki L, Zhu TS, et al. NOTCH pathway blockade depletes CD133-positive glioblastoma cells and inhibits growth of tumor neurospheres and xenografts. *Stem Cells* 2010;28:5-16.

Gedye C, Hill RP, Ailles L. Final thoughts: complexity and controversy surrounding the "cancer stem cell" paradigm cancer stem cells in solid tumors. In: Allan AL, ed. *Cancer Stem Cells in Solid Tumors.* New York, NY: Humana Press; 2011:433-464.

Grudzien P, Lo S, Albain KS, et al. Inhibition of Notch signaling reduces the stem-like population of breast cancer cells and prevents mammosphere formation. *Anticancer Res* 2010;30: 3853-3867.

Gunther HS, Schmidt NO, Phillips HS, et al. Glioblastoma-derived stem cell-enriched cultures form distinct subgroups according to molecular and phenotypic criteria. *Oncogene* 2008;27:2897-2909.

Gupta P, Onder T, Jiang G, et al. Identification of selective inhibitors of cancer stem cells by high-throughput screening. *Cell* 2009;138: 645-659.

Guzman ML, Rossi RM, Neelakantan S, et al. An orally bioavailable parthenolide analog selectively eradicates acute myelogenous leukemia stem and progenitor cells. *Blood* 2007;110:4427-4435.

Hamburger AW, Salmon SE. Primary bioassay of human tumor stem cells. *Science* 1977;197:461-463.

Hermann PC, Huber SL, Herrler T, et al. Distinct populations of cancer stem cells determine tumor growth and metastatic activity in human pancreatic cancer. *Cell Stem Cell* 2007;1:313-323.

Hewitt H. A critical examination of the foundations of immunotherapy for cancer. *Clin Radiol* 1979;30:361-369.

Hill RP. Identifying cancer stem cells in solid tumors: case not proven. *Cancer Res* 2006;66:1891-1895.

Hope KJ, Jin L, Dick JE. Acute myeloid leukemia originates from a hierarchy of leukemic stem cell classes that differ in self-renewal capacity. *Nat Immunol* 2004;5:738-743.

Hung JJ, Yang MH, Hsu HS, et al. Prognostic significance of hypoxia-inducible factor-1alpha, TWIST1 and Snail expression in resectable non-small cell lung cancer. *Thorax* 2009;64: 1082-1089.

Ishizawa K, Rasheed ZA, Karisch R, et al. Tumor-initiating cells are rare in many human tumors. *Cell Stem Cell* 2010;7:279-282.

Jeter CR, Badeaux M, Choy G, et al. Functional evidence that the self-renewal gene NANOG regulates human tumor development. *Stem Cells* 2009;27:993-1005.

Ji J, Ng SH, Sharma V, et al. Elevated coding mutation rate during the reprogramming of human somatic cells into induced pluripotent stem cells. *Stem Cells* 2012;30:435-440.

Jin L, Hope KJ, Zhai Q, Smadja-Joffe F, Dick JE. Targeting of CD44 eradicates human acute myeloid leukemic stem cells. *Nat Med* 2006;12:1167-1174.

Jones S, Chen WD, Parmigiani G, et al. Comparative lesion sequencing provides insights into tumor evolution. *Proc Natl Acad Sci U S A* 2008;105:4283-4288.

Kalluri R, Weinberg RA. The basics of epithelial-mesenchymal transition. *J Clin Invest* 2009;119:1420-1428.

Kim M, Gans JD, Nogueira C, et al. Comparative oncogenomics identifies NEDD9 as a melanoma metastasis gene. *Cell* 2006;125: 1269-1281.

Kong DS, Kim MH, Park WY, et al. The progression of gliomas is associated with cancer stem cell phenotype. *Oncol Rep* 2008;19: 639-643.

Korkaya H, Paulson A, Charafe-Jauffret E, et al. Regulation of mammary stem/progenitor cells by PTEN/Akt/β-catenin signaling. *PLoS Biol* 2009;7:e1000121.

Kucherlapati R, Wheeler DA, et al. for The Cancer Genome Atlas Network. Comprehensive molecular characterization of human colon and rectal cancer. *Nature* 2012;487:330-337.

Lagadec C, Vlashi E, Della Donna L, et al. Survival and self-renewing capacity of breast cancer initiating cells during fractionated radiation treatment. *Breast Cancer Res* 2010;12:R13.

Lander A. The "stem cell" concept: is it holding us back? *J Biol* 2009;8:70.

Lapidot T, Sirard C, Vormoor J, et al. A cell initiating human acute myeloid leukaemia after transplantation into SCID mice. *Nature* 1994;367:645-648.

Lee J, Kotliarova S, Kotliarov Y, et al. Tumor stem cells derived from glioblastomas cultured in bFGF and EGF more closely mirror the phenotype and genotype of primary tumors than do serum-cultured cell lines. *Cancer Cell* 2006;9:391-403.

Lenkiewicz M, Li N, Singh SK. Culture and isolation of brain tumor initiating cells. *Curr Protoc Stem Cell Biol* 2009;Chapter 3:Unit 3.3.

Lessard J, Sauvageau G. Bmi-1 determines the proliferative capacity of normal and leukaemic stem cells. *Nature* 2003;423:255-260.

Li C, Heidt DG, Dalerba P, et al. Identification of pancreatic cancer stem cells. *Cancer Res* 2007;67:1030-1037.

Li X, Lewis MT, Huang J, et al. Intrinsic resistance of tumorigenic breast cancer cells to chemotherapy. *J Natl Cancer Inst* 2008;100: 672-679.

Liu G, Yuan X, Zeng Z, et al. Analysis of gene expression and chemoresistance of CD133+ cancer stem cells in glioblastoma. *Mol Cancer* 2006;5:67.

Liu R, Wang X, Chen GY, et al. The prognostic role of a gene signature from tumorigenic breast-cancer cells. *N Engl J Med* 2007;356:217-226.

Liu W, Laitinen S, Khan S, et al. Copy number analysis indicates monoclonal origin of lethal metastatic prostate cancer. *Nat Med* 2009;15:559-565.

Luzzi KJ, MacDonald IC, Schmidt EE, et al. Multistep nature of metastatic inefficiency: dormancy of solitary cells after successful extravasation and limited survival of early micrometastases. *Am J Pathol* 1998;153:865-873.

Ma I, Allan AL. The role of human aldehyde dehydrogenase in normal and cancer stem cells. *Stem Cell Rev* 2011;7:292-306.

Ma S, Chan K-W, Hu L, et al. Identification and characterization of tumorigenic liver cancer stem/progenitor cells. *Gastroenterology* 2007;132:2542-2556.

Macfarlan TS, Gifford WD, Driscoll S, et al. Embryonic stem cell potency fluctuates with endogenous retrovirus activity. *Nature* 2012;487:57-63.

Majeti R, Chao MP, Alizadeh AA, et al. CD47 Is an adverse prognostic factor and therapeutic antibody target on human acute myeloid leukemia stem cells. *Cell* 2009;138:286-299.

Mani SA, Guo W, Liao M-J, et al. The epithelial-mesenchymal transition generates cells with properties of stem cells. *Cell* 2008; 133:704-715.

McDermott SP, Wicha MS. Targeting breast cancer stem cells. *Mol Oncol* 2010;4:404-419.

Merlos-Suarez A, Barriga Francisco M, Jung P, et al. The intestinal stem cell signature identifies colorectal cancer stem cells and predicts disease relapse. *Cell Stem Cell* 2011;8:511-524.

Mikami S, Katsube K, Oya M, et al. Expression of Snail and Slug in renal cell carcinoma: E-cadherin repressor Snail is associated with cancer invasion and prognosis. *Lab Invest* 2011;91:1443-1458.

Moore KA, Lemischka IR. Stem cells and their niches. *Science* 2006; 311:1880-1885.

Mueller MT, Hermann PC, Witthauer J, et al. Combined targeted treatment to eliminate tumorigenic cancer stem cells in human pancreatic cancer. *Gastroenterology* 2009;137:1102-1113.

Naugler C. Population genetics of cancer cell clones: possible implications of cancer stem cells. *Theor Biol Med Model* 2010;7:42.

Navin N, Hicks J. Future medical applications of single-cell sequencing in cancer. *Genome Med* 2011;3:31.

Nes JH, Kruijf E, Putter H, et al. Co-expression of SNAIL and TWIST determines prognosis in estrogen receptor-positive early breast cancer patients. *Breast Cancer Res Treat* 2012;133:49-59.

Ning N, Pan Q, Zheng F et al. Cancer stem cell vaccination confers significant antitumor immunity. *Cancer Res* 2012;72:1853-1864.

Notta F, Mullighan CG, Wang JCY, et al. Evolution of human BCR-ABL1 lymphoblastic leukaemia-initiating cells. *Nature* 2011;469:362-367.

Nowell P. The clonal evolution of tumor cell populations. *Science* 1976;194:23-28.

O'Brien CA, Pollett A, Gallinger S, Dick JE. A human colon cancer cell capable of initiating tumour growth in immunodeficient mice. *Nature* 2007;445:106-110.

Paget S. The distribution of secondary growths in cancer of the breast. *Lancet* 1889;1:571-573.

Palmon A, David R, Neumann Y, et al. High-efficiency immunomagnetic isolation of solid tissue-originated integrin-expressing adult stem cells. *Methods* 2012;56:305-309.

Park JH, Tallman MS. Managing acute promyelocytic leukemia without conventional chemotherapy: is it possible? *Expert Rev Hematol* 2011;4:427-436.

Patrawala L, Calhoun T, Schneider-Broussard R, et al. Highly purified CD44+ prostate cancer cells from xenograft human tumors are enriched in tumorigenic and metastatic progenitor cells. *Oncogene* 2006;25:1696-1708.

Peacock CD, Wang Q, Gesell GS, et al. Hedgehog signaling maintains a tumor stem cell compartment in multiple myeloma. *Proc Natl Acad Sci U S A* 2007;104:4048-4053.

Pece S, Tosoni D, Confalonieri S, et al. Biological and molecular heterogeneity of breast cancers correlates with their cancer stem cell content. *Cell* 2010;140:62-73.

Piccirillo SG, Reynolds BA, Zanetti N, et al. Bone morphogenetic proteins inhibit the tumorigenic potential of human brain tumour-initiating cells. *Nature* 2006;444:761-765.

Pierce GB, Speers WC. Tumors as caricatures of the process of tissue renewal: prospects for therapy by directing differentiation. *Cancer Res* 1988;48:1996-2004.

Pierce GB, Wallace C. Differentiation of malignant to benign cells. *Cancer Res* 1971;31:127-134.

Pollard SM, Yoshikawa K, Clarke ID, et al. Glioma stem cell lines expanded in adherent culture have tumor-specific phenotypes and are suitable for chemical and genetic screens. *Cell Stem Cell* 2009;4:568-580.

Prince ME, Sivanandan R, Kaczorowski A, et al. Identification of a subpopulation of cells with cancer stem cell properties in head and neck squamous cell carcinoma. *Proc Natl Acad Sci U S A* 2007;104:973-978.

Quintana E, Shackleton M, Foster HR, et al. Phenotypic heterogeneity among tumorigenic melanoma cells from patients that is reversible and not hierarchically organized. *Cancer Cell* 2010;18:510-523.

Quintana E, Shackleton M, Sabel MS, et al. Efficient tumour formation by single human melanoma cells. *Nature* 2008;456: 593-598.

Rawlins EL, Hogan BLM. Ciliated epithelial cell lifespan in the mouse trachea and lung. *Am J Physiol Lung Cell Mol Physiol* 2008;295:L231-L234.

Reim F, Dombrowski Y, Ritter C, et al. Immunoselection of breast and ovarian cancer cells with trastuzumab and natural killer cells: selective escape of CD44high/CD24low/HER2low breast cancer stem cells. *Cancer Res* 2009;69:8058-8066.

Reya T, Morrison SJ, Clarke MF, Weissman IL. Stem cells, cancer, and cancer stem cells. *Nature* 2001;414:105-111.

Reynolds BA, Weiss S. Generation of neurons and astrocytes from isolated cells of the adult mammalian central nervous system. *Science* 1992;255:1707-1710.

Ricci-Vitiani L, Lombardi DG, Pilozzi E, et al. Identification and expansion of human colon-cancer-initiating cells. *Nature* 2007;445:111-115.

Ricci-Vitiani L, Pallini R, Biffoni M, et al. Tumour vascularization via endothelial differentiation of glioblastoma stem-like cells. *Nature* 2010;468:824-828.

Roesch A, Fukunaga-Kalabis M, Schmidt EC, et al. A temporarily distinct subpopulation of slow-cycling melanoma cells is required for continuous tumor growth. *Cell* 2010;141:583-594.

Ryu HS, Park DJ, Kim HH, Kim WH, Lee HS. Combination of epithelial-mesenchymal transition and cancer stem cell-like phenotypes has independent prognostic value in gastric cancer. *Hum Pathol* 2012;43:520-528.

Sanders MA, Majumdar AP. Colon cancer stem cells: implications in carcinogenesis. *Front Biosci* 2011;16:1651-1662.

Schatton T, Murphy GF, Frank NY, et al. Identification of cells initiating human melanomas. *Nature* 2008;451:345-349.

Scheel C, Weinberg RA. Phenotypic plasticity and epithelial-mesenchymal transitions in cancer and normal stem cells? *Int J Cancer* 2011;129:2310-2314.

Shackleton M, Quintana E, Fearon ER, Morrison SJ. Heterogeneity in cancer: cancer stem cells versus clonal evolution. *Cell* 2009;138:822-829.

Sharma SV, Lee DY, Li B, et al. A chromatin-mediated reversible drug-tolerant state in cancer cell subpopulations. *Cell* 2010; 141:69-80.

Singh SK, Clarke ID, Terasaki M, et al. Identification of a cancer stem cell in human brain tumors. *Cancer Res* 2003;63:5821-5828.

Singh SK, Hawkins C, Clarke ID, et al. Identification of human brain tumour initiating cells. *Nature* 2004;432:396-401.

Soda Y, Marumoto T, Friedmann-Morvinski D, et al. Transdifferentiation of glioblastoma cells into vascular endothelial cells. *Proc Natl Acad Sci U S A* 2011;108: 4274-4280.

Somervaille TC, Matheny CJ, Spencer GJ, et al. Hierarchical maintenance of MLL myeloid leukemia stem cells employs a transcriptional program shared with embryonic rather than adult stem cells. *Cell Stem Cell* 2009;4:129-140.

Stewart JM, Shaw PA, Gedye C, et al. Phenotypic heterogeneity and instability of human ovarian tumor-initiating cells. *Proc Natl Acad Sci U S A* 2011;108:6468-6473.

Stoletov K, Kato H, Zardouzian E, et al. Visualizing extravasation dynamics of metastatic tumor cells. *J Cell Sci* 2010;123:2332-2341.

Tarin D. The fallacy of epithelial mesenchymal transition in neoplasia. *Cancer Res* 2005;65:5996-6001.

Tassone P, Neri P, Carrasco DR, et al. A clinically relevant SCID-hu in vivo model of human multiple myeloma. *Blood* 2005;106: 713-716.

Tehranchi R, Woll PS, Anderson K, et al. Persistent malignant stem cells in del(5q) myelodysplasia in remission. *N Engl J Med* 2010; 363:1025-1037.

Till JE, McCulloch EA. A direct measurement of the radiation sensitivity of normal mouse bone marrow cells. *Radiat Res* 1961;14:213-222.

Todaro M, Alea MP, Di Stefano AB, et al. Colon cancer stem cells dictate tumor growth and resist cell death by production of interleukin-4. *Cell Stem Cell* 2007;1:389-402.

Todaro M, D'Asaro M, Caccamo N, et al. Efficient killing of human colon cancer stem cells by gammadelta T lymphocytes. *J Immunol* 2009;182:7287-7296.

Uchida N, Buck DW, He D, et al. Direct isolation of human central nervous system stem cells. *Proc Natl Acad Sci U S A* 2000;97: 14720-14725.

van Staveren WC, Solis DY, Hebrant A, et al. Human cancer cell lines: experimental models for cancer cells in situ? For cancer stem cells? *Biochim Biophys Acta* 2009;1795:92-103.

Vargaftig J, Taussig DC, Griessinger E, et al. Frequency of leukemic initiating cells does not depend on the xenotransplantation model used. *Leukemia* 2012;26:858-860.

Wang R, Chadalavada K, Wilshire J, et al. Glioblastoma stem-like cells give rise to tumour endothelium. *Nature* 2010;468: 829-833.

Wang Z, Li Y, Ahmad A, et al. Targeting miRNAs involved in cancer stem cell and EMT regulation: An emerging concept in overcoming drug resistance. *Drug Resist Updat* 2010;13: 109-118.

Xiang R, Liao D, Cheng T, et al. Downregulation of transcription factor SOX2 in cancer stem cells suppresses growth and metastasis of lung cancer. *Br J Cancer* 2011;104:1410-1417.

Yaddanapudi K, Mitchell RA, Putty K, et al. Vaccination with embryonic stem cells protects against lung cancer: is a broad-spectrum prophylactic vaccine against cancer possible? *PLoS ONE* 2012;7:e42289.

Yang M-H, Hsu DS-S, Wang H-W, et al. Bmi1 is essential in Twist1-induced epithelial-mesenchymal transition. *Nat Cell Biol* 2010;12:982-992.

Yang ZF, Ngai P, Ho DW, et al. Identification of local and circulating cancer stem cells in human liver cancer. *Hepatology* 2008;47: 919-928.

Yilmaz OH, Valdez R, Theisen BK, et al. Pten dependence distinguishes haematopoietic stem cells from leukaemia-initiating cells. *Nature* 2006;441:475-482.

Zhang S, Balch C, Chan MW, et al. Identification and characterization of ovarian cancer-initiating cells from primary human tumors. *Cancer Res* 2008;68:4311-4320.

Zhao C, Blum J, Chen A, et al. Loss of [beta]-catenin impairs the renewal of normal and CML stem cells in vivo. *Cancer Cell* 2007; 12:528-541.

Zhou J, Zhang H, Gu P, et al. NF-kappaB pathway inhibitors preferentially inhibit breast cancer stem-like cells. *Breast Cancer Res Treat* 2008;111:419-427.

14

Imaging in Oncology

David A. Jaffray

14.1 INTRODUCTION

The need to detect and characterize cancer in an individual has resulted in a dramatic increase in the use of imaging over the last 20 years. Clinical imaging is now a routine part of diagnosis, staging, guiding localized therapy, and assessing response to treatment. Cancers occur anatomically among surrounding normal tissues, including critical structures, such as major vessels and nerves, and delineation of the extent of malignant and nonmalignant tissues is essential for planning surgery and radiation therapy. Cancers also have morphological, physiological, and biochemical heterogeneity (see Chaps. 10 and 12), which is important in understanding their biology and response to treatment. The ability to explore and define this heterogeneity with modern imaging methods, as well as serum and tissue-derived metrics, will enable "personalized cancer medicine."

Imaging is diverse in that it offers an "anatomical image" of a mass on a computed tomography (CT) or a magnetic resonance (MR) image, a "functional image" of disease status in positron emission tomography (PET) images of glucose metabolism, and a "microscopic image" used during classification of histological type and grade. Imaging is applied at these multiple levels to help characterize, understand, and treat cancer (Fig. 14–1) and there is general acceptance that advances in imaging are central in the fight against cancer. This chapter provides a brief introduction to the rapidly evolving field of oncological imaging by presenting both the physical principles underlying the most common imaging modalities and their clinical and research applications in oncology.

14.2 GENERAL CONCEPTS RELATING TO CANCER IMAGING

Imaging is a broad science that encompasses the design, development, evaluation, and application of technologies that allow spatial and temporal characterization of an object; ideally, with a minimum of invasion. When using imaging, it is important to understand what *signal* is being detected and how this signal relates to the underlying *biological processes* or *structural elements*. Imaging signals can be broadly classified as *endogenous or exogenous. Endogenous signals* are those associated with the intrinsic characteristics of the body and how these characteristics affect the imaging modality. For example, a chest x-ray detects a lung lesion because of the intrinsic difference in the x-ray attenuation coefficient of the lung and the tissue of the tumor. Similarly in the MR image of a brain tumor, increased swelling (edema) alters the environment of the protons in water and results in an altered MR signal around the tumor. *Exogenous signals* are those that arise from the introduction of an imaging agent (eg, injecting an iodinated x-ray-absorbing contrast agent for CT scanning or injecting a radiolabeled

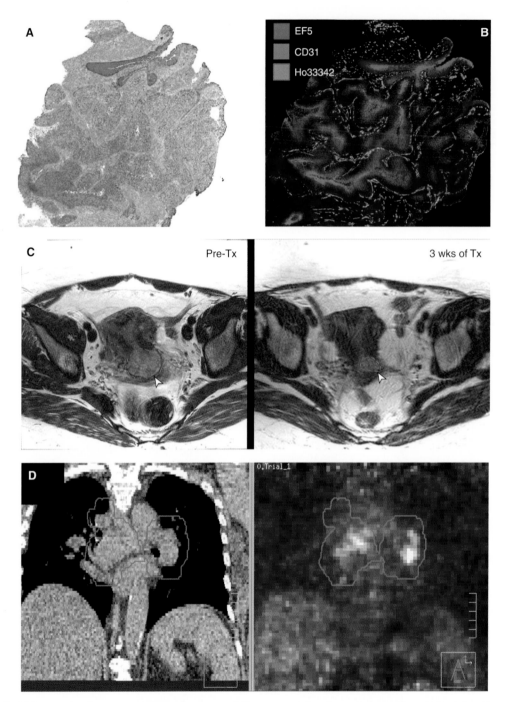

FIGURE 14-1 **Different visual representations of cancer at different spatial scales and time points. A)** Traditional hematoxylin and eosin (H&E) staining of a cervix cancer xenograft. These stains highlight the cellular architecture and are used to assess histological type and grade of cancer. **B)** More advanced immunohistochemical staining of the same tumor demonstrating the complex microenvironment with the tumor. Substantial variation in microvasculature (CD31, green) and oxygen tension (EF5, red) are seen despite the evidence that the tumor is perfused (indicated by the injected Hoechst 33342 dye, blue). **C)** T$_2$-weighted MR image of a cancer of the cervix before (left) and during (right) radiotherapy (after 48 Gy) showing regression of the tumor as outlined in red. **D)** Slice taken from a CT image of a lung cancer patient being planned for radiation therapy. The corresponding fluorodeoxyglucose (FDG)-PET image is on the right. Functional and anatomical information are often complementary in describing the extent and nature of the cancer. The purple outlines demonstrate the volume to be irradiated as part of the radiation treatment.

sugar analog for PET imaging of metabolism) that alters or generates the image signal in a manner that can be distinguished from normal, endogenous signals.

Advances in molecular biology have stimulated the development of a variety of targeted molecular imaging agents whose distribution in the body reflects the regional differences in biological avidity or expression of the targets to which they bind. This field is referred to as *molecular imaging*. Multimodal imaging procedures, hybrid imaging devices, and probes that allow the use of many different imaging (endogenous and exogenous) signals to be acquired and coregistered may also be used to provide a more complete characterization of the cancer. The development of combination PET and CT scanners highlights the value of combining 2 modalities wherein the specificity of disease detection was improved through the combination of anatomical and functional information in a single representation. The complexity of biological, structural, and microenvironmental factors (eg, stroma, blood vessels, hypoxia, interstitial fluid pressure) within solid cancers (see Chaps. 10, 11 and 12) is likely to require the use of many imaging modalities to fully characterize the multiple biological states of an individual's cancer (see Fig. 14–1).

Modern imaging systems are largely digital and allow separation of the image signals into many adjacent spatial compartments called *pixels* or *voxels* (see PET image in Fig. 14–1*D* for a "pixelated" image). Systems capable of generating images with smaller pixels or voxels do not necessarily have higher resolution. The ability of an imaging system to resolve the spatial detail of the underlying image signal is referred to as its *limiting spatial resolution*, and this is determined by the physics of signal formation. For example, a large x-ray focal spot in a chest radiography machine causes a blur in the image as a result of x-rays emanating from different positions in the focal spot creating an image of the same anatomical structure at slightly different, overlapping positions. This limits the spatial resolution or detail contained in the resulting chest radiograph. Similarly in the case of a PET image, the range (a few mm) travelled by the positrons, emitted by the radiolabeled molecule in the tissue, before they annihilate with an electron and create the parallel-opposed 511 keV γ-rays that are detected by the scanner (see Sec. 14.3.3), limits the PET scanner's ability to resolve fine detail in the heterogeneity in uptake within a tumor.

In addition to spatial resolution, the underlying signal needs to be detected in each voxel with a sufficient level of precision to make the image of value. The ratio of the signal in a voxel to the variation in signal found in its neighbors (or to itself over time) is a metric referred to as the *signal-to-noise ratio (SNR)*. This is an important metric in characterizing the performance of an imaging system under specific conditions. Although it is almost always desirable to increase the SNR, this typically comes at a cost through either increased imaging time, increased radiation exposure, a loss in resolution, or, in the context of exogenous imaging agents, toxicity associated with a larger quantity of the imaging agent injected.

14.3 IMAGING TECHNOLOGIES

Imaging methods employ different forms of energy to probe and detect anatomy and biological processes. Figure 14–2 presents these energy forms together with an overlay of exogenous imaging agents. In the following sections, the dominant imaging modalities used in cancer are reviewed in terms of the process of signal formation, as well as a synopsis of their more interesting applications in oncology.

14.3.1 X-ray–Based Systems: Radiography and Computed Tomography

X-ray imaging is based upon the differential attenuation of x-rays within different tissues in the body. The discovery of x-rays by Roentgen in 1895 revealed the value of noninvasive imaging and its clinical applications were immediate. Despite 100 years in advancing this technology, the main methods of x-ray generation and detection have not changed substantially: a vacuum x-ray tube and a 2-dimensional (2D) detector on either side of the subject have remained the central elements. Although the chest x-ray is still a useful tool, x-ray–based CT has become a standard technology to detect and stage cancer since its invention in the 1960s by Hounsfield and Cormack (for which they shared the 1979 Nobel Prize in Physiology or Medicine). The basic process for image generation is shown in Figure 14–3*A*. Briefly, a highly efficient 2D array of x-ray detectors is located opposite a powerful x-ray tube operating in excess of one hundred thousand volts (~120 kVp). The gantry rotates through 360 degrees over a period of less than 0.5 seconds while acquiring hundreds of digital radiographs of the patient. A computerized process of digital filtering and back-projection allows an estimate of the x-ray attenuation coefficient of each voxel in a "slice" (1 to 5 mm thick) through the patient to be estimated (Kak et al, 1988). Modern CT scanners can acquire multiple slices simultaneously and images of the entire body can be acquired by moving the patient through the CT scanner during rotation. Computerized postprocessing of the individual voxels then allows reconstruction of an image in any plane desired.

The CT image signal is measured in Hounsfield units (HU), a linear measure of the attenuation coefficient of the tissue relative to water (water is 0 HU and air is−1000 HU). Images formed at typical imaging doses would have approximately 1% noise (10 HU) and percent differences in HU between tissues such as fat and muscle are only approximately 5% (corresponding to a differential of ~50 HU). It was originally hoped that quantifying the CT signal could be used to classify normal tissue and disease, but the lack of specificity of the CT signal has resulted in little progress on this front. However, the recent development of dual-energy CT imaging systems provides a much higher fidelity in characterizing tissues, and these systems will revitalize the concept of tissue classification (Gupta et al, 2010). High-atomic-number contrast agents (eg, iodinated molecules) are used routinely in CT imaging to increase the contrast-to-noise ratio of various structures and are used in bolus studies with fast (2 to 3 images per second) repetitive scanning to study the permeability of tissues perfusion (Miles, 1991). Xenon gas has also been explored as an agent that is inhaled to assess lung ventilation and as an agent to measure tissue blood flow in hepatocellular carcinoma (Murakami et al, 2004).

CT has the advantage that it achieves high spatial resolution (<1 mm), soft-tissue discrimination, is highly reproducible, and can be employed quantitatively for measuring tumor size and detecting response. However, the image quality in terms

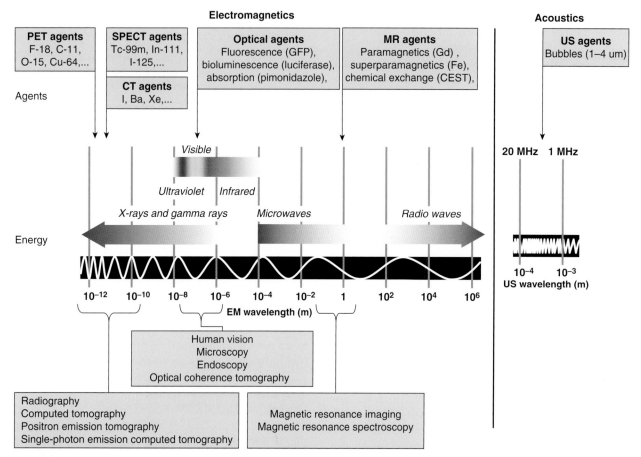

FIGURE 14–2 **Images can be developed from endogenous signals or from exogenous signals induced by the introduction of contrast agents or molecular probes.** The detection of these signals is through either electromagnetic or acoustic energy transfer. Imaging agents are designed to either produce the detected signal (eg, radiolabeled PET/single-photon emission computed tomography [SPECT]) or to alter the interaction between the object and the applied energy (eg, high atomic number materials such as iodine, barium, or xenon in radiography and CT, paramagnetic agents in MR, bubbles in ultrasound). Optical imaging operates at energies corresponding to biological processes and can therefore provide insight into active biological processes (eg, detection of bioluminescent signals). Similarly, MR offers insight into the chemical activity in the body by exploiting effects related to the impact of chemical milieu on nuclear magnetic resonance to create image-like maps of these effects. This is referred to as MR spectroscopy imaging (MRSI). Chemical milieu can also be probed through the exchange of protons between specific chemical species (CEST).

of SNR is related to the applied dose of ionizing radiation—typical CT imaging doses range from 1 to 10 cGy (see Chap. 15, Sec. 15.2.2 for definition of radiation dose). As the first soft-tissue volumetric imaging modality, CT transformed oncological imaging and is used routinely for detection and diagnosis of cancer, as well as for monitoring patients that have undergone therapy. The clinical impact is seen in the management of the patient through noninvasive cancer staging (see Chap. 10, Sec. 10.3.1 for brief description of TNM staging), which has led to a reduction in the frequency of exploratory laparoscopic surgery. Characterization of regional extent of disease is undertaken using pretreatment, posttreatment, and follow-up CT imaging. CT also has a major role in directing therapy, including its use in directing radiofrequency ablation of liver metastases by interventional radiologists, assisting surgeons in head and neck surgery, and delineating lung tumors for image-guided stereotactic radiotherapy. There is widespread use of CT-guidance in interventional radiology and radiation therapy.

CT is used to screen for lung cancer in higher risk populations (see Chap. 22, Sec. 22.3.3) and randomized clinical trials have demonstrated its ability to improve outcome for people with lung cancer (Aberle et al, 2011). The value of CT screening for cancer in other sites has not been established and there are concerns about potential health effects and secondary malignancies relating to the use of CT scanning for screening the general public (Brenner et al, 2007; see Chap. 16, Sec. 16.8).

Recent interest in characterizing the vascularity of tumors has spurred the use of dynamic CT imaging (multiple slices/volumes per second) in which CT scanning is undertaken with a bolus intravenous (IV) injection of a low-molecular-weight-iodinated agent to characterize the vascularity and permeability of cancer lesions as it passes through the patient's tissues. This is referred to as *perfusion CT, functional CT*, or, more recently, *dynamic contrast-enhanced computed tomography (DCE-CT)*. One application of these methods is to detect response of hepatocellular carcinoma to antiangiogenic

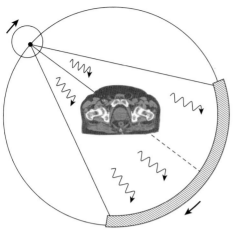

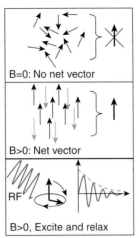

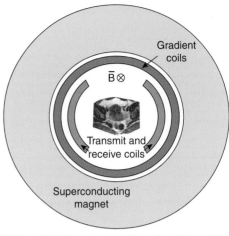

CT signal: Attenuation of x-rays within the patient

MR Signal: Variations in relaxation of certain nuclei in a magnetic field (eg, hydrogen protons in water)

A

B

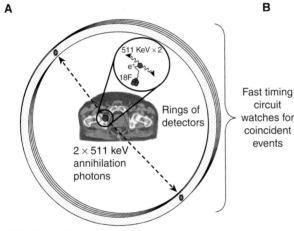

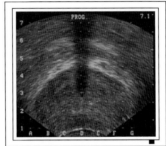

PET Signal: Detection of decaying nuclei through detection of coincident positron annihilation events

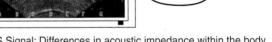

US Signal: Differences in acoustic impedance within the body

C

D

FIGURE 14–3 **Imaging technologies used in oncology. A)** In a modern CT imaging system, a multirow detector and high-power x-ray source rotate about the patient at high speed (>2 revolutions per second). Thousands of "projections" are collected as the patient advances through the scanner and computers are used to "reconstruct" multiple imaged slices representing the attenuation characteristics of the patient. This is presented in grayscale form as the CT image. **B)** An MR image signal has many forms, but relies largely on the excitation and relaxation of a population of field-aligned magnetic dipoles associated with protons (hydrogen nuclei) in water. MR imaging systems consist of a large superconducting magnet that maintains the static field (typically 1.5 Tesla), that causes the field alignment of the magnetic dipoles of hydrogen nuclei of the water molecules, and a set of gradient-inducing coils that manipulate the magnetic field throughout the volume. The radiofrequency transmit and receive coils are responsible for perturbing the hydrogen nuclei and then recording their relaxation back to the ground state in the presence of the magnetic field. **C)** PET imaging is often used in conjunction with a CT system (called a PET-CT scanner). PET image formation is achieved through detection of positron-emitting decay events that ultimately produce pairs of 511 keV photons at approximately 180 degrees from each other. This image is then superimposed on the CT image generated at the same time by the dual-purpose scanner. **D)** Ultrasound (US) imaging systems exploit variations in acoustic impedance within the body to generate images. Ultrasound waves are reflected at boundaries between tissues of differential impedance (eg, fat, muscle, bladder wall). In this figure, an axial ultrasound image of the prostate is shown as generated by a transrectal ultrasound probe (see illustration).

therapies. DCE-CT is sensitive to vascular changes that occur before conventional size-related measures of tumor response (Jiang et al, 2011).

14.3.2 Magnetic Resonance Imaging

The MR image signal arises from the following 5 concepts (see Fig. 14–3B): (a) a large ensemble of nuclear magnetic moments

or "tiny bar magnets" (eg, hydrogen nuclei in water) are contained within the human body; (b) an applied, static magnetic field (eg, 1.5 Tesla [T]) sets a slight bias in their orientation—the higher the field, the larger the bias; (c) the application of an external radiofrequency field to perturb the moments from this bias; (d) the surrounding chemical and physical microenvironment impacts the time required (T1) to return to alignment (relax) with the static field; and (e) the ability of the ensemble to induce a measureable current in a detecting antenna (conducting loop) exterior to the object. Protons (and other atomic nuclei possessing a magnetic moment) within tissues oscillate, or precess, in this magnetic field (B) at a frequency (w) given by $w = \gamma B$ where the proportionality constant γ is called the *gyromagnetic ratio*; γ is specific for each nucleus and depends on the magnetic moment of the nucleus.

Damadian (1971) first proposed that the rate of relaxation of protons in water could distinguish normal from tumor tissue and demonstrated that tumors (sarcomas and hepatomas) had differing T1 relaxation times that were 1.5 to 2 times longer than in normal tissues in the same animal. These differences in relaxation times are a reflection of the different environments in which the protons relax to alignment with the static field—the presence of cancer alters this environment compared to that found in normal tissue.

The development of methods to generate images of nominal relaxation times followed from the work of Lauterbur (1973) and Mansfield (Mansfield and Maudsley, 1977) for which they received the Nobel Prize in Medicine in 2003. MR imaging (MRI) systems are now widely used in cancer detection and diagnosis. Figure 14–3*B* demonstrates the central components: A static magnetic field (typically 1.5 Tesla or 15,000 times the earth's field) is generated by a superconducting magnet; the patient is placed within the magnet; gradient coils are used to create slight differences in magnetic field across the patient to encode for location; and, finally, a pair of antennae is responsible for exciting the nuclei and detecting the electromagnetic signal that they induce as they return to their ground states. Spatial information that allows the formation of images is obtained by slightly varying the applied magnetic field across the body in 3 orthogonal directions using the gradient coils.

In a 1.5-Tesla magnetic field, the precession frequency of water protons is 64 MHz. Radiofrequency (RF) pulses of energy applied at this frequency alter the angle at which the protons are precessing around the magnetic field lines. Once a 90-degree pulse is switched off, the protons gradually return to alignment with the static field. The time taken for the return to alignment (the T_1 signal, also called the *spin-lattice relaxation time*) is one metric of the local chemical and physiological environment of the protons and can provide contrast between tissues. Similarly, the phase of their precession can be synchronized within the transverse plane (through a 180-degree pulse). When the RF is switched off, dephasing gradually occurs and the time to reduce the transverse magnetization is referred to as T_2. This dephasing is associated with both molecular effects and inhomogeneity in the magnetic field; T_2 is used commonly to distinguish soft tissues and is called the *spin-spin relaxation time*.

Because complete isolation of T_1 and T_2 signals is challenging, images are typically T_1 or T_2 "weighted" depending on the RF pulse sequence applied. Specifically, by varying the repetition time (TR) between RF pulse cycles and the time to sample the resulting signal or the echo time (TE), it is possible to "weight" the image. There are 3 basic weightings used

in clinical practice: T_1, T_2, and proton-density weighting. In general, T_1 weighting provides anatomical detail, while T_2-weighted images give elevated signal for tissues with a higher content of free unbound water and are essential in imaging inflammation or "neoplastic" tissue. Proton density simply reflects the density of water protons available for signal production in the voxel.

MR can be used to explore other tissue parameters, such as changes in local transport of water in tissue that may reflect cellular sensitivity to treatment. This can be characterized by exposing excited nuclei in tissue to variations in a magnetic field and examining the rate of signal loss; this is referred to as *apparent diffusion coefficient* (ADC) imaging (Le Bihan et al, 1986). Figure 14–4*A* illustrates the process used in MR to estimate the diffusion of water within a voxel (Hagmann et al, 2006). In brief, a conventional spin-echo sequence is modified by applying 2 gradient pulses before and after the 180-degree pulse to encode the degree of proton mobility (ie, diffusion) into a loss in recovered signal as a result of transport-induced imperfections in rephasing of the spins. Figure 14–4*B* presents diffusion-weighted images of a patient before and after treatment for lymphoma.

Exogenous agents can be applied to alter the MR signal. Spin-lattice relaxation time (T_1) and spin-spin relaxation time (T_2) may be shortened considerably in the presence of paramagnetic species (eg, gadolinium), which have unpaired electrons. Stable agents that contain gadolinium are used in the clinical setting (eg, gadopentate dimeglumine or gadolinium-diethylenetriamine pentaacetic acid [Gd-DPTA]; gadoteridol [Gd-HP-D03A]), and there is growing interest in iron oxides, for detection and characterization of nodal disease (Harisinghani et al, 2006) or for use in cell "tracking" studies in animal research (Heyn et al, 2006). New MR contrast agents are being developed, including some that rely on the rapid exchange of protons between molecular environments to describe the chemical milieu (Sherry and Woods, 2008) and some that can increase the polarization of specific nuclei to enhance the MR signal by several orders of magnitude (Golman, Ardenkjaer-Larsen et al, 2003).

Magnetic resonance spectroscopy imaging (MRSI) involves the extension of nuclear magnetic resonance (NMR) techniques employed in chemistry to the concepts of imaging. Spectra associated with the chemical shift in resonance peaks for various biomolecules in small regions of interest can be acquired on MRI systems. Collecting a number of spectra in adjacent regions in a rectilinear array (Fig. 14–5*A*) and generating a coarse image is referred to as *MRSI* or *chemical shift imaging* (CSI). MRSI can be applied to protons in water or other nuclei with a magnetic moment such as ^{31}P, ^{13}C, and ^{19}F. Figure 14–5*B* illustrates the nature of the spectra produced on a clinical 1.5-Tesla MR scanner when imaging the prostate; the poorly resolved spectra are reduced to ratios of peaks to form a color-coded image of disease burden. Adoption of higher field (3 Tesla) MR scanners will enable greater spectral separation of the peaks and may lead to accelerated adoption of these techniques (Glunde et al, 2011).

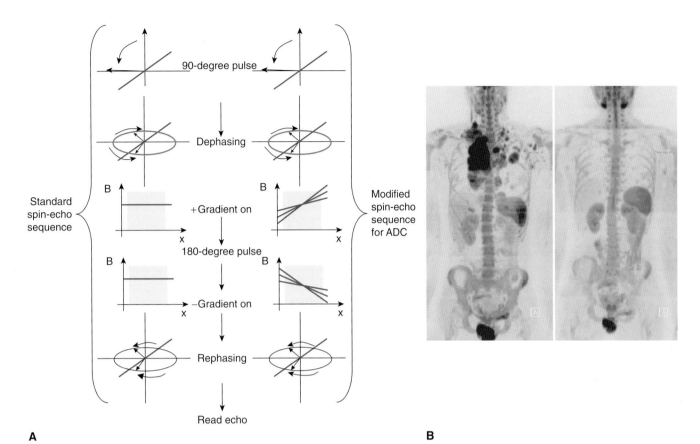

A

B

FIGURE 14–4 **A) The ADC (or diffusion-weighted imaging [DWI]) imaging technique seeks to measure the diffusion of water within a voxel by exposing the excited water protons to a spatial gradient during their dephasing to encode for their diffusive transport.** This exposure is done before and after a 180-degree spin-echo pulse. Voxels that contain spins exposed to differential fields because of diffusive transport will have a reduced echo following the 180-degree rephasing pulse. Those that are stationary will be refocused to within normal T_2 losses. **B)** DWI is also of interest in assessing total cancer burden, as these techniques can also be used to image the entire body. In their review of DWI in oncology, Padhani et al (2011) demonstrate DWI in the assessment of pretreatment disease burden and its response to chemotherapy in a patient with Hodgkin lymphoma. The 2 panels show pre- and posttreatment DWI images. (Reproduced with permission from Padhani et al, 2011.)

The excellent soft-tissue discrimination of MR makes it well-suited to oncology and MRI has a role in the diagnosis, staging, and management of many solid cancer. For example, MR has become the dominant imaging method for cancers of the central nervous system where the high T_1 contrast and sensitivity of T_2 to changes in edema delineate the extent of disease and allow understanding of the patterns of spread. Its role in evaluating metastatic lesions in the spinal column, including those requiring urgent treatment because of spinal cord compression is definitive. MRSI is also employed in neurooncology as an additional classifier of disease prior to surgical intervention (Hollingworth et al, 2006). Although use of MR in breast screening or directing surgery is controversial, it is useful as a screening method for women at high risk (~20% probability) of developing breast cancer (Lehman et al, 2009). Dynamic contrast-enhanced magnetic resonance (DCE-MR) (conceptually equivalent to DCE-CT) is emerging as a biomarker of drug activity in breast cancer (Moon et al, 2009) and is being used in clinical trials that assess response of disease to antivascular agents (Yankeelov and Gore, 2009) and

to radiation therapy (Cao, 2011). There is a growing interest in the development of dedicated MRI systems to guide cancer therapy; this includes the direction of high-intensity focused ultrasound (HIFU), neurosurgery, and MR-guided radiotherapy (Lagendijk et al, 2008). Until recently, the relatively slow acquisition times have limited the use of MRI in sites influenced by motion (eg, chest), but this is changing rapidly with the development of faster imaging techniques that employ multiple channels. The progression to higher field strength (3 Tesla) offers increases in SNR and spatial resolution, and MR is attractive in that there is no exposure of subjects to ionizing radiation and hence to risk of second (radiation-induced) malignancies (see Chap. 16, Sec. 16.8).

14.3.3 Single-Photon and Positron Emission Tomography

Unstable nuclei that emit high-energy gamma-rays or positrons provide a powerful tool in probing the nature of cancer and contribute to its management. Molecules containing such

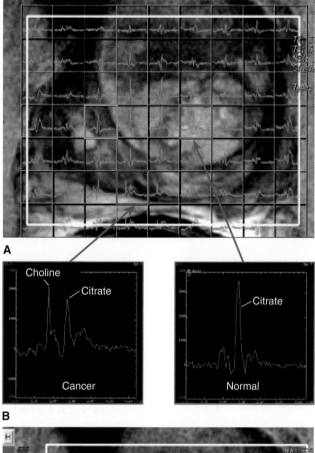

A

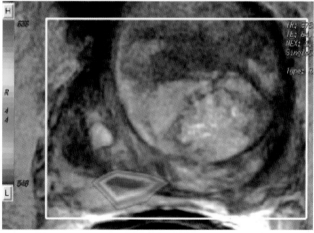

B

C

FIGURE 14–5 **Magnetic resonance spectroscopy (MRS) offers the potential for metabolic imaging by detecting molecular environment-induced frequency shifts in the resonance of nuclei. A)** A set of MR spectra acquired in a rectilinear array and overlaid on the conventional MR image of the prostate (1.5 Tesla with endorectal coil). The spectra contain a citrate peak present in normal and disease tissues, while the elevated choline peak corresponds to disease (**B**). **C)** Spectral analysis in these studies consists of calculating ratios of signal over specific frequency intervals or peak heights estimated from peak-fitting algorithms (eg, Cho/Cit ratios). These ratios are then converted to a color-coded pattern and overlaid on the MR image to identify regions of elevated disease burden.

nuclei can be injected into the body and accumulate through a variety of processes that reflect different metabolic aspects of the disease state. Single-photon emission computed tomography (SPECT) imaging operates on the principle of emission of gamma-rays in the range of 100 keV that are detected by a collimated crystal (gamma camera) that encodes for direction and location in the field of view. The gamma camera images are then used to reconstruct an estimate of the distribution of the gamma-ray emitters in the body. SPECT is heavily utilized in cancer for the staging and assessment of cancer progression in the form of a "bone scan." In this technique, the patient is injected with a small amount of radioactive material such as technetium-99m (^{99m}Tc)-labeled medronic acid (a bisphosphonate) and then scanned with a gamma or 3-dimensional (3D) SPECT camera. The accumulation of the medronic acid in regions of bone remodeling is a sensitive detector of metastasis to bone.

In contrast to SPECT, PET employs radioisotopes that emit a positron upon decay. For example, a radioactive isotope of fluorine (^{18}F) emits a positron that annihilates through interaction with an electron to produce a pair of annihilation photons (511 keV each), which are emitted at approximately 180 degrees to each other. Figure 14–3C illustrates the coincident detection of the event in detectors distributed on multiple rings around the patient. Large numbers of these coincident events are then used to generate (or reconstruct) an image of the spatial distribution of the annihilation events, which represents the distribution of the ^{18}F-labelled agent. The most widely used PET agent is a radiolabeled sugar that becomes trapped within cells that have active glucose metabolism, as is the case for malignant tumors (see Chap. 12, Sec. 12.3.1). ^{18}F-Fluorodeoxyglucose (FDG) is injected intravenously into the body and allowed to circulate and metabolize for approximately 45 minutes. The patient is then positioned in the PET scanner and images are collected to image the whole body for regions of elevated uptake.

There are advantages and disadvantages to the SPECT and PET approaches. The ability to integrate radioisotopes directly into a molecule of interest minimizes impact on the pharmacokinetics of the agent itself. Moreover agents can be designed to target many aspects of tumor cell metabolism and the tumor microenvironment. However, the half-life of the probe needs to be selected for the specific objective: the radioactive half-life needs to be longer than the half-life of the physical process that one is interested in characterizing, but it shouldn't be much longer, or the radiation dose delivered would be excessive. Some positron-emitting radioisotopes (^{15}O, ^{11}C) can be readily integrated into various molecules but have very short half-lives and require production in a cyclotron that is adjacent to the radiochemistry laboratory and the imaging suite. ^{18}F, the most commonly used positron-emitting radioisotope, has a half-life of 110 minutes and therefore can be shipped from remote sources within a few hours with sufficient activity for imaging purposes. ^{99m}Tc is the most commonly used SPECT isotope and is a daughter product of a molybdenum generator that can be located within the local SPECT laboratory.

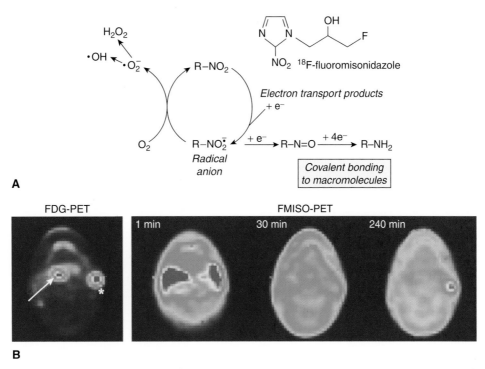

FIGURE 14–6 **A) Hypoxia results in the accumulation of FMISO in the cell through a process that is dependent on reduction of the nitro (NO_2) group by 1 e– nitroreductases.** If O_2 is not present, the tracer is sequentially further reduced to an alkylating agent and is bound in the cell. In the presence of oxygen, the initial reduction step is back-oxidized to recreate the original molecule, which can diffuse out of the cell again (Mason et al, 2010). **B)** This illustrative figure adapted from Padhani et al (2007), with permission, shows an FDG-PET image (bottom left) with increased uptake in both the oropharyngeal tumor (arrow) and in the left neck nodal metastasis (asterisk). The FMISO-PET images (bottom right series) were selected from the dynamic acquisition after 1 minute, 30 minutes, and 240 minutes. The early distribution (1 minute) shows hyperperfusion in the region of the primary tumor and metastasis. However, only the left neck nodal metastasis is shown to retain FMISO (and hence is suspected of containing hypoxic cells) after 240 minutes.

The development of combined PET-CT and SPECT-CT systems was motivated by the advantages of using CT to correct for attenuation by the patient's anatomy in reconstruction of the image (Townsend et al, 2003), but it is now recognized that the additional imaging information provided from the CT is also beneficial. FDG-PET is employed in detecting regional disease and metastatic lesions in people with cancer; it increases the accuracy of staging and thereby promises to lead to better outcomes (Al-Ibraheem et al, 2009). The role of FDG-PET images for target delineation in radiotherapy is a topic of intense research with its value varying with disease site (Gregoire et al, 2007). In addition to imaging metabolism, PET has been employed to characterize the degree of hypoxia in solid cancers (see Chap. 12, Sec. 12.2.1 and Chap. 16, Sec. 16.4). F-misonidazole (FMISO)-PET and ^{18}F-fluoroazomycin arabinoside (FAZA)-PET are hypoxia localizing agents that become trapped in cells as a result of reduction in the absence of oxygen, so that accumulation occurs only in cells that have low oxygen concentration (Padhani et al, 2007; Krohn et al, 2008). Figure 14–6A illustrates the process of trapping of FMISO in the cell under conditions of hypoxia. The dynamics of agent delivery can also be used to examine perfusion of the tissues (Fig. 14–6B; Thorwarth et al, 2005). Numerous cancer-related PET agents are in development, but FDG remains the only one

in routine use: Challenges to bringing additional agents to the clinical domain include cost, the requirement for validation studies, regulatory constraints, and difficulty integrating the new image-based information into clinical use.

14.3.4 Ultrasound Imaging

Ultrasound imaging utilizes the variations in acoustic impedance in the different tissues of the body to generate anatomic images. Figure 14–3D illustrates a modern ultrasound probe configuration for transrectal ultrasound of the prostate. Piezoelectric crystals are capable of generating very high-frequency acoustic waves (ultrasonic) in the range of 1 to 20 MHz and correspond to short wavelengths given the speed of sound in tissue (~1500 m/s). The ultrasound image is formed through careful manipulation of the acoustic source and detection of the reflected acoustic pressure wave. Although ultrasound is limited in its depth of penetration (1 to 15 cm), it has many useful advantages including low cost, adaptability to small probes for directing minimally invasive biopsy procedures (eg, endobronchial ultrasound, prostate biopsy) and use in tissues that are relatively homogenous (eg, liver imaging). In addition to structural information, ultrasound also offers accurate assessment of flow rates in large vessels using the

Doppler phenomenon, in which, the relative motion of the blood induces frequency shifts in the reflected sound waves. Ultrasound can also be applied with contrast agents, such as, microbubbles (Wilson and Burns, 2001) that reflect the sound waves producing very-high-contrast signals. This technique has been used to study tissue perfusion in organs and neoplastic lesions (Delorme et al, 2006). Researchers are also applying molecular imaging approaches to specifically target the bubbles to endothelial cell surface receptors to allowing imaging of the density of such receptors in normal tissue or tumor blood vessels (Caskey et al, 2011).

In the clinic, ultrasound is used widely in the detection, diagnosis, clinical staging, and treatment of cancer. Ultrasound has proven useful in the characterization of lesions in the breast, liver, and kidney, and recent use of ultrasonic contrast agents such as bubbles has improved this performance substantially (Quaia et al, 2006). In addition to diagnosis, ultrasound is used for directing biopsies, providing information in the surgical management of prostate or pancreatic lesions, and is also employed for localizing structures during radiation therapy. For example, transabdominal ultrasound imaging is used in daily radiation treatments to localize the prostate and adjust the patient position just prior to treatment. In the context of brachytherapy of prostate cancer using permanent radioactive seed implants, transrectal ultrasound is used to localize both the gland and the seeds as they are placed in the gland by the oncologist.

14.3.5 Optical Imaging

Optical imaging continues to play an expanding role in characterization and management of cancer. The development of endoscopic systems has been accelerated by advances in fiberoptic and camera technologies that permit high-quality optical imaging to be applied within the body's orifices and luminal structures (eg, colonoscopy, bronchoscopy, and cystoscopy). High-definition video capture, integration of channels for biopsy/resection, and the development of navigation technologies is increasing the application of these systems. These systems can collect light over a wide spectrum from near infrared to blue or operate on a narrow band. In addition, they can be used with different light sources ranging from white light to higher-frequency stimulating sources to generate fluorescence. The endogenous absorption of light in tissue provides significant signal for the detection and characterization of disease by these methods. Although optical imaging suffers from scattering and absorption within the body, it has several advantages, including the high detection efficiency of optical detectors, the abundance of light photons that can be generated and interact without harm to tissue, and the potential to support molecular imaging. The potential for optical imaging to increase the sensitivity of detecting lesions on luminal structures (eg, colon, glottis, esophagus) has resulted in substantial research in this area. The detection of autofluorescence demonstrating increased sensitivity to cancer lesions in the oral cavity is a very promising example

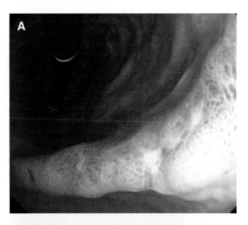
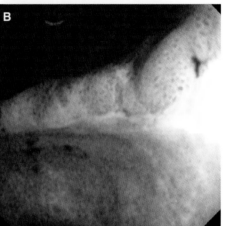
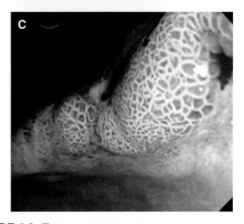

FIGURE 14–7 **Endoscopic techniques continue to evolve as demonstrated in this series of images from Filip et al (2011).** Endoscopy of an early gastric adenocarcinoma at the level of the gastric angle reveals (**A**) an irregular ulcer visualized in white-light endoscopy and (**B**) autofluorescence images showing in magenta the neoplastic margins and a larger lesion extension, as compared with white-light endoscopy. Further advances in resolution and selection of a narrow wavelength band (**C**) shows a modified pit pattern, with irregular and distorted vascular pattern in the center suggesting high-grade dysplasia/early cancer.

(Poh et al, 2006). This is illustrated in Figure 14–7 where (a) white light, (b) autofluorescence, and (c) narrowband imaging each provide increasing detail in the characterization of a gastric adenocarcinoma.

Endoscopic imaging is a heavily used imaging modality in cancer detection and in the context of colon cancer, colonoscopy is now a recommended procedure for patients over the age of 50 years as part of a broader screening program. The same tools are used to direct the biopsy and remove suspicious lesions. Challenges persist in the characterization of flat lesions and the introduction of optical imaging techniques beyond that of white light is a current area of research. Endoscopy is also a routine part of cancer management of many other sites including cancer of the head and neck, lung, and esophagus. The low cost and adaptability of endoscopes has resulted in other uses, including the design of radiation therapy treatments (Weersink et al, 2011) and the assessment of the response of tissue to cancer therapeutics. Georg et al (2009) have correlated rectal endoscopy scores with the volume of rectal tissue receiving elevated doses during radiation therapy of the cervix. The continued advances in endoscope technology and advances in optical imaging probes make this a particularly promising area of development for cancer imaging.

14.4 IMAGING OF ANIMAL MODELS IN ONCOLOGY

With the growing use of small animal models of disease in cancer research, there has been a corresponding growth in the use of small animal imaging systems to characterize the disease with the aim of understanding cancer in these animal models and its response to novel therapies. Imaging is forming an effective bridge between the clinical and preclinical domains as investigators relate image-based observations from the clinic to the biological basis of the disease in pertinent genetically engineered animals or human tumor xenografts (see Chap. 2, Sec. 2.4.5). Preclinical models of cancer typically include human tumor xenografts (primary or serially transplanted) and genetically engineered murine or rat models. The use of imaging technologies (micro-MRI, -PET, -CT, -SPECT, and optical imaging) can interrogate local tumor growth, metastatic progression, tumor metabolism, and treatment response to allow for the design and testing of novel clinical regimens (Weissleder et al, 2008). The use of multiple preclinical, noninvasive imaging techniques also allows the choice of the best way to address a particular oncology question, something that cannot be easily done in the clinic because of cost and patient inconvenience.

The scaling of CT systems from man to mouse was made possible by the creation of high-resolution digital detectors (~0.1 mm resolution) for radiography and fluoroscopy, as conventional CT detectors (~1 mm resolution) would be of limited use in a mouse model. In addition to the challenges of achieving higher resolution, there is concern associated with the radiation dose necessary to maintain a good signal to noise ratio (SNR) at the required resolution. In CT, the SNR in a cubic voxel depends on the square of the voxel dimension. Thus, achieving 50-μm images with a SNR comparable to that found in human CT imaging (500-μm images) would

require the imaging dose to be increased 100-fold. Although this has been a concern, this technology has been applied with a compromise between noise and acceptable imaging doses (~5 to 30 cGy), and preclinical CT systems with spatial resolution as low as 18 μm are available (Marxen et al, 2004). These preclinical CT systems have been applied for purposes similar to those used for human imaging—measuring tumor growth, assessing bone injury in metastatic models of disease, and even mimicking the DCE-CT techniques used in clinical oncology. For example, rat brain CT perfusion studies with a resolution of approximately 150 μm have been achieved with these systems (Greschus et al, 2005). As with clinical CT, the excellent geometric integrity can be used to guide microenvironmental probes to specific locations within the imaged subject, and to direct biopsies (Waspe et al, 2010). Robotic systems directed under preclinical CT can achieve targeted biopsies with mean errors of less than 100 μm. Similarly, cone-beam CT systems have been integrated with irradiation systems to direct small radiation beams (<2 mm in diameter) to treat xenograft tumor models in mice (Clarke et al, 2009).

The powerful soft-tissue imaging capabilities of MR has driven the development of high-field MR scanners to enable high-resolution, low-noise imaging of small animals. For example, DCE-MR methods have been adapted to these platforms for quantitative, multiparametric evaluation of treatment response. This has been of particular interest to those examining the optimization of treatment protocols that employ antivascular agents. The creation of a "preclinical mimic" of clinical imaging techniques is an attractive development to allow preclinical evaluation of therapies that would benefit from an image-based biomarker of response.

The ability to monitor noninvasively chemical interactions within the body would reveal a great deal about cancer biology. Concentrations of highly polarized ^{13}C nuclei (10^5 times higher signal than water-based MR) produce sufficient signal to map molecular distributions of injected ^{13}C within organs for several seconds after injection (Golman, Olsson et al, 2003). Through frequency selection and careful design of pulse sequences, different metabolic species (eg, ^{13}C pyruvate) can be monitored as the ^{13}C is transported through metabolic processes. Figure 14–8 demonstrates the capabilities of MRI techniques when combined with high-contrast metabolically active agents (Kurhanewicz et al, 2008). These techniques bring a powerful new perspective for understanding cancer metabolism and are being advanced into the clinical setting.

Preclinical SPECT and PET imaging systems are routinely employed in preclinical oncological research. Figure 14–9 illustrates the result of an FDG-PET imaging study in a mouse tumor model. The close proximity of the detectors to the animal permits higher resolution imaging than achieved in clinical systems and illustrates heterogeneity in FDG uptake across the tumor. The preclinical systems are used to evaluate novel PET probes, such as hypoxia agents, which need to be cross-calibrated against other measures of the partial pressure of oxygen (pO_2) (Busk, Horsman, Jakobsen et al, 2008).

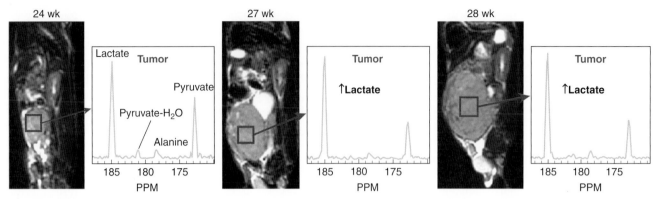

FIGURE 14–8 **The development of 3D MRSI with hyperpolarized ^{13}C is an exciting development for oncology imaging.** Postinjection rapid MR spectroscopy (14 seconds/spectrum over a 0.135 cm^3 region within the tumor) can be used to monitor the signal from injected ^{13}C-pyruvate and its metabolic derivatives, including lactate and alanine. In this transgenic model of prostate cancer (TRAMP), Kurhanewicz et al (2008) demonstrate high levels of lactate were produced from hyperpolarized ^{13}C-pyruvate and that lactate production (relative to the pyruvate signal) in the tumor increased as the tumor progressed from the 24th to the 27th and 28th week postimplantation.

PET and SPECT systems are also very useful in evaluating the performance of novel targeted therapies by tracking accumulation of radiolabeled therapeutics (Pinchuk et al, 2006), probing molecular markers of cancer during therapy (McLarty et al, 2009), and for assessment of drug or vehicle delivery (Harrington et al, 2001).

Ultrasound systems have also been adapted to support very-high-frequency probes for preclinical studies and ultrasound microscopy (Foster et al, 2009; Knspik et al, 2000). Ultrasound is being employed to characterize growth delay in tumor models following therapy, assess the impact of antivascular therapies (Cheung et al, 2007), and measure cellular responses to

treatment, such as apoptosis (Czarnota et al, 2002). Preclinical ultrasound is used to evaluate the development of novel ultrasound contrast agents that are actively targeted or can be used in synergy with other therapeutic agents.

Development of optical imaging technologies in the preclinical domain include flat-field bioluminescent and fluorescent imaging systems, as well as the development of 3D systems to allow more quantitative measures (Graves et al, 2004). These systems rely on high-performance cameras that incorporate charge-coupled devices and multichannel plate technology to achieve low-noise images of the emitted optical signal. The development of bioluminescent technologies, such as transfection of fluorescent proteins or luciferase into cells, has enhanced the usefulness of these devices. Endoscopic confocal microscopes with resolutions of approximately 5 μm now allow visualization of biological processes in real-time (Lin et al, 2008). The creation of these preclinical tools has spurred the initiation of research in optical tracers and probes that is likely to have a profound impact on the role of optical imaging in the clinic.

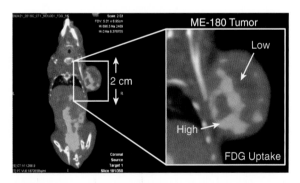

FIGURE 14–9 **PET imaging can also be applied in the preclinical setting to increase our understanding of the underlying biology, as well as inform the design of clinical imaging studies.** In this example, an FDG-PET image is acquired of a subcutaneous tumor (ME-180, cancer cervix model). The accumulation of FDG is seen to be quite heterogeneous within the mass. The generation of such a high-resolution image would be challenging on a clinical PET scanner because of the detector geometry. The use of a preclinical system helps to inform our understanding of a clinical FDG image and how it relates to the very-high-resolution microscopy demonstrated in Figure 14–1A. (Image courtesy of STTARR Facility, Toronto, Canada.)

14.5 NEW DIRECTIONS IN ONCOLOGY IMAGING

14.5.1 Quantitative Methods and Quality Assurance

The promise of using imaging for noninvasive characterization of disease requires that the measurement systems are accurate and provide fidelity of the spatial distribution. For example, it is well-known that the resolution of the FDG-PET imaging system can reduce the accuracy of the specific uptake value (SUV) estimation (Erdi et al, 1997), but this knowledge is not routinely applied in assessing clinical response. Similar issues are found in MRI, wherein, changes to an imaging sequence or modification of the MR scanner can introduce spurious results into longitudinal imaging studies designed to monitor response. The National Institutes of Health in the United States has embarked on an effort to increase the quantitative performance of clinical imaging (Clarke et al, 2009). The Quantitative Imaging Network (QIN) aims to "promote research and development of quantitative imaging methods for the measurement of tumor response to therapies in clinical trial settings, with the overall goal of facilitating clinical decision making" (NCI/NIH, 2009). This program for coordinated imaging in clinical trials is also establishing a qualification program that includes standardized operating procedures for quality assurance, patient preparation, imaging, and image analysis. In conjunction with these efforts, there has been an increased use of test phantoms for evaluating both static and dynamic imaging sequences, as well as evaluating the dose delivered during CT imaging studies. These efforts will help transform clinical CT, MR, and PET scanners from simply being "imaging systems" to become quantitative measurement tools that can be used to make certified measurements to direct cancer care.

14.5.2 Automated Analysis Methods: Improving on RECIST Criteria

Although the generation of the image is often the focus of imaging research, the extraction of relevant information for use in directing therapy or correlative studies is of equivalent importance. For example, the Response Evaluation Criteria in Solid Tumors (RECIST) was published in 2000 as a consensus among European, American, and Canadian cancer research groups (Therasse et al, 2000). The fundamental measure in RECIST is the longest diameter of the target lesion(s) and its change during therapy (ie, 30% decrease for response, 20% increase for progressive disease). Given the wealth of information collected by imaging methods described in this chapter, the RECIST measure is a remarkable reduction of information. RECIST criteria are heavily used in current clinical trials despite their known weaknesses (Therasse et al, 2006). The development of quantitative imaging metrics beyond tumor size should allow more advanced analysis of tumor response to treatment. The introduction of functional measures such as FDG-PET, the use of contrast agents, and the broader use of MRI in assessment of response (eg, DCE-MR) is raising concerns about the relevance of the RECIST criteria (Tuma, 2006). While it is recognized that RECIST needs to evolve, it should be done with appropriate levels of standardization and validation, and there has been substantial effort put toward automated segmentation algorithms with the objective of developing efficient 3D measurements (Marten et al, 2007; Farmaki et al, 2010) and voxel-based measures of response using MR (Moffat et al, 2005). The continued growth of uni- and multimodal image sets will require automated algorithms to assist in observer-independent interpretation and efficient reporting if the impact of imaging on cancer is going to reach its full potential.

14.5.3 Images and Biological Information Combined for Discovery

There has been a substantial shift in the past decade toward using multiple modalities for the characterization of cancer. The combination of molecular and anatomical imaging, such as PET and CT, allows 3D quantitative analysis of a molecular imaging signal. While PET-CT was motivated by the advantages of using CT for correction of attenuation, it has proven to be even more valuable as a result of improvements in specificity achieved when both images, perfectly registered, are presented to the nuclear medicine physician. Research groups are developing combined MR-PET imaging systems with the expectation of further gains, but these remain to be proven (Schlemmer et al, 2009). There are ongoing efforts to integrate optical and CT systems in the preclinical domain to allow optical systems to be more quantitative (da Silva et al, 2007). Challenges for multimodal imaging in the clinical domain have stimulated development of software to allow images collected at various time points and by various modalities to be integrated, and corrected for variations in anatomical position (Brock, 2007). This remains an area of significant research and development.

There is an ongoing challenge of quantifying and relating image signals to the underlying cellular and biological properties of tissue, as traditionally characterized by morphological or molecular pathology (Busk, Horsman, Overgaard et al, 2008). There has been an increased focus on histopathological validation of image signals; for example, Daisne et al (2004) studied the extent of disease in head and neck patients by examining clinical images and pathology sections. They were able to compare the relative performance of CT, MR, and FDG-PET in delineating tumor extent. The development of large field-of-view microscopes, registration/deformation software algorithms, and standardized tissue-handling protocols for these activities are slowly advancing the field. In addition to comparison with resected whole-mount specimens, targeted biopsy of tissue within MR and ultrasound images has been undertaken as a means of generating histopathological validation of the complexity of information achieved with multimodality imaging (Bax et al, 2008; Susil et al, 2006).

Most recently, the fusion of imaging information with genomic information has developed as an area of cancer research. In these studies, the image signals are employed in the bioinformatics framework to identify correlations between specific imaging signals/textures and the gene expression profiles of the associated tissues collected through surgery or biopsy. This is referred to as "radiogenomics" or "radiomics" (Lambin et al, 2012). Figure 14–10 demonstrates such an analysis linking radiologist classification of MR images of brain tumors with various tissue-derived microarray signatures. More recently, morphologically relevant MRI signatures have been correlated with specific genes and microRNAs that are associated with mesenchymal transformation and invasion (Zinn et al, 2011). This type of research will help bridge the molecular–clinical gap of translational cancer medicine, with imaging being a powerful research tool with a subsequent role in clinical applications of image-based personalized cancer medicine.

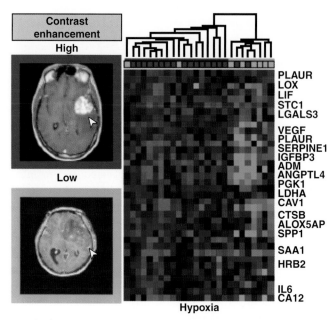

Contrast enhancement
High
Low
Hypoxia

PLAUR
LOX
LIF
STC1
LGALS3

VEGF
PLAUR
SERPINE1
IGFBP3
ADM
ANGPTL4
PGK1
LDHA
CAV1

CTSB
ALOX5AP
SPP1

SAA1

HRB2

IL6
CA12

FIGURE 14–10 Radiomics or radiogenomics involves the integration of imaging signals or "image-based biomarkers" into the bioinformatics framework being developed for genetic profiling and correlations with outcome. Imaging also brings distinct spatial information, such as size and invasiveness, and can be remeasured during the course of therapy. Diehn et al (2008) examined the gene-expression surrogates for traits in MR images as shown. MR image signal phenotypes (10 types defined by expert radiologists) were defined and hierarchical clustering of the gene expression profiles of 32 samples, including glioblastoma multiforme and normal brain specimens, was performed and tested for statistical significance. The results specific to contrast accumulation in the brain and hypoxia have been selected for presentation shown here.

SUMMARY

- Imaging provides a means to characterize the dynamic, heterogeneous nature of cancer through morphological and biological signals.
- Advances in CT, MR, and ultrasound imaging technologies allow detection and delineation of disease in the context of screening, design of treatment, and assessment of response to therapy.
- Injecting exogenous agents that interact with specific biological processes enables "molecular imaging" of cancer. These approaches require highly sensitive imaging instruments such as PET and SPECT systems or novel approaches to MR.
- The potential to use these comprehensive imaging measures in the "personalized cancer medicine" paradigm to tune each patient's treatment is one of the most exciting prospects in cancer treatment.
- Substantial effort is required to validate the measured image signals, to develop standards for their consistent deployment across multiple institutions, and to bring them to evaluation through clinical trials.

- Imaging researchers are pushing the limits of imaging science, establishing image-based studies of cancer biology, and linking preclinical and clinical models to accelerate translation of their work.
- Although imaging is an important tool in cancer management and research, it will be used in conjunction with other measures, such as genomic analyses, to advance our understanding of cancer and the development of new treatments.

REFERENCES

Aberle DR, Adams AM, Berg CD, et al. Reduced lung-cancer mortality with low-dose computed tomographic screening. *N Engl J Med* 2011;365:395-409.

Al-Ibraheem A, Buck A, Krause BJ, et al. Clinical Applications of FDG PET and PET/CT in Head and Neck Cancer. *J Oncol* 2009; 2009:208725.

Bax J, Cool D, Gardi L, et al. Mechanically assisted 3D ultrasound guided prostate biopsy system. *Med Phys* 2008;35:5397-5410.

Brenner DJ, Hall EJ. Computed tomography—an increasing source of radiation exposure. *N Engl J Med* 2007;357:2277-2284.

Brock KK. Image registration in intensity-modulated, image-guided and stereotactic body radiation therapy. *Front Radiat Ther Oncol* 2007;40:94-115.

Busk M, Horsman MR, Jakobsen S, et al. *Int J Radiat Oncol Biol Phys* 2008;70(4):1202-1212. doi: 10.1016/j.ijrobp.2007.11.034.

Busk M, Horsman MR, Overgaard J. Resolution in PET hypoxia imaging: voxel size matters. *Acta Oncol* 2008;47:1201-1210.

Cao Y. The promise of dynamic contrast-enhanced imaging in radiation therapy. *Semin Radiat Oncol* 2011;21:147-156.

Caskey CF, Hu X, Ferrara KW. Leveraging the power of ultrasound for therapeutic design and optimization. *J Control Release* 2011; 156:297-306.

Cheung AM, Brown AS, Cucevic V, et al. Detecting vascular changes in tumour xenografts using micro-ultrasound and micro-ct following treatment with VEGFR-2 blocking antibodies. *Ultrasound Med Biol* 2007;33:1259-1268.

Clarke LP, Croft BS, Nordstrom R, et al. Quantitative imaging for evaluation of response to cancer therapy. *Transl Oncol* 2009;2: 195-197.

Czarnota GJ, Kolios MC, Hunt JW, et al. Ultrasound imaging of apoptosis. DNA-damage effects visualized. *Methods Mol Biol* 2002;203:257-277.

da Silva A, Bordy T, Debourdeau M, et al. Coupling X-ray and optical tomography systems for in vivo examination of small animals. *Conf Proc IEEE Eng Med Biol Soc* 2007;2007:3 335-3338.

Daisne JF, Duprez T, Weynand B, et al. Tumor volume in pharyngolaryngeal squamous cell carcinoma: comparison at CT, MR imaging, and FDG PET and validation with surgical specimen. *Radiology* 2004;233:93-100.

Damadian R. Tumor detection by nuclear magnetic resonance. *Science* 1971;181:1151-1153.

Delorme S, Krix M. Contrast-enhanced ultrasound for examining tumor biology. *Cancer Imaging* 2006;6:148-152.

Diehn M, Nardini C, Wang DS, et al. Identification of noninvasive imaging surrogates for brain tumor gene-expression modules. *Proc Natl Acad Sci U S A* 2008;105:5213-5218.

Erdi YE, Mawlawi O, Larson SM, et al. Segmentation of lung lesion volume by adaptive positron emission tomography image thresholding. *Cancer* 1997;80:2505-2509.

Farmaki C, Marias K, Sakkalis V, et al. Spatially adaptive active contours: a semi-automatic tumor segmentation framework. *Int J Comput Assist Radiol Surg* 2010;5:369-384.

Filip M, Iordache S, Saftoiu A, et al. Autofluorescence imaging and magnification endoscopy. *World J Gastroenterol* 2011;17:9-14.

Foster FS, Mehi J, Lukacs M, et al. A new 15-50 MHz array-based micro-ultrasound scanner for preclinical imaging. *Ultrasound Med Biol* 2009;35:1700-1708.

Georg P, Kirisits C, Goldner G, et al. Correlation of dose-volume parameters, endoscopic and clinical rectal side effects in cervix cancer patients treated with definitive radiotherapy including MRI-based brachytherapy. *Radiother Oncol* 2009; 91:173-180.

Glunde K, Bhujwalla ZM. Metabolic tumor imaging using magnetic resonance spectroscopy. *Semin Oncol* 2011;38:26-41.

Golman K, Ardenkjaer-Larsen JH, Petersson JS, et al. Molecular imaging with endogenous substances. *Proc Natl Acad Sci U S A* 2003;100:10435-10439.

Golman K, Olsson LE, Axelsson O, et al. Molecular imaging using hyperpolarized 13C. *Br J Radiol* 2003;76 Spec No 2:S118-S127.

Graves EE, Weissleder R, Ntziachristos V. Fluorescence molecular imaging of small animal tumor models. *Curr Mol Med* 2004;4: 419-430.

Gregoire V, Haustermans K, Geets X, et al. PET-based treatment planning in radiotherapy: a new standard? *J Nucl Med* 2007; 48(suppl 1):68S-77S.

Greschus S, Kiessling F, Lichy MP, et al. Potential applications of flat-panel volumetric CT in morphologic and functional small animal imaging. *Neoplasia* 2005;7:730-740.

Gupta RT, Ho LM, Marin D, et al. Dual-energy CT for characterization of adrenal nodules: initial experience. *AJR Am J Roentgenol* 2010;194:1479-1483.

Hagmann P, Jonasson L, Maeder P, et al. Understanding diffusion MR imaging techniques: from scalar diffusion-weighted imaging to diffusion tensor imaging and beyond. *Radiographics* 2006; 26(suppl 1):S205-S223.

Harisinghani MG, Saksena MA, Hahn PF, et al. Ferumoxtran-10-enhanced MR lymphangiography: does contrast-enhanced imaging alone suffice for accurate lymph node characterization? *AJR Am J Roentgenol* 2006;186:144-148.

Harrington KJ, Mohammadtaghi S, Uster PS, et al. Effective targeting of solid tumors in patients with locally advanced cancers by radiolabeled pegylated liposomes. *Clin Cancer Res* 2001;7:243-254.

Heyn C, Ronald JA, Ramadan SS, et al. In vivo MRI of cancer cell fate at the single-cell level in a mouse model of breast cancer metastasis to the brain. *Magn Reson Med* 2006;56: 1001-1010.

Hollingworth W, Medina LS, Lenkinski RE, et al. A systematic literature review of magnetic resonance spectroscopy for the characterization of brain tumors. *AJNR Am J Neuroradiol* 2006;27:1404-1411.

Jiang T, Kambadakone A, Kulkarni NM, et al. Monitoring response to antiangiogenic treatment and predicting outcomes in advanced hepatocellular carcinoma using image biomarkers,

CT perfusion, tumor density, and tumor size (RECIST). *Invest Radiol* 2011;47:11-17.

Kak AC, Slaney M. *Principles of Computerized Tomographic Imaging.* New York, NY: IEEE Press; 1988.

Knspik DA, Starkoski B, Pavlin CJ, et al. A 100-200 MHz ultrasound biomicroscope. *IEEE Trans Ultrason Ferroelectr Freq Control* 2000; 47:1540-1549.

Krohn KA, Link JM, Mason RP. Molecular imaging of hypoxia. *J Nucl Med* 2008;49(suppl 2):129S-148S.

Kurhanewicz J, Bok R, Nelson SJ, et al. Current and potential applications of clinical 13C MR spectroscopy. *J Nucl Med* 2008;49:341-344.

Lagendijk JJ, Raaymakers BW, Raaijmakers AJ, et al. MRI/linac integration. *Radiother Oncol* 2008;86:25-29.

Lambin P, Rios-Velazquez E, Leijenaar R, et al. Radiomics: Extracting more information from medical images using advanced feature analysis. *Eur J Cancer* 2012;48:441-446.

Lauterbur P. Image formation by induced local interactions: examples employing nuclear magnet resonance. *Nature* 1973;242:190-191.

Le Bihan D, Breton E, Lallemand D, et al. MR imaging of intravoxel incoherent motions: application to diffusion and perfusion in neurologic disorders. *Radiology* 1986;161:401-407.

Lehman CD, Smith RA. The role of MRI in breast cancer screening. *J Natl Compr Canc Netw* 2009;7:1109-1115.

Lin KY, Maricevich M, Bardeesy N, et al. In vivo quantitative microvasculature phenotype imaging of healthy and malignant tissues using a fiber-optic confocal laser microprobe. *Transl Oncol* 2008;1:84-94.

Mansfield P, Maudsley AA. Medical imaging by NMR. *Br J Radiol* 1977;50:188-194.

Marten K, Auer F, Schmidt S, et al. Automated CT volumetry of pulmonary metastases: the effect of a reduced growth threshold and target lesion number on the reliability of therapy response assessment using RECIST criteria. *Eur Radiol* 2007;17:2561-2571.

Marxen M, Thornton MM, Chiarot CB, et al. MicroCT scanner performance and considerations for vascular specimen imaging. *Med Phys* 2004;31:305-313.

Mason RP, Zhao D, Pacheco-Torres J, et al. Multimodality imaging of hypoxia in preclinical settings. *Q J Nucl Med Mol Imaging* 2010;54:259-280.

McLarty K, Cornelissen B, Cai Z, et al. Micro-SPECT/CT with 111In-DTPA-pertuzumab sensitively detects trastuzumab-mediated HER2 downregulation and tumor response in athymic mice bearing MDA-MB-361 human breast cancer xenografts. *J Nucl Med* 2009;50:1340-1348.

Miles KA. Measurement of tissue perfusion by dynamic computed tomography. *Br J Radiol* 1991;64:409-412.

Moffat BA, Chenevert TL, Lawrence TS, et al. Functional diffusion map: a noninvasive MRI biomarker for early stratification of clinical brain tumor response. *Proc Natl Acad Sci U S A* 2005; 102:5524-5529.

Moon M, Cornfeld D, Weinreb J. Dynamic contrast-enhanced breast MR imaging. *Magn Reson Imaging Clin N Am* 2009;17:351-362.

Murakami T, Hori M, Kim T, et al. Xenon-inhalation computed tomography for noninvasive quantitative measurement of tissue blood flow in hepatocellular carcinoma. *Invest Radiol* 2004;39:210-215.

NCI/NIH. *Quantitative Imaging for Evaluation of Responses to Cancer Therapies (U01).* http://imaging.cancer.gov/ programsandresources/SpecializedInitiatives/qin.

Padhani AR, Koh DM, Collins DJ. Whole-body diffusion-weighted MR imaging in cancer: current status and research directions. *Radiology* 2011;261:700-718.

Padhani AR, Krohn KA, Lewis JS, et al. Imaging oxygenation of human tumours. *Eur Radiol* 2007;17:861-872.

Pinchuk AN, Rampy MA, Longino MA, et al. Synthesis and structure-activity relationship effects on the tumor avidity of radioiodinated phospholipid ether analogues. *J Med Chem* 2006;49:2155-2165.

Poh CF, Zhang L, Anderson DW, et al. Fluorescence visualization detection of field alterations in tumor margins of oral cancer patients. *Clin Cancer Res* 2006;12:6716-6722.

Quaia E, D'Onofrio M, Palumbo A, et al. Comparison of contrast-enhanced ultrasonography versus baseline ultrasound and contrast-enhanced computed tomography in metastatic disease of the liver: diagnostic performance and confidence. *Eur Radiol* 2006;16:1599-1609.

Schlemmer HP, Pichler BJ, Krieg R, et al. An integrated MR/PET system: prospective applications. *Abdom Imaging* 2009;34:668-674.

Sherry AD, Woods M. Chemical exchange saturation transfer contrast agents for magnetic resonance imaging. *Annu Rev Biomed Eng* 2008;10:391-411.

Susil RC, Menard C, Krieger A, et al. Transrectal prostate biopsy and fiducial marker placement in a standard 1.5T magnetic resonance imaging scanner. *J Urol* 2006;175:113-120.

Therasse P, Arbuck SG, Eisenhauer EA, et al. New guidelines to evaluate the response to treatment in solid tumors. European Organization for Research and Treatment of Cancer, National Cancer Institute of the United States, National Cancer Institute of Canada. *J Natl Cancer Inst* 2000;92:205-216.

Therasse P, Eisenhauer EA, Verweij J. RECIST revisited: a review of validation studies on tumour assessment. *Eur J Cancer* 2006;42:1031-1039.

Thorwarth D, Eschmann SM, Scheiderbauer J, et al. Kinetic analysis of dynamic 18F-fluoromisonidazole PET correlates with radiation treatment outcome in head-and-neck cancer. *BMC Cancer* 2005;5:152.

Townsend DW, Beyer T, Blodgett TM. PET/CT scanners: a hardware approach to image fusion. *Semin Nucl Med* 2003;33:193-204.

Tuma RS. Sometimes size doesn't matter: reevaluating RECIST and tumor response rate endpoints. *J Natl Cancer Inst* 2006;98:1272-1274.

Waspe AC, McErlain DD, Pitelka V, et al. Integration and evaluation of a needle-positioning robot with volumetric microcomputed tomography image guidance for small animal stereotactic interventions. *Med Phys* 2010;37:1647-1659.

Weersink RA, Qiu J, Hope AJ, et al. Improving superficial target delineation in radiation therapy with endoscopic tracking and registration. *Med Phys* 2011;38:6458-6468.

Weissleder R, Pittet MJ. Imaging in the era of molecular oncology. *Nature* 2008;452:580-589.

Wilson SR, Burns PN. Liver mass evaluation with ultrasound: the impact of microbubble contrast agents and pulse inversion imaging. *Semin Liver Dis* 2001;21:147-159.

Yankeelov TE, Gore JC. Dynamic contrast enhanced magnetic resonance imaging in oncology: theory, data acquisition, analysis, and examples. *Curr Med Imaging Rev* 2009;3:91-107.

Zinn PO, Mahajan B, Sathyan P, et al. Radiogenomic mapping of edema/cellular invasion MRI-phenotypes in glioblastoma multiforme. *PLoS One* 2011;6:e25451.

Molecular and Cellular Basis of Radiotherapy

Shane M. Harding, Richard P. Hill, and Robert G. Bristow

15.1 INTRODUCTION

Since their discovery by Roentgen more than a century ago, x-rays have played a major role in modern medicine. The first recorded use of x-rays for the treatment of cancer occurred within 1 year of their discovery. Subsequently there has been intensive study of x-rays and other ionizing radiations, and their clinical application to cancer treatment has become increasingly sophisticated. This chapter and Chapter 16 review the biological effects of ionizing radiation and the application of that knowledge to cancer treatment.

The present chapter begins with a review of the physical properties of ionizing radiations, their interactions within the cell (membrane, cytoplasm, and nucleus), and the molecular and cellular processes that ensue. The effect of energy deposition in tissue is discussed with emphasis on the pathways that control cellular proliferation following exposure to ionizing radiation. Finally, various genetic and epigenetic factors known to influence the radiosensitivity of normal and tumor cells are described in the context of using molecularly-based targets for designing treatment and predicting response to radiotherapy.

15.2 INTERACTION OF RADIATION WITH MATTER

15.2.1 Types of Radiation, Energy Deposition, and Measurements of Radiation Dose

X- and γ-rays constitute part of the continuous spectrum of electromagnetic (EM) radiation that includes radio waves, heat, and visible and UV light (Fig. 15–1). All types of EM radiation can be considered as moving packets (quanta) of energy called *photons*. The amount of energy in each individual photon defines its position in the EM spectrum. For example, x- or γ-ray photons carry more energy than heat or light photons and are at the high-energy end of the EM spectrum. Individual photons of x-rays are sufficiently energetic that their interaction with matter can result in the complete displacement of an electron from its orbit around the nucleus of an atom. Such an atom (or molecule) is left with a net (positive) charge and is thus an ion; hence the term *ionizing radiation*. Typical binding energies for electrons in biological material are in the neighborhood of 10 eV (electron volts). Thus photons with energies

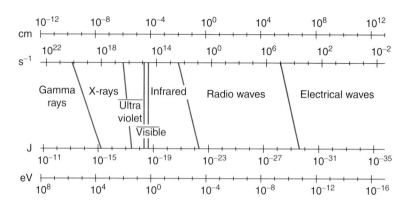

FIGURE 15–1 EM spectrum showing the relationship of photon wavelength in centimeters (cm) to its frequency in inverse seconds (s⁻¹) and to its energy in joules (J) and electron volts (eV). The various bands in the spectrum are indicated. Slanted lines between bands indicate the degree of overlap in the definition of the various bands.

greater than 10 eV are considered to be ionizing radiation, while photons with energies of 2 to 10 eV are in the UV range and are nonionizing. An interaction that transfers energy, but does not completely displace an electron, produces an "excited" atom or molecule and is called an *excitation*.

UV radiation is split into 3 general classes, UV-C, UV-B, and UV-A, corresponding to wavelengths of 200 to 290 nm, 290 to 320 nm and greater than 320 nm, respectively. UV-C and UV-B irradiation can be absorbed by DNA in cells leading to the production of various photoproducts, notably 6-4 photoproducts (6-4PPs) and interstrand crosslinks in the form of cyclobutane pyrimidine dimers. Such lesions may be repaired by a number of processes including nucleotide excision repair (see Chap. 5, Sec. 5.3.3). Because of the limited penetration of UV radiation through tissue, its effects in humans are primarily associated with the skin.

X-rays are produced when accelerated electrons hit a tungsten target and then decelerate emitting a spectrum of *Bremsstrahlung* radiation. The resulting spectrum is filtered to produce a clinically useful beam with minimal x-ray scatter from the axis of the central beam. When x-ray photons interact with tissue, they give up energy by 1 of 3 processes: the photoelectric effect, the Compton effect, or pair production. In the energy range most widely used in radiotherapy (100 keV to 25 MeV), the Compton effect is the most important mechanism leading to deposition of energy in tissue. This energy-transfer process involves a collision between the photon and an outer orbital electron of an atom, with partial transfer of energy to the electron and scattering of the photon into a new direction. The electron (and the photon) can then undergo further interactions, causing more ionizations and excitations, until its energy is dissipated. All 3 of the interaction processes mentioned above result in the production of energetic electrons that, in turn, lose energy by exciting and ionizing target atoms and molecules and setting more electrons in motion.

Modern clinical radiotherapy uses ionizing radiation to treat cancer patients and can be delivered to tissues by external beam radiotherapy using linear accelerators (ie, high-energy x-rays and electron beams), ⁶⁰Co sources (γ-rays produced by radioactive decay as a result of unstable nuclei), or charged particle accelerators. Clinical radiotherapy can also be given using brachytherapy, which delivers highly localized radiation dose from within an organ or tissue using isotopes such as ¹³¹I, ¹²⁵I, and ¹⁰³Pd following radioactive decay (see Chap. 16,

Sec. 16.2.3). The choice of the type of delivery of radiotherapy depends on tumor type and location within the body.

Because of their initial attenuation within the first few millimeters of tissue, low-energy x-ray beams (50 to 250 keV) deposit most of their energy close to the skin surface, and are therefore typically used to treat skin cancers or skin metastases. In contrast, high-energy x-ray beams (18 or 25 MeV) are less attenuated at the skin surface (ie, are "skin-sparing") and deposit most of their energy at a greater depth within the body.

Charged particles can also be used for clinical radiotherapy and include electrons, *light particles* such as protons, and *heavy particles* such as carbon ions. Typically, electron beams are used to treat superficial tumors that require a uniform "skin to specific depth" dose distribution starting right from the outer skin surface while particle beams have been used for high-precision radiotherapy to treat tumors deep within the body because a monoenergetic particle beam has sharply defined edges and depth of penetration into tissue. Neutrons have also been used in radiotherapy. They have no charge and deposit energy by collision with nuclei, particularly hydrogen nuclei (protons), thereby transferring their energy to create moving charged particles capable of both ionization and excitation. In contrast to electromagnetic (EM) forms of radiotherapy in which the radiotherapy dose falls off exponentially over the depth of tissue treated, particle-based radiotherapy deposits its energy at a depth within a Bragg peak (see Fig. 15–2 and Chap. 16, Fig. 16–3A).

Radiation dose is measured in terms of the amount of energy (joules) absorbed per unit mass (kg) and is quoted in grays (1 Gy is equivalent to 1 J/kg). It is not the total amount of energy absorbed that is critical for the biological effect of ionizing radiation. For example, a whole-body dose of 8 Gy would result in the death (caused by bone marrow failure) of many animals, including humans, yet the amount of energy deposited, if evenly distributed, would cause a temperature rise of only about 2×10^{-3} °C. It is the size and localized nature of the individual energy-deposition events caused by ionizing radiations that is the reason for their efficacy in damaging biological systems.

15.2.2 Linear Energy Transfer and Energy Absorption

The deposition of energy in matter by moving charged particles is chiefly a result of electrical field interactions and

TABLE 15–1 Linear energy transfer of various radiations.

Radiation	LET (keV/μm)
Photons	
⁶⁰Co (~1.2 MeV)	0.3
200-keV x-ray	2.5
Electrons	
1 Mev	0.2
100 keV	0.5
10 keV	2
1 keV	10
Charged particles	
Proton 2 MeV	17
Alpha 5 MeV	90
Carbon 100 MeV	160
Neutrons	
2.5 MeV	15 to 80
14.1 MeV	3 to 30

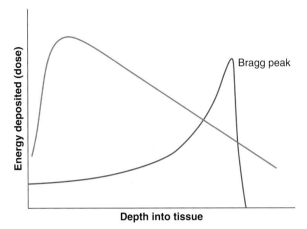

FIGURE 15–2 Schematic of the energy deposition by electromagnetic (EM) photon radiotherapy (pink curve) versus a charged particle along its track in tissue (red curve). The particle has a high velocity at the left-hand side of the figure, but as it loses energy, it slows down until it comes to rest in the region of the Bragg peak. In contrast, the electromagnetic (EM) form of photon radiotherapy leads to absorbed dose that falls off exponentially over the depth of tissue treated.

depends both on the velocity and on the charge of the particle. As a charged particle moves through matter, it transfers energy by a series of interactions that occur at random. The particle's energy loss *dE*, along a portion of its track *dx*, is dependent on its velocity *v*, charge *Z*, and the electron density of the target *ρ* as indicated by mathematical relationship as Equation 15.1:

$$\frac{dE}{dx} \propto \frac{Z^2 \rho}{v^2} \qquad [15.1]$$

The efficiency with which different types of ionizing radiation cause biological damage varies, even though photons, charged particles, and neutrons ultimately all set electrons in motion. The important difference between different types of radiation is the average density of energy loss *along* the track of the particle. The average energy lost by a particle over a given track length is known as the *linear energy transfer* (LET). The units of LET are given in terms of energy lost per unit path-length, for example, keV/μm. Table 15–1 provides some representative values of LET for different particles. Because the energy of the particle depends on its mass (m) and velocity (E = mv²), it can be seen from Equation 15.1 that as a particle slows down, it loses energy more and more rapidly and reaches a maximum rate of energy loss (the Bragg peak) just before it comes to rest (Fig. 15–2). The LET of an individual charged particle thus varies along the length of its track.

The biological effect of a dose of radiation depends on its LET; it is therefore necessary to know the LET at each point in an irradiated volume to predict the biological response accurately. When EM radiation (eg, *low-LET* 6-MV photons,

produced by a linear accelerator) is used to irradiate tissue, electrons are set in motion in the tissue. Because of their small mass (1/1860 of the mass of a proton), they are easily deflected and their track through the tissue is tortuous. Each electron track has a Bragg peak at its termination and a range of LET values along its track, but both the initiation and termination points of the electron tracks occur at random in the tissue, so that the LET spectrum is similar at all depths. A similar result occurs if the irradiation is with a primary electron beam. In contrast, if a beam of monoenergetic heavier-charged particles (eg, high-energy protons or carbon nuclei) is used to irradiate the tissue, the tracks of the particles are much straighter because their much larger mass (than the electrons in the tissue with which they mostly interact) reduces the chance of significant deflection. The Bragg peak then occurs at a similar depth in the tissue for all particles. Thus, there is a region in the tissue where a relatively large amount of energy is deposited. This feature of irradiation with *high-LET* particles makes them potentially attractive because the beam can be designed to deposit most of its energy in a deep-seated tumor (see Chap. 16, Sec. 16.2.4).

15.2.3 Radiation Damage within the Cell

The interactions leading to energy deposition in tissue occur very rapidly and generate chemically reactive free electrons and free radicals (molecules with unpaired electrons). Many different molecules in cells are altered either as a result of *direct* energy absorption or as a result of energy transfer from one molecule to another, giving rise to *indirect* effects (Fig. 15–3). Most of the energy deposited in cells is absorbed initially in water (because the cell is approximately 80% water), leading to the rapid (ie, within 10^{-14} to 10^{-4} s) production of reactive intermediates (oxidizing and reducing radicals), which, in turn, can interact

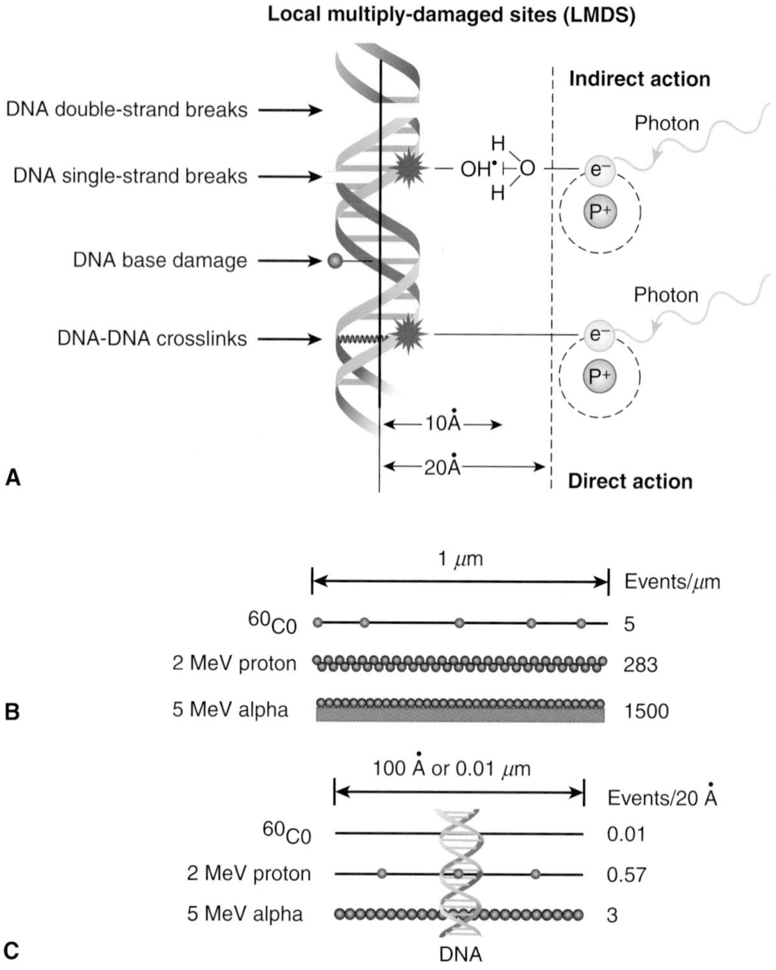

FIGURE 15–3 A) Direct and indirect effects of ionizing radiation on DNA. In the indirect model, chemically reactive free radicals are produced during ionization of water molecules in close proximity (ie, 10 to 20 angstroms [Å]) to the DNA helix. These free radicals, such as the hydroxyl radical, OH·, can react chemically with DNA to produce DNA damage. In the direct model, absorption of the energetic electron occurs directly within the DNA causing localized damage without an intermediate free radical step. Indirect and direct damage can lead to clusters of DNA single-strand and double-strand breaks, DNA base damage, DNA–DNA or DNA–protein crosslinks. These can occur as local multiply-damaged sites (LMDS). (Adapted from Hall, 2000.) **B)** and (**C**) The frequency of primary energy-loss events along the tracks of various radiations of widely differing linear energy transfer. B) Schematic of primary energy-loss events over a distance of 1 μm. C) Primary energy-loss events over 0.01 μm or 100 Å, depending on type of radiation. The dimensions of a DNA double helix are illustrated.

with other molecules in the cell (indirect effect). The hydroxyl [OH·] radical, an oxidizing agent, is probably the most damaging. The cell contains naturally occurring thiol compounds such as glutathione, cysteine, cysteamine, and metallothionein, whose sulfhydryl (SH) groups can react chemically with the free radicals to decrease their damaging effects. Other antioxidants include the vitamins C and E and intracellular manganese superoxide dismutase (MnSOD). The intracellular levels of thiols and antioxidative molecules may differ between normal and tumor tissues, and their manipulation may offer a clinical strategy to protect normal tissues from radiotherapy-induced damage. One example is the use of the thiol-containing drug, amifostine to protect against radiotherapy-induced xerostomia (ie, dry mouth) after irradiation of salivary glands (see Chap. 16, Sec. 16.5.7).

The random nature of the energy-deposition events means that radiation-induced changes can occur in any molecule in a cell. DNA is a major target of ionizing radiation, because of its biological importance to the cell. Even relatively small amounts of DNA damage can lead to cell lethality. It has been estimated that approximately 10^5 ionizations can occur within a diploid cell per gray of absorbed radiation dose, leading to approximately 1000 to 3000 DNA–DNA or DNA–protein crosslinks, 1000 damaged DNA bases, 500 to 1000 single-strand and 25 to 50 double-strand DNA breaks (ie, the vast majority of the

ionization events do not cause DNA damage). Focal areas of DNA damage can arise because of the clustering of ionizations within a few nanometers of the DNA (Ward, 1994). These "local multiply damaged sites" (LMDS; see Fig. 15–3) include combinations of single- or double-strand breaks in the sugar-phosphate backbone of the molecule, alteration or loss of DNA bases, and formation of crosslinks (between the DNA strands or between DNA and chromosomal proteins). Most DNA lesions can be repaired by DNA repair pathways (see Chap. 5, Sec. 5.3) probably acting together to repair clustered LMDS-associated lesions. High LET irradiation causes an increase in both the number and complexity of DNA clustered lesions and is more difficult to repair.

Most studies suggest that cell death following radiation is correlated with either initial or residual levels of DNA double-strand breaks (Jeggo and Lavin, 2009). Table 15–2 outlines evidence to support the role of damage to DNA as a crucial type of cellular damage in relation to cell killing.

The reactive oxygen species (ROS) induced by ionizing radiation can also interact with proteins in the cell membrane, some of which may be involved in signal transduction. This can lead to apoptosis in certain cell types (eg, endothelial cells) by activation in the membrane of a ceramide-sphingomyelin pathway (see Sec. 15.3.2; Fuks et al, 1995). Furthermore, preincubation

TABLE 15–2 **Evidence supporting DNA as a critical target for radiation-induced lethality.**

1. Microbeam irradiation demonstrates the cell nucleus to be much more sensitive than the cytoplasm.
2. Radioisotopes with short-range emissions (eg, ^{3}H, ^{125}I) incorporated into DNA cause cell killing at much lower absorbed doses than those incorporated into the cellular cytoplasm.
3. Incorporation of thymidine analogs (eg, iododeoxyuridine [IUdR] or bromodeoxyuridine [BUdR]) into DNA modifies cellular radiosensitivity.
4. The level of chromatid and chromosomal aberrations following ionizing radiation correlates with cell lethality.
5. The number of unrepaired DNA double-strand breaks correlates with cell lethality following ionizing radiation in many cells.
6. For different types of radiation, cell lethality correlates best with the level of radiation-induced DNA double-strand breaks rather than with other types of damage.
7. The extreme radiosensitivity of some mutant cells is a result of defects in DNA repair (see Chap. 5, Secs. 5.3 and 5.5).

of cells with agents capable of altering either protein function or lipid peroxidation within the cell membrane, including anticeramide antibodies, can also modify the level of radiation-induced apoptosis (Fuks et al, 1995; Rotolo et al, 2012). Overall,

the cellular response to ionizing radiation is mediated both by the direct damage to DNA and a complex interaction between proteins located within the plasma membrane, cytoplasm, and nucleus of the cell (see Sec. 15.3.2).

15.2.4 Genetic Instability, Chromosomal Damage, and Bystander Effects

Many human cancers contain chromosomal rearrangements, including chromosomal translocations, deletions, and amplifications. Chromosome rearrangements can also be observed in cells after irradiation, and if nonlethal, may contribute to the carcinogenic properties of ionizing radiation (see Chap. 16, Sec. 16.8). Chromosomal instability following irradiation has been demonstrated using a variety of techniques including spectral karyotyping (SKY) and fluorescence in situ hybridization (FISH) (see Chap. 2, Sec. 2.2.6). DNA double-strand breaks can lead to chromosomal rearrangements at the first mitosis after exposure to ionizing radiation and the type of aberration (ie, chromosomal versus chromatid types of rearrangements; Fig. 15–4) reflects the cell-cycle phase at the time of irradiation. Pathways for rejoining of DNA double-strand breaks in mammalian cells, include homologous recombination and nonhomologous end-joining (see Chap. 5, Sec. 5.3),

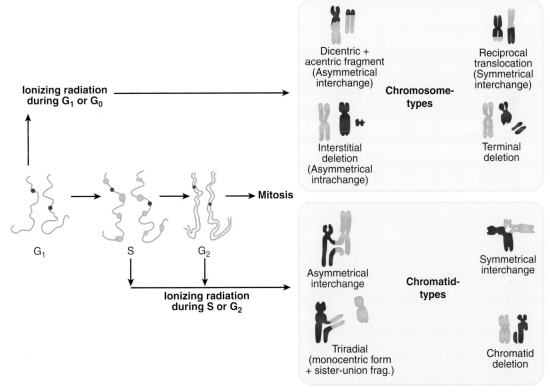

FIGURE 15–4 **Chromosomal versus chromatid types of radiation-induced damage as a function of cell-cycle phase during irradiation.** If a cell is irradiated during the G_1 or early S phase when only 1 chromosomal homolog exists, a nonrepaired DNA-DSB (double-strand break) can lead to dicentrics, reciprocal translocations and acentric fragments. During irradiation in late S and G_2 phases, sister chromatids have duplicated and the DNA-DSB gives rise to interchanges, triradials, or a chromatid deletion. Consequently, the type of chromosomal damage observed may also reflect the relative ability of cells to utilize the nonhomologous end-joining (optimally used during G_1) or homologous recombination (optimal in S and G_2) repair pathways to correct the DNA-DSB. (From Nagasawa et al, 2010.)

but it is unclear which factors determine whether or not an induced break will lead to a chromosomal rearrangement.

Examination of the break points in very large deletions often show that novel chromosomal fragments found in rearrangements are derived from other chromosomal sites of radiation damage in the same cell; they can arise from complex interactions between a number of damaged sites in the cellular DNA (Singleton et al, 2002). These rearrangements occur preferentially between genomic regions that are located in a similar vicinity in the nucleus (Misteli, 2009). Furthermore, if a cell survives and proliferates after irradiation, delayed chromosomal instability can be observed in the descendants of the exposed cell. Such radiation-induced chromosomal instability may be secondary to a breakage-fusion-bridge cycle (see Chap. 5, Sec. 5.7) or to *epigenetic effects* which perpetuate the unstable phenotype in irradiated cells (Huang et al, 2003).

Reactive oxygen species (ROS) or other factors may be released from an irradiated cell to cause damage to neighboring nonirradiated cells (ie, *bystander* cells). Thus, media transfer from irradiated cells to an unirradiated cell population can lead to cell death in the nonirradiated cells. Similarly, targeting of 10% to 30% of a cell population with high LET irradiation using a focused microbeam can lead to cell death in the nontargeted surrounding cells within the culture dish (Fig. 15–5). The mechanisms for these nontargeted effects of radiation and their importance for radiation effects in vivo remain uncertain but appear to involve stress signaling pathways. This

is a developing area of radiobiological study, particularly since bystander effects of radiation have implications for assessment of radiation effects in multicellular organisms and for health risks associated with radiation exposure (Morgan and Sowa, 2009; Blyth and Sykes, 2011; Mothersill and Seymour, 2012).

15.3 CELL DEATH RESPONSES TO IONIZING RADIATION

15.3.1 In Vitro and In Vivo Assays for Radiation Cell Survival

Inhibition of the continued reproductive ability of cells is an important consequence of the molecular and cellular responses to radiation, as it occurs at relatively low doses (a few grays) and it is the major aim of clinical radiotherapy. A tumor is controlled if its stem cells are prevented from continued proliferation. A cell that retains unlimited proliferative capacity after radiation treatment is regarded as having *survived* the treatment. In contrast, a cell that has lost the ability to generate a "clone" or *colony* is regarded as having been killed, even though it may undergo a few divisions or remain intact for a substantial period before it lyses and is lost from the cell population. Colony formation following irradiation is thus an important end point, because it relates to a cell's ability to repopulate normal or tumor tissues following exposure to ionizing radiation (see also Chap. 17, Sec. 17.4.1). In the assay that is used most often to assess colony formation, cells grown in culture are irradiated either before or after preparation of a suspension of single cells and plated at low concentration in tissue-culture dishes. Following irradiation, the cells are incubated for a number of days, and those that retain proliferative capacity divide repeatedly to form discrete colonies of cells (Fig. 15–6). After incubation, the colonies are fixed and stained so that they can be counted.

Cells that do not retain proliferative capacity following irradiation (ie, are killed) may divide a few times, but form only very small "abortive" colonies. If a colony contains more than 50 cells (ie, derived from a single cell by at least 6 division cycles), it is usually capable of continued growth and can be regarded as having arisen from a surviving cell. The plating efficiency (PE) of the cell population is calculated by dividing the number of colonies formed by the number of cells plated. The ratio of the PE for the irradiated cells to the PE for control cells is calculated to give the fraction of cells surviving the treatment (*cell survival/surviving fraction*). If a range of radiation doses is used, then these cell-survival values can be plotted to give a *survival curve*, such as the ones shown in Figures 15–7 and 15–8. Cells taken directly from animal or human tumors can also be grown in culture, allowing the in vitro assay to be extended to study the radiation sensitivity of tumor cells treated in vivo (see Fig. 15–6). Untreated cells rarely have a PE of 1 (more usually it is 0.5 to 0.8 for cells passaged for many generations and much lower for cells derived from spontaneous tumors).

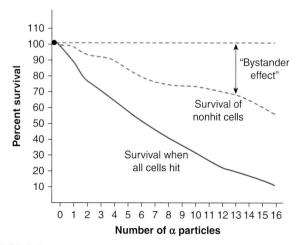

FIGURE 15–5 The radiation bystander effect. Direct single-cell irradiation of V79 cells with α particles can be accomplished using a specialized targeting microbeam in which the irradiation and fate of single cells can be tracked postirradiation. It was observed that cells that were not targeted by the α particles can also be killed (ie, they do not form colonies). This *radiation bystander effect* may be secondary to factors released by Irradiated cells into the surrounding media. In the plot shown, direct cell kill increases with increasing α-particle dose following single-cell irradiation. However, the death of nonirradiated cells also increases as a function of dose. The difference between an expected survival of 100% for nonirradiated cells and the actual survival observed, reflects the extent of cell kill by the bystander effect. (Adapted from Hall and Hei, 2003.)

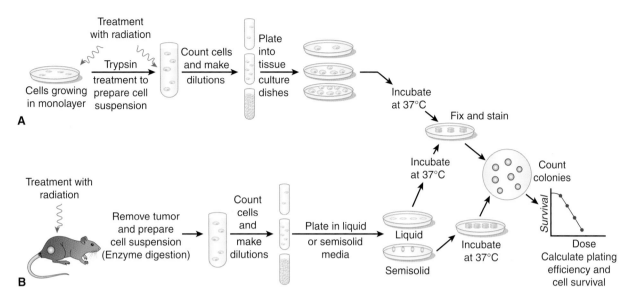

FIGURE 15–6 **Schematic of in vitro plating assays to assess cell survival. A)** Assay for the radiation sensitivity of cells growing in culture. **B)** In vivo–in vitro assay for the sensitivity of tumor cells grown and irradiated in vivo.

The techniques described above have been used to obtain survival curves for a wide range of malignant and normal cell populations. In general, for low-LET radiation (eg, X- or γ-rays), these curves have the shape(s) illustrated in Figure 15–7, when cell survival is plotted on a log scale as a function of dose plotted on a linear scale. At low doses, there is evidence of a shoulder region; but at higher doses, the curve either becomes steeper and straight so that survival decreases

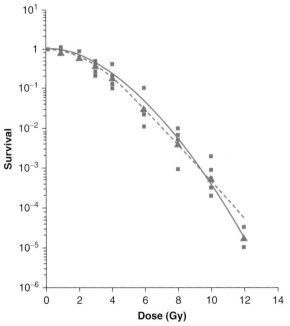

FIGURE 15–7 **Survival data for a murine melanoma cell line treated with low-LET (γ-rays) radiation.** The survival is plotted on a logarithmic scale against dose plotted on a linear scale. The data from 5 independent survival experiments are shown as the small squares, with the geometric mean value at each dose shown as the large triangles. The survival curves shown are the result of fitting the data to target theory (dashed line) or linear quadratic (solid line) models (Appendix 15.1). (Adapted from Bristow et al, 1990.)

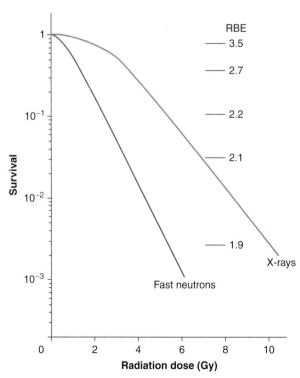

FIGURE 15–8 **Comparison of survival curves for low-LET (x-ray) and high-LET (fast-neutron) radiation.** The RBE (relative biological effectiveness) is calculated as indicated in the text and varies at different levels of survival.

exponentially with dose (dotted line in Fig. 15–7) or appears to be continually bending downward on the semilogarithmic plot (solid line in Fig. 15–7). There is greater variation in the low-dose or shoulder region of the radiation survival curves obtained for mammalian cells as compared to the variation in the slopes of the high-dose region of the curves (see Chap. 16, Sec. 16.3.2).

Figure 15–8 illustrates the difference in survival curves for X- or γ-rays (low-LET) and for fast-neutron (high-LET) irradiation. In general, the shoulder of the survival curve is reduced for higher-LET radiation and the curve is steeper. The biological effectiveness (RBE) of different types of radiation can be defined as the ratio of the dose of a standard type of radiation to that of the test radiation that gives the same biological effect. The standard type of radiation was originally taken as 200- or 250-kVp x-rays. Cobalt-60 γ-rays are also used as a standard for comparison studies, although their RBE relative to 250-kVp x-rays is approximately 0.9. Because the shoulder of the survival curve is reduced for high-LET radiation, the RBE varies with the dose or the survival level at which it is determined (see Fig. 15–8).

Many different mathematical models have been used to produce equations that can fit survival-curves to data within the limits of experimental error. Two commonly used models are the *target-theory* and *linear-quadratic* models of cell survival (explained in detail in Appendix 15.1) from which parameters (D_0, n, or α and β respectively) can be used to describe the shape of the low-dose and high-dose regions of mammalian clonogenic cell survival curve. The accuracy of the data is usually such that either shape could fit the data adequately over the first few decades of survival, as illustrated in Figure 15–7. However, such descriptions are useful when comparing cellular radiosensitivity amongst a variety of cell types or when the shape of the survival curve is altered following treatment with drugs or changes in the environment (eg, hypoxia; see Chap. 16, Sec. 16.4.1).

Nonclonogenic assays have also been used to estimate the relative radiosensitivity of cells, although assays that measure short-term growth or programmed cell death/apoptosis (see Chap. 17, Sec. 17.4.1 and Sec. 15.3.2) often do not correlate with colony-forming assays. Assays for apoptosis may predict clonogenic survival for lymphoma and testicular cancer cell lines, as these cell types tend to die uniformly by apoptosis following irradiation. Assays that evaluate cellular growth for a short period (eg, 1 to 5 days) following radiation, such as the *MTT (3-[4,5-dimethylthiazol-2-yl]-2,5 diphenyl tetrazolium bromide) (or similar) assay* that determines cellular viability by colorimetric assessment of the reduction of a tetrazolium compound, are also useful primarily for cells that die by apoptosis. They are of limited value for radiosensitivity studies of other cell types because they usually do not reflect the later death (following a few cell divisions) that is detected with a colony-forming assay. Such assays also have a limited range and it is rarely possible to assess more than one decade of cell kill. At present, clonogenic survival remains the "gold standard" for determining the radiosensitivity of cells in vitro.

Methods have been developed for assessing the ability of cells to form colonies in vivo. One of these is the spleen-colony method, which has been used to assess both the radiation and drug sensitivity of specific bone marrow (stem) cells (McCulloch and Till, 1962). In this assay, bone marrow from treated animals is injected into irradiated new hosts and colonies from surviving bone marrow (spleen colony-forming) cells can be then counted in the spleen. Initially these cells were thought to be hematopoietic stem cells but it is now known that they are downstream of the true hematopoietic stem cells in the maturation hierarchy (see Chap. 17, Fig. 17–10). In an analogous method, the lung-colony assay, tumor cells from treated animals are injected intravenously and form colonies in the lungs of syngeneic mice (Hill and Bush, 1969). Other colony-forming assays have been developed to study the radiation response of stem cells in situ in certain proliferative tissues, including skin, and gastrointestinal tract (see Chap. 16, Sec. 16.5.1).

15.3.2 Radiation-Induced Cell Death: Apoptosis, Autophagy, Mitotic Catastrophe, and Terminal Growth Arrest

Table 15–3 outlines mechanisms of cell death following irradiation. Many types of cells do not show morphological evidence of radiation damage until they attempt to divide. The morphology of the cell at the time of cell lysis following irradiation can be apoptotic or necrotic (see Chap. 9, Sec. 9.4.1). Following doses of less than approximately 10 Gy, lethally damaged cells may: (a) undergo a permanent (terminal) growth arrest, (b) undergo interphase death and lysis as a result of radiation-induced apoptosis or necrosis, or (c) undergo up to 4 abortive mitotic cycles and then finally undergo cell lysis as a result of mitotic catastrophe. The process of autophagy, which is primarily a cell-survival mechanism (see Chap. 12, Sec. 12.3.7), may also contribute to overall cell death within

TABLE 15–3 Characteristics of different modes of cell death following cellular exposure to ionizing radiation.

Cell Death Type	Description
Apoptosis	Programmed cell death controlled by molecular signaling
Necrosis	Passive death resulting from membrane breakdown by poorly understood mechanisms
Mitotic catastrophe	Multiple abortive mitoses and mitotic spindle abnormalities may take place when lethally irradiated cells attempt to divide with unrepaired DNA damage
Terminal growth arrest (senescence)	Molecularly controlled exit from the cell cycle where cells do not maintain capacity to divide but remain metabolically active

Data from Brown and Attardi, 2005.

an irradiated population (Chaachouay et al, 2011; Anbalagan et al, 2012; Speirs et al, 2012).

A radiation survival curve based on a clonogenic assay represents the total or cumulative cell death within an irradiated cell population as a result of all types of cell death. The biochemical and morphological differences observed for cells undergoing these processes are reviewed in Chapters 9 (Sec. 9.4) and 12 (Sec. 12.3.7). They can be related to loss of reproductive integrity defined by a colony-forming assay to determine the dominant mode of radiation-induced cell death within a given cell type.

For the majority of normal and tumor cells, death secondary to mitotic catastrophe accounts for most of the cell kill following irradiation. However, in some radiosensitive cells and the cancers that arise from them—notably lymphocytes, spermatocytes, thymocytes, and salivary gland epithelium—irradiation causes the cells to undergo an early (within a few hours) interphase death. This death is associated with the biochemical and morphological characteristics of apoptosis (ie, cell membrane blebbing, the formation of nuclear apoptotic bodies, and specific DNA fragmentation patterns). Depending on the type of cell, the intracellular target(s) for the induction of the apoptotic response may be either the cell membrane or the DNA or both. The reasons why some cell types undergo extensive radiation-induced apoptosis within a few hours after irradiation, while others do not, remains uncertain but may relate to the relative expression and function of proteins which trigger an apoptotic response. For example, in hematopoietic cells, radiation can lead to upregulation of genes (such as *fas, bax,* and *caspase-3),* which can facilitate apoptosis and/or downregulation of genes (such as *bcl-2),* which act to prevent apoptosis (Kitada et al, 1996).

Ionizing radiation can also initiate a sphingomyelin-dependent signaling pathway within the cell membrane, which can induce apoptosis in the absence of DNA damage (Ruiter et al, 1999; Kolesnick and Fuks, 2003). Ceramide is generated from sphingomyelin (SM) by the action of acid sphingomyelinase (ASM), or by de novo synthesis coordinated through the enzyme ceramide synthase. In endothelial, lymphoid, and hematopoietic cells, ceramide mediates apoptosis, whereas in other cells, ceramide may play no role in the death response. The ceramide-mediated apoptotic response to radiation can be inhibited by basic fibroblast growth factor (bFGF) or by genetic mutation of *ASM.* Radiation-induced crypt damage, organ failure, and death from the GI syndrome were reduced when apoptosis of supporting vascular endothelial cells was inhibited by intravenous bFGF or by deletion of the *ASM* gene (Paris et al, 2001). In animal studies, sphingosine 1-phosphate preserved fertility in irradiated female mice without propagating genomic damage in offspring, suggesting it might have a role to reduce radiotherapy-induced sterility during clinical treatment (Paris et al, 2002).

Some tumors may evade radiation-induced apoptosis by carrying *p53* gene mutations or by lacking p53 expression or function, suggesting that restoration of wild-type p53 function using gene therapy might potentiate radiation cell kill (Ma et al, 2003). However, the level of radiation-induced apoptosis does not correlate with cell survival as measured by colony-forming assays for most types of tumor, so this approach is likely to have limited application (Brown and Wouters, 2001).

Autophagy is an important process responsible for degrading and recycling long-lived proteins, cellular aggregates and damaged organelles. A number of cellular stressors can activate autophagy in tumor cells leading to the process of selective cellular self-consumption (see Chap. 12, Sec. 12.3.7). One such stress is hypoxia (see Chap. 16, Sec. 16.4.1) and autophagy-mediated survival of hypoxic cells may affect tumor response to irradiation (Kim et al, 2009; White and DiPaola, 2009). Inhibitors of autophagy might be useful in augmenting radiation-induced cell death (Kim et al, 2009).

Most tumor cell lines retain the capacity of normal cells to undergo accelerated senescence after irradiation, and although the p53 and p21 genes act as positive regulators of treatment-induced senescence, they are not required for this response in tumor cells (Chang et al, 2000). Senescent or terminally-arrested cells are metabolically active but do not proliferate and do not form colonies following irradiation; they eventually undergo necrosis days to weeks following irradiation (ie, they are already dead in the clonogenic sense). This may explain the relatively slow resolution, yet ultimate cure, of some tumors following radiotherapy. Treatments that differentially increase terminal arrest in tumor cells might sensitize tumors to radiotherapy. For example, differentiation agents (eg, retinoids) have been used to induce a senescence-like phenotype and can radiosensitize both breast cancer and head and neck cancer cells in vitro and in vivo (Ma et al, 2003).

15.4 MOLECULAR AND CELLULAR RESPONSES TO IONIZING RADIATION

15.4.1 Cell-Cycle Sensitivity and DNA Damage Checkpoints

Mammalian cells respond to ionizing radiation by delaying their progression through the cell cycle. Such delays allow for the repair of DNA damage in cells prior to undergoing either DNA replication or mitosis and are thought to prevent genetic instability in future cell generations (Kastan and Bartek, 2004). There is a rapid decrease in the mitotic index in an irradiated cell population, as both lethally damaged and surviving cells ceased to enter mitosis, while cells already in mitosis continued to progress to the G_1 phase. After a period of time, which depends on both the cell type and the radiation dose, surviving cells reenter mitosis (Fig. 15–9); this time is known as the *mitotic delay.* Mitotic delay appears to be due largely to a block of cell-cycle progression in G_2 phase, although cells in G_1 and S phases are also delayed to a lesser extent in their progression through the cell cycle. There is typically 3 to 4 hours of G_2 delay per 1 Gy radiation in diploid cells. Cells may continue to experience delays in their progression through the next and subsequent cell cycles. As a result of radiation-induced delays

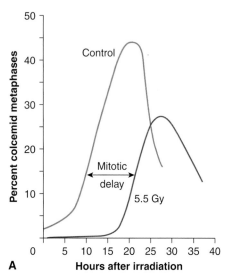
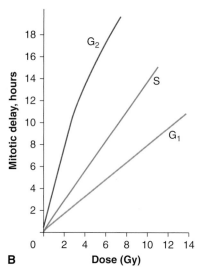

FIGURE 15–9 **The effects of radiation on the progression of cells into mitosis after the treatment. A)** At time zero, the cells are placed in medium containing colcemid, a drug that arrests cells in mitosis, and the percentage of cells that accumulate in mitosis is plotted as a function of time. The decline in the curves at late times is a result of cells escaping the drug-induced block or dying. The mitotic delay caused by a radiation dose of 5.5 Gy displaces the curves for the radiation-treated cells to the right. **B)** Cells are irradiated when in different phases of the cell cycle and the mitotic delay observed is plotted as a function of radiation dose. (Whitmore GF, Till JE & Gulyas S, unpublished data.)

in the cell cycle, cell populations can be partially synchronized by irradiation.

Cells in different phases of the cell cycle have different radiosensitivity (Terasima and Tolmach, 1961; Wilson, 2004). This is illustrated for Chinese hamster cells by the survival curves shown in Figure 15–10A. If a single radiation dose is given to cells in different phases (ie, a vertical cut is taken through the curves in Fig. 15–10A), then a pattern of cell survival as a function of cell-cycle position is obtained (Fig. 15–10B). Figure 15–10 shows that Chinese hamster cells in late S phase have the highest probability of survival after radiation (ie, are the most resistant), and that cells in mitosis (M phase) are the most sensitive. Although many cell lines appear to have a resistant period in S phase following irradiation in vitro, cell lines have variability in sensitivity just before mitosis in the G_2 phase of the cell cycle (Wilson, 2004). For example, some oncogene-transfected cells show increased resistance in the G_2 phase, whereas other cells, including DNA repair-deficient cells, show similar sensitivity throughout all phases of the cell cycle (Kao et al, 2001).

The molecular biology of the mammalian cell cycle and its response to DNA damage (including that of ionizing radiation) is discussed in detail in Chapter 5, Section 5.4 and Chapter 9, Section 9.3. The ATM (ataxia-telangiectasia mutated) protein plays a role in initiating checkpoint pathways in all 3 cell-cycle phases (Shiloh, 2003). G_1 cell-cycle arrest following irradiation centers around an intact ATM-p53/CDC25A-RB pathway and decreased activity of CYCLIN D and E complexes. This leads to continued hypophosphorylation of the retinoblastoma (RB) protein at the G_1–S interface and blocking of the initiation of DNA replication. Consequently, radiation-induced G_1 arrest is abrogated in cells that lack functional p53, ATM, or

RB proteins (Fei and El-Deiry, 2003; Cuddihy and Bristow, 2004). Although somewhat controversial, it is likely that loss of p53 protein function (and an abrogated G_1 checkpoint) do not lead to radiosensitivity or radioresistance in comparison with those cells having normal p53 protein function; in contrast, mutant p53 has been reported to confer a radiosensitive phenotype (Choudhury et al, 2006). The S-phase checkpoint is controlled though ATM-mediated phosphorylation of the BRCA1, NBS1, and FANCD2 proteins that modify the activity of transcription factors (ie, E2F) and DNA replication proteins (RPA [replication protein A], PCNA [proliferating cell nuclear antigen]) during S-phase and DNA replication (Iliakis et al, 2003; see Chap. 5, Sec. 5.4).

There are 2 "checkpoints" in irradiated G_2 cells. The G_2/M checkpoint occurs early after radiation, is transient, is ATM-dependent and dose-independent (between 1 and 10 Gy). This checkpoint controls the entry into mitosis of cells that were in G_2-phase at the time of irradiation. The "G_2 accumulation checkpoint" is independent of ATM, but dependent on dose and ensures that cells that pass through earlier cell-cycle phases with DNA damage do not enter mitosis (Xu et al, 2002) The G_2 arrest following exposure to ionizing radiation probably allows damaged DNA to be repaired prior to mitosis since DNA repair activity has been detected during the radiation-induced G_2 delay and has been related to cellular radiosensitivity (Nagasawa et al, 1994; Kao et al, 2001). Molecular alterations that have been associated with the onset and duration of the G_2 delay following radiation treatment include (a) cytoplasmic sequestration or decreased expression and stability of the CYCLIN-B protein and (b) inhibitory phosphorylation of the $p34^{CDC2}$ protein after inactivation of the CDC25C phosphatase following radiation-induced activation of CHK1

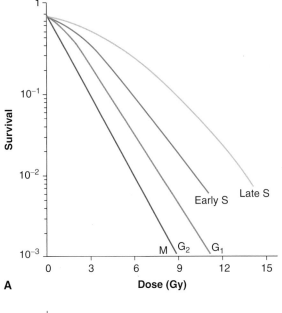

A

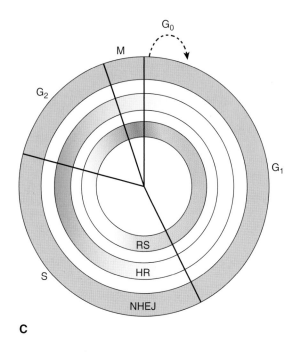

C

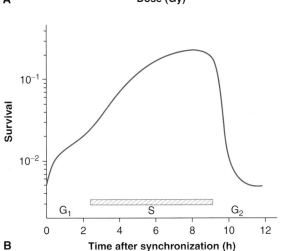

B

FIGURE 15–10   The effect of position in the cell cycle on cellular radiosensitivity. A) Survival curves for Chinese hamster cells irradiated in different phases of the cell cycle. **B)** Cells were selected in mitosis and irradiated with a fixed dose as a function of time of incubation after synchronization. The pattern of cell survival reflects the changing cellular sensitivity as the cells move through the cell cycle. **C)** Diagram indicating the active repair mechanisms during the various cell cycle phases and relative radiosensitivity. *HR,* Homologous recombination which occurs during the S and G_2 phases of the cell cycle; *NHEJ,* nonhomologous end-joining recombination that occurs in all phases of the cell cycle; *RS,* relative radiosensitivity. Dark shading indicates activity of the particular repair pathway. Dark red shading indicates most radiosensitive portions of the cell cycle. (From Rothkamm et al, 2003.)

or CHK2. These effects result in prevention of the formation of nuclear cyclin-B-p34^{CDC2} complexes, which are required for G_2 progression (see Chap. 9, Sec. 9.2.3). Cells lacking either ATM or ATR-CHK1 function exhibit a defective G_2 checkpoint after irradiation (Xu et al, 2002 and Chap. 5, Sec. 5.4).

Tumor cells often exhibit an aberrant G_1 cell-cycle checkpoint because of defects in the ATM-p53-RB pathways, while the G_2 cell-cycle checkpoints remain intact. There have been attempts to develop drugs that abrogate the G_2 checkpoint (eg, caffeine, methylxanthines, or 7-hydroxystaurosporine [UCN-01]) in tumor cells to potentiate the cytotoxicity of ionizing radiation over that of normal cells. These drugs lead to the induction of premature mitosis and mitotic catastrophe in the treated cells. For example, UCN-01 preferentially sensitizes p53-mutated, radioresistant tumor cells to ionizing radiation. Identification of the targets of caffeine and UCN-01 (ie, ATM/ATR and CHK1/2) has led to interest in the development of this class of agent for the radiosensitization of tumors (Tenzer and Pruschy, 2003; Choudhury et al, 2006; Mitchell et al, 2010).

15.4.2 Cellular and Molecular Repair

The repair of cellular damage between radiation doses is the major mechanism underlying the clinical observation that a larger total dose can be tolerated when the radiation dose is fractionated. The shoulder of the survival curve reflects accumulation of *sublethal damage* that can be repaired (Elkind and Sutton, 1960; Fig. 15–11). When Chinese hamster cells were incubated at 37°C (98.6°F) for 2.5 hours between the first and second radiation treatments, the original shoulder of the survival curve was partially regenerated, and it was completely regenerated when the cells were incubated for 23 hours between the treatments (Fig. 15–11A). When the interval between 2 fixed doses of radiation was varied (Fig. 15–11B), there was a rapid rise in survival as the interval was increased from zero (single dose) to about 2 hours. This was followed by a decrease before the survival rose again to a maximum level after about 12 hours. This pattern of recovery is a result of 2 processes. *Repair of sublethal damage (SLDR)* accounts for the early rise in survival. Because cells that survive radiation

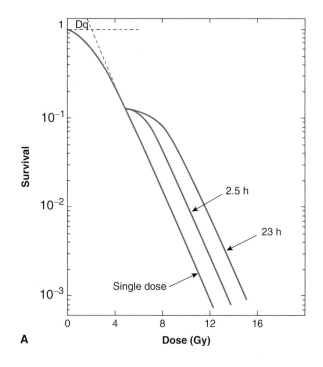

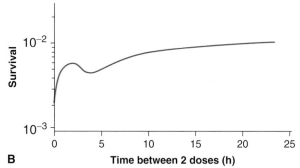

FIGURE 15–11   Illustration of the repair of sublethal damage that occurs between 2 radiation treatments. A) Survival curves for a single-dose treatment or for treatments involving a fixed first dose followed, after 2.5 or 23 hours of incubation (at 37°C), by a range of second doses. **B)** Pattern of survival observed when 2 fixed doses of irradiation are given with a varying time interval of incubation (at 37°C) between them. (Adapted from Elkind and Sutton, 1960.)

tend to be synchronized in the more resistant phases of the cell cycle, their subsequent progression (inevitably into more sensitive phases) leads to a reduction in survival at 4 hours. Continued repair and repopulation explain the increases in survival at later times (see Chap. 16, Sec. 16.6). This pattern of *SLDR* has been demonstrated for a wide range of cell lines.

The repair capacity of the cells of many tissues in vivo has been demonstrated using cell survival and functional assays in vivo (Withers and Mason, 1974). An increase in total dose is required to give the same level of biological damage when a single dose (D_1) is split into 2 doses (total dose D_2) with a time interval between them (Fig. 15–12). The difference in dose ($D_2 - D_1$) is a measure of the repair by the cells in the tissue. The capacity of different cell populations to undergo *SLDR* is reflected by the width of the shoulder on their survival

curve—that is, the D_q or $D_2 - D_1$ value. Survival curves for bone marrow cells have little to no shoulder, presumably because of their propensity to undergo radiation-induced apoptosis. Cells that demonstrate little or no evidence of cellular repair and that do not undergo radiation-induced apoptosis (such as fibroblasts derived from the radiosensitive disorders ataxia telangiectasia [AT] and Nijmegen breakage syndrome [NBS]; see Chap. 5, Sec. 5.5) also lack a shoulder to their survival curve and accumulate increased levels of DNA breaks (Fig. 15–13A) (Shiloh, 2003; Jeggo and Lavin, 2009). This relationship is shown in Figure 15–13 where the increased radiosensitivity is associated with an increased accumulation of residual and lethal DNA double strand breaks. Other cells (eg, jejunal crypt cells) can demonstrate a large *SLDR for* repair capacity ($D_2 - D_1$ value of 4 to 5 Gy – see Fig. 15–12A).

The effect of a given dose of radiation on human tissues and cells differs widely for exposures given over a short time (acute irradiation) and over an extended period of time (chronic irradiation given at a low-dose rate). Dose rates above approximately 1 Gy/min can be regarded as acute (single-dose) treatment and result in survival curves similar to that in Figure 15–7. As the total dose of X- or γ-rays is delivered at decreasing dose rates, the DNA damage in the cell diminishes progressively because of repair of the damage during the treatment. As a result, the shape of the radiation survival curve changes from one exhibiting a shoulder at high dose rates to one approaching linearity at low dose rates (Fig. 15–14A, B).

The magnitude of the *dose-sparing effect* may be calculated as the relative survival under conditions of low-dose rate irradiation compared to survival under conditions of acute-dose rate irradiation. Cell lines with a greater capacity to repair sublethal damage will demonstrate a large dose-sparing effect relative to those cells that have limited capacity to repair the damage. In addition to cellular repair, low-dose rate irradiation can trigger the G_1, S, and G_2 checkpoints, slowing down the progression of the cells through the cycle. However, if the dose rate is low enough, the cells will continue to divide and repopulate. Because cells in late S phase are often the most radioresistant, they will preferentially survive, but eventually will move into the more sensitive phases of the cell cycle during radiation, a process termed *redistribution*. The process of repopulation leads to relative radioresistance of the cell population whereas cell-cycle redistribution leads to relative radiosensitization. Most of the effect of cellular repair occurs in the range of dose rates of 1.0 to 0.01 Gy/min. Below approximately 0.1 Gy/min, the effects of cell-cycle progression (redistribution and the G_2 block; see Sec. 15.4.1) become apparent; below approximately 0.01 Gy/min, the effects of cell repopulation will start to become evident as the radiation damage is not severe enough to trigger cell-cycle arrest (see Fig. 15–14C). Repair, repopulation, and redistribution are important for understanding dose fractionation in clinical radiotherapy, as described in Chapter 16, Section 16.6.

Cell survival can be increased by holding cells after irradiation under conditions of suboptimal growth, such as low

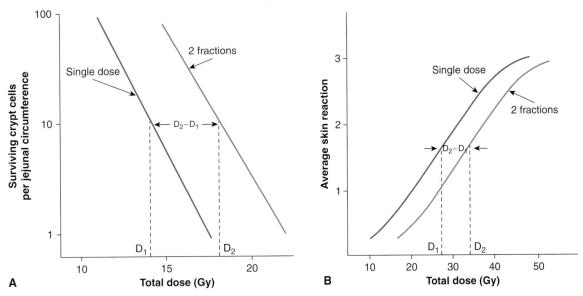

FIGURE 15–12 Repair of radiation damage in vivo. A) Survival curves for murine intestinal crypt cells γ-irradiated in situ with a single dose (red line) or with 2 equal fractions given 3 hours apart (blue line). (Modified from Withers and Mason, 1974.) **B)** Average skin reaction following x-irradiation of mouse skin with a single dose (red line) or 2 fractions given 24 hours apart (blue line). In both cases, an increase in total dose is required to give the same level of biological damage when a single dose (D_1) is split into 2 doses (total dose D_2) with a time interval between them. The difference in dose ($D_2 - D_1$) is a measure of the repair by the cells in the tissue.

temperature, nutrient deprivation, or high cell density. The latter conditions may reflect those experienced by G_0-G_1 populations of cells in growth-deprived regions of tumors (Malaise et al, 1989; see Chap. 12, Secs. 12.2 and 12.3). The

property is a result of the repair of *potentially lethal damage (PLDR)*, which usually results in a change in the slope of the cell-survival curve. Such repair may contribute to increased radiation survival observed in vivo for some transplantable

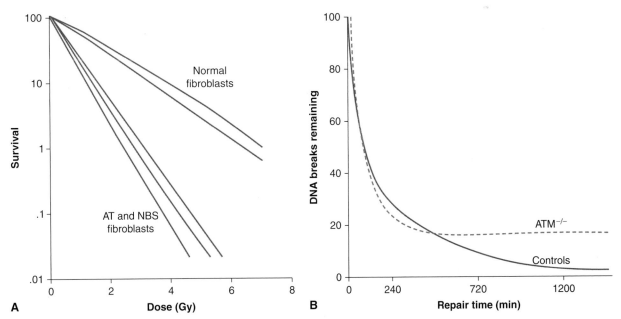

FIGURE 15–13 The relationship between radiosensitivity and DNA double strand breaks. In addition to aberrant cell-cycle checkpoints, increased radiosensitivity and subtle DNA double-strand break repair defects are associated with the AT and NBS disorders. Shown in (**A**) is the relative radiation survival for normal diploid fibroblasts versus that of AT or NBS fibroblasts. Note increased radiosensitivity following clinically relevant doses of 1 to 2 Gy. Shown in (**B**) are the DNA double-strand break rejoining curves (based on pulse-field gel electrophoresis) for AT cells relative to normal cells. The number of DNA double-strand breaks remaining is plotted against time following irradiation. Although the 2 sets of data initially have similar rates of DNA rejoining, the AT cells have increased numbers of residual DNA double-strand breaks relative to controls at later times postirradiation. (Modified from Girard et al, 2000.)

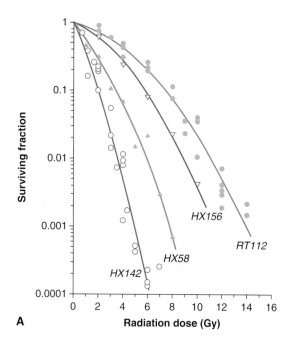

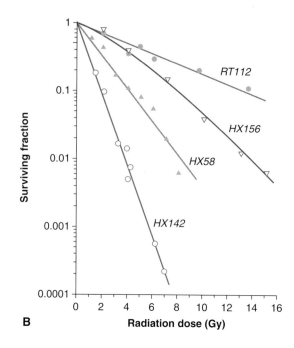

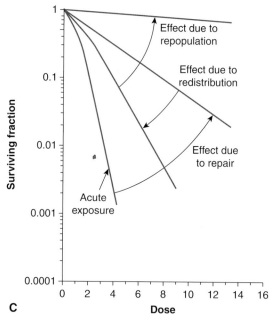

FIGURE 15–14 **Survival curves for a series of human cancer cells lines irradiated under acute (high; >1 Gy/min) (A) or continuously (low; ~1Gy/h) (B) dose rates.** (From Steel, 1991.) **C)** Schematic to illustrate the influence on the survival curve following continuous low-dose rate irradiation, of the processes of cellular repair, redistribution, and repopulation. (Data compiled by Dr. J.D. Chapman, Fox Chase Cancer Center, Philadelphia.)

cell lines when compared to the radiosensitivity of the same cells growing in vitro.

The molecular components of DNA repair pathway(s) are described in Chapter 5, Section 5.3. Data from a number of studies indicate that double-strand breaks (DSBs) are responsible for the majority of lethal damage induced by ionizing radiation (Jeggo and Lavin, 2009). The main pathways of repair of DNA-DSBs include homologous recombination (HR), which is maximally operational during S- and G_2-phases, and nonhomologous end-joining (NHEJ), which is operational throughout the cell cycle (Rothkamm et al, 2003; Valerie and Povirk, 2003), as diagrammed in Figure 15–10.

There is no simple relationship between expression of DNA repair genes and relative radiosensitivity amongst normal or tumor cells that do not have a recognized genetic defect in DNA repair (Jeggo and Lavin, 2009). However, DNA repair capacity can influence cellular radiosensitivity, as indicated by the extreme radiosensitivity of cells from patients with DNA repair deficiency syndromes such as AT and the NBS (see Fig. 15–13 and Chap. 5, Sec. 5.5). Similarly, cells deficient in the BRCA1 or BRCA2 proteins, can have decreased HR-related repair and cell survival following radiation (Powell and Kachnic, 2003). A reduced capacity for repair of DNA DSBs is also observed among (radiosensitive) fibroblasts derived from severe combined immunodeficiency (SCID)

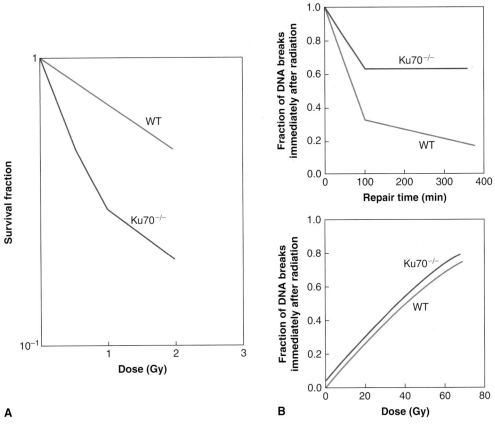

FIGURE 15–15 **The role of NHEJ in DNA DSB repair and cellular radiosensitivity. A)** The Ku70 protein, with the Ku80 and DNA-PKcs proteins, forms an important DNA-PK complex that initially catalyzes the repair of DNA-DSBs (see Chap. 5, Sec. 5.3.5 for details). As shown in (*A*), cells that are deficient in NHEJ proteins (eg, Ku70$^{-/-}$ fibroblasts) show exquisite radiosensitivity relative to normal wild-type (WT) cells. This is also true for Ku80- and DNA-PKcs-deficient cells. This increased radiosensitivity is a result of a reduced capacity for DNA break rejoining such that NHEJ-deficient cells have increased residual DNA breaks following irradiation leading to increased cell killing. This is illustrated in (**B**) (upper panel) where the number of remaining DNA DSBs at 400 minutes following irradiation is increased in Ku70$^{-/-}$ cells relative to WT cells. This is consistent with a DNA rejoining defect in the Ku70$^{-/-}$ cells. Note that the induction of DNA DSBs is similar between the 2 types of cells (lower panel), which, shows the number of DNA breaks induced for a given dose measured immediately following irradiation. (Modified from Ouyang et al, 1997.)

mice in which deficient NHEJ is caused by a mutation in the enzyme DNA-PKcs, which is involved in recruiting repair proteins to the break site (see Chap. 5, Sec. 5.3.5). Indeed, mouse cells made deficient for NHEJ (ie, mouse knockouts for DNA-PKcs or Ku70 genes) have exquisite radiosensitivity and defective rejoining of DNA-DSBs (see Fig. 15–15).

Broadly, cells can fall into 3 categories of sensitivity to ionizing radiation (Fig. 15–16*A*): Group I represents the "normal" case and Li-Fraumeni cells with p53-mutations and cells from patients with defects in DNA repair pathways not involved in DSB repair, such as nucleotide excision repair (NER), fall in this category. The G_1/S checkpoint may be lost owing to p53-mutations, but this has no effect on the sensitivity of most cells to IR. Group II includes cells that have defects in HR or in "mediator" proteins, such as RNF168 (see Chap. 5, Sec. 5.5 and Table 5–1). Group III is the most radiosensitive and includes cells with defects in NHEJ and with mutations in the NBS1, ATM, or DNA ligase IV genes from DNA repair disorders (Girard et al, 2000). These cells are sensitive as a consequence of errors in end-processing and end-joining

of DSB, defects in chromatin modifications that prevent efficient rejoining of DSBs, and inefficient ATM-mediated G_2/M-checkpoints (Beucher et al, 2009) (see Chap. 5, Sec. 5.5 and Table 5–1).

Most cells that show sensitivity to IR are not sensitive to UV radiation. Cells derived from people with Cockayne syndrome or xeroderma pigmentosum patients with NER defects are exquisitely sensitive to UV irradiation (Fig. 15–16*B*). This is consistent with the different types of damage caused by IR versus UV radiation and the different DNA repair pathways that are used (eg, DNA DSBs and single-strand breaks, repaired by HR and NHEJ versus cyclobutane pyrimidine dimers (CPDs) and 6-4PPs repaired by NER, respectively (see Chap. 5, Sec. 5.3 for details). It also highlights the repair of DSBs as the primary determinant of survival following IR.

Greater understanding of the relationship between deficient DNA repair and radiosensitivity has led to strategies designed to radiosensitize tumor cells. In human fibroblasts, small silencing RNAs (siRNAs; see Chap. 2, Sec. 2.4.3) or small molecule inhibitors have been used to decrease expression of

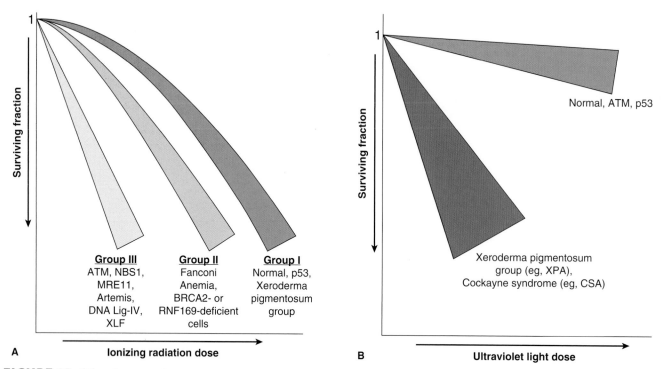

FIGURE 15–16 Schematic of clonogenic survival curves showing differences in survival following IR (A) and UV (B) radiation for cells deficient in genes involved in DNA repair or DNA damage signaling. These data are derived from experiments using DNA repair-deficient cells from DNA instability syndromes (details of these syndromes are as discussed in Chapter 5 [see Sec. 5.3.5]).

endogenous DNA-PKcs or ATM, which results in defective DSB repair and an increase in residual (unrejoined) DNA DSBs, which leads to increased radiation cell killing (Peng et al, 2002; Thoms and Bristow, 2010). Similarly antisense RNA or pharmacological approaches (ie, the drug imatinib, which inhibits the interaction between the protein product of the *c-abl* oncogene and the DNA repair protein RAD51; see Chap. 17, Sec. 17.3.1) have been used to decrease expression of DNA repair proteins with resultant radiosensitization (Collis et al, 2001). Inhibiting the repair of DNA base damage and single-strand DNA breaks with inhibitors of poly (ADP-ribose) polymerase (PARP; see Chap. 17; Sec. 17.3.2) can also lead to radiosensitization (Chalmers et al, 2010). However, the degree of radiosensitization and DSB repair may differ in vitro and in vivo because of the additional effects of the microenvironment, which may lead to differential DSB induction and altered expression and function of DSB repair pathways (Chan et al, 2009; Jamal et al, 2010).

There may be a therapeutic advantage to targeting DNA repair in combination with radiotherapy in that cell kill in tumor cells can be increased relative to cell kill in normal tissues. In some tumor cells, DNA repair pathways may be nonfunctional so that the tumor cells are radiosensitized if there are tumor-specific defects in HR or NHEJ. Furthermore, some drugs, such as PARP inhibitors, may be selectively toxic to HR-defective tumor cells based on synthetic lethality, which could be used to decrease the number of tumor clonogens prior to or during radiotherapy (Thoms and Bristow, 2010).

15.4.3 Intracellular Signaling, Gene Expression, and Radiosensitivity

Intrinsic changes in gene expression in tumors can influence response to radiation, and irradiation can modify the expression of some genes. Biochemical processes in cells, such as DNA, RNA, or protein synthesis, respiration, or other metabolism can be inhibited by irradiation, but this usually requires quite large doses of the order of 10 to 100 Gy. Clinical doses of radiation can affect the expression of a number of genes involved in the response of cells to stress and this may change their properties. Aberrant expression of oncogenes or tumor-suppressor genes may increase the intrinsic cellular radioresistance of human and rodent cells (Haffty and Glazer, 2003). For example, increased radiation survival has been observed in selected cell lines following the transfection of a single oncogene, such as activated *Ras, Src,* or *Raf* (Kasid et al, 1996; Gupta et al, 2001). This has led to studies designed to radiosensitize tumor cells by the inhibition of oncogene function using inhibitors of intracellular signaling pathways or antisense RNA to decrease oncogene overexpression (Kasid and Dritschilo, 2003). Figure 15–17 indicates pathways that may be targeted and the preclinical and clinical data to support such targeting in tumor cell radiosensitization strategies (Begg et al, 2011)

When the *Ras* oncogene undergoes mutation, it is permanently activated in the guanosine triphosphate (GTP)-bound signaling state, providing proliferative signals in the absence of growth factor ligands, leading to altered cell growth, transformation, and, occasionally, radioresistance

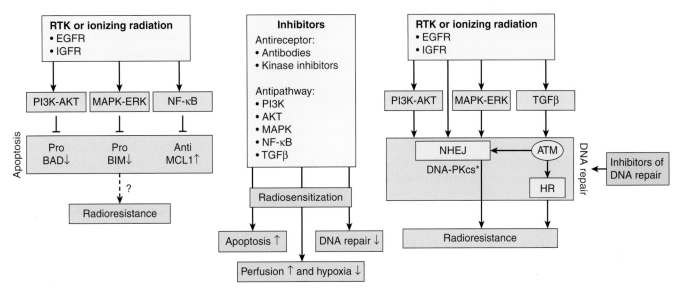

FIGURE 15–17 **Targeting signal transduction.** Growth factor receptor activation by mutation or overexpression, or mutations in oncogenes (such as *RAS*) or tumor suppressor genes (such as *PTEN*) can lead to signaling through the phophatidylinositol-3 kinase (PI3K)-AKT, mitogen-activated protein kinase (MAPK)-extracellular signal regulated kinase (ERK), nuclear factor-κB (NF-κB), and transforming growth factor-β (TGFβ) pathways. Such signaling can affect radiosensitivity by decreasing apoptosis (left) or increasing DNA repair (right). AKT, MAPK, and NF-κB signaling can all lead to phosphorylation and inactivation of proapoptotic proteins or activation of antiapoptotic proteins. Altering apoptosis does not always lead to changes in clonogenic cell survival (dashed arrow with question mark). Activation of the AKT and MAPK pathways leads to the activation of the catalytic subunit of DNA-dependent protein kinase (DNA-PKcs), a central protein in DSB repair by NHEJ. Direct inhibition of DNA repair may also lead to radiosensitization by targeting the ATM and DNA-PKcs kinases or PARP proteins. DNA-PKcs can also be activated by the receptor tyrosine kinase (RTK) epidermal growth factor receptor (EGFR) after it is translocated to the nucleus. There is a strong correlation between DNA repair capacity, particularly for DSBs, and radiosensitivity. Ionizing radiation can also activate the PI3K, MAPK, and NF-κB pathways. Inhibition of signaling pathways following irradiation can therefore reverse (Begg et al, 2011) tumor cell radioresistance. Some inhibitors have also been shown to affect tumor vasculature, leading to improved perfusion and reduced hypoxia (see also Chap. 16, Sec. 16.2.5). Asterisk indicates activation. (Taken from Begg et al, 2011.)

(see Chap. 8, Sec. 8.2.3). However, increased radioresistance is more commonly observed in cells transfected with an activated *Ras* gene in combination with a nuclear cooperating oncogene, such as c-*Myc* or mutant *p53* (McKenna et al, 1990; Bristow et al, 1996). Downstream to RAS, the RAS-MEK-ERK and phosphatidylinositol-3 kinase (PI3K)-AKT/PKB pathways (see Chap. 8, Sec. 8.2.5) have been linked to tumor radioresistance (Bussink et al, 2008). Using antisense oligonucleotides or silencing RNA against human *Raf* leads to increased cancer cell radiosensitivity (Woods Ignatoski et al, 2008; Kidd et al, 2010). RAS-mediated radioresistance in rat cells appears to be dependent on PI3K and RAF signaling pathways, and less on the MEK signaling pathway (Affolter et al, 2012). Inhibitors of RAS and PI3K signaling, such as LY294002 and wortmannin, significantly enhanced the response to radiation in lung, bladder, colon, breast, prostate, head and neck squamous cell carcinoma (HNSCC), and cervical cancer cells (Xiao et al, 2010). Although inhibitors of RAS protein prenylation or function (farnesyl transferase inhibitors) have been reported to enhance radiation-induced cytotoxicity among preclinical models of human breast, lung, colon, and bladder cancer cells expressing mutated *H-* or *K-ras* genes, the use of these agents in the clinic has been limited by the lack of biomarkers that reflect a precise drug targeting of RAS versus other intercommunicating signaling pathways (Rengan et al, 2008).

Activation of the PI3K-AKT/PKB pathway is associated with 3 major mechanisms of tumor radioresistance: intrinsic radioresistance, tumor-cell proliferation, and hypoxia. Activation of this pathway can be caused by stimulation of receptor tyrosine kinases, such as epidermal growth factor receptor (EGFR; see Chap. 8, Sec. 8.2.1). In clinical trials, an independent association has been noted between expression of activated AKT and outcome of treatment of head and neck cancer with radiotherapy (Bussink et al, 2008). More recent data implicate the *Akt* gene in DSB repair, as AKT can stimulate the accumulation of DNA-PKcs at DNA-DSBs and promote DNA-PKcs activity during NHEJ, and itself can bind to DSBs in vitro following irradiation (Fraser et al, 2011; Toulany et al, 2012). Consequently, there is interest in the use of AKT inhibitors as clinical radiosensitizers given the overexpression of activated AKT in many tumors.

Tyrosine kinase activity of EGFR is increased following cellular exposure to radiation and addition of exogenous epidermal growth factor (EGF) to cell culture renders cells relatively radioresistant. Both EGFR and the related HER-2/neu receptor are overexpressed in a wide variety of epithelial tumors (head and neck squamous cell cancers (HNSCC), gliomas, breast, lung, colorectal and prostate cancers) and this overexpression has been associated with poor clinical outcome following radiotherapy due in part to increased tumor cell repopulation during therapy (Verheij et al, 2010). Targeting EGFR or human epidermal growth receptor 2 (HER-2)/neu signaling using monoclonal antibodies or specific inhibitors (eg, cetuximab-EGFR or trastuzumab-HER-2) leads to radiosensitization, in vitro and in vivo. These drugs are being tested in combination with radiotherapy and chemotherapy in randomized, multicenter clinical trials (Verheij et al, 2010; see Chap. 16, Sec. 16.2.5). Nuclear EGFR is now thought to also be part of the DNA-damage repair complex that interacts with proteins involved with the NHEJ repair pathway during ATM activation and chromatin relaxation during the sensing and repair of DSBs. Thus, inhibition of EGFR signaling during radiotherapy may lead to both decreased tumor cell repopulation and increased cell kill as a consequence of defective DSB repair (Dittmann et al, 2011; Yu et al, 2012).

The radiosensitivity of cells may be influenced by the addition of exogenous growth factors or hormones in receptor-positive cells before or after irradiation. The insulin-like growth factor-1 receptor (IGF-1R) is a cell-surface receptor with tyrosine kinase activity that has been linked to increased radioresistance. IGF-1R is expressed at low levels in AT cells; this may, in part, contribute to their radiosensitivity, as reintroduction of IGF-1R, or addition of exogenous insulin-like growth factor (IGF), can increase their radioresistance (Peretz et al, 2001). Other data implicate a role for IGF-1R directly in DSB repair, at least in part via the HR pathway and small molecule IGF-1R kinase inhibitors can decrease radioresistance in tumor cells (Turney et al, 2012).

15.4.4 Radiation-Induced Changes in Gene Expression

Irradiation can modify intracellular signaling through modification of the activity of tyrosine kinases, mitogen-activated protein (MAP)-kinases, stress-activated protein (SAP)-kinases, and RAS-associated proteins (Ruiter et al, 1999; Dent et al, 2003; Schmidt-Ullrich et al, 2003). Tyrosine phosphorylation is involved in several DNA damage response pathways; an example is activation of the c-ABL pathway, which phosphorylates RAD51, a DNA repair protein at sites of DNA damage. Genes induced by radiation include those encoding cell-cycle-related proteins (eg, growth arrest after DNA damage [GADD] genes, p34^{CDC2}, CYCLIN B, p53), growth factors, and cytokines (eg, platelet-derived growth factor [PDGF], transforming growth factor beta [TGF-β], bFGF, tumor necrosis factor alpha [TNF-α]), and enzymes (eg, plasminogen activator). Liberation of inflammatory cytokines such as TNF-α and interleukin-1 (IL-1) by cells following radiation damage may lead to a continuing cascade of cytokine production, which may be responsible for the acute inflammation and late-onset fibrosis observed in some irradiated tissues (see Chap. 16, Sec. 16.5.3).

Induction of the expression of early response genes (ie, within seconds to minutes) by irradiation can be initiated by damage to the plasma membrane or to nuclear DNA (Criswell et al, 2003). Some early response genes, such as the early growth response factor (EGR-1) and p21 Cdk-inhibitor proteins (see Chap. 9, Secs. 9.2 and 9.3), contain radiation-responsive regulatory domains in their promoter regions, which can facilitate

their rapid induction by radiation (Hallahan et al, 1995). These sequences might be used in radiation-induced gene therapy as vectors to drive expression of suicide genes (eg, TNF-α) for tumor therapy. Synthetic enhancers of gene expression designed for use with radiation utilize short motifs of sequence CC(A/T)$_6$GG (ie, radiation-responsive elements) derived from the EGR-1 gene (Datta et al, 1992; Marples et al, 2002). Such constructs can be responsive to radiation at doses of 1 to 5 Gy. These tumor-targeting vectors might be used in clinical situations where the radiation volume can be tightly controlled to spare normal tissues using conformal radiotherapy (see Chap. 16, Sec. 16.2.2) and have shown promise in animal models (Mauceri et al, 2009).

Approaches using complementary DNA (cDNA) microarrays (see Chap. 2, Sec. 2.2.12) have led to the discovery that radiation-induced gene expression can be cell-type specific and while induction of some genes is dose-dependent across a range of doses, others are activated specifically at either low (ie, 1 to 3 Gy) or high doses (ie, 10 Gy) (Khodarev et al, 2001; Nuyten and van de Vijver, 2008; Rashi-Elkeles et al, 2011). Furthermore, gene expression following a given radiation dose can be substantially higher when solid tumors are irradiated in vivo than when the same cell line is irradiated in culture. However, studies of biopsies from human tumors have demonstrated that differences in radiation-induced gene expression are greater between patients' tumors than within the tumor of a given patient (Hartmann et al, 2002). This observation supports the concept that "molecular profiling" of the tumors and normal tissues in individual patients may be able to predict radiation response.

MicroRNAs (miRNAs) are emerging as a class of endogenous gene modulators that control protein levels, thereby adding a new layer of regulation to the DNA damage response (see Chap. 2, Sec. 2.4.3). There is increasing interest in an association between miRNA expression in tumors and chemo- and radiosensitivity, both with regards to predicting and modulating sensitivity. These include the miRNAs of the Let-7 family, miR-21 and miR-200b, as inhibition of these miRNAs leads to increased radiosensitivity (Hu and Gatti, 2010).

The translation of preclinical to clinical testing for molecularly-based compounds is limited by multiple factors including the appropriate scheduling and toxicity of the agent, the interpatient and intratumoral variability of the expression of the molecular target and its role as a predictor of treatment response, and molecular crosstalk among redundant, parallel intracellular signaling pathways (Haffty and Glazer, 2003). Some of these limitations might be bypassed by simultaneous determination of multiple pathways using genomic and proteomic analyses (see Chap. 2) of both normal and tumor tissues as the basis for selection of the best molecular agents to be combined with radiation treatments (Ma et al, 2003; Ishkanian et al, 2010; Begg, 2012). The majority of proteins involved in DNA repair undergo posttranslational modification or novel protein–protein interactions following irradiation at sites of DNA damage. Because such modifications would not be detected using cDNA microarray analyses, which detect alteration of messenger RNA expression rather than altered protein levels, proteomic anaysis (see Chap. 2, Sec. 2.5) of tissue samples or sera may be required to determine molecular pathways that lead to radio-response in patients (Bentzen et al, 2008).

SUMMARY

- Ionizing radiation causes damage to cells and tissues by depositing energy as a series of discrete events.
- Different types of radiation have different abilities to cause biological damage because of the different densities of the energy deposition events produced.
- The RBE of densely ionizing (high-LET) radiation is greater than that of low-LET radiation. Radiation can cause damage to any molecule in a cell, but damage to DNA is most crucial in causing cell lethality expressed by loss of proliferative potential.
- Depending on cell type, cells may die by a permanent (terminal) growth arrest, undergo interphase death or lysis during radiation-induced apoptosis, or undergo up to 4 abortive mitotic cycles before mitotic catastrophe.
- Several assay procedures have been developed for assessing the clonogenic capacity of both normal and malignant cells, and these have been used to obtain radiation survival curves for a wide range of cell types.
- For x- and γ-rays, survival curves for most mammalian cells have a shoulder region at low doses, while at higher doses the survival decreases approximately exponentially with dose.
- Following treatment with low-LET radiation, cells can repair some of their damage over a period of a few hours; thus if the treatment is prolonged or fractionated, it is less effective than if given as a single acute dose.
- Cells in S phase are often more resistant than cells in the G_2/M phases, but there is variability between cell types.
- The accurate and timely rejoining of DNA DSBs are correlated to the relative radiation survival of both normal and tumor cells. Defects in the DNA repair pathways in tumor cells may be useful in targeting repair-defective cancer cells using synthetic lethality or molecular-targeting treatment strategies.
- Cell-cycle checkpoints in cells are activated following irradiation (to allow time for DNA repair) and the molecular events relating to G_1- and G_2-phase cell-cycle arrest appear to involve ATM, p53, and CYCLIN-CDK complexes that are associated with cell-cycle regulation.
- There is an association between the aberrant expression of RAS, RAF, and p53 proteins and cellular response to radiation.
- Future treatments involving radiation will increasingly utilize molecular-targeted drugs that increase tumor radiosensitivity by interfering with the G_1, S, and G_2 cell-cycle checkpoints, or modify intracellular signaling following DNA damage. Genomic and proteomic assays may be useful to discover abnormal signaling pathways in tumors to help use molecular-targeted drugs for radiosensitization in selected patients.

REFERENCES

Affolter A, Drigotas M, Fruth K, et al. Increased radioresistance via G12S K-Ras by compensatory upregulation of MAPK and PI3K pathways in epithelial cancer. *Head Neck* 2012 doi: 10.1002/hed.22954. [Epub ahead of print]

Anbalagan S, Pires IM, Blick C, et al. Radiosensitization of renal cell carcinoma in vitro through the induction of autophagy. *Radiother Oncol* 2012;103:388-393.

Begg AC. Predicting recurrence after radiotherapy in head and neck cancer. *Semin Radiat Oncol* 2012;22:108-118.

Begg AC, Stewart FA, Vens C. Strategies to improve radiotherapy with targeted drugs. *Nat Rev Cancer* 2011;11:239-253.

Bentzen SM, Buffa FM, Wilson GD. Multiple biomarker tissue microarrays: bioinformatics and practical approaches. *Cancer Metastasis Rev* 2008;27:481-494.

Beucher A, Birraux J, Tchouandong L, et al. Atm and Artemis promote homologous recombination of radiation-induced DNA double-strand breaks in G2. *EMBO J* 2009;28: 3413-3427.

Blyth BJ, Sykes PJ. Radiation-induced bystander effects: what are they, and how relevant are they to human radiation exposures? *Radiat Res* 2011;176:139-157.

Bristow RG, Benchimol S, Hill RP. The p53 gene as a modifier of intrinsic radiosensitivity: implications for radiotherapy. *Radiother Oncol* 1996;40:197-223.

Bristow RG, Hardy PA, Hill RP. Comparison between in vitro radiosensitivity and in vivo radioresponse of murine tumor cell lines. I: Parameters of in vitro radiosensitivity and endogenous cellular glutathione levels. *Int J Radiat Oncol Biol Phys* 1990;18: 133-145.

Brown JM, Attardi LD. The role of apoptosis in cancer development and treatment response. *Nat Rev Cancer* 2005;5:231-237.

Brown JM, Wouters BG. Apoptosis: mediator or mode of cell killing by anticancer agents? *Drug Resist Updat* 2001;4:135-136.

Bussink J, Van Der Kogel AJ, Kaanders JH. Activation of the PI3-K/AKT pathway and implications for radioresistance mechanisms in head and neck cancer. *Lancet Oncol* 2008;9:288-296.

Chaachouay H, Ohneseit P, Toulany M, Kehlbach R, Multhoff G, Rodemann HP. Autophagy contributes to resistance of tumor cells to ionizing radiation. *Radiother Oncol* 2011;99: 287-292.

Chalmers AJ, Lakshman M, Chan N, Bristow RG. Poly(ADP-ribose) polymerase inhibition as a model for synthetic lethality in developing radiation oncology targets. *Semin Radiat Oncol* 2010; 20:274-281.

Chan N, Koch CJ, Bristow RG. Tumor hypoxia as a modifier of DNA strand break and cross-link repair. *Curr Mol Med* 2009;9: 401-410.

Chang BD, Watanabe K, Broude EV, et al. Effects of p21Waf1/Cip1/Sdi1 on cellular gene expression: implications for carcinogenesis, senescence, and age-related diseases. *Proc Natl Acad Sci U S A* 2000;97:4291-4296.

Choudhury A, Cuddihy A, Bristow RG. Radiation and new molecular agents part I: targeting ATM-ATR checkpoints, DNA repair, and the proteasome. *Semin Radiat Oncol* 2006; 16:51-58.

Collis SJ, Tighe A, Scott SD, Roberts SA, Hendry JH, Margison GP. Ribozyme minigene-mediated RAD51 down-regulation increases radiosensitivity of human prostate cancer cells. *Nucleic Acids Res* 2001;29:1534-1538.

Criswell T, Leskov K, Miyamoto S, Luo G, Boothman DA. Transcription factors activated in mammalian cells after clinically relevant doses of ionizing radiation. *Oncogene* 2003;22:5813-5827.

Cuddihy AR, Bristow RG. The p53 protein family and radiation sensitivity: yes or no? *Cancer Metastasis Rev* 2004;23:237-257.

Datta R, Rubin E, Sukhatme V, et al. Ionizing radiation activates transcription of the EGR1 gene via CArG elements. *Proc Natl Acad Sci U S A* 1992;89:10149-10153.

Dent P, Yacoub A, Fisher PB, Hagan MP, Grant S. MAPK pathways in radiation responses. *Oncogene* 2003;22:5885-5896.

Dittmann K, Mayer C, Fehrenbacher B, Schaller M, Kehlbach R, Rodemann HP. Nuclear epidermal growth factor receptor modulates cellular radio-sensitivity by regulation of chromatin access. *Radiother Oncol* 2011;99:317-322.

Elkind MM, Sutton H. Radiation response of mammalian cells grown in culture. 1. Repair of X-ray damage in surviving Chinese hamster cells. *Radiat Res* 1960;13:556-593.

Fei P, El-Deiry WS. P53 and radiation responses. *Oncogene* 2003; 22:5774-5783.

Foray N, Badie C, Alsbeih G, Fertil B, Malaise EP. A new model describing the curves for repair of both DNA double-strand breaks and chromosome damage. *Radiat Res* 1996;146:53-60.

Fraser M, Harding SM, Zhao H, Coackley C, Durocher D, Bristow RG. MRE11 promotes AKT phosphorylation in direct response to DNA double-strand breaks. *Cell Cycle* 2011;10:2218-2232.

Fuks Z, Haimovitz-Friedman A, Kolesnick RN. The role of the sphingomyelin pathway and protein kinase C in radiation-induced cell kill. *Important Adv Oncol* 1995;19-31.

Girard PM, Foray N, Stumm M, et al. Radiosensitivity in Nijmegen breakage syndrome cells is attributable to a repair defect and not cell cycle checkpoint defects. *Cancer Res* 2000;60:4881-4888.

Gupta AK, Bakanauskas VJ, Cerniglia GJ, et al. The Ras radiation resistance pathway. *Cancer Res* 2001;61:4278-4282.

Haffty BG, Glazer PM. Molecular markers in clinical radiation oncology. *Oncogene* 2003;22:5915-5925.

Hall EJ. *Radiobiology for the Radiologist*, 5th ed. Philadelphia: Lippencott, Williams & Wilkins; 2000.

Hall EJ, Hei TK. Genomic instability and bystander effects induced by high-LET radiation. *Oncogene* 2003;22:7034-7042.

Hallahan DE, Dunphy E, Virudachalam S, Sukhatme VP, Kufe DW, Weichselbaum RR. C-jun and Egr-1 participate in DNA synthesis and cell survival in response to ionizing radiation exposure. *J Biol Chem* 1995;270:30303-30309.

Hartmann KA, Modlich O, Prisack HB, Gerlach B, Bojar H. Gene expression profiling of advanced head and neck squamous cell carcinomas and two squamous cell carcinoma cell lines under radio/chemotherapy using cDNA arrays. *Radiother Oncol* 2002; 63:309-320.

Hill RP, Bush RS. A lung-colony assay to determine the radiosensitivity of cells of a solid tumour. *Int J Radiat Biol Relat Stud Phys Chem Med* 1969;15:435-444.

Hu H, Gatti RA. MicroRNAs: new players in the DNA damage response. J Mol Cell Biol 2010;3:151-158.

Huang L, Snyder AR, Morgan WF. Radiation-induced genomic instability and its implications for radiation carcinogenesis. *Oncogene* 2003;22:5848-5854.

Iliakis G, Wang Y, Guan J, Wang H. DNA damage checkpoint control in cells exposed to ionizing radiation. *Oncogene* 2003; 22:5834-5847.

Ishkanian AS, Zafarana G, Thoms J, Bristow RG. Array CGH as a potential predictor of radiocurability in intermediate risk prostate cancer. *Acta Oncol* 2010;49:888-894.

Jamal M, Rath BH, Williams ES, Camphausen K, Tofilon PJ. Microenvironmental regulation of glioblastoma radioresponse. *Clin Cancer Res* 2010;16:6049-6059.

Jeggo P, Lavin MF. Cellular radiosensitivity: how much better do we understand it? *Int J Radiat Biol* 2009;85:1061-1081.

Kao GD, Mckenna WG, Yen TJ. Detection of repair activity during the DNA damage-induced G2 delay in human cancer cells. *Oncogene* 2001;20:3486-3496.

Kasid U, Dritschilo A. RAF antisense oligonucleotide as a tumor radiosensitizer. *Oncogene* 2003;22:5876-5884.

Kasid U, Suy S, Dent P, Ray S, Whiteside TL, Sturgill TW. Activation of Raf by ionizing radiation. *Nature* 1996;382:813-816.

Kastan MB, Bartek J. Cell-cycle checkpoints and cancer. *Nature* 2004;432:316-323.

Khodarev NN, Park JO, Yu J, et al. Dose-dependent and independent temporal patterns of gene responses to ionizing radiation in normal and tumor cells and tumor xenografts. *Proc Natl Acad Sci U S A* 2001;98:12665-12670.

Kidd AR 3rd, Snider JL, Martin TD, Graboski SF, Der CJ, Cox AD. Ras-related small GTPases RalA and RalB regulate cellular survival after ionizing radiation. *Int J Radiat Oncol Biol Phys* 2010; 78:205-212.

Kim KW, Moretti L, Mitchell LR, Jung DK, Lu B. Combined Bcl-2/mammalian target of rapamycin inhibition leads to enhanced radiosensitization via induction of apoptosis and autophagy in non-small cell lung tumor xenograft model. *Clin Cancer Res* 2009; 15:6096-6105.

Kitada S, Krajewski S, Miyashita T, Krajewska M, Reed JC. Gamma-radiation induces upregulation of Bax protein and apoptosis in radiosensitive cells in vivo. *Oncogene* 1996;12:187-192.

Kolesnick R, Fuks Z. Radiation and ceramide-induced apoptosis. *Oncogene* 2003;22:5897-5906.

Ma BB, Bristow RG, Kim J, Siu LL. Combined-modality treatment of solid tumors using radiotherapy and molecular targeted agents. *J Clin Oncol* 2003;21:2760-2776.

Malaise EP, Deschavanne PJ, Fertil B. The relationship between potentially lethal damage repair and intrinsic radiosensitivity of human cells. *Int J Radiat Biol* 1989;56:597-604.

Marples B, Greco O, Joiner MC, Scott SD. Molecular approaches to chemo-radiotherapy. *Eur J Cancer* 2002;38:231-239.

Mauceri HJ, Beckett MA, Liang H, et al. Translational strategies exploiting TNF-alpha that sensitize tumors to radiation therapy. *Cancer Gene Ther* 2009;16:373-381.

McCulloch EA, Till JE. The sensitivity of cells from normal mouse bone marrow to gamma radiation in vitro and in vivo. *Radiat Res* 1962;16:822-832.

McKenna WG, Weiss MC, Endlich B, et al. Synergistic effect of the v-myc oncogene with H-ras on radioresistance. *Cancer Res* 1990; 50:97-102.

Misteli T. Self-organization in the genome. *Proc Natl Acad Sci U S A* 2009;106:6885-6886.

Mitchell JB, Choudhuri R, Fabre K, et al. In vitro and in vivo radiation sensitization of human tumor cells by a novel checkpoint kinase inhibitor, AZD7762. *Clin Cancer Res* 2010; 16:2076-2084.

Morgan WF, Sowa MB. Non-targeted effects of ionizing radiation: implications for risk assessment and the radiation dose response profile. *Health Phys* 2009;97:426-432.

Mothersill C, Seymour C. Changing paradigms in radiobiology. *Mutat Res* 2012;750:85-95.

Nagasawa H, Brogan JR, Peng Y, Little JB, Bedford JS. Some unsolved problems and unresolved issues in radiation cytogenetics: a review and new data on roles of homologous recombination and non-homologous end joining. *Mutat Res* 2010;701:12-22.

Nagasawa H, Keng P, Harley R, Dahlberg W, Little JB. Relationship between gamma-ray-induced G2/M delay and cellular radiosensitivity. *Int J Radiat Biol* 1994;66:373-379.

Nuyten DS, van de Vijver MJ. Using microarray analysis as a prognostic and predictive tool in oncology: focus on breast cancer and normal tissue toxicity. *Semin Radiat Oncol* 2008;18:105-114.

Ouyang H, Nussenzweig A, Kurimasa A, et al. Ku70 is required for DNA repair but not for T cell antigen receptor gene recombination in vivo. *J Exp Med* 1997;186:921-929.

Paris F, Fuks Z, Kang A, et al. Endothelial apoptosis as the primary lesion initiating intestinal radiation damage in mice. *Science* 2001; 293:293-297.

Paris F, Perez GI, Fuks Z, et al. Sphingosine 1-phosphate preserves fertility in irradiated female mice without propagating genomic damage in offspring. *Nat Med* 2002;8:901-902.

Peng Y, Zhang Q, Nagasawa H, Okayasu R, Liber HL, Bedford JS. Silencing expression of the catalytic subunit of DNA-dependent protein kinase by small interfering RNA sensitizes human cells for radiation-induced chromosome damage, cell killing, and mutation. *Cancer Res* 2002;62:6400-6404.

Peretz S, Jensen R, Baserga R, Glazer PM. ATM-dependent expression of the insulin-like growth factor-I receptor in a pathway regulating radiation response. *Proc Natl Acad Sci U S A* 2001;98:1676-1681.

Powell SN, Kachnic LA. Roles of BRCA1 and BRCA2 in homologous recombination, DNA replication fidelity and the cellular response to ionizing radiation. *Oncogene* 2003;22:5784-5791.

Rashi-Elkeles S, Elkon R, Shavit S, et al. Transcriptional modulation induced by ionizing radiation: p53 remains a central player. *Mol Oncol* 2011;5:336-348.

Rengan R, Cengel KA, Hahn SM. Clinical target promiscuity: lessons from ras molecular trials. *Cancer Metastasis Rev* 2008;27:403-414.

Rothkamm K, Kruger I, Thompson LH, Lobrich M. Pathways of DNA double-strand break repair during the mammalian cell cycle. *Mol Cell Biol* 2003;23:5706-5715.

Rotolo J, Stancevic B, Zhang J, et al. Anti-ceramide antibody prevents the radiation gastrointestinal syndrome in mice. *J Clin Invest* 2012;122:1786-1790.

Ruiter GA, Zerp SF, Bartelink H, Van Blitterswijk WJ, Verheij M. Alkyl-lysophospholipids activate the SAPK/JNK pathway and enhance radiation-induced apoptosis. *Cancer Res* 1999;59: 2457-2463.

Schmidt-Ullrich RK, Contessa JN, Lammering G, Amorino G, Lin PS. ERBB receptor tyrosine kinases and cellular radiation responses. *Oncogene* 2003;22:5855-5865.

Shiloh Y. ATM and related protein kinases: safeguarding genome integrity. *Nat Rev Cancer* 2003;3:155-168.

Singleton BK, Griffin CS, Thacker J. Clustered DNA damage leads to complex genetic changes in irradiated human cells. *Cancer Res* 2002;62:6263-6269.

Speirs CK, Hwang M, Kim S, et al. Harnessing the cell death pathway for targeted cancer treatment. *Am J Cancer Res* 2012; 1:43-61.

Steel GG. Cellular sensitivity to low dose-rate irradiation focuses the problem of tumour radioresistance. *Radiother Oncol* 1991;20:71-83.

Tenzer A, Pruschy M. Potentiation of DNA-damage-induced cytotoxicity by G2 checkpoint abrogators. *Curr Med Chem Anticancer Agents* 2003;3:35-46.

Terasima T, Tolmach LJ. Changes in x-ray sensitivity of HeLa cells during the division cycle. *Nature* 1961;190:1210-1211.

Thoms J, Bristow RG. DNA repair targeting and radiotherapy: a focus on the therapeutic ratio. *Semin Radiat Oncol* 2010;20: 217-222.

Toulany M, Lee KJ, Fattah KR, et al. Akt promotes post-irradiation survival of human tumor cells through initiation, progression, termination of DNA-PKcs-dependent DNA double-strand break repair. *Mol Cancer Res* 2012;10:945-957.

Turney BW, Kerr M, Chitnis MM, et al. Depletion of the type 1 IGF receptor delays repair of radiation-induced DNA double strand breaks. *Radiother Oncol* 2012;103:402-409.

Valerie K, Povirk LF. Regulation and mechanisms of mammalian double-strand break repair. *Oncogene* 2003;22:5792-5812.

Verheij M, Vens C, Van Triest B. Novel therapeutics in combination with radiotherapy to improve cancer treatment: rationale, mechanisms of action and clinical perspective. *Drug Resist Updat* 2010;13:29-43.

Ward JF. The complexity of DNA damage: relevance to biological consequences. *Int J Radiat Biol* 1994;66:427-432.

White E, Dipaola RS. The double-edged sword of autophagy modulation in cancer. *Clin Cancer Res* 2009;15:5308-5316.

Wilson GD. Radiation and the cell cycle, revisited. *Cancer Metastasis Rev* 2004;23:209-225.

Withers HR, Mason KA. The kinetics of recovery in irradiated colonic mucosa of the mouse. *Cancer* 1974;34(suppl):896-903.

Woods Ignatoski KM, Grewal NK, Markwart SM, et al. Loss of Raf kinase inhibitory protein induces radioresistance in prostate cancer. *Int J Radiat Oncol Biol Phys* 2008;72:153-160.

Xiao H, Zhang Q, Shen J, Bindokas V, Xing HR. Pharmacologic inactivation of kinase suppressor of Ras1 sensitizes epidermal growth factor receptor and oncogenic Ras-dependent tumors to ionizing radiation treatment. *Mol Cancer Ther* 2010;9: 2724-2736.

Xu B, Kim ST, Lim DS, Kastan MB. Two molecularly distinct G(2)/M checkpoints are induced by ionizing irradiation. *Mol Cell Biol* 2002;22:1049-1059.

Yu YL, Chou RH, Wu CH, et al. Nuclear EGFR suppresses ribonuclease activity of polynucleotide phosphorylase through DNAPK-mediated phosphorylation at serine 776. *J Biol Chem* 2012;287:31015-31026.

APPENDIX 15.1 MATHEMATICAL MODELS USED TO CHARACTERIZE RADIATION CELL SURVIVAL

Appendix 15.1.1 Target Theory

The target-theory model was based on the hypothesis that a number of critical targets had to be inactivated for cells to be killed. Cell killing by radiation is now recognized to be more complex, but the equation and parameters derived from the model are still used to describe the shape of cell survival curves. The number of targets (dN) inactivated by a small dose of radiation (dD) should be proportional to the initial number of targets N and dD, so that

$$dN \propto N \cdot dD \quad or \quad dN = -\frac{N \cdot dD}{D_0} \qquad \text{[Appendix Eq. 15.1]}$$

where $1/D_0$ is a constant of proportionality and the negative sign is introduced because the number of active targets N decreases with increasing dose. This equation can be integrated to give

$$N = N_0 \cdot e^{-D/D_o} \qquad \text{[Appendix Eq. 15.2]}$$

where N_0 is the number of active targets present at zero dose. If it is assumed that cells contain only a single target that must be inactivated for them to be killed, then the fractional survival (S) of a population of cells is represented by

$$S = \frac{N}{N_0} = e^{-D/D_0} \qquad \text{[Appendix Eq. 15.3]}$$

where N_0 and N are the initial and final number of cells surviving a radiation dose D. This also represents the probability that any individual cell will survive the radiation dose D. Appendix Equation 15.3 gives a *single-hit, single-target* survival curve that is a straight line on a semilogarithmic plot originating at a surviving fraction of 1 at zero dose (Appendix Fig. 15–1, *line a*). Survival curves of this shape have been obtained for viruses and bacteria, for radiosensitive normal and malignant cells (ie, cells in the bone marrow or lymphoma cells), and for many types of cells treated with high-LET radiation. The term D_0 represents the dose required to reduce the surviving fraction to 0.37 and is a measure of the slope of *line a* in Appendix Figure 15–1. It can be shown mathematically that the radiation dose required to kill 90% of the initial number of cells, termed the D_{10} value, is equivalent to $2.3 \times D_0$ (where 2.3 is the natural logarithm of 10).

If, instead of one target, it is assumed that a cell contains n identical targets, *each of which* must be inactivated (by a single hit) to cause cell death, then the *multitarget, single-hit* cell survival equation can be represented by

$$S = \frac{N}{N_0} = 1 - (1 - e^{-D/D_0})^n \qquad \text{[Appendix Eq. 15.4]}$$

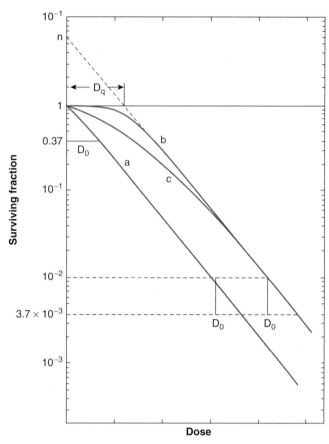

APPENDIX FIGURE 15–1 Survival curves defined by the single-hit and multitarget models of cell killing discussed in the text. *Curve a.* Single-hit (single-target) survival curve defined by Appendix Equation 15.3. *Curve b.* Multitarget survival curve defined by Appendix Equation 15.4. *Curve c.* Composite (2-component) survival curve resulting from both multitarget and single-hit components. Also shown is how the parameters D_0, n, and D_q can be derived from the survival curves.

Again, this equation represents the probability that any individual cell will survive a dose D. A plot of this equation leads to a survival curve with a shoulder at low doses and a straight-line section on a semilogarithmic plot, as shown in Appendix Figure 15–1, *line b*. The parameters D_0, n, and D_q can be determined for this curve as shown. At doses that are large compared to D_0 (ie, $D \gg D_0$), Appendix Equation 15.4 reduces to $S = n \exp - (D/D_0)$, which is similar to Appendix Equation 15.3. The straight-line part of the survival curve thus extrapolates to a value n at zero dose and has a slope defined by D_0. As indicated previously, the D_0 value is the dose required to reduce cell survival from S to $0.37S$ in the *straight-line region* of the survival curve. The quasithreshold dose D_q, is the dose at which the extrapolated straight-line section of the survival curve crosses the dose axis (survival = 1) and quantitatively describes the size of the shoulder. It can be calculated by $D_q = D_0 \ln n$. For this model, the size of the shoulder is regarded as giving an indication of the repair capacity of cells.

One limitation of Appendix Equation 15.4 is that it predicts that a certain amount of damage must be accumulated in a cell before it is killed—that is, at very low doses, the survival curve should be parallel to the dose axis or have an initial slope of zero. This is contrary to much experimental data, which indicate that, for cell populations irradiated with X- or γ-rays, the survival curve often has a finite initial slope (Appendix Fig. 15–1, *line c*).

Appendix 15.1.2 The Linear-Quadratic Model

The linear-quadratic model is based on the concept that multiple lesions, induced by radiation, interact in the cell to cause cell killing. The lesions that interact could be caused by a single ionizing track, giving a direct dependence of cell killing on dose, or by 2 or more separate tracks, giving a dependence of lethality on higher powers of dose. The assumption that 2 lesions must interact to cause cell killing gives an equation that can fit most experimental survival curves, at least over the first few decades of survival, and is given by

$$S = N/N_0 = exp - (\alpha D - \beta D^2) \qquad \text{[Appendix Eq. 15.5]}$$

The parameters α and β represent the probability of the interacting lesions being caused by energy-deposition events as a result of a single charged-particle track or by 2 independent tracks, respectively. The linear-quadratic equation defines a survival curve that is concave downward on a semilogarithmic plot and never becomes strictly exponential (see red line – Appendix Fig. 15–2). However, the curvature is usually small at high doses. The α component can be regarded as describing cell inactivation by nonrepairable damage, while the β component describes cell inactivation by accumulation of repairable damage (blue dashed lines – Appendix Fig. 15–2). The values for α and β vary considerably for different types of mammalian cells both in vitro and in vivo. Typical values of α are in the range 1 to 10^{-1} Gy^{-1} and of β in the range 10^{-1} to 10^{-2} Gy^{-2}.

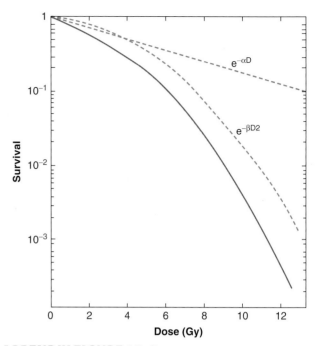

APPENDIX FIGURE 15–2 Survival curve (*red line*) as defined by the linear-quadratic model of cell killing, **Appendix Equation 15.5.** The curves defined by the 2 components of the equation are shown separately as the blue dashed lines.

Alternative equations similar to the linear-quadratic equation can be derived by making various biological assumptions, for example, concerning the capacity of cells to repair radiation damage and the effect of radiation treatment on that capacity (Foray et al, 1996). It should be stressed that a good fit of a given equation to the survival data does not validate the underlying biological assumptions of the model. However, these modeling approaches can be useful in altering radiotherapy fractionation schedules (discussed in Chap. 16, Sec. 16.7.3).

Tumor and Normal Tissue Response to Radiotherapy

16

Richard P. Hill and Robert G. Bristow

16.1 INTRODUCTION

The dose of radiation that can be delivered to a tumor is limited by the damage caused to surrounding normal tissues and the consequent risk of complications. Whether a certain risk of developing complications is regarded as acceptable depends both on the function of the tissue(s) and the severity of the damage involved. This risk must be compared to the probability of benefit (ie, eradicating the tumor) to determine the overall gain from the treatment. This gain can be estimated for an average group of patients, but it may vary for individual patients, depending on the particular characteristics of their tumors and the normal tissues at risk. The balance between the probabilities for tumor control and normal tissue complications gives a measure of the therapeutic ratio of a treatment

(see Sec. 16.5.8). The therapeutic ratio can be improved either by increasing the effective radiation dose delivered to the tumor relative to that given to surrounding normal tissues, or by increasing the biological response of the tumor relative to that of the surrounding normal tissues (see Figs. 16–1 to 16–3).

External beam radiation therapy is usually delivered in relatively small daily doses over the course of several weeks. The empiric development of such multifractionated treatments, which involve giving fractions of approximately 1.8 to 3 Gy daily for 5 to 8 weeks, is an example of exploiting biological factors to improve the therapeutic ratio. More recently, technical improvements in the physical aspects of radiation therapy have allowed an increase in the effective dose of radiation to deep-seated tumors without increasing the dose to normal tissues. Further improvements are occurring with the use of

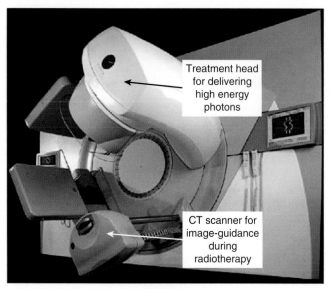

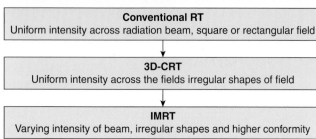

Conventional RT
Uniform intensity across radiation beam, square or rectangular field

↓

3D-CRT
Uniform intensity across the fields irregular shapes of field

↓

IMRT
Varying intensity of beam, irregular shapes and higher conformity

↓

IGRT
IMRT which changes to follow changes in size, shape, and location of tumor and other organs

FIGURE 16–1 **The evolution of modern radiotherapy planning techniques from conventional radiotherapy (RT) to 3-dimensional conformal radiotherapy (3D-CRT), to IMRT, and, finally, to image-guided radiotherapy (IGRT).** For many tumor sites, IMRT and IGRT improve the therapeutic ratio by allowing for increased radiotherapy dose to tumor and decreased dose to normal tissues.

more sophisticated treatment planning methods, allowing for *3-dimensional (3D) conformal radiotherapy (3D-CRT), intensity-modulated radiation therapy (IMRT),* and *stereotactic* treatments (Fig. 16–1). These new methods limit the volume of normal tissues irradiated to high doses and allow escalated doses to the tumor. *Stereotactic body/brain radiation therapy (SBRT)* uses a specially designed coordinate system for the exact localization of the tumor in the body so as to treat it with limited, but highly precise, treatment fields. SBRT involves the delivery of a single high-dose radiation treatment or a few (large-dose) fractionated radiation treatments (usually up to 5 treatments). A highly potent biological dose of radiation is delivered to the tumor over this period and has been used for individual brain or vertebral metastases or for small lung tumors (Milano et al, 2008). Finally, low-dose-rate and high-dose-rate brachytherapy can highly conform dose by placing radioactive sources directly within or adjacent to tumors (see Fig. 16–2). Although these newer treatment strategies

improve the efficiency of radiation therapy delivery, they may also provide opportunities to exploit biological factors. Examples are the continuing exploration of ways to exploit the oxygen effect to cause greater tumor cell killing and more recent efforts to develop drugs that can protect normal tissue from effects of irradiation (without affecting tumor response). Biological factors that may influence the outcome of radiation therapy and their exploitation to improve therapy are discussed in this chapter.

16.2 PRINCIPLES OF CLINICAL RADIOTHERAPY

16.2.1 Radiotherapy Dose

As discussed in Chapter 15, radiotherapy involves both external-beam radiotherapy and brachytherapy; treatment choice depends on the type of tumor and location within the body. The dose of radiation is determined by the intent of the therapy (ie, curative or palliative), the volume of tumor, the relative radiosensitivity of the tumor cells and expected toxicity to the surrounding normal tissues. Other factors relate to the condition of the patient, including age and other health problems that might increase the side effects of radiotherapy (eg, inflammatory and connective tissue disorders). The acute and chronic side effects that may occur following local radiotherapy are linked to the normal structures and tissues within the irradiated volume (Table 16–1); these effects increase with the volume of the irradiated field and with the size of the dose fractions. For example, head and neck irradiation can lead to altered swallowing or a dry mouth (xerostomia), whereas irradiation of pelvic structures may lead to a change in bladder and bowel function. Whole-body radiotherapy, which is sometimes given in addition to chemotherapy during bone marrow transplantation, can lead to nausea and vomiting, decreased blood counts, and altered humoral and cell-mediated immune responses (see Sec. 16.5; Chap. 21, Secs. 21.2 and 21.3).

Most curative radiotherapy regimens consist of daily treatments or fractions in the range of 1.8 to 3 Gy per day over a period of 5 to 8 weeks. The intent is to achieve local control of the tumor, thereby preventing local tissue destruction, organ failure, and the seeding of secondary metastases. Using modern planning techniques (see Sec. 16.2.2) doses up to approximately 75 Gy to the tumor can usually be achieved without causing severe side effects. There are substantial data to indicate that increased radiotherapy dose is associated with increased local control (Armstrong, 2002; Suit, 2002). Typically, the dose to normal tissues is limited so that severe complications occur in no more than 5% of the surviving patients after a period of 5 years (known as the *TD5/5* value). However, this dose limit may be increased if radiotherapy is the only curative treatment option for the patient. Palliative radiotherapy is given when the disease is incurable but there is a need to achieve better pain control, to control bleeding, or

TABLE 16–1 Severe acute and chronic side effects of radiotherapy.*

Irradiation Site	Tissues at Risk	Acute Effect	Chronic Effect[†]
Brain	Brain; neural structures (eye, brainstem)	Drowsiness, hair loss	Cognitive dysfunction and decreased visual acuity
Head and neck	Oral mucosa, salivary glands, skin	Oral inflammation (mucositis), xerostomia (dry mouth), erythema (skin redness)	Permanent xerostomia, decreased ability to open mouth (trismus), dental caries, skin fibrosis
Thorax	Esophageal mucosa, lung, skin	Esophagitis, pneumonitis	Lung fibrosis, esophageal stricture, skin fibrosis
Abdomen	Intestine, pancreas, liver, spleen, kidneys	Nausea, hepatitis, diarrhea	Renal compromise, liver fibrosis, intestinal obstruction
Pelvis	Bladder, rectum, prostate	Increased frequency and dysuria, diarrhea	Bladder or rectal bleeding or rectal ulceration, impotence

*Acute and chronic (late) effects will be idiosyncratic to the patient, the total dose, the dose fractionation, and the irradiation volume.
[†]Severe chronic effects observed in less than 5% of population at 5 years.

to prevent tissue destruction or ulceration. These radiotherapy treatments are usually of short duration and consist of 1 to 3 fractions of 5 to 8 Gy or 5 to 10 fractions of 3 to 4 Gy.

16.2.2 Radiotherapy Planning and Dose Delivery

Conformal radiotherapy employs 3D treatment planning using a series of specific radiation beams given from different angles to maximize tumor dose while minimizing normal tissue irradiation. IMRT is an alternative method that uses a computerized algorithm to design optimal beam orientations and intensities. With IMRT, the individual radiation beams are shaped using special collimators that move during the time of irradiation, so that relatively high-dose volumes of irradiation are contoured to treat the tumor. The combination of multiple beams then allows for better dose distributions resulting in a decreased volume of normal tissue in the high dose region (Bauman et al, 2012).

Both types of planning use magnetic resonance imaging (MRI) or computed tomography (CT) scans or other imaging to localize the tumor and critical normal tissues (see Chap. 14, Sec. 14.3). The energy type (see Chap. 15, Sec. 15.2) and number of radiation beams and their orientation are then chosen. Successful delivery is tracked during treatment using verification images. The extent of the tumor is defined as the *gross tumor volume (GTV)*, but the final radiation plan will deliver the maximum dose to a slightly larger radiation volume (the *planning target volume [PTV]*). The PTV accounts for microscopic disease just beyond the detectable edge of the tumor, for body or organ movement, and for dose gradients that occur at the edge of the radiation beam (the "penumbra") where the dose decreases rapidly. Special techniques and markers are sometimes used to track organ movement within the body (eg, movement of a lung tumor during normal breathing), thereby increasing the accurate targeting of the radiation dose. This type of *image-guided radiation therapy (IGRT)* uses serial 2- and 3-dimensional imaging

to optimize the treatment coordinates during a course of radiation treatment (Dawson and Sharpe, 2006). For small, anatomically accessible tumors, high doses of finely localized irradiation can also be delivered through the use of brachytherapy (Fig. 16–2; discussed in Sec. 16.2.3) or stereotactic body or brain radiosurgery. The latter uses highly focused irradiation beams of charged particles (eg, proton beams; see Sec. 16.2.4), γ-rays, or high-energy x-rays precisely targeted to the tumor site.

Determination of the relationship between normal tissue response and dose is often confounded by the nonuniform dose distribution within the normal organs. However, a dose-volume histogram (DVH) can be generated as part of a modern radiotherapy plan for each exposed organ in a patient (see Sec. 16.2.4 and Fig. 16–3). Several models have been proposed for predicting normal tissue response to radiotherapy using such histograms. However, the quality of clinical data available for such predictions is rarely sufficient to alter radiotherapy practice. Nonetheless, in prostate cancer radiotherapy, for example, DVH plots can be used to show that the volume of the anterior rectum irradiated to high doses is directly correlated to late complications within the rectum (Bauman et al, 2012; Budaus et al, 2012). One important complexity with IMRT plans is that increased volumes of normal tissue are exposed to lower doses and this raises concerns about increased radiation-induced second malignancies (see Sec. 16.8).

16.2.3 Brachytherapy, Radionucleotides, and Radioimmunotherapy

Low-dose rate (LDR; dose rates of up to ~2 Gy/h) radiation sources placed into or beside the tumor (known as brachytherapy) can be used, either alone or in combination with external beam radiotherapy, to treat accessible tumors such as those of the cervix, prostate, head and neck, breast, bladder, lung, esophagus, and some sarcomas. Close to the implanted brachytherapy source the radiation dose is high,

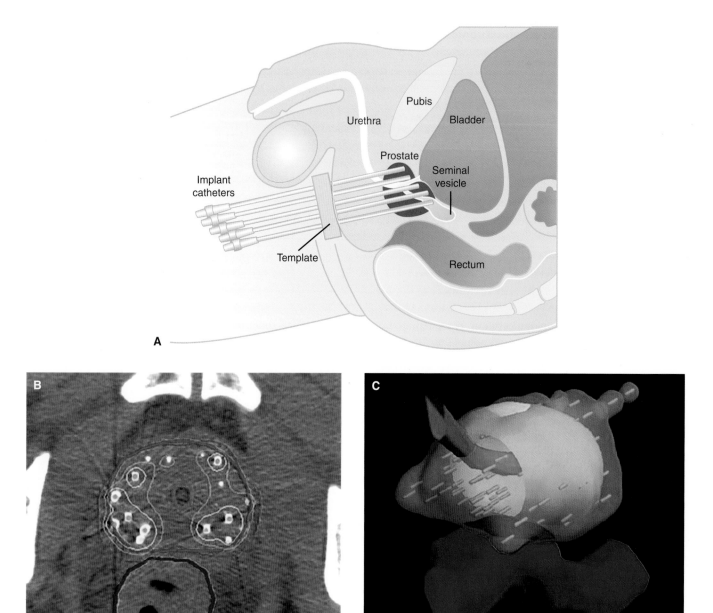

FIGURE 16–2 **Images of a prostate gland treated with high-dose rate radiotherapy using catheters placed into the prostate gland (A) through the patient's perineum. B)** CT image near middle of prostate overlaid with contours delineating prostate (red), urethra (green), and rectum (dark blue). Also shown are isodose lines corresponding to 100% (red), 150% (orange), and 200% (yellow) of the prescribed dose of 145 Gy. **C)** 3D rendering of the 145-Gy isodose surface (translucent orange) covering the prostate.

leading to effective killing of tumor cells, whereas normal cell killing is less at increasing distances from the source as a result of lower doses (and dose rates) (see Fig. 16–2). The cellular effects of continuous LDR irradiation (described in Chap. 15, Sec. 15.4.2) are similar to those of reducing fraction size and thereby allow for cellular repair in normal tissues (see Sec. 16.6.1 and Fig. 16–20). Computer-controlled brachytherapy systems can deliver radiation doses as short high-dose pulses (pulsed-dose brachytherapy) or with a high-dose rate (HDR brachytherapy; rate of dose delivery exceeds 12 Gy/h). The high-dose source travels along a catheter track

within the tumor. By varying the position and dwell time of the radiation source, the dose is neatly sculpted to conform to the shape of the target. The patient typically receives the total dose in a series of 1 to 10 treatments. HDR brachytherapy uses a relatively intense source of radiation (eg, iridium 192) delivered through temporarily placed applicators. The benefits of HDR brachytherapy, compared to manual-loaded brachytherapy techniques, can include treatments being planned after the applicator placement, but before radiation delivery, helping to improve treatment efficacy and safety, and a rapid dose delivery, which can lead to decreased outpatient visits for treatments. Radiobiological modeling suggests that the acute and late reactions with pulsed-dose brachytherapy are similar to traditional (continuous) brachytherapy as long as the gaps between pulses are less than 1 hour (Brenner and Hall, 1991).

The use of injected radionucleotides to treat cancer is based on their selective uptake by tumors or adjacent normal tissues, so that local irradiation may lead to death of the tumor cells. Examples are ^{131}I to treat well-differentiated thyroid cancer, radiolabeled somatostatin analogs for the treatment of neuroendocrine tumors, and ^{89}Sr or [223]Ra to treat bone metastases, mainly in prostate cancer (Autio et al, 2012); the latter isotopes are chemically similar to calcium and thus taken up selectively into bone where they can irradiate and cause death of neighboring cancer cells. The conjugation of radioisotopes to specific antibodies or to agents that bind to receptors on cancer cells allows targeted radiotherapy to tumors expressing the relevant antigens or receptors and is termed *radioimmunotherapy (RIT)*. Optimal radioisotopes are those emitting *a*-particles and short-range electrons (ie, β-particles) resulting in the killing of cells within a radius of 1 to 3 cell diameters of the bound isotope (eg, [111]Indium). In animal models, RIT was found to kill disseminated solid tumor cells and small metastases when targeting differentiation antigens (eg, CD20 or CD21) on lymphomas, somatostatin receptors on neuroendocrine tumors, or epidermal growth factor receptors (EGFRs) on certain breast cancers. However, in patients, this approach has been limited by the lack of specific uptake in tumor cells when compared to normal cells and the attendant difficulty of accurate dosimetry and treatment planning. Clinical success has so far been achieved mostly with radiolabeled antibodies against CD20 (^{131}I-tositumomab and ^{90}Y-ibritumomab) for the treatment of relapsed or refractory CD20+ follicular B-cell non-Hodgkin lymphoma or consolidation therapy in patients with follicular non-Hodgkin lymphoma that achieve a partial or complete response to first-line chemotherapy. The predominant complication of RIT is hematological toxicity, but this is usually manageable (Pouget et al, 2011).

16.2.4 High Linear Energy Transfer Radiotherapy: Protons and Carbon Ions

Particle therapy is a form of external-beam radiotherapy using beams of energetic protons, neutrons, or positive ions for cancer treatment. The most common type of particle therapy is proton therapy. Particle therapies may have high linear energy transfer (LET) and might contribute to improvements in the therapeutic ratio in several ways. First, because much of the energy of particle beams is deposited in tissue at the end of particle tracks (Fig. 16–3) (ie, in the region of the Bragg peak; see Chap. 15, Sec. 15.2.2), they can give improved depth-dose distributions for deep-seated tumors. Neutron beams do not demonstrate a Bragg peak and depth-dose distributions are similar to those for low-LET radiation. Heavy ion therapy, for example, using carbon ions, is being investigated in a number of centers across the world. These beams have higher LET than protons and increased relative biological effectiveness (RBE; see Chap. 15, Sec. 15.3.1).

The therapeutic ratio may also be improved by particle therapies because the oxygen enhancement ratio (OER) is reduced at high LET (see Sec. 16.4.1), so that hypoxic cells in tumors are protected to a lesser degree. The variation in radiosensitivity with position in the cell cycle (see Chap. 15, Sec. 15.4.1) is also reduced for high-LET radiation and, in general, there is reduced variability in response between different cells. This is partly because cells exhibit reduced capacity for repair following high-LET radiation relative to that following low-LET radiation, leading to an increase in RBE (see Chap. 15, Sec. 15.3.1). Compared to protons, carbon ions have the disadvantage that beyond the Bragg peak, the dose does not decrease to zero, because nuclear reactions between the carbon ions and the atoms of the tissue lead to production of lighter ions that have increased range.

One potential difficulty in using high-LET radiation is that because late-responding tissues demonstrate greater repair capacity than early responding tissues (see Secs. 16.7.1 and 16.7.2), the reduction in repair capacity following high-LET irradiation will result in relatively higher RBE values for late-responding normal tissues. However, the ability to deliver dose in a finely focused manner using protons or heavy ions combined with IMRT planning techniques reduces the volume of normal tissue exposed to high doses, limiting this concern. Results with protons demonstrate an advantage for treatment of some tumors, such as choroidal melanomas and skull-base tumors (Suit, 2002), that require precise treatment of a highly localized lesion, and in pediatric tumors where the dose to normal structures should be decreased as much as possible to avoid developmental side-effects during development (DeLaney, 2011).

There have been extensive clinical studies using high-energy neutrons, but such treatments have been associated with an increase in complications, particularly subcutaneous fibrosis, and randomized trials have not demonstrated therapeutic gain (Fowler, 1988; Raju, 1996); thus there is limited current use of such therapy. An alternative approach is boron neutron capture therapy (BNCT), in which compounds enriched with [10]B are administered prior to irradiation with a lower-energy (thermal) neutron beam. Neutrons interact preferentially with the [10]B atoms in the tumors, and, a fission reaction produces high-energy charged particles ([7]Li and [4]He), resulting in tumor cell killing. For an improved therapeutic ratio with BNCT, relatively high concentrations of [10]B must be achieved in the tumor, with low concentrations in normal tissues. New boronated compounds and new strategies for delivering them are needed to improve the differential concentrations achievable in tumors and surrounding normal tissues, but encouraging results have been obtained, particularly for the treatment of brain tumors (Yamamoto et al, 2008; Barth, 2009). However, the depth-dose distribution for the thermal neutron beam is relatively poor and this remains a serious limitation in the clinical use of this treatment for deep-seated tumors.

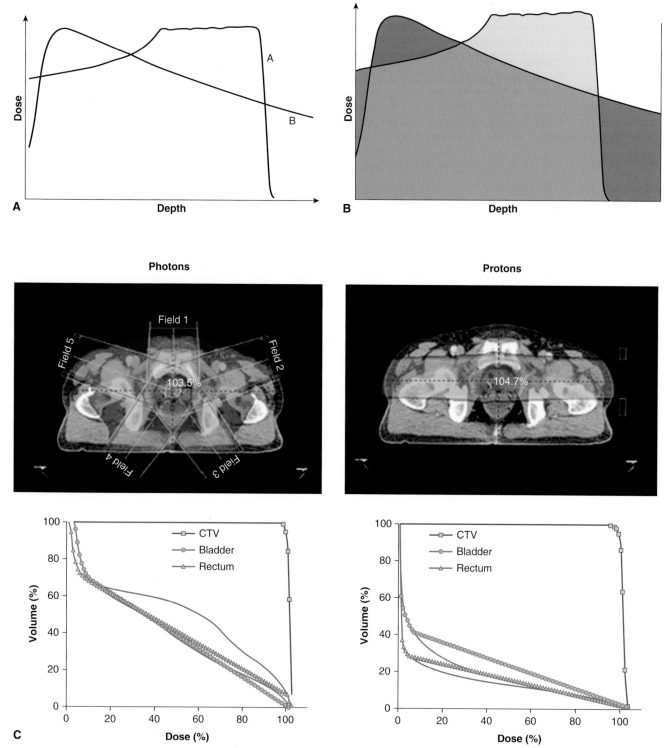

FIGURE 16–3 **A) Generalized depth dose curves for a high-energy photon (6MV or above) and a modulated-energy proton beam.**
The proton beam (A) delivers its dose at increased depth as compare to a high-energy photon beam (B). **B)** Illustration of differences between
photon and proton depth dose distribution (red, dose delivered by the photon beam that is greater than that delivered by the proton beam;
green, same dose from both photon and proton beams; blue, dose delivered by proton beam but not photon beam; gold, dose delivered to
defined target by protons but not by photons). **C)** Comparison of isodose distributions and dose volume histograms (DVH) for protons versus
photons for a typical prostate cancer radiotherapy plan. The 5-beam photon plan shows increased volumes (*y*-axis on plot) of bladder and
rectum being irradiated for increasing percentage of the total dose delivered (*x*-axis on plot) when compared to the use of a 2-beam proton
plan (*CTV*, clinical tumor volume to be treated with the total radiotherapy dose).

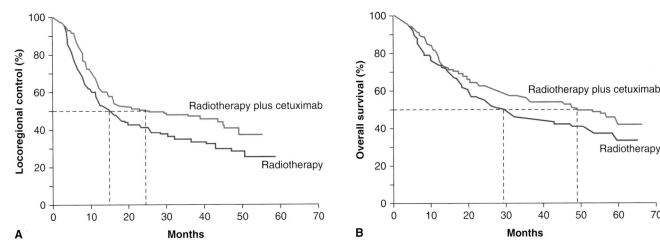

FIGURE 16–4 Kaplan-Meier estimates of (A) locoregional control and (B) overall survival among all patients randomly assigned to radiotherapy plus cetuximab or radiotherapy alone. (Redrawn from Bonner et al, 2006 with permission.)

16.2.5 Combining Radiotherapy with Other Cancer Treatments

Radiotherapy is increasingly used with other cancer treatments, including surgery and drug therapy with hormones, chemotherapy, or molecular targeted agents. Combining radiotherapy with surgery can improve outcome by sterilizing microscopic or residual disease within, and just beyond, the surgical bed. Alternatively, surgery can be used as salvage therapy in patients where the use of radiotherapy alone was not sufficient to control the tumor locally. Concomitant chemotherapy is used for treatment of locally advanced head and neck, lung, and cervical cancers to increase the probability of cure or local control by radiotherapy, and concomitant hormone therapy is used to improve survival of men with locally advanced prostate cancer. Results from preclinical local tumor control experiments suggest that multiple radiobiological mechanisms might contribute to an improved therapeutic ratio with this approach, including the prevention of tumor cell repopulation, decreased number of clonogenic tumor cells, increased cellular radiation sensitivity, improved reoxygenation of clonogenic tumor cells during the combined treatment, and killing of circulating endothelial precursor cells that might replace tumor vasculature destroyed during radiotherapy (Zips et al, 2008; Ahn and Brown, 2009; Begg et al, 2011). Important interactions between radiation and chemotherapy in tumor and normal tissues are reviewed in Chapter 17, Section 17.6.4.

Increasingly, molecular-targeted agents that can sensitize tumors to radiotherapy are being combined with radiotherapy; this is discussed in Chapter 15, Section 15.4. A specific example of the clinical application of such an approach is the phase III randomized study that demonstrated that the EGFR inhibitor cetuximab given concomitantly with radiotherapy for head and neck cancer, improved locoregional control and overall survival without increasing mucosal toxicity (Fig. 16–4) when compared to radiotherapy alone (Bonner et al, 2010). The use of an EGFR inhibitor was thought to combat tumor cell repopulation during radiotherapy as the basis for the improved therapeutic

ratio for this combination (Zips et al, 2008). Newer Phase III clinical trials are assessing the benefit of adding cetuximab to the current standard regimen of cisplatin and radiotherapy, but increased toxicity of the 3 agents when combined may limit this modality approach (Walsh et al, 2011). Other trials are assessing the benefit of chemotherapy and or/cetuximab added to radiotherapy for human papillomavirus (HPV)-positive versus HPV-negative cancers, given the reported increased sensitivity of HPV-positive head and neck cancers to fractionated radiotherapy (Ang et al, 2010). Biomarkers that reflect the HPV status of the tumor (eg, HPV viral or P16[INK4a] gene expression) predict patients with differing prognosis following radical radiotherapy (Ang and Sturgis, 2012).

In another example, histone deacetylase (HDAC) inhibitors, such as vorinostat, that have shown radiosensitizing activity in preclinical tumor models are being assessed in patients. A recent Phase I study has shown that vorinostat can be safely combined with short-term pelvic palliative radiotherapy and may therefore be of benefit in long-term curative pelvic radiotherapy as a component of preoperative chemoradiotherapy for rectal cancer (Ree et al, 2010). Similar efforts are ongoing across many tumor types receiving radiotherapy in Phase I to III trials, where the effectiveness of a molecular-targeted agent is being matched to a biomarker of radioresistance (Begg et al, 2011). Any benefit of combined modality therapy will be predicated on improving the therapeutic ratio in which the molecular agent does not add radiotoxicity to normal tissues.

16.3 TUMOR CONTROL FOLLOWING RADIOTHERAPY

16.3.1 Dose Response and Tumor Control Relationships

The emphasis in Chapter 15 on the molecular and cellular effects of radiation treatment reflects a view that the response

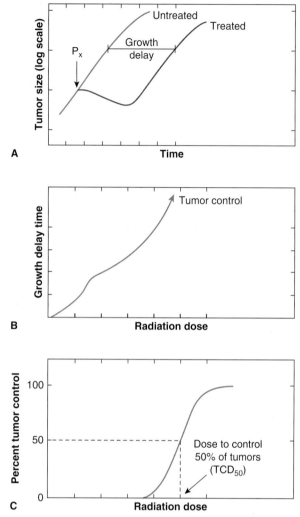

FIGURE 16–5 **Illustration of 2 assays for tumor response.** In (**A**), growth curves for groups of treated and untreated tumors are shown and the measurement of growth delay indicated. Growth delay is plotted as a function of radiation dose in (**B**). At large doses, some of the tumors may not regrow and the percentage of controlled tumors can be plotted as a function of dose as in (**C**).

of tumors can be understood largely in terms of the sensitivity of the cancer cells within those tumors. However, there is increasing evidence that the extracellular environment in tumors can play a substantial role in their response to treatment (Hanahan and Weinberg, 2011). For radiation, hypoxia is known to play an important role in tumor response (see Sec. 16.4.2; Chap. 12, Sec. 12.2). Consequently, techniques that assess tumor response in situ rather than measuring the survival of tumor cells after removing and dissociating the tumor are important (Fig. 16–5). The size of untreated and irradiated tumors can be measured as a function of time to allow the generation of growth curves (Fig. 16–5A). The delay in growth is the difference in time for treated and untreated tumors to grow to a defined size, and this time difference can be plotted as a function of radiation dose, as shown for single-dose treatments in Figure 16–5B. The curve shown in Figure 16–5B is

drawn to show a change in slope, consistent with the presence of a fraction of hypoxic cells in the tumor (see Sec. 16.4.2). At higher radiation doses, some tumors will be permanently controlled. If groups of animals receive different radiation doses to their tumors, the percentage of controlled tumors can be plotted as a function of dose to give a dose-control curve as shown in Figure 16–5C.

The concept that tumors contain a fraction of cells that have unlimited proliferative capacity (ie, cancer stem cells [CSCs]) was introduced in Chapter 13. As discussed in that chapter, there are uncertainties about the properties of such cells and about the plasticity of the CSC phenotype, but, because cells expressing a CSC phenotype are the ones that can regenerate the tumor after treatment, their radiosensitivity is critical to achieving tumor control. For a simple model, which assumes that the response of a tumor to radiation depends on the individual responses of the cells within it, the dose of radiation required to control a tumor only depends on (a) the radiation sensitivity of the CSCs and (b) their number. From a knowledge of the sensitivity of the CSCs in a tumor, it is possible to predict the expected level of survival following a given single radiation dose. A simple calculation, using Appendix Equation 15.4 in Appendix 15.1 (see Chap. 15) and typical survival curve parameters for well-oxygenated cells (D_0 = 1.3 Gy, D_q = 2.1 Gy), indicates that a single radiation dose of 26 Gy might be expected to reduce the probability of survival of an individual cell to approximately 10^{-8}. For a tumor containing 10^8 CSCs, this dose would thus leave, on average, 1 surviving CSC. Because of the random nature of radiation damage there will be statistical fluctuation around this value. The statistical fluctuation expected from random cell killing by radiation follows a Poisson distribution; the probability (P_n) of a tumor having n surviving CSCs when the average number of CSCs surviving is a is given by:

$$P_n = (a^n e^{-a})/n!$$ [Eq. 16.1]

For tumor control, the important parameter is P_0, which is the probability that a tumor will contain no surviving CSCs (ie, $n = 0$). From Equation 16.1:

$$P_0 = e^{-a}$$ [Eq. 16.2]

For $a = 1$, as in the example above, the probability of control would be $e^{-1} = 0.37$. Different radiation doses will, of course, result in different values of a and it is possible to construct a theoretical curve relating the probability of tumor control with dose, which shows a sigmoid relationship (Fig. 16–6, solid lines).

The central red curve in Figure 16–6 represents a group of identical tumors each containing 10^8 CSCs. For tumors containing 10^7 or 10^9 CSCs, the curves will be displaced (to smaller (blue) or larger (green) doses, respectively) by a dose sufficient to reduce survival by a factor of 10. These dose-control curves illustrate the concept that the dose of radiation required to control a tumor depends on the number of CSCs that it contains, although as noted above, the uncertainties

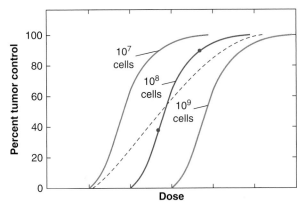

FIGURE 16-6 **Percentage tumor control plotted as a function of dose for single radiation treatments.** Theoretical curves for groups of tumors containing different numbers of tumor stem cells are shown. The points on the red curve labeled "10⁸ cells" are derived as discussed in the text. The composite curve (dashed) was obtained for a group containing equal proportions from the 3 individual groups.

about the identification of such cells and the plasticity of their phenotype may make it difficult to determine the number of cells with CSC potential in an individual tumor.

The above discussion also assumes that the CSCs exhibit a uniform radiosensitivity within a tumor. Recent studies suggest the possibility that CSCs may be more resistant to radiation than other (progenitor) cell populations in a tumor (Krause et al, 2011). Also, the microenvironment of the CSCs in the tumor can affect their sensitivity to radiation and there may also be differences as a result of genetic or epigenetic heterogeneity among the tumor cells. The role of hypoxia is well documented (see Sec. 16.4.2), but there may also be interactions of the cells with the extracellular matrix (ECM) and/or interactions with growth factors, such as transforming growth factor β (TGF-β1), which may influence cellular sensitivity and tumor response (Bouquet et al, 2011). Interactions between the tumor cells and the ECM can also influence cellular signaling, such as the EGFR/MEK/ERK (extracellular signal regulated kinase) or phosphatidylinositol-3 kinase (PI3K)/AKT pathways (see Chap. 8, Sec. 8.2.5) that can affect cellular sensitivity to radiation (see Chap. 15, Sec. 15.4.3). Knowledge of the role that such factors may play in tumor response is limited, but there is increasing evidence that cell contact and expression of certain integrins can affect the radiation sensitivity of cells (Eke and Cordes, 2011). Also, vascular damage and radiation-induced apoptosis of endothelial cells in tumors may play a role in response to radiation treatment (Garcia-Barros et al, 2010) through (opposing) effects of death of tumor cells from nutrient deprivation, or increase in hypoxia and radioresistance of surviving tumor cells. Recent work also points to the possibility that bone-marrow derived myeloid populations of cells, particularly monocytes/macrophages, may play a role in repair of the vasculature in tumors, thereby increasing their resistance to irradiation (Kioi et al, 2010; Zaleska et al, 2011).

16.3.2 Predicting the Response of Tumors

Even tumors of the same size and histopathological type are likely to vary in their proportion of CSCs. Thus, a dose-control curve for a group of human tumors will be a composite of the simple ones shown in Figure 16–6; the slope of the composite dose-control curve will be less than that for the individual simple curves (see Fig. 16–6, dashed line). Fractionation of the radiation treatment (see Sec. 16.6) and heterogeneity in the radiosensitivity of CSCs (either intrinsic or as a result of their microenvironment) will also result in a decrease in the slope of the dose-control curve. Thus, the slope of the dose-control curve derived from a clinical study is likely to be quite shallow. It is therefore desirable to seek a way of assigning the tumors to more homogeneous groups, so that patients with differences in prognosis can be identified. This is a major motivation for attempts to develop predictive assays. In vitro studies of a wide range of cell lines derived from human tumors have shown intrinsic variations in radiation sensitivity. Survival curves can vary considerably even for cells of similar histopathological types, particularly in the width of the shoulder region (Fig. 16–7). Even small differences in the shoulder region can be important because they are magnified during the multiple fractionated daily doses of 1.8 to 2 Gy given in clinical radiotherapy. Estimates of the surviving fraction following a dose of 2 Gy for different human tumor cell lines growing in culture may be grouped according to histopathological type and compared with the likelihood that such tumors will be controlled by radiation treatment (Table 16–2). There is a trend toward higher levels of survival at 2 Gy for the cells from tumor groups that, by experience, are less radiocurable.

The concept that tumor response for an individual patient can be predicted has been tested using the survival following 2 Gy (SF2) for cells from primary human cervix tumor biopsies grown in soft agar. West et al (1997) found that patients with tumors containing radioresistant cells (SF2 > median) had significantly worse local control and survival than those with tumors containing more radiosensitive cells (SF2 < median; Fig. 16–8) and similar results were reported for head and neck cancers (Bjork-Eriksson et al, 2000). However, other groups have had difficulty confirming the generality of these findings. Furthermore, the widespread application of such assays has been limited by technical problems; for example, the soft agar assay requires 5 to 6 weeks before scoring, and measurements could not be obtained in 25% to 30% of tumors. Other potential limitations of such assays are (a) they do not account for microenvironmental factors influencing radiosensitivity; (b) tumors may contain clonogenic (CSC) subpopulations of different intrinsic radiosensitivity; (c) the assay relies on colony formation in agarose to identify CSCs, and many of them may not proliferate in this artificial environment; and (d) if other (progenitor) tumor cells can also form small colonies, the assay may not be measuring the radiosensitivity of the CSCs alone.

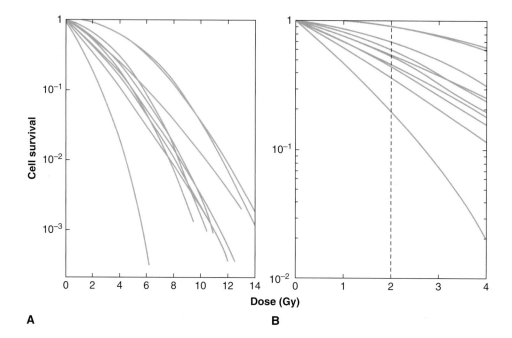

FIGURE 16-7 A) Survival curves for a number of different human melanoma cell lines. The lines were drawn to be continuously curving and conform to the linear-quadratic model (see Chap. 15, Appendix 15.1). **B)** The low-dose region of the curves is illustrated, demonstrating the range of cell survival values at 2 Gy. (Adapted from Fertil and Malaise, 1981.)

More recently, genetic profiling is being investigated as an approach to prediction of treatment response and identification of possible therapeutic targets to enhance response (eg, Miyamoto and Harris, 2011; Settle and Sulman, 2011). Mutations associated with DNA repair (such as ATM [ataxia-telangiectasis mutated]) can affect radiation sensitivity, and

as discussed in Chapter 5, Section 5.4, inhibitors of DNA repair in combination with radiotherapy might be used to take advantage of inherent defects in DNA repair in tumor cells. This field is evolving rapidly and studies have identified other pathways such as PI3K/AKT in cervix cancer that might be predictive of response to radiotherapy (Schwarz et al, 2012). A potential problem is that most genetic analyses are being undertaken on the bulk tumor population and largely reflect changes in the majority population of tumor cells, and thus may miss critical changes in a small proportion of the tumor cells, particularly populations of CSCs.

TABLE 16-2 Values of the surviving fraction (cell survival) at 2 Gy for human tumor cell lines.

Tumor Cell Type*	Number of Lines	Mean Survival at 2 Gy (Range)
1. Lymphoma Neuroblastoma Myeloma Small-cell lung cancer Medulloblastoma	14	0.20 (0.08 to 0.37)
2. Breast cancer Squamous-cell cancer Pancreatic cancer Colorectal cancer Non–small-cell lung cancer	12	0.43 (0.14 to 0.75)
3. Melanoma Osteosarcoma Glioblastoma Hypernephroma	25	0.52 (0.20 to 0.86)

*Tumor types are grouped (1 to 3) approximately in decreasing order of their likelihood of local control by radiation treatment.

Source: Modified from Deacon et al, 1984.

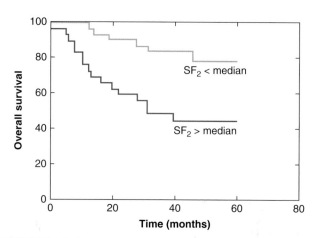

FIGURE 16-8 Actuarial survival in patients with cervical cancer treated by radical radiotherapy as a function of intrinsic radiosensitivity of tumors stratified as above (red line) or below (blue line) the median survival following 2 Gy (SF2) of 0.41. Overall survival and local control (not shown) are significantly worse for patients with SF2 > 0.41. (Redrawn from Levine et al, 1995.)

16.4 HYPOXIA AND RADIATION RESPONSE

16.4.1 The Oxygen Effect and Radiosensitivity

The biological effects of radiation on cells are enhanced by oxygen. The primary mechanism (called the *oxygen fixation hypothesis*) is believed to be that oxygen can interact with (secondary) radicals, on cellular molecules such as DNA, formed by their interaction with the (primary) hydroxyl radicals produced by radiation effects on water in the cell (Fig. 16–9A). These interactions result in damage to DNA that is initially permanent or "fixed" and must be repaired by the cell enzymatically. For this effect, oxygen must be present in the cells at the time of or within a few milliseconds of the radiation exposure (because of the short lifetime of the radicals). At low levels of oxygen, free sulfhydryls in the cells can effectively compete with oxygen to interact with the radicals and can cause an immediate chemical repair. Cells irradiated in the presence of air are about 3 times more sensitive than cells irradiated under conditions of severe acute hypoxia (Fig. 16–9B). The sensitizing effect of different concentrations of oxygen is shown in Figure 16–9C. At very low levels of oxygen the cells are resistant but, as the level of oxygen increases, their sensitivity rises rapidly to almost maximal levels at oxygen concentrations

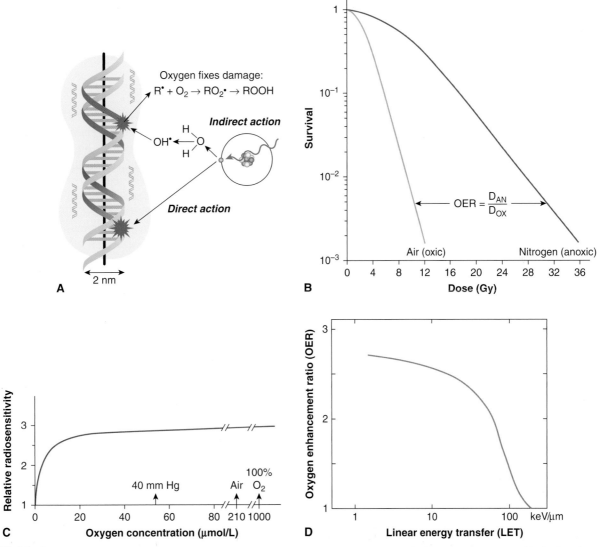

FIGURE 16–9 **Effect of oxygen as a radiosensitizer. A)** Illustration of oxygen interacting with damage to DNA caused by hydroxyl (OH) radicals created by the effects of radiation on water molecules (Modified from Hall, 2000). **B)** Survival curves obtained when cells are treated with low-LET radiation in the presence (air) or absence (nitrogen) of oxygen. The OER is calculated as indicated (D_{OX} = dose in air, D_{AN} = dose in nitrogen) and as described in the text. **C)** The relative radiosensitivity of cells is plotted as a function of oxygen concentration in the surrounding medium to illustrate the dependence of the sensitizing effect on oxygen concentration. (Adapted from Chapman et al, 1974.) **D)** Illustration of the dependence of the OER on the LET of the radiation.

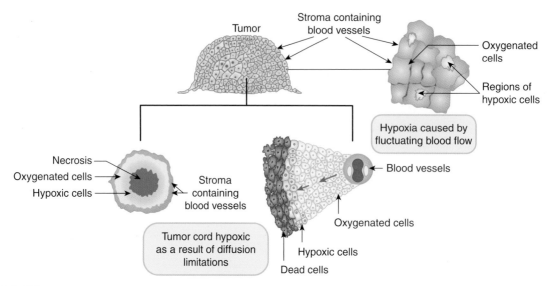

FIGURE 16–10 **Schematic of 2 models for the development of hypoxia in tumors.** Hypoxia may arise as a result of fluctuating blood flow (as illustrated in the diagram on the upper right) or as a result of diffusion limitations in the tumor cord model (inward or outward diffusion from vessels as illustrated in the lower 2 diagrams).

above approximately 35 μmoles/L (equivalent oxygen partial pressure ~25 mm of mercury [mm Hg]). The oxygen concentration at which the sensitizing effect is one-half of maximum (the Km value) varies among cell lines (probably as a result of free sulfhydryl levels in the cells) but is usually in the region 5 to 15 μmoles/L (4 to 12 mm Hg equivalent partial pressure).

The degree of sensitization afforded by oxygen is characterized by the OER, which is defined (see Fig. 16–9B) as the ratio of doses required to give the same biological effect in the absence or the presence of oxygen. For doses of X- or γ-radiation greater than approximately 3 Gy, the OER for a wide range of cell lines in vitro, and for most tissues in vivo, is in the range of 2.5 to 3.3. For X- or γ-ray doses less than approximately 3 Gy (ie, in the shoulder region of the survival curve), the OER is reduced in a dose-dependent manner. A reduction of the OER at low doses is clinically important because the individual treatments of a fractionated course of treatment are usually 2 Gy or less. The OER is also dependent on the type of radiation, declining to a value of 1 for radiation with LET values greater than approximately 200 kiloelectron volts per micrometer (keV/μm) (see Fig. 16–9D).

16.4.2 Tumor Hypoxia

The cells in a tumor are influenced both by their interactions with the ECM (see Chap. 10, Sec. 10.2), and by their microenvironment, which is characterized by regions of nutrient deprivation, low extracellular pH, high interstitial fluid pressure (IFP), and hypoxia (see Chap. 12, Sec. 12.2). The oxygen level (pO$_2$) in most normal tissues ranges between approximately 20 and 80 mm Hg, whereas tumors often contain regions where the pO$_2$ is less than 5 mm Hg. These conditions in solid tumors are primarily caused by the abnormal vasculature

that develops during tumor angiogenesis (see Chap. 11). The blood vessels in solid tumors have highly irregular architecture, and are more widely separated than in normal tissues. A proportion of tumor cells may lie in chronically hypoxic regions beyond the diffusion distance of oxygen (Fig. 16–10; see also Chap. 12, Figs. 12–5 and 12–6). Tumor cells may also be exposed to shorter (often fluctuating) periods (minutes to a few hours) of acute hypoxia as a result of intermittent flow in individual blood vessels (see Fig. 16–10). Tumor hypoxia has been observed in a majority of tumors both human and experimental (see Sec. 16.4.3 and Chap. 12, Sec. 12.2.1), but has been found to be very heterogeneous both within and among tumors, even those of similar histopathological type, and it does not correlate simply with standard prognostic factors such as tumor size, stage, and grade (Vaupel et al, 2001). Acute and chronic hypoxia can coexist in the same tumor and hypoxic regions in tumors are often diffusely distributed throughout the tumor (see Fig. 16–10) and are rarely concentrated only around a central core of necrosis.

Evidence that cells in the hypoxic regions of tumors growing in experimental animals are viable and capable of regrowing the tumor is provided by analysis of cell survival curves generated by irradiating the tumor in situ and then plating the cells in vitro. For most tumors the terminal slope of such curves is characteristic of that for hypoxic cells (Fig. 16–11). The proportion of viable hypoxic cells in tumors can be estimated (Fig. 16–11) from the ratio (S$_{Air}$/S$_{Anox}$) of the cell survival obtained for tumors in air-breathing animals irradiated with a large dose to the cell survival obtained for tumors irradiated with the same dose under anoxic conditions (eg, tumor blood supply clamped). As discussed below, substantial levels of hypoxia in human tumors have been shown to be a poor prognostic indicator. However, cells exposed to acute versus chronic

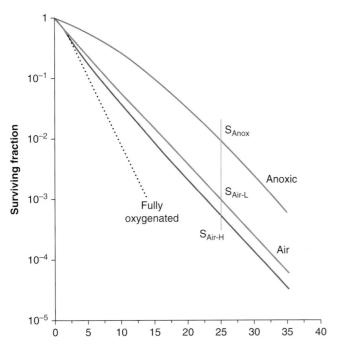

FIGURE 16-11 The influence of a subpopulation of hypoxic cells on the survival curve obtained for an irradiated tumor. The 4 curves shown are for a well-oxygenated population of cells (dotted line), 2 curves derived from tumors irradiated under air-breathing conditions, and a curve for tumors irradiated under anoxic conditions (blue line). The 2 curves for irradiation under air-breathing conditions are for tumors in animals with high (H-red line) or low (L-green line) hemoglobin levels. The hypoxic fraction can be estimated by taking the ratio of the survival obtained under air-breathing conditions (S_{Air}) to that obtained under anoxic conditions (S_{Anox}) at a dose level where the survival curves are parallel, as illustrated. For the tumors in animals with a high hemoglobin this value is approximately 0.06 (6%) and for the tumors in animals with low hemoglobin it is approximately 0.12 (12%). (Modified from Hill et al, 1971.)

hypoxia in the tumor may exhibit different degrees of resistance. In cells exposed to longer periods of (chronic) hypoxia, gene expression changes may occur (see Chap. 12, Sec. 12.2.3) which can reduce the OER value as a consequence of a reduced ability to repair radiation-induced DNA damage. Thus acutely hypoxic cells may be the more resistant of the hypoxic cell populations in tumors. Hypoxia may play an important role in treatment outcome for many tumor types and can affect the metastatic ability of some tumor cells (see Chap. 10, Sec. 10.5.7) as well as the response of the primary tumor to treatment.

16.4.3 Measuring Hypoxia in Tumors

Table 16-3 lists techniques to determine oxygenation in individual tumors. A common method for human tumors has been polarographic oxygen electrodes (eg, the Eppendorf oxygen electrode) to measure microregional pO_2 (estimated to be in a volume equivalent to approximately 500 cells) in multiple locations. This technology has revealed wide pO_2 variations both within and between tumors (Fig. 16-12 *A, B*).

Results from clinical studies in cervix and head and neck carcinomas (see Fig. 16-12C and Chap. 12, Fig. 12-8) treated by radiotherapy indicate that hypoxic tumors have a worse prognosis (Nordsmark et al, 2005; Fyles et al, 2006). It should be noted that hypoxic cervix tumors treated by surgery also had a worse prognosis, consistent with the fact that hypoxic tumors tend to be more aggressive and have increased metastasis (Hockel et al, 1996). The oxygen electrode has the disadvantage that it is invasive and it is difficult to distinguish between measurements made in viable versus nonviable tissue regions.

More recent studies have focussed on noninvasive imaging or immunohistochemical (IHC) staining of biopsies using extrinsic or intrinsic markers of hypoxia. Commonly used extrinsic markers are pimonidazole and [¹⁸F]-labeled nitroimidazoles such as [¹⁸F]-misonidazole or [¹⁸F]-fluoroazomycinarabinofuranoside ([¹⁸F]FAZA), which can be injected into patients and form protein adducts within hypoxic regions in the tumor. To assess the regions of hypoxia in the tumor the [¹⁸F]-labeled compounds can be imaged with positron emission tomography (PET; see Chap. 14, Sec. 14.3.3), while staining with antibodies to the (pimonidazole) adducts is used on tissue sections (Ljungkvist et al, 2007; Chitneni et al, 2011). Both pimonidazole and another nitroimidazole (EF5) have also been used widely in animal models. Such studies have provided evidence for substantial heterogeneity in hypoxia both within and between tumors. A recent study in laryngeal cancer using pimonidazole has reported poorer locoregional control in patients with more hypoxic tumors (Janssens et al, 2012). Intrinsic markers of hypoxia (such as hypoxia inducible factor-1a [HIF-1a], glucose transporter-1 [GLUT-1], carbonic anhydrase-9 [CA-9] and osteopontin [OPN]; see Chap. 12, Sec. 12.2.3) are proteins that are upregulated in the cells exposed to hypoxia and can be detected by IHC staining with appropriate antibodies. Intrinsic markers have the advantage that they can be applied to existing tissue blocks for retrospective analysis of previous clinical studies, but because their expression can be affected by other mechanisms in the cell, they have imperfect correlation with hypoxic regions identified with extrinsic markers. Increased levels of these various markers have, however, been associated with poorer treatment outcome in different tumor types (Bussink et al, 2003; Vordermark and Brown, 2003; Lim et al, 2012).

The heterogeneity in levels of hypoxia throughout tumors poses a problem for techniques using tissue sections, as assessment of multiple biopsies is necessary to achieve an overall assessment of hypoxia in the tumor. PET imaging of the binding of radiolabelled nitroimidazoles can be used to evaluate the whole tumor, although the volume resolution of such imaging is much lower than that achieved in tissue sections (see Chap. 14, Sec. 14.3.3). Use of this technique in patients with head and neck tumors was predictive for treatment outcome with radiochemotherapy (Rischin et al, 2006).

The recent development of whole-genome analysis has allowed for the identification of specific gene signatures associated with hypoxia. Initial studies suggest that such signatures can have predictive power for radiation treatment of

TABLE 16–3 Assays for intratumoral hypoxia.

Technique	Principle	Advantages	Disadvantages
Histomorphometric assays	Measures distance between blood vessels and zones of necrosis. Measures vascular density.	Simple. Can be applied on archived tissue. Can be combined with cryospectrophotometry to measure hemoglobin saturation within frozen tissue section.	Indirect measure of tumor oxygenation. Does not take into account perfusion in blood vessels.
Oxygen electrode measurements	pO_2 electrode is stepped through tissue and electrode signals are converted to pO_2 values.	Provides real-time measure of tissue oxygenation with multiple sampling.	Invasive. Does not differentiate pO_2 values in necrotic versus viable regions or between tumor and normal tissue. pO_2 probe consumes oxygen, preventing measurements over time in same location.
Luminescent probe	Probe is inserted into the tissue and interrogated with light pulses to measure lifetime of luminescence, which is proportional to O_2 concentration.	Precalibrated probe does not consume oxygen. This allows for measurements of pO_2 over time in the same location.	Invasive. Does not differentiate pO_2 values in necrotic versus viable regions or between tumor and normal tissue.
DNA strand-break assays	Comet assay to measure DNA strand breaks in irradiated tumor cells. Hypoxic cells exhibit fewer breaks.	Direct assay to measure DNA damage in cells under hypoxia conditions in situ.	Invasive and indirect. Requires rapid preparation of a cell suspension from a tissue biopsy postirradiation. Subject to sampling errors.
Extrinsic hypoxic cell markers	Preferential binding/uptake by hypoxic cells of radioactive or fluorescent compounds (eg, nitroimidazoles). Imaged by MRS, PET, SPECT, or fluorescence microscopy.	Detection of the hypoxic cells is noninvasive with external scanning procedures. Microscopy can visualize the hypoxic cells at the cellular level.	Requires the injection or ingestion of the marker drug. Binding can be affected by metabolic factors and diffusion limitations. Microscopic analysis subject to sampling error.
Intrinsic hypoxic cell markers	Antibody staining of proteins upregulated in cells by hypoxic exposure (eg, HIF-1α, CA-9, GLUT-1, VEGF)	Markers can be assessed in archived tissue.	Markers may be upregulated by factors other than hypoxia. Uniform fixation of tissue important for reliable quantitation.
Imaging of blood oxygenation and flow	MRI-BOLD (blood oxygen level dependent) imaging or functional MRI or CT using contrast agents introduced into the blood. Near-infrared light spectroscopy. Measures HbO_2 saturation by absorption at different wavelengths.	Noninvasive.	Does not measure tumor oxygenation directly. Relatively poor spatial resolution.

Abbreviations: CA-9, Carbonic anhydrase 9; GLUT-1, glucose transporter 1; HIF-1α, hypoxia-inducible factor 1α; HbO₂, oxyhemoglobin; MRS, magnetic resonance spectroscopy; PET, positron emission tomography; SPECT, single-photon emission computed tomography; VEGF, vascular endothelial growth factor.

HPV-negative head and neck cancer (Toustrup et al, 2011; see Fig. 16–12D) and other cancers (Buffa et al, 2010).

16.4.4 Targeting Hypoxic Cells in Tumors

Because hypoxic cells represent a radiation-resistant subpopulation in tumors that is not present in most normal tissues, the therapeutic ratio might be improved by techniques to reduce the influence of hypoxic cells on tumor response. Various approaches have been investigated over the last 50 years, including (a) attempts to increase oxygen delivery to tumors; (b) use of drugs to modify oxygen consumption of the tumor cells to increase oxygen diffusion distances in the tumor; (c) use of drugs that mimic the radiosensitizing properties of oxygen; (d) use of drugs that are specifically toxic to hypoxic cells; (e) use of high-LET radiations that have a reduced OER (see Sec. 16.4.1 and Fig. 16–9D); and (f) use of drugs that exploit the reduced DNA repair capacity of chronically hypoxic cells. Some of these approaches are discussed in this section.

16.4.4.1 Increasing Oxygen Delivery Clinical studies demonstrate the negative effect of anemia on prognosis (Fyles et al, 2000; Hoff et al, 2011), and blood transfusions are often used to maintain patients at normal hemoglobin levels during

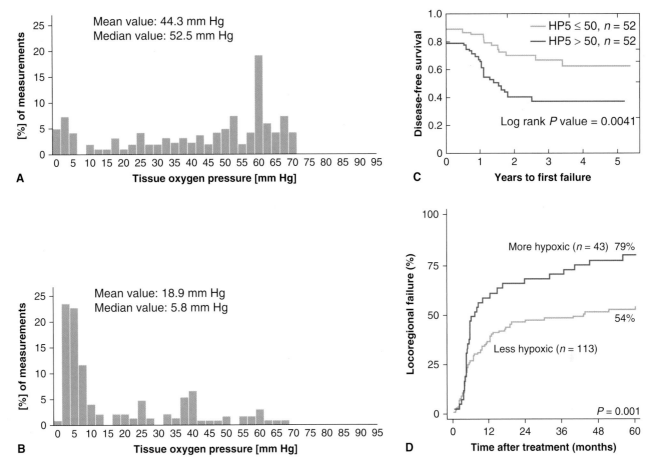

FIGURE 16–12 Distribution of tumor pO_2 in 2 human cervix carcinomas as measured by the Eppendorf oxygen electrode and treatment outcome for patients with high/low levels of hypoxia in their tumors. **(A, B)** Each distribution represents 160 individual measurement points in the tumor. Tumor in **(A)** is less hypoxic and shows fewer regions with low pO_2 measurements than tumor in **(B)** (courtesy of Fyles, unpublished). Panel **(C)** shows results for cancer of the cervix treated with radiotherapy and demonstrates that patients with tumors with a higher degree of hypoxia (HP5 > 50%) have poorer disease-free survival. HP5 is the percentage of pO_2 measurements in the tumor that were below 5 mm Hg. (Redrawn from Fyles, Milosevic, Hedley et al, 2002.) Panel **(D)** shows the cumulative incidence of locoregional tumor failure in head and neck cancer patients treated with conventional radiotherapy alone and separated into "more" and "less" hypoxic tumors by a 15-gene hypoxia signature. (Reprinted by permission from the American Association for Cancer Research: Toustrup et al, 2011.)

radiotherapy. A small randomized study in patients with carcinoma of the cervix showed improvement of local control with blood transfusions (Bush, 1986) but this was not observed in head and neck cancers (Hoff et al, 2011). The administration of erythropoietin has also been used to correct anemia (Seidenfeld et al, 2001), but there is little evidence that it can improve local control or disease-free survival following radiotherapy (Henke et al, 2003). Experimental studies suggest that carbon monoxide in cigarette smoke, which can reduce the oxygen-carrying and -unloading capacity of the blood, may result in reduced tumor oxygenation. Patients with head and neck cancer who continue to smoke during radiotherapy have decreased local control and survival after radiation treatment (Hoff et al, 2012), although results in cervix cancer were not significant (Fyles, Voduc et al, 2002).

Oxygen delivery to tumor cells may be increased by giving animals or patients oxygen under hyperbaric conditions (200 to 300 kPa) during radiation treatment and early clinical studies with high-pressure oxygen (HPO) as an adjuvant to

radiation therapy did demonstrate significant improvement in local tumor control and survival for patients with cancers of the head and neck and cervix (Table 16–4), but this has not been observed in the limited studies of tumors at other sites (Overgaard and Horsman, 1996). The technical difficulties of giving modern radiation treatments with the patient in an HPO chamber have led to this technique being abandoned in favor of other strategies. One such strategy is the use of a combination of nicotinamide, which has been shown to increase tumor perfusion, and carbogen (95% O_2 and 5% CO_2) breathing. This combination has been reported recently to improve local outcome in laryngeal and bladder cancers treated with radiation therapy (Hoskin et al, 2010; Janssens et al, 2012).

Paradoxically, there is evidence in animal tumor models that treatment with antiangiogenic agents (see Chap. 11, Sec. 11.7.1) can improve oxygenation in some tumors, possibly as a result of regularization of the vasculature. Studies combining such agents with radiation treatment of experimental tumors have indicated improved treatment response

TABLE 16–4 **Summary of clinical trials testing sensitization of hypoxic cells.**

Sensitizing Agent	Number of Trials	Significant Benefit	Nonsignificant Trend for Benefit	No Benefit
Hyperbaric oxygen	15	3	6	6
Misonidazole	39	4	4	31

Source: From Dische and Saunders, 1989.

Head and Neck Cancer Metaanalysis: Hypoxic Modification of Radiotherapy

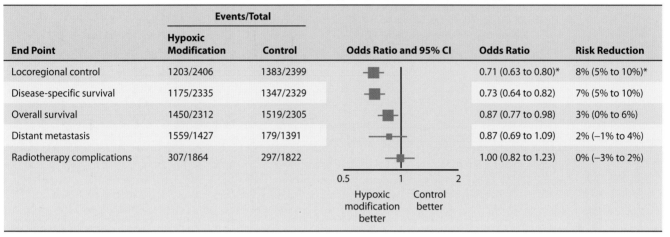

End Point	Events/Total		Odds Ratio and 95% CI	Odds Ratio	Risk Reduction
	Hypoxic Modification	Control			
Locoregional control	1203/2406	1383/2399		0.71 (0.63 to 0.80)*	8% (5% to 10%)*
Disease-specific survival	1175/2335	1347/2329		0.73 (0.64 to 0.82)	7% (5% to 10%)
Overall survival	1450/2312	1519/2305		0.87 (0.77 to 0.98)	3% (0% to 6%)
Distant metastasis	1559/1427	179/1391		0.87 (0.69 to 1.09)	2% (−1% to 4%)
Radiotherapy complications	307/1864	297/1822		1.00 (0.82 to 1.23)	0% (−3% to 2%)

*95% CI.

Source: From Overgaard, 2011.

(Goel et al, 2011). It remains uncertain whether these improved responses are a result of improved oxygenation or of factors such as direct tumor cell kill induced by the antiangiogenic treatment. Reducing oxygen consumption in cells by modifying mitochondrial respiration has been demonstrated to increase oxygenation of tumors in experimental models, and this might be an effective way to decrease hypoxia in tumors (Secomb et al, 2004; Diepart et al, 2011).

16.4.4.2 Hypoxic Cell Sensitizers and Cytotoxins The development of drugs that mimic the radiosensitizing properties of oxygen, known as *hypoxic cell radiosensitizers*, was based on the idea that the radiosensitizing properties of oxygen are a consequence of its electron affinity and that other electron-affinic compounds might act as sensitizers. Certain nitromidazoles, such as misonidazole, were able to sensitize hypoxic cells both in vitro and in animal tumors. The extent of the sensitization can be assessed in terms of a sensitizer enhancement ratio (SER) that is analogous to the OER discussed in Section 16.4.1. SERs depend on the drug concentration in the tumor at the time of radiation. There is a good correspondence between the values obtained for tumors and the results from in vitro studies. If misonidazole is combined with fractionated radiation doses, the SER is reduced both because of reoxygenation occurring between the fractions (see Sec. 16.6.4) and because lower individual doses of the drug are tolerated when it is given as multiple doses during fractionated treatment.

The results from the clinical trials using misonidazole were disappointing (see Table 16–4), possibly because the dose of

misonidazole was limited by dose-dependent peripheral neuropathy, although many of the individual trials had small numbers of patients included, and therefore low statistical power to detect differences in outcome (see Chap. 22, Sec. 22.2.6). Studies using the less-toxic drug, nimorazole, have been associated with improved tumor control in head and neck cancer in the Danish Head and Neck Cancer Study (DAHANCA) trial (Overgaard et al, 1998). Furthermore, a recent metaanalysis of results for patients with head and neck cancer treated in randomized trials, using radiotherapy with HPO or hypoxic cell sensitizers (see Table 16–4) has indicated a small but significant improvement in local control and survival (Overgaard, 2011). Greater benefits might have been observed if there had been selection of patients with high levels of hypoxia in their tumors; reanalysis of a trial using plasma osteopontin levels as an intrinsic marker for hypoxia suggested that only the one-third of patients with the most hypoxic tumors benefitted from treatment with nimorazole (Overgaard et al, 2005).

Another approach to reducing the influence of hypoxia on the radiation response of tumors has been to use (bioreductive) drugs that are toxic under hypoxic conditions (see Chap. 19; Sec. 19.3.2). The most extensively studied of these drugs is tirapazamine, which is cytotoxic to hypoxic cells at oxygen concentrations up to approximately 10 µmoles/L (equivalent partial pressure of approximately 7 mm Hg) (Brown, 1999). Under hypoxia, tirapazamine is metabolized to an agent that produces DNA damage, including double-strand breaks, probably by interacting with topoisomerases. In the presence of oxygen, the active form is converted (by oxidation) back to the parent compound. The drug also interacts with the chemotherapeutic agent cisplatin to increase its toxicity. Tirapazamine has shown efficacy in some clinical trials when used with cisplatin, but a large randomized Phase III trial of tirapazamine with chemoradiotherapy for head and neck cancers failed to show significant benefit, although this may have been related to the quality of the radiotherapy delivered (Peters et al, 2010; Rischin et al, 2010). This trial did not select for patients with more hypoxic tumors and analysis of a small subset in whom hypoxia imaging was performed suggested benefit only for those with the most hypoxic tumors (Rischin et al, 2006), similar to the retrospective analysis for nimorazole described above. This has important implications for clinical studies of other hypoxic cytotoxins currently under development (Wilson and Hay, 2010). One such drug is TH-302, a 2-nitroimidazole with a bromoisophosphoramide mustard side chain that is released following reduction under hypoxic conditions to give a diffusible toxic product that can diffuse to kill less hypoxic (bystander) cells as well as the producing cell. Studies in animal tumor models with this agent in combination with conventional chemotherapy have shown promising results and clinical studies are in progress (Liu et al, 2012).

16.5 NORMAL TISSUE RESPONSE TO RADIOTHERAPY

16.5.1 Cellular and Tissue Responses

Radiation treatment can cause loss of function in normal tissues. In renewal tissues, such as skin, bone marrow, and the gastrointestinal mucosa, loss of function may be correlated with loss of proliferative activity of stem cells. In these and other tissues, loss of function may also occur through damage to more mature cells and/or through damage to supporting stroma and vasculature, the influx of immune cells, and the induction of inflammatory responses (Stewart and Dorr, 2009). Traditionally, the effects of radiation treatment on normal tissues has been divided, based largely on directly observable functional and histopathological end points, into early (or acute) responses, which occur within 3 months of radiation treatment, and late responses that may take many months or years to develop. It should be noted that such end-points do not assess early changes in gene expression associated with irradiation that occur in all tissues (see below). Acute responses occur primarily in tissues where rapid cell renewal is required to maintain the function of the organ. Because many cells express radiation damage during mitosis, there is early death and loss of cells killed by the radiation treatment. Late responses tend to occur in organs whose parenchymal cells divide infrequently (eg, liver or kidney) or rarely (eg, central nervous system or muscle) under normal conditions. Depletion of the parenchymal cell population as a result of entry of cells into mitosis, with the resulting expression of radiation damage and cell death, will thus be slow. Damage to the connective tissue and vasculature of the organ (which also proliferates slowly under normal conditions) may

lead to progressive impairment of its circulation and secondary parenchymal cell death may occur as a consequence of nutrient deprivation. The loss of functional cells may induce other parenchymal cells to divide, causing further cell death as they express their radiation damage, leading eventually to functional failure of the organ. Consequential late effects may also occur where severe early reactions have led to impaired tissue recovery and/or development of infection. Several systems for documenting normal tissue responses (side effects) to irradiation in patients have been developed to facilitate cross-comparisons between investigators and institutions. These include the Radiation Therapy Oncology Group (RTOG)/European Organization for Research and Treatment of Cancer (EORTC) classification, the Common Terminology Criteria for Adverse Events (CTCAE v4) scale devised by the National Cancer Institute (NIH/NCI, 2009) and the Late Effects Normal Tissue Task Force Subjective, Objective, Management, and Analytic (LENT/SOMA) system, specifically designed to score late reactions (Hoeller et al, 2003).

The radiosensitivity of the cells of some normal tissues can be determined directly using in situ assays that allow the observation of proliferation from single surviving cells in vivo. One such assay determines the fraction of regenerating crypts in the small intestine following radiation doses sufficient to reduce the number of surviving stem cells per crypt to 1 or less, and analysis of the results allows the generation of a survival curve (Tucker et al, 1991). Survival curves obtained for the cells of different normal tissues in mice and rats are shown in Figure 16–13. Considerable variability in sensitivity is apparent, and as with tumor cells, most of the difference appears to

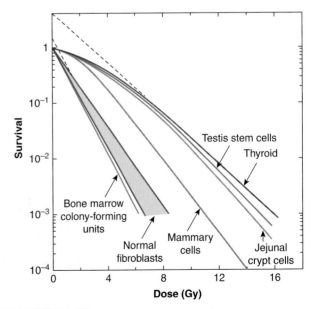

FIGURE 16–13 Survival curves for cells from some normal tissues. Most of the curves are for cells from rodent tissues and the curves were produced using in vivo or in situ clonogenic assays. Survival curves for normal human fibroblasts are for cultured cell strains. (Data compiled by Dr. J.D. Chapman, Fox Chase Cancer Center, Philadelphia.)

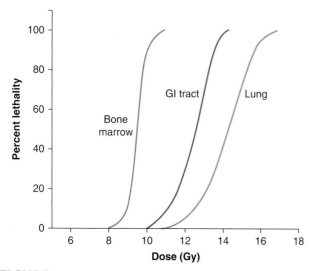

FIGURE 16–14 **Three different curves indicating percentage lethality plotted as a function of radiation dose for the same strain of mouse.** The "bone marrow" (blue) and "GI tract" (red) curves were obtained using whole-body irradiation and assessing lethality prior to day 30 or prior to day 7, respectively, because death as a result of damage to the gastrointestinal tract occurs earlier than that as a result of bone marrow failure. The green curve labeled "lung" was obtained by assessing lethality 180 days after local irradiation to the thorax.

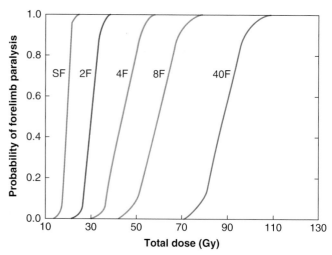

FIGURE 16–15 **Dose-response curves for forelimb paralysis following fractionated radiation treatments to the rat spinal cord.** The fractions (F) were given once daily to allow for repair of radiation damage between fractions. *SF*, Single fraction. (Redrawn from Wong et al, 1992.)

be in the shoulder region of the survival curve, suggesting differences in repair capacity.

Alternative experimental analyses of normal tissue radiation damage most often use functional assays. The crudest functional assay is the determination of the dose of radiation given either to the whole body or to a specific organ that will cause lethality in 50% of the treated animals within a specified time (LD_{50}). The relationship between lethality and single radiation dose is usually sigmoidal in shape, and some experimentally derived relationships for different normal tissues in mice are shown in Figure 16–14.

For individual organs, a level of functional deficit is defined and the percentage of irradiated subjects that express at least this level of damage following different radiation doses is plotted as a function of dose. A tolerance dose for a specific organ can be defined as the dose above which more than 5% of patients express that level of functional deficit (TD5). In animal models, complete dose-response curves have usually been obtained and an example for the rat spinal cord using forelimb paralysis as the end point is shown in Figure 16–15. These curves are sigmoidal in shape and generally quite steep. Similar results have been reported for specific functional deficits in many other tissues (eg, increased breathing rate in lung, reduced flexibility as a result of increased fibrosis in subcutaneous tissue, elevated clearance rates in kidney).

An influx of immune cells (macrophages, lymphocytes, and neutrophils) into irradiated tissue and increased cytokine and chemokine expression have been observed within hours after irradiation when there are no apparent functional changes, and aspects of this inflammatory response may persist over months as the irradiated tissue transits to regeneration and

repair (Schaue and McBride, 2010). Early increases in cytokine expression can occur after low doses of radiation (~1 Gy), but longer-term changes have been observed after larger doses (5 to 25 Gy). A wide range of cytokines is involved including pro- and anti-inflammatory factors, such as tumor necrosis factor alpha (TNF-α), interleukin 1 (IL-1α and IL-1β), and TGF-β. In specific tissues, the response to radiation may include other growth factors that are associated with collagen deposition, fibrosis, inflammation, and aberrant vascular growth. These inflammatory factors may induce production of damaging radicals, such as reactive oxygen species, independently of those caused directly by the radiation treatment. The interplay between cell killing, cell repopulation, cytokine production, vascular damage, and immune cells infiltrates in producing the overall tissue damage remains poorly understood and is likely to vary from one organ to another (Stewart and Dorr, 2009).

16.5.2 Acute Tissue Responses

Acute radiation responses occur mainly in renewal tissues and have been related to death of critical cell populations such as the stem cells in the crypts of the small intestine, in the bone marrow, or in the basal layer of the skin. These responses occur within 3 months of the start of radiotherapy (in humans) but are not usually limiting for fractionated radiotherapy because of the ability of the stem cells in the tissue to undergo rapid repopulation to regenerate the transit and end cell populations. Radiation-induced cell death in normal tissues generally occurs when the cells attempt mitosis, thus the tissue tends to respond on a time scale similar to the normal rate of loss of functional cells in that tissue and the demand for proliferation of the supporting stem cells. Radiation-induced apoptosis can also be detected in many tissues, but is usually a minor factor in overall radiation-induced cell death, except in lymphoid and myeloid tissue.

Endothelial cells in the vasculature supporting the crypts and villi of the small intestine of mice have been reported to be prone to radiation-induced apoptosis, and prevention of this effect by treatment with basic fibroblast growth factor can protect the animals against radiation-induced gastrointestinal injury, suggesting that dysfunction of the vasculature can reduce the ability of the crypts to regenerate (Paris et al, 2001). Contrary to most cell killing, which involves DNA damage, radiation-induced apoptosis of endothelial cells can occur via a cell membrane effect leading to activation of the ceramide pathway (see Chap. 15, Sec. 15.3.2) (Kolesnick and Fuks, 2003), and blocking this effect can protect the intestine from radiation damage (Rotolo et al, 2012). These effects appear to be more prominent following larger radiation doses (>10 Gy) such as those used in stereotactic body radiotherapy (SBRT) than at the doses used commonly for fractionated radiation therapy (~2 Gy).

Following irradiation of mucosa (and skin), there is early erythema within a few days of irradiation as a result of increased vascular permeability related to the release of 5-hydroxytryptamine by mast cells. Similar mechanisms may lead to early nausea and vomiting observed following irradiation of the intestine. Expression of further acute mucositis (or moist desquamation in skin) and ulceration depends on the relative rates of cell loss and cell proliferation of the transit cells and the (basal) stem cells in the tissue. The time of expression for this damage depends on the time over which (intensity of) the dose is received (Fig. 16–16), and the extent of these reactions and the length of time for recovery is dependent on the total dose received and the volume (area) of mucosa (or skin) irradiated. Early recovery depends on the number of surviving basal stem cells that are needed to repopulate the tissue and these cells can migrate from undamaged areas into the irradiated area. Erythema occurs in humans at single doses greater than 24 Gy in 2 Gy fractions, whereas mucositis occurs after fractionated doses above approximately 50 Gy in 2 Gy fractions. Severe skin reactions in patients are relatively uncommon as high-energy radiation beams have a build-up region that results in a reduced dose at the skin surface (see Sec. 16.2.4 and Fig. 16–3A), but oral mucositis is prevalent during radiation treatment of head and neck cancers.

16.5.3 Late Tissue Responses

Late tissue responses occur in organs whose parenchymal cells normally divide infrequently and hence do not express mitosis-linked death until later times when called upon to divide. They also occur in tissues that manifest early reactions, such as skin/subcutaneous tissue and intestine, but these reactions (subcutaneous fibrosis, intestinal stenosis) are quite different from early reactions in these tissues. Late responses (usually regarded as those which occur more than 3 months after treatment) usually limit the dose of radiation that can be delivered to a patient during radiotherapy. Damage can be expressed as diminished organ function, such as radiation-induced nephropathy (symptoms of hypertension or increased serum creatinine) or myelopathy following spinal cord damage, as illustrated in Figure 16–15, and is usually progressive over time. The nature and timing of late reactions depends on

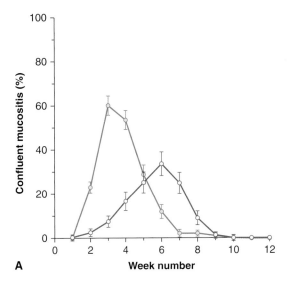

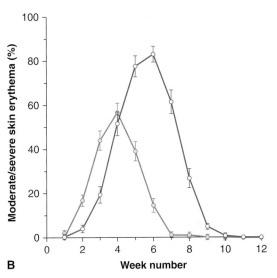

FIGURE 16–16 Estimated prevalence of confluent mucositis (**A**) or moderate to severe skin reactions (**B**) in patients following conventional radiotherapy over 5 to 6 weeks (red lines) or accelerated radiotherapy in less than 2 weeks (blue lines) in the CHART (Continuous Hyperfractionated Accelerated Radiotherapy) study. (Modified from Bentzen et al, 2001.)

the tissue involved. Damage to stromal and vascular elements of the tissue and the influx of inflammatory cells may cause secondary parenchymal cell death, resulting in increased cell proliferation and further death of parenchymal cells as they attempt mitosis. The latent period to manifestation of organ dysfunction depends on the dose received, because the higher the initial dose the smaller the fraction of surviving parenchymal cells that can repopulate the tissue.

One common late reaction is the slow development of tissue fibrosis that occurs in many tissues (eg, subcutaneous tissue, muscle, lung, gastrointestinal tract), often several years after radiation treatment. Radiation-induced fibrosis is associated with a chronic inflammatory response following irradiation, the aberrant and prolonged expression of the growth factor TGF-β and radiation-induced differentiation of fibroblasts

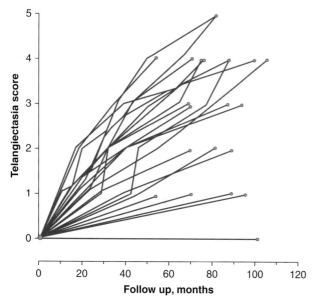

FIGURE 16–17 **Clinical manifestations of skin telangiectasis.** Progression of telangiectasia in individual patients treated with 5 fractions of 1.8 Gy/wk to a total of 35 fractions. (Redrawn from Turesson, 1990.)

of microvasculature leading to atrophy (and fibrosis) that is manifest in skin and other tissues. Figure 16–17 shows the development of telangiectasia in patients following fraction-ated treatment and illustrates that heterogeneity in response between different patients is not limited to tumors but can also occur with normal tissue effects (Turesson et al, 1990).

The lung is an important site of late radiation damage. There are 2 types of reactions: pneumonitis that occurs 2 to 6 months after irradiation, and fibrosis that usually occurs more than 1 year after irradiation. These reactions can cause increases in tissue density on CT scans (see Chap. 14, Sec. 14.3.1) and increases in breathing rate if severe. Measuring changes in breathing rate has been used extensively to assay the dose–response relationship for radiation-induced lung damage in rats and mice, particularly the development of pneumonitis. Studies in rodents have documented that inflammatory cells and inflammatory cytokines play a major role in lung response to irradiation injury (Fig. 16–18), but the relationship between this inflammatory response and the later development of func-tional symptoms is unclear. Studies in lung cancer patients suggest that increases in TGF-β levels in plasma following radiotherapy can contribute to the likelihood of developing lung complications (Anscher et al, 1998; Evans et al, 2006).

The dose required to cause functional impairment in lung depends on the volume irradiated, with small volumes being able to tolerate quite large doses (Marks, Bentzen et al, 2010); this is a result of the functional reserve of the remaining lung because the irradiated region will develop fibrosis. Studies in rodents, using the dose required to cause an increased breathing frequency in 50% of animals (ED_{50}) as an end point, have defined a relationship between ED_{50} and lung volume

into fibrocytes that produce collagen (Hakenjos et al, 2000; Martin et al, 2000). Transforming growth factor-β also plays a major role in wound healing and the development of radia-tion fibrosis has similarities to the healing of chronic wounds (Denham and Hauer-Jensen, 2002). Another common late reaction is progressive vascular damage, including telan-giectasia that can be observed in skin and mucosa, and loss

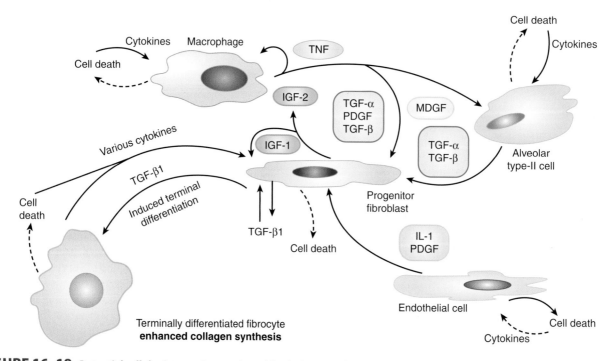

FIGURE 16–18 **Potential cellular interactions and cytokine induction after irradiation of lung tissue.** The various cell populations and some of the cytokines induced potentially leading to fibrosis (increased collagen levels) are illustrated. (Modified from Rodemann and Bamberg, 1995.)

irradiated, which indicates that the base of the lung is more sensitive than the apex (Travis et al, 1997). The underlying mechanisms may relate to the functional reserve in different regions of the lung and/or to the extent of cytokine production following irradiation of different regions of the lung. There is also evidence for regional effects following irradiation of human lung (Marks, Bentzen et al, 2010).

A theoretical framework introduced by Withers et al (1988b) suggests that late responding tissues can be considered as arrays of functional subunits (FSU) containing groups of cells that are critical for function (eg, bronchioli in lung, nephrons in the kidney). These FSU were postulated to be able to be regenerated from a single surviving tissue stem cell. Furthermore, tissues were considered to have these FSU operating in parallel to achieve overall tissue function (such as occurs in lung, kidney, liver) or in series (such as in spinal cord or intestine) in analogy with electrical circuits. Tissues with a parallel structure of FSU have substantial reserve capacity and, although damage to a small volume may completely inactivate this volume, the remaining regions can maintain function and/or may undergo hypertrophy to replace any loss of function (eg, kidney and liver). Tissues with a series structure of FSU may cease to function if even a small region of the tissue is irreparably damaged, such as may occur in the spinal cord where localized injury can cause complete tissue dysfunction and myelopathy, or in the intestine if severe stenosis causes obstruction. In practice, tissues do not fall neatly into these 2 categories for various reasons, including the common role of the vasculature, the development of inflammatory responses that may extend beyond the treatment field, because FSU may require more than one type of undamaged stem cells for repair and these stem cells may migrate into areas of damage either locally or via the circulation. However, the concept that the volume irradiated to high dose is critical to tissue response and that this varies for different organs is well established and used in mathematical models designed to predict normal tissue complication probabilities (NTCP) (Bentzen et al, 2010; Marks, Yorke et al, 2010).

16.5.4 Whole-Body Irradiation

The response of animals to single-dose whole-body irradiation can be divided into 3 separate syndromes (hematological, gastrointestinal, and neurovascular) that manifest following different doses and at different times after irradiation (Mettler and Voelz, 2002; Dainiak et al, 2003). The neurovascular syndrome occurs following large doses of radiation (>20 Gy) and usually results in rapid death (hours to days) as a consequence of cardiovascular and neurological dysfunction. The gastrointestinal syndrome occurs after doses greater than approximately 5 to 15 Gy and, in rodents, doses at the upper end of this range usually result in death at about 1 week after irradiation as a consequence of severe damage to the mucosal lining of the gastrointestinal tract; this causes a loss of the protective barrier with consequent infection, loss of electrolytes, and fluid imbalance. Intensive nursing with antibiotics, fluid, and electrolyte

replacement can prevent early death from this syndrome in human victims of radiation accidents, but these patients may die later as a result of damage to other organs, particularly skin, if large areas are exposed. The hematopoietic syndrome occurs at doses in the range of 2 to 8 Gy in humans (3 to 10 Gy in rodents) and is caused by severe depletion of blood elements as a result of killing of precursor cells in the bone marrow. This syndrome causes death in rodents (at the higher dose levels) between approximately 12 to 30 days after irradiation, and somewhat later in larger animals, including humans. Death can sometimes be prevented by bone marrow transplantation (BMT) and cytokine therapy (eg, GM-CSF [granulocyte-macrophage colony-stimulating factor], G-CSF [granulocyte colony-stimulating factor], stem cell factor) provided that the radiation exposure is not too high when damage to other organs may become lethal. Following the Chernobyl accident, 28 of the emergency workers (of 104 identified as showing symptoms of acute radiation syndrome) died within 4 months. Most of these workers received bone marrow doses greater than 4 Gy and much higher doses to the skin (10 to 30 times). Bone marrow failure was the primary cause of death, particularly for those dying within the first 2 months. Although 13 of these patients had BMT, most died, probably because of serious radiation damage to the skin (UNSCEAR, 2008). There are substantial differences in the doses required to induce death from the hematopoietic syndrome (ie, LD_{50} value) between different species of animals and even between different strains of the same species. The LD_{50} value for humans has been estimated at 4 to 7 Gy, depending on the available level of supportive care (excluding BMT). Following doses greater than approximately 2 Gy, humans will develop early nausea and vomiting within hours of irradiation (prodromal syndrome), which may be controlled with 5-hydroxytryptamine antagonists.

16.5.5 Retreatment Tolerance

Although tissues may repair damage and regenerate after irradiation, previously irradiated tissues may have a reduced tolerance for subsequent radiation treatments, indicating the presence of residual injury. For tissues that undergo only an early response to radiation, there is almost complete recovery in a few months, so that a second high dose of radiation can be tolerated. For late-responding tissue damage, the extent of the residual injury depends on the level of the initial damage and is tissue dependent. There is substantial recovery in skin, mucosa, spinal cord, and lung over a period of 3 to 6 months, but kidney and bladder show little evidence of recovery (Stewart and Dorr, 2009). Clinical studies have demonstrated that retreatment to high doses with curative intent is possible depending on the tissues involved but usually entails increased risk of normal tissue damage.

16.5.6 Predicting Normal Tissue Response

Patients receiving identical radiation treatments may experience differing levels of normal tissue injury (see, eg, Fig. 16–17).

Thus predictive assays might be useful in identifying those patients who are at greater risk of experiencing the side effects of radiotherapy. The enhanced radiosensitivity of patients with ataxia telangiectasia (AT) and other DNA repair-deficiency syndromes (see Chap. 5, Sec. 5.5) supports a genetic contribution to individual variability in radiosensitivity, although other factors, such as diet or environment, could also play a role. Studies of women with breast cancer show individual correlation of acute and late skin reactions in one treatment field with those in a different treatment field (Bentzen et al, 1993). Several studies have quantified the in vitro radiosensitivity of fibroblasts and peripheral lymphocytes as a potential predictive assay for normal tissue damage. These studies show variations in the radiosensitivity of fibroblasts from individual patients, but are inconsistent in predicting late radiation fibrosis (Russell and Begg, 2002). Fibroblasts from people who are heterozygous for mutations in the *ATM* gene are reported to have increased radiosensitivity, but it has not been possible to directly link severity of normal tissue reactions to heterozygosity in this gene. Thus, although cellular sensitivity is an important contributor to normal tissue damage, other factors, such as cytokine induction and the response of the tissue stroma and vasculature, likely also play an important role in normal tissue injury. In rodents, genetic differences associated with different strains have been reported to influence the development of normal tissue damage, for example, pneumonitis and fibrosis following lung irradiation, although these factors do not affect the radiosensitivity of lung fibroblasts directly (Haston et al, 2002). Extensive genetic screening of large populations is underway to identify genetic alterations or gene signatures that may predict patients predisposed to differential responses to irradiation (West et al, 2010).

16.5.7 Radioprotection

Many agents can protect against radiation damage to cells in culture (Weiss and Landauer, 2009). These include agents that can scavenge radiation-produced radicals, such as dimethyl sulfoxide (DMSO), or the superoxide dismutase enzymes (SODs), or sulfhydryl-containing compounds, such as glutathione, and cysteine. These latter compounds can also donate a hydrogen atom back to a radical site created on a macromolecule such as DNA by hydroxyl radicals produced by water radiolysis. Because of the short lifetimes of radiation-induced radicals, exogenously added agents have to be present in the cell at the time of the irradiation. They are equally effective for tumor and normal cells in vitro; thus specificity for therapeutic application in vivo depends largely on preferential uptake of such agents into the normal tissue. One agent that appears to fulfill this criterion is amifostine, a prodrug that is converted into a sulfhydryl-containing compound in vivo by the action of alkaline phosphatases. The selective activity of this compound in normal tissue is believed to be a result of poor penetration from tumor blood vessels and reduced levels of alkaline phosphatase in tumors. Amifostine was shown to protect a variety of normal tissues with variable, mostly small, protection of tumors in animal models (for review, see

Lindegaard and Grau, 2000). Studies in patients with head and neck and lung cancers show substantial protection of normal tissue, including salivary gland, lung, and mucosa, without detectable change in tumor response (Brizel et al, 2000; Antonadou et al, 2003), although the compound is not widely used clinically because of unrelated toxicities.

Another strategy for protection of normal tissue is to block the development of late radiation effects with treatment given after the end of the radiation. The use of steroids after irradiation to prevent lung injury is an example, although this treatment appears to delay the development of symptoms rather than prevent them. Agents that block angiotensin-converting enzyme (ACE) activity (eg, captopril, enalapril) or that block directly the action of angiotensin II mitigate the development of radiation-induced pulmonary fibrosis and nephropathy, respectively (Cohen et al, 2011). Various strategies, including antiinflammatory agents and antioxidants, are being studied in patients to determine whether they can reverse the progressive nature of radiation-induced fibrosis and necrosis (Delanian and Lefaix, 2007; Delanian et al, 2011). Extensive efforts are underway to develop agents to mitigate multiple organ damage in cases of accidental radiation exposure (Williams and McBride, 2011).

16.5.8 Therapeutic Ratio

The concept of therapeutic ratio is illustrated in Figure 16–19, which shows theoretical dose–response curves for tumor control and normal tissue complications as described in Sections 16.3.1 and 16.5.1 (see also similar curves for systemic therapy in Chap. 17, Fig. 17–9). Tumor-control curves (red lines) tend to be shallower than those for normal tissue response (blue lines) because of the large heterogeneity among tumors as discussed in Section 16.3.1. The therapeutic ratio is often defined as the percentage of tumor cures that are obtained at a given level of normal tissue complications (ie, by taking a vertical cut through the 2 curves at a tolerance dose, eg, at 5% complications after 5 years). In experimental studies, an alternative approach is to define the therapeutic ratio as the ratio of radiation doses D_n/D_t required to produce a given percentage of complications and tumor control (usually 50%). It is then a measure of the horizontal displacement between the 2 curves. It remains imprecise, however, because it depends on the shape of the dose–response curves for tumor control and normal tissue complications. The curves shown in Figure 16–19A depict a situation in which the therapeutic ratio is favorable because the tumor-control curve is displaced to the left of that for normal tissue damage. The greater this displacement, the more radiocurable the tumor. Because the tumor-control curve is shallower than that for normal tissue damage, the therapeutic ratio tends to be favorable only for low and intermediate tumor-control levels. If the 2 curves are close together or the curve for tumor control is displaced to the right of that for complications (Fig. 16–19B), the therapeutic ratio is unfavorable because a high level of complications must be accepted to achieve even a minimal level of tumor control.

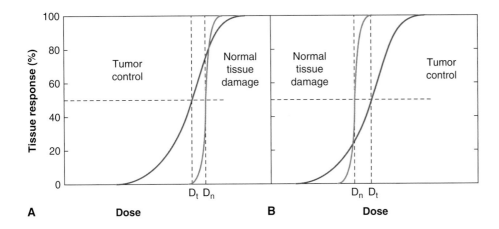

FIGURE 16–19 **Illustration of the concept of a therapeutic ratio in terms of dose–response relationships for tumor control and normal tissue damage.** The red curves represent dose response for tumor control, and the blue curves represent dose response for critical normal tissue damage. See the text for specific discussion of the 2 parts of the figure.

16.6 RADIOTHERAPY FRACTIONATION

It is generally accepted that the therapeutic ratio is improved by fractionating radiation treatments. Many of the underlying biological effects occurring during fractionated radiation treatment have been identified, and improvement of the therapeutic ratio may be explained in terms of the biological response of tissue. The most important biological factors influencing the responses of tumors and normal tissues to fractionated treatment are often called the "five Rs": radiosensitivity, repair, repopulation, redistribution, and reoxygenation. These biological factors were introduced in Chapter 15, and radiosensitivity of tumors and normal tissues is discussed in Sections 16.3 and 16.5 above. Here these concepts are discussed further in the context of fractionated irradiation.

16.6.1 Repair

The shoulder on a survival curve after single radiation doses is usually indicative of the capacity of the cells to accumulate and repair radiation damage. If multiple doses are given with sufficient time between the fractions for repair to occur (4 to 24 hours, depending on the cells or tissue involved) survival curves for cells treated with fractionated irradiation will be similar to those illustrated in Figure 16–20. The dashed lines in this figure represent the effective survival curves for different fractionated treatments. The effective slope depends on the size of the individual dose fractions, becoming shallower as the fraction size is reduced (eg, blue curve vs green curve). This effect is also illustrated by the dose–response curves shown in Figure 16–15 for forelimb paralysis of rats following irradiation with different numbers of fractions to the spinal cord, where the curves for higher numbers of (smaller) fractions are displaced to higher total doses.

The single-dose (red) survival curve for most cells has a finite initial slope, apparently as a result of a nonrepairable component of radiation damage (see Chap. 15, Appendix 15.1), so there is a limit below which further reduction of the fraction size will no longer reduce the effective slope of the survival curve (see orange curve in Fig. 16–20); this limit differs among cell populations. When the size of the individual dose fraction

is such that survival is represented by the curvilinear shoulder region of the survival curve, as for most dose fractions used clinically, then repair will be maximal when equal-sized dose fractions are given. Thus, if a certain total dose is given with unequal fraction sizes, it would produce more damage than the same total dose given in equal fraction sizes.

16.6.2 Repopulation

In both tumors and in normal tissues, proliferation of surviving cells may occur during the course of fractionated treatment.

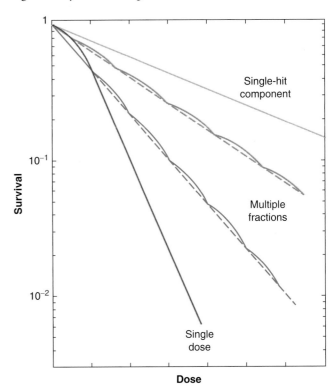

FIGURE 16–20 **The influence of fractionating the radiation treatment on the shape of cell-survival curves.** When repair occurs between the fractions, the shoulder of the survival curve is repeated for every fraction resulting in curves that are shallower for smaller fraction sizes (eg, blue vs green curves). The curve labeled "single-hit component" (orange curve) is discussed in the text.

Furthermore, as cellular damage and cell death occur during the course of the treatment, the tissue may respond with an increased rate of proliferation of the surviving cells. The effect of this cell *repopulation*, will be to increase the number of surviving cells during the course of the treatment and reduce the overall response to irradiation. This effect is most important in early responding normal tissues (eg, skin, gastrointestinal tract) or in tumors whose stem cells are capable of rapid proliferation. In contrast, it will be of little consequence in late-responding, slowly proliferating tissues (eg, kidney, liver, spinal cord), which do not suffer much early cell death and hence do not produce an early proliferative response to the radiation treatment. Figure 16–21 illustrates the effect of repopulation for early skin reactions versus (lack of repopulation) for late kidney response. Regenerative responses are particularly important in reducing acute normal tissue responses during prolonged treatments, such as those involving a period without irradiation (split-course treatment), but this effect can also be important in decreasing tumor response as discussed below.

Repopulation is likely to be more important toward the end of a course of treatment, when sufficient damage has accumulated (and cell death occurred) to induce a robust regenerative response. This is consistent with clinical observations that oral mucosa can start to heal toward the end of a 6- to 7-week course of therapy, despite the continued treatment, because of rapid proliferation of basal (stem) cells in the mucosa. Similar increases in proliferation of surviving (stem) cells can

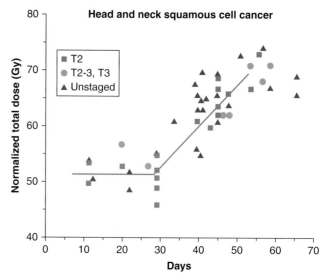

FIGURE 16–22 **Estimated total doses of fractionated irradiation required to achieve 50% probability of tumor control for squamous cell carcinomas of the head and neck (various stages) plotted as a function of the overall treatment time.** Each point is for a different group of patients and is obtained from published results. The actual doses used to treat the different groups of patients were normalized to a standard schedule of 2 Gy per fraction using the technique described in Section 16.7.3. (Modified from Withers et al, 1988a.)

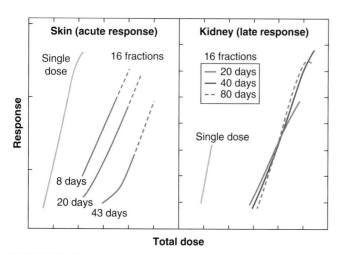

FIGURE 16–21 **Illustration of the effect of repopulation during fractionated treatment of skin or kidney.** Treatment was a single dose or 16 equal fractions given in different overall times as indicated. Acute skin response was assessed using a numerical scoring technique and kidney response was determined by reduction in ethylenediaminetetraacetic acid (EDTA) clearance. For both tissues the fractionated treatment results in the curves moving to the right (higher doses) due to repair. For the acute skin reactions, extending the time over which a course of 16 fractions is given (from 8 days to 43 days) results in a further increase in the total dose required for a given level of response (isoeffective dose). In contrast, for late response of kidney there is no change in the isoeffective dose for 16 fractions regardless of whether the treatment is given over 20 or 80 days. (Modified from Denekamp, 1986.)

also occur in tumors. Evidence that accelerated repopulation can occur in human tumors during a course of fractionated therapy is shown in Figure 16–22. Here the (normalized) total dose required to give 50% control of head and neck cancers is plotted as a function of the overall duration of the fractionated treatment. For overall times less than approximately 3 to 4 weeks, there is little change in the dose required for 50% tumor control; at longer times, however, there is a substantial increase in the total dose required as the duration of treatment increases. This observation suggests that the initial part of the fractionated therapy has resulted in increased proliferation of the surviving tumor stem cells, which for head and neck tumors becomes apparent at 3 to 4 weeks after the start of the treatment. The data are consistent with an (accelerated) doubling time of approximately 4 days for the clonogenic tumor cells, compared to a median volume doubling time of approximately 2 to 3 months for unperturbed tumor growth (see Chap. 12, Sec. 12.1.1). Repopulation of tumor cells during a conventional course of radiotherapy is an important factor influencing local tumor control in patients with rapidly growing tumors and is the reason why it is preferable to avoid treatment delays during therapy. Repopulation provides the biological rationale for accelerated fractionated radiation therapy (see Sec. 16.7.4). Overall treatment time would be expected to be less important for slower-growing tumors such as prostate or breast cancer.

Attempts to predict the effects of accelerated repopulation in tumors have focused on measurements of the potential doubling time (T_{pot}), which assesses the underlying rate at which new tumor cells are added to the tumor cell population, ignoring cell loss. Values of T_{pot} for human tumors can be estimated using methods described in Chapter 12, Section 12.1.2; such values vary widely for different tumors, but the median is in the range of 4 to 5 days (Begg, 1995). The pretreatment T_{pot} might reflect the proliferative rate of the surviving tumor cells following radiotherapy, and a trend for an adverse treatment outcome associated with short T_{pot} values has been reported in patients with head and neck cancer and cervical cancer. However, subsequent studies have not confirmed its utility in predicting the benefit of reducing overall treatment time (Begg et al, 1999; Wilson, 2007), perhaps because the assay measures the proliferation of all the cells (both progenitor and stem cells) and may thus not assess the proliferation of the cell population critical for tumor control. In the context of individualized therapy, new approaches to directly measure tumor stem cell proliferation may help to identify which patients have tumors needing accelerated therapy. An alternative approach may be combination with systemic therapy (see Sec. 16.2.5 and Chap. 17, Sec. 17.6.4) to reduce repopulation during treatment, although this may exacerbate early normal tissue reactions.

16.6.3 Redistribution

Variation in the radiosensitivity of cells in different phases of the cell cycle results in the cells in the more resistant phases being more likely to survive a dose of radiation (see Chap. 15, Sec. 15.4.1). Two effects can make the cell population more sensitive to a subsequent dose of radiation. Some of the cells will be blocked in the later (sensitive) part of G_2 phase and some of the (more resistant) surviving cells will redistribute into other parts of the cell cycle (which by definition are more sensitive). Both effects will tend to make the whole population more sensitive to fractionated treatment as compared with a single dose. Because redistribution inevitably involves cell proliferation, cell survival also will be influenced (in the opposite direction) by repopulation. Both redistribution and repopulation are important primarily in proliferating cell populations. Also, not all cell lines show large differences in radiosensitivity between different cell-cycle phases, and the effect of redistribution will be correspondingly less for these types of cells. In many normal tissues (and probably in some tumors), stem cells can be in a resting phase (G_0) but can be recruited into the cell cycle to repopulate the tissue. There is some evidence that cells in cycle are slightly more sensitive to radiation than G_0 cells, possibly because G_0 cells may repair more potentially lethal damage (see Chap. 15, Sec. 15.4.2). Recruitment of resting cells into the proliferative cycle during the course of fractionated treatment may, therefore, tend to increase the sensitivity of the whole population. Neither recruitment nor redistribution would be expected to have much influence on late responses, as these occur predominantly as a result of injury to tissues in which the proportion of cells in proliferative phases of the cell cycle is low.

16.6.4 Reoxygenation

The response of tumors to large single doses of radiation is dominated by the presence of hypoxic cells within them, even if only a very small fraction of the tumor stem cells are hypoxic (see Sec. 16.4.2). Because hypoxic cells are resistant

to radiotherapy, the proportion of the surviving cells (those retaining long-term proliferative ability; see Chap. 15, Sec. 15.3.1) that is hypoxic will be elevated immediately after a dose of radiation. However, with time, some of the surviving hypoxic cells may gain access to oxygen (*reoxygenate*) and become more sensitive to a subsequent radiation treatment. Reoxygenation can result in a substantial increase in the sensitivity of tumors during fractionated treatment. The survival curve following fractionated irradiation for a tumor containing 10% hypoxic cells that do not reoxygenate would be dominated at higher doses by the radioresistant hypoxic cells (Fig. 16–23, blue (b) and green (a) dashed lines), whereas that for a tumor cell population that has complete reoxygenation between dose fractions (Fig. 16–23, turquoise (d) dashed line) lies close to the curve for a fully oxygenated population. In practice there will also be many cells at intermediate oxygen levels in tumors, and as seen in Fig. 16–23 (orange (c) dashed line) these cells will dominate the survival curve when

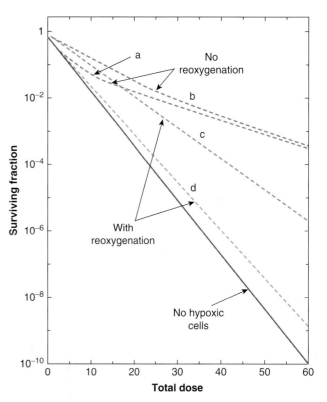

FIGURE 16–23 Theoretical survival curves calculated to illustrate the influence of reoxygenation on the level of cell killing in a tumor following treatment with 2-Gy fractions. The solid red line illustrates the expected survival curve for a tumor with no hypoxic cells. For a tumor with hypoxic cells, it was assumed that the tumor initially had 10% hypoxic cells and either 90% well-oxygenated cells (green (a) and turquoise (d) dashed lines representing survival without and with reoxygenation respectively) or a proportion of well-oxygenated cells and cells at intermediate oxygen concentrations calculated using a radial diffusion model (blue (b) and orange (c) dashed lines representing survival without and with reoxygenation respectively). It was assumed that reoxygenation was sufficient to maintain the same proportions of hypoxic cells among the surviving cells during the fractionated treatment. (Redrawn from Wouters and Brown, 1997.)

reoxygenation occurs during fractionated treatment (Wouters and Brown, 1997). Reoxygenation has been shown to occur in almost all rodent tumors that have been studied, but the extent and timing of reoxygenation are variable. One mechanism for this effect is the fluctuations of blood flow and the resulting short-term (acute) hypoxia that is caused (see Sec. 16.4.2). Cells that were (acutely) hypoxic at the time of the radiation will be reoxygenated by this process, probably within a few hours. Other potential mechanisms include reduced oxygen utilization by radiation-damaged cells, or rapid death and removal of radiation-damaged cells so that the hypoxic cells become closer to functional blood vessels.

It is probable that reoxygenation is a major reason why fractionating treatment leads to an improvement in therapeutic ratio (as compared to a few large doses) in clinical radiotherapy. There is limited direct information about reoxygenation of cells in human tumors during treatment, but measurements of the pO_2 in human tumors using Eppendorf oxygen electrodes (see Sec. 16.4.3) during fractionated radiotherapy have demonstrated increasing oxygen levels in some tumors (Dunst et al, 1999). Although this is consistent with reoxygenation, these measurements do not distinguish between oxygen levels of surviving cells and those of cells already inactivated by the treatment. Evidence that the oxygen status of tumors can predict treatment outcome following radiation therapy (see Sec. 16.4.3) suggests that reoxygenation is inadequate to eliminate the effects of hypoxia during standard fractionated treatment for at least some tumors (eg, head and neck cancers) in humans. Shortening treatment schedules as in stereotactic body radiotherapy (SBRT) (see Sec. 16.1) may exacerbate this problem as data from animal models demonstrate that treatments with larger fraction sizes are more prone to the protective effects of hypoxia. Administration of hypoxic cell sensitizers might enhance such treatments.

16.7 MODELING THE EFFECTS OF FRACTIONATION

16.7.1 Time and Dose Relationships

Repair and repopulation increase the total dose required to achieve a given level of biological damage (an isoeffect) from a course of fractionated radiation treatment. In contrast, redistribution and reoxygenation would be expected to reduce the total dose required for an isoeffect. It is often difficult to dissect the influence of these factors, but reoxygenation applies mostly to tumors (because they contain hypoxic cells), whereas repopulation and redistribution apply both to tumors and proliferating normal tissues. Repair is an important factor in the response of virtually all tissues. Experimental studies from 50 years ago, examining acute reactions in pig skin, established that fraction number (reflecting repair of sublethal damage between fractions) was a more important factor than overall treatment time (reflecting repopulation) in determining isoeffect in fractionation schedules extending out to 4 weeks (Fowler

and Stern, 1963). Further studies established that fraction size (which is linked to fraction number in therapy regimes) is the critical parameter regarding normal tissue response, as illustrated for cell killing in Figure 16–20. For early normal tissue reactions (and tumors) the contribution of repopulation increases as the fractionated treatment is extended to longer times, as illustrated in Figures 16–21 and 16–22. Repopulation makes a lesser contribution for late normal tissue reactions but repair plays the major role, as illustrated in Figure 16–21 and discussed in Section 16.6.2. Redistribution reduces the effect of repopulation, but is probably a minor factor affecting tissue response to fractionated treatment, as discussed in Section 16.6.3.

That the biological effect of radiation depends on the fractionation schedule has important clinical implications for the planning of therapy. To obtain the maximum dose to a tumor while minimizing dose to surrounding normal tissue, modern radiotherapy will often use a number of overlapping radiation beams. The dose at any given location will be calculated by summing the doses given by the various individual beams, and the dose distribution will be represented by a series of isodose curves (like contours on a map) joining points that are expected to receive equal percentages of the dose at a particular point. As noted in Section 16.6.1, equal-size dose fractions allow for maximum repair; thus, if different beams are delivered over times sufficient for significant repair to occur (0.5 to 5.0 hours depending on the tissue) the tissues that receive unequal contributions from different beams (usually normal tissue surrounding the tumor) would have less-optimal repair than those where the contributions from the different beams are equal (usually the tumor). Thus the biological effect could be different at different points on the same isodose line; that is, isodose does not necessarily imply isoeffect.

16.7.2 Isoeffect Curves

Different fractionation schedules that give the same level of biological effect can be presented in the form of an isoeffect curve. Isoeffect curves are generated by plotting the total radiation dose to give a certain biological effect against the overall treatment time, fraction number, or fraction size, as illustrated in Figure 16–24. Experimental studies, performed mainly in rodents, have established isoeffect curves for different normal tissues using end points of either early or late radiation damage. Some of these isoeffect curves are shown in Figure 16–25, with the dashed blue lines representing early tissue responses and the red solid lines late responses. The isoeffect lines for late responses are steeper than those for early responses, meaning that a larger increase in total dose is required to give the same level of late toxicity as the dose per fraction is reduced and the number of fractions increased. This implies a greater capacity for the repair of damage in tissues where it is expressed late than for damage in tissues where it is expressed early after radiation treatment. Possible reasons for this difference include a greater contribution of potentially lethal damage repair because of limited proliferation early after treatment in late responding tissues (see Chap. 15, Sec. 15.4.2) but exact reasons remain

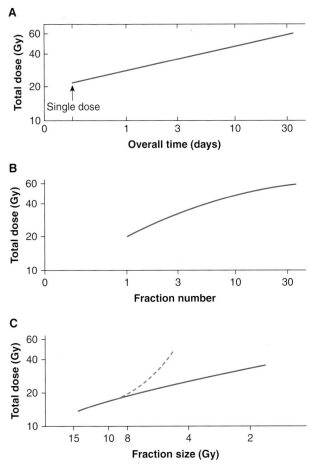

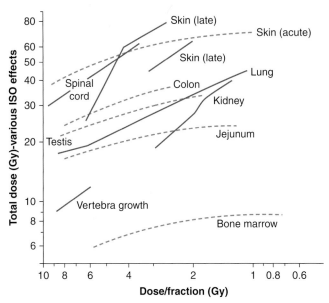

FIGURE 16–25 Isoeffect curves for a number of rodent tissues obtained using a variety of different cell survival or functional assays. The total dose required to obtain a fixed level of tissue damage is plotted as a function of the dose/fraction. The displacement of the curves on the vertical axis is a result of the fact that different isoeffective end points were used for the different tissues. (Modified from Thames et al, 1982.)

FIGURE 16–24 Isoeffect curves for fractionated treatments plotted in three different formats. A) Line plotted by Strandqvist, (1944) to define normal tissue tolerance and control of carcinoma of the skin and lip using the axes of total dose and overall treatment time. B) Isoeffect curve for damage to pig skin plotted as total dose versus number of fractions. (Adapted from Fowler, 1971.) C) Isoeffect curve for the crypt cells of the mouse intestine plotted as total dose versus fraction size using an inverted scale. The solid (red) line is for fractions given 3 hours apart and the dashed (blue) line for fractions given 24 hours apart. All three curves illustrate that the total (isoeffective) dose increases with fractionated treatment. (Adapted from Withers and Mason, 1974.)

unclear and may differ for different tissues. Nevertheless, the observation that late-responding normal tissues demonstrate greater repair capacity than early responding normal tissues is a fundamental radiobiological principle underlying altered fractionation schedules using multiple daily fractions in clinical radiotherapy. This is discussed in more detail in Section 16.7.4.

16.7.3 The Linear Quadratic Equation and Models for Isoeffect

Modeling isoeffect relationships (particularly for normal tissues) can allow appropriate choice of dose and schedule when changing fractionation schedules. Several models have been proposed, but most modeling is currently based on the linear-quadratic (LQ) equation (see Chap. 15, Appendix 15.1). In using

the LQ model, it is assumed that each fraction has an equal effect, thus for a fractionated regime (n fractions of size d):

$$SF = [e^{-(\alpha d + \beta d^2)}]^n \qquad [\text{Eq. 16.3}]$$

where SF = surviving fraction. This reduces to:

$$-\ln SF = n(\alpha d + \beta d^2) \qquad [\text{Eq. 16.4}]$$

It is further assumed that if different fractionation regimes (eg, n_1 fractions of size d_1 and n_2 fractions of size d_2) are isoeffective for a given tissue, they lead to the same SF. Thus we have:

$$\text{Isoeffect } (E) = -\ln SF = n_1(\alpha d_1 + \beta d_1^2)$$
$$= n_2(\alpha d_2 + \beta d_2^2) \qquad [\text{Eq. 16.5}]$$

Equation (16.5) can then be simplified to give:

$$n_1 d_1 / n_2 d_2 = (\alpha + \beta d_2)/(\alpha + \beta d_1) \qquad [\text{Eq. 16.6}]$$

From this relationship and knowing the values of n_1, d_1, n_2, and d_2, the constant α/β can be determined for a particular tissue and used in the equation to predict other isoeffective treatment schedules.

Data similar to those shown in Figure 16–25 have been used to estimate α/β values for different normal tissues in rodents. In general, late-responding normal tissues have α/β values in the range of 2 to 5 Gy, while early responding normal tissues have α/β values in the range of 8 to 12 Gy. Tumors generally have values similar to or greater than early responding normal tissues. The available data for human tissues suggest values in the same ranges but confidence limits are large and the available data suggest that grouping the responses of different tissues as described above is an oversimplification. Similarly there are exceptions to the general rule that all tumors have α/β values similar to or greater than those for early responding tissues as some (slowly growing) tumors, for example, prostate cancer, may have low α/β values between 1 and 3 Gy, suggesting a large repair capacity (see Bentzen and Joiner, 2009).

Critical to the original derivation of the LQ model was the underlying assumption that the primary factor underlying normal tissue responses to irradiation was killing of the relevant parenchymal cell population. As discussed in Section 16.5, normal tissue response to irradiation is now recognized as multifactorial, and this assumption is unlikely to be correct. Nevertheless, the model has proven to be valuable in the clinic provided that it is not extrapolated to predict the effects of fractionation schedules that are very different from clinical experience (eg, fraction sizes outside the range of 1 to 5 Gy). In the original model, there was no consideration of the effect of treatment time: This is a limitation that applies primarily to early normal tissue (and tumor) responses, where repopulation plays a substantial role. In the original LQ model, it was also assumed that there is complete repair between the fractions, which is incorrect when the interfraction interval is too short or where repair of sublethal damage is slow, as occurs in some late-responding tissues, such as neural tissues. Modifications to the model allow corrections to be made for these factors, but there remains uncertainty in their ability to predict outcome when dose and schedule are modified. More detailed discussion can be found in the books listed in the bibliography.

16.7.4 Altered Fractionation Schedules

The possibility of obtaining a therapeutic gain by exploiting the higher capacity for repair of radiation damage in late-responding normal tissues, as compared with early responding normal tissues and many tumors, has been investigated by reducing the fraction size below that used conventionally (from approximately 2 Gy to 1 to 1.5 Gy) and increasing the number of fractions. The increase in dose that can be tolerated at the isoeffective level of late normal tissue damage should be greater than that required to maintain the same level of tumor control, meaning that the tumor would receive a larger biologically effective dose and hence the control rate should be higher. The larger number of fractions required must be given more than once per day (or over weekends) if the treatment time is not to be prolonged. Such a treatment protocol is termed *hyperfractionation*. Clinical trials for patients with head and neck cancers evaluating a larger total dose delivered by hyperfractionation (2 fractions per day with 4- to 6-hour intervals) have reported an increase in local control with no difference in late normal tissue damage (see Horiot et al, 1992), although others (Fu et al, 2000) reported increased late effects as well as improved tumor control in their study.

The intent of hyperfractionation is to reduce late effects while achieving the same or better tumor control and the

same or slightly increased early effects. The time interval between the fractions must be sufficiently long to allow for complete repair to occur. Repair kinetics have been estimated in normal rodent tissues, and half-times for repair ranged from 0.5 hours in jejunum to 1 to 2 hours in skin, lung, and kidney, so that repair will be complete in most normal tissues after an interfraction interval of 6 to 8 hours. However, for some late-responding tissues in humans, including nervous tissue, estimated repair half-times are in the range of 3 to 5 hours, so repair may not be complete even with an interfraction interval of 8 hours (Bentzen et al, 1999; Lee et al, 1999). Thus, an increase in late morbidity would be expected when multiple fractions per day are given to fields that include the spinal cord, as was observed in the CHART (Continuous Hyperfractionated Accelerated Radiotherapy) trials in which patients were given 3 fractions per day (Dische and Saunders, 1989). An increase in early normal tissue reactions would be expected with hyperfractionation because the larger α/β value for early responding tissues implies a smaller change in the amount of repair as fraction size is reduced relative to that occurring in late-responding tissues (that have smaller α/β values). Severe mucositis was observed in the CHART trial (see Fig. 16–16), but it is likely that this was a result of the very short total treatment time limiting the possibility for repopulation to occur in the mucosa.

Shortening of the overall treatment time has also been investigated as an approach to improving the therapeutic ratio because it reduces the time for repopulation to occur in the tumor during treatment (see Sec. 16.6.2). A similar effect might be achieved by blocking growth factors or their receptors, which are required for tumor cell proliferation (see Sec. 16.2.5). The tolerance of late-responding normal tissues should be little affected because cell proliferation is slow within them. Reduced treatment time is achieved by giving more than 1 fraction per day with standard dose fractions of 1.8 to 2.5 Gy, usually given 6 to 8 hours apart to allow for repair (although these time intervals may be insufficient to allow full repair in some late-responding tissues, as discussed above). This strategy is called *accelerated fractionation*. Randomized trials of accelerated compared to conventional fractionation for treatment of head and neck cancer have provided evidence supporting the importance of repopulation as a cause of treatment failure. A CHART study gave a reduced total dose in the experimental arm of the study, but maintained the same tumor control level, with a slight reduction in late morbidity (Dische et al, 1997). A second study, which gave a similar total dose in both arms, reported increased tumor control in the accelerated fractionation arm, but there was also increased late toxicity (Horiot et al, 1997). This increased toxicity was likely a result of the short (4-hour) interfraction interval, which was probably not sufficient to allow for complete repair between the fractions. Table 16–5 outlines factors relating to altered fractionation schedules. A metaanalysis of studies of altered fractionation regimes in head and neck squamous cell cancers concluded that hyperfractionation had a greater benefit than accelerated fractionation (Bourhis et al, 2006).

TABLE 16–5 Summary of normal tissue responses to altered schedules of fractionated radiation.

Normal Tissue Reaction*	Acute	Late	Consequential
Tissues	Skin, oral mucosa, GI mucosa	Liver, kidney, spinal cord, lung or skin fibrosis, muscle	Skin, mucosa
Time of onset	<3 months	>6 months	>6 months
α/β values	~8 to 12 Gy	~2 to 4 Gy	??
Fractionation response	Hyperfractionated ⇔ Accelerated ⇑	Hyperfractionated ⇓ Accelerated ⇔	Hyperfractionated ⇓ Accelerated ⇑

*See Sec. 16.5.1 for definition of normal tissue reactions.

Accelerated radiotherapy, carbogen, and nicotinamide (ARCON) protocols involve accelerated radiotherapy combined with carbogen (95% oxygen plus 5% carbon dioxide) breathing and nicotinamide and are designed to limit repopulation and decrease the influence of hypoxia, because reoxygenation may be less during short treatment schedules. Phase I and II clinical trials showed the feasibility of ARCON therapy and produced promising results in terms of tumor control in cancers of the head and neck and bladder. A Phase III trial in larynx cancer has been completed and an initial report indicates that the early toxicities associated with the treatment are not significantly enhanced, whereas local tumor outcome is improved (Janssens et al, 2012).

A more extreme form of accelerated therapy involves stereotactic radiosurgery (SBRT) to treat some tumors, including those in the brain, in which large single doses or a few large fractions are given (3 to 5 fractions of 8 to 20 Gy each). This technique has been applied for localized treatments of small primary lesions and isolated metastases, particularly in the lung. Such treatments are expected to cause complete loss of normal tissue function in the high-dose region of the beam, and tolerability of such treatments depends on the small volume irradiated, its location, and the reserve capacity of the normal tissues involved (see Sec. 16.5.3). Results and appropriate applications of this accelerated form of radiation treatment have been reviewed (Kavanagh et al, 2011).

16.8 RADIATION-INDUCED SECOND MALIGNANCIES

As cancer patients treated with radiotherapy can be cured or may have prolonged survival after treatment, an effect of increasing concern is the induction of second malignancies. Most information about radiation-induced cancers has come from the long-term life span study (LSS), set up in 1950, that is tracking cancer incidence and mortality in a cohort of more than 85,000 Japanese atomic (A)-bomb survivors who were exposed in 1945. Cancer survivors, nuclear workers, uranium miners, and people exposed during radiation accidents, such as that at Chernobyl, have been, and are being, followed to provide better assessments of risk.

The most recent analysis of results from the LSS of the A-bomb survivors is *Report 14*, which covers the period from 1950 to 2003 (Ozasa et al, 2012). Subjects of this study were estimated to have received doses of less than 4 Gy, with most receiving doses of less than 0.2 Gy. This report indicates that the incidence of most types of solid cancers is elevated with a linear dose–response relationship up to a dose of approximately 3 Gy (Fig. 16–26). Radiation risk is defined as the increase in the number of cancer deaths over that expected for an unirradiated population. Excess absolute risk (EAR) is expressed as the increased number of cancers per 10^4 person-years after exposure to 1 Sievert (1 Sv is equivalent to 1 Gy of X- or γ-radiation). Excess relative risk (ERR) is the increase in cancers above that expected in an unirradiated population expressed as a fraction of the level in the unirradiated population. There was elevated risk for all doses of radiation in the A-bomb survivors with no evidence for a threshold. The effects are dependent on sex, age at exposure, and attained age (Fig. 16–27), with females and those exposed at younger ages showing higher ERR. The EAR increases throughout life and was 0.42 for all solid cancer at age 70 years, after exposure

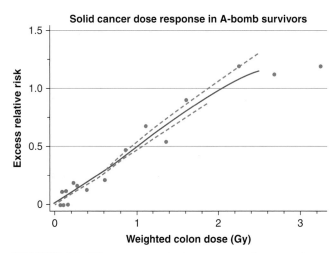

FIGURE 16–26 Incidence of solid cancer as a function of dose from the A-Bomb survivor incidence data. The solid (red) line is the estimated gender-averaged excess relative risk (ERR) at age 70 years after exposure at age 30 years. The blue dashed lines are 1 standard error above or below the line. (Redrawn from Preston et al, 2007.)

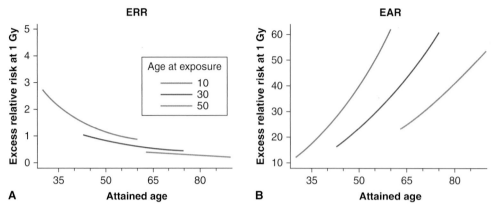

FIGURE 16–27 **Effects of age at exposure on the excess risks of solid cancers.** Panel (**A**) shows the excess relative risk (ERR) gender-average for exposure to 1 Gy and panel (**B**) shows the excess absolute risk (EAR) for the same groups. (Redrawn from Preston et al, 2007.)

at age 30 years based on a linear model. There was also an increased risk of other diseases, including those of the circulatory, respiratory, and digestive systems. An analysis of mortality as a consequence of leukemia in the A-bomb survivors over the period 1950 to 2000 demonstrated a curvilinear (LQ) dose–response relationship with an estimated ERR at 1 Sv of 4.7 (Richardson et al, 2009). Again, the risk was age- and dose-dependent and much higher for those exposed at younger than 10 years of age. The predominant type of leukemia was acute myeloid leukemia (AML) and the relative risk rose rapidly in the first 5 to 10 years after exposure and then declined, so that after 25 years the excess risk was small. General observations from the LSS are that radiation tends to increase the incidence of tumors, which arise naturally in the population and the increased incidence is seen primarily at ages when spontaneously arising tumors of the same type would occur.

The risk of second malignancies in cancer survivors has been reviewed by a number of groups over the last few years. A metaanalysis of 26 studies of childhood cancer survivors demonstrated induction of different types of cancer and estimated an overall ERR of second malignancy of 0.6 (Doi et al, 2011). A report from the Childhood Cancer Survivor Study (CCSS) reported a cumulative incidence at 30 years after diagnosis of childhood cancer of 20.5%, with the most frequent being non-melanoma skin cancers and breast cancer. A specific analysis of thyroid cancer from this study demonstrated that the relative risk increased up to (fractionated) doses of 20 to 25 Gy and then declined at higher doses (Fig. 16–28).

A detailed report on cancer survivors of all ages by the National Council on Radiation Protection and Measurements (NCRP) showed an elevated risk of breast and lung cancers in particular for patients treated for Hodgkin lymphoma (Travis et al, 2012). The increased risk for breast cancer extends to at least 30 years after treatment, with incidence rising to 20% to 30% of patients given radiotherapy. There is dependence on dose to the breast and age at treatment with greater risk for women who received radiation at young ages; incidence is lower in patients who received only chemotherapy. Some of the increased incidence of second cancers may be a result

of underlying genetic predisposition, as may occur with BRCA1/2 carriers, but this does not account for the majority of such second malignancies. A population of patients that may be at increased risk are patients treated with the newer IMRT techniques rather than 3D conformal therapy. Their risk was estimated to be almost 2-fold higher, because IMRT requires many more fields from different angles than conformal therapy and a larger volume of normal tissue is exposed to radiation (Hall, 2006). However, it will require 1 to 2 decades of careful follow-up to see if this is the case and assays to determine genetic predisposition to undergo radiation-induced carcinogenesis would be required to assess individual patient risk (Hussein et al, 2012).

The first 20 years of studies of carcinogenesis in people exposed to fallout after the Chernobyl accident in 1986 show

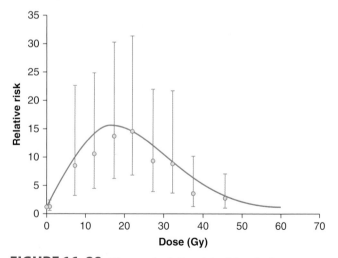

FIGURE 16–28 **Observed relative risk of developing secondary thyroid cancer in childhood cancer survivors as a function of mean radiation dose to the thyroid during radiotherapy for the initial cancer.** Line is based on a model adjusted for attained age, sex, and type of first cancer. The points represent the dose categories and are shown with 95% confidence intervals. (Modified from Bhatti et al, 2010.)

a large increase in the incidence of thyroid cancers in young people (Williams, 2008), most of whom have been treated successfully. There was early incidence (within 4 years) in those exposed at a very young age and longer latency for those exposed at older ages. These tumors are associated with exposure to radioactive iodine, much of it probably ingested from contaminated milk. Iodine is concentrated in the thyroid, giving much higher exposures to the gland (~1000-fold the average whole-body dose). The developing thyroid gland is more sensitive than the mature gland in older children and adults, probably because of a higher level of proliferation. Most of these tumors are associated with rearrangements in chromosome 10 involving the *RET* oncogene, which differ for early (*RET-PTC-3* involving the *ELE-1* gene) and later (*RET-PTC1* involving the *H4* gene) incidence tumors; mutations of the *BRAF* gene (see Chap. 7, Sec. 7.5.5) have also been observed. No increases in other malignancies have yet been associated unequivocally with radiation exposure as a consequence of the Chernobyl fallout, although there is some indication of increases in breast cancer incidence in young women. Experience from the LSS study indicates that longer follow-up will be necessary to assess how radiation-induced cancer incidence varies with the different types of exposures involved (acute single external exposures for the A-bomb survivors vs. prolonged exposures to ingested radioisotopes for the Chernobyl survivors).

Experimental models to evaluate carcinogenic effects of ionizing radiation are based on concepts similar to those for the study of chemical carcinogens, particularly the multistep carcinogenesis model (see Chap. 4, Sec. 4.2.1). Radiation is both an initiator and promoter of carcinogenesis. Single doses of X- or γ-rays in the range of 0.25 to 8 Gy given to the whole body increase the frequency of tumors in irradiated animals. Different tissues have different sensitivities for tumor induction, and genetic characteristics, age, environment, dietary factors, and modifying agents all affect the incidence of radiation-induced cancers in animals (Kennedy, 2009). The relationship between tumor induction and radiation dose given to the whole body appears to be sigmoid (Fig. 16–29): At low doses there is little induction, but as the dose increases there is a steep increase in the number of tumors followed by saturation or a decrease at high doses likely caused by cell killing (red line). High LET radiations are more effective (green line) and fractionation of low LET exposure is less effective in inducing cancer (blue line).

The initial effect of radiation is assumed to be induction of genetic instability associated with DNA damage, which can result in genetic changes in the descendants of irradiated cells including (a) mutations in genes involved in control of DNA synthesis or DNA repair; (b) the induction of chromosome instability; (c) persisting aberrant production of oxygen radicals that can damage DNA; (d) prolonged inflammatory processes in tissues; (e) epigenetic effects (Aypar et al, 2011; Mukherjee et al, 2012). These "initiator" effects would allow for a higher probability of developing further "rare" mutations, leading to malignant transformation by the activation of (proto)oncogenes or inactivation of tumor-suppressor genes.

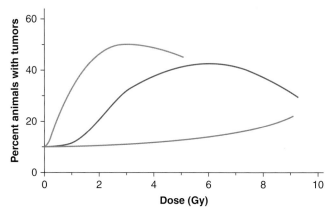

FIGURE 16–29 **Schematic of induction of a specific tumor type in mice exposed to various doses of ionizing radiation given to the whole body based on a review of a number of different in vivo results.** *Red curve:* Tumors induced by single acute doses of low-LET radiation. *Green curve:* Tumors induced by single acute doses of high-LET radiation. *Blue curve:* Tumors induced by fractionated doses (eg, 1 Gy/day) of low-LET radiation.

The observations that radiation tends to increase the incidence of tumors that arise naturally, and that the increased incidence is seen primarily at ages when spontaneously arising tumors of the same type would occur, are consistent with radiation acting to induce an increased likelihood of the occurrence of processes that naturally lead to cancer development, such as activation of oncogenes or inactivation of suppressor genes. However, in irradiated cultured cell populations, genetic instability has been detected over many generations and can apparently arise de novo, supporting the idea of late secondary effects (and possibly bystander effects; see Chap. 15, Sec. 15.2.4). Furthermore, so-called clastogenic factors, molecules that can induce chromosome damage in unirradiated cells (and may reflect aberrant production of oxygen radicals and underlying chronic inflammatory processes), have been detected in the blood of radiotherapy patients, Japanese A-bomb survivors, and the Chernobyl liquidators. This suggests a prolonged effect of irradiation that is also consistent with a classic promoter role.

SUMMARY

- Radiotherapy for cancer has developed empirically and usually involves giving 25 to 40 individual dose fractions of approximately 2 Gy once daily, over a period of 5 to 8 weeks.
- Improvements in technology have led to the introduction of conformal and intensity-modulated radiotherapy, allowing a decrease in normal tissue dose (and, hence, side effects) with dose escalation to tumor tissues.
- Other radiotherapy technologies that have improved the therapeutic ratio through physical means for some types of tumors include high-LET irradiation, brachytherapy, and changes in fractionation.

- Five biological factors (the "5 Rs") influence response to fractionated treatment and the therapeutic ratio. These are radiosensitivity, repair of radiation damage, repopulation of damaged tissues by proliferation of surviving cells, redistribution of proliferating cells through the cell cycle, and reoxygenation of hypoxic cells. Repair and repopulation are the reasons why normal tissues can tolerate a larger total dose when it is fractionated and repair is the main process influencing late radiation damage that is often dose limiting. Repopulation by tumor cells during the latter part of conventional (5- to 7-week) fractionated treatments increases the dose required for tumor control. Reoxygenation in tumors contributes to the improved therapeutic ratio obtained with fractionated treatment.

- Both tumor and normal tissue responses to irradiation are complex. Radiation can kill individual tumor and normal cells directly and this can be expressed as mitosis-linked cell death or, in a few tissues, as early apoptosis. Damage to vasculature may lead to secondary death of cells. Particularly in normal tissues, there are other indirect effects, such as the induction of cytokines and inflammation that can influence early and late tissue responses.

- Tumor control requires the killing of all the tumor stem cells but there is heterogeneity in cellular radiosensitivity in tumors as a result of microenvironmental factors such as hypoxia, and possibly also as a result of the presence of subpopulations because of genetic instability.

- Different fractionated schedules that give an equal level of normal tissue response or tumor control can be expressed in the form of isoeffect relationships described by the parameters α and β of the LQ model. Late-responding tissues tend to have smaller α/β values than early responding tissues, implying greater capacity for repair of damage that leads to late effects, but there is uncertainty about values for specific tissues and damage.

- A therapeutic gain can be achieved by using hyperfractionation, where treatment with smaller dose fractions is given 2 or 3 times per day, but if the time between fractions is too short, increased late normal tissue damage may occur.

- Giving treatments more than once per day with the aim of reducing overall treatment time (accelerated fractionation) can also lead to a therapeutic gain if repopulation occurs more rapidly in the tumors than in the dose-limiting normal tissues and sufficient time is allowed between the fractions for full repair to occur.

- Despite increasing knowledge of biological factors that influence the response of tissues and tumors to fractionated irradiation, prediction of treatment outcome for individual patients is not possible except for those with known mutations in DNA repair genes and, to a limited extent, from measurements of tumor hypoxia. Genetic analyses of tumors and normal cells of patients may lead to better predictive assays.

- Despite its ability to successfully treat cancers, radiation is also a carcinogen, most probably because of induction of genetic instability in cells. The risk of cancer development following irradiation has been extensively documented, particularly in the Japanese A-bomb survivors, in cancer survivors treated with radiation, and following various radiation accidents. The risk is higher for people exposed at a younger age and increases with attained age. Initially, risk increases with the dose received (with no evidence for a low-dose threshold), but may decline at higher doses.

REFERENCES

Ahn GO, Brown JM. Influence of bone marrow-derived hematopoietic cells on the tumor response to radiotherapy: experimental models and clinical perspectives. *Cell Cycle* 2009;8:970-976.

Ang KK, Harris J, Wheeler R, et al. Human papillomavirus and survival of patients with oropharyngeal cancer. *N Engl J Med* 2010;363:24-35.

Ang KK, Sturgis EM. Human papillomavirus as a marker of the natural history and response to therapy of head and neck squamous cell carcinoma. *Semin Radiat Oncol* 2012;22:128-142.

Anscher MS, Kong FM, Andrews K, et al. Plasma transforming growth factor beta1 as a predictor of radiation pneumonitis. *Int J Radiat Oncol Biol Phys* 1998;41:1029-1035.

Antonadou D, Throuvalas N, Petridis A, Bolanos N, Sagriotis A, Synodinou M. Effect of amifostine on toxicities associated with radiochemotherapy in patients with locally advanced non-small-cell lung cancer. *Int J Radiat Oncol Biol Phys* 2003;57:402-408.

Armstrong J. Three-dimensional conformal radiation therapy: evidence-based treatment of prostate cancer. *Radiother Oncol* 2002;64:235-237.

Autio KA, Scher HI, Morris MJ. Therapeutic strategies for bone metastases and their clinical sequelae in prostate cancer. *Curr Treat Options Oncol* 2012;13:174-188.

Aypar U, Morgan WF, Baulch JE. Radiation-induced genomic instability: are epigenetic mechanisms the missing link? *Int J Radiat Biol* 2011;87:179-191.

Barth RF. Boron neutron capture therapy at the crossroads: challenges and opportunities. *Appl Radiat Isot* 2009;67:S3-S6.

Bauman G, Rumble RB, Chen J, Loblaw A, Warde P. Intensity-modulated radiotherapy in the treatment of prostate cancer. *Clin Oncol (R Coll Radiol)* 2012;24:461-473.

Begg AC. The clinical status of Tpot as a predictor? Or why no tempest in the Tpot! *Int J Radiat Oncol Biol Phys* 1995;32:1539-1541.

Begg AC, Haustermans K, Hart AA, et al. The value of pretreatment cell kinetic parameters as predictors for radiotherapy outcome in head and neck cancer: a multicenter analysis. *Radiother Oncol* 1999;50:13-23.

Begg AC, Stewart FA, Vens C. Strategies to improve radiotherapy with targeted drugs. *Nat Rev Cancer* 2011;11:239-253.

Bentzen S, Joiner M The linear-quadratic approach in clinical practice. In: Joiner M, Van der Kogel A, eds. *Basic Clinical Radiobiology.* 4th ed. London, UK: Edward Arnold; 2009;120-134.

Bentzen SM, Constine LS, Deasy JO, et al. Quantitative analyses of normal tissue effects in the clinic (QUANTEC): an introduction to the scientific issues. *Int J Radiat Oncol Biol Phys* 2010; 76:S3-S9.

Bentzen SM, Overgaard M, Overgaard J. Clinical correlations between late normal tissue endpoints after radiotherapy: implications for predictive assays of radiosensitivity. *Eur J Cancer* 1993;29A:1373-1376.

Bentzen SM, Saunders MI, Dische S. Repair halftimes estimated from observations of treatment-related morbidity after CHART or conventional radiotherapy in head and neck cancer. *Radiother Oncol* 1999;53:219-226.

Bentzen SM, Saunders MI, Dische S, Bond SJ. Radiotherapy-related early morbidity in head and neck cancer: quantitative clinical radiobiology as deduced from the CHART trial. *Radiother Oncol* 2001;60:123-135.

Bhatti P, Veiga LH, Ronckers CM, et al. Risk of second primary thyroid cancer after radiotherapy for a childhood cancer in a large cohort study: an update from the childhood cancer survivor study. *Radiat Res* 2010;174:741-752.

Bjork-Eriksson T, West C, Karlsson E, Mercke C. Tumor radiosensitivity (SF2) is a prognostic factor for local control in head and neck cancers. *Int J Radiat Oncol Biol Phys* 2000; 46:13-19.

Bonner JA, Harari PM, Giralt J, et al. Radiotherapy plus cetuximab for locoregionally advanced head and neck cancer: 5-year survival data from a phase 3 randomised trial, and relation between cetuximab-induced rash and survival. *Lancet Oncol* 2010;11:21-28.

Bonner JA, Harari PM, Giralt J, et al. Radiotherapy plus cetuximab for squamous-cell carcinoma of the head and neck. *N Engl J Med* 2006;354:567-578.

Bouquet F, Pal A, Pilones KA, et al. TGFbeta1 inhibition increases the radiosensitivity of breast cancer cells in vitro and promotes tumor control by radiation in vivo. *Clin Cancer Res* 2011;17: 6754-6765.

Bourhis J, Overgaard J, Audry H, et al. Hyperfractionated or accelerated radiotherapy in head and neck cancer: a meta-analysis. *Lancet* 2006;368:843-854.

Brenner DJ, Hall EJ. Conditions for the equivalence of continuous to pulsed low dose rate brachytherapy. *Int J Radiat Oncol Biol Phys* 1991;20:181-190.

Brizel DM, Wasserman TH, Henke M, et al. Phase III randomized trial of amifostine as a radioprotector in head and neck cancer. *J Clin Oncol* 2000;18:3339-3345.

Brown JM. The hypoxic cell: a target for selective cancer therapy—eighteenth Bruce F. Cain Memorial Award lecture. *Cancer Res* 1999;59:5863-5870.

Budaus L, Bolla M, Bossi A, et al. Functional outcomes and complications following radiation therapy for prostate cancer: a critical analysis of the literature. *Eur Urol* 2012;61:112-127.

Buffa FM, Harris AL, West CM, Miller CJ. Large meta-analysis of multiple cancers reveals a common, compact and highly prognostic hypoxia metagene. *Br J Cancer* 2010;102: 428-435.

Bush RS. The significance of anemia in clinical radiation therapy. *Int J Radiat Oncol Biol Phys* 1986;12:2047-2050.

Bussink J, Kaanders JH, van der Kogel AJ. Tumor hypoxia at the micro-regional level: clinical relevance and predictive value of exogenous and endogenous hypoxic cell markers. *Radiother Oncol* 2003;67:3-15.

Chapman JD, Dugle DL, Reuvers AP, Meeker BE, Borsa J. Letter: studies on the radiosensitizing effect of oxygen in Chinese hamster cells. *Int J Radiat Biol Relat Stud Phys Chem Med* 1974;26:383-389.

Chitneni SK, Palmer GM, Zalutsky MR, Dewhirst MW. Molecular imaging of hypoxia. *J Nucl Med* 2011;52:165-168.

Cohen EP, Bedi M, Irving AA, et al. Mitigation of late renal and pulmonary injury after hematopoietic stem cell transplantation. *Int J Radiat Oncol Biol Phys* 2011;83:292-296.

Dainiak N, Waselenko JK, Armitage JO, MacVittie TJ, Farese AM. The hematologist and radiation casualties. *Hematology Am Soc Hematol Educ Program* 2003:473-496.

Dawson LA, Sharpe MB. Image-guided radiotherapy: rationale, benefits, and limitations. *Lancet Oncol* 2006;7:848-858.

Deacon J, Peckham MJ, Steel GG. The radioresponsiveness of human tumours and the initial slope of the cell survival curve. *Radiother Oncol* 1984;2:317-323.

DeLaney TF. Proton therapy in the clinic. *Front Radiat Ther Oncol* 2011;43:465-485.

Delanian S, Chatel C, Porcher R, Depondt J, Lefaix JL. Complete restoration of refractory mandibular osteoradionecrosis by prolonged treatment with a pentoxifylline-tocopherol-clodronate combination (PENTOCLO): a phase II trial. *Int J Radiat Oncol Biol Phys* 2011;80:832-839.

Delanian S, Lefaix JL. Current management for late normal tissue injury: radiation-induced fibrosis and necrosis. *Semin Radiat Oncol* 2007;17:99-107.

Denekamp J. Cell kinetics and radiation biology. *Int J Radiat Biol Relat Stud Phys Chem Med* 1986;49:357-380.

Denham JW, Hauer-Jensen M. The radiotherapeutic injury—a complex "wound." *Radiother Oncol* 2002;63:129-145.

Diepart C, Karroum O, Magat J, et al. Arsenic trioxide treatment decreases the oxygen consumption rate of tumor cells and radiosensitizes solid tumors. *Cancer Res* 2011;72:482-490.

Dische S, Saunders M, Barrett A, Harvey A, Gibson D, Parmar M. A randomised multicentre trial of CHART versus conventional radiotherapy in head and neck cancer. *Radiother Oncol* 1997;44: 123-136.

Dische S, Saunders MI. Continuous, hyperfractionated, accelerated radiotherapy (CHART): an interim report upon late morbidity. *Radiother Oncol* 1989;16:65-72.

Doi K, Mieno MN, Shimada Y, Yonehara H, Yoshinaga S. Meta-analysis of second cancer risk after radiotherapy among childhood cancer survivors. *Radiat Prot Dosimetry* 2011;146: 263-267.

Dunst J, Hansgen G, Lautenschlager C, Fuchsel G, Becker A. Oxygenation of cervical cancers during radiotherapy and radiotherapy + cis-retinoic acid/interferon. *Int J Radiat Oncol Biol Phys* 1999;43:367-373.

Eke I, Cordes N. Radiobiology goes 3D: how ECM and cell morphology impact on cell survival after irradiation. *Radiother Oncol* 2011;99:271-278.

Evans ES, Kocak Z, Zhou SM, et al. Does transforming growth factor-beta1 predict for radiation-induced pneumonitis in patients treated for lung cancer? *Cytokine* 2006;35:186-192.

Fertil B, Malaise EP. Inherent cellular radiosensitivity as a basic concept for human tumor radiotherapy. *Int J Radiat Oncol Biol Phys* 1981;7:621-629.

Fowler JF. Experimental animal results relating to time-dose relationships in radiotherapy and the "ret" concept. *Br J Radiol* 1971;44:81-90.

Fowler JF. What to do with neutrons in radiotherapy: a suggestion. *Radiother Oncol* 1988;13:233-235.

Fowler JF, Stern BE. Fractionation and dose-rate. II. Dose-time relationships in radiotherapy and the validity of cell survival curve models. *Br J Radiol* 1963;36:163-173.

Fu KK, Pajak TF, Trotti A, et al. A Radiation Therapy Oncology Group (RTOG) phase III randomized study to compare hyperfractionation and two variants of accelerated fractionation to standard fractionation radiotherapy for head and neck squamous cell carcinomas: first report of RTOG 9003. *Int J Radiat Oncol Biol Phys* 2000;48:7-16.

Fyles A, Milosevic M, Hedley D, et al. Tumor hypoxia has independent predictor impact only in patients with node-negative cervix cancer. *J Clin Oncol* 2002;20:680-687.

Fyles A, Milosevic M, Pintilie M, et al. Long-term performance of interstitial fluid pressure and hypoxia as prognostic factors in cervix cancer. *Radiother Oncol* 2006;80:132-137.

Fyles A, Voduc D, Syed A, Milosevic M, Pintilie M, Hill R. The effect of smoking on tumour oxygenation and treatment outcome in cervical cancer. *Clin Oncol (R Coll Radiol)* 2002;14:442-446.

Fyles AW, Milosevic M, Pintilie M, Syed A, Hill RP. Anemia, hypoxia and transfusion in patients with cervix cancer: a review. *Radiother Oncol* 2000;57:13-19.

Garcia-Barros M, Thin TH, Maj J, et al. Impact of stromal sensitivity on radiation response of tumors implanted in SCID hosts revisited. *Cancer Res* 2010;70:8179-8186.

Goel S, Duda DG, Xu L, et al. Normalization of the vasculature for treatment of cancer and other diseases. *Physiol Rev* 2011;91:1071-1121.

Hakenjos L, Bamberg M, Rodemann HP. TGF-beta1-mediated alterations of rat lung fibroblast differentiation resulting in the radiation-induced fibrotic phenotype. *Int J Radiat Biol* 2000;76:503-509.

Hall EJ. Intensity-modulated radiation therapy, protons, and the risk of second cancers. *Int J Radiat Oncol Biol Phys* 2006;65:1-7.

Hall EJ. *Radiobiology for the Radiologist.* 5th ed. Philadelphia: Lippencott, Williams & Wilkins; 2000.

Hanahan D, Weinberg RA. Hallmarks of cancer: the next generation. *Cell* 2011;144:646-674.

Haston CK, Zhou X, Gumbiner-Russo L, et al. Universal and radiation-specific loci influence murine susceptibility to radiation-induced pulmonary fibrosis. *Cancer Res* 2002;62:3782-3788.

Henke M, Laszig R, Rube C, et al. Erythropoietin to treat head and neck cancer patients with anaemia undergoing radiotherapy: randomised, double-blind, placebo-controlled trial. *Lancet* 2003;362:1255-1260.

Hill RP, Bush RS, Yeung P. The effect of anaemia on the fraction of hypoxic cells in an experimental tumour. *Br J Radiol* 1971;44:299-304.

Hockel M, Schlenger K, Aral B, Mitze M, Schaffer U, Vaupel P. Association between tumor hypoxia and malignant progression in advanced cancer of the uterine cervix. *Cancer Res* 1996;56:4509-4515.

Hoeller U, Tribius S, Kuhlmey A, Grader K, Fehlauer F, Alberti W. Increasing the rate of late toxicity by changing the score? A comparison of RTOG/EORTC and LENT/SOMA scores. *Int J Radiat Oncol Biol Phys* 2003;55:1013–1018.

Hoff CM, Grau C, Overgaard J. Effect of smoking on oxygen delivery and outcome in patients treated with radiotherapy for head and neck squamous cell carcinoma—a prospective study. *Radiother Oncol* 2012;103:38-44.

Hoff CM, Lassen P, Eriksen JG, et al. Does transfusion improve the outcome for HNSCC patients treated with radiotherapy? Results from the randomized DAHANCA 5 and 7 trials. *Acta Oncol* 2011;50:1006-1014.

Horiot JC, Bontemps P, van den Bogaert W, et al. Accelerated fractionation (AF) compared to conventional fractionation (CF) improves loco-regional control in the radiotherapy of advanced head and neck cancers: results of the EORTC 22851 randomized trial. *Radiother Oncol* 1997;44:111-121.

Horiot JC, Le Fur R, N'Guyen T, et al. Hyperfractionation versus conventional fractionation in oropharyngeal carcinoma: final analysis of a randomized trial of the EORTC cooperative group of radiotherapy. *Radiother Oncol* 1992;25:231-241.

Hoskin PJ, Rojas AM, Bentzen SM, Saunders MI. Radiotherapy with concurrent carbogen and nicotinamide in bladder carcinoma. *J Clin Oncol* 2010;28:4912-4918.

Hussein M, Aldridge S, Guerrero Urbano T, Nisbet A. The effect of 6 and 15 MV on intensity-modulated radiation therapy prostate cancer treatment: plan evaluation, tumour control probability and normal tissue complication probability analysis, and the theoretical risk of secondary induced malignancies. *Br J Radiol* 2012;85:423-432.

Janssens GO, Rademakers SE, Terhaard CH, et al. Accelerated radiotherapy with carbogen and nicotinamide for laryngeal cancer: results of a phase III randomized trial. *J Clin Oncol* 2012;30:1777-1783.

Kavanagh BD, Timmerman R, Meyer JL. The expanding roles of stereotactic body radiation therapy and oligofractionation: toward a new practice of radiotherapy. *Front Radiat Ther Oncol* 2011;43:370-381.

Kennedy AR. Factors that modify radiation-induced carcinogenesis. *Health Phys* 2009;97:433-445.

Kioi M, Vogel H, Schultz G, Hoffman RM, Harsh GR, Brown JM. Inhibition of vasculogenesis, but not angiogenesis, prevents the recurrence of glioblastoma after irradiation in mice. *J Clin Invest* 2010;120:694-705.

Kolesnick R, Fuks Z. Radiation and ceramide-induced apoptosis. *Oncogene* 2003;22:5897-5906.

Krause M, Yaromina A, Eicheler W, Koch U, Baumann M. Cancer stem cells: targets and potential biomarkers for radiotherapy. *Clin Cancer Res* 2011;17:7224-7229.

Lee AW, Sze WM, Fowler JF, Chappell R, Leung SF, Teo P. Caution on the use of altered fractionation for nasopharyngeal carcinoma. *Radiother Oncol* 1999;52:207-211.

Levine EL, Renehan A, Gossiel R, et al. Apoptosis, intrinsic radiosensitivity and prediction of radiotherapy response in cervical carcinoma. *Radiother Oncol* 1995;37:1-9.

Lim AM, Rischin D, Fisher R, et al. Prognostic significance of plasma osteopontin in patients with locoregionally advanced head and neck squamous cell carcinoma treated on TROG 02.02 phase III trial. *Clin Cancer Res* 2012;18:301-307.

Lindegaard JC, Grau C. Has the outlook improved for amifostine as a clinical radioprotector? *Radiother Oncol* 2000;57:113-118.

Liu Q, Sun JD, Wang J, et al. TH-302, a hypoxia-activated prodrug with broad in vivo preclinical combination therapy efficacy: optimization of dosing regimens and schedules. *Cancer Chemother Pharmacol* 2012;69:1487-1498.

Ljungkvist AS, Bussink J, Kaanders JH, van der Kogel AJ. Dynamics of tumor hypoxia measured with bioreductive hypoxia cell markers. *Radiat Res* 2007;167:127-145.

Marks LB, Bentzen SM, Deasy JO, et al. Radiation dose-volume effects in the lung. *Int J Radiat Oncol Biol Phys* 2010;76:S70-S76.

Marks LB, Yorke ED, Jackson A, et al. Use of normal tissue complication probability models in the clinic. *Int J Radiat Oncol Biol Phys* 2010;76:S10-S19.

Martin M, Lefaix J, Delanian S. TGF-beta1 and radiation fibrosis: a master switch and a specific therapeutic target? *Int J Radiat Oncol Biol Phys* 2000;47:277-290.

Mettler FA Jr, Voelz GL. Major radiation exposure—what to expect and how to respond. *N Engl J Med* 2002;346:1554-1561.

Milano MT, Katz AW, Schell MC, Philip A, Okunieff P. Descriptive analysis of oligometastatic lesions treated with curative-intent stereotactic body radiotherapy. *Int J Radiat Oncol Biol Phys* 2008;72:1516-1522.

Miyamoto DT, Harris JR. Molecular predictors of local tumor control in early-stage breast cancer. *Semin Radiat Oncol* 2011;21:35-42.

Mukherjee D, Coates PJ, Lorimore SA, Wright EG. The in vivo expression of radiation-induced chromosomal instability has an inflammatory mechanism. *Radiat Res* 2012;177:18-24.

NIH/NCI Common Terminology Criteria for Adverse Events V 4: 2009; http://evs.nci.nih.gov/ftp1/CTCAE/CTCAE_4.03_2010-06-14_QuickReference_5x7.pdf.

Nordsmark M, Bentzen SM, Rudat V, et al. Prognostic value of tumor oxygenation in 397 head and neck tumors after primary radiation therapy. An international multi-center study. *Radiother Oncol* 2005;77:18-24.

Overgaard J. Hypoxic modification of radiotherapy in squamous cell carcinoma of the head and neck—a systematic review and meta-analysis. *Radiother Oncol* 2011;100:22-32.

Overgaard J, Eriksen JG, Nordsmark M, Alsner J, Horsman MR. Plasma osteopontin, hypoxia, and response to the hypoxia sensitiser nimorazole in radiotherapy of head and neck cancer: results from the DAHANCA 5 randomised double-blind placebo-controlled trial. *Lancet Oncol* 2005;6:757-764.

Overgaard J, Hansen HS, Overgaard M, et al. A randomized double-blind phase III study of nimorazole as a hypoxic radiosensitizer of primary radiotherapy in supraglottic larynx and pharynx carcinoma. Results of the Danish Head and Neck Cancer Study (DAHANCA) Protocol 5-85. *Radiother Oncol* 1998;46:135-146.

Overgaard J, Horsman MR. Modification of hypoxia-induced radioresistance in tumors by the use of oxygen and sensitizers. *Semin Radiat Oncol* 1996;6:10-21.

Ozasa K, Shimizu Y, Suyama A, et al. Studies of the mortality of atomic bomb survivors, Report 14, 1950-2003: an overview of cancer and noncancer diseases. *Radiat Res* 2012;177:229-243.

Paris F, Fuks Z, Kang A, et al. Endothelial apoptosis as the primary lesion initiating intestinal radiation damage in mice. *Science* 2001;293:293-297.

Peters LJ, O'Sullivan B, Giralt J, et al. Critical impact of radiotherapy protocol compliance and quality in the treatment of advanced head and neck cancer: results from TROG 02.02. *J Clin Oncol* 2010;28:2996-3001.

Pouget JP, Navarro-Teulon I, Bardies M, et al. Clinical radioimmunotherapy—the role of radiobiology. *Nat Rev Clin Oncol* 2011;8:720-734.

Preston DL, Ron E, Tokuoka S, et al. Solid cancer incidence in atomic bomb survivors: 1958-1998. *Radiat Res* 2007;168:1-64.

Raju MR. Particle radiotherapy: historical developments and current status. *Radiat Res* 1996;145:391-407.

Ree AH, Dueland S, Folkvord S, et al. Vorinostat, a histone deacetylase inhibitor, combined with pelvic palliative radiotherapy for gastrointestinal carcinoma: the Pelvic Radiation and Vorinostat (PRAVO) phase 1 study. *Lancet Oncol* 2010;11:459-464.

Richardson D, Sugiyama H, Nishi N, et al. Ionizing radiation and leukemia mortality among Japanese Atomic Bomb Survivors, 1950-2000. *Radiat Res* 2009;172:368-382.

Rischin D, Hicks RJ, Fisher R, et al. Prognostic significance of [18F]-misonidazole positron emission tomography-detected tumor hypoxia in patients with advanced head and neck cancer randomly assigned to chemoradiation with or without tirapazamine: a substudy of Trans-Tasman Radiation Oncology Group Study 98.02. *J Clin Oncol* 2006;24:2098-2104.

Rischin D, Peters LJ, O'Sullivan B, et al. Tirapazamine, cisplatin, and radiation versus cisplatin and radiation for advanced squamous cell carcinoma of the head and neck (TROG 02.02, HeadSTART): a phase III trial of the Trans-Tasman Radiation Oncology Group. *J Clin Oncol* 2010;28:2989-2995.

Rodemann HP, Bamberg M. Cellular basis of radiation-induced fibrosis. *Radiother Oncol* 1995;35:83-90.

Rotolo J, Stancevic B, Zhang J, et al. Anti-ceramide antibody prevents the radiation gastrointestinal syndrome in mice. *J Clin Invest* 2012;122:1786-1790.

Russell NS, Begg AC. Editorial radiotherapy and oncology 2002: predictive assays for normal tissue damage. *Radiother Oncol* 2002;64:125-129.

Schaue D, McBride WH. Links between innate immunity and normal tissue radiobiology. *Radiat Res* 2010;173:406-417.

Schwarz JK, Payton JE, Rashmi R, et al. Pathway-specific analysis of gene expression data identifies the PI3K/Akt pathway as a novel therapeutic target in cervical cancer. *Clin Cancer Res* 2012;18:1464-1471.

Secomb TW, Hsu R, Dewhirst MW. Synergistic effects of hyperoxic gas breathing and reduced oxygen consumption on tumor oxygenation: a theoretical model. *Int J Radiat Oncol Biol Phys* 2004;59:572-578.

Seidenfeld J, Piper M, Flamm C, et al. Epoetin treatment of anemia associated with cancer therapy: a systematic review and meta-analysis of controlled clinical trials. *J Natl Cancer Inst* 2001;93:1204-1214.

Settle SH, Sulman EP. Tumor profiling: development of prognostic and predictive factors to guide brain tumor treatment. *Curr Oncol Rep* 2011;13:26-36.

Stewart FA, Dorr W. Milestones in normal tissue radiation biology over the past 50 years: from clonogenic cell survival to cytokine networks and back to stem cell recovery. *Int J Radiat Biol* 2009;85:574-586.

Strandqvist M. Studien Uber die kumulative Wirkung der Rontgenstrahlen bei Fracktionierung. *Acta Radiologica* (old series) 1944;25, suppl 55;1-300.

Suit H. The Gray Lecture 2001: coming technical advances in radiation oncology. *Int J Radiat Oncol Biol Phys* 2002;53:798-809.

Thames HD Jr, Withers HR, Peters LJ, Fletcher GH. Changes in early and late radiation responses with altered dose fractionation: implications for dose-survival relationships. *Int J Radiat Oncol Biol Phys* 1982;8:219-226.

Toustrup K, Sorensen BS, Nordsmark M, et al. Development of a hypoxia gene expression classifier with predictive impact for hypoxic modification of radiotherapy in head and neck cancer. *Cancer Res* 2011;71:5923-5931.

Travis EL, Liao ZX, Tucker SL. Spatial heterogeneity of the volume effect for radiation pneumonitis in mouse lung. *Int J Radiat Oncol Biol Phys* 1997;38:1045-1054.

Travis LB, Ng AK, Allan JM, et al. Second malignant neoplasms and cardiovascular disease following radiotherapy. *J Natl Cancer Inst* 2012;104:357-370.

Tucker SL, Thames HD, Brown BW, Mason KA, Hunter NR, Withers HR. Direct analyses of in vivo colony survival after single and fractionated doses of radiation. *Int J Radiat Biol* 1991;59: 777-795.

Turesson I. Individual variation and dose dependency in the progression rate of skin telangiectasia. *Int J Radiat Oncol Biol Phys* 1990;19:1569-1574.

UNSCEAR. *Sources and Effects of Ionizing Radiation Report to the General Assembly: Volume II: Annex D: Health Effects Due to Radiation from the Chernobyl Accident.* New York, NY: United Nations; 2008.

Vaupel P, Kelleher DK, Hockel M. Oxygen status of malignant tumors: pathogenesis of hypoxia and significance for tumor therapy. *Semin Oncol* 2001;28:29-35.

Vordermark D, Brown JM. Endogenous markers of tumor hypoxia predictors of clinical radiation resistance? *Strahlenther Onkol* 2003;179:801-811.

Walsh L, Gillham C, Dunne M, et al. Toxicity of cetuximab versus cisplatin concurrent with radiotherapy in locally advanced head and neck squamous cell cancer (LAHNSCC). *Radiother Oncol* 2011;98:38-41.

Weiss JF, Landauer MR. History and development of radiation-protective agents. *Int J Radiat Biol* 2009;85:539-573.

West C, Rosenstein BS, Alsner J, et al. Establishment of a radiogenomics consortium. *Int J Radiat Oncol Biol Phys* 2010;76:1295-1296.

West CM, Davidson SE, Roberts SA, Hunter RD. The independence of intrinsic radiosensitivity as a prognostic factor for patient response to radiotherapy of carcinoma of the cervix. *Br J Cancer* 1997;76:1184-1190.

Williams D. Radiation carcinogenesis: lessons from Chernobyl. *Oncogene* 2008;27 Suppl 2:S9-S18.

Williams JP, McBride WH. After the bomb drops: a new look at radiation-induced multiple organ dysfunction syndrome (MODS). *Int J Radiat Biol* 2011;87:851-868.

Wilson GD. Cell kinetics. *Clin Oncol (R Coll Radiol)* 2007;19: 370-384.

Wilson WR, Hay MP. Targeting hypoxia in cancer therapy. *Nat Rev Cancer* 2010;11:393-410.

Withers HR, Mason KA. The kinetics of recovery in irradiated colonic mucosa of the mouse. *Cancer* 1974;34(suppl):896-903.

Withers HR, Taylor JM, Maciejewski B. The hazard of accelerated tumor clonogen repopulation during radiotherapy. *Acta Oncol* 1988a;27:131-146.

Withers HR, Taylor JM, Maciejewski B. Treatment volume and tissue tolerance. *Int J Radiat Oncol Biol Phys* 1988b;14:751-759.

Wong CS, Minkin S, Hill RP. Linear-quadratic model underestimates sparing effect of small doses per fraction in rat spinal cord. *Radiother Oncol* 1992;23:176-184.

Wouters BG, Brown JM. Cells at intermediate oxygen levels can be more important than the "hypoxic fraction" in determining tumor response to fractionated radiotherapy. *Radiat Res* 1997;147:541-550.

Yamamoto T, Nakai K, Matsumura A. Boron neutron capture therapy for glioblastoma. *Cancer Lett* 2008;262:143-152.

Zaleska K, Bruechner K, Baumann M, Zips D, Yaromina A. Tumour-infiltrating CD11b+ myelomonocytes and response to fractionated irradiation of human squamous cell carcinoma (hSCC) xenografts. *Radiother Oncol* 2011;101:80-85.

Zips D, Krause M, Yaromina A, et al. Epidermal growth factor receptor inhibitors for radiotherapy: biological rationale and preclinical results. *J Pharm Pharmacol* 2008;60:1019-1028.

BIBLIOGRAPHY

Hall EJ, Giaccia AJ. *Radiobiology for the Radiologist.* 7th ed. Philadelphia, PA: Lippincott; 2010.

Joiner M, van der Kogel A, eds. *Basic Clinical Radiobiology.* 4th ed. London, UK: Arnold; 2009.

Discovery and Evaluation of Anticancer Drugs

17

Aaron D. Schimmer and Ian F. Tannock

17.1 INTRODUCTION

Chemotherapy is used primarily as (a) the major treatment modality for a few types of malignancies, such as Hodgkin disease and other hematopoietic cancers, acute leukemia in children, and testicular cancer in men; (b) palliative treatment for many types of advanced cancers; and (c) adjuvant treatment before, during, or after local treatment (surgery and/or radiotherapy) with the aim of both eradicating occult micrometastases and of improving local control of the primary tumor. Such treatments usually involve a combination of drugs. The most important factors underlying the successful use of drugs in combination are (a) the ability to combine drugs at close to full tolerated doses with additive effects against tumors and less-than-additive toxicities to normal tissues, and (b) the expectation that drug combinations will include at least 1 drug to which the tumor is sensitive. Since the first documented clinical use of chemotherapy in 1942, when the alkylating agent nitrogen mustard was used to obtain a brief clinical

remission in a patient with lymphoma, about 45 cytotoxic drugs or biological agents (excluding hormonal agents) have been licensed for use in North America, and several more are undergoing clinical trials. The pharmacology of many of these agents is described in Chapter 18. In recent years, new types of anticancer agents have been developed, including monoclonal antibodies (eg, rituximab, trastuzumab, and bevacizumab) that target cell-surface receptors, and small molecules that interact with various cell signaling pathways (eg, imatinib). These newer agents represent a substantial shift in emphasis in anticancer drug therapy. In contrast to conventional cytotoxic agents, which usually target proliferating cells and interact with DNA, the newer agents target specific metabolic pathways that interfere with various functions of the cell, including those that promote cell division (trastuzumab, imatinib) or contribute to immune-mediated cellular damage (rituximab). Other agents, such as those that inhibit angiogenesis (eg, bevacizumab; see Chap. 11, Sec. 11.7.1) act indirectly to inhibit tumor growth.

This chapter deals with the scientific basis of cancer drug discovery. It introduces the concepts of how cancer drug targets are identified and some of the approaches used to discover and design new drugs. The chapter also discusses the biological properties of important anticancer drugs, experimental methods used to determine their activity, their toxicity to normal tissues and the concept of therapeutic index, and the biological basis of using drugs in combination and with radiotherapy. Chapter 18 addresses the pharmacology of anticancer drugs and Chapter 19 describes the many causes of drug resistance.

17.2 STRATEGIES TO DEVELOP ANTICANCER DRUGS

17.2.1 Gene Expression and Identification of Potential Targets for Anticancer Drugs

Although many chemotherapy drugs were developed by observing the ability of compounds to kill cancer cells in culture and in experimental animals without knowledge of a specific molecular target, modern drug discovery begins typically with the identification of a therapeutic target. To identify novel targets, a variety of strategies can be employed, including a survey of the expression of genes within a cancer cell to identify dysregulated genes, gene families, or pathways. DNA microarray analysis can measure the expression of messenger RNA (mRNA) in samples derived from cell lines or primary tissues of patients (Fig. 17–1). Microarray analysis is described in detail in Chapter 2, Section 2.7. The essence of the procedure is that it detects the presence of mRNA transcripts and assesses their relative abundance in the cancer tissue analyzed. Using bioinformatics, computer software, and advanced

statistical analysis, patterns of dysregulated genes and pathways can be identified that can be targeted to develop new cancer drugs. How drugs are developed to inhibit these new targets is discussed in Section 17.2.4.

17.2.2 High-Throughput DNA Sequencing

Cancer drug targets can also be identified by high-throughput DNA sequencing of cell lines or primary patient samples (Hudson et al, 2010). Advances in DNA sequencing have increased the speed and throughput of sequencing and decreased the cost (see Chap. 2, Sec. 2.2.10). These advances have allowed sequencing of primary tumors and normal tissues from multiple patients with malignancy and have identified mutations in oncogenes or tumor-suppressor genes that are prognostic markers and/or potential therapeutic targets. For example, through a focused sequencing effort in patients with acute myeloid leukemia (AML), activating mutations in the FLT3 kinase have been identified. Activation of the membrane-based FLT3 tyrosine kinase is important for the expansion and proliferation of normal early hematopoietic cells. In AML, internal tandem duplication of the juxtamembrane domain results in constitutive activation of this kinase leading to increased proliferation of the leukemic blasts. FLT3 internal tandem duplications are found in 20% to 30% of adult patients with AML and are associated with a higher rate of relapse and worse overall survival (Kottaridis et al, 2001; Thiede et al, 2002). Specific mutations in the coding region of the FLT3 kinase in patients with AML have also been demonstrated to result in its constitutive activation (Frohling et al, 2007). Inhibitors of FLT3 kinase, such as midostaurin and AC220, are being evaluated in clinical trials for patients with AML. Patients with either FLT3 internal tandem duplications or mutations in the coding region are eligible for inclusion in these studies.

FIGURE 17–1 Microarray analysis to study gene expression. mRNA is isolated from cells and is reverse transcribed to complementary DNA (cDNA), which is fluorescently labeled. The cDNA is then hybridized to a microarray chip into which cDNA probe sequences representing tens of thousands of genes in the human genome have been embedded. After hybridization, the chip is washed to remove cDNA that has been bound nonspecifically, and fluorescent signal on each spotted gene is measured. The intensity of the fluorescent signal is proportionate to that amount of bound labeled cDNA and thus the amount of target mRNA in the cell. Using bioinformatics, computer software, and advanced statistical analysis, the abundance of mRNA sequences can be compared between groups of cells. These groups of cells can represent different cell lines, tissues, or treatments. As shown in this example, the mRNA from 1 sample is hybridized to 1 chip. Alternatively, 2 samples labeled with fluorescent probes of different colors can be hybridized to the same chip. See also Chapter 2.

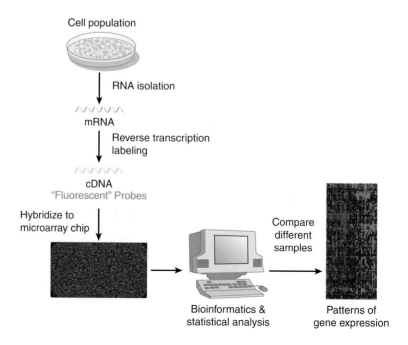

The International Cancer Genome Consortium (ICGC) is undertaking high-throughput sequencing of the entire genomes of approximately 500 tumors from 50 different types and subtypes of cancer, along with normal tissue controls, to identify tumor-specific mutations (Hudson et al, 2010). These studies are expected to identify mutations that contribute to (and are critical for) cancer development and/or growth, known as *driver mutations*, and mutations not associated with cancer development or growth, known as *passenger mutations*. Differentiating between drivers and passengers is a complex process and can require use of advanced statistical analysis, structural studies to investigate the impact of the mutation on the protein structure, and molecular studies to demonstrate transformation as a result of overexpression of the mutant gene (Torkamani et al, 2009). Driver mutations can then be targeted to develop new cancer drugs.

17.2.3 RNA Interference Screening

Potential targets of anticancer drugs can also be identified through RNA interference (RNAi) screening. The introduction of double-stranded RNA sequences leads to degradation of homologous host mRNA sequences with subsequent reductions in expression levels of the target protein (Fig. 17–2; Chap. 2, Sec 2.4.3) through

mechanisms that have not been fully elucidated. However, it appears that upon entry of double-stranded RNA into cells, the endogenous enzyme Dicer digests that RNA into short sequences of approximately 21 nucleotides. These short sequences then interact with the RISC (RNA-induced silencing complex) that matches these sequences to complementary endogenous mRNA. Upon binding, the endogenous mRNA target is degraded leading to reduction in target protein levels. Using this approach, the functional importance of individual gene knockdown can be ascertained. When combined with high-throughput screening, the functional significance of knocking down thousands of genes in the human genome can be evaluated. For example, high-throughput screens have identified kinases critical for the growth of myeloma cell lines such as GRK6 (Tiedemann et al, 2010); inhibitors of such kinases can then be developed and evaluated in clinical trials for patients with multiple myeloma. Similar approaches can be used to identify synergistic therapeutic approaches. Here combinations of drug and RNAi can identify genes whose mutation or knockdown can sensitize cells to the drug of interest. For example, a genome-wide RNAi screen was performed to identify synthetic lethal interactions with the *KRAS* oncogene. The screen identified the kinase PLK1 whose depletion induced death preferentially in *KRAS* mutant cells. Thus, these results suggest that PLK1 inhibitors could be useful in *KRAS* mutant tumors.

17.2.4 Identification of Active Drugs

Once a therapeutic target has been identified several approaches can be used to develop or select for inhibitors of this target.

Chemical libraries can be used for high-throughput screening of large libraries of compounds to identify small molecule leads for novel anticancer drugs. These screens can identify chemical compounds that inhibit the desired target in cell-free assays, by using enzymatic methods or physical binding. Fluorescent polarization is a common high-throughput assay to evaluate drug–target binding; in this method, polarized light is used to measure the speed of rotation or "tumbling time" of a fluorescently labeled molecule. Under fluorescent polarization, the speed of rotation of the molecule is coupled to the emission of light in a polarized plane; small molecules rotate faster and larger molecules rotate more slowly. When the fluorescently labeled molecule (probe) interacts with its target protein, the molecule tumbles more slowly. Drug screening assays search for chemicals that disrupt the interaction between the fluorescently labeled probe and target protein thereby increasing the tumbling of the fluorescent probe. The lead compounds are then investigated for their effects on intact cells.

Alternatively, cell-based screens can be conducted to identify chemical compounds that alter a cancer-associated phenotype of the cells such as their viability, or their ability to migrate or invade in tissue culture models. Follow-up studies are then required to identify the targets and mechanisms

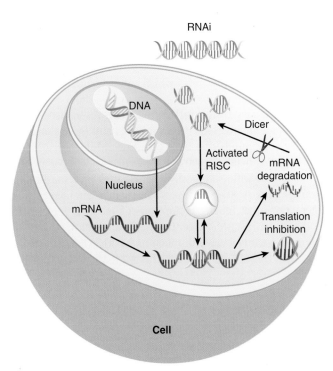

FIGURE 17–2 Proposed mechanism of action of RNAi to silence gene expression. Upon entry of double-stranded RNA into the cytoplasm, the endogenous enzyme Dicer cleaves the RNA into short sequences of approximately 21 nucleotides. These short sequences then interact with the RISC (RNA-inducing silencing complex) that matches these sequences to complementary endogenous mRNA. Upon binding, the endogenous mRNA target is degraded leading to eventual reduction in target protein levels or inhibition of translation by complementary base pairing to the mRNA transcript.

of action of the lead compounds. The chemicals present in these large libraries are usually synthetic compounds that represent diverse types of chemical structures. Smaller and more focused chemical libraries can also be developed to provide more in-depth coverage of a specific type of chemical structure. These focused libraries are useful to help identify more active analogs of compounds identified from a larger screen.

Natural product libraries can also be fruitful sources of leads for novel therapeutic agents. Natural products from, for example, plants and marine life, are isolated initially as extracts containing multiple compounds. Later, the individual chemical compounds are identified and purified, and methods to isolate individual compounds from extracts have improved. In addition, advances in medicinal and synthetic chemistry permit modification of natural products to improve their utility as anticancer agents. Natural products offer some potential advantages over synthetic chemical compounds. For example, they may have unique physical and chemical structures that cannot easily be synthesized. Some extracts from natural products may be sufficiently active to permit their direct evaluation in clinical trials. Multiple chemotherapeutic agents in clinical use are natural products or are derived from them; for example, paclitaxel is a chemotherapeutic agent isolated from the bark of the yew tree. Likewise, the irreversible proteasome inhibitor NPI-0052 is derived from the marine bacterium *Salinispora tropica* and is being investigated in clinical trials for patients with advanced malignancies (Chauhan et al, 2008; Singh et al, 2010).

Libraries of known drugs are another potential source of new anticancer agents. Old drugs with previously unrecognized anticancer activity can be rapidly incorporated in cancer treatments by relying on their prior safety, pharmacokinetic, solubility, and stability data (Table 17–1). A classic example is the development of thalidomide as a novel antimyeloma therapy. Thalidomide was developed initially as a therapy for nausea during pregnancy, but was withdrawn from the market in 1961 because of teratogenicity. In 1999, thalidomide was reported to be active in multiple myeloma and produced a 32% response rate in patients with refractory disease (Sinha et al, 1999). Subsequently, thalidomide in combination with

melphalan and prednisone was shown to prolong survival of older patients when compared to melphalan and prednisone alone (Palumbo et al, 2006). The success of thalidomide led to the development of the second-generation analog lenalidomide that also improves outcomes in patients with multiple myeloma as well as other hematological malignancies, such as myelodysplasia (List et al, 2005; Dimopoulos et al, 2007). The identification of old drugs with unrecognized anticancer activity has been largely serendipitous, but more recently, academics as well as industry have taken a systematic approach to their identification by compiling libraries of on-patent and off-patent drugs and screening these libraries for unrecognized anticancer activity.

Rational drug design can be used to develop therapeutic agents if the 3-dimensional structure of a target is known. These structure-based studies can be used to follow-up on screens of available molecules or can be the starting point to develop the initial lead compounds. Guided by the crystal structure of a protein target, small molecules that bind the active site of the target can be synthesized. These initial compounds are then tested for activity in cell-free and cell-based assays and refinements are made to the chemical structure to improve potency, stability, specificity, and solubility. Thus, through an iterative process, potent and selective drugs are developed. Often, the selection of compounds can be aided by virtual modeling, where chemical structures are docked into target proteins using computer software that recreates 3-dimensional images of the molecule and its protein target. Million-compound libraries can be screened in virtual docking studies to identify "hits," which can be validated in physical binding studies.

Binding assays using nuclear magnetic resonance (NMR) can evaluate interactions between drugs and targets, and can identify compounds that bind with low affinity. Small libraries of approximately 10,000 low-molecular-weight compounds are incubated with isotopically labeled target proteins. Binding of fragments is assessed by NMR, which can detect weak interactions that require concentrations of the 2 components in the 20 to 100 µM range. By chemically linking 2 binding fragments, a molecule with much higher (nM) affinity can be generated (Fig. 17–3). Through this approach, small molecule

TABLE 17–1 Examples of drug repositioning for new anticancer indications.

Drug	Initial Indication	New Anticancer Indication	Stage of Development (in 2012)
Thalidomide	Nausea during pregnancy	Multiple myeloma Myelodysplasia	FDA approved
Celecoxib	Arthritis	Familial adenomatous polyposis	FDA approved
Ketoconazole	Antifungal	Prostate cancer	Phase III trials
Ribavirin	Antiviral	Acute myeloid leukemia	Phase II trials
Clioquinol	Antiparasitic	Myeloma and leukemia	Phase I trials
Ciclopirox olamine	Antifungal	Myeloma and leukemia	Phase I trials

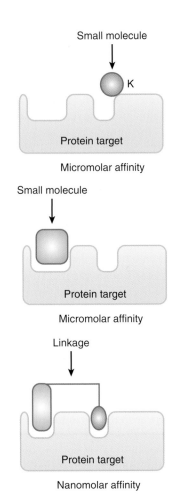

Small molecule

K

Protein target

Micromolar affinity

Small molecule

Protein target

Micromolar affinity

Linkage

Protein target

Nanomolar affinity

FIGURE 17–3 **Methods for evaluation of interactions between a putative drug and its target.** NMR binding studies can aid in the development of novel therapeutic agents for cancer. Using NMR, small fragment-based chemical libraries can be screened searching for small molecules that bind with micromolar affinity. When such fragments bind the target protein in close proximity, the molecules can be linked together chemically to create a new molecule that binds much more avidly with nanomolar affinity.

inhibitors of BCL-2 were developed to promote apoptosis (see Chap. 9, Sec. 9.4.2); this strategy has proven to be capable of inducing regression in experimental models of cancer and one such inhibitor (ABT-263 or navitoclax) is being evaluated in clinical trials (Wilson et al, 2010).

17.3 NEW STRATEGIES FOR CANCER TREATMENT

As discussed above, newer anticancer agents entering clinical use tend to be targeted to specific molecular targets in the cancer cell. These new therapeutic strategies include small molecules that target transmembrane and intracellular kinases, small molecules targeting other intracellular enzymes, antibodies that inhibit or activate cell-surface proteins, small molecules that disrupt protein–protein interactions, and gene knockdown with antisense oligonucleotides or RNAi.

17.3.1 Small Molecule Tyrosine Kinase Inhibitors

Multiple small molecules that target the adenosine triphosphate (ATP)-binding pocket of intracellular kinases have been developed. The first protein tyrosine kinase inhibitor to enter routine clinical use was imatinib, which was developed as an inhibitor of the ABL tyrosine kinase that is dysregulated as a result of the *BCR-ABL* fusion gene (Druker et al, 2001; see Chap. 7; Sec. 7.5.1). This agent, therefore, has activity in tumors that carry abnormalities in these genes and has found initial clinical application in the management of chronic myeloid leukemia (which expresses *BCR-ABL*) where it can induce remission in a large proportion of patients. Mutations in the active site of the ABL kinase can render chronic myeloid leukemia (CML) cells resistant to imatinib and lead to disease progression. Other drugs that inhibit ABL with greater potency than imatinib (eg, nilotinib), and drugs with a wider kinase inhibitory profile (eg, dasatinib) have been developed and approved for the treatment of imatinib-resistant CML (Hochhaus et al, 2007; le Coutre et al, 2008). These agents are superior to imatinib in their ability to induce a major molecular response at 12 months in previously untreated patients with CML, and as a result, this is now the front-line treatment of this disease (Kantarjian et al, 2010; Saglio et al, 2010). Imatinib also inhibits the tyrosine kinases of KIT, the product of the *c-kit* oncogene, and the platelet-derived growth factor receptor (PDGFR). Consistent with this activity, imatinib has activity against gastrointestinal stromal tumors, the majority of which express *c-kit*, and eosinophilic syndromes that have defects in PDGFR signaling.

Although drugs like imatinib highlight the attractiveness of highly specific kinase inhibitors, a growing trend has seen the development of kinase inhibitors that inhibit multiple targets. Examples of such multikinase inhibitors are sunitinib and sorafenib, which inhibit RAF, vascular endothelial growth factor receptor (VEGFR), PDGFR, and c-KIT kinases. These drugs have been shown to provide clinical benefit in the treatment of advanced renal cell and hepatocellular carcinoma (Escudier et al, 2007; Motzer et al, 2007; Llovet et al, 2008).

Small molecules have also been developed that target transmembrane kinases. For example, activation of the transmembrane epidermal growth factor receptor (EGFR) leads to cellular proliferation by activating RAS/RAF/MAPK (mitogen-activated protein kinase), PI3K (phosphatidylinositol-3 kinase)/AKT, and STAT (signal transducer and activator of transcription) signaling pathways (see Chap. 8, Secs. 8.2.4 and 8.2.5). EGFR is mutated or overexpressed in a variety of solid tumors, including non–small cell lung cancer, and this dysregulation contributes to pathogenesis and progression of the disease. Two inhibitors that interact with the ATP-binding pocket of the EGFR kinase have been developed and approved for the treatment of non–small cell lung cancer, gefitinib and erlotinib (Fig. 17–4; Grünwald and Hidalgo, 2003). Predicting which patients are

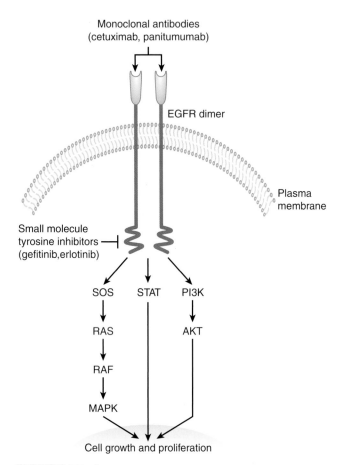

FIGURE 17–4 **Cellular targets for anticancer drugs.**
Targeting the EGFR signaling pathway to develop novel therapeutic agents. Activation of the EGFR signaling pathway promotes cellular proliferation and survival by signaling through the RAS/RAF/MAPK, PI3K/AKT, and STAT pathways. Small-molecule ATP mimics (gefitinib and erlotinib) have been developed that bind and inhibit the enzymatic site of the EGFR kinase. Likewise, humanized monoclonal antibodies (cetuximab and panitumumab) bind the EGFR receptor and inhibit signaling through this pathway.

most and least likely to respond to these newer therapies is an important component of the rational prescription of anticancer therapy. Studies demonstrate that tumors with mutations in *KRAS* have little chance of responding to EGFR inhibitors as the *KRAS* mutation leads to constitutive activation of the signaling pathway downstream of the EGFR receptor (Eberhard et al, 2005; Zhu et al, 2008). Thus, testing for *KRAS* mutations prior to treatment with EGFR inhibitors should help to identify patients most likely to respond.

17.3.2 Enzyme Inhibitors

Small molecules that bind and inhibit the active sites of enzymes important for tumor growth and proliferation have also been developed and are in clinical use. Proteasome inhibitors are an example of this class of agent. The 26S proteasome has as its major function the degradation of cellular proteins, including damaged, misfolded, and regulatory

proteins. Tumor cells require proteasome-dependent turnover of many cell-cycle proteins to complete mitosis successfully (see Chap. 9, Fig. 9–4B), and proteasome inhibitors may induce cell death. Such inhibition can lead to induction of endoplasmic reticulum (ER) stress with activation of the unfolded protein response, inhibition of the nuclear factor-κB (NFκB) inflammatory pathway, increased generation of reactive oxygen species, and activation of Caspase-8 and apoptosis (Hideshima et al, 2001; Chauhan et al, 2005; Bazzaro et al, 2006; Meister et al, 2007). Bortezomib is a covalently bound but reversible inhibitor of the β5-subunit of the proteasome that is used for the treatment of multiple myeloma and mantle cell lymphoma. Additional proteasome inhibitors are under development. Some of these newer proteasome inhibitors are oral agents, and some inhibit the proteasome through mechanisms distinct from bortezomib. For example, carfilzomib inhibits the active site of the proteasome irreversibly; this drug is more potent than bortezomib and can produce clinical responses in bortezomib-resistant patients (Kuhn et al, 2007; Parlati et al, 2009).

Histone deacetylase (HDAC) catalyzes the removal of acetyl groups from lysine residues of nucleosomal histones. The acetylation status of histones influences the regulation of transcriptional activity of some genes, and aberrant activity of HDAC is associated with the development of some malignancies. HDAC inhibitors have been developed that bind the zinc ion in the active site of HDAC, thereby inhibiting its enzymatic function. The HDAC inhibitors vorinostat and romidepsin are used for the treatment of cutaneous T-cell lymphoma (Olsen et al, 2007). These and other HDAC inhibitors are under investigation for the treatment of various malignancies, including AML and myelodysplasia.

Inhibition of the enzyme poly (ADP)-ribose polymerase (PARP), which is involved in DNA repair (see Chap. 5, Sec. 5.8) represents an approach to the development of agents that lead to synthetic lethality—2 genes or pathways are in a synthetic–lethal relationship if mutations or lack of function in either of them alone is not lethal but mutations or lack of function in both of them produce cell death (Fig. 17–5; Table 17–2; Kaelin, 2005; Iglehart and Silver, 2009). Cancers in patients with *BRCA1* and *BRCA2* mutations develop from cells that undergo loss of heterozygosity at these sites. Cells bearing these mutations have impaired DNA repair because of defects in homologous recombination and become dependent on a second mechanism of DNA repair, base-excision repair, for their survival (see Chap. 5, Secs. 5.3.2 and 5.3.4). A key enzyme in this process is PARP, and when PARP inhibitors are given to these patients, both mechanisms of DNA repair are impaired, and cancer cells undergo cell death particularly if exposed to agents that cause DNA damage such as platinum compounds or irradiation (Fig. 17–5; Turner et al, 2004; Iglehart and Silver, 2009). In the clinical development of these compounds, short-interference RNA (siRNA) libraries were used to identify genes that mediate sensitivity to PARP inhibitors including *BRCA1* and *BRCA2* (Turner et al, 2008). The PARP inhibitor

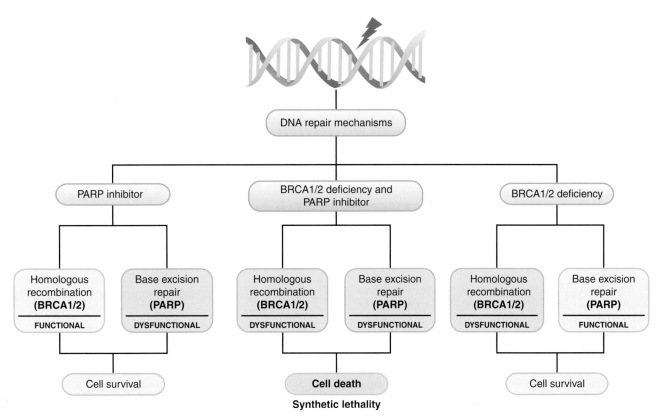

FIGURE 17–5 The concept of synthetic lethality. Cells with BRCA1 or BRCA2 deficiency lack the ability to repair DNA lesions by homologous recombination. Application of a PARP inhibitor, which inhibits the alternative pathway of base excision repair, is then selectively lethal to such cells, which are dependent on this pathway, especially after application of an agent that induces lesions in DNA such as chemotherapy with platinum-containing drugs or radiation. (Adapted from Amir et al, 2010 with permission.)

olaparib was also evaluated in transgenic mice that mimic basal-like human breast cancer, a type of tumor with alterations in DNA-repair mechanisms and with enrichment of *BRCA1* mutations (Rottenberg et al, 2008). Promising results with these compounds have been reported in several tumor types with these molecular alterations. Recent experimental studies also suggest that exposure of cells to prolonged hypoxia, as can occur in tumors, results in reduced DNA repair capacity and the potential for synthetic lethality with PARP inhibitors (Bristow and Hill, 2008).

TABLE 17–2 Properties of tumor cells that could be exploited to provide therapeutic advantage from the combined use of two drugs or of radiation and drugs.

Property	Effect of Combined Treatment
Genetic instability of tumors, leading to different mechanisms of resistance for different clones	Killing of resistant cells by one agent, and removal of surviving cells by the second agent *if* mechanisms of resistance are independent
Two genes or pathways are in a synthetic- lethal relationship if mutations or lack of function in either of them is not lethal but mutations or lack of function in both of them produce cell death	Each agent inhibits the complementary gene or pathway, leading to synthetic lethality
DNA repair	One agent inhibits repair of DNA damage caused by the other; synthetic lethality is a special case where there is inhibition of complementary repair pathways
Differences in cell proliferation between tumor and normal tissue	Selective uptake of radiosensitizing nucleosides (eg, iododeoxyuridine [IUdR])
Differences in repopulation during radiation treatment for tumor and normal tissue	Inhibition of repopulation by drugs could lead to therapeutic advantage *if* repopulation were faster in the tumor
Environmental factors such as hypoxia and acidity, which are usually confined to tumors	Beneficial effects from combining radiotherapy or drugs with greater activity for cycling cells with drugs that have selective toxicity for hypoxic and/or acidic cells

17.3.3 Antibody-Based Anticancer Therapies

Specific inactivating antibodies against the extracellular portion of a membrane-based receptor tyrosine kinase provide an alternative to small-molecule kinase inhibitors that inhibit signaling pathways. One such receptor is human epidermal growth factor receptor-2 (HER2), which does not have a known growth factor ligand, but whose constitutive activity provides intracellular signals leading to cell proliferation. HER2 is amplified or overexpressed in approximately 20% of breast cancers, and is associated with more aggressive disease and a worse prognosis (see Chap. 20, Sec. 20.3.3). In vitro experiments demonstrated that murine monoclonal antibodies directed against the extracellular domain of HER2 were able to inhibit the growth of HER2 overexpressing cell lines, but not of cells expressing normal amounts of the receptor. A humanized form of the most effective of these murine antibodies was developed, in an attempt to prevent the development of neutralizing antibodies, and thus allow long-term use in humans. This compound, trastuzumab, produces a prolongation in survival when used in conjunction with chemotherapy in women with HER2 overexpressing metastatic breast cancer (Slamon et al, 2001), and when used as adjuvant therapy after surgery (Piccart-Gebhart et al, 2005; Romond et al, 2005). To improve the efficacy of these antibodies, conjugates with chemotherapy have also been developed. For example, trastuzumab has been conjugated to the microtubule-disrupting drug DM1 and the conjugate (TDM1) has led to improved survival in women with HER2 positive breast cancer (Verma et al, 2012).

Structurally related to HER2 are the other EGFRs (HER1 or EGFR, HER3, and HER4; see Chap. 7, Sec. 7.5.3). The same approach as described above has been exploited in the development of cetuximab and panitumumab, which are humanized monoclonal antibodies that bind the extracellular domain of the EGFR receptor and prevent EGFR ligands from binding and activating the receptor (Fig. 17–4; Grunwald and Hidalgo, 2003). These antibodies are used for the treatment of advanced colon and head and neck cancer.

Other inhibitor antibodies include bevacizumab, which is a recombinant humanized monoclonal antibody directed against VEGF (Ferrara, 2004). Bevacizumab prevents the ligand VEGF from binding to its receptor, and thereby blocks its action in stimulating angiogenesis (see Chap. 11, Sec. 11.7.1). This drug has clinical efficacy in the treatment of colorectal and several other solid tumors, but clinical benefit is limited, probably because there are multiple alternative signaling pathways that can stimulate angiogenesis. Small molecule inhibitors of VEGF or its receptor such as sunitinib and sorafenib have also been developed and are in clinical use for treatment of kidney cancer.

Activating or agonistic antibodies are also being developed as anticancer agents. Activation of the death receptor pathway of Caspase activation with TRAIL (TNF-related apoptosis-inducing ligand) induces cell death by apoptosis (see Chap. 9, Sec. 9.4.4), and this effect may be greater in malignant cells where there is a high baseline level of cell death. Consequently, humanized monoclonal activating antibodies directed against the DR4 and DR5 TRAIL receptors have been developed and are being evaluated in clinical trials in combination with cytotoxic agents (Buchsbaum et al, 2007).

Other antibody-based therapies target cell-surface proteins that are overexpressed by the tumor cell, but do not activate or inhibit the targets. For example, rituximab is a chimeric monoclonal antibody that binds to the CD20 protein found on the surface of chronic lymphocytic leukemia (CLL) and lymphoma cells, and has clinical benefit when used as a single agent or in combination with chemotherapy. Binding of rituximab to CD20 does not impact the function of this protein, but rather leads to elimination of the malignant cells through a variety of mechanisms, including promotion of antibody- and complement-mediated cytotoxicity (see Chap. 21, Sec. 21.5.2) and induction of apoptosis. Based on the success of rituximab, antibodies directed against other cell-surface proteins have been developed, including alemtuzumab that targets CD52, which is approved for the treatment of T-cell lymphoma and CLL. These antibodies can also be conjugated to radioisotopes to improve their ability to kill the tumor cells.

17.3.4 Disrupting Protein–Protein Interactions

Protein–protein interactions play a critical role in most cellular functions and the development of inhibitors of these interactions for critical proteins is an attractive therapeutic strategy. Vinblastine and vincristine are established cancer therapies that work by this mechanism as they disrupt the interaction between α- and β-tubulin. The relatively large surface area involved in protein–protein interactions has made the development of specific inhibitors of such interactions challenging, but when critical contacts can be localized to small areas of the protein, the development of these inhibitors can be successful. For example, binding assays identified the small molecules ABT-263 and ABT-737 (see Sec. 17.2.4), which binds BCL-2 and its family members in the BH3 pocket and prevents these antiapoptotic proteins from binding to and inhibiting their proapoptotic binding partners (see Chap. 9, Sec. 9.4.2; Kang and Reynolds, 2009). This agent and obatoclax mesylate, a compound with similar activity, are being evaluated for anticancer activity in clinical trials. Small molecules that bind the caspase inhibitor XIAP (X-linked inhibitor of apoptosis) and prevent it from binding to and inhibiting caspases 3 and 9, which are important mediators of apoptosis (see Chap. 9, Sec. 9.4.2), have also been developed and have advanced into clinical trial (Rajapakse, 2007).

17.3.5 Antisense Oligonucleotides and RNAi

Antisense oligonucleotides and RNAi (see Chap. 2, Sec. 2.4.3) act by binding to specific target mRNAs in cancer cells and promoting their degradation. Although RNAi is more effective than antisense oligonucleotides at knocking down protein expression, antisense technology was discovered first and is more advanced in clinical development. Antisense molecules such as oblimersen sodium that target BCL-2 are being evaluated in late-stage Phase III clinical trials for both solid tumors and hematological malignancies (Kang and Reynolds, 2009), but as yet none has been approved for routine clinical use. RNAi therapeutics are also being advanced into clinical trials, but are at an earlier stage of development.

17.3.6 Directed Drug Delivery

A major limitation to the use of nontargeted chemotherapy is lack of selectivity for tumor cells. As new targets that are expressed selectively on tumor cells are characterized, a potential method for increasing the therapeutic index of conventional drugs is to link them to a carrier that may be targeted to tumor cells. Such carriers may include liposomes and other types of nanoparticles, as well as monoclonal antibodies.

A large body of research relates to the entrapment of anticancer drugs in nanoparticles (Petros and DiSimone, 2010), and several agents have now been approved for clinical use. For example pegylated liposomal doxorubicin improved the outcome of patients with Kaposi sarcoma compared to conventional chemotherapy (Northfelt et al, 1998), and it also reduced cardiac toxicity when compared to conventional doxorubicin for treatment of metastatic breast cancer (Batist et al, 2001). Nanoparticle albumin-bound paclitaxel (nab-paclitaxel) may also improve outcome for women with metastatic breast cancer as compared to conventional taxanes (Gradishar et al, 2009). These approved agents are not targeted specifically against molecules expressed selectively on cancer cells, but there are several mechanisms whereby drugs associated with liposomes or other nanoparticles might lead to improvement in therapeutic index relative to free drug: (a) slow, continuous release of the anticancer drug into the circulation, which may protect against organ-specific toxicity (eg, cardiotoxicity caused by doxorubicin) and/or lead to improvement in antitumor effects; (b) fusion of liposomes with cell membranes, leading to efficient internal delivery of drugs, which may overcome drug resistance caused by impaired uptake of free drug; and (c) selective deposition of nanoparticles in tumor tissue, because of their enhanced permeability and retention as a result of the abnormal vasculature of tumors (see Chap. 11, Sec. 11.5.1). Many laboratories are trying to improve on these therapeutic results through the incorporation of molecules that target human cancer cells, but at present this research remains largely preclinical (eg, Byrne et al, 2008; Hirsjärvi et al, 2011).

Several anticancer drugs, as well as potent toxins such as *Pseudomonas* exotoxin, diphtheria toxin, and ricin, have been linked to monoclonal antibodies directed against tumor-associated receptors or other antigens (Teicher, 2009). Several problems have slowed development of this approach, including use of mouse monoclonal antibodies that were immunogenic, insufficient potency because of limited ability to bind sufficient toxins or chemotherapy, and instability of the linkage leading to release of drug or toxin in the circulation with accompanying toxicity. However, trastuzumab emtansine (TDM1), in which the anti-HER2 monoclonal antibody trastuzumab is bound to the microtubule-disrupting drug DM1, has improved survival of women with HER2–positive metastatic breast cancer (Verma et al, 2012).

17.4 PRECLINICAL EVALUATION OF POTENTIAL ANTICANCER DRUGS

Compounds identified through any of the above drug-discovery platforms need to be evaluated in preclinical studies for both their ability to inhibit their putative targets and their potential anticancer effects. There are multiple steps in the evaluation of a potential anticancer drug, and only a small proportion of such agents will eventually enter clinical trials (Ocana et al, 2011; Fig. 17–6). These steps involve identification and verification of the target and mechanism of action, evaluation for activity against cultured tumor cells, and evaluation of activity and toxicity in various in vivo models. It is important to verify the specificity of the target molecule or pathway in animal models and in early clinical trials, as putative targeted agents may sometimes have unexpected toxic effects that are independent of inhibition of the target for which they were designed.

17.4.1 Evaluation of Drugs for Activity Against Cultured Cells

An important phase of preclinical testing involves evaluating whether the candidate agent can either kill or inhibit the proliferation of cancer cells. Screening of candidate drugs requires an initial assay of activity that is rapid and can be automated. Some measures of cell damage that have been used employ dyes such as methyl thiazole tetrazolium (MTT), which depends on the reduction of a tetrazolium-based compound to a blue formazan product by living, but not dead, cells. The amount of reduced product is quantified in an automated system using multiple tissue-culture wells in which cells have been exposed to a range of doses of the drugs under test. Another dye that is useful in quantifying cell number is sulforhodamine B, a pink anionic dye that binds to basic amino acids of fixed cells such that dye intensity is linearly related to the number of cells. These tests assess the number of metabolically active cells in the culture at the time of analysis and hence largely track the effects of the treatment to induce rapid cell death and/or reduced proliferation. In general, they are useful for assessing changes in the number of metabolically active cells by a factor of 10 to 20 (ie, reductions down to 5-10% of control).

Following treatment with drugs, tumor cells may undergo programmed cell death or apoptosis (see Chap. 9, Sec. 9.4.2; Schimmer, 2007; Kang and Reynolds, 2009). Apoptosis can be quantified by various methods (eg, by annexin V and TUNEL [terminal deoxynucleotidyl transferase-mediated

FIGURE 17–6 Preclinical to clinical evaluation of candidate anticancer drugs.
Selected steps in development of anticancer drugs. Drugs are usually evaluated first for activity against cultured cells, followed by solid tumor models in order to reflect the microenvironment of solid tumors. This step is usually followed by demonstration of activity against xenografts generated from implantation of selected human tumor cell lines into immune-deficient mice; xenografts better reflect the properties of the corresponding human tumor if grown in the same tissue of origin (ie, implanted orthotopically). Use of genetically modified (transgenic or knockout) mice allows information about the relation between drug activity and expression of potential target genes. Finally, the drug is evaluated in Phase I studies in humans, which traditionally encompassed a simple evaluation of tolerance and pharmacokinetics and has expanded to provide further information about the molecular target and to identify and validate biomarkers that correlate with drug activity. *MTD*, Maximum tolerated dose. (Adapted from Ocana et al, 2011.)

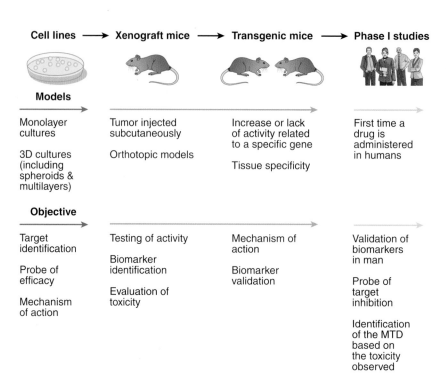

deoxyuridine triphosphate-biotin nick-end labeling] staining) to provide an estimate of the number of cells undergoing apoptosis or an apoptotic index. This index generally increases after drug treatment of tumors, and the proportion of cells undergoing apoptosis may give a broad indication of drug effectiveness. However, there is evidence that radiation and many drugs often kill cancer cells by mechanisms other than apoptosis, and that assays of apoptosis correlate poorly with cell killing assessed by colony-forming assays (Brown and Attardi, 2005). Even where apoptosis is an important mechanism leading to drug-induced cell death, it is a dynamic process whose assessment can be very dependent on when measurements are made during or after treatment.

The important activity of an effective anticancer drug is to cause tumor cells to lose their capacity for indefinite proliferation, and therefore the ability to regenerate the tumor. The above assays, as well as other short-term methods for evaluation of drug effects, including induced morphological changes, or other properties of cancer cells, such as changes in DNA, RNA, or protein synthesis, all suffer from the fundamental limitation that they apply to an unselected population of cells and have limited correlation with loss of reproductive potential of the cells.

Colony-forming assays can be performed following exposure to potential anticancer drugs of established cell lines derived from tumors, primary malignant cells derived from patient samples or normal hematopoietic and other cells (see also Chap. 15, Sec. 15.3.1). In such assays, candidate cells are exposed to various doses of the agent of interest for a fixed time, or to a fixed dose (that is expected to be achievable in vivo) for varying times. The drug is then washed out and

different numbers of cells are evaluated for colony formation in a new environment. If the assay is performed in tissue culture, the number of colonies per cell plated is called the *plating efficiency*, and the ratio of the plating efficiency from drug-treated cells to untreated cells is the *surviving fraction*. The surviving fraction (plotted on a logarithmic scale) can then be plotted against drug dose (for a fixed time exposure) or against time (for exposure to a fixed drug concentration) to produce a survival curve. This assay can usually assess cell surviving fractions down to 10^{-3} to 10^{-4} of control.

Figure 17–7 shows an example of a survival curve. The survival curve is analogous to survival curves generated to describe the dose response to radiation (see Chap. 15, Figs. 15–6 and 15–7), although there is rarely an exponential decrease in cell survival with increasing drug dose as may be observed for radiation. Many chemotherapy drugs (eg, antimetabolites such as cytosine arabinoside and methotrexate) are relatively specific in killing cells in a given phase of the cell cycle (usually S-phase) so there is an initial steep fall in survival as the sensitive cells are killed, but then a flattening of the survival curve. Survival may be further decreased by more prolonged exposure to the drug, although such drugs often also retard entry of cells into the drug sensitive phase. Most drugs, including molecular-targeted agents, are more active against rapidly proliferating cells, even if they are not cell-cycle-phase specific. For these drugs, also, there will be a trend for cell-survival curves to be concave upward, as in Figure 17–7, as higher doses interact with progressively more resistant, slowly proliferating cells.

Drug activity may depend critically on cell–cell interactions, and such interactions are lost when potential drugs

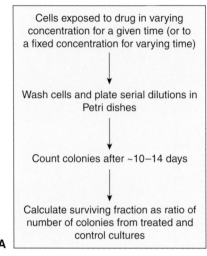
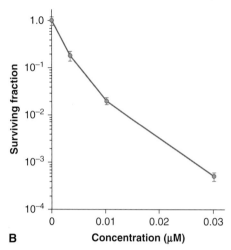

FIGURE 17–7 **Cell survival curves. A)** Cells are exposed either in monolayer or in suspension culture to different doses of a drug for a given time, or to a single dose of the drug for a variable time. The cells are then washed in fresh medium and serial dilutions are plated in Petri dishes; colonies formed from surviving cells are counted, usually 10 to 14 days later. **B)** Experimentally determined cell survival curve for murine EMT6 cells exposed to the drug mitoxantrone. Note that surviving fraction is plotted using a logarithmic scale against dose on a linear scale.

are evaluated against dispersed cells in culture. One model that preserves some of these interactions uses coculture of myeloma plasma cells and stromal bone marrow cells from myeloma patients (Mitsiades et al, 2008). Assays of antimyeloma drugs that determine their ability to preserve activity in this environment are informative about the potentially protective action of stromal components on drug-induced cell death, and about relative effects of the treatment to kill myeloma cells in their microenvironment. Other models that include in vitro-generated blood vessels, or coincubation with immune cells, may offer clues as to antiangiogenic or immunomodulatory properties of the compound of interest. The tumor microenvironment is particularly important for development of drugs with activity against solid tumors. Contact between cells in solid tumors can mediate drug resistance. To be effective drugs must penetrate tissue from blood vessels to reach all of the target tumor cells and achieve a toxic concentration, and should be active under microenvironmental conditions (hypoxia, acidity) that inhibit tumor cell proliferation (see Chap. 12, Sec. 12.2.1 and Chap. 19, Sec. 19.3; Minchinton and Tannock, 2006). Evaluation of drugs in monolayer cell cultures has a limited ability to predict responsiveness in solid tumors, but in vitro models, including tumor spheroids and multilayered cell cultures, can reproduce important properties of solid tumors, such as cellular contact and an extracellular matrix, as well as gradients of nutrient distribution, cell proliferation, and drug access (see Chap. 19, Sec. 19.3.1).

If a potential drug shows activity as assessed by 1 or more of the above assays, it is important to determine its target and mechanism of action. If the agent is designed to target a certain molecule, such as a receptor tyrosine kinase, it is important to show that the agent does, in fact, bind to its target, and that it inhibits downstream signaling from that

target at a concentration that might reasonably be expected to be achieved in subsequent in vivo studies. Helpful strategies might include comparing the sensitivity of cells selected for the presence of, and/or dependence on a particular target or pathway, and of genetically modified cells that are not dependent on the target or pathway. Likewise, insights into mechanism of action can be derived by selecting populations of cells resistant to the drug and using genetic approaches, including gene expression profiling or genetic sequencing to identify mechanism of resistance. In the absence of such evaluation, agents might display nonspecific toxicity that is unlikely to lead to selective antitumor effects in vivo.

17.4.2 Evaluation of Potential Anticancer Drugs In Vivo

The in vitro assays described in the preceding sections assess directly the sensitivity of cultured tumor cells to drug treatment, but they do not assess the impact of the drug's pharmacokinetics or its toxicity to normal cells, both of which are important determinants of the clinical efficacy of a cancer drug. Assays that have been used to assess the effects of drugs on tumors in animals include drug-induced delay in tumor growth and evaluation of colony formation in vitro following treatment of tumors and excision and plating of the tumor cells. Comparison of tumor growth in treated and untreated animals is used most frequently to evaluate drug effects against solid tumors that are transplanted into animals (Fig. 17–8). Tumor shrinkage and delay of regrowth are used to model the clinical assessment of tumor remission, and this approach is relatively humane because animals can be killed painlessly before tumors are sufficiently large to cause discomfort. Drugs that appear promising in in vitro screens are usually evaluated against

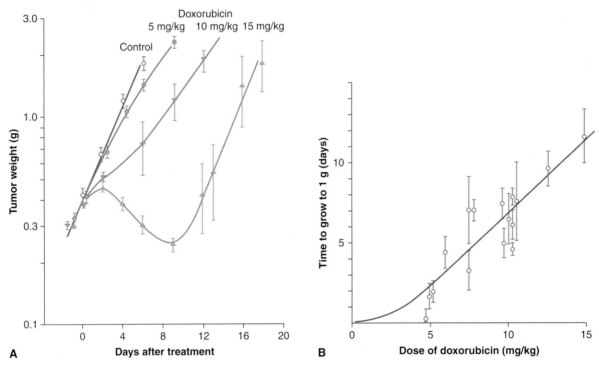

FIGURE 17–8 Tumor growth curve, and dose response relationship. A) Illustration of tumor growth curves for treatment of an experimental tumor with doxorubicin. Tumor weight was estimated by prior calibration with measurements of tumor diameter and is plotted on a logarithmic scale against time on a linear scale. Straight lines then represent exponential growth, and tumor doubling time can be determined from the slope. Note that growth curves after drug treatment are not always parallel to the growth curve for controls and that interanimal variation may lead to large standard errors. **B)** Dose–response curve relating drug dose to the time for tumors to grow from size at treatment (~0.4 g) to 1 g.

syngeneic tumors transplanted into inbred mice, and in xenografts where human tumor cell lines are implanted into immune-deficient mice.

The most widely used host for xenografting of human tumors is the congenitally athymic nude mouse (so called because they lack fur). The nude mouse is not a perfect host because it may produce antibodies and also has large numbers of natural killer cells that may inhibit tumor growth. Alternative hosts include mice with severe combined immune deficiency (SCID) or SCID mice with further mutations to reduce further their ability to reject foreign tissue grafts. These mice may be better recipients for transplanted human tissues and have allowed the establishment of grafts of lymphoid and hemopoietic tissues, as well as of solid tumors. Xenografts possess the advantage that they may have characteristics more similar to those of the human tumors from which they are derived (eg, enzyme activities), as compared to tumors of murine origin. However, xenograft models have several limitations for evaluation of potential new drugs. Firstly, the stromal component of a xenograft is not human, so it is difficult to evaluate the effect of the microenvironment on drug response, or to evaluate drugs such as monoclonal antibodies that may target only human proteins (eg, bevacizumab, which targets human VEGF and does not recognize murine VEGF). Secondly, the rate of growth of xenografts derived from serially transplanted human tumor cell lines is often very rapid (typical doubling times of a few days) compared with that of primary human tumors (typical doubling times of 1 to 3 months), and they are more likely to respond to antiproliferative agents. Thirdly, the animal is immune-compromised so testing of agents with immunomodulatory effects is difficult or impossible. Finally, it may be difficult to select for resistance to drugs using xenograft models, thereby limiting the use of these in vivo models for studying mechanisms of drug resistance.

Transplantation of tumor cells into subcutaneous sites of mice allows easy evaluation of tumor size, but there is evidence that the molecular profile and microenvironment of the tumors is more similar to their human counterpart if they are transplanted orthotopically (eg, mammary tumors are implanted in the mammary fat-pad of female mice, or pancreatic tumors are transplanted into the pancreas of mice) (Nakamura et al, 2007). Humanized mouse models have also been developed; for example, human mammary cells and/or fibroblasts have been transplanted into a cleared mouse mammary gland. Evaluation of tumor growth (or shrinkage after treatment) is more difficult in orthotopic than subcutaneous sites, but is facilitated by a variety of methods for imaging of small animals (see Chap. 14, Sec. 14.4). Also, a gene encoding a marker such as green fluorescent protein (GFP) or luciferase may be introduced and stably expressed in the malignant cells, allowing them to be detected and quantified by optical imaging in the whole animal. This approach allows estimation not only of tumor volume in the primary site, but also enables the following of metastatic spread and the influence of treatment.

Genetically engineered mouse models (GEMMs), in which the expression of a protein is temporally and/or spatially controlled by genetic manipulation, are being used to better assess transformation events and potential anticancer activity related to their inhibition (Sharpless and Depinho, 2006). These transgenic mouse models (see Chap. 2, Sec. 2.4.5) can simulate some aspects of human cancer by introducing alterations in oncogenes or tumor-suppressor genes in germlines of mice. The GEMM can be used in 2 ways in the evaluation of preclinical agents: the treatment of an established tumor, and their effects on tumor prevention. For example administration of the anti-EGFR/HER2 tyrosine kinase inhibitor lapatinib prevents tumor initiation in MMTV (mouse mammary tumor virus)-erbB2 transgenic mice (Strecker et al, 2009), while the mammalian target of rapamycin (mTOR) inhibitor everolimus prevents the formation of colonic adenomas in the Apc(Delta716) heterozygous mouse, which is a model for human familial adenomatous polyposis (Fujishita et al, 2008). Evidence of activity of a drug to prevent or delay tumor formation in the GEMM can give important insight into mechanisms of activity, and may indicate molecular properties of a tumor (ie, biomarkers; see Fig. 17–6) that may correlate with increased likelihood of activity. However, activity of a drug in the GEMM does not necessarily imply that the drug will also be active in treating tumors with similar types of genetic change.

The benefits of the GEMM for preclinical evaluation of potential anticancer drugs include: (a) that the tumor has developed in an immune-competent animal, and (b) genetic alterations can be modified in a time- and tissue-specific manner. For example, regulatory elements in the inserted transgenic DNA that are sensitive to tetracycline or tamoxifen can be incorporated in these mouse models, so that administration of these well-tolerated drugs to the mice can turn on or off specific molecular pathways (Kistner et al, 1996). However, GEMMs are imperfect models for human tumors, where there are often multiple genetic abnormalities, because the initial molecular alterations in the mice are limited to the ones that have been introduced. However, further mutations in GEMMs may restore activity of a defective molecular pathway. Also the stroma and other normal tissue elements are derived from the rodent, and usually have the same genetic alteration as the tumor. To avoid these potential caveats, some investigators have transplanted the tumors generated in the transgenic mice subsequently into wild-type mice. Transplantation also offers the possibility of shortcutting the long latency for appearance of spontaneous tumors and the possibility of treating genetically similar transplants with different drugs. Thus far, GEMMs have been used more often for the study of the transformation process than for evaluation of novel drugs.

A limitation of most of the above in vitro and in vivo assays of drug activity is that they evaluate relatively short-term effects against cells that have been selected to grow in culture or in mice. However, there is evidence, described in Chapter 13, that tumors may contain a small population of cells with indefinite proliferation, or *tumor stem cells*, and if so, it is these cells that are the appropriate targets of therapy that may lead to long-term remission or cure. Recently, there have been attempts to screen drugs for activity against tumor cells bearing cell-surface markers that indicate an enriched stem cell population, and compounds with selective activity against such cells were identified (Hassane et al, 2008; Gupta et al, 2009). One approach to evaluating the ability of a drug to target the stem cell fraction is to treat the cells in culture or in immunodeficient mice with the drug or buffer control and then inject the treated tumor cells into further immunodeficient mice. The primary transplants, along with secondary transplants where cells from the primary mice are injected into secondary recipients, can be used to evaluate the effects of the drug on the stem cell fraction. When the stem cells are targeted and killed, the treated tumor cells do not engraft in the secondary mice (Jin et al, 2006).

17.4.3 Relationship Between Tumor Remission and Cure

For most solid tumors the limit of clinical and/or radiological detection is about 1 g of tissue (10^9 cells). If therapy can reduce the number of malignant cells below this limit of detection, the patient will be described as being in complete clinical remission. Surgical biopsy of sites that were known to be involved with tumor previously may lower the limit of detection, especially if immunohistochemistry is used to identify specific markers on tumor cells, but a pathologist is unlikely to detect sporadic tumor cells present at a frequency of less than 1 in 10,000 normal cells. Therefore, even a surgically confirmed complete remission may be compatible with the remaining presence of a large number of tumor cells (up to 10^5/g tissue). Tumor cure requires eradication of all tumor cells that have the capacity for tumor regeneration. The proportion of such stem cells among those of the tumor population is unknown, but clinical and even surgically confirmed complete remissions are compatible with the presence of a substantial residual population of surviving tumor stem cells.

High doses of radiation therapy may lead to local tumor control (or to cure in the absence of metastasis) and small groups of mice can be treated with different doses of radiation to their tumors and assayed for tumor remission and long-term recurrence; this approach allows identification of the dose of radiation that will control 50% of the tumors (tumor control dose 50% [TCD_{50}], see Chap. 16, Sec. 16.3.1). Only rarely can tolerated doses of systemic agents cure tumors in mice, and multiple treatments are usually necessary, but when that is possible related experiments can be formulated to define the dose and schedule that leads to cure in 50% of the animals. An advantage of such assays is that they evaluate drug effects against tumor stem cells.

17.5 TOXICITY OF ANTICANCER DRUGS

17.5.1 The Concept of Therapeutic Index

In addition to their antitumor effects, all anticancer drugs are toxic at some level to normal tissues, and it is this toxicity that limits the dose of drugs that can be administered to patients. The relationship between the probability of a biological effect of a drug and the administered dose is usually described by a sigmoid curve (Fig. 17–9), although it is possible that for targeted agents there is an optimal dose where the target is completely inhibited and using higher doses only augments the toxicity. If the drug is to be useful, the curve describing the probability of antitumor effect (eg, complete clinical remission) must be displaced toward lower doses as compared with the curve describing the probability of major toxicity to normal tissues (eg, myelosuppression leading to infection). The *therapeutic index* (or *therapeutic ratio*) may be defined from such curves as the ratio of the dose required to produce a given probability of toxicity and the dose required to give a defined effect against the tumor. The therapeutic index in Figure 17–9 might be represented by the ratio of the drug dose required for a 5% level of probability of severe toxicity (sometimes referred to as toxic dose 05 [TD_{05}]) to that required for 50% probability of antitumor effect (ie, effective dose 50 [ED_{50}]). Any stated levels of probability might be used. The appropriate end points of tumor response and toxicity will depend on the limiting toxicity of the drug and the intent of treatment (ie, cure versus palliation). Improvement in the therapeutic index is the goal of systemic treatment. However, although dose–response curves similar to those of Figure 17–9 have been defined in animals, they have rarely been obtained for drug effects in humans. They emphasize the important concept that any modification in treatment that leads to increased killing of tumor cells in tissue culture or animals must be assessed for its effects on critical normal tissues prior to therapeutic trials.

Toxicity to normal tissues limits both the dose and frequency of drug administration. Many drugs cause toxicity because of their preferential activity against rapidly proliferating cells, and this is especially true for chemotherapy, but also for some targeted agents—normal adult tissues that maintain a high rate of cellular proliferation include the bone marrow, intestinal mucosa, hair follicles, and gonads (see Chap. 12, Sec. 12.1.3). Nausea, vomiting, fatigue, and carcinogenic effects are also common side effects of many drugs. In addition, several drug-specific toxicities to other tissues of the body may be observed. The biological basis for toxic damage to normal tissues that may occur through a common mechanism is discussed below, whereas toxic effects specific for individual drugs are described in Chapter 18. Targeted agents, in particular, may cause a variety of side effects that are not specific to rapidly proliferating tissues.

17.5.2 Toxicity to Bone Marrow and Scheduling of Treatment

Within the bone marrow there is evidence for a pluripotent stem cell that under normal conditions proliferates slowly to replenish cells in the myelocytic, erythroid, and megakaryocytic lineages (Fig. 17–10A). Lineage-specific precursors proliferate more rapidly than stem cells, whereas the morphologically recognizable but immature precursor cells (eg, myeloblasts) have a very rapid rate of cell proliferation. Beyond a certain stage of maturation, proliferation ceases and the cells mature into circulating blood cells. The relationship between proliferation and maturation in bone marrow precursor cells provides a plausible explanation for the observed fall and recovery of blood granulocytes (and more rarely of platelets) that follows treatment with most chemotherapy drugs (Fig. 17–10B). Proliferation-dependent cytotoxic drugs, including most types of chemotherapy, deplete the rapidly proliferating cells in the earlier part of the maturation series, with minimal effects against the more mature nonproliferating cells and against slowly proliferating stem cells. Blood counts may remain in the normal range while the more mature surviving cells continue to differentiate but will then fall rapidly at a time when the cells depleted earlier would normally have completed maturation. A substantial decrease in the number of mature cells is common for granulocytes because their lifetime is only 1 to 2 days, less common for platelets (lifetime of a few days), and rare for red blood cells (mean lifetime of approximately 120 days), but it may also be influenced by differences in the intrinsic sensitivities of their precursor cells for different drugs. The number of mature granulocytes usually

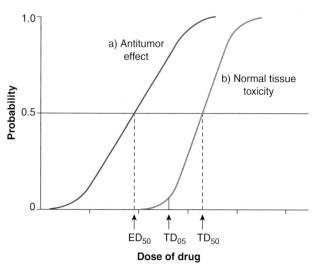

FIGURE 17–9 Concept of Therapeutic Index. Schematic relationship between dose of a drug and the probability of a given measure of antitumor effect (*curve a*), and the probability of a given measure of normal-tissue toxicity (*curve b*). Heterogeneity among tumors often leads to a shallower slope of the line representing tumors, as shown in red. The therapeutic index might be defined as the ratio of doses to give 50% probabilities of normal-tissue damage and antitumor effects. However, if the end point for toxicity is severe (eg, sepsis as a result of bone marrow suppression), it would be more appropriate to define the therapeutic index at a lower probability of toxicity (eg, toxic dose [TD_{05}]/effective dose [ED_{50}]).

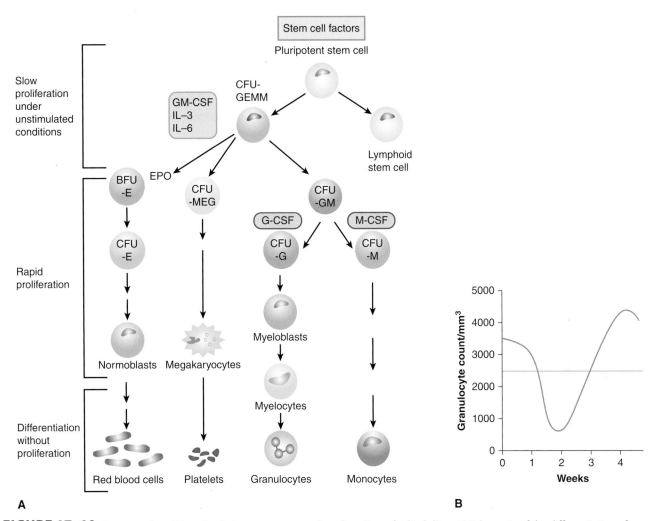

FIGURE 17–10 **Pattern of proliferation in bone marrow and explanation of scheduling. A)** Schematic of the differentiation of hematopoietic precursor cells in the bone marrow, leading to the production of red blood cells, platelets, granulocytes, and monocytes. *CFU,* colony-forming unit; *BFU,* blast-forming unit; *E,* erythroid; *MEG,* megakaryocytic; *G,* granulocytic; *M,* monocytic. Various cells are stimulated to proliferate and/or differentiate by the growth factors interleukin (IL)-3 and -6, granulocyte-macrophage colony-stimulating factor (GM-CSF), granulocyte colony-stimulating factor (G-CSF), monocyte colony-stimulating factor (M-CSF), erythropoietin (EPO), stem cell factors (eg, Sox2, Klf4, Nanog), and others; only their main target cells are indicated here. Under normal conditions, the early precursor cells proliferate slowly, intermediate precursors proliferate rapidly (in the megakaryocytic series there is nuclear replication without cell division) to expand the population, and later precursors of the functional cells differentiate without further cell division. **B)** Fall and recovery of the peripheral granulocyte count after chemotherapy. For most drugs the count falls to a nadir at 10 to 14 days after treatment, with complete recovery by 3 to 4 weeks.

decreases at 8 to 10 days after treatment with drugs such as cyclophosphamide, doxorubicin, or paclitaxel, but may do so earlier for other drugs (eg, vinblastine). The variation in time from treatment to the fall in peripheral blood counts for different drugs probably reflects their different effects on the rate of cell maturation. When the peripheral granulocyte count falls, proliferation of stem cells is mediated by release of growth factors, with subsequent recovery of the entire bone marrow population. Administration of growth factors (eg, granulocyte colony-stimulating factor [G-CSF]) after chemotherapy can accelerate the reappearance of mature cells in the peripheral blood and decrease the possibility of infection that can occur in the absence of mature granulocytes. For many drugs (eg, cyclophosphamide, doxorubicin, taxanes), recovery of

peripheral blood counts is complete at approximately 3 weeks after therapy (or at ~2 weeks if growth factors are given), and further treatment may be given with little or no evidence of residual damage to bone marrow.

Following treatment with some drugs, such as melphalan, or with wide-field radiation to a high proportion of the bone marrow, recovery of mature granulocytes and platelets to normal levels is slower, usually requiring approximately 6 weeks after treatment. Drugs that produce prolonged myelosuppression cause direct damage to slowly or nonproliferating stem cells. Thus recovery is delayed because of repopulation from a smaller number of bone marrow stem cells, and some damage may be permanent because of incomplete repopulation of the stem cell pool.

Recovery of blood counts after treatment with anticancer drugs is the usual determinant of the interval between courses of chemotherapy. If myelosuppressive drugs are given when peripheral blood counts are low, they will not only delay recovery and increase the chance of infection and bleeding, but will also have a higher chance of depleting the stem cell population, because it is likely to be proliferating rapidly. Drug administration can be repeated up to 1 week after initial treatment, before the decrease in mature granulocytes and platelets is observed; this schedule has been incorporated into several drug regimens where anticancer drugs are given on days 1 and 8 of a 21- or 28-day cycle. Some drugs (eg, bleomycin, vincristine, and many of the newer targeted agents) cause only minimal toxicity to bone marrow, probably because of intrinsic resistance of the precursor cells; they can be given when peripheral granulocyte and platelet counts are low following the use of myelosuppressive agents.

Red blood cells have a long lifetime, which usually prevents the rapid development of anemia following initiation of chemotherapy. However, repeated courses of chemotherapy cause repeated interruptions of red blood cell production so that the serum level of hemoglobin tends to decrease slowly, leading to anemia and contributing to fatigue. This effect can occur with all types of drug therapy, but occurs more rapidly following the use of some drugs, such as cisplatin. Injection of erythroid-stimulating agents, which are analogs of the growth factor erythropoietin, can be used to stimulate production of red blood cells, thus minimizing the effects of chemotherapy to cause anemia and reducing the associated fatigue. However, these agents must be used with caution, as some tumor cells may also express the erythropoietin receptor and be stimulated by these agents, and they have also been shown to induce thrombosis in people with near-normal levels of hemoglobin, which may be life-threatening (Hadland and Longmore, 2009).

Chemotherapy is scheduled most often using intermittent large doses, but there is evidence that continuous daily administration of low doses of drugs (known as *metronomic therapy*) can give superior effects in animal models, perhaps because of superior effects against tumor blood vessels (Kerbel and Kamen, 2004). Although such schedules can have activity (and low toxicity) against some human tumors, there is no evidence as yet that they provide better long-term outcomes.

Many of the molecular-targeted agents described in Section 17.3 require chronic administration to provide sustained inhibition of their target receptor or pathway. Monoclonal antibodies such as trastuzumab or cetuximab have long half-lives in the circulation, and sustained levels can be achieved by dosing at weekly intervals or less often. However, most inhibitors of receptor tyrosine kinases are small molecules that are given orally (eg, everolimus, an inhibitor of mTOR) and these agents are most often given on a continuous daily schedule. Many of these agents inhibit pathways that stimulate proliferation of cancer (and other cells) and although when used alone they do not usually lead to myelosuppression, they can add substantially to this and other toxicities when used in combination with chemotherapy, and a dose reduction of both agents is then generally required.

17.5.3 Toxicity of Drugs to Other Proliferative Tissues

Ulceration of the mucosa in the mouth, throat, esophagus, or intestine may also occur after treatment with antiproliferative drugs, and can lead to soreness, intestinal bleeding, and diarrhea. It is caused by interruption of the production of new cells that normally replace the mature cells continually being sloughed into the intestine (see Chap. 12, Fig. 12–4). Damage to bone marrow is more commonly dose-limiting in humans, but mucosal ulceration may occur after treatment with several drugs, including methotrexate, 5-fluorouracil, bleomycin, and cytosine arabinoside; it may also occur after treatment with several targeted agents, including sunitinib and sorafenib, presumably because they inhibit proliferation and maturation in mucosal epithelium. Mucosal damage usually begins approximately 5 days after treatment, and its duration increases with the severity. Full recovery is usually possible if the patient can be supported through this period; recovery is analogous to that in the bone marrow, with repopulation from slowly proliferating stem cells.

Partial or complete hair loss is common after treatment with many anticancer drugs and is a result of lethal effects of drugs against proliferating cells in hair follicles; this usually begins approximately 2 weeks after treatment. Full recovery usually occurs after cessation of treatment, suggesting the presence of slowly proliferating precursor cells. In some patients, regrowth of hair is observed despite continued treatment with the agent that initially caused its loss. Regrowth of hair might reflect a compensating proliferative process that increases the number of stem cells, or may represent the development of drug resistance in a normal tissue akin to that which occurs in tumors.

Spermatogenesis in men and formation of ovarian follicles in women both involve rapid cellular proliferation and are susceptible to the toxic effects of many anticancer drugs. Men who receive chemotherapy often have decreased production of sperm and consequent infertility. Testicular biopsy usually demonstrates a loss of germinal cells within the seminiferous tubules, presumably because of drug effects against these rapidly proliferating cells. Antispermatogenic effects may be reversible after lower doses of chemotherapy, but some men remain permanently infertile; it is now usual to recommend sperm banking for young men who undergo intensive chemotherapy for potentially curable malignancies such as Hodgkin disease or testicular cancer. Chemotherapy given to premenopausal women often leads to temporary or permanent cessation of menstrual periods and to menopausal symptoms, and is accompanied by a fall in serum levels of estrogen. Reversibility of this effect depends on age, the types of drug used, and the duration and intensity of chemotherapy. Biopsies taken from the ovaries have shown failure of formation of ovarian follicles, sometimes with ovarian fibrosis. The pathological findings are consistent with a primary effect of drugs against the proliferating germinal epithelium.

17.5.4 Nausea, Vomiting, and Other Common Toxicities

Nausea and vomiting are frequent during the first few hours after treatment with many types of chemotherapy, but occur rarely after use of targeted agents. Drug-induced vomiting may occur because of direct stimulation of chemoreceptors in the brainstem, which then emit signals via connecting nerves to the neighboring vomiting center, thus eliciting the vomiting reflex. Major evidence for this mechanism comes from studies in animals, where induction of vomiting by chemotherapy is prevented by removal of the chemoreceptor zone. In addition to a central mechanism, some chemotherapeutic agents exert direct effects on the gastrointestinal tract that may contribute to nausea and vomiting. Several neurotransmitters, such as serotonin (5-HT$_3$) and substance P are involved in transmitting signals involved in producing nausea and vomiting. Medications have been developed that inhibit nausea and vomiting after chemotherapy. The most effective of these are the serotonin antagonists (such as ondansetron, tropisetron, and granisetron), which block 5-HT$_3$ receptors, and the neurokinin 1 (NK1) receptor antagonists (such as aprepitant), which block substance P.

Some drugs can produce diarrhea without directly damaging the intestinal mucosa. For example, irinotecan can produce diarrhea soon after administration as a consequence of a direct cholinergic effect on the cells of the intestinal mucosa. This type of diarrhea may be prevented through the use of anticholinergic drugs. A second form of diarrhea, secretory in nature, may occur several days following administration of irinotecan, and may be a result of damage to the mucosa coupled with cytokine release causing fluid secretion (see Chap. 18, Sec. 18.4.1).

Fatigue is a common side effect of both the presence of cancer and its treatment, and several types of chemotherapy (eg, taxanes) and targeted agents that inhibit multiple receptors (eg, sunitinib, sorafenib, and pazopanib) can cause profound fatigue. Unfortunately there are no pharmacological treatments that have been found to relieve fatigue, and the only strategy of proven benefit is exercise, possible only for select patients with metastatic cancer.

The hand-foot syndrome (or palmar-plantar erythrodysesthesia) may occur during treatment with several types of chemotherapy (eg, capecitabine) and with targeted agents such as sunitinib and sorafenib (Lipworth et al, 2009). Patients have redness and pain on the palms of the hands and soles of the feet, sometimes with blistering and desquamation, which can be quite disabling. The condition responds to reduction of dose of the anticancer drug. The cause of this condition is uncertain, although it might relate in part to sensitivity of proliferating cells in the basal layer of the skin in these sites.

Subtle cognitive dysfunction has also been identified as a side effect of chemotherapy, especially in women who are receiving adjuvant chemotherapy for breast cancer (Ahles et al, 2007; Vardy et al, 2007). The mechanisms underlying these effects are unknown; they may be mediated in part by changes in the levels of sex hormones and induction of menopausal symptoms, but are probably also a result of direct effects of anticancer drugs on the brain.

17.5.5 Drugs as Carcinogens

Many anticancer drugs cause toxic damage through effects on DNA; they can also cause mutations and chromosomal damage. These properties are shared with known carcinogens (see Chap. 4), and patients who are long-term survivors of such chemotherapy may be at an increased risk for developing a second malignancy. This effect has become apparent only under conditions where chemotherapy has resulted in long-term survival for some patients with drug-sensitive diseases (eg, Hodgkin disease, other lymphomas, testicular cancer) or where it is used as an adjuvant to decrease the probability of recurrence of disease following local treatment (eg, breast cancer). Many of the second malignancies are acute leukemias, and their most common time of presentation is 2 to 6 years after initiation of chemotherapy. Increased incidence of solid tumors may also be observed after longer periods of follow up. Alkylating agents are the drugs most commonly implicated as the cause of second malignancy, and there is increased risk if patients also receive radiation. It is often difficult to separate an increase in the probability of second malignancy that may be associated with the primary neoplasm (eg, in a patient with lymphoma) or with a shared etiological factor, either environmental or as a result of genetic predisposition, from that associated with treatment.

Comparisons of the incidence of leukemia and other malignancies in clinical trials that randomize patients to receive adjuvant chemotherapy or no chemotherapy after primary treatment have given conclusive evidence of the carcinogenic potential of some drugs. The relative risk of leukemia in drug-treated, as compared with control patients, was increased in women receiving adjuvant therapy for breast cancer that included an alkylating agent (especially when melphalan was used) but for modern regimens that include conventional dose cyclophosphamide there is no significant increase in relative risk (Curtis et al, 1992). There is a 2- to 3-fold increased relative risk of endometrial cancer following use of tamoxifen, but the absolute risk is below 1% and most are curable by surgery (Matesich and Shapiro, 2003). Drugs that target topoisomerase II (eg, doxorubicin, epirubicin, mitoxantrone, and etoposide; see Chap. 18, Sec. 18.4) have also been identified as causes of treatment-related leukemia, with a relative risk of approximately 1.5 compared to those not receiving this treatment (Patt et al, 2007). Leukemias that occur following treatment with these drugs have a limited number of characteristic chromosomal translocations that distinguishes them from those that occur following alkylating agents, and they tend to occur after a shorter latent period of 1 to 3 years after treatment of their primary cancer (Mistry et al, 2005).

The risk of second solid tumors following treatment with chemotherapy is far lower than that of leukemia. Nonetheless, a 4.5-fold increase in the risk of transitional cell carcinoma of the urothelium has been demonstrated in patients who had received cyclophosphamide for the treatment of non-Hodgkin lymphoma (Travis et al, 1995), and there is an increased risk of breast and other cancers in patients who are treated for Hodgkin lymphoma with radiotherapy or chemotherapy, and especially in those receiving both treatments. The absolute risk of second malignancy is small compared with the potential benefits in treating curable cancers but care is needed in using carcinogenic drugs as adjuvant chemotherapy for malignancies where benefit is minimal.

17.5.6 Determinants of Normal-Tissue Toxicity

When chemotherapy is given to a patient, a drug dose is selected on the basis of early phase clinical trials that have determined the *average* dose (usually per unit of body surface area) that gives some toxicity, but at an acceptable level. At this dose, there may be a small proportion of patients, who experience severe, potentially lethal toxicity. Multiple factors influence the distribution of drugs to tissues in the body (see Chap. 18, Sec. 18.1) and the response of normal cells to these drugs. Some patients have genetically determined traits that influence drug metabolism or excretion, and the study of genetically determined factors that influence the probability of drug toxicity is known as pharmacogenetics (see Chap. 3, Sec. 3.6.2 and Chap. 18, Sec. 18.3.1). For example, patients who lack the enzyme dihydropyrimidine dehydrogenase (DPD), which catabolizes 5-fluorouracil show extreme sensitivity to this drug (see Chap. 18, Sec. 18.3.2; Milano et al, 1999). Genetic abnormalities that give rise to the DPD-deficient phenotype have been identified, and screening tests can identify susceptible individuals. Changes in the activity of enzymes that metabolize other drugs, either genetically determined or induced by concomitant medications, may also have a profound effect on drug-induced toxicity.

Because lethal damage caused by chemotherapy results most often from interaction of drugs with DNA, patients with deficiencies in DNA repair (see Chap. 5, Sec. 5.5) are very sensitive to anticancer drugs, as they are to radiation. People who are heterozygous for such gene mutations (eg, xeroderma pigmentosum or ataxia telangiectasia) may also be at high risk for severe toxicity if treated by chemotherapy. Predictive assays, based on assessing chromosomal damage in lymphocytes, are being developed that could allow identification of individuals who may exhibit extreme radio- (and possibly chemo-) sensitivity (Pfuhler et al, 2011). However, the clinical utility of such tests will need to be evaluated carefully, given the low prevalence of the abnormalities being tested, although such individuals may be overrepresented among cancer patients (see also Chap. 5, Table 5–1).

17.6 TREATMENT WITH MULTIPLE AGENTS

17.6.1 Influence on Therapeutic Index

Patients are treated frequently with drug combinations or with drugs and radiation therapy. When 2 or more agents are combined to give an improvement in the therapeutic index, this implies that the increase in toxicity to critical normal tissues is less than the increase in damage to tumor cells. Because the dose-limiting toxicity to normal tissues may vary for different drugs and for radiation, 2 agents are often combined with only minimal reduction in doses as compared with those that would be used if either agent were given alone. Additive effects against a tumor with less than additive toxicity for normal tissue may then lead to a therapeutic advantage. Mechanisms by which different agents may give therapeutic benefit when used in combination have been classified by Steel and Peckham (1979) as follows: (a) independent toxicity, which may, for example, allow combined use of anticancer drugs at full dosage; (b) spatial cooperation, whereby disease that is missed by one agent (eg, local radiotherapy) may be treated by another (eg, chemotherapy); (c) protection of normal tissues; and (d) enhancement of tumor response, where there is selective sensitization of effects of one agent against tumor cells by another.

The above mechanisms suggest guidelines for choosing drugs that might be given in combination. Most drugs exert dose-limiting toxicity for the bone marrow, but this is not the case for vincristine (dose-limiting neurotoxicity), cisplatin (nephrotoxicity), or bleomycin (mucositis and lung toxicity). Some (but not all) of these drugs can be combined with myelosuppressive agents at close to full dosage and have contributed to the therapeutic success of drug combinations used to treat lymphoma and testicular cancer. Most trials of combined chemotherapy and targeted agents have led to increased toxicity and a requirement for dose reduction, even though the targets of the drugs are different. Most such combinations have employed concurrent treatment, which is conceptually counterintuitive: targeted agents often act initially to inhibit proliferation of target cells, which might then protect them from cycle-active chemotherapy. A more logical schedule may be to use chemotherapy and targeted agents in sequence, and might have the added advantage of inhibiting tumor cell repopulation in the intervals between chemotherapy (see Chap. 19, Sec. 19.3.4; Kim and Tannock, 2005).

17.6.2 Synergy and Additivity

Claims are made frequently that 2 agents are synergistic, implying that the 2 agents given together are more effective than would be expected from their individual activities. Confusion has arisen because of disagreement as to what constitutes an expected level of effect when 2 noninteracting agents are combined. The use of multiple agents may lead to an increase in the therapeutic index, but it is rare that a claim for synergy of effects against a single population of mammalian cells can be substantiated (Ocana et al, 2012). Two methods have been used to evaluate possible synergy, additivity, or antagonism between 2 agents: isobologram analysis as proposed by Steel and Peckham (1979) and calculation of an "interaction index," based on the median effect principle (Chou and Talalay, 1984; Lee et al, 2007).

The above concepts require consideration of the dose–response relationship following treatment of a single population of cells either in a tumor or in a normal tissue, by either agent alone, or of a combination of the two agents. Thus, suppose a given dose of agent A gives a surviving fraction of cells (S_A), that a surviving fraction (S_B) follows treatment with a given dose of agent B, and a combination of the agents gives a surviving fraction (S_{AB}; Fig. 17–11). Claims for synergy are often made if S_{AB} is less than the product $S_A \times S_B$. This conclusion is correct only if cell survival is exponentially related to dose for both agents. If the survival curves have an initial shoulder, as in Figure 17–11, then combined treatment will be expected to lead to a lower level of survival if, after treatment with the first agent, A, the survival falls exponentially with dose (in the absence of a shoulder effect) for the second agent, B (Fig. 17–11). The fallacy of defining this lower level of survival as a synergistic effect can be illustrated by replacing agent B with a second, equivalent dose of agent A given immediately after the first dose: the combined survival curve then follows that for agent A (Fig. 17–11A). If agent A has a survival

curve with an initial shoulder, one would then conclude erroneously that agent A was synergistic with itself.

The above discussion implies that there is a range over which 2 agents can produce additive effects. Isobologram analysis provides a method for defining this range of additivity (Steel and Peckham, 1979). Dose–response curves are first generated for each agent used alone. These dose–response curves are then used to generate isoeffect plots (known as *isobolograms*). These curves relate the dose of agent A to the dose of agent B that would be predicted, when used in combination, to give a constant level of biological effect (eg, cell survival) for the assumptions of (a) independent damage and (b) overlapping damage (Fig. 17–12). These curves define an envelope of additivity. If, when the 2 agents are given together, the doses required to give the same level of biological effect lie within the envelope, the interaction is said to be *additive*. If they lie between the lower isobologram and the axes (ie, the combined effect is caused by lower doses of the 2 agents than predicted) the interaction is *supraadditive* or synergistic. If the required doses of the 2 agents in combination lie above the envelope of additivity (ie, the effect is caused by higher doses than predicted), the interaction is *subadditive* or antagonistic (Fig. 17–12).

The median effect principle represents an alternative method of evaluating additivity or synergy between agents and a simplified explanation of the principle has been provided (Chou, 2010). The method also depends on the availability of a

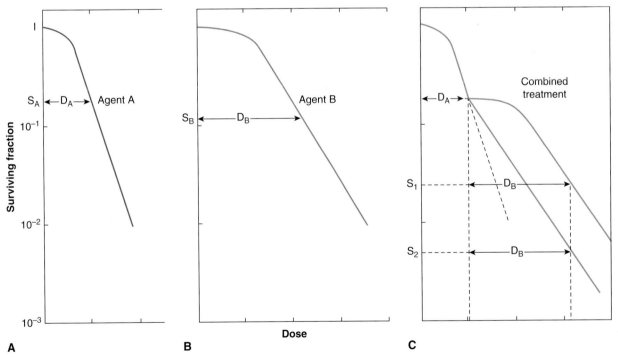

FIGURE 17–11 **Interaction of 2 agents A and B. A, B)** Cell survival (S_A or S_B) is indicated following treatment with either of 2 agents, A and B, each of which has a survival curve characterized by an initial shoulder followed by an exponential fall with increasing dose. **C)** Survival (S_{AB}) after combined use of dose D_A of agent A and dose D_B of agent B will be equal to $S_1 = (S_A \times S_B)$ if there is no overlap of damage, and the "shoulder" representing accumulation of sublethal damage is retained for the second agent. Survival after combined treatment (S_{AB}) will be equal to S_2 if cells have accumulated maximum sublethal damage from the first agent A, and the "shoulder" of the curve is lost for the second agent, B.

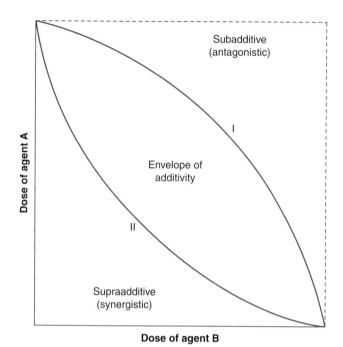

FIGURE 17–12 Isobologram analysis. Isobologram relating the doses of 2 agents that would be expected to give a constant level of biological effect when used together. It was generated from dose–response curves for each agent separately. Assumptions about overlap or non-overlap of damage (see Fig. 17–11) lead to the generation of 2 isobologram curves (I and II) that describe an envelope of additive interaction. Experimental data falling outside this envelope may indicate synergistic or antagonistic interactions, as shown. (Adapted from Steel and Peckham, 1979.)

dose–effect relationship for each of the agents used alone, and for both agents in combination, and relies on the calculation of a "combination index" (CI); a computer program is available to facilitate this calculation. A CI of 1 represents additivity, a CI greater than 1 represents synergy, and a CI less than 1 represents antagonism. The method can also be used to plot a normalized isobologram, and although the mathematical formulation is more complex, it is in conceptual agreement with the representation described in Figures 17–11 and 17–12.

Demonstration that 2 or more agents have a supraadditive or synergistic interaction has been used as a rationale for their inclusion in clinical protocols (Ocana et al, 2012). This rationale is valid only if the interaction leads to a greater effect against the tumor as compared with that against limiting normal tissues (ie, if it leads to an improvement in therapeutic index; see Sec. 17.5.1). It is theoretically possible that antagonistic agents (subadditive interaction) could improve therapeutic index provided that there was greater antagonism of toxic effects for normal tissues as compared to toxicity for the tumor, or they have non-overlapping toxicities.

17.6.3 Modifiers of Drug Activity or Toxicity

Some drugs with little or no toxicity for tumor cells may modify the action of anticancer drugs to produce increased antitumor effect or may protect normal tissue. Examples of interactions that might lead to therapeutic benefit through increased antitumor effects include (a) the use of doxorubicin with agents such as verapamil, cyclosporine, or their analogs (which inhibit multidrug resistance; see Chap. 19, Sec. 19.2.3.4), and (b) use of folinic acid with 5-fluorouracil (5-FU), which may provide a necessary cofactor for inhibition of the target enzyme thymidylate synthase (see Chap. 18, Sec. 18.3.2). Alternatively, reduction of the toxic effects of chemotherapy against bone marrow may be achieved by coadministration of growth factors such as G-CSF, which can stimulate earlier recovery of mature granulocytes after bone marrow suppression by chemotherapy, or after stem cell transplantation (see Sec. 17.5.2). G-CSF is used commonly in situations where reduction in dosage of chemotherapy might lead to a decrease in the probability of cure or long-term survival of patients. Growth factors are also being developed to protect against the effects of chemotherapy (and radiotherapy) on other body systems. For example, recombinant human thrombopoietin, and other agents that stimulate platelet production, have shown activity in clinical trials (Vadhan-Raj, 2010). Also palifermin (recombinant keratinocyte growth factor), can stimulate proliferation of the oral and gastrointestinal mucosa, and has been used in selected patients to decrease mucosal injury following chemotherapy (Vadhan-Raj et al, 2010).

Two other agents that may protect normal tissues from damage caused by chemotherapy are dexrazoxane and amifostine. Dexrazoxane is a prodrug with an active form that chelates iron. Because complexes between iron and anthracyclines, such as doxorubicin (and the consequent formation of free radicals), appear to mediate cardiac toxicity but not antitumor effects, dexrazoxane may decrease cardiac toxicity of these drugs and increase their therapeutic index (Speyer et al, 1988; Venturini et al, 1996). Amifostine is also a prodrug that is converted to a sulfhydryl-containing active form. Amifostine is localized selectively in normal tissues, probably because of increased activity of the activating enzyme alkaline phosphatase on the membranes of normal cells. Therefore, it may offer selective protection against a variety of drugs (and radiation) that damage cells by producing reactive intermediates that bind to sulfhydryl groups (Kemp et al, 1996). There remain concerns, however, that these agents might also provide some protection of tumor cells from drug effects.

The crucial test for all modifiers is the demonstration in well-designed clinical trials that higher doses of chemotherapy given with the modifier improve therapeutic index (for example, by increasing the probability or duration of tumor response with no increase in toxicity) as compared to lower doses of chemotherapy used alone.

17.6.4 Drugs and Radiation

Many patients receive treatment with both drugs and radiation, and there is evidence that concurrent treatment with radiation and drugs such as cisplatin leads to improvement in therapeutic index in a variety of cancer sites such as the head and neck and uterine cervix. Here, radiation therapy is the primary treatment and local failure is a major problem that can be decreased with use of concurrent chemotherapy. Mechanisms of interaction between drugs and radiation at the cellular level may be evaluated from cell survival curves for radiation obtained in the presence or absence of the drug (Fig. 17–13). Drugs may influence the survival curve in at least 3 ways: (a) the curve may be displaced downward by the amount of cell kill caused by the drug alone; (b) the shoulder on the survival curve may be lost, suggesting an inability to repair radiation damage in the presence of the drug; and (c) the slope of the exponential part of the survival curve may be changed, indicating sensitization or protection by the drug. Most drugs influence survival curves according to the first 2 patterns; this effect corresponds to the limits of additivity defined in Section 17.6.2, where sublethal damage may be independent or overlapping. The third pattern, leading to a change in slope of the dose response curve, defines agents that are radiation sensitizers or protectors (see Chap. 16, Secs. 16.4.4.2 and 16.5.7). Sensitization of this type has been reported inconsistently for cisplatin and for prolonged exposure to 5-FU after radiation.

Improvement in therapeutic index from use of drugs and radiation requires selective effects to increase damage to tumor cells as compared to those in normal tissues. One mechanism by which combined treatment with radiation and drugs leads to therapeutic advantage arises when radiation is used to provide effective treatment for sites of bulky disease (usually the primary tumor) and drugs are used to treat metastatic sites containing smaller numbers of cells. This spatial cooperation (see Sec. 17.6.1) requires no interaction of the 2 modalities, but involves different dose-limiting toxicities. There are also mechanisms whereby the combined use of radiation and drugs might be used to

obtain therapeutic advantage for treatment of a primary tumor. Table 17–2 lists some properties of cells that might be exploited to give therapeutic advantage for the combined use of radiation and drugs.

Genetic instability in tumors often leads to the presence of sub-clones, which coexist in the tumor with different levels of sensitivity to drugs and to radiation (see Chap. 5, Sec. 5.2). When therapy is applied, any resistant cells that are present will have a selective survival advantage and will determine tumor response; thus, heterogeneity in therapeutic response may tend to make tumors more resistant to treatment than normal tissues. Combined treatment with radiation and drugs might then lead to improved therapeutic index if radiation can eradicate small populations of drug-resistant cells, or if drugs can eliminate populations that are relatively resistant to radiation therapy. This cooperative effect requires that mechanisms of resistance to the 2 therapeutic agents are independent. Mechanisms (other than hypoxia) that convey clinical resistance to radiotherapy remain poorly understood, but probably include enhanced ability to repair damage to DNA, increased levels of sulfhydryl compounds such as glutathione (or of associated glutathione S-transferase enzymes) that scavenge free radicals (especially in hypoxic cells), and decreased ability to undergo apoptosis. These mechanisms may also convey resistance to some anticancer drugs, whereas many other mechanisms of drug resistance (see Chap. 18) are unlikely to cause resistance to radiation. Resistance to any given drug may be caused by multiple mechanisms so that a radiation–drug combination that provides therapeutic advantage for one tumor may not do so for another if different mechanisms of drug resistance are dominant. Effective use of combined treatment would be facilitated by rapid pretreatment assays that give insight into mechanisms of resistance prior to initiation of therapy.

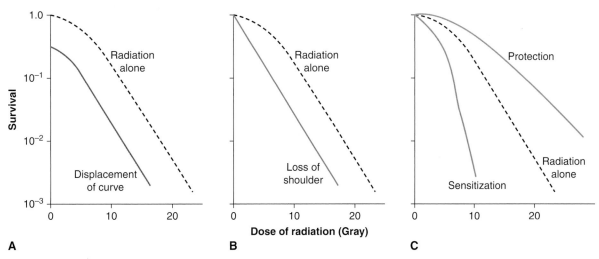

FIGURE 17–13 Drugs and radiation. Possible influences of drug treatment on the relationship between radiation dose and cell survival: (**A**) displacement of curve; (**B**) loss of shoulder, indicating effects of drug on the repair of sublethal radiation damage; (**C**) change in the slope of the curve, indicating sensitization or protection.

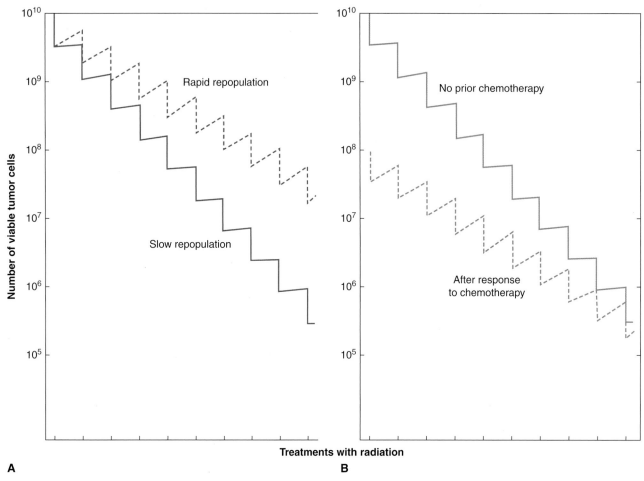

FIGURE 17–14 **Schematic illustrating the effect of repopulation in a tumor during a course of fractionated irradiation.** Each radiation fraction is assumed to kill the same fraction of tumor cells. In (**A**), the effect of different rates of repopulation is illustrated. In (**B**), it is assumed that prior chemotherapy kills 99% of the cells but induces "accelerated" repopulation by the survivors. Response to radiation treatment alone (solid line) or radiation treatment following the chemotherapy (dashed line) is illustrated. The accelerated repopulation induced by the prior drug treatment may rapidly negate the extra cell kill achieved by the drug treatment.

Proliferation of surviving cells during a course of fractionated radiation (ie, repopulation; see Chap. 19, Sec. 19.3.4) acts to increase the total number of cells that must be killed. Anticancer drugs given *during* the course of fractionated radiation might be expected to inhibit repopulation (Fig 17–14). Combined treatment may then convey therapeutic advantage if the rate of repopulation is greater for the tumor cells than it is for normal tissues within the radiation field. Greater specificity would be expected for agents that inhibit specifically the proliferation of tumor cells; this might be achieved through use of hormonal agents (tamoxifen, antiandrogens) used concurrently with radiation for treatment of breast or prostate cancer (see Chap. 20, Sec. 20.4), or through use of molecular-targeted agents. Improved survival of patients with head and neck cancer treated with radiotherapy and concurrent cetuximab, an inhibitor of EGFR, as compared to radiotherapy alone (Bonner et al, 2010), is most likely a result of inhibition of repopulation of tumor cells during the course of radiotherapy, although it is not clear that

this targeted agent provides better therapeutic outcome than concurrent cisplatin.

Repopulation during fractionated radiation therapy might also be influenced by prior treatment with neoadjuvant chemotherapy. Such chemotherapy may cause tumor shrinkage, followed by improved nutrition of surviving cells, with consequent stimulation of cell proliferation (Withers et al, 1988). If there is increased repopulation of surviving cells during the subsequent course of fractionated radiation therapy, any advantage from initial shrinkage of the tumor caused by chemotherapy may be lost or reversed because of the decreased net effectiveness of subsequent radiation treatment (Fig. 17–14).

Regrowth of tumors following radiotherapy depends on maintenance of a vascular supply to provide nutrients to surviving cells. Clinical courses of radiotherapy are likely to lead to killing of endothelial and other cells that constitute the preexisting vasculature and it has been proposed that tumor regeneration depends on recruitment of circulating myeloid precursors that form new blood vessels in irradiated tumors

(Ahn and Brown, 2009). These circulating precursors might be killed or suppressed by chemotherapy given concurrently with radiation, or by agents that target them more specifically (Ahn et al, 2010).

A fourth mechanism that has potential for exploitation through combined use of radiation and drugs depends on the presence of a hypoxic microenvironment within solid tumors (see Chap. 12, Sec. 12.2). An hypoxic environment conveys resistance to radiation because cell killing is dependent in part on the presence of oxygen (see Chap. 16, Sec. 16.4). Several drugs have been developed that require bioreduction under hypoxic conditions for activity, and therefore have selective toxicity for hypoxic cells; effective drugs may also diffuse to influence neighboring aerobic regions (Brown, 1999). Such drugs would be expected to have fewer effects against normal tissues, where adequate vasculature usually prevents development of a hypoxic microenvironment, although there is evidence for hypoxic regions in bone marrow and some other normal tissues (Parmar et al, 2007). Hypoxia-selective drugs might augment both the effects of radiation, and of conventional chemotherapy, whereas hypoxic cells and their neighbors might be spared because of limited drug distribution within solid tumors and their low proliferative rate (Minchinton and Tannock, 2006; see Chap. 19, Sec. 19.3.2). The first-generation hypoxia-selective agent, tirapazamine, has been evaluated with cisplatin with and without radiotherapy for patients with lung or head and neck cancer (von Pawel et al, 2000; Rischin et al, 2010). Despite some positive effects especially in tumors selected for hypoxia (Rischin et al, 2006), this drug adds toxicity without long-term benefit but more promising hypoxia-activated pro-drugs, such as TH-302, are being evaluated in clinical trials.

Whenever radiation and drugs are used together or in sequence, there is potential for increased damage to normal tissues in the radiation field. Some of the effects of combined treatment may lead to changes in function that occur months to years after treatment. Both clinical experience and studies in animals have shown that most anticancer drugs can increase the incidence of toxicity from radiation, sometimes in organs (eg, the kidney) where the drugs alone rarely cause overt toxicity (von der Maase, 1986). The effect of a drug on radiation toxicity to any organ may be expressed in terms of a dose-enhancement ratio (DER), which is the dose of radiation to produce a given effect when used alone divided by the dose of radiation that gives the same effect when combined with the drug. For acute effects of radiation on normal tissues of mice, typical values of DER range from 1.0 to 1.5, depending on the drug and normal tissue; maximum interaction occurs when drug and radiation are administered within a short time span (von der Maase, 1986). The therapeutic gain factor equals the ratio of DER for the tumor to the DER for the dose-limiting normal tissue in the radiation field. In experimental systems, this ratio may vary widely depending on the drug used, the doses of drug and radiation, and the treatment sequence. Thus, it is difficult to predict the dose schedules that are likely to lead to therapeutic gain in patients.

SUMMARY

- The discovery of novel anticancer drugs begins with the identification of potential therapeutic targets. Molecular characterization of events in cellular transformation and tumor progression is being used to identify new targets for anticancer agents.
- Modern approaches use gene expression profiling, high-throughput genetic sequencing, and RNAi technology to knockdown the genetic target and thereby determine whether it is essential for tumor growth.
- After a target is selected, drug candidates are developed using a variety of approaches including automated physical screens and structure-guided rational drug design with x-ray crystallography and NMR.
- Drug candidates are evaluated in preclinical models using cell culture systems and animal models. Drugs that display efficacy in preclinical models and a probable therapeutic window advance into clinical trials for definitive assessments of toxicity and efficacy.
- Characterization of molecular targets coupled with new approaches to drug discovery has generated therapeutic agents that are more selective for cancer cells as compared to normal cells. Such agents include small molecules and monoclonal antibodies that inhibit membrane-based tyrosine kinases or critical intracellular enzymes.
- RNAi-based therapeutics are in early development, but hold promise for cancer therapy as gene targets important for cancer growth and proliferation can be suppressed specifically.
- Many anticancer drugs, both chemotherapy and targeted agents, act primarily to inhibit cell proliferation, and may share common toxicities against proliferating cells in normal tissues such as the bone marrow and intestine.
- Other frequent toxicities include nausea, vomiting, and fatigue, and several agents can also act as carcinogens.
- Improvement in treatment requires an improvement in therapeutic index, a measure of the relative toxic effects against a tumor as compared to the dose-limiting normal tissue(s).
- Anticancer drugs are used frequently in combination with each other and with radiation. Analysis of interactions between different agents is complex and claims for synergy need to be validated experimentally.
- Mechanisms that may lead to therapeutic advantage from combined use of radiation and drugs include (a) spatial cooperation, whereby radiation is used to treat bulk disease and chemotherapy to treat metastases; (b) use of each modality to kill tumor cells that have developed resistance to the other; (c) inhibition by drugs of repopulation of surviving cells during fractionated radiotherapy; (d) killing of myeloid precursor cells that can form new blood vessels in irradiated tumors; and (e) use of drugs that are selective for hypoxic cells that are resistant to radiation.

REFERENCES

Ahles TA, Saykin AJ. Candidate mechanisms for chemotherapy-induced cognitive changes. *Nat Rev Cancer* 2007;7:192-201.

Ahn GO, Brown JM. Influence of bone marrow-derived hematopoietic cells on the tumor response to radiotherapy: experimental models and clinical perspectives. *Cell Cycle* 2009;8:970-976.

Ahn GO, Tseng D, Liao CH, et al. Inhibition of Mac-1 (CD11b/CD18) enhances tumor response to radiation by reducing myeloid cell recruitment. *Proc Natl Acad Sci U S A* 2010;107:8363-8368.

Amir E, Seruga B, Serrano R, Ocana A. Targeting DNA repair in breast cancer: a clinical and translational update. *Cancer Treat Rev* 2010;36:557-565.

Batist G, Ramakrishnan G, Rao CS, et al. Reduced cardiotoxicity and preserved antitumor efficacy of liposome-encapsulated doxorubicin and cyclophosphamide compared with conventional doxorubicin and cyclophosphamide in a randomized, multicenter trial of metastatic breast cancer. *J Clin Oncol* 2001;19:1444-1454.

Bazzaro M, Lee MK, Zoso A, et al. Ubiquitin-proteasome system stress sensitizes ovarian cancer to proteasome inhibitor-induced apoptosis. *Cancer Res* 2006;66:3754-3763.

Bonner JA, Harari PM, Giralt J, et al. Radiotherapy plus cetuximab for locoregionally advanced head and neck cancer: 5-year survival data from a phase 3 randomised trial, and relation between cetuximab-induced rash and survival. *Lancet Oncol* 2010;11:21-28.

Bristow RG, Hill RP. Hypoxia and metabolism. Hypoxia, DNA repair and genetic instability. *Nat Rev Cancer* 2008;8:180-192.

Brown JM. The hypoxic cancer cell: a target for selective cancer therapy - eighteenth Bruce F Cain Memorial Award lecture. *Cancer Res* 1999;59:5863-5870.

Brown JM, Attardi LD. The role of apoptosis in cancer development and treatment response. *Nat Rev Cancer* 2005;5:231-237.

Buchsbaum DJ, Forero-Torres A, LoBuglio AF. TRAIL-receptor antibodies as a potential cancer treatment. *Future Oncol* 2007;3:405-409.

Byrne JD, Betancourt T, Brannon-Peppas L. Active targeting schemes for nanoparticle systems in cancer therapeutics. *Adv Drug Deliv Rev* 2008;60:1615-1626.

Chauhan D, Catley L, Li G, et al. A novel orally active proteasome inhibitor induces apoptosis in multiple myeloma cells with mechanisms distinct from Bortezomib. *Cancer Cell* 2005;8:407-419.

Chauhan D, Singh A, Brahmandam M, et al. Combination of proteasome inhibitors bortezomib and NPI-0052 trigger in vivo synergistic cytotoxicity in multiple myeloma. *Blood* 2008;111:1654-1664.

Chou TC. Drug combination studies and their synergy quantification using the Chou-Talalay method. *Cancer Res* 2010;70:440-446.

Chou TC, Talalay P. Quantitative analysis of dose-effect relationships: the combined effects of multiple drugs or enzyme inhibitors. *Adv Enzyme Regul* 1984;22:27-55.

Curtis RE, Boice JD Jr, Stovall M, et al. Risk of leukemia after chemotherapy and radiation treatment for breast cancer. *N Engl J Med* 1992;326:1745-1751.

Dimopoulos M, Spencer A, Attal M, et al. Lenalidomide plus dexamethasone for relapsed or refractory multiple myeloma. *N Engl J Med* 2007;357:2123-2132.

Druker BJ, Talpaz M, Resta DJ, et al. Efficacy and safety of a specific inhibitor of the BCR-ABL tyrosine kinase in chronic myeloid leukemia. *N Engl J Med* 2001;344:1031-1037.

Eberhard DA, Johnson BE, Amler LC, et al Mutations in the epidermal growth factor receptor and in KRAS are predictive and prognostic indicators in patients with non-small-cell lung cancer treated with chemotherapy alone and in combination with erlotinib. *J Clin Oncol* 2005;23:5900-5909.

Escudier B, Eisen T, Stadler WM, et al. Sorafenib in advanced clear-cell renal-cell carcinoma. *N Engl J Med* 2007;356:125-134.

Ferrara N. Vascular endothelial growth factor as a target for anticancer therapy. *Oncologist* 2004;9 Suppl 1:2-10.

Frohling S, Scholl C, Levine RL, et al. Identification of driver and passenger mutations of FLT3 by high-throughput DNA sequence analysis and functional assessment of candidate alleles. *Cancer Cell* 2007;12:501-513.

Fujishita T, Aoki K, Lane HA, et al. Inhibition of the mTORC1 pathway suppresses intestinal polyp formation and reduces mortality in ApcDelta716 mice. *Proc Natl Acad Sci U S A* 2008;105, 13544-13549.

Gerhold DL, Jensen RV, Gullans SR. Better therapeutics through microarrays. *Nat Genet* 2002;32 Suppl:547-551.

Gradishar WJ, Krasnojon D, Cheporov S, et al., Significantly longer progression-free survival with nab-paclitaxel compared with docetaxel as first-line therapy for metastatic breast cancer. *J Clin Oncol* 2009;27:3611-3619.

Grünwald V, Hidalgo M. Developing inhibitors of the epidermal growth factor receptor for cancer treatment. *J Natl Cancer Inst* 2003;95:851-867.

Gupta PB, Onder TT, Jiang G, et al. Identification of selective inhibitors of cancer stem cells by high-throughput screening. *Cell* 2009;138:645-659.

Hadland BK, Longmore GD. Erythroid-stimulating agents in cancer therapy: potential dangers and biologic mechanisms. *J Clin Oncol* 2009;27:4217-4226.

Hassane DC, Guzman ML, Corbett C, et al. Discovery of agents that eradicate leukemia stem cells using an in silico screen of public gene expression data. *Blood* 2008;111:5654-5662.

Hideshima T, Richardson P, Chauhan D, et al. The proteasome inhibitor PS-341 inhibits growth, induces apoptosis, and overcomes drug resistance in human multiple myeloma cells. *Cancer Res* 2001;61:3071-3076.

Hirsjärvi S, Passirani C, Benoit JP. Passive and active tumour targeting with nanocarriers. *Curr Drug Discov Technol* 2011;8:188-196.

Hochhaus A, Kantarjian HM, Baccarani M, et al. Dasatinib induces notable hematologic and cytogenetic responses in chronic-phase chronic myeloid leukemia after failure of imatinib therapy. *Blood* 2007;109:2303-2309.

Hudson TJ, Anderson W, Artez A, et al. International network of cancer genome projects. *Nature* 2010;464:993-998.

Iglehart JD, Silver DP. Synthetic lethality—a new direction in cancer-drug development. *N Engl J Med* 2009;361:189-191.

Jin L, Hope KJ, Zhai Q, et al. Targeting of CD44 eradicates human acute myeloid leukemic stem cells. *Nat Med* 2006;12:1167-1174.

Kaelin WG Jr. The concept of synthetic lethality in the context of anticancer therapy. *Nat Rev Cancer* 2005;5:689-698.

Kang MH, Reynolds CP. Bcl-2 inhibitors: targeting mitochondrial apoptotic pathways in cancer therapy. *Clin Cancer Res* 2009;15:1126-1132.

Kantarjian H, Shah NP, Hochhaus A, et al. Dasatinib versus imatinib in newly diagnosed chronic-phase chronic myeloid leukemia. *N Engl J Med* 2010;362:2260-2270.

Kemp G, Rose P, Lurain J, et al. Amifostine pretreatment for protection against cyclophosphamide-induced and cisplatin-induced toxicities: results of a randomized control trial in patients with advanced ovarian cancer. *J Clin Oncol* 1996; 14:2101-2112.

Kerbel RS, Kamen BA. The anti-angiogenic basis of metronomic chemotherapy. *Nat Rev Cancer* 2004;4:423-436.

Kim JJ, Tannock IF. Repopulation of cancer cells during therapy: an important cause of treatment failure. *Nat Rev Cancer* 2005;5: 516-525.

Kistner A, Gossen M, Zimmermann F, et al. Doxycycline-mediated quantitative and tissue-specific control of gene expression in transgenic mice. *Proc Natl Acad Sci U S A* 1996;93:10933-10938.

Kottaridis PD, Gale RE, Frew ME, et al. The presence of a FLT3 internal tandem duplication in patients with acute myeloid leukemia (AML) adds important prognostic information to cytogenetic risk group and response to the first cycle of chemotherapy: analysis of 854 patients from the United Kingdom Medical Research Council AML 10 and 12 trials. *Blood* 2001;98: 1752-1759.

Kuhn DJ, Chen Q, Voorhees PM, et al. Potent activity of carfilzomib, a novel, irreversible inhibitor of the ubiquitin-proteasome pathway, against preclinical models of multiple myeloma. *Blood* 2007;110:3281-3290.

le Coutre P, Ottmann OG, Giles F, et al. Nilotinib (formerly AMN107), a highly selective BCR-ABL tyrosine kinase inhibitor, is active in patients with imatinib-resistant or -intolerant accelerated-phase chronic myelogenous leukemia. *Blood* 2008;111:1834-1839.

Lee JJ, Kong M, Ayers GD, Lotan R. Interaction index and different methods for determining drug interaction in combination therapy. *J Biopharm Stat* 2007;17:461-480.

Lipworth AD, Robert C, Zhu AX. Hand-foot syndrome (hand-foot skin reaction, palmar-plantar erythrodysesthesia): focus on sorafenib and sunitinib. *Oncology* 2009;77:257-271.

List A, Kurtin S, Roe DJ, et al. Efficacy of lenalidomide in myelodysplastic syndromes. *N Engl J Med* 2005;352:549-557.

Llovet JM, Ricci S, Mazzaferro V, et al. Sorafenib in advanced hepatocellular carcinoma. *N Engl J Med* 2008;359:378-390.

Matesich SM, Shapiro CL Second cancers after breast cancer treatment. *Semin Oncol* 2003;30:740-748.

Meister S, Schubert U, Neubert K, et al. Extensive immunoglobulin production sensitizes myeloma cells for proteasome inhibition. *Cancer Res* 2007;67:1783-1792.

Milano G, Etienne MC, Pierrefite V, et al. Dihydropyrimidine dehydrogenase deficiency and fluorouracil-related toxicity. *Br J Cancer* 1999;79:627-630.

Minchinton AI, Tannock IF. Drug penetration in solid tumours. *Nat Rev Cancer* 2006;6:583-592.

Mistry AR, Felix CA, Whitmarsh RJ, et al. DNA topoisomerase II in therapy-related acute promyelocytic leukemia. *N Engl J Med* 2005;352:1529-1538.

Mitsiades CS, Ocio EM, Pandiella A, et al. Aplidin, a marine organism-derived compound with potent antimyeloma activity in vitro and in vivo. *Cancer Res* 2008;68:5216-5225.

Motzer RJ, Hutson TE, Tomczak P, et al. Sunitinib versus interferon alfa in metastatic renal-cell carcinoma. *N Engl J Med* 2007;356: 115-124.

Nakamura T, Fidler IJ, Coombes KR. Gene expression profile of metastatic human pancreatic cancer cells depends on the organ microenvironment. *Cancer Res* 2007;67:139-148.

Northfelt DW, Dezube BJ, Thommes JA, et al. Pegylated-liposomal doxorubicin versus doxorubicin, bleomycin, and vincristine in the treatment of AIDS-related Kaposi's sarcoma: results of a randomized phase III clinical trial. *J Clin Oncol* 1998;16: 2445-2451.

Ocana A, Amir E, Yeung C, Seruga B, Tannock IF. How valid are claims for synergy in published clinical studies? *Ann Oncol* 2012; 23:2161-2166.

Ocana A, Pandiella A, Siu LL, Tannock IF. Preclinical development of molecular targeted agents for cancer. *Nat Rev Clin Oncol* 2011; 8:200-209.

Olsen EA, Kim YH, Kuzel TM, et al. Phase IIb multicenter trial of vorinostat in patients with persistent, progressive, or treatment refractory cutaneous T-cell lymphoma. *J Clin Oncol* 2007;25: 3109-3115.

Oltersdorf T, Elmore SW, Shoemaker AR, et al. An inhibitor of Bcl-2 family proteins induces regression of solid tumours. *Nature* 2005;435:677-681.

Palumbo A, Bringhen S, Caravita T, et al. Oral melphalan and prednisone chemotherapy plus thalidomide compared with melphalan and prednisone alone in elderly patients with multiple myeloma: randomised controlled trial. *Lancet* 2006; 367:825-831.

Parlati F, Lee SJ, Aujay M, et al. Carfilzomib can induce tumor cell death through selective inhibition of the chymotrypsin-like activity of the proteasome. *Blood* 2009;114:3439-3447.

Parmar K, Mauch P, Vergilio JA, et al. Distribution of hematopoietic stem cells in the bone marrow according to regional hypoxia. *Proc Natl Acad Sci U S A* 2007;104:5431-5436.

Patt DA, Duan Z, Fang S, et al. Acute myeloid leukemia after adjuvant breast cancer therapy in older women: understanding risk. *J Clin Oncol* 2007;25:3871-3876.

Petros RA, DeSimone JM. Strategies in the design of nanoparticles for therapeutic applications. *Nat Rev Drug Discov* 2010;9: 615-627.

Pfuhler S, Fellows M, van Benthem J, et al. In vitro genotoxicity test approaches with better predictivity: summary of an IWGT workshop. *Mutat Res* 2011;723:101-107.

Piccart-Gebhart MJ, Procter M, Leyland-Jones B, et al. Trastuzumab after adjuvant chemotherapy in HER2-positive breast cancer. *N Engl J Med* 2005;353:1659-1672.

Rajapakse HA.Small molecule inhibitors of the XIAP protein-protein interaction. *Curr Top Med Chem* 2007;7:966-971.

Rischin D, Hicks RJ, Fisher R, et al; Prognostic significance of [18F]-misonidazole positron emission tomography-detected tumor hypoxia in patients with advanced head and neck cancer randomly assigned to chemoradiation with or without tirapazamine: a substudy of Trans-Tasman Radiation Oncology Group Study 98.02. *J Clin Oncol* 2006;24:2098-2104.

Rischin D, Peters LJ , O'Sullivan B, et al. Tirapazamine, cisplatin, and radiation versus cisplatin and radiation for advanced squamous cell carcinoma of the head and neck (TROG 02.02, HeadSTART): A phase III trial of the Trans-Tasman Radiation Oncology Group. *J Clin Oncol* 2010;28:2989-2995.

Romond EH, Perez EA, Bryant J, et al. Trastuzumab plus adjuvant chemotherapy for operable HER2-positive breast cancer. *N Engl J Med* 2005;353:1673-1684.

Rottenberg S, Jaspers JE, Kersbergen A, et al. High sensitivity of BRCA1-deficient mammary tumors to the PARP inhibitor AZD2281 alone and in combination with platinum drugs. *Proc Natl Acad Sci U S A* 2008;105:17079-17084.

Saglio G, Kim DW, Issaragrisil S, et al. Nilotinib versus imatinib for newly diagnosed chronic myeloid leukemia. *N Engl J Med* 2010; 362:2251-2259.

Sandler A, Gray R, Perry MC, et al. Paclitaxel-carboplatin alone or with bevacizumab for non-small-cell lung cancer. *N Engl J Med* 2006;355:2542-2550.

Schimmer AD. Novel therapies targeting the apoptosis pathway for the treatment of acute myeloid leukemia. *Curr Treat Options Oncol* 2007;8:277-286.

Seidenfeld J, Piper M, Flamm C, et al. Epoetin treatment of anemia associated with cancer therapy: a systematic review and meta-analysis of controlled clinical trials. *J Natl Cancer Inst* 2001;93: 1204-1214.

Sharpless NE, DePinho RA. The mighty mouse: genetically engineered mouse models in cancer drug development. *Nat Rev Drug Discov* 2006;5:741-754.

Singh AV, Palladino MA, Lloyd GK, et al. Pharmacodynamic and efficacy studies of the novel proteasome inhibitor NPI-0052 (marizomib) in a human plasmacytoma xenograft murine model. *Br J Haematol* 2010;149:550-559.

Sinha S, Anderson J, Barbour R, et al. Purification and cloning of amyloid precursor protein ß-secretase from human brain. *Nature* 1999;402:537-540.

Slamon DJ, Leyland-Jones B, Shak S, et al. Use of chemotherapy plus a monoclonal antibody against HER2 for metastatic breast cancer that overexpresses HER2. *N Engl J Med* 2001;344:783-792.

Speyer JL, Green MD, Kramer E, et al. Protective effect of the bispiperazinedione ICRF-187 against doxorubicin-induced cardiac toxicity in women with advanced breast cancer. *N Engl J Med* 1988;319:745-752.

Steel GG, Peckham MJ. Exploitable mechanisms in combined radiotherapy-chemotherapy: the concept of additivity. *Int J Radiat Oncol Biol Phys* 1979;5:85-91.

Strecker TE, Shen Q, Zhang Y, et al. Effect of lapatinib on the development of estrogen receptor-negative mammary tumors in mice. *J Natl Cancer Inst* 2009;101:107-113.

Teicher BA. Antibody-drug conjugate targets. *Curr Cancer Drug Targets* 2009;9:982-1004.

Thiede C, Steudel C, Mohr B, et al. Analysis of FLT3-activating mutations in 979 patients with acute myelogenous leukemia: association with FAB subtypes and identification of subgroups with poor prognosis. *Blood* 2002;99:4326-4335.

Tiedemann RE, Zhu YX, Schmidt J, et al. Kinome-wide RNAi studies in human multiple myeloma identify vulnerable kinase targets, including a lymphoid-restricted kinase, GRK6. *Blood* 2010;115:1594-1604.

Torkamani A, Verkhivker G, Schork NJ. Cancer driver mutations in protein kinase genes. *Cancer Lett* 2009;281:117-127.

Travis LB, Curtis RE, Glimelius B, et al. Bladder and kidney cancer following cyclophosphamide therapy for non-Hodgkin's lymphoma. *J Natl Cancer Inst* 1995;87:524-530.

Turner NC, Lord CJ, Iorns E, et al. A synthetic lethal siRNA screen identifying genes mediating sensitivity to a PARP inhibitor. *EMBO J* 2008;27:1368-1377.

Turner N, Tutt A, Ashworth A. Hallmarks of "BRCAness" in sporadic cancers. *Nat Rev Cancer* 2004;4:814-819.

Vadhan-Raj S. Clinical findings with the first generation of thrombopoietic agents. *Semin Hematol* 2010;47:249-257.

Vadhan-Raj S, Trent J, Patel S, et al. Single-dose palifermin prevents severe oral mucositis during multicycle chemotherapy in patients with cancer: a randomized trial. *Ann Intern Med* 2010;21:153:358-367.

Vardy J, Rourke S, Tannock IF. Evaluation of cognitive function associated with chemotherapy: a review of published studies and recommendations for future research. *J Clin Oncol* 2007; 25:2455-2463.

Verma S, Miles D, Gianni L, et al. Trastuzumab emtansine for HER2-positive advanced breast cancer. *N Engl J Med* 2012; 367:1783-1791.

Venturini M, Michelotti A, Del Mastro L, et al. Multicenter randomized controlled clinical trial to evaluate cardioprotection of desrazoxane versus no cardioprotection in women receiving epirubicin chemotherapy for advanced breast cancer. *J Clin Oncol* 1996;14:3112-3120.

von der Maase. Experimental studies on interactions of radiation and cancer chemotherapeutic drugs in normal tissues and a solid tumour. *Radiother Oncol* 1986;7:47-68.

von Pawel J, von Roemeling R, Gatzemeier U, et al. Tiripazamine plus cisplatin in advanced non-small cell lung cancer. A report of the international CATAPULT 1 study group. Cisplatinum and tiripazamine in subjects with advanced previously untreated non-small-cell lung tumors. *J Clin Oncol* 2000;18:1351-1359.

Wilson WH, O'Connor OA, Czuczman MS, et al. Navitoclax, a targeted high-affinity inhibitor of BCL-2, in lymphoid malignancies: a phase 1 dose-escalation study of safety, pharmacokinetics, pharmacodynamics, and antitumour activity. *Lancet Oncol* 2010;11:1149-1159.

Withers HR, TaylorJM, Maciejewski B. The hazard of accerated tumor clonogen repopulation during radiotherapy. *Acta Oncol* 1988;27:131-146.

Zhu CQ, da Cunha Santos G, Ding K, et al. Role of KRAS and EGFR as biomarkers of response to erlotinib in National Cancer Institute of Canada Clinical Trials Group Study BR.21. *J Clin Oncol* 2008;26:4268-4275.

Pharmacology of Anticancer Drugs

Eric X. Chen

18.1 GENERAL PRINCIPLES OF PHARMACOLOGY

In this chapter, general principles of pharmacology relevant to anticancer drugs are presented. The specific properties of the most important anticancer drugs in clinical use are reviewed, with emphasis on their structure, mechanism of action, pharmacokinetics, and toxicity. In systemic cancer therapy, it is common to combine several drugs. Drugs in such combinations generally have different mechanisms of action, and different toxicity profiles, so that each drug can be administered at close to its maximally tolerated dose. Combination therapy may overcome tumor resistance to an individual drug, and is generally more efficacious than a single drug. It is also common to combine surgery, radiation, and chemotherapy in treatment. Adjuvant chemotherapy and/or radiation are usually given after the definitive management of the primary cancer through surgery. The purpose of adjuvant chemotherapy is to eradicate micrometastatic disease, and reduce the risk of tumor recurrence. Adjuvant chemotherapy is given for a defined period of time, generally 4 to 6 months. Neoadjuvant chemotherapy refers to chemotherapy given before the definitive management of the primary cancer, and is given to reduce the size of the primary tumor for better cosmetic and functional outcomes.

18.1.1 Pharmacokinetics and Pharmacodynamics

Pharmacokinetics is the study of the time course of drug and metabolite levels in different body fluids and tissues, including absorption, distribution, metabolism, and elimination. The study of the relationship between drug effect and its concentration is known as *pharmacodynamics*. Alterations in pharmacokinetic properties of a drug may result in different drug concentrations over time at tissue levels. Understanding the pharmacodynamics of the drug can help to account for subsequent differences in drug effect or response.

Although most anticancer drugs are administered intravenously and drug absorption is not a therapeutic concern, many newer agents are given orally. Oral drug administration is convenient for patients, but it requires patient compliance and depends on efficient absorption from the gastrointestinal tract. For an orally administered drug, only a proportion may be delivered to the systemic circulation intact and become available for potential therapeutic effects. The term *bioavailability* refers to the amount of a drug that is available after oral administration compared to that after intravenous administration. Factors influencing the bioavailability of a drug include patient compliance, disintegration of a capsule or a tablet, dissolution of drug into gastrointestinal fluid, stability of the drug in the gastrointestinal tract, absorption through the gastrointestinal mucosa, and first-pass metabolism in the liver. Problems seen in cancer patients, such as changes in gastrointestinal motility, mucosal damage from cancer therapy, and the use of other medications, can also affect bioavailability. Absorption of a drug may vary among patients receiving the same treatments, or within 1 patient from one course of treatment to another. This variability can account for some differences in toxicity, and possibly in tumor response. In most cases, such variations in drug bioavailability are not detected clinically because routine pharmacokinetic measurements are not made in patients.

Once in the blood, the distribution of a drug within the body is governed by factors such as blood flow to different organs, protein and tissue binding, lipid solubility, diffusion, and carrier-mediated transport. In general, drugs with extensive protein–tissue binding or with high lipid solubility will tend to exhibit prolonged elimination phases because the release of bound drug from tissues is slow.

Metabolism of drugs takes place primarily in the liver and consists of oxidative, reductive, and hydrolytic reactions via the superfamily of cytochrome P450 (Phase I) and conjugation (Phase II) enzymes. Phase I reactions can produce metabolites that retain therapeutic activity or convert an inactive prodrug (eg, cyclophosphamide) to an active moiety. Phase II reactions generally produce inactive metabolites that can be eliminated from the body by biliary or renal excretion. Many anticancer drugs have active metabolites, and this introduces additional complexity into understanding the relationship between drug pharmacokinetics and pharmacodynamics. There are genetic polymorphisms that can affect the activity of many of the drug-metabolizing enzymes (Paugh et al, 2011). As well, acquired changes as a result of hepatic impairment or the use of other medications may affect their activity. Unfortunately, simple tests of liver function, such as serum levels of bilirubin or transaminases, have not proved useful in predicting hepatic metabolic activity because the decline in activity of metabolizing enzymes varies in the setting of hepatic dysfunction.

Most drugs are eventually eliminated from the body by the kidney or through the biliary tract. Renal excretion can either be of the active drug or of metabolites. Impairment of renal function will influence drug clearance and may enhance toxicity for drugs that are eliminated unchanged in the urine, such as carboplatin and methotrexate. Dosage reductions proportionate to the decline in creatinine clearance (a common measure of kidney function) are usually required. Several chemotherapy drugs are also toxic to the kidney (eg, cisplatin and high-dose methotrexate), and combinations of these drugs with others that are eliminated by the kidney require extra caution and maintenance of a high urinary output.

Cancer patients frequently take multiple other medications for relief of pain, nausea, and other symptoms. Interaction between drugs may influence each of the processes of absorption, metabolism, distribution, and excretion. For example, patients receiving warfarin (to prevent blood clotting) require increased monitoring if they are also receiving fluoropyrimidines because of such interactions. Possible interactions between anticancer drugs, and between such drugs and other medications, are common (Riechelmann et al, 2008), but have not been investigated extensively.

The concentration of most anticancer drugs can be measured in the blood or in the tissue of a patient. If a drug is measured in blood or tissue over time, then a curve relating drug concentration to time can be defined. The area-under-the-concentration-time curve (AUC) is a commonly used measure of total systemic drug exposure. For drugs like cisplatin, their effect in killing of tumor cells or toxicity to normal tissues is related directly to the AUC; whereas for other drugs, such as taxanes, the duration of exposure above a threshold concentration may be more important than the AUC.

The concentration-time curve (Fig. 18–1) can be modeled mathematically. Table 18–1 lists some important terms derived from such modeling. Clearance (CL) is the proportionality factor that relates the rate of elimination of a drug from the body and its plasma concentration:

$$\text{Rate of elimination} = \text{CL} \times \text{plasma concentration}$$

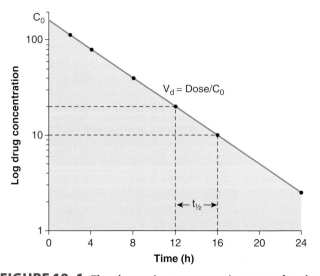

FIGURE 18–1 **The plasma time-concentration curve after the intravenous bolus administration of a drug.** Drug concentrations are measured every 2 hours. In this case, the drug is eliminated via a first-order process with the elimination half-life ($t_{1/2}$) being 4 hours. The shaded area is the AUC. Volume of distribution (V_d) can be calculated by dividing dose by the concentration at time 0 (C_0) which can be obtained by extrapolating the curve to time 0.

TABLE 18-1 Glossary of terms used commonly in pharmacokinetics.

Pharmacokinetic Term	Definition
AUC	Area under the plasma concentration-time curve, either from zero to infinity (AUC_{inf}) or from zero to the last point of blood sampling (AUC_t)
$C(t)$	Drug concentration in plasma at time t
CL	Clearance, the proportionality factor that relates the rate of elimination of a drug from the body and its plasma concentration
C_{ss}	Steady-state plasma drug concentration
$t_{1/2}$	Half-life, the time required for the drug concentration to decrease by 50%
V_d	Volume of distribution, a hypothetical volume required to dissolve the total amount of drug at the same concentration as is found in blood immediately after intravenous administration

Clearance can be represented by a volume from which the drug is totally eliminated in a unit of time, such as liters per hour. The AUC of a drug is related to its dose and clearance:

$$AUC = Dose/CL$$

Thus, if the clearance of a drug declines (eg, in the setting of renal or hepatic dysfunction), its AUC will increase without an adjustment in dose, resulting in increased toxicities. Similarly, individual variability in drug clearance will manifest as differences in AUC and in effect. Clearance is independent of dose unless there is saturation of drug metabolizing enzymes in which case the AUC will increase at a greater rate than dose and severe toxicities can result.

The volume of distribution (V_d) represents a hypothetical volume of body fluid that would be required to dissolve the total amount of drug at the same concentration as that found in blood immediately after intravenous administration. A large V_d (a value larger than the total volume of the body water is possible) represents extensive binding of drug in tissue (eg, vinca alkaloids). Curves relating drug concentration in blood with time after administration often have components that are approximately exponential (see Fig. 18-1). The half-life ($t_{1/2}$) of a drug is the time required for the drug concentration to decrease by half, and different values of $t_{1/2}$ (labeled α, β, and γ) can be used to characterize successive exponential components of the clearance curve; the last of these is commonly referred to as the elimination half-life. The elimination half-life is useful in estimating the time required for a drug to reach a steady state (where the amount of drug being eliminated from the body is equal to the amount being added after multiple administrations such that the plasma concentration remains constant).

18.1.2 Dosing of Chemotherapy in Individual Patients

Most anticancer drugs have a low therapeutic index (ie, a small difference between doses that cause anticancer effects and those that cause toxicity) and are given at close to the maximum tolerated dose (MTD) (see Chap. 22, Sec. 22.2.1). There is a need to reduce interindividual variability to have a consistent response and to minimize toxicity. Efforts in relating drug concentration to effects have generally been unsuccessful. The majority of chemotherapeutic agents are dosed on the basis of body surface area (BSA) by tradition on the premise that the factors relevant in pharmacokinetics, such as cardiac output, body fat, and creatinine clearance, are all related to body size. BSA dosing is useful in interspecies comparisons as MTD remains relatively constant between different animals when expressed as milligrams per square meter, and it may have value in pediatric patients where they may be large ranges in body size. Many reports have questioned the convention of calculating the dose of chemotherapy in adults on the basis of BSA (Ratain, 1998). Multiple studies show that there is no reduction in pharmacokinetic variability when compared to a standard dose or dose based on body weight. Furthermore, BSA based dosing makes drug administration unnecessarily complex and more subject to human error.

Factors within an individual that may account for variability in pharmacokinetics and pharmacodynamics are still poorly understood. The usual approach is to use a standard starting dose (in mg/m²) and then modify subsequent doses based upon the observed toxicity. An exception is the dosing of carboplatin, where a relationship between kidney functions and clearance of carboplatin has been demonstrated and carboplatin dose is calculated on the basis of the creatinine clearance (Calvert et al, 1989). The approach to dose modification will also be influenced by the goals of therapy. In a setting where treatment is curative (eg, testicular cancer), the drug doses are usually maintained despite severe toxicity, often with administration of G-CSF (see Chap. 17, Sec. 17.5.2), whereas in a palliative situation (eg, 5-fluorouracil [5-FU] for advanced colon cancer) dose reductions are appropriate for even moderate toxicity. The approach to dose reduction is usually empiric with fractional dose reductions of one or more of the drugs thought to be causing the toxicity.

Many of the newer anticancer drugs, especially molecular-targeted agents, are administered orally. Therapy is usually initiated at a fixed dose regardless of height or weight.

18.1.3 Pharmacogenetics

Pharmacogenetics refers to the study of how genetic features of the patient (and their tumor) will influence response and toxicity. In the broadest sense, pharmacogenetics seeks to explain phenotypic differences in response on the basis of differences in the activity of genes that are involved in drug metabolism and are related to specific mutations or polymorphisms (Paugh et al, 20011). In the past, this was done by defining a particular phenotype following drug exposure (eg, serious toxicity, second malignancy) and then looking for changes at the genetic level that might account for this phenotype. This could be a result of determinants of drug pharmacokinetics, such as the function of drug-metabolizing enzymes, to genetic factors that would influence pharmacodynamics or even to genetic polymorphisms that might relate to the development of cancers (see Chap. 3, Sec. 3.6.2).

An early example of the effect of pharmacogenetics on response and toxicity is the use of 5-FU in the treatment of colorectal cancer. Approximately 80% of intravenously administered 5-FU is catabolized to an inactive metabolite through the enzyme, dihydropyrimidine dehydrogenase (DPD) (van Kuilenburg, 2004; see Fig. 18–9). Although DPD activity is present in different tissues and organs, including the gastrointestinal mucosa, the liver is the major site of 5-FU catabolism. The DPD gene is present as a single copy on chromosome 1p22, and consists of 23 exons. Mutations and polymorphism can lead to a deficiency of DPD activity. Although this deficiency does not lead to any detectable problems under normal circumstances, patients with this deficiency are subjected to increased toxicity when they are exposed to 5-FU. The most common mutation identified in patients who experienced severe 5-FU toxicity is a G-to-A mutation in the invariant GT splice donor site, which results in skipping of exon 14 immediately upstream. It is estimated that approximately 25% of patients with grade 3/4 5-FU toxicity are homozygous or heterozygous for this mutation (van Kuilenburg, 2004). This mutation is commonly detected in northern European patients, but, it has not been reported in Japanese or African Americans.

There are several other examples of genetic polymorphisms leading to alterations in drug toxicity, most of them relating to individual differences in drug metabolizing enzymes. The topoisomerase I inhibitor, irinotecan, is partially metabolized to SN-38, an active metabolite, through carboxylesterase. SN-38, when excreted unconjugated in the biliary tract, can cause damage to the gastrointestinal mucosa, resulting in diarrhea. Polymorphisms of uridine diphosphate glucuronosyltransferase (UGT)-1A1, the enzyme involved in conjugation of SN-38, have been identified and those leading to a reduced rate of conjugation are associated with higher risk of irinotecan toxicity, such as neutropenia and diarrhea (Mathijssen et al, 2001, 2003).

Several drugs rely on enzymes to be converted to active metabolites. Reduced enzyme activity as a result of genetic polymorphism would lead to lower levels of metabolites, resulting in lower therapeutic effects. Tamoxifen, which has a major role in endocrine therapy for breast cancer, is converted to an active metabolite, endoxifen, through the cytochrome P450 family of enzymes, in particular, CYP2D6 (see Chap. 20, Sec. 20.5.2). So far, more than 100 genetic variants in CYP2D6 have been identified, and patients can be grouped into 4 groups based on CYP2D6 activity: ultrahigh, normal, reduced, and no activity (Schroth et al, 2009). Some, but not all, studies suggest that patients with reduced CYP2D6 activity are at higher risks of failing to respond to tamoxifen, compared to those with normal CYP2D6 activity.

18.2 ALKYLATING AGENTS

Alkylating agents were the first drugs introduced for the systemic therapy of cancer. They are a chemically diverse group of drugs, but they all contain alkyl groups (eg, $-CH_2Cl$). In vivo, the alkyl groups generate highly reactive, positively charged intermediates, which then combine with an electron-rich nucleophilic group, such as an amino, phosphate, sulfhydryl, or hydroxyl moieties, on intracellular macromolecules, such as DNA. Although nucleophilic groups occur on almost all biological molecules, alkylation of bases in DNA appears to be the major cause of lethal toxicity.

Alkylating agents may contain 1 or 2 reactive groups and are thus classified as monofunctional or bifunctional, respectively. Bifunctional alkylating agents have the ability to form crosslinks between DNA strands and are the most clinically useful of these agents. Interstrand crosslinking of DNA, which prevents cell replication, unless repaired, seems to be the major mechanism of cytotoxicity for bifunctional alkylating agents, whereas the toxicity of monofunctional alkylating agents is probably related to single-strand breaks in DNA or to damaged bases. Mechanisms of resistance of alkylating agents include decreased transport across the cell membrane, increased intracellular thiol concentrations (eg, glutathione); such compounds react with alkylating agents and thus reduce the likelihood of interaction with DNA (see Chap. 19, Sec. 19.2.4), increased enzymatic detoxification of reactive intermediates, and alterations in DNA repair enzymes.

Because alkylating agents bind directly to DNA, they lack cell-cycle specificity, although they may have greater toxicity for proliferating cells. Common toxicities include myelosuppression, immunosuppression, hair loss, nausea, and vomiting. Some alkylating agents have long-term effects, such as infertility and carcinogenesis caused by long-lasting DNA damage. Nitrogen mustard, melphalan, and nitrosoureas are associated with an increased incidence of acute myelogenous leukemia, whereas cyclophosphamide is associated with irritation of the bladder and rarely development of bladder cancer. Mechanisms of resistance to alkylating agents include decreased transport across the cell membrane, increased intracellular thiol concentration leading to reduced DNA interactions, increased enzymatic detoxification of reactive intermediates, and alterations in DNA repair enzymes such as guanine-O[6]-alkyltransferase (Pegg, 1990; see Chap. 19, Sec. 19.2.6).

18.2.1 Nitrogen Mustards, Nitrosoureas, and Others

The development of nitrogen mustard and related compounds as anticancer drugs originated from the observation of lymphoid aplasia in men exposed to the more reactive, but chemically similar, sulfur mustard gas during World War II.

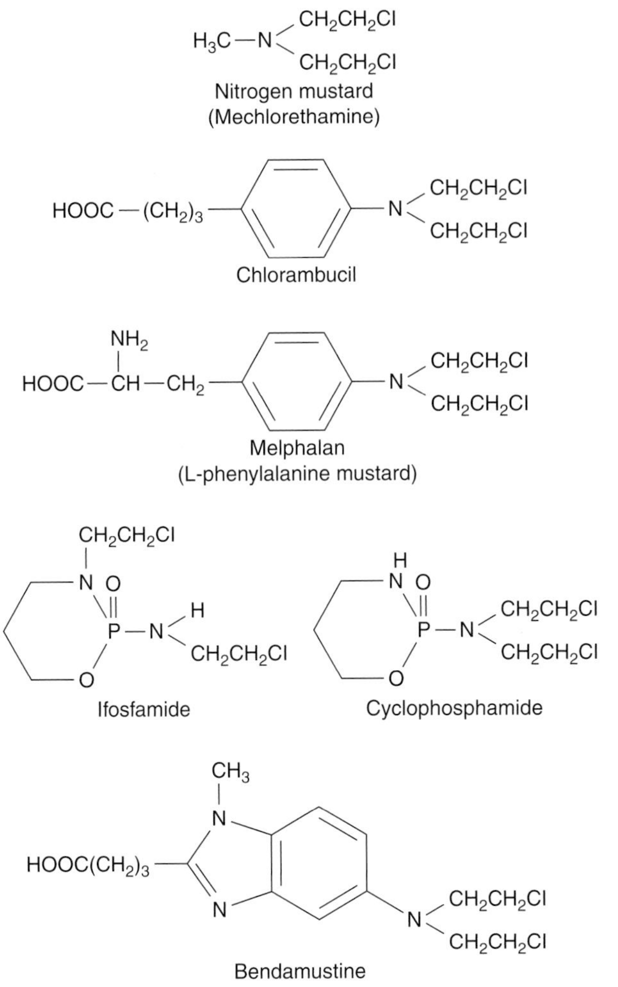

FIGURE 18-2 Structures of clinically used alkylating agents of the nitrogen mustard family.

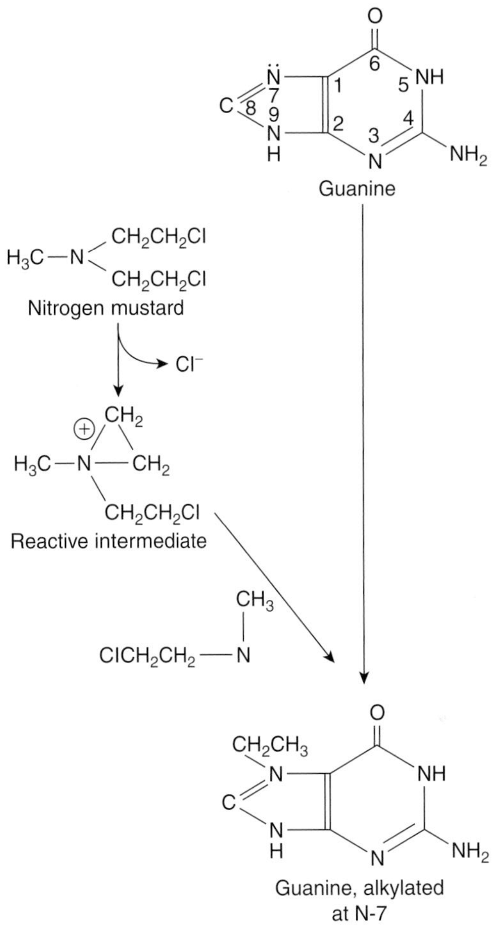

FIGURE 18-3 Reactions leading to alkylation at the N-7 position of guanine by nitrogen mustard.

This family of drugs, all chemically derived from nitrogen mustard (mechlorethamine) contains several drugs in common clinical use. The structures of these drugs are shown in Figure 18-2; each is bifunctional, with 2 chloroethyl groups that form the reactive electron-deficient groups responsible for alkylation of DNA.

The most common site of alkylation of DNA by nitrogen mustards is the N-7 position on the base guanine (Fig. 18-3). First, one of the chloroethyl side chains releases a chloride ion, resulting in a highly reactive, positively charged intermediate. This intermediate then binds covalently with the electronegative N-7 group on a guanine base, resulting in alkylation. Alkylation of guanine leads to mispairing with thymine or to strand breakage. The second chloroethyl side chain of nitrogen mustard may undergo a similar reaction, leading to covalent binding with another base on the opposite strand of DNA and thus to formation of an interstrand crosslink.

Mechlorethamine was the first anticancer drug introduced to clinical use. However, it is chemically unstable, and undergoes spontaneous hydrolysis. A large number of analogs have been synthesized and 5 of them (chlorambucil, melphalan, cyclophosphamide, ifosfamide, and bendamustine) have largely replaced mechlorethamine, which is only used clinically as part of the MOPP protocol (mechlorethamine, Oncovin [vincristine], procarbazine, prednisone) for Hodgkin disease. The addition of ring structures to the nitrogen mustard molecule confers increased stability, such that these agents can be administered orally.

Chlorambucil is a well-absorbed oral drug with a narrow spectrum of activity, and is used mainly in slowly progressive neoplasms, such as low-grade lymphomas and chronic lymphocytic leukemia. Oral melphalan is used for treatment of plasma cell myeloma and in some high-dose bone marrow transplantation protocols. Absorption of melphalan is variable and unpredictable; some patients with no effect after oral administration may respond when melphalan is given intravenously. Both chlorambucil and melphalan are almost equally toxic to cycling and noncycling cells, and may lead to delayed and/or cumulative effects on bone marrow because of their toxicity to hematopoietic stem cells.

Cyclophosphamide is the alkylating agent in widest clinical use and is part of treatment protocols for breast,

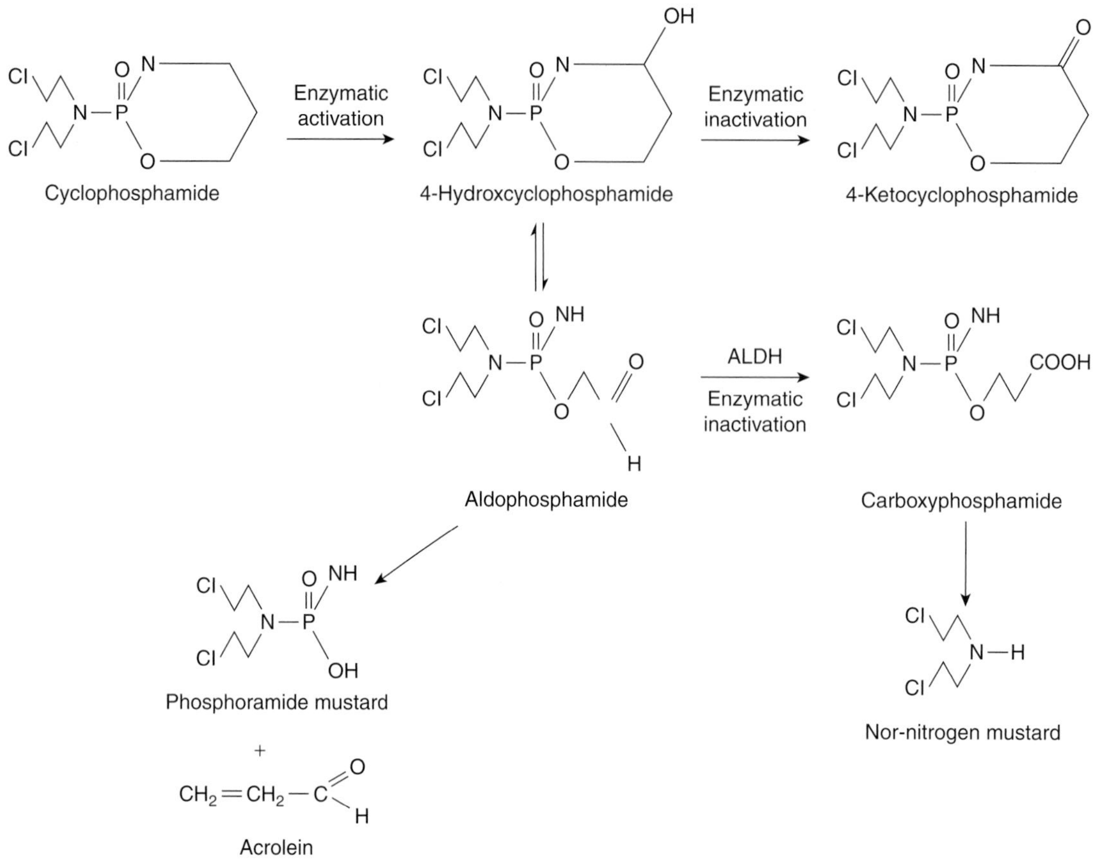

FIGURE 18–4 **The metabolism of cyclophosphamide.** *ALDH,* aldehyde dehydrogenase.

lymphatic, gynecological and pediatric tumors, in high-dose chemotherapy regimens, and for a number of autoimmune diseases. Cyclophosphamide is well absorbed after oral administration; however, the parent compound is inactive, requiring metabolism by hepatic mixed-function oxidases to form the alkylating intermediate phosphoramide mustard (Fig. 18–4). Hepatic microsomal enzymes metabolize cyclophosphamide to 4-hydroxycyclophosphamide, which exists in equilibrium with its acyclic isomer aldophosphamide. 4-Hydroxycyclophosphamide enters cells and spontaneously decomposes to form phosphoramide mustard and acrolein, or it is inactivated by aldehyde dehydrogenase. Elimination of cyclophosphamide and its metabolites is mainly by renal excretion. Cyclophosphamide induces cytochrome P450 enzymes, and hence its own metabolism with repeated administration. This alters the rate but not the absolute amount of phosphoramide mustard formation, so no dose adjustment is required.

The dose of cyclophosphamide given to patients ranges from 100 to 200 mg/m^2 per day given orally, to 600 to 1000 mg/m^2 given intravenously every 3 to 4 weeks. Very high doses are used in preparation for bone marrow transplantation. The dose in this setting is limited by irreversible damage to the heart, which occurs with single doses greater than 60 mg/kg (approximately 2500 mg/m^2). The usual dose-limiting toxicity is myelosuppression, and cyclophosphamide causes a fall in granulocyte count with rapid recovery by 3 to 4 weeks after administration (see Chap. 17, Sec. 17.5.2). There is relative sparing of stem cells and platelets, which may be a result of the higher concentrations of aldehyde dehydrogenase in early progenitor cells. Cyclophosphamide causes hemorrhagic cystitis with chronic use or at higher doses because of the direct irritative effect of acrolein on the bladder mucosa.

Ifosfamide is an analog of cyclophosphamide that differs in the presence of only 1 chloroethyl group on the oxazaphosphorine ring. It is used in the treatment of testicular cancer and sarcoma. Hemorrhagic cystitis is more common as a result of increased production of acrolein, such that all patients receiving ifosfamide should be given a sulfhydryl-containing compound, such as 2-mercaptoethane sulfonate (Mesna), which conjugates with acrolein in the urinary tract and renders it inactive. As Mesna dimerizes to an inactive metabolite in blood, and is hydrolyzed to its active form only in urine, it does not affect the cytotoxicity of cyclophosphamide or ifosfamide at other sites. Neurotoxicity, manifesting as changes in mental status including confusion, hallucination, cerebellar dysfunction, seizures, and coma, may occur with higher doses of ifosfamide, but not cyclophosphamide. Risks for ifosfamide neurotoxicity include low serum albumin, elevated creatinine and prior cisplatin treatment (Pratt et al, 1990; David and Picus, 2005).

Bendamustine is the newest bifunctional mechlorethamine derivative introduced into clinical practice. It is indicated for patients with chronic lymphocytic leukemia and indolent non-Hodgkin lymphoma.

The chloroethylnitrosoureas, BCNU (carmustine) and CCNU (lomustine), are lipid-soluble drugs that can penetrate into the central nervous system (CNS). These drugs have limited clinical application because they cause prolonged myelosuppression and are leukemogenic, likely because of direct effects on bone marrow stem cells. Streptozotocin, a methylnitrosourea, is used mainly in the treatment of pancreatic islet-cell tumors; it has less hematological toxicity than other nitrosoureas.

Busulfan, an alkyl alkane sulfonate, has a different mechanism of alkylation from the nitrogen mustards. It reacts more extensively with thiol groups of amino acids and proteins, but its ability to crosslink DNA is uncertain. Busulfan has selective effects on hematopoietic stem cells, and is now used mainly in high-dose bone marrow transplantation regimens. Busulfan is eliminated via hepatic metabolism, and the higher doses of busulfan used in marrow transplantation may cause hepatic venoocclusive disease in patients who metabolize the drug slowly.

A group of other compounds, with diverse chemical structures, that are also capable of forming covalent crosslink with intracellular macromolecules includes procarbazine, dacarbazine (DTIC), and temozolomide. Procarbazine is a synthetic derivative of hydrazine that was used in combination to treat lymphoma, including Hodgkin disease. It undergoes extensive metabolism to produce alkylating species, although details of its metabolism and mechanism of action remain unclear. It has largely been replaced by other alkylating agents. DTIC was synthesized originally as an antimetabolite to inhibit purine synthesis, but is believed to function through formation of methylcarbonium ions with alkylating properties. DTIC is metabolized by CYP450 enzymes to MTIC ([methyl-triazene-1-yl]-imidazole-4-carboxamide) which alkylates DNA at the O^6 and N^7 guanine positions (Marchesi et al, 2007). DTIC is sensitive to light, but is stable in neutral solutions away from light. Temozolomide is a prodrug that is stable under acidic conditions but undergoes rapid, spontaneous, nonenzymatic conversion to MTIC at pH levels greater than 7 (Marchesi et al, 2007); it is rapidly and completely absorbed after oral administration with a $t_{1/2}$ of 1 to 2 hours. Temozolomide is indicated for patients with newly diagnosed or recurrent malignant glioma, and has also shown activity in melanoma.

18.2.2 Platinating Agents

The prototype agent is cisplatin (cis-diamminedichloroplatinum II; Fig. 18–5), a drug whose discovery followed an observation that an electric current delivered to bacterial culture via platinum electrodes led to inhibition of bacterial growth. The active compound was identified as cisplatin, and it was shown subsequently to exert broad cytotoxic activity. Cisplatin is one of the most useful anticancer agents and is part of first-line therapy for testicular, urothelial, lung, gynecological,

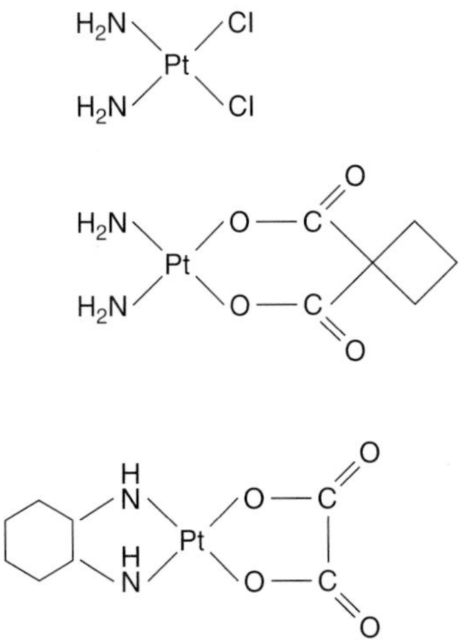

FIGURE 18–5 **Structure of platinum agents.**

and other cancers. It is also associated with substantial toxicity, which limits both the number of patients who are able to receive the drug, as well as the cumulative dose that can be given. There has been a major effort to identify other platinum analogs, either to reduce the toxicity while maintaining efficacy, or to expand the use of these compounds to tumors resistant to cisplatin. The 2 analogs in routine clinical usage are carboplatin and oxaliplatin (Fig. 18–5).

Platinum drugs can exist in a 2+ (II) or 4+ (IV) oxidation state, with 4 or 6 bonds linking the platinum atom, respectively. All currently used platinum drugs are platinum II compounds that exhibit a planar structure and have 4 attached chemical groups. The nature of these groups dictates the efficacy and pharmacokinetic properties of these compounds. Two of the groups are considered carrier groups, and are chemically inert, whereas the 2 leaving groups are available for substitution and reaction with molecules such as DNA.

Cisplatin acts by a mechanism that is similar to that of classical alkylating agents. The chlorine atoms are leaving groups that may be compared to those of nitrogen mustards; these atoms may be displaced directly by nucleophilic groups in DNA or indirectly after chloride ions are replaced by hydroxyl groups through reaction of the drug with water. These reactions occur more readily in environments where the chloride concentration is low, such as within the cell. The preferred sites for binding of cisplatin to DNA are the 7 positions of the guanine and adenine bases. The fact that structurally similar analogs, such as transplatin, will produce DNA binding but are devoid of cytotoxicity suggests that the stereochemistry of the compound is critical. Cisplatin binds to 2 sites on DNA and 95% of the binding produces intrastrand crosslinkages, usually between 2 adjacent guanine bases or adjacent guanine and adenine sites, with the remainder being interstrand guanine crosslinkages. The binding of platinum compounds to DNA is responsible for their cytotoxicity, although the mechanism whereby this leads to cell death is not clear.

Carboplatin is an analog of cisplatin with substitution of cyclobutanedicarboxylate for the chloride leaving groups.

This leads to a less-reactive compound that also has less toxicity but either comparable or slightly reduced efficacy to cisplatin. Oxaliplatin is one of a series of analogs with a substitution of a diaminocyclohexane (DACH) for the amine carrier groups (see Fig. 18–5). The DACH analogs have a different efficacy profile from cisplatin and have shown activity in tumors resistant to cisplatin, such as colorectal cancer. Carboplatin and oxaliplatin produce the same types of DNA adducts as cisplatin, although a higher concentration of carboplatin is required to produce a comparable number of adducts to cisplatin. Adducts formed by oxaliplatin are more likely to cause cell death, probably because of the different 3-dimensional structure that results from the DACH groups.

The pharmacokinetic differences between cisplatin and its analogs are a result of the differences in the leaving groups. Cisplatin is the most reactive and, following administration, it is rapidly and irreversibly bound to plasma proteins, with greater than 90% of free cisplatin lost in the first 2 hours. Total cisplatin (free and bound) disappears more slowly from plasma, with a prolonged $t_{1/2}$ of 2 to 3 days. Cisplatin is excreted mainly via the urine, and 15% to 30% of the administered dose is excreted during the first 24 hours. Carboplatin is more stable in plasma and is excreted primarily unchanged by the kidney, with 90% of administered dose excreted within 24 hours. The clearance of carboplatin is predicated by creatinine clearance; therefore, it is possible to determine the dose of carboplatin based on the desired carboplatin AUC and creatinine clearance (Calvert et al, 1989):

$$\text{Carboplatin dose (mg)} = \text{AUC} \times (\text{creatinine clearance} + 25)$$

Similar to cisplatin, oxaliplatin also binds to plasma proteins, although at a somewhat slower rate; it is also excreted primarily by the kidney.

Cisplatin causes little toxicity to bone marrow as a single agent, but can add to the toxic effects of other drugs, and may lead to anemia. Its major dose-limiting toxicities are nausea and vomiting, and damage to the kidney, to nerves, and to the ear with resulting loss of hearing. Vigorous intravenous hydration and maintaining a rapid urine output during and after drug administration minimize the effects on the kidneys; there is no known method for reducing the auditory or neurotoxicity.

Carboplatin has comparable activity to cisplatin against ovarian and lung tumors but is less active against urothelial and testicular cancers. Carboplatin has a better overall toxicity profile, which may make it preferable in palliative treatment regimens. There is minimal nephrotoxicity, and the drug causes less nausea and vomiting than cisplatin, but bone marrow suppression, particularly thrombocytopenia, is the dose-limiting toxicity. Carboplatin is used in some high-dose regimens prior to stem cell transplantation because its toxicities other than myelosuppression are relatively mild.

Oxaliplatin is used mainly in the treatment of colorectal cancer; it has minimal renal toxicity, and causes less vomiting than cisplatin and no ototoxicity. Oxaliplatin causes a unique spectrum of sensory neurotoxicity, ranging from acute neuropathy (paresthesia, muscle spasm and fasciculations or muscle twitching) immediately after infusion with marked sensitivity to the cold, particularly in the oropharynx, to a late cumulative dose-limiting sensory neuropathy resulting in sensory ataxia and functional impairment. Coadministration of calcium and magnesium may delay the onset of neuropathy and reduce its severity (Gamelin et al, 2008).

Resistance to platinating agents can be a result of reduced platinum-DNA adduct formation, or of increased repair or tolerance of the platinum-DNA adduct. Decreased uptake or increased binding to intracellular scavengers can result in reduced platinum-DNA adduct formation (Koberle et al, 2010).

18.3 ANTIMETABOLITES

Antimetabolites are drugs that interfere with normal cellular functions, particularly the synthesis of DNA that is required for cell replication. Many of the clinically useful agents are purine or pyrimidine analogs that either inhibit the formation of the normal nucleotides or interact with DNA and prevent further extension of the new DNA strand, leading to inhibition of cell division. The antifolates (eg, methotrexate) are not nucleoside analogs; they prevent the formation of reduced folates, which are required for the synthesis of DNA.

Most antimetabolites are cell-cycle specific; their toxicity relates to effects on proliferating cells and is primarily seen in bone marrow and gastrointestinal mucosa. As they do not interact directly with DNA, they do not cause the later problems of carcinogenesis seen with alkylating agents. The effects of these drugs are dependent upon the schedule of administration. For many drugs the duration of exposure above a critical threshold required to inhibit an enzyme is more important than the peak concentration. Therefore, although large doses may be tolerated if the drug is given as a single intravenous injection, a much lower dose is required if the drug is given repeatedly or by continuous infusion.

18.3.1 Antifolates

Methotrexate is an analog of the vitamin folic acid (Fig. 18–6). Reduced folate is required for transfer of methyl groups in the biosynthesis of purines and in the conversion of deoxyuridine monophosphate (dUMP) to thymidine monophosphate (dTMP), a reaction catalyzed by thymidylate synthase. Reduced folate becomes oxidized in the latter reaction; its regeneration is dependent on the enzyme dihydrofolate reductase (DHFR) for reduction to its active form. Methotrexate competitively inhibits DHFR and prevents the formation of reduced folate (Fig. 18–7). The result of this inhibition may be cessation of DNA synthesis because of nonavailability of dTMP and/or purines, leading to cell death.

Methotrexate enters the cell primarily by active transport. However, its uptake may be by passive diffusion at high drug concentrations. Intracellular metabolism of methotrexate leads to addition of glutamic acid residues to the initial

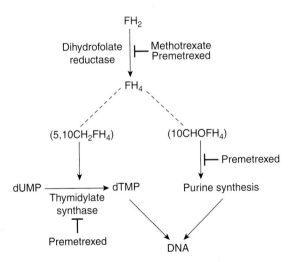

FIGURE 18–6 **Structures of folic acid, methotrexate, and pemetrexed.**

glutamate residue of the drug, a process known as *polygluta-mation*. Methotrexate polyglutamates cannot be transported across the cell membrane, so their formation prevents efflux of the drug, and they appear to be more effective than metho-trexate itself in inhibiting the activity of DHFR. The cytotoxic action of methotrexate depends critically on the duration of exposure of tissue to levels of drug above a certain threshold,

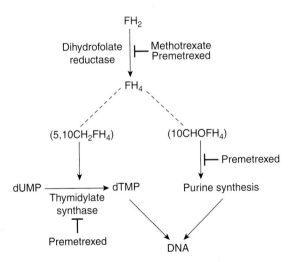

FIGURE 18–7 **Influence of methotrexate on cellular metabolism.** Methotrexate competitively inhibits DHFR and depletes the pools of reduced folates (FH$_4$): 5,10-methylene tetrahydrofolate (5,10CH$_2$FH$_4$) and 10 formyltetrahydrofolate (10CHOFH$_4$). Reduced folates are required in the conversion of dUMP to dTMP and for purine synthesis, respectively. Interruption of these processes leads to inhibition of DNA synthesis.

rather than on the peak levels of drug in the tissue. For many tissues, the threshold concentration for cytotoxicity appears to be in the range of 10^{-8} to 10^{-7} M. Methotrexate has selective toxicity for cells synthesizing DNA, and prolonged treatment with the drug may cause toxicity to more cells as they enter the S-phase of the cell cycle.

The toxicity of methotrexate may be reversed by adminis-tration of thymidine and exogenous purines or by a source of reduced folate. These agents circumvent the effects of metho-trexate by providing products of the interrupted metabolism (see Fig. 18–7). They have been used clinically to reverse the activity of methotrexate following a defined period of expo-sure (usually 24 to 36 hours) to methotrexate at high doses. Reduced folate in the form of 5-formyltetrahydrofolate (also known as leucovorin or folinic acid) has been used in many clinical protocols and has allowed the administration of doses of methotrexate that are increased by factors of 10 to 100 over conventional doses. The arguments put forward for such high-dose methotrexate treatment include (a) selective uptake by tumor cells, (b) better CNS penetration, and (c) lack of myelo-suppression. This type of protocol allows for frequent admin-istration of methotrexate and retained therapeutic efficacy with little or no toxicity in many patients. However, responses to treatment are observed only rarely in patients who are refractory to conventional doses of methotrexate given with-out leucovorin rescue. Although toxicity is often lower with the use of high doses of methotrexate and leucovorin, an occa-sional patient may experience life-threatening toxicity, usually as a consequence of damage to the kidney or sequestration in fluid-filled spaces (eg, ascites, pleural effusions) and conse-quently delayed drug clearance. Methotrexate can cause renal dysfunction during infusion, and this is thought to be a result of precipitation of methotrexate and its metabolites in acidic urine. Therefore, most protocols of high-dose methotrexate mandate vigorous hydration and alkylation of the urine. Methotrexate infusion should not start until the urine output is more than 100 mL/h, and urine pH is 7.0 or higher.

Methotrexate can be given orally, intramuscularly, intravenously, and intrathecally (ie, into the cerebrospinal fluid that surrounds the brain and spinal cord). It crosses the blood–brain barrier but achieves cytotoxic concentrations in the CNS only with intrathecal or high-dose intravenous administration. It accumulates in fluid-filled spaces such as pleural effusions, from which it is released slowly. The parent compound and hepatic metabolites are excreted by the kidney. This excretion can be inhibited by the presence of weak organic acids such as aspirin or penicillin. Aspirin may also displace methotrexate from its binding sites on plasma albumin, and these 2 effects of aspirin can increase the toxicity of methotrexate. Methotrexate dose needs to be reduced in patients with renal dysfunction. The $t_{1/2}$ of methotrexate ranges from 3 to 10 hours.

Methotrexate has a wide spectrum of clinical activity and may be curative for women with choriocarcinoma, a tumor derived from fetal elements. Its major toxicities are myelosuppression and inflammation of the oral and gastrointestinal mucosa; these toxicities are usually observed within 5 to 7 days of administration, earlier than for many other drugs. Rarer toxicities include damage to liver, lung, and brain, the latter occurring most frequently after intrathecal administration. In general, the drug is well tolerated compared with many other anticancer drugs.

Pemetrexed is a folate-based potent inhibitor of thymidylate synthase (TS) with glutamic acid at one end of the molecule (see Fig. 18–6). Similar to methotrexate, pemetrexed can be polyglutamated for increased retention in cells and increased potency of TS inhibition. In addition to targeting TS, pemetrexed inhibits DHFR and glycinamide ribonucleotide formyltransferase (GARFT); the latter is a folate-dependent enzyme involved in purine synthesis. Pemetrexed has activity in non–small cell lung cancer and mesothelioma; it is administered intravenously and renal excretion is the major route of elimination with a $t_{1/2}$ of 3 to 4 hours. The main toxicities are myelosuppression, inflammation of the oral and gastrointestinal mucosa, and skin rash. Treatment with pemetrexed requires supplementation with folic acid and vitamin B_{12}.

Raltitrexed is another inhibitor of TS with similar mechanisms of action to pemetrexed. Although it was initially thought to be as active as 5-FU in the treatment of colorectal cancer, subsequent studies showed increased mortality related to raltitrexed . Its use is limited to patients who are intolerant of 5-FU.

18.3.2 5-Fluoropyrimidines

5-FU is a drug that resembles the pyrimidine bases uracil and thymine, which are components of RNA and DNA, respectively (Fig. 18–8). It penetrates rapidly into cells, where it is metabolized to nucleosides by addition of ribose or deoxyribose; these

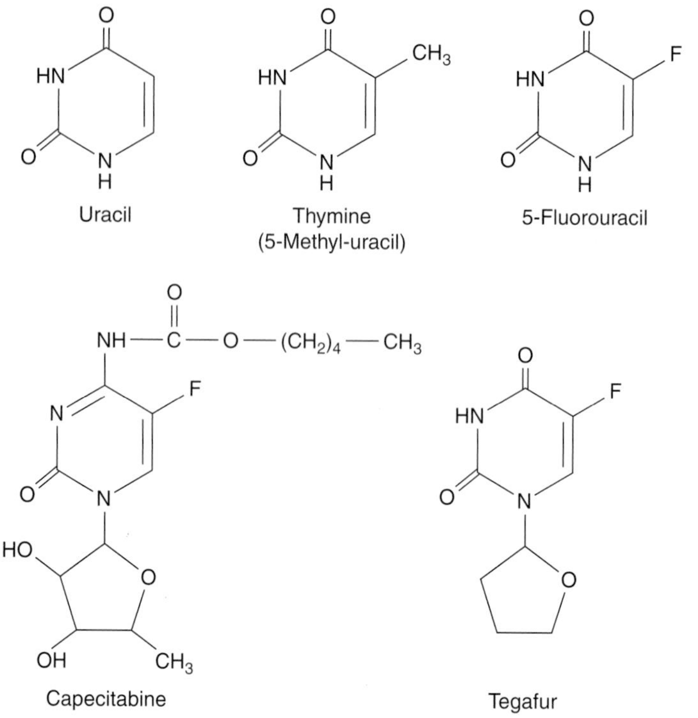

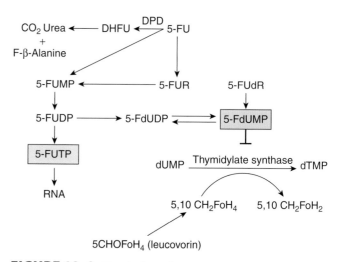

FIGURE 18–8 Structures of uracil, thymine, 5-FU, capecitabine, and tegafur.

reactions are catalyzed by enzymes that normally act on uracil and thymine. Phosphorylation then leads to the active fluorinated nucleotides 5-fluoro-uridine-triphosphate (5-FUTP) and 5-fluoro-deoxyuridine-monophosphate (5-FdUMP) (Fig. 18–9). 5-FUTP can be incorporated into RNA in place of UTP (uridine triphosphate); this leads to inhibition of the nuclear processing of ribosomal and messenger RNA and may cause

FIGURE 18–9 Metabolic pathways of 5-fluorouracil (5-FU). Fo is used here to distinguish 'Folate' from 'F, Fluorine'. *DHFU*, dihydrofluorouracil; *DPD*, dihydropyrimidine dehydrogenase; *5-FdUDP*, 5-fluorouridine diphosphate; *5-FdUMP*, 5-fluorodeoxyuridine monophosphate; *5-FUDP*, 5-fluorouridine diphosphate; *5-FUMP*, 5-fluorouridine monophosphate; *5-FUR*, 5-Fluorouridine.

other errors of base pairing during transcription of RNA. 5-FdUMP binds irreversibly to, and inhibits, the enzyme TS, leading to depletion of dTMP (thymidine monophosphate), which is required for DNA synthesis.

Approximately 80% of 5-FU administered is catabolized to CO_2, urea, and α-fluro-β-alanine, mainly in the liver. The rate-limiting step in 5-FU catabolism is mediated by the enzyme DPD. The catabolism of 5-FU appears to be an important determinant of normal-tissue toxicity. Although DPD deficiency does not lead to any detectable problems in healthy individuals, patients with a partial or complete deficiency of DPD are at risk for severe toxicity from the drug (see Chap. 3, Sec. 3.6.2 and Chap. 18, Sec. 18.1.3).

Inhibition of TS by FdUMP is dependent on the presence of the cofactor 5,10-methyl-N-tetrahydrofolate, which combines with TS and FdUMP to form a covalent ternary complex. The dissociation rate of this complex is decreased in the presence of excess cofactor, which led to studies showing that addition of the prodrug 5-formyltetrahydrofolate (5-CHOFH$_4$, leucovorin or folinic acid) increased the cytotoxicity of 5-FU (see Fig. 18–8). Clinical studies demonstrate that this combination has greater activity in the treatment of patients with metastatic colorectal cancer than 5-FU alone.

5-FU is used most commonly for treatment of breast and gastrointestinal cancers. It is administered intravenously because bioavailability after oral administration is low and variable. 5-FU is eliminated rapidly from plasma with a $t_{1/2}$ of a few minutes. This agent demonstrates nonlinear pharmacokinetics because of a saturation of metabolism at higher concentrations, which may be seen when it is given by bolus injection, but not when given by infusion. This difference in pharmacokinetic behavior under the 2 conditions of administration may explain why the dose-limiting toxicity is to bone marrow for bolus injection and to mucous membranes if the drug is given over 4 to 5 days by continuous infusion. Rarer toxicities include skin rashes, conjunctivitis, ataxia as a result of effects on the cerebellum, and cardiotoxicity. Prolonged low-dose infusion of 5-FU can be administered with a decrease in some of the above toxicities, but they are associated with changes in sensation as well as with redness and peeling of the skin on the palms of the hands and the soles of the feet, referred to as *palmar-plantar erythrodysesthesia*, or *the hand-foot syndrome*. There is limited evidence that this method of 5-FU administration results in improvement of antitumor effects when compared with 5-FU given by bolus injection.

Several oral fluoropyrimidine derivatives have been developed to provide a convenient route of administration and sustained drug exposure. Capecitabine is absorbed unchanged from the gastrointestinal tract, metabolized in the liver by carboxylesterase to 5′-deoxy-5-fluorocytidine (5′-DFCR), which is then converted to 5′-deoxy-5-fluorouridine (5′-DFUR) by cytidine deaminase, mainly located in the liver and tumor tissues. Further metabolism of 5′-DFUR to the cytotoxic moiety 5-FU occurs at the site of the tumor by thymidine phosphorylase, an enzyme present in higher concentrations in tumor cells, resulting in levels considerably higher in tumor tissues

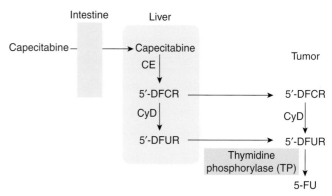

FIGURE 18–10 **Enzymatic activation of capecitabine.** *CE*, carboxyesterase; *CyD*, cytidine deaminase.

compared to normal tissues (Fig. 18–10; Miwa et al, 1998). The toxicity profile of capecitabine is similar to that of prolonged low-dose infusion of 5-FU, with lower frequencies of myelosuppression and stomatitis, but higher incidence of palmar-plantar erythrodysesthesia than intravenous bolus 5-FU. Capecitabine has demonstrated efficacy in breast and colorectal malignancies. Randomized Phase III trials comparing capecitabine to intravenous 5-FU plus leucovorin have shown equivalent efficacy in patients with metastatic colorectal cancer.

Tegafur is a prodrug of 5-FU. Although it is absorbed orally, tegafur needs to be administered at high doses to produce sufficiently high plasma 5-FU levels, and, unfortunately, high doses of tegafur are associated with a high incidence of CNS toxicity. UFT is a combination formulation of uracil and tegafur at a 4:1 ratio. The excess uracil competes with 5-FU for DPD, thereby inhibiting 5-FU catabolism and resulting in sustained and sufficiently high plasma 5-FU levels. S-1 is another oral combination formulation consisting of tegafur, 5-chloro-2,4-dihydroxypyridine (an inhibitor of DPD), and potassium oxonate (an inhibitor of orotate phosphoribosyltransferase, which phosphorylates 5-FU in the intestine resulting in diarrhea) in a 1:0.4:1 ratio. S-1 has similar efficacy, but a better toxicity profile compared to 5-FU (Ajani et al, 2010).

18.3.3 Cytidine Analogs

Nucleoside analogs compete with their physiological counterparts for incorporation into DNA and RNA, thereby exerting their cytotoxicity. Cytosine arabinoside (ara-C) differs from the nucleoside deoxycytidine only by the presence of a β-hydroxyl group on the 2-position of the sugar, so that the sugar moiety is arabinose instead of deoxyribose (Fig. 18–11). Ara-C penetrates cells rapidly by a carrier-mediated process shared with deoxycytidine and is phosphorylated to ara-CTP. Ara-CTP is a competitive inhibitor of DNA polymerase, an enzyme necessary for DNA synthesis, and has similar affinity for this enzyme to the normal substrate dCTP. When ara-CTP binds to this enzyme, DNA synthesis is arrested and S-phase cells may die. In addition, Ara-CTP is incorporated into elongating DNA strands, resulting in DNA chain termination.

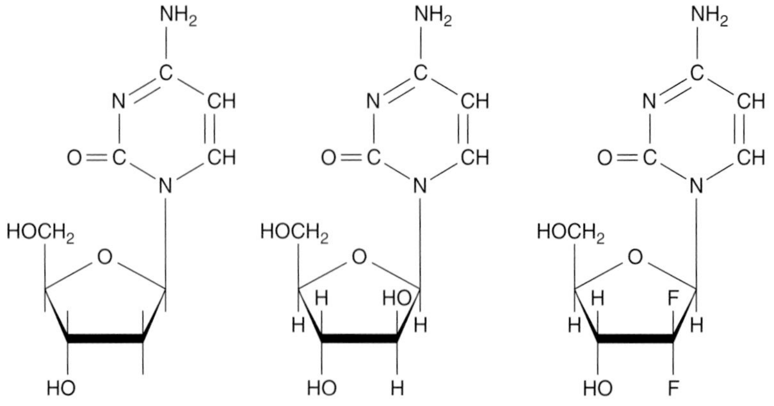

FIGURE 18–11 Structures of deoxycytidine and its analogs.

Deoxycytidine   Cytosine arabinoside   Gemcitabine

The availability of ara-CTP for cytotoxic activity depends critically on the balance between kinases that activate the drug and deaminases that degrade it. The activity of these enzymes varies greatly among different types of cells, leading to different rates of generation of ara-CTP. Resistance to the action of ara-C may occur by mutations that lead to deficiency in deoxycytidine kinase or to cells with an expanded pool of dCTP that competes with the active metabolite ara-CTP and regulates enzymes involved in activation and degradation of the drug. Ara-C is specific in its activity for cells synthesizing DNA. Because it is rapidly degraded in plasma with a $t_{1/2}$ of 7 to 20 minutes, it must be given intravenously by frequent injections or by continuous infusion. The drug is used primarily for treatment of acute leukemia. Myelosuppression and gastrointestinal toxicity are the major side effects, but abnormal behavior and thought processes may also occur after high doses.

Gemcitabine (2′,2′-difluorodeoxycytidine) is a cytosine analog with structural similarities to ara-C (see Fig. 18–11). Unlike ara-C, gemcitabine has activity against a variety of solid tumors. Like ara-C, gemcitabine requires intracellular activation to its triphosphate derivative dFdCTP, which is then incorporated into DNA and inhibits further DNA synthesis. Although gemcitabine is less effective than ara-C in DNA chain termination, a favorable pharmacokinetic characteristic of gemcitabine is the prolonged retention of dFdCTP in cells, with a $t_{1/2}$ as long as 72 hours. Gemcitabine has other intracellular effects that may contribute to its cytotoxic activity including inhibition of ribonucleotide reductase, stimulation of deoxycytidine kinase, and inhibition of cytidine deaminase. Through inhibition of ribonucleoside reductase, gemcitabine affects DNA synthesis by preventing de novo synthesis of the deoxyribonucleoside triphosphate precursors. Gemcitabine has activity against non-small cell lung cancer, pancreatic cancer, breast cancer, bladder cancer, and nasopharyngeal cancer. Toxicity is primarily myelosuppression, especially, thrombocytopenia.

18.3.4 Purine Antimetabolites

There are 2 adenosine analogs in clinical use (Fig. 18–12). Fludarabine is a derivative that is resistant to deamination and has activity against low-grade lymphoma, chronic lymphocytic leukemia, hairy cell leukemia, and Waldenström macroglobulinemia. After administration, fludarabine is rapidly dephosphorylated to 2-fluoro-ara-A, which then is transported into cells and converted to the active triphosphate derivative. Mechanisms of cytotoxicity include inhibition of DNA polymerase and termination of DNA and RNA replication. Because 2-fluoro-ara-A is excreted primarily unchanged in the urine, dose reduction is necessary in the setting of renal insufficiency. Fludarabine can be administered either intravenously or orally with a $t_{1/2}$ of approximately 20 hours. The

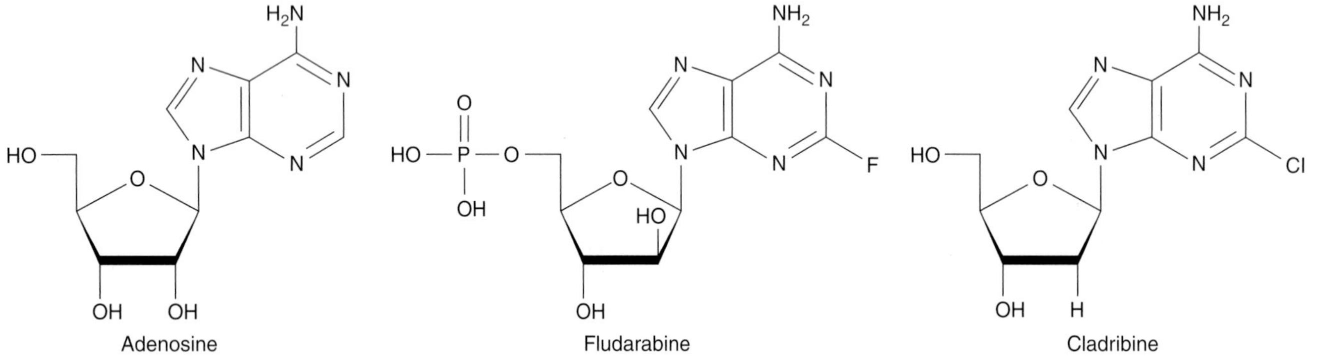

Adenosine   Fludarabine   Cladribine

FIGURE 18–12 Structures of adenosine and analogs.

major toxicity of fludarabine is myelosuppression and immunosuppression. Rarely, fludarabine is associated with development of autoimmune disease, such as hemolytic anemia and autoimmune thrombocytopenia, and CNS toxicity.

Cladribine (2CdA) is a potent chlorinated adenosine that is also resistant to deamination. It has a similar spectrum of clinical activity and toxicity to fludarabine. Cladribine is administered intravenously with a $t_{1/2}$ of 5 hours.

18.4 TOPOISOMERASE INHIBITORS

DNA topoisomerases are ubiquitous nuclear enzymes that relax supercoiled double-stranded DNA to allow DNA replication and RNA transcription. Torsional strain is relieved via the formation of a single-strand nick (topoisomerase I) or a double-strand nick (topoisomerase II), followed by swiveling of DNA at the nick(s) and subsequent religation (Fig. 18–13; see also Chap. 19, Sec. 19.2.5). Topoisomerase inhibitors bind to and stabilize the DNA/topoisomerase cleavable complex, thus preventing the religation of DNA strands. Irreversible damage results when an advancing DNA replication fork encounters the drug-stabilized cleavable complex, ultimately leading to lethal double-stranded breaks and cell death.

18.4.1 Topoisomerase I Inhibitors

Camptothecin is an extract from the wood of the Chinese tree *Camptotheca acuminate* (Fig. 18–14). Camptothecin affects only topoisomerase I activity; cells in S-phase are very sensitive, possibly because the process of DNA replication requires topoisomerase I activity and because the topoisomerase-associated single-strand breaks are converted into double-strand breaks. Initial Phase I studies conducted in the early 1970s were terminated because of poor solubility and severe and unpredictable toxicity, mainly hemorrhagic cystitis and gastroenteritis. Several analogs of camptothecin have been synthesized to improve solubility and reduce toxicity after the elucidation of its mechanism of action. These analogs all have a basic heterocyclic 5-ring structure with a lactone moiety and a hydroxyl moiety on the E ring (see Fig. 18–14). Substitutions on the A ring tend to increase the aqueous solubility while retaining cytotoxicity. All camptothecins can undergo a rapid, reversible, pH-dependent, nonenzymatic hydrolysis of the closed lactone ring to yield an open-ring carboxylate form. The carboxylate form is more water soluble than the lactone; it predominates at physiological pH, but is much less active as an inhibitor of topoisomerase I.

Topotecan can be given orally or intravenously. It does not undergo any appreciable metabolism and is primarily

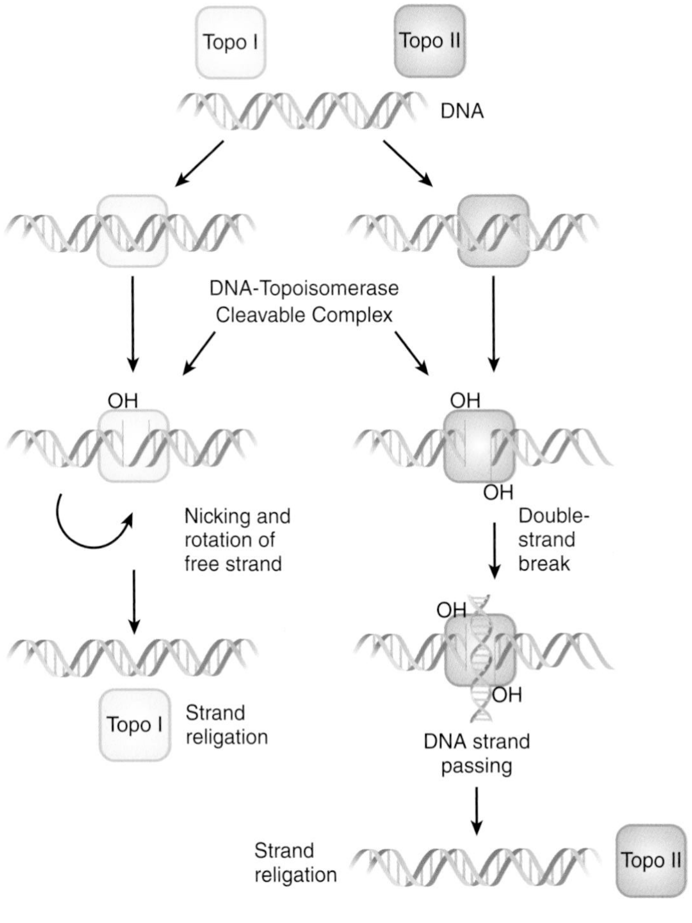

FIGURE 18–13 Topoisomerase (Topo) I and II enzymes form single-strand nicks and double-strand nicks, respectively. Swiveling of supercoiled DNA then occurs at the nick(s), followed by religation to relieve torsional strain.

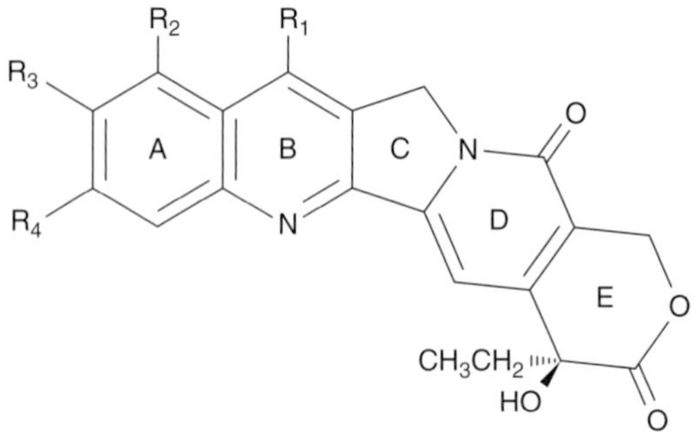

Compound	Molecular weight	R_1	R_2	R_3	R_4
Camptothecin	348	—H	—H	—H	—H
Topotecan	421	—H	—CH₂N(CH₃)₂	—OH	—H
Irinotecan	587	—CH₂CH₃	—H	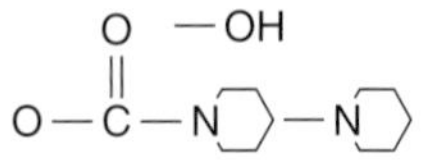 (carbamate-piperidine-piperidine group)	—H
SN-38	392	—CH₂CH₃	—H	—OH	—H

FIGURE 18–14 Structures of camptothecin and its derivatives.

eliminated unchanged by the kidneys. Therefore, dose reduction is required in patients with renal dysfunction. The dose-limiting toxicity is myelosuppression. It is used as treatment for ovarian cancer and small cell lung cancer.

Irinotecan (CPT-11) requires esterification by serum and tissue carboxylesterases to an active metabolite SN-38. SN-38 is subsequently inactivated through glucuronidation by the enzyme uridine diphosphate (UDP)-glucuronosyltransferase 1A1 (UGT1A1) into SN-38G, and excreted into bile and the intestine. Dose-limiting toxicity consists of myelosuppression and diarrhea. Irinotecan can produce an early cholinergic syndrome consisting of abdominal cramps, diarrhea, and diaphoresis that typically occurs acutely during or immediately after infusion, and prompt resolution can be obtained with intravenous or subcutaneous atropine. Patients who experience this reaction may benefit from prophylactic atropine prior to subsequent irinotecan infusions. A second distinct type of diarrhea is associated with irinotecan, typically with a delayed onset. This type of diarrhea tends to be more severe and protracted and is believed to be a result of damage to the gastrointestinal mucosa by SN-38. Severe late-onset diarrhea, especially in the setting of myelosuppression, can be life-threatening and can be managed with high-dose loperamide (Rothenberg et al, 2001). Genetic polymorphism in the UGT1A1 gene can result in reduced activity, and increased levels of SN-38. The most common variant is the UGT1A1*28 variant, which contains 7 TA repeats in the TATA repeat box instead of the normal 6 TA repeats. Patients who are homozygous or heterozygous for the UGT1A1*28 allele have reduced UGT1A1 activity, and are therefore at increased risk of neutropenia and diarrhea, and the irinotecan dose should be reduced (van der Bol et al, 2010). Irinotecan is approved for the treatment of advanced colorectal cancer, where it has been shown to improve survival when used in combination with 5-FU and leucovorin.

18.4.2 Epipodophyllotoxins

Etoposide (VP-16) and teniposide (VM-26) are semisynthetic glycoside derivatives of podophyllotoxin, an antimitotic agent derived from the mandrake plant (Fig. 18–15). Although podophyllotoxin binds to tubulin and inhibits its polymerization, etoposide and teniposide act through inhibition of DNA topoisomerase II. These agents are substrates for P-glycoprotein, and drug resistance can thus be mediated by the multidrug-resistant mechanism (see Chap. 19, Sec. 19.2.3). Etoposide is a component of first-line treatment regimens in small cell lung cancer, testicular cancer, pediatric cancers, and malignant lymphomas. Teniposide has a more limited role and is used mainly in the treatment of childhood leukemia. The effectiveness of

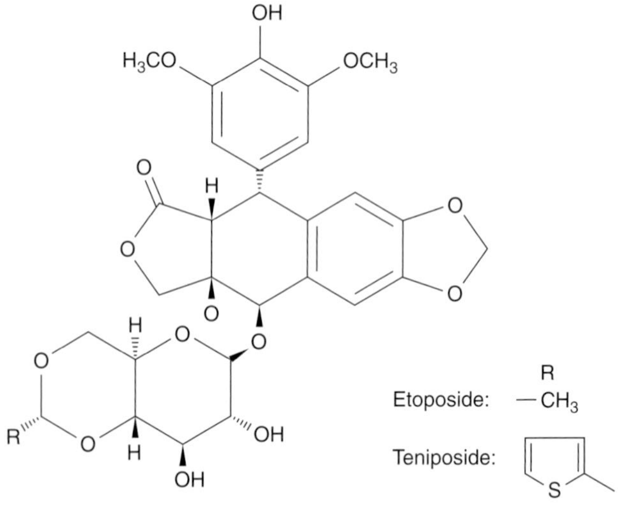

FIGURE 18–15 Structures of etoposide and teniposide. Solid and broken tapered arrows indicate bonds above and below the plane of the rest of the molecule, respectively.

etoposide is markedly schedule dependent, with repeated daily doses providing greater activity than a single intravenous administration. Etoposide can be administered orally, with a bioavailability of approximately 50% but considerable interindividual variability. Following intravenous administration, etoposide is eliminated by hepatic glucuronidation, but approximately 40% of the drug is excreted unchanged in the urine. The toxicity of etoposide at standard doses is myelosuppression and hair loss, with other side effects being uncommon. This toxicity profile makes etoposide ideal for high-dose transplantation regimens, and at these higher doses, mucositis becomes dose-limiting. An association between the use of etoposide and a secondary leukemia with a characteristic 11q23 translocation has been described. In contrast to secondary leukemia arising from the use of alkylating agents, which occur with a latency of up to 10 years, those arising from etoposide tend to occur sooner, with a median latent period of approximately 2 to 3 years after drug administration. Most cases of etoposide-induced secondary leukemia are monocytic and myelomonocytic (FAB M-4 and M-5), with no antecedent pancytopenia before the development of frank leukemia.

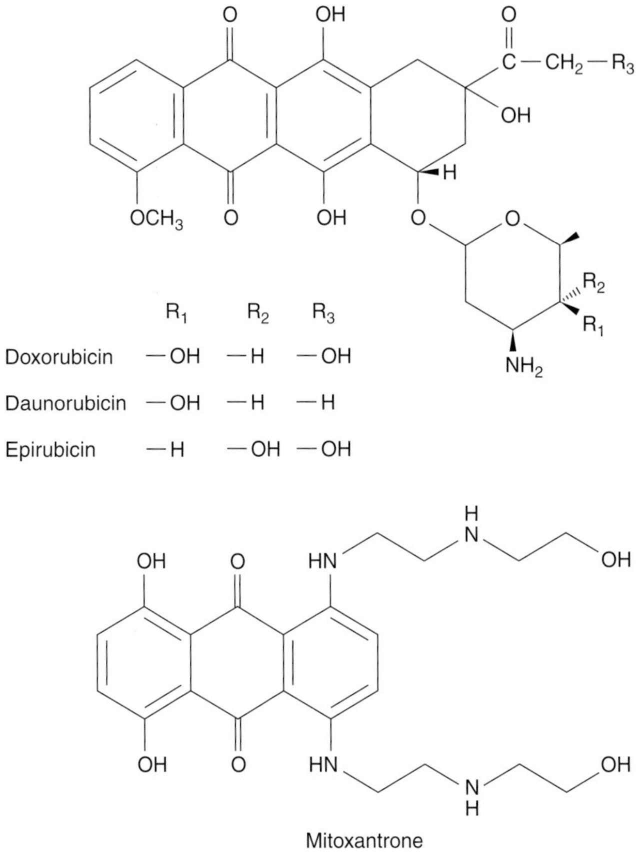

18.4.3 Anthracyclines and Anthracenediones

The original anthracycline, daunorubicin, is a product of a *Streptomyces* species isolated from an Italian soil sample in 1958. The drug has a high activity against acute leukemia and remains a component of many current protocols for acute myelogenous leukemia. Modifications of the structure of daunorubicin led to the identification of doxorubicin, an analog with greater activity against many solid tumors and one of the most active anticancer drugs in clinical practice (Fig. 18–16). The success of doxorubicin led to synthesis of other analogs, but of the hundreds developed and tested, only 2 are used currently; both have only marginal advantages. Idarubicin can be given orally and has similar activity against acute leukemia. Epirubicin differs from doxorubicin only in its 3-dimensional configuration; it has equal activity and possibly less toxicity.

Several mechanisms may contribute to the cytocidal effect of doxorubicin and related drugs, including interaction with topoisomerase II, DNA intercalation, formation of free radicals, and effects on the cell membrane. Doxorubicin can interact with topoisomerase II by binding directly with the enzyme and preventing resealing of topoisomerase II-induced DNA cleavage, ultimately leading to cytocidal DNA breaks (see Fig. 18–13). Doxorubicin can also intercalate between base pairs perpendicular to the long axis of the double helix. However, much of the DNA is organized and folded into chromatin and may be protected from this type of drug interaction. Also the concentration of doxorubicin required to intercalate into DNA and to cause inhibition of DNA and RNA polymerase cannot be achieved in vivo without excessive toxicity.

Doxorubicin may undergo metabolism of its quinone ring to a semiquinone radical (ie, a group containing an unpaired electron) that, in turn, reacts rapidly with oxygen to yield

	R_1	R_2	R_3
Doxorubicin	—OH	—H	—OH
Daunorubicin	—OH	—H	—H
Epirubicin	—H	—OH	—OH

Mitoxantrone

FIGURE 18–16 Structures of doxorubicin, daunorubicin, epirubicin, and mitoxantrone.

superoxide, O_2^-. The superoxide radical is known to undergo several reactions that can lead to cell death, including oxidative damage of cell membranes and DNA (Gewirtz, 1999). There is evidence that free radical formation accounts for the cardiac toxicity of anthracyclines, but the contribution of free radicals to the killing of cancer cells is uncertain. Resistance to anthracyclines has been associated with an increase in the free radical scavenger system (glutathione and related compounds), but doxorubicin retains toxicity under hypoxic conditions, when superoxide radicals cannot be formed. Another mechanism of resistance is increased drug efflux caused by overexpression of P-170 glycoprotein and other multidrug resistant proteins (Broxterman et al, 2009; see Chap. 19, Sec. 19.2.3).

With the exception of idarubicin, anthracyclines are administered intravenously, because oral absorption is poor. They are widely distributed in the body, with significant binding to plasma proteins and tissue. Doxorubicin is metabolized in the liver to doxorubicinol, which retains some cytotoxic activity, and to several other metabolites; the drug and its metabolites are excreted via the bile. Thus, dosage reduction is required for patients with hepatic dysfunction or biliary obstruction.

The acute toxicities of doxorubicin include myelosuppression, total loss of hair, nausea, vomiting, mucositis, and local tissue necrosis following leakage of drug at the injection site. Repeated administration is limited by a chronic irreversible cardiomyopathy that occurs with increasing frequency once a total dose of approximately 500 mg/m^2 has been given. The mechanism of cardiotoxicity is probably related to damage to sarcoplasmic reticulum mediated by the formation of free radicals within cardiac muscle. Patients with preexisting cardiac disease or those who have received mediastinal radiation are more likely to develop this problem. Cardiac toxicity appears to be more related to peak concentration of drug than to overall exposure, so that infusional or repeated lower-dose administration will reduce the chances of its occurrence. Dexrazoxane, an iron-chelating agent, reduces cardiac toxicity by binding free iron and prevents oxidative stress on cardiac tissues. Doxorubicin efficacy is not compromised when dexrazoxane is administered (Marty et al, 2006).

Pegylated liposomal doxorubicin is a formulation where doxorubicin is confined in liposomes that are coated with polyethylene glycol to resist degradation by the endoreticular system. As a result, it has a long half-life, approximately 70 hours, compared to less than 10 minutes when doxorubicin alone is administered intravenously. The long circulating half-life promotes preferential uptake into tumor tissues and reduces uptake by normal tissues. It has been shown that pegylated liposomal doxorubicin reduces cardiac toxicity, myelosuppression, and nausea, but maintains a comparable efficacy with doxorubicin. However, pegylated liposomal doxorubicin increases the risk of skin toxicity, with 20% of patients developing grade 3 hand-foot syndrome (Gordon et al, 2001).

Mitoxantrone is an anthracenedione that differs from the anthracyclines in lacking the sugar and the tetracyclic ring (see Fig. 18–16). It is a synthetic drug with 3 planar rings that intercalates into DNA, with a preference for guanine-cytosine base pairs. It may function as an alternative to anthracyclines in the treatment of acute myelogenous leukemia, breast cancer, and prostate cancer. Although generally less active than doxorubicin, it causes less nausea, vomiting, mucositis, and hair loss, and has found a role in the palliative treatment of cancers of the breast and prostate. Mitoxantrone can also cause cardiac toxicity leading to heart failure. Anthracyclines and mitoxantrone are also (like etoposide) associated with the rare development of secondary leukemia.

18.5 ANTIMICROTUBULAR AGENTS

18.5.1 Vinca Alkaloids

The vinca alkaloids, vinblastine, vincristine, and vinorelbine, are naturally occurring or semisynthetic derivatives from the periwinkle plant. These compounds bind to the protein tubulin and inhibit its polymerization to form microtubules. Microtubules have several important cellular functions, including formation of the mitotic spindle responsible for separation of chromosomes, and structural and transport functions in axons of nerves. Microtubules are in a state of dynamic equilibrium, with continuous formation and degradation from cytoplasmic tubulin. This process is interrupted by vinca alkaloids, and lethally damaged cells may be observed to enter an abortive metaphase

and then lyse. However, experiments with synchronized cells have demonstrated that maximum lethal toxicity for vinblastine and vincristine occurs when cells are exposed during the period of DNA synthesis; presumably the morphological expression of that damage is observed in the attempted mitosis.

Vincristine and vinblastine are structurally similar, differing only in a substitution on the central rings (Fig. 18–17). Vinca alkaloids have large volumes of distribution, indicating a high degree of tissue binding, and are eliminated mainly by hepatic metabolism and biliary excretion. Consequently, dose reduction should be considered in patients with elevated bilirubin. The elimination half-lives of vinca alkaloids are approximately 20 hours.

Despite similarities in their structures, these drugs differ in both their clinical spectra of activity and their toxicities. Vinblastine is an important drug in combination chemotherapy of testicular cancer, whereas vincristine is a mainstay of treatment for childhood leukemia. Both drugs have been combined with other cytotoxic agents to treat lymphomas or various solid tumors. Vinorelbine has activity against non–small cell lung cancer and breast cancer.

Vinblastine causes major toxicity to bone marrow, with some risk of autonomic neuropathy, leading to constipation. The dose of vincristine is limited by its toxicity to peripheral nerves, and this damage relates to the duration of treatment as well as to the total dose of vincristine used. This neurotoxicity probably occurs because of damage to the microtubules in axons. The dose-limiting toxicity of vinorelbine is myelosuppression. Neurotoxicity can occur but is less common than with vincristine, possibly because of a lower affinity for axonal microtubules.

18.5.2 Taxanes

Paclitaxel and docetaxel are plant alkaloids derived from the bark of the Pacific yew tree *Taxus brevifolia*, and the needles of the European yew tree *Taxus baccata*, respectively (Fig. 18–18). Paclitaxel was identified as an anticancer drug more than 30 years ago, but its clinical development was hampered by a limited supply, as the Pacific yew tree is relatively rare. Subsequent discovery of an intermediary from the relatively abundant needles of the yew tree made it possible to produce large quantities for clinical evaluation and application.

Taxanes bind to tubulin at a site different from that of the vinca alkaloids. In contrast to the vinca alkaloids, taxanes are believed to inhibit microtubular disassembly, which then prevents the normal growth and breakdown of microtubules that is required for cell division. However, the classic view of vinca alkaloids depolymerizing microtubules and taxanes stabilizing microtubules has been challenged. It has been suggested that both classes of agents may have a similar mechanism of action, involving the modulation of microtubule dynamics (Jordan and Wilson, 2004).

The pharmacokinetics of paclitaxel and docetaxel are characterized by a large volume of distribution with extensive tissue binding, elimination by hepatic metabolism, and elimination half-lives of 10 to 12 hours. As hepatic metabolism to

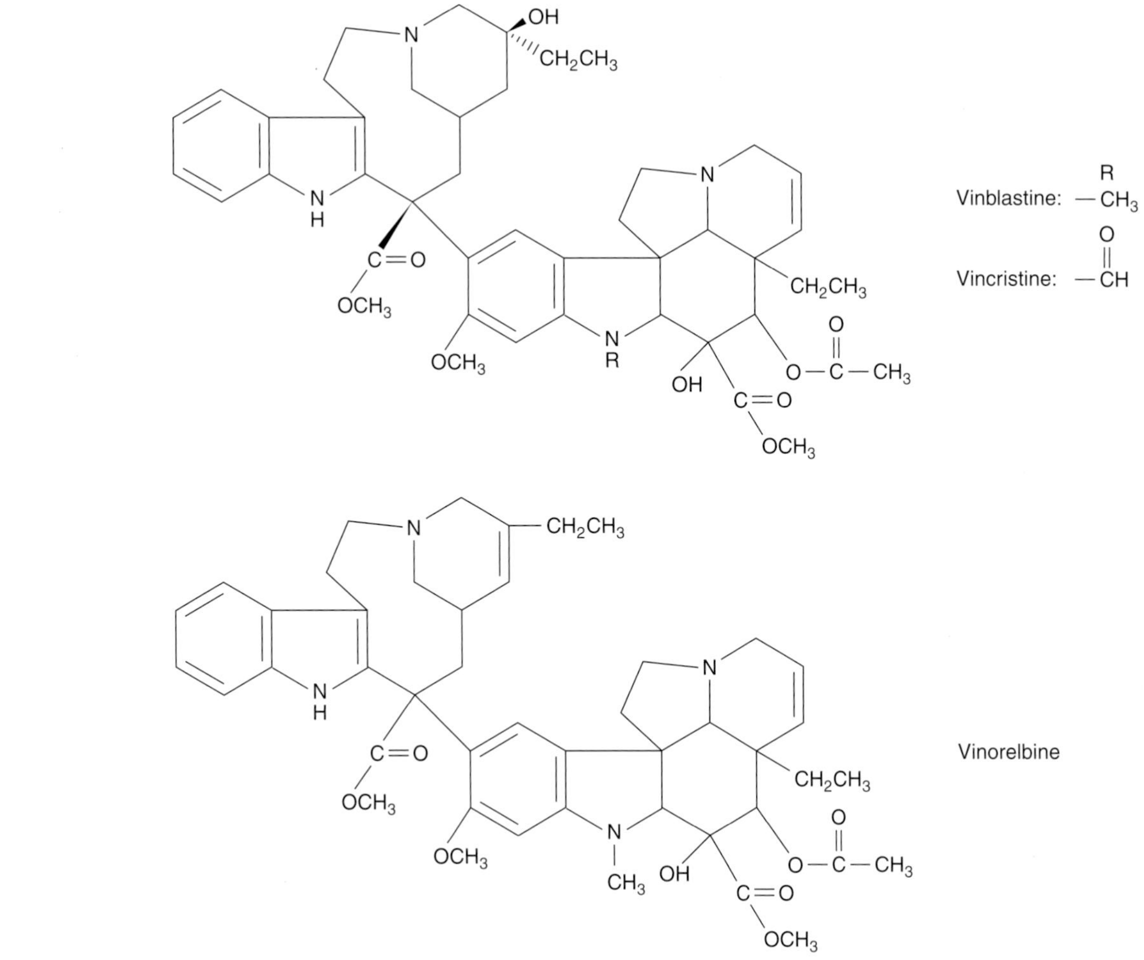

Vinblastine: —CH$_3$

Vincristine:

Vinorelbine

FIGURE 18-17 Structures of vinblastine, vincristine, and vinorelbine.

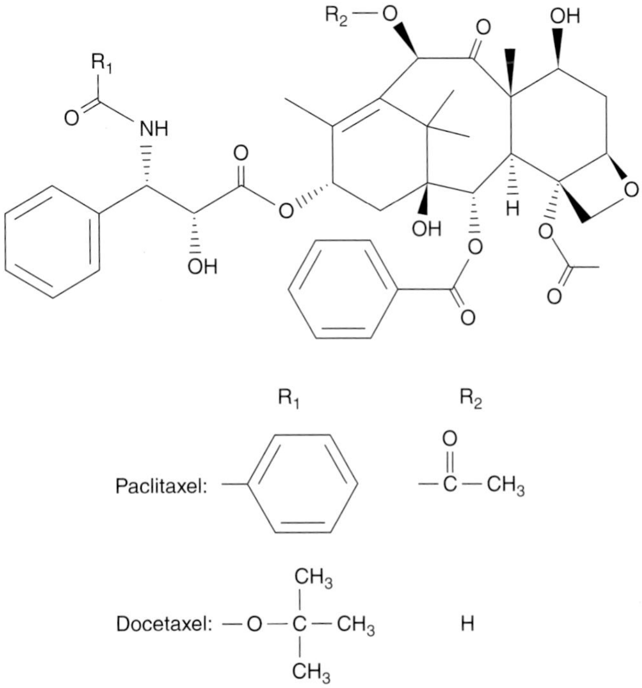

Paclitaxel:

Docetaxel:

FIGURE 18-18 Structures of paclitaxel and docetaxel.

inactive metabolites is mediated through cytochrome P450 enzymes, agents that influence cytochrome P450 can modify the clearance and toxicity of the taxanes; for example, patients on anticonvulsants have demonstrated increased clearance and reduced toxicity.

Paclitaxel and docetaxel share many common toxicities. The dose-limiting toxicity is myelosuppression, mainly neutropenia. For paclitaxel, the severity of neutropenia correlates best with the duration that plasma concentration exceeds a critical threshold level ranging from 0.05 to 0.1 μmol/L. Both drugs can cause hypersensitivity reactions with bronchial constriction, allergic skin reactions such as urticaria, and hypotension. This problem has been reduced substantially by prophylactic treatment with steroids and histamine antagonists. The vehicles in which the taxanes are formulated have been implicated as possible causes of the hypersensitivity reactions, but different vehicles are used for paclitaxel (Cremophor EL) and for docetaxel (polysorbate 80). A sensory peripheral neuropathy can occur with repeated or high-dose administration. Docetaxel can also cause fluid retention and skin and nail changes over time. These drugs have activity against ovarian, breast, lung, and prostate cancers. Alterations of microtubule structures as a result of mutations can result in altered microtubule dynamics or impaired binding of taxanes to tumors, leading to resistance. Increased expression of the multidrug-resistance gene, *MDR1* can also result in resistance (Trock et al, 1997).

Nab-paclitaxel is a novel formulation of nanometer-sized albumin-bound paclitaxel particles. It allows preferential delivery of paclitaxel to tumor tissues by taking advantage of the increased delivery of albumin to tumors through receptor-mediated transport and enhanced passage of these particles through larger gaps between capillary endothelial cells. The absence of Cremophor EL reduces toxicity. Nab-paclitaxel is indicated for the treatment of advanced breast cancer.

18.6 MISCELLANEOUS CYTOTOXIC DRUGS

Bleomycin consists of a family of molecules with a complex structure; it is derived from fungal culture, the dominant active component being known as bleomycin A2. Bleomycin causes DNA double-stranded breaks through a complex sequence of reactions involving the binding of a bleomycin–ferrous iron complex to DNA. This binding leads to insertion of the drug between base pairs (intercalation) and unwinding of the double helix. A second step in the formation of DNA strand breaks may involve the reduction of molecular oxygen to superoxide or hydroxyl radicals, catalyzed by the bleomycin–ferrous iron complex. However, like doxorubicin, bleomycin retains some of its lethal activity under hypoxic conditions. Bleomycin may exert preferential toxicity in the G_2-phase of the cycle, but also has toxicity for slowly proliferating cells in plateau-phase cell culture. Bleomycin is a large molecule that crosses cell membranes slowly. Once within the cell, it can be activated or broken down by bleomycin hydrolase; cellular sensitivity to bleomycin has been found to correlate inversely with the concentration of this enzyme.

After intravenous injection, most of the administered drug is eliminated unchanged in the urine with a $t_{1/2}$ of 4 to 8 hours. The major use of bleomycin is in combination with other drugs for the curative therapy of testicular cancer and lymphomas. Bleomycin has little toxicity to the bone marrow but may cause fever, chills, and damage to skin and mucous membranes. The most serious toxicity is interstitial fibrosis of the lung leading to shortness of breath and death of some patients; its incidence is related to cumulative dose, age, renal function, and the use of other agents that may damage the lung, such as high oxygen supplementation or radiation therapy.

Mitomycin C is derived from a streptomyces species and is a quinine-containing compound that requires activation to an alkylating metabolite by reductive metabolism. Because of the requirement for reductive metabolism, the drug is more active against hypoxic than aerobic cells, at least in tissue culture. Mitomycin C causes delayed and rather unpredictable myelosuppression. More seriously, the drug can produce kidney failure through a hemolytic-uremic syndrome, which is usually fatal and is probably caused by small-vessel endothelial damage. Another potential lethal effect is interstitial lung disease with progression to pulmonary fibrosis. It is sometimes instilled into the bladder by a catheter to treat superficial bladder cancer and is also used with radiation therapy to treat cancer of the anal canal.

18.7 MOLECULAR-TARGETED AGENTS

Advances in molecular biology have provided a better understanding of intricate cellular pathways that are critical to tumor formation and growth. New classes of anticancer drugs have been developed that target aberrant expression or alterations in molecular pathways rather than DNA, as is the case for most drugs discussed above. Molecular-targeted agents offer greater specificity and different toxicity as these aberrant expressions or alterations are more common in tumors than in normal tissues (see Chap. 17, Sec. 17.3).

18.7.1 Inhibitors of Angiogenesis

A rate-limiting step in tumor growth is angiogenesis. Without neovascularization, tumor growth is limited and some cells in the tumor become hypoxic, resulting in increased production of proangiogenic factors (see Chap. 11, Sec. 11.4; Folkman, 1971). A dominant factor that stimulates angiogenesis is vascular endothelial growth factor (VEGF). There are 5 isoforms of VEGF, and they bind to 3 main subtypes of cell surface receptors (VEGFR). Binding of VEGF to VEGFR leads to dimerization, phosphorylation of intracellular tyrosine kinases, and subsequent activation of downstream signal cascades. There are 2 approaches to inhibit the VEGF signaling pathway: antibodies that bind to circulating VEGF to prevent its binding to VEGFR, and small molecules to inhibit intracellular tyrosine kinase activity.

Bevacizumab is a humanized monoclonal antibody against VEGF-A. It has limited anticancer effects when administered alone, but has shown activity when given together with cytotoxic chemotherapies in the treatment of advanced colorectal cancer, and other cancers (Hurwitz et al, 2004; Escudier, Pluzanska et al, 2007). It is hypothesized that agents such as bevacizumab cause a temporary normalization of poorly formed and more permeable tumor vasculature, leading to increased blood flow to tumor and reduced interstitial pressure. As a result, there may be enhanced delivery of cytotoxic chemotherapies to tumor sites. Bevacizumab is administered at 2- to 3-week intervals because the elimination $t_{1/2}$ is approximately 20 days. Adverse events associated with bevacizumab include hypertension, bleeding, proteinuria, would healing complications, thromboembolic events, and perforation of the gastrointestinal tract. A rare syndrome of reversible posterior leukoencephalopathy has been reported in patients receiving bevacizumab (Marinella and Markert, 2009).

Several inhibitors of membrane-based tyrosine kinases have activity against human cancer (Fig. 18–19; see Chap. 17, Sec. 17.3.1). Sunitinib inhibits multiple receptor tyrosine kinases, including those associated with VEGFR,

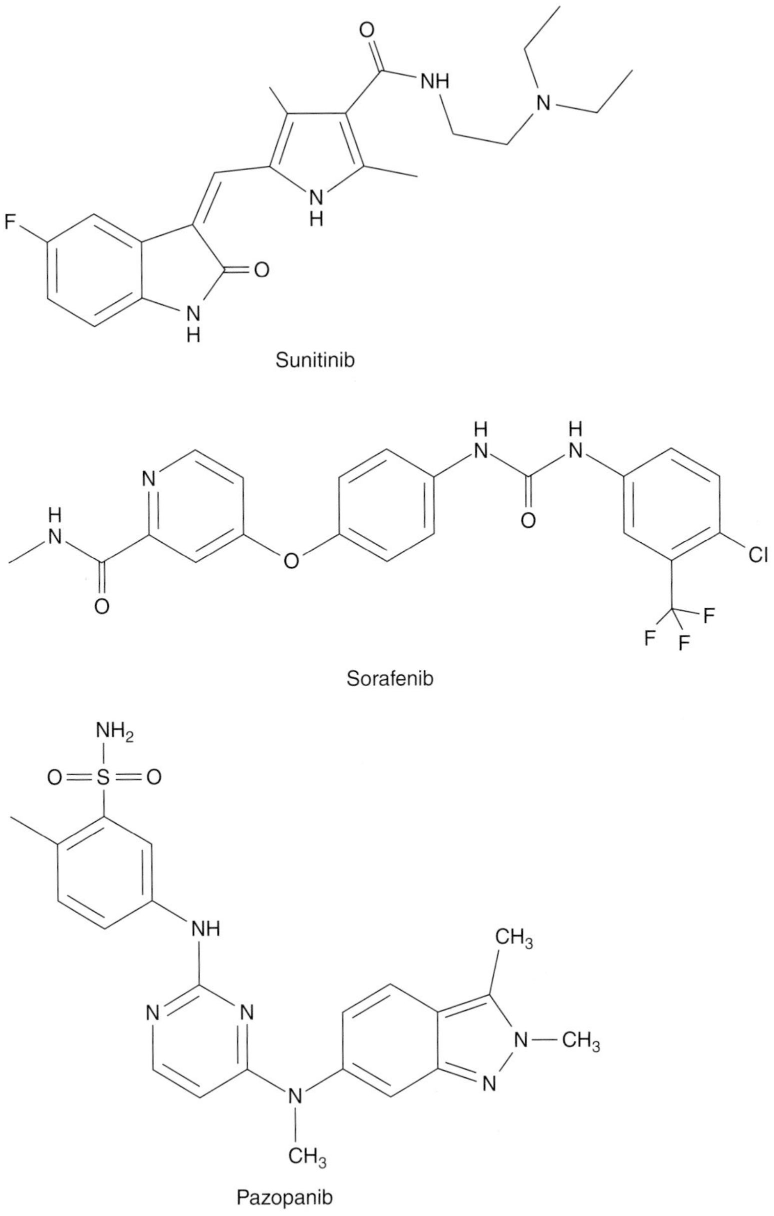

FIGURE 18–19 **Structures of sunitinib, sorafenib, and pazopanib.**

platelet-derived growth factor receptor (PDGFR), and c-kit (Mendel et al, 2003). It is an oral agent and is usually administered daily for 4 out of 6 weeks, although its $t_{1/2}$ ranges from 40 to 60 hours. Sunitinib undergoes hepatic metabolism via cytochrome P450 system, mainly CYP3A4; hence, the dosage of sunitinib requires adjustment in patients taking strong CYP3A4 inhibitors. Common adverse effects of sunitinib include fatigue, diarrhea, hypertension, thyroid dysfunction, and hand-foot syndrome. Sunitinib is approved for the treatment of advanced renal cell carcinoma and gastrointestinal stromal tumors (GISTs) (Demetri et al, 2006; Motzer et al, 2007).

Sorafenib inhibits tyrosine kinases associated with cell-surface receptors, including VEGFR, PDGFR, and c-kit. It also inhibits intracellular raf kinases. Approximately 40% of sorafenib is absorbed when administered orally, and its bioavailability is further decreased when it is taken together with a high-fat meal. Sorafenib is administered twice daily

on a continuous basis, even though its $t_{1/2}$ is approximately 40 hours. Adverse events caused by sorafenib are similar to those associated with sunitinib. Sorafenib is used in treating advanced hepatocellular carcinoma and renal cell carcinoma (Escudier et al, 2007; Llovet et al, 2008).

Like sunitinib and sorafenib, pazopanib inhibits tyrosine kinases associated with multiple cell-surface receptors. It is given orally and its bioavailability is increased when given together with food or if the tablet is crushed. Pazopanib is administered once daily continuously and its $t_{1/2}$ is approximately 30 hours. Pazopanib is also used for treating advanced renal cell carcinoma (Sternberg et al, 2010).

Thalidomide (Fig. 18–20) was first developed in 1950s as treatment for pregnancy-associated nausea and vomiting. However, it was soon withdrawn from market with the recognition that thalidomide use was associated with teratogenicity leading to a defect in the development of limbs.

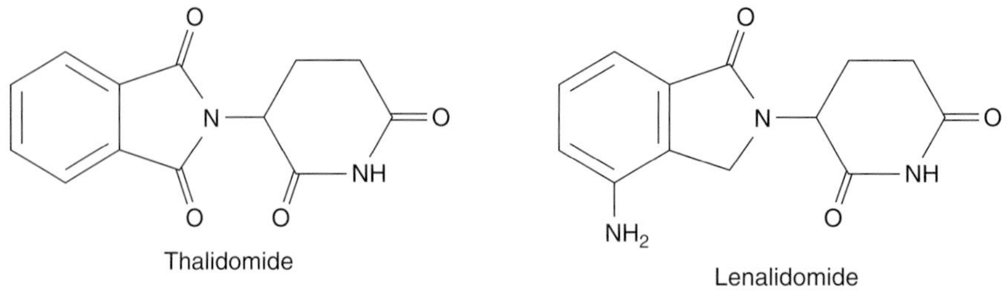

FIGURE 18–20 Structures of thalidomide and lenalidomide.

Thalidomide   Lenalidomide

The interest in thalidomide and related drugs was rekindled in the 1980s because of anecdotal reports of activity in a number of conditions such as erythema nodosum leprosum (ENL). Several studies confirmed that thalidomide has activity in advanced multiple myeloma (Singhal et al, 1999). Although thalidomide is thought to inhibit angiogenesis, its precise mechanism of anticancer effects is not known. Because of its potential teratogenic effects, thalidomide can only be prescribed under strict guidance, particularly for female patients who are premenopausal and male patients whose partner is of childbearing age. Thalidomide is orally administered and undergoes nonenzymatic hydrolysis to form multiple inactive metabolites. Side effects include fluid retention, fatigue, skin toxicities, thromboembolic events, and peripheral sensory neuropathy.

Lenalidomide is an analog of thalidomide (see Fig. 18–20), and also has activity in multiple myeloma (Badros, 2012). Unlike thalidomide which undergoes extensive metabolism, lenalidomide is excreted mostly unchanged in urine. Patients with renal dysfunction require dose reduction. The $t_{1/2}$ of lenalidomide is approximately 3 hours in patients with normal renal function, and 9 hours in patients with moderate-to-severe renal impairment. It is readily absorbed after oral administration and is given daily for 21 days followed by 7 days of rest. Lenalidomide is also teratogenic, and its use must be strictly monitored in women of child-bearing potential similar to thalidomide. Lenalidomide is also associated with increased risks of thromboembolic events.

18.7.2 Inhibitors of Epidermal Growth Factor Receptors

The epidermal growth factor receptor (EGFR) is composed of an extracellular ligand-binding domain, a transmembrane region, and an intracellular domain with tyrosine kinase activity. Activation of the EGFR pathway initiates cascades of intracellular RAS-RAF-MAPK (mitogen-activated protein kinase) and phophatidylinositol-3 kinase (PI3K)-AKT signaling pathways, which, in turn, stimulate transcription of genes that promote cell proliferation and survival (see Chap. 8, Sec. 8.2). Aberrant signaling through the EGFR pathway induces tumorigenesis with cell proliferation, angiogenesis, invasion, and metastasis, as well as inhibition of apoptosis. There are 2 approaches to inhibit EGFR-related pathways: antibodies against the cell surface receptors, or small molecules to inhibit the intracellular tyrosine kinases. Inhibiting

EGFR causes diarrhea and skin toxicities. Skin toxicities initially manifest as an acneiform skin rash involving the face and upper trunk, and over time progress to dry skin, fissures, and infection around nail beds (Lacouture et al, 2010).

Cetuximab is a chimeric monoclonal antibody against EGFR, whereas panitumumab is a fully humanized monoclonal antibody against EGFR. The half-lives of cetuximab and panitumumab are approximately 7 days, and they are administered intravenously weekly or every 2 weeks. Large, randomized trials have confirmed that cetuximab and panitumumab can prolong overall survival and progression-free survival in patients with advanced colorectal cancer compared to best supportive care. The Ras protein is involved early in the EGFR signaling pathway, and mutations in the Ras gene can result in constitutive activation, thereby abrogating blockage of the EGFR pathway. Up to 40% of patients with advanced colorectal cancer may carry a mutated Ras gene, and multiple studies have confirmed that anti-EGFR antibodies are only effective in patients with wild-type *KRAS* (Amado et al, 2008; Karapetis et al, 2008). Other mutations in the EGFR signaling pathway, such as *BRAF*, may affect therapeutic response, and these are active areas of investigation. Hypomagnesemia is a common side effect with EGFR inhibition since EGFR is also involved in regulating magnesium reabsorption in renal tubules. Cetuximab has a slight risk of hypersensitivity reaction, which can be prevented by antihistamines and corticosteroids. Recent data suggest that prophylactic measures, such as skin moisturizers, sunscreen, topical steroids, and oral antibiotics (doxycycline/minocycline) can reduce the severity of skin toxicities without affecting treatment efficacy.

Erlotinib and gefitinib are 2 small-molecule inhibitors of EGFR-associated tyrosine kinases (Fig. 18–21). Both agents are administered orally. Food increases the bioavailability of erlotinib from 60% to almost 100%, whereas gefitinib is absorbed slowly with peak concentrations at 3 to 7 hours after drug administration and the bioavailability is approximately 60%. Both erlotinib and gefitinib are extensively metabolized, primarily via CYP3A4, and metabolites are excreted through the biliary system. Their half-lives range from 30 to 40 hours, and both are administered on a continuous basis. Gefitinib is indicated for patients with advanced non–small cell lung cancer after progression on platinum or docetaxel therapies. A large, randomized study showed that gefitinib is superior to carboplatin-paclitaxel as an initial treatment for pulmonary adenocarcinoma among nonsmokers or former light smokers in East Asia (Mok et al, 2009). Furthermore, the presence in

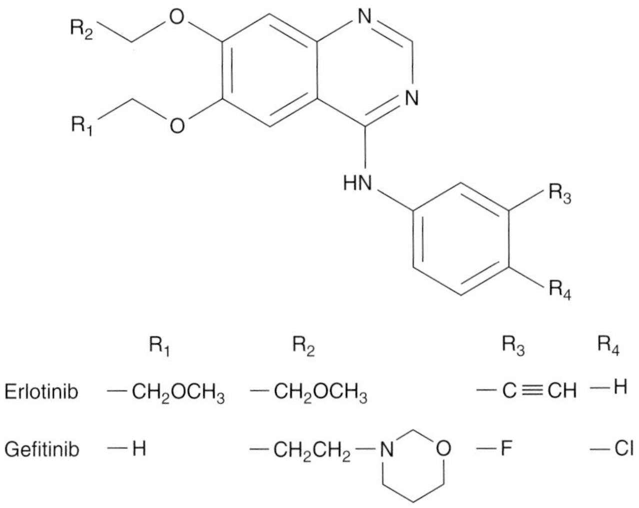

	R_1	R_2	R_3	R_4
Erlotinib	$-CH_2OCH_3$	$-CH_2OCH_3$	$-C\equiv CH$	$-H$
Gefitinib	$-H$	$-CH_2CH_2-N{\bigcirc}O$	$-F$	$-Cl$

FIGURE 18–21 Structures of erlotinib and gefitinib.

the tumor of a mutation of the *EGFR* gene is a strong predictor of a better outcome with gefitinib. In addition to non–small cell lung cancer, erlotinib provides a small survival advantage when used as first-line treatment for locally advanced or metastatic pancreatic cancer in combination with gemcitabine (Moore et al, 2007).

The HER-2 oncogene encodes a transmembrane receptor with tyrosine kinase activity belonging to the EGFR family of receptors (King et al, 1985). Amplication of HER-2 or overexpression of its protein product occurs in approximately 20% of patients with breast cancer, and is a strong predictor of therapeutic response to anti–HER-2 agents (see Chap. 20, Sec. 20.3.3). Trastuzumab is a monoclonal antibody against HER-2, and is indicated as adjuvant therapy for HER-2 overexpressing early breast cancer or as therapy for metastatic breast cancer alone or in combination with other drugs (Baselga et al, 2005; Robert et al, 2006; Romond et al, 2005). Trastuzumab is associated with reduction in left ventricular ejection fraction and, less commonly, heart failure. Patients with preexisting heart disease, previous radiation, and concomitant administration or prior exposure to anthracyclines are at increased risks of heart failure with trastuzumab therapy. In addition, there is an increased risk of pulmonary toxicity. Other antibodies directed against HER-2, such as pertuzumab, and trastuzumab emtansine (TDM-1), in which the cytotoxic agent emtansine is linked to trastuzumab, may further improve therapy for HER-2-positive breast cancer (Baselga et al, 2012; Verma et al, 2012).

Lapatinib is a small-molecule inhibitor of tyrosine kinase activity associated with HER-2. It is administered orally and its bioavailability is improved with high-fat food (Ratain and Cohen, 2007). It undergoes extensive metabolism mediated by CYP3A4 and CYP3A5. It is indicated with capecitabine for patients with HER-2 overexpressing advanced breast cancer. Like trastuzumab, lapatinib causes cardiac and pulmonary toxicities. In addition, lapatinib is occasionally associated with severe hepatotoxicity.

18.7.3 Mammalian Target of Rapamycin Inhibitors

The mammalian target of rapamycin (mTOR) pathway is downstream of the PI3KAkt pathway which is regulated by PTEN (Wullschleger et al, 2006; see Chap. 7, Sec. 7.6.2). The mTOR pathway is aberrantly activated in many cancers. The first agent targeting the mTOR pathway, rapamycin (sirolimus), is a macrocyclic isolated from *Streptomyces hygroscopicus* in a soil sample from Britain. It binds to an intracellular protein, FKBP-12, and forms a stable complex to inhibit mTOR kinase activity. Sirolimus is an immunosuppressant and is used to prevent organ rejection in transplant recipients. Several analogs of rapamycin have been developed (Fig. 18–22). Temsirolimus is an intravenously administered rapamycin analog. It is metabolized via CYP3A4 to its major active metabolite, sirolimus. The dose of temsirolimus should be reduced in patients with liver dysfunction. Common side effects include skin toxicity; metabolic disorders such as hyperglycemia, hypercholesterolemia, and hyperlipidemia; gastrointestinal toxicities, such as mucositis, nausea, and vomiting; and hematological toxicities, mainly anemia and lymphopenia. Uncommon but potentially life-threatening toxicities include hypersensitivity reaction and pneumonitis. Temsirolimus is used in the treatment of advanced renal cell cancer (Hudes et al, 2007).

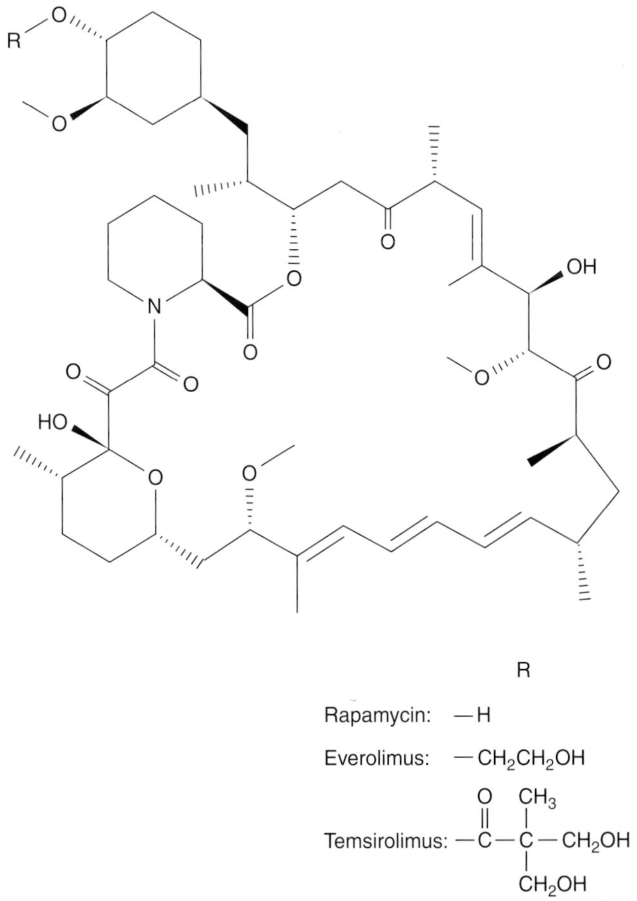

	R
Rapamycin:	$-H$
Everolimus:	$-CH_2CH_2OH$
Temsirolimus:	$-\overset{O}{\underset{\parallel}{C}}-\overset{CH_3}{\underset{\underset{CH_2OH}{\mid}}{C}}-CH_2OH$

FIGURE 18–22 Structures of rapamycin and analogs.

Because of the relatively long $t_{1/2}$ of sirolimus (approximately 50 hours), temsirolimus is given weekly.

Unlike temsirolimus, everolimus is rapidly absorbed orally with a bioavailability of approximately 30% and its $t_{1/2}$ is approximately 30 hours. Everolimus is administered daily and its dose should be reduced in patients with moderate to severe hepatic dysfunction. In a Phase III study, everolimus significantly prolonged progression-free survival for patients with advanced renal cell carcinoma who had progressive disease on or shortly after therapy with VEGF tyrosine kinase inhibitors (Motzer et al, 2008). Common side effects include metabolic disorders (hyperglycemia, hypercholesterolemia, and hyperlipidemia), hematological toxicities (anemia and lymphopenia), and gastrointestinal toxicities, such as mucositis, nausea, and diarrhea. Everolimus is also associated with pulmonary toxicity.

18.7.4 Miscellaneous Agents

Imatinib is an orally available tyrosine kinase inhibitor. It inhibits the tyrosine kinase activity of the constitutively active fusion protein BCR-ABL arising from the Philadelphia (Ph) chromosome (see Chap. 7, Sec. 7.5.1) of chronic myelogenous leukemia (CML) through competitive inhibition at the adenosine triphosphate (ATP) binding site. The discovery and the successful treatment of CML with imatinib ushered in the era of cancer therapy with drugs targeting signaling pathways (Druker et al, 2001). Resistance to imatinib results from mutations that alter amino acids at the imatinib binding site or prevent BCR-ABL from achieving the inactive conformation that is required for imatinib binding (Shah et al, 2002). Imatinib also inhibits the tyrosine kinase activity of c-KIT (CD-117) which is overexpressed in 80% of GISTs and a related tyrosine kinase receptor, PDGFR. Treatment with imatinib leads to rapid and sustained clinical effects and has revolutionized the management of CML and GIST (Blanke et al, 2008). Although all GIST patients with KIT mutation are likely to respond to imatinib therapy, those with an exon 11 mutation have a more prolonged response than those with an exon 9 mutation. However, patients with exon 9 mutations can still respond with higher doses of imatinib. Imatinib is rapidly and completely absorbed, and undergoes hepatic metabolism via CYP3A4 enzymes. Imatinib is generally well tolerated with mild nausea, diarrhea, fluid retention, muscle cramps and fatigue.

Dasatinib inhibits BCR-ABL kinases among others, and has shown activity in patients who are resistant or intolerant to imatinib therapy (Apperley et al, 2009; Kantarjian et al, 2010). Dasatinib undergoes extensive metabolism and is mainly excreted through the biliary system.

Nilotinib is another inhibitor of multiple kinases, including BCR-ABL, c-KIT, and PDGFR kinases (Saglio et al, 2010). It is designed to fit into the ATP binding site of BCR-ABL with higher affinity than imatinib. It is also active in the presence of multiple mutations that lead to resistance to imatinib. Nilotinib is usually taken on an empty stomach because food may increase its bioavailability, and patients with hepatic dysfunction require dose reduction because nilotinib undergoes extensive metabolism. Nilotinib can cause changes in the electrocardiogram and electrolyte imbalance, such as hypokalemia and hypomagnesemia, which require correction before initiation of therapy. It is contraindicated in patients with long QT syndrome.

SUMMARY

- Anticancer drugs are grouped according to their mechanisms of action.
- Although traditional agents cause damage to DNA, either directly or indirectly, resulting in cell death, newer agents target specific aberrant molecular pathway changes in tumors. These agents have improved specificity, but are associated with toxicities such as hypertension, heart failure, and skin changes.
- The efficacy of anticancer drugs depends on drug concentration and time of exposure, which, in turn, depend on absorption, metabolism, distribution, and excretion. Understanding of the pharmacology of these agents is essential for their effective and safe usage in clinical practice.
- Advances in pharmacogenetics and cancer biology could provide further insights to explain interpatient variability in efficacy and toxicity, and allow therapy to be personalized based on molecular properties of the patient and the patient's tumor.

REFERENCES

Ajani JA, Rodriguez W, Bodoky G, et al. Multicenter phase III comparison of cisplatin/S-1 with cisplatin/infusional fluorouracil in advanced gastric or gastroesophageal adenocarcinoma study: the FLAGS trial. *J Clin Oncol* 2010;28:1547-1553.

Amado RG, Wolf M, Peeters M, et al. Wild-type KRAS is required for panitumumab efficacy in patients with metastatic colorectal cancer. *J Clin Oncol* 2008;26:1626-1634.

Apperley JF, Cortes JE, Kim DW, et al. Dasatinib in the treatment of chronic myeloid leukemia in accelerated phase after imatinib failure: the START a trial. *J Clin Oncol* 2009;27:3472-3479.

Badros AZ. Lenalidomide in myeloma—a high-maintenance friend. *N Engl J Med* 2012;366:1836-1838.

Baselga J, Carbonell X, Castaneda-Soto NJ, et al. Phase II study of efficacy, safety, and pharmacokinetics of trastuzumab monotherapy administered on a 3-weekly schedule. *J Clin Oncol* 2005;23: 2162-2171.

Baselga J, Cortes J, Kim S-B, et al. Pertuzumab plus trastuzumab plus docetaxel for metastatic breast cancer. *N Engl J Med* 2012;366:109-119.

Blanke CD, Rankin C, Demetri GD, et al. Phase III randomized, intergroup trial assessing imatinib mesylate at two dose levels in patients with unresectable or metastatic gastrointestinal stromal tumors expressing the kit receptor tyrosine kinase: S0033. *J Clin Oncol* 2008;26:626-632.

Broxterman HJ, Gotink KJ, Verheul HM. Understanding the causes of multidrug resistance in cancer: a comparison of doxorubicin and sunitinib. *Drug Resist Updat* 2009;12:114-126.

Calvert AH, Newell DR, Gumbrell LA, et al. Carboplatin dosage: prospective evaluation of a simple formula based on renal function. *J Clin Oncol* 1989;7:1748-1756.

David KA, Picus J. Evaluating risk factors for the development of ifosfamide encephalopathy. *Am J Clin Oncol* 2005;28:277-280.

Demetri GD, van Oosterom AT, Garrett CR, et al. Efficacy and safety of sunitinib in patients with advanced gastrointestinal stromal tumour after failure of imatinib: a randomised controlled trial. *Lancet* 2006;368:1329-1338.

Druker BJ, Talpaz M, Resta DJ, et al. Efficacy and safety of a specific inhibitor of the BCR-ABL tyrosine kinase in chronic myeloid leukemia. *N Engl J Med* 2001;344:1031-1037.

Escudier B, Eisen T, Stadler WM, et al. Sorafenib in advanced clear-cell renal-cell carcinoma. *N Engl J Med* 2007;356:125-134.

Escudier B, Pluzanska A, Koralewski P, et al. Bevacizumab plus interferon alfa-2a for treatment of metastatic renal cell carcinoma: a randomised, double-blind phase III trial. *Lancet* 2007;370:2103-2111.

Folkman J. Tumor angiogenesis: therapeutic implications. *N Engl J Med* 1971;285:1182-1186.

Gamelin L, Boisdron-Celle M, Morel A, et al. Oxaliplatin-related neurotoxicity: interest of calcium-magnesium infusion and no impact on its efficacy. *J Clin Oncol* 2008;26:1188-1189; author reply 1189-1190.

Gewirtz DA. A critical evaluation of the mechanisms of action proposed for the antitumor effects of the anthracycline antibiotics Adriamycin and daunorubicin. *Biochem Pharmacol* 1999;57:727-741.

Gordon AN, Fleagle JT, Guthrie D, Parkin DE, Gore ME, Lacave AJ. Recurrent epithelial ovarian carcinoma: a randomized phase III study of pegylated liposomal doxorubicin versus topotecan. *J Clin Oncol* 2001;19:3312-3322.

Hudes G, Carducci M, Tomczak P, et al. Temsirolimus, interferon alfa, or both for advanced renal-cell carcinoma. *N Engl J Med* 2007;356:2271-2281.

Hurwitz H, Fehrenbacher L, Novotny W, et al. Bevacizumab plus irinotecan, fluorouracil, and leucovorin for metastatic colorectal cancer. *N Engl J Med* 2004;350:2335-2342.

Jordan MA, Wilson L. Microtubules as a target for anticancer drugs. *Nat Rev Cancer* 2004;4:253-265.

Kantarjian H, Shah NP, Hochhaus A, et al. Dasatinib versus imatinib in newly diagnosed chronic-phase chronic myeloid leukemia. *N Engl J Med* 2010;362:2260-2270.

Karapetis CS, Khambata-Ford S, Jonker DJ, et al. K-ras mutations and benefit from cetuximab in advanced colorectal cancer. *N Engl J Med* 2008;359:1757-1765.

King CR, Kraus MH, Aaronson SA. Amplification of a novel v-erbB-related gene in a human mammary carcinoma. *Science* 1985;229:974-976.

Koberle B, Tomicic MT, Usanova S, Kaina B. Cisplatin resistance: preclinical findings and clinical implications. *Biochim Biophys Acta* 2010;1806:172-182.

Lacouture ME, Maitland ML, Segaert S, et al. A proposed EGFR inhibitor dermatologic adverse event-specific grading scale from the MASCC skin toxicity study group. *Support Care Cancer* 2010;18:509-522.

Llovet JM, Ricci S, Mazzaferro V, et al. Sorafenib in advanced hepatocellular carcinoma. *N Engl J Med* 2008;359:378-390.

Marchesi F, Turriziani M, Tortorelli G, Avvisati G, Torino F, De Vecchis L. Triazene compounds: mechanism of action and related DNA repair systems. *Pharmacol Res* 2007;56:275-287.

Marinella MA, Markert RJ. Reversible posterior leucoencephalopathy syndrome associated with anticancer drugs. *Intern Med J* 2009;39:826-834.

Marty M, Espie M, Llombart A, Monnier A, Rapoport BL, Stahalova V. Multicenter randomized phase III study of the cardioprotective effect of dexrazoxane (Cardioxane) in advanced/metastatic breast cancer patients treated with anthracycline-based chemotherapy. *Ann Oncol* 2006;17:614-622.

Mathijssen RH, Marsh S, Karlsson MO, et al. Irinotecan pathway genotype analysis to predict pharmacokinetics. *Clin Cancer Res* 2003;9:3246-3253.

Mathijssen RH, van Alphen RJ, Verweij J, et al. Clinical pharmacokinetics and metabolism of irinotecan (CPT-11). *Clin Cancer Res* 2001;7:2182-2194.

Mendel DB, Laird AD, Xin X, et al. In vivo antitumor activity of SU11248, a novel tyrosine kinase inhibitor targeting vascular endothelial growth factor and platelet-derived growth factor receptors: determination of a pharmacokinetic/pharmacodynamic relationship. *Clin Cancer Res* 2003;9:327-337.

Merry S, Courtney ER, Fetherston CA, Kaye SB, Freshney RI. Circumvention of drug resistance in human non-small cell lung cancer in vitro by verapamil. *Br J Cancer* 1987;56:401-405.

Miwa M, Ura M, Nishida M, et al. Design of a novel oral fluoropyrimidine carbamate, capecitabine, which generates 5-fluorouracil selectively in tumours by enzymes concentrated in human liver and cancer tissue. *Eur J Cancer* 1998;34:1274-1281.

Mok TS, Wu YL, Thongprasert S, et al. Gefitinib or carboplatin-paclitaxel in pulmonary adenocarcinoma. *N Engl J Med* 2009;361:947-957.

Moore MJ, Goldstein D, Hamm J, et al. Erlotinib plus gemcitabine compared with gemcitabine alone in patients with advanced pancreatic cancer: a phase III trial of the National Cancer Institute of Canada Clinical Trials Group. *J Clin Oncol* 2007;25:1960-1966.

Motzer RJ, Escudier B, Oudard S, et al. Efficacy of everolimus in advanced renal cell carcinoma: a double-blind, randomised, placebo-controlled phase III trial. *Lancet* 2008;372:449-456.

Motzer RJ, Hutson TE, Tomczak et al. Sunitinib versus interferon alfa in metastatic renal-cell carcinoma. *N Engl J Med* 2007;356:115-124.

Paugh SW, Stocco G, McCorkle JR, Diouf B, Crews KR, Evans WE. Cancer pharmacogenomics. *Clin Pharmacol Ther* 2011;90:461-466.

Pegg AE. Mammalian O6-alkylguanine-DNA alkyltransferase: regulation and importance in response to alkylating carcinogenic and therapeutic agents. *Cancer Res* 1990;50:6119-6129.

Pratt CB, Goren MP, Meyer WH, Singh B, Dodge RK. Ifosfamide neurotoxicity is related to previous cisplatin treatment for pediatric solid tumors. *J Clin Oncol* 1990;8:1399-1401.

Ratain MJ. Body-surface area as a basis for dosing of anticancer agents: science, myth, or habit? *J Clin Oncol* 1998;16:2297-2298.

Ratain MJ, Cohen EE. The value meal: how to save $1,700 per month or more on lapatinib. *J Clin Oncol* 2007;25:3397-3398.

Riechelmann RP, Zimmermann C, Chin SN, et al. Potential drug interactions in cancer patients receiving supportive care exclusively. *J Pain Symptom Manage* 2008;35:535-543.

Robert N, Leyland-Jones B, Asmar L, et al. Randomized phase III study of trastuzumab, paclitaxel, and carboplatin compared with trastuzumab and paclitaxel in women with HER-2-overexpressing metastatic breast cancer. *J Clin Oncol* 2006;24:2786-2792.

Romond EH, Perez EA, Bryant J, et al. Trastuzumab plus adjuvant chemotherapy for operable HER2-positive breast cancer. *N Engl J Med* 2005;353:1673-1684.

Rothenberg ML, Meropol NJ, Poplin EA, Van Cutsem E, Wadler S. Mortality associated with irinotecan plus bolus fluorouracil/leucovorin: summary findings of an independent panel. *J Clin Oncol* 2001;19:3801-3807.

Saglio G, Kim DW, Issaragrisil S, et al. Nilotinib versus imatinib for newly diagnosed chronic myeloid leukemia. *N Engl J Med* 2010;362:2251-2259.

Schroth W, Goetz MP, Hamann U, et al. Association between CYP2D6 polymorphisms and outcomes among women with early stage breast cancer treated with tamoxifen. *JAMA* 2009;302:1429-1436.

Shah NP, Nicoll JM, Nagar B, et al. Multiple BCR-ABL kinase domain mutations confer polyclonal resistance to the tyrosine kinase inhibitor imatinib (STI571) in chronic phase and blast crisis chronic myeloid leukemia. *Cancer Cell* 2002;2:117-125.

Singhal S, Mehta J, Desikan R, et al. Antitumor activity of thalidomide in refractory multiple myeloma. *N Engl J Med* 1999;341:1565-1571.

Sternberg CN, Davis ID, Mardiak J, et al. Pazopanib in locally advanced or metastatic renal cell carcinoma: results of a randomized phase III trial. *J Clin Oncol* 2010;28:1061-1068.

Trock BJ, Leonessa F, Clarke R. Multidrug resistance in breast cancer: a meta-analysis of MDR1/gp170 expression and its possible functional significance. *J Natl Cancer Inst* 1997;89:917-931.

van der Bol JM, Mathijssen RH, Creemers GJ, et al. A CYP3A4 phenotype-based dosing algorithm for individualized treatment of irinotecan. *Clin Cancer Res* 2010;16:736-742.

van Kuilenburg AB. Dihydropyrimidine dehydrogenase and the efficacy and toxicity of 5-fluorouracil. *Eur J Cancer* 2004;40:939-950.

Verma S, Miles D, Gianni L, et al. Trastuzumab emtansine for HER2-positive advance breast cancer. *N Engl J Med* 2012;367:1783-1791.

Wullschleger S, Loewith R, Hall MN. TOR signaling in growth and metabolism. *Cell* 2006;124:471-484.

Drug Resistance

Susan P.C. Cole and Ian F. Tannock

19.1 INTRODUCTION

A major problem with systemic treatment of cancers is the presence or induction of drug resistance in the tumor cells. In practice many types of cancer that occur commonly in humans (eg, colon cancer, most types of non–small cell lung cancer, pancreatic cancer) have a limited response to treatment with current anticancer drugs. Other human tumors (eg, breast cancer, ovarian cancer, or small cell lung cancer) often respond to initial treatment, but acquired resistance to further therapy usually prevents drug treatment from being curative. Resistance to chemotherapy may have multiple causes, and the most widely studied of these are genetically determined mechanisms that lead to resistance of the individual tumor cells. Sensitivity to drugs may differ widely among cell populations from tumors and normal tissues and also among the cells of a single tumor. The selection or induction of a drug resistant subpopulation in human tumors is a major factor limiting the efficacy of clinical chemotherapy. Even if drug-resistant cells are present initially only at low frequency (eg, 1 drug resistant cell per 10^5 drug-sensitive cells), their selective advantage during drug treatment will lead to their rapid emergence as the dominant cell population, giving the clinical impression of "acquired resistance."

There is substantial evidence, reviewed below, that drug resistance may occur through mutation, deletion, or amplification of genes that influence the uptake, metabolism, and efflux of anticancer drugs from target cells. Factors other than genetically determined mechanisms of resistance can lead to clinical resistance of human tumors to anticancer drugs (Sharma et al, 2010). Transient changes in cellular phenotype may occur through epigenetic mechanisms (see Chap. 2, Sec. 2.3): These mechanisms influence the expression of genes (and hence of the proteins encoded by them) as compared to genetic resistance which relates to information transmitted by the DNA sequence of a gene.

The activity of many drugs is dependent on the proliferative status of the cells, and for many of them, on the phase of the cell cycle (see Chap. 17, Sec. 17.5.2). Thus a tumor may appear resistant if many of its constituent cells are nonproliferating or are spared in a drug-resistant phase of the cell cycle. Rapid proliferation of surviving tumor cells (ie, repopulation) between courses of chemotherapy can counter the effects of cell killing and lead to effective resistance. Cure or long-term remission of tumors may be governed by a small population of cells with high proliferative potential (although not necessarily high proliferative rate), so called *tumor stem cells* (see Chap. 13, Sec. 13.4), and it is the sensitivity of these cells that may ultimately determine success of chemotherapy.

Sensitivity to drugs may depend not only on the intrinsic sensitivity of the constituent tumor cells, but also on the microenvironment and on contact between the tumor cells.

Drugs can only exert their lethal effects if they reach the cells at a sufficient concentration to cause lethality. Thus limited vascular access and the requirement to diffuse through tissue from tumor blood vessels are additional causes of drug resistance in solid tumors.

This chapter provides a review of the various mechanisms that lead to clinical resistance of human tumors, as well as potential strategies that might be used to overcome them. These studies are not only important in providing leads for improving therapeutic outcome, but have also contributed to knowledge about the biology of tumors. They have provided information about tumor progression, heterogeneity of the properties of constituent cells, mechanisms of gene regulation and amplification, and mechanisms of transmembrane transport of cellular nutrients and signaling molecules.

19.2 CAUSES OF CELLULAR DRUG RESISTANCE

19.2.1 Molecular Mechanisms of Drug Resistance

A wide range of changes in the properties of tumor cells may lead to resistance to specific drugs; Table 19–1 summarizes some of the underlying mechanisms, which are described

TABLE 19–1 Cellular mechanisms associated with resistance to anticancer drugs.*

Mechanism	Drugs
Decreased uptake	Methotrexate, other antimetabolites, cisplatin, nitrogen mustard
Increased efflux	Anthracyclines, Vinca alkaloids, etoposide, taxanes, methotrexate, 5-FU, TKIs
Decrease in drug activation	Many antimetabolites (eg, 5-FU, ara-C, gemcitabine)
Increase in drug catabolism	Many antimetabolites (eg, 5-FU, ara-C)
Increase or decrease in target enzyme levels	Methotrexate, topoisomerase inhibitors, 5-FU, TKIs
Alterations in target protein (eg, changes in affinity)	Methotrexate, other antimetabolites, topoisomerase inhibitors, TKIs
Inactivation by binding to sulfhydryls (eg, glutathione, metallothionein)	Alkylating agents, cisplatin
Increased DNA repair	Alkylating agents, cisplatin, anthracyclines
Decreased ability to undergo apoptosis	Alkylating agents, cisplatin, anthracyclines, etoposide, anthracyclines, etc

Abbreviations: ara-C, Cytosine arabinoside; *5-FU*, 5-fluorouracil; *TKIs*, tyrosine kinase inhibitors.

*Additional mechanisms include those that lead to drug resistance that is expressed selectively in a solid tumor environment (see Sec. 19.3).

in detail in the following sections. Multiple mechanisms of resistance may emerge in response to exposure to a single class of drugs. For example, resistance to several antimetabolite drugs can result from impaired drug uptake into cells, overproduction or reduced affinity of the drug target, upregulation of alternative metabolic pathways, impaired activation or increased inactivation of the antimetabolite, as well as increased drug (or metabolite) efflux. The folic acid analog methotrexate is an example of a drug that can be rendered ineffective by all of these mechanisms (Fig. 19–1; Chap. 18, Sec. 18.3.1). Thus the action of methotrexate depends on active uptake into cells mediated by a membrane transporter, its conversion to more stable intracellular polyglutamated metabolites, and its binding to its target enzyme, dihydrofolate reductase (DHFR), which leads to inhibition of thymidylate and purine biosynthesis, and induction of apoptosis (Fig. 19–1). Similarly, resistance to cisplatin can occur because of changes in processes (drug uptake, drug efflux, and/or intracellular drug sequestration) that prevent adequate levels of the drug reaching its DNA target, or by enhanced activity of processes that repair the DNA after it has been modified by the drug (Fig. 19–2; Chap. 18, Sec. 18.2.2; Kelland, 2007). Because multiple mechanisms may contribute to resistance to every anticancer drug, it is not surprising that initial or acquired drug resistance is observed after treatment of most cell populations.

The following evidence indicates that many types of drug resistance are genetic in origin:

1. Characteristics of drug-resistant cells (ie, their phenotypes) are often inherited in the absence of the selecting drug.
2. Drug-resistant cells are generated spontaneously at a rate that is consistent with known rates of genetic mutation.
3. Generation of drug-resistant cells is increased by exposure to compounds that cause mutations in genes or facilitate gene amplification (increased gene copy number). This property has been used to generate and select drug-resistant variant cells that have been used to study resistance phenotypes. Because of the genomic instability of tumor cells and the interaction of many anticancer drugs with DNA, drug treatment may itself accelerate the development of resistance.
4. Altered drug-target proteins that are the products of mutated genes have been identified in many drug-resistant cells.
5. Drug-resistant phenotypes have been transferred to drug-sensitive cells by transfer of genes (see Chap. 2, Sec. 2.2.3).

The presence of drug-resistant cells among the cells in human tumors has implications for planning optimal chemotherapy. Goldie and Coldman (1984) first used mathematical modeling to suggest that the probability of there being at least 1 drug-resistant cell in a tumor population is dependent on tumor size and will increase from near zero to near unity over a small range of tumor sizes (6 doublings), with the critical size depending on the rate of mutation to drug

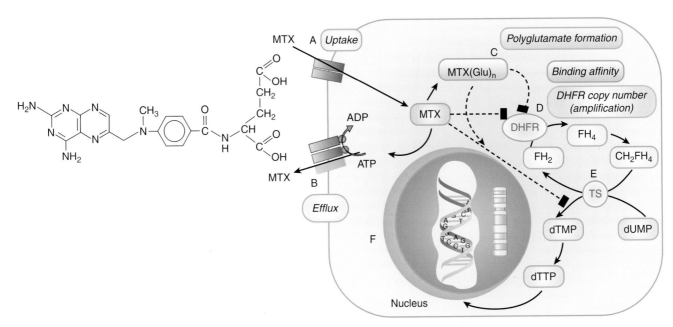

FIGURE 19–1 Multiple molecular mechanisms underlying cellular resistance to methotrexate. Methotrexate (MTX) uptake into cells can be limited by mutations in the reduced folate carrier (*RFC1/SLC 19A1*) (*A*). Resistance can also be observed when intracellular levels of MTX are reduced by the action of 1 or more drug efflux pumps such as P-glycoprotein or MRP1 (*B*). Changes in polyglutamylation of MTX (*C*) can reduce cellular sensitivity to this drug as MTX and its polyglutamates inhibit the enzyme dihydrofolate reductase (DHFR), causing a block in the conversion of dihydrofolate (FH$_2$) to tetrahydrofolate (FH$_4$), which ultimately results in a reduction in DNA synthesis and cell death. Binding of MTX and its polyglutamates can also be diminished by mutations in DHFR (*D*). MTX and its polyglutamates inhibit thymidylate synthesis (TS) (*E*), which also reduces DNA synthesis; drug resistance can occur because of changes in the levels or affinity of this enzyme. Finally, drug resistance may develop when the number of copies of the *DHFR* gene on chromosome 5 is increased through gene amplification (*F*).

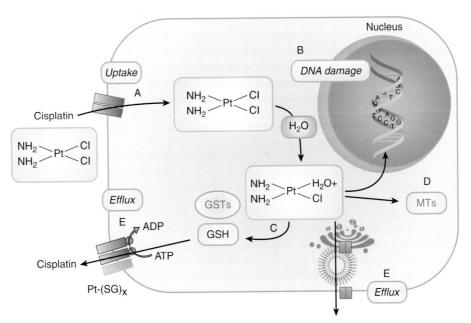

FIGURE 19–2 Multiple molecular mechanisms underlying cellular resistance to cisplatin. Cisplatin uptake into cells can be limited by mutations in the uptake transporter CTR1 (*SLC31A1*) resulting in drug resistance (*A*). Once inside the cell, one of the 2 Cl groups is replaced by water producing a reactive nucleophilic species that enters the nucleus where it can covalently modify DNA (primarily by intrastrand binding to adjacent guanines) and cause cell death. Resistance can occur when the damaged DNA is repaired (eg, nucleotide excision repair) or the damaged DNA is "tolerated" (eg, loss of mismatch repair or downregulation of apoptotic pathways) (*B*). Prior to entering the nucleus, conjugation of the activated cisplatin with glutathione (GSH) by GSH *S*-transferases (GSTs) (*C*), or interaction with the sulfhydryl-containing metallothioneins (*D*) can result in reduced drug efficacy. Finally, resistance can occur if intracellular levels of cisplatin or its metabolites are reduced by the efflux activity of several membrane transporters, including the MRP2 (*ABCC2*) efflux pump and the ATP7B P-type adenosine triphosphatase (ATPase) transporter (*E*).

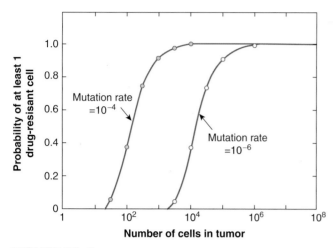

FIGURE 19–3 **Probability that there will be at least 1 drug-resistant cell in a tumor containing varying numbers of cells, based on rates of mutation of 10^{-6} (open symbols) and 10^{-4} (closed symbols) per cell per generation.** Note that this probability increases from low to high values over a relatively short period in the life history of the tumor and that drug-resistant cells are likely to be established prior to clinical detection.

resistance (Fig. 19–3). The Goldie-Coldman model implies a greater chance of cure if therapy is begun early, when only microscopic foci of tumor cells are present, and also predicts a better therapeutic effect when 2 equally effective and "noncrossresistant" drugs are alternated rather than given sequentially, as this minimizes the emergence of cell populations that are resistant to both drugs. Treatment of micrometastatic disease is the principal underlying adjuvant therapy in patients without evident metastatic disease after surgery, which has improved the cure rate for multiple cancers, but it has been difficult to demonstrate benefit from alternate use of noncrossresistant drugs.

Although drug resistance in many cultured tumor cell lines is caused by gene mutation or amplification, the relevance of these mechanisms to clinical drug treatments is variable. In earlier studies, one method used to select drug-resistant cells was to expose cells to mutagens, followed by selection in high concentrations of drug. This likely predisposed to selection of cells with genetically based drug resistance. However, exposure of cells to lower concentrations of drugs, without prior exposure to mutagens, can also lead to cells that show resistance that may be either stable or transient; transient resistance of some cells in the population may also occur spontaneously, without prior drug exposure.

Mechanisms underlying unstable drug resistance may include transient amplification of genes, changes in patterns of DNA methylation, and other factors that influence gene expression (so-called epigenetic mechanisms). Methylation of cytosines located within CpG dinucleotides is a frequent epigenetic modification in human DNA (see Chap. 2, Sec. 2.3.2; Sharma et al, 2010). CpG-rich regions (so-called CpG islands) are found typically in the proximal promoter regions of genes,

and in normal cells are usually unmethylated. In tumor cells, such regions are more often methylated and transcription of the affected gene may be impaired. Gene inactivation by hypermethylation can have consequences on virtually all pathways in the cell. However, when genes encoding DNA repair enzymes (such as *MGMT* and *hMLH1*; Sec. 19.2.6; see Chap. 5, Sec. 5.3), drug transporters (such as the adenosine triphosphate [ATP]-dependent drug efflux transporter *ABCG2*; Sec. 19.2.3), or proteins that regulate the cell cycle (eg, *CDKN2/p16INK4a*; see Chap. 9, Sec. 9.2.2) and apoptosis (see Sec. 19.2.8) are hypermethylated, the response to antineoplastic agents can be markedly altered.

Another epigenetic mechanism of gene regulation that can influence the drug sensitivity of tumor cells is acetylation and deacetylation of histones, nuclear proteins closely associated with DNA (see Chap. 2, Sec. 2.3.1; Muller and Kramer, 2010). Hyperacetylated histones are associated with an open chromatin configuration and they permit transcription of genes to occur. Responses to drugs can be modulated if the gene affected is a known determinant of drug sensitivity. For example, leukemia cells treated with a histone deacetylase (HDAC) inhibitor showed an increased expression of the nuclear drug target, topoisomerase II (see Sec. 19.2.5) and an acquired hypersensitivity to etoposide (Kurz et al, 2001). When combined, inhibitors of DNA methylation and histone acetylation can be particularly effective in restoring drug sensitivity even in solid tumors, at least in experimental systems (Steele et al, 2009). Finally, genes involved in drug sensitivity and resistance can also be regulated by a process known as *RNA interference* (RNAi). This involves naturally occurring small RNA molecules, known as microRNAs (miRNAs), which can "silence" genes, typically by binding to complementary sequences in the 3'-untranslated regions of target messenger RNA (mRNA) transcripts followed by translational repression or mRNA degradation (Boni et al, 2010; see Chap. 2, Sec. 2.4.3).

19.2.2 Resistance Caused by Impaired Drug Uptake

Drug uptake into cells occurs by one of the following mechanisms: (a) passive diffusion, in which the drug enters the cell by an energy- and temperature-*independent* process without interacting with specific constituents in the cell membrane; (b) facilitated diffusion, in which the drug interacts in a chemically specific manner with a transport carrier in the cell membrane and is translocated into the cell in an energy- and temperature-*independent* process; (c) binding of drug to a cell surface receptor that is then internalized; and (d) active transport, in which the drug is actively transported by a carrier-mediated process that is both temperature- and energy-*dependent* (Sugano et al, 2010). All mechanisms allow for drug entry into cells down a concentration gradient, but the fourth mechanism can also lead to transport against a concentration gradient.

A common mechanism of resistance is impaired unidirectional drug influx. Cellular uptake of hydrophilic drugs is commonly mediated by members of the solute carrier (SLC) superfamily (gene symbol *SLC*) of membrane transport proteins. This superfamily contains more than 300 proteins organized into 47 families whose major physiological function is to import nutrients and other naturally occurring metabolites into cells.

Many of the SLC importers that have been implicated in the drug sensitivity of malignant and normal cells have a common core structure typified by 2 membrane-spanning domains each containing 6 transmembrane α-helices that form a pore through the membrane. The polytopic SLC proteins mediate the cellular import of a wide range of hydrophilic anticancer drugs that often resemble the natural physiological substrates of the transporter itself. For example, methotrexate is imported across the plasma membrane primarily by an energy-dependent folic acid uptake system, the reduced folate carrier RFC1 (*SLC19A1*). Drug-resistant cells may have impaired methotrexate uptake into the cell as a result of point mutations in *RFC1/SLC19A1* (see Fig. 19–1; Drori et al, 2000); this mechanism of acquired resistance has been found in patients with acute leukemia (Ashton et al, 2009). Similarly, cellular uptake of purine and pyrimidine nucleoside analogs, such as gemcitabine, cladribine, fludarabine, and cytarabine, occurs primarily via membrane transport carriers such as the nucleoside transporters CNT1 and CNT3, which belong to the *SLC28* subfamily, and ENT1 and ENT2, which belong to the *SLC29* subfamily. Cisplatin and other platinum-containing drugs may be taken up into cells by membrane proteins encoded by the *SLC7A11* or *CTR1/SLC31A1* genes, which normally import amino acids and copper, respectively. Cells deficient in these carrier proteins are often resistant to these drugs, at least in vitro (see Fig. 19–2; Zhang et al, 2007; Howell et al, 2010). Naturally occurring genetic polymorphisms that result in downregulation or upregulation of these *SLC* genes in normal and/or tumor cells may also contribute to variation in systemic and intracellular levels of (and hence response to) their drug substrates (Yee et al, 2010).

19.2.3 Multiple Drug Resistance Caused by Enhanced Drug Efflux

Drug accumulation in side cells is determined by the balance between drug uptake and drug efflux. Many anticancer drugs, particularly natural products or their derivatives (eg, doxorubicin, vincristine, etoposide, and paclitaxel), and drug metabolites are effluxed from cells by one or more ATP-binding cassette (ABC) transporters. ABC proteins are found throughout nature from mammals to plants, marine organisms, and prokaryotes, where they carry out many important functions, including the export of potential toxins from cells. Most ABC transporters move one or more molecules (which can range from ions to sugars to small peptides) across biological membranes, a process powered by energy derived from binding and hydrolysis of ATP.

The human ABC superfamily contains 48 proteins, which are organized into 7 subfamilies (*A* through *G*) based on

TABLE 19–2 ABC transporters that confer multiple drug resistance in human tumors and their specificity for individual cytotoxic anticancer drugs.

P-Glycoprotein	MRP1	ABCG2/BCRP
Doxorubicin	Doxorubicin	Doxorubicin
Daunorubicin	Daunorubicin	Daunorubicin
Epirubicin	Epirubicin	Mitoxantrone
Mitoxantrone		
Vinblastine	Vinblastine*	
Vincristine	Vincristine	
Etoposide	Etoposide	
Methotrexate	Methotrexate	Methotrexate
Paclitaxel	Paclitaxel*	
	Camptothecin derivatives	Camptothecin derivatives
	SN-38	SN-38
	Topotecan	Topotecan
	Flutamide	Gefitinib
	Hydroxyflutamide	

*Low level.

the relative similarities of their amino acid sequences (Dean and Allikmets, 2001). Twelve of the 48 ABC transporters are known to efflux drugs and other xenobiotics (or their metabolites) at least in vitro but only 3 of them appear relevant to clinical drug resistance in human tumors and have the ability to export a wide range of structurally diverse anticancer drugs (Table 19–2). The first of these clinically relevant multidrug efflux pumps to be described (in 1976) was P-glycoprotein: human P-glycoprotein is encoded by the *ABCB1* gene (formerly known as the *MDR1* gene) (Gottesman et al, 2002; Leslie et al, 2005). Multidrug resistance protein 1 (MRP1; gene symbol *ABCC1*), was described by Cole et al. (1992), while the ABCG2 protein (formerly known as the breast cancer resistance protein [BCRP]) was described by Doyle et al. (1998). These 3 ABC transporters are detected consistently in drug-resistant malignant cells from patients.

In normal cells, P-glycoprotein, MRP1, ABCG2, and several other clinically relevant MRP-related drug transporters are often expressed in a polarized manner and contribute to drug absorption (bioavailability), distribution (limiting drug access to so-called pharmacological sanctuaries such as the brain, cerebral spinal fluid, and testes), and elimination (efflux into bile or urine) (Fig. 19–4). In contrast to the SLC uptake transporters which generally display specificity for a single class of drugs, the clinically relevant ABC drug efflux pumps typically recognize and transport a structurally diverse array of molecules in addition to the anticancer drugs listed in Table 19–2. It is still not well understood how a single membrane protein can recognize so many structurally dissimilar chemical entities.

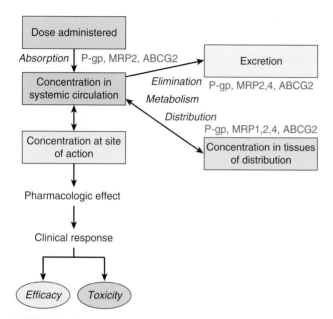

FIGURE 19–4 Multiple roles of the ABC transporters. ABC transport proteins as determinants of drug efficacy and toxicity. While the ABC transporters P-glycoprotein, MRP1, and ABCG2/BCRP have been widely detected in drug-resistant tumor cells, these transporters (together with MRP2 and MRP4) are also now known to affect drug sensitivity and resistance by virtue of their influence on drug absorption (P-glycoprotein, MRP2, ABCG2) and tissue distribution (P-glycoprotein, MRP1, MRP2, MRP4, ABCG2/BCRP), as well as elimination of drugs and their metabolites through the bile, kidney, or other excretory tissue. In tumor cells, the ABC transporters are all found on the plasma membrane. In normal polarized epithelial and endothelial cells in tissues such as the gut, liver, kidney, and brain which are important for drug absorption, distribution and elimination, P-glycoprotein, MRP2, and ABCG2 are found on apical membranes while MRP1 is found on basolateral membranes. MRP4 is unusual in that its localization depends on the tissue in which it is expressed (eg, apical in kidney, brain; basolateral in prostate, liver). *P-gp*, P-glycoprotein. (Slot et al, 2011).

19.2.3.1 P-Glycoprotein

In humans, ABCB1 (formerly MDR1) has been mapped to chromosome 7, and its gene product, P-glycoprotein, is a relatively large phosphoglycoprotein of molecular weight 170 kDa. It contains 2 homologous halves, each of which is comprised of 6 transmembrane α-helices followed by a cytosolic nucleotide (ATP)-binding domain. Thus, like most ABC proteins, P-glycoprotein has a typical 4-domain structure (Fig. 19–5A) and all 4 domains are required for its full activity. The drug-binding sites of P-glycoprotein are generally found in the 2 hydrophobic membrane-spanning domains, which together also form the drug translocation pathway through the membrane (Fig. 19–5A). Structural evidence indicates that for transport to occur, these hydrophobic domains are coupled with the 2 energy-providing ATP-binding domains (NBD1/2), and this coupling is mediated by the cytoplasmic loops that connect the transmembrane helices to one another. The details by which this coupling of substrate transport to the adenosine triphosphatase (ATPase) activity of these

drug efflux pumps occurs are not completely understood but are thought to be common among all ABC proteins (Hollenstein et al, 2007).

P-glycoprotein confers resistance against a wide spectrum of complex heterocyclic hydrophobic, antineoplastic drugs mostly derived from natural products that include the anthracycline antibiotics, the *Vinca* alkaloids, and the taxanes (see Table 19–2). Other substrates include the tyrosine kinase inhibitors gefitinib and imatinib (see Chap. 17, Sec. 17.3.1). P-glycoprotein also mediates the cellular efflux of other drugs used with cancer chemotherapy, such as ondansetron and granisetron, that are used to control emesis. Certain fluorescent chemicals (eg, rhodamine 123) and radiopharmaceuticals used in imaging (eg, ^{99m}Tc-sestamibi) are also P-glycoprotein substrates and are being investigated for their ability to detect clinical drug resistance mediated by this transporter, the latter by external imaging.

In vitro studies show that single amino acid substitutions can markedly alter the substrate specificity of P-glycoprotein (Loo and Clarke, 2005). Furthermore, a naturally occurring polymorphism in the *ABCB1* gene has been described that affects the ability of P-glycoprotein to recognize some of its drug substrates (Kimchi-Safarty et al, 2007).

In addition to being expressed at elevated levels in certain tumor types, P-glycoprotein is also found in normal tissues, such as the kidney and adrenal gland, as well as the lung, liver, and gastrointestinal tract. P-glycoprotein is localized to the apical surface of polarized cells that line the tubules or ducts or lumen of these organs, and thus provides such cells with a mechanism for extruding xenobiotic molecules that are recognized by the transporter, or for impeding uptake of these molecules (delaying absorption) (see Fig. 19–4; Leslie et al, 2005). P-glycoprotein is also expressed on the apical membrane of endothelial cells lining the blood–brain barrier, where it excludes toxic natural products from the central nervous system. Strong evidence for the function of P-glycoprotein as a regulator of drug uptake comes from studies of mice in which these genes have been disrupted by homologous recombination (see Chap. 2, Sec. 2.4.5). These P-glycoprotein *Abcb1* knockout mice display a marked increase in sensitivity to the neurotoxic side effects of several different drugs (Lagas et al, 2009). Such animals also show enhanced oral absorption (bioavailability) of certain drugs, and this appears also to be true in humans when P-glycoprotein is inhibited.

Many investigators have measured levels of P-glycoprotein in human tumors, both before and after treatment with anticancer drugs (Gottesman et al, 2002). Elevated P-glycoprotein has been found in sarcomas and in cancers of the colon, adrenal, kidney, liver, and pancreas. All these tumors tend to be resistant to chemotherapy. Elevated levels of P-glycoprotein have also been detected following relapse after chemotherapy in more drug-sensitive tumors, including multiple myeloma and cancers of the breast and ovary. These findings suggest that P-glycoprotein may contribute to clinical drug resistance. Increased P-glycoprotein has also been reported to correlate

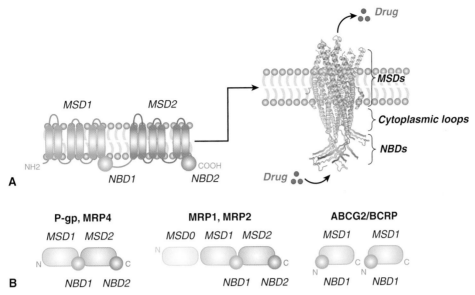

FIGURE 19–5 **General structure of ABC membrane drug efflux pumps. A)** *(left)* Shown is a linear topological cartoon of the core structure of ABC transporters such as P-glycoprotein showing the 2 cytoplasmic nucleotide-binding domains (NBDs) and 12 transmembrane (TM) helices (here shown as cylinders) equally distributed between 2 membrane-spanning domains (MSDs). *(right)* Shown is a 3D homology model of the core structure of MRP1 (lacking MSD0, see Fig 19–5B) generated using the crystal structure of *Staphylococcus aureus* Sav1866 as template (Hollenstein et al, 2007; DeGorter et al, 2008). The α-carbon backbone in ribbon representation of the core structure (MSD1-NBD1-MSD2-NBD2) is viewed from the plane perpendicular to the membrane bilayer (DeGorter et al, 2008). Homology models of P-glycoprotein, MRP4 and other ABC transporters look very similar. The 2 NBDs form a "sandwich" dimer for the effective binding and hydrolysis of 2 molecules of ATP, providing the energy for the transport process. Signaling between the MSDs (translocation pathway through the membrane) and the NBDs (which provide the energy for transport) is mediated by specific sequences in the cytoplasmic loops. Substrates that enter the cell by diffusion or active transport, or are formed in the cell by conjugation, are thought to be exported from the cell either directly through the pore from the cytoplasm, or in the case of hydrophobic drugs, are taken up from the inner leaflet of the membrane lipid bilayer. **B)** Domain organization of ABC transporter drug (and drug metabolite) efflux pumps implicated in drug resistance in malignant cells. P-glycoprotein and the MRPs are encoded as multidomain single polypeptides containing MSDs and NBDs in the orientations shown, while ABCG2/BCRP is encoded as a "half-transporter" and 2 identical subunits assemble together to form a functional transporter. Each of the MSDs contains 6 transmembrane segments (α-helices) except for MSD0 of MRP1 and MRP2 which contains just 5. *P-gp*, P-glycoprotein.

with a poor prognosis in children with neuroblastoma, rhabdomyosarcoma, and osteogenic sarcoma.

19.2.3.2 Multidrug Resistance Proteins

A second multidrug transporter, now known as MRP1 (gene symbol ABCC1), was cloned originally from a drug-selected cell line derived from human small cell lung cancer that did not express P-glycoprotein but did contain multiple gene copies of ABCC1 (Cole et al, 1992; Fig. 19–6). Although P-glycoprotein and MRP1 are both members of the ABC superfamily, the 2 proteins share only 15% amino acid sequence identity and differ in several significant structural and pharmacological ways (Leslie et al, 2005). The *ABCC1* gene is located on chromosome 16p13.1 and encodes a 190-kDa phosphoglycoprotein with 17 transmembrane α-helices, 5 more than P-glycoprotein. These extra transmembrane helices of MRP1 form a third NH$_2$-proximal membrane-spanning domain, MSD0 (see Fig. 19–5B). The role of this NH$_2$-terminal hydrophobic extension has not been elucidated, but it appears important for the transport of some MRP1 substrates and has been implicated in stabilizing expression of this transporter at the plasma membrane (Deeley et al, 2006).

As for P-glycoprotein, increased expression of MRP1 leads to a net decrease in cellular accumulation of a variety of anticancer drugs, including both natural products and the folic acid analog methotrexate (see Table 19–2). The spectrum of drugs that MRP1 transports is slightly different from P-glycoprotein in that MRP1 confers at most low levels of resistance to the hydrophobic paclitaxel and vinblastine. Also, transport of some drugs (eg, vincristine, daunorubicin) by MRP1 depends on the presence of the antioxidant glutathione (GSH) or a tripeptide analog (Fig. 19–7A; Rappa et al, 1997; Loe et al, 1998). In vitro, GSH causes changes in the conformation of the MRP1 protein, which increases its affinity for some of its drug substrates (Cole and Deeley, 2006; Rothnie et al, 2006), but GSH may also influence MRP1 function in other ways.

In addition to its ability to confer resistance to anticancer drugs in both malignant and normal cells, MRP1 transports a broad spectrum of organic anions, another property not shared by P-glycoprotein. For example, metabolites of drugs and other xenobiotics that are conjugated to GSH, glucuronide, or sulfate (the products of Phase II drug metabolism; see Fig. 19–7A), are frequently effluxed by MRP1 but not by P-glycoprotein. Conjugates of endogenous metabolites are

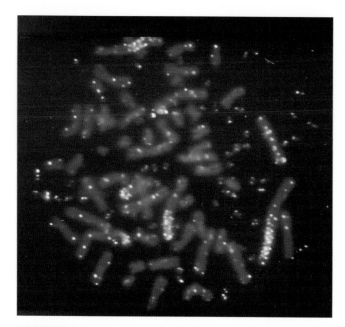

FIGURE 19–6 Metaphase spread of a highly drug-resistant lung cancer cell that contains approximately 100 copies of the *ABCC1* gene. Fluorescent in situ hybridization analysis of *ABCC1*, the gene encoding the drug efflux pump MRP1. The normal cellular locus of *ABCC1* is chromosome 16p13.1. However, in many drug-resistant cell lines where expression of MRP1 is elevated, *ABCC1* has been amplified. The figure shows a metaphase spread of a highly drug-resistant lung cancer cell that contains approximately 100 copies of the *ABCC1* gene. Note that the fluorescently labeled *ABCC1* probe has hybridized to several homogeneously staining regions (HSRs) and multiple double minute chromosomes (DMs). (From Slovak et al, 1993).

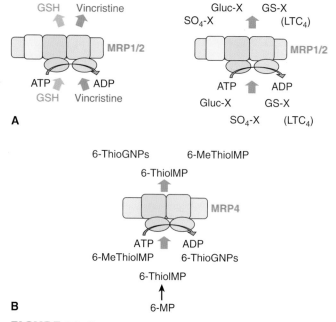

FIGURE 19–7 Transport of conjugated and unconjugated drugs by "long" and "short" MRPs across cell membranes. A) Efflux of several natural product drugs (eg, vincristine and doxorubicin) by the "long" MRP1 or MRP2 is dependent on the presence of reduced GSH, which is cotransported with the drug (*left*). Transport of drug metabolites, including those conjugated to glutathione (GS-X), glucuronide (Gluc-X), and sulphate (SO$_4$-X) (*right*) by MRP1 (and MRP2) usually does not require GSH. The major physiological metabolite transported by MRP1 is the GSH-conjugated leukotriene C$_4$ (LTC$_4$). **B)** Efflux of the active metabolites of 6-mercaptopurine (6-MP) by the "short" MRP4.

also transported by MRP1, most notably the cysteinyl leukotriene, LTC$_4$, a potent mediator of inflammation. Thus, mice bearing a disrupted *Abcc1* gene exhibit enhanced sensitivity of tissues such as seminiferous tubules and the oropharyngeal cavity to anticancer agents like etoposide, but also an impaired response to proinflammatory stimuli associated with diminished LTC$_4$ secretion from mast cells (Wijnholds et al, 1997; Lagas et al, 2009). Other potential physiological substrates of MRP1 include the conjugated estrogens estradiol glucuronide and estrone sulfate, folic acid, GSH and its prooxidant metabolite GSH disulfide (GSSG) (see Fig. 19–7A). MRP1 also transports several fluorescent organic anions, such as calcein, which facilitates measurement of the activity of this transport protein in clinical and experimental studies. Thus the substrates of MRP1 are more diverse than those of P-glycoprotein (Leslie et al, 2005; Slot et al, 2011).

MRP1 has been detected in a wide variety of human tumors and normal tissues (Deeley et al, 2006). Increased expression has been observed in several types of drug-resistant human tumors, such as lung cancer and some leukemias, and in many cell lines derived from human tumors. In children with neuroblastoma, expression of MRP1 was correlated with expression of the *N-MYC* oncogene and predicted poor survival (Haber et al, 2006). In vitro, certain mutations in *ABCC1* cause

changes in the substrate specificity of MRP1, such as substitution of Trp[1246], which results in total loss of drug resistance (Ito et al, 2001). In primary neuroblastoma, the naturally occurring ABCC1 polymorphism G2012T is associated with patient outcome and altered stability of the *ABCC1* gene transcript (Pajic et al, 2011).

Eight additional MRP-related proteins have been described, 5 of which have been shown to transport one or more drugs, at least in vitro, but have no significant role in tumor cell resistance (Deeley et al, 2006; Slot et al, 2011). Despite the fact it is rarely found in tumors, however, MRP2 in normal cells may impact drug sensitivity because it can influence the distribution and elimination (and hence pharmacokinetics) of some anticancer drugs and their metabolites (see Fig. 19–4). MRP2 is structurally very similar to MRP1, but unlike MRP1, it is expressed predominantly on apical membranes of the bile canaliculus, renal epithelium, and intestinal enterocytes. Thus, MRP2 plays a role in the oral bioavailability and elimination of drugs and their metabolites that are substrates of this transport protein (Table 19–3; Nies and Keppler, 2007).

MRP4 (gene symbol *ABCC4*) is a "short" MRP because it lacks the third NH$_2$-terminal membrane-spanning domain of MRP1 and MRP2 (Slot et al, 2011) and thus is a 4-domain ABC transporter like P-glycoprotein. MRP4 can transport

TABLE 19–3 Drugs and drug metabolites that interact with MRP2 and MRP4 that may be important for drug disposition and elimination.

	Drugs/Metabolites
MRP2	cisplatin, anthracyclines, *Vinca* alkaloids, etoposide, camptothecin, irinotecan, SN-38, methotrexate *(short exposure);* organic anions (glutathione-, glucuronide-, sulphate-conjugated drug metabolites); As, Sb oxyanions
MRP4	methotrexate, monophosphorylated metabolites of 6-mercaptopurine, 6-thioguanine *(thiopurines);* topotecan, irinotecan

topotecan and the monophosphorylated, bioactive forms of the antimetabolites 6-mercaptopurine and 6-thioguanine, as well as nucleotide analogs used to treat patients with viral infections (Leggas et al, 2004; Russel et al, 2008; see Fig. 19–7B and Table 19–3). However, like MRP2, increased levels of MRP4 have only rarely been detected in tumor samples from patients. In contrast, a role for MRP4 in drug disposition/elimination (pharmacokinetics) and adverse drug reactions has been revealed by studies of *Abcc4⁻/⁻* mice. Topotecan accumulation in both brain tissue and in cerebrospinal fluid is enhanced in *Abcc4⁻/⁻* mice, reflecting the unusual dual localization of MRP4 at the basolateral membrane of the choroid plexus epithelium, and at the apical membrane of the endothelial cells of the brain capillaries (Leggas et al, 2004). Renal elimination of many drugs (or their metabolites) is also reduced in *Abcc4⁻/⁻* mice, consistent with a protective role for MRP4 in the kidney. Common nonsteroidal antiinflammatory drugs (NSAIDs) (eg, celecoxib) inhibit transport by MRP4, which may contribute to renal toxicity when a cytotoxic agent such as methotrexate is coadministered with NSAIDs (El-Sheikh et al, 2007). *Abcc4⁻/⁻* mice are also more sensitive to the hematopoietic toxicity of thiopurines. In humans, a polymorphism in *ABCC4* encodes a nonfunctional MRP4 transporter and the generally greater sensitivity of Japanese patients to thiopurines may reflect the greater frequency (>18%) of this polymorphism in the Japanese population (Krishnamurthy et al, 2008).

19.2.3.3 *ABCG2* The third ABC drug efflux pump of clinical relevance in drug resistance of tumor cells is ABCG2 (formerly BCRP), which was first cloned from a drug-resistant breast cancer cell line that expressed neither P-glycoprotein nor MRP1 (Doyle et al, 1998). The *ABCG2* gene has been mapped to chromosome 4q22 and encodes a protein containing just 655 amino acids, compared to 1280 amino acids for P-glycoprotein and 1531 amino acids for MRP1. ABCG2 is comprised of only a single membrane-spanning domain and nucleotide-binding domain, and is often referred to as a "half-transporter": 2 ABCG2 proteins must come together to form a functional 4-domain transporter (see Fig. 19–5B).

When overexpressed, ABCG2 can render tumor cells resistant to a variety of clinically important drugs, including mitoxantrone, doxorubicin, daunorubicin, topotecan, and SN-38 (the

active metabolite of irinotecan), as well as the epidermal growth factor receptor (EGFR) inhibitor gefitinib (see Table 19–2) (Doyle et al, 1998; Vlaming et al, 2009). Thus despite substantial differences in their amino acid sequences and structural organization, ABCG2 can efflux some of the same drugs as P-glycoprotein and MRP1. Like P-glycoprotein and MRP1, ABCG2 also transports some fluorescent molecules, which facilitates detection of this transporter in clinical samples.

ABCG2 is widely expressed in normal tissues and, like P-glycoprotein and MRP2, is present on apical membranes of polarized endothelial and epithelial cells, and has been implicated in the absorption, distribution and elimination of certain xenobiotics. In a mouse model, Abcg2 has been shown to contribute to the blood–brain, blood–testis, and blood–fetal barriers (Vlaming et al, 2009). Efflux of the fluorescent dye Hoechst 33342 has been reported in the so-called side-population of bone marrow cells that are highly enriched for undifferentiated stem cells. This ABC transporter might serve to extrude a metabolite(s) from embryonic stem cells that helps prevent differentiation (Sarkadi et al, 2010). ABCG2 likely also serves a protective role in these cells against damage by xenobiotics.

19.2.3.4 Reversal or Circumvention of Drug Resistance Mediated by ABC Transporters Many agents have been identified that inhibit the function of P-glycoprotein and increase the sensitivity of drug-resistant tumor cells in culture (eg, Gottesman et al, 2002). Some of these agents are themselves substrates for P-glycoprotein and competitively inhibit the efflux of anticancer drugs, but noncompetitive mechanisms have also been implicated. Multiple clinical trials have assessed the potential of P-glycoprotein antagonists to increase the sensitivity of human tumors to anticancer drugs such as doxorubicin and vinorelbine. Some patients with hematological malignancies that were drug resistant responded to the same anticancer drugs when an inhibitor of P-glycoprotein was added to the drug regimen, but the results of studies with solid tumors have been disappointing. There are several possible reasons for the inconclusive outcomes of many of these clinical trials (Gottesman et al, 2002; Yu et al, 2012), including poor trial design, resistance because of mechanisms in addition to or other than P-glycoprotein, and failure to achieve adequate levels of the reversing agent in the tumor tissue. Several "third-generation" P-glycoprotein reversal agents with higher affinity and greater potency and specificity are under investigation.

Agents such as verapamil and cyclosporine, which may reverse drug resistance as a result of P-glycoprotein in cell culture, have much less effect on drug resistance because of MRP1. The cysteinyl leukotriene receptor antagonist MK-571 was identified as a relatively potent inhibitor of MRP1-mediated transport, but suffers from a lack of specificity. High-throughput screening has identified more potent and specific agents that antagonize the drug efflux activity of MRP1, but these have not yet been widely tested in humans (Boumendjel et al, 2005; Burkhart et al, 2009). In cultured cells, resistance to some (but not all) drugs caused by MRP1 can be reversed by using agents that deplete cellular GSH, but it is not yet known if this is the case in humans (Cole and Deeley, 2006).

The search for modulators of drug efflux mediated by ABCG2 has been less extensive, although several highly specific inhibitors have been identified by high-throughput screens of large chemical libraries (Vlaming et al, 2009). Although these agents have been shown to be effective in vitro and in mice bearing drug-resistant human tumors, none thus far have been tested in clinical trials.

Novel agents that inhibit the transport function of P-glycoprotein (as well as MRP1, MRP2, MRP4, and ABCG2) are also being investigated for their ability to improve oral absorption of antineoplastic drugs or enable better penetration of drugs into pharmacological sanctuaries (eg, the central nervous system), tissues that are normally protected by these transporters (Leslie et al, 2005; Matsson et al, 2009). These studies reflect a growing appreciation of the role that transporters in normal cells may play in the clinical efficacy and toxicity of drugs as well as drug–drug interactions (see Fig. 19–4). The ability of these ABC proteins to confer drug resistance has also led to exploration of the use of vectors to deliver genes encoding these transporters into bone marrow and other drug-sensitive normal tissues to protect them from the toxic side effects of chemotherapy.

19.2.4 Resistance Caused by Decreased Drug Activation or Increased Drug Inactivation

Many antineoplastic drugs, and in particular the antimetabolites, must be converted to a pharmacologically active form after cellular uptake in order to exert their cytotoxic effects (see Chap. 18, Sec. 18.3). Resistance to these agents can occur when there is a decrease in activity or levels of the activating enzyme(s), or an increase in the activity or levels of an enzyme that is responsible for detoxifying the active form of the drug. For example, drug-resistant leukemia cells may show a decrease in polyglutamylation of intracellular methotrexate as a result of either decreased activity of the synthetic enzyme, folylpolyglutamate synthase, or increased activity of the catabolic enzyme, folylpolyglutamate hydrolase (see Fig. 19–1). Resistance to the pyrimidine analog cytosine arabinoside (ara-C) may occur as a result of decreased activation by various kinases, such as deoxycytidine kinase and/or enhanced inactivation by deaminases. Similarly, resistance to the pyrimidine analog, 5-fluorouracil (5-FU), is associated with alterations in the enzymes (eg, uridine monophosphate [UMP] kinase) responsible for its activation (Humeniuk et al, 2009), or of its catabolism (eg, dihydropyrimidine dehydrogenase; Yang et al, 2011).

Many anticancer drugs and carcinogens cause cellular damage by the production of chemically reactive electrophilic intermediates, especially reactive oxygen species (see Chap. 4, Sec. 4.2.3). Similar processes are involved during the interaction of ionizing radiation with tissue (see Chap. 15, Sec. 15.2.3). One mechanism by which cells can

protect themselves from damage caused by reactive agents is by upregulating the synthesis of sulfhydryl-containing molecules, especially the nucleophilic tripeptide GSH, which can form conjugates with the electrophilic metabolites and render them less reactive and thus nontoxic. The importance of GSH in the protection of normal cells is reflected in its widespread distribution and its relatively high intracellular concentration (>1 mM in many tissues). GSH can inactivate peroxides and free radicals, which may be produced by drugs such as etoposide and the anthracyclines (eg, doxorubicin). It can also react with positively charged electrophilic molecules, such as the active groups of cisplatin and alkylating agents, rendering them less toxic and more easily excreted. These reactions are catalyzed, respectively, by the enzymes GSH peroxidase and GSH S-transferase (GST) (see Fig. 19–2).

By conjugating GSH to various drugs or their active metabolites, GSTs appear to play a role in the development of cellular resistance to some antineoplastic agents (Townsend and Tew, 2003; Sau et al, 2010). The cytosolic GSTs are a highly polymorphic multigene family of enzymes that are often classified by their isoelectric points, as well as by their relative sequence homology: the major classes are the basic (α class), neutral (μ class), and acidic (π class) GSTs. Each functional GST enzyme is a homo- or heterodimer made up of subunits encoded by gene loci from within a given class. Not all cell lines selected for resistance to alkylating agents have shown increases in GST protein levels or activity, but several lines of evidence support a role for GSTs in resistance to alkylating and platinum-containing agents:

1. Nitrogen mustards can form GSH conjugates in reactions catalyzed by GSTs.
2. Human tumors and tumor cell lines often overexpress GST isozymes.
3. GST inhibitors can sometimes sensitize cultured tumor cells to cisplatin and alkylating agents (Pasello et al, 2008; see Fig. 19–2).
4. Cell-cycle–dependent sensitivity to melphalan correlates with the cell-cycle–dependent expression of certain GSTs.
5. Transfection of complementary DNAs (cDNAs) encoding certain GST isoforms can confer resistance to alkylating agents (Smitherman et al, 2004).
6. Elevation of GST can occur within several days of exposure to chlorambucil as part of the normal cellular response.

In addition to their conjugating activities, the π and μ classes of GSTs have an antiapoptotic function because of their regulatory role in the mitogen-activated protein (MAP) kinase pathway via inhibitory interactions with c-Jun N-terminal kinase 1 (JNK1) and ASK1 (apoptosis signal-regulating kinase) (Townsend and Tew, 2003; Sau et al, 2010; see Chap. 8, Sec. 8.2.4). Thus GSTs may contribute to resistance by facilitating drug detoxification as well as by acting as an inhibitor of the MAP kinase pathway.

Drugs conjugated to GSH, glucuronide, or sulfate groups are negatively charged and these conjugated organic anions are extruded from cells by an energy-dependent process.

GSH-conjugate export carriers (known variably as *GS-X pumps* or *multispecific organic anion transporters*) are involved, and this export function is undertaken, in large part, by the ABC transporters MRP1 and MRP2 (Cole and Deeley, 2006; Sec. 19.2.3). Although conjugated metabolites are usually less reactive, the active efflux of conjugated metabolites by the MRP transporters prevents their intracellular accumulation, thereby reducing the possibility of hydrolytic enzymes causing the regeneration of the active parent compound. However, some conjugated metabolites can be directly cytotoxic because of their ability to inhibit enzymes important for cell viability, as well as by inhibition of the conjugating enzymes. Thus, elimination of conjugated metabolites from the cell is an important component of the detoxification process (Leslie et al, 2005).

Resistance to cisplatin and alkylating agents also is associated with increased levels of metallothioneins, proteins rich in sulfhydryl-containing cysteine residues (see Fig. 19–2). The presumed mechanism is "neutralization" of the toxic electrophilic drugs or their metabolites, by their interaction with these proteins; indeed, each molecule of metallothionein can bind up to 10 platinum atoms. Nevertheless, although cells transfected with a human metallothionein gene can acquire resistance to cisplatin and alkylating agents (Kelley et al, 1988), and cells that do not produce metallothionein show increased chemosensitivity (Kondo et al, 1995), there is no in vivo evidence to support a major role for metallothioneins in clinical drug resistance.

19.2.5 Resistance Caused by Altered Levels or Modification of the Drug Target

To exert their cytotoxicity, antineoplastic agents must interact efficiently with their intracellular protein targets. Changes may occur such that levels of the target protein are increased, thus requiring increased concentrations of drug to elicit cytotoxicity. Alternatively, the gene encoding the protein can acquire a mutation such that it retains its normal physiological activity but exhibits reduced affinity for drugs. These resistance mechanisms reduce the effectiveness of both conventional (below) and novel targeted therapeutic agents (see Sec. 19.2.7).

19.2.5.1 Resistance to Drugs Targeting Enzymes Involved in Folate Metabolism and DNA Synthesis
Among the multiple mechanisms of resistance to 5-FU, is the acquisition of mutations in thymidylate synthase, the target of its active metabolite 5-FdUMP (5-fluoro-deoxyuridine-monophosphate; see Chap. 18, Sec. 18.3.2). Similarly, resistance to methotrexate may occur because of the production of variant forms of DHFR, the target enzyme for this drug (see Fig. 19–1). Variant enzymes have been found that retain adequate function for reduction of their normal substrate (dihydrofolate) but have decreased affinity for methotrexate.

Another mechanism leading to methotrexate resistance is elevated production of DHFR resulting from an increase in the number of copies of the *DHFR* gene (gene amplification)

(see Fig. 19–1; Schimke, 1984). High levels of methotrexate resistance in cultured cells is usually observed after stepwise increases in the drug concentration in the medium, and this may lead to as many as 100 to 1000 copies of the *DHFR* gene. Amplification of *DHFR* has also been observed in human lung tumors from patients treated with methotrexate.

Although gene amplification has been studied most extensively in relation to methotrexate resistance, there is increasing evidence for the importance of this mechanism in determining resistance to several other drugs, including upregulation of the target enzyme for the active metabolite of 5-FU (thymidylate synthetase) (Watson et al, 2010). Amplification of genes encoding 1 or more of the ABC drug efflux pumps (P-glycoprotein, MRP1, or ABCG2/BCRP), can also lead to multidrug resistance phenotypes (Cole et al, 1992; see Fig. 19–6), although amplification of these *ABC* genes is rarely detected in patient samples (see Sec. 19.2.3).

Drug resistance caused by gene amplification may be either stable or unstable when cells are grown in the absence of the drug. Stable amplification is typically associated with a chromosomal location of the amplified genes, often seen as *homogeneously staining regions (HSRs)* in stained chromosome preparations. Unstable amplification is usually associated with location of the genes in extrachromosomal chromatin structures known as *double minutes (DMs)*. Multiple gene copies at both locations may be evident during selection for drug resistance (see Fig. 19–6).

19.2.5.2 Resistance to Drugs Targeting the DNA Topoisomerases
DNA topoisomerases are nuclear enzymes that catalyze topological changes of DNA structure required for recombination and replication of DNA and for transcription of RNA. These enzymes also play a central role in chromosome structure, condensation/decondensation, and segregation (Nitiss, 2009; Pommier, 2009). Under physiological conditions, these covalent enzyme-DNA cleavage complexes are short-lived intermediates present at low concentration that are well tolerated by the cell. Topoisomerases serve as cellular targets for several important antineoplastic agents, some of which appear to stabilize the DNA-enzyme complex, leading to increased DNA strand cleavage, and thereby mediating, at least in part, the cytocidal activity of these compounds (see Chap. 18, Sec. 18.4). Other drugs targeted to topoisomerases act as conventional enzyme inhibitors and do not require that the topoisomerase be bound to DNA to be toxic (Nitiss, 2009; Pommier, 2009).

Camptothecin and its close structural analogs topotecan and CPT-11 exert their antitumor activity by inhibiting the 100-kDa topoisomerase I (see Chap. 18, Sec. 18.4.1). Under physiological conditions, the enzyme produces transient single-strand breaks in DNA and binds covalently to the 3′-phosphoryl end of DNA at the break site through a tyrosine residue at position 723 in the COOH-terminus. It then facilitates passage of an intact DNA strand through the break site, followed by religation of the cleaved DNA. Camptothecin (and its analogs) form a reversible complex with topoisomerase I and DNA, which shifts the equilibrium reaction markedly in the direction of cleavage. This results in increased DNA damage and, ultimately, cell death. Downregulation and production of mutant forms of topoisomerase I have been reported in cells resistant to these drugs (Pommier, 2009). Point mutations involving amino acid residues 361-364 appear particularly critical for resistance to camptothecin and its derivatives. Analyses of the topoisomerase I crystal structure indicate that this region is important for hydrogen bonding to camptothecin and it is close to the catalytic tyrosine residue and the bound DNA (Urasaki et al, 2001).

All vertebrates have 2 forms of topoisomerase II: an α-isoform (170 kDa), encoded by the human *TOP2A* gene on chromosome 17q21-22, and a β-isoform (180 kDa), encoded by the *TOP2B* gene on chromosome 3p24. Both enzymes function as homodimers and the mechanisms by which they alter the topology of double-stranded DNA, like topoisomerase I, require a catalytic tyrosine residue in each topoisomerase II subunit for binding to DNA. Distinct from topoisomerase I, the catalytic cycle of topoisomerase II is ATP-dependent.

Drugs that target topoisomerase II are divided into 2 broad classes (see Chap. 18, Sec. 18.4). One class includes the clinically important etoposide, doxorubicin, and mitoxantrone, and these drugs "convert" topoisomerase II into a DNA-damaging agent by increasing the levels of topoisomerase II/DNA covalent complexes and DNA double-stranded breaks (DSBs). The DSBs caused by drug-stabilized topoisomerase II-linked DNA, although often repaired by a complex array of nucleolytic and proteolytic pathways (see Chap. 5, Sec. 5.3), may lead to cell death. Decreases in topoisomerase IIα content or activity caused by alterations in *TOP2A* transcription or increased protein degradation, as well as point mutations and small deletions that alter the enzyme's ability to bind DNA and/or drug, are associated with resistance to topoisomerase II poisons in numerous cultured cell lines. Mutations associated with resistance to the topoisomerase "poisons" cluster around the ATP-binding site or around the catalytic tyrosine residue in the DNA-binding region of topoisomerase II. The prevalence of these *TOP2A* mutations in clinical samples is not known, but several studies suggest it is low. Conversely, a good correlation with increased sensitivity to anthracyclines has been found in human tumors where *TOP2A* has been coamplified with the nearby *ERBB2/NEU* on chromosome 17 (Mano et al, 2007).

Although closely related in amino acid sequence homology (>70%), topoisomerase IIα and β differ in biochemical and biophysical characteristics as well as in their tissue-specific expression, subcellular localization, cell-cycle dependence, and sensitivity to some antineoplastic agents (Nitiss, 2009). Nevertheless, many drugs target both isoenzymes, which may have implications for reducing the risk of acquiring resistance because 2 targets are involved. Targeting the β-isoform is associated with induction of cardiotoxicity and secondary malignancies, and likely provides less benefit than targeting the α-isoform. This has prompted a search for topoisomerase IIα-specific drugs which might have greater antitumor activity and reduced toxicity.

19.2.5.3 Resistance to Agents Targeting Microtubules Microtubules are dynamic polymeric structures comprised of heterodimers of α- and β-tubulin (each with several subtypes) that are assembled and disassembled as required during many cellular events, including cell movement and intracellular transport, and are particularly important regulators of cell-cycle progression. Thus microtubules play a critical role in mitosis and drugs that bind to tubulin may cause mitotic arrest and cell death. These drugs may be classified according to where they bind: the *Vinca* alkaloids bind to the ends of microtubules, while taxanes bind along the interior surface of the microtubules (Dumontet and Jordan, 2010; see Chap. 18, Sec. 18.5). The mechanisms underlying resistance to the microtubule-destabilizing *Vinca* alkaloids vincristine and vinblastine, and the microtubule-stabilizing taxanes (eg, paclitaxel) are not fully understood. Mutations in βI-tubulin are found commonly in drug-resistant cell lines, but their clinical relevance appears questionable (Kavallaris, 2010). Abnormal high levels of expression of βIII-tubulin have been detected in drug-resistant solid tumors, including both lung and ovarian carcinomas. How elevated βIII-tubulin mediates resistance and enhances cell survival is complex, but this tubulin subunit helps to protect cells against the genotoxic stress induced by cytotoxic drugs. Microtubule-associated proteins have also been observed in drug-resistant cells. Microtubule-associated proteins (eg, tau) can bind to and stabilize microtubules against depolymerization. Binding of tau to the outer microtubule wall probably results in limited access of drugs, such as paclitaxel, to the inner luminal surface of the microtubule (Ferlini et al, 2007).

19.2.6 Drug Resistance and Repair of Drug-Mediated DNA Damage

DNA is constantly being subjected to damage by both exogenous and endogenous molecules. Many chemotherapeutic agents cause a variety of toxic DNA lesions that lead to cell death unless the damage is repaired. Detection and repair of drug-induced DNA lesions is carried out by lesion-specific DNA repair pathways (Helleday et al, 2008; see Chap. 5, Sec. 5.3). Resistance to DNA-damaging agents may occur because DNA repair processes in the tumor cells have become more efficient.

Cisplatin induces cell death by forming DNA-platinum adducts and interstrand DNA crosslinks but resistance can ensue if the lesions are repaired. Repair of platinum-modified DNA often involves nucleotide excision repair (NER; see Chap. 5, Sec. 5.3.3) and variations in NER activity can be an important determinant of drug sensitivity and resistance. For example, elevated levels of the excision repair cross-complementation group 1 (ERCC1) enzyme, which plays a rate-limiting role in the NER pathway, has been correlated with increased responsiveness to cisplatin-based adjuvant therapy in lung cancer patients (Olaussen et al, 2006). Conversely, defective NER has been implicated in the relative sensitivity of testicular cancer to cisplatin therapy.

Alkylating agents such as temozolomide also exert their cytotoxicity, at least in part, by binding to the guanine bases in DNA (see Chap. 18, Sec. 18.2.1). O^6-methylguanine-DNA methyltransferase (MGMT) (also known as O^6-alkylguanine DNA alkyltransferase) is one of the enzymes responsible for the repair of alkylated DNA. MGMT removes adducts from the O^6 position of guanine and transfers the alkyl group to a specific cysteine residue ("acceptor site") on the enzyme (Fig. 19–8). Because this transfer and alkylation of MGMT renders the enzyme inactive, the enzyme is considered to act by a "suicide" mechanism. Levels of MGMT or the methylation status of the *MGMT* promoter (which controls the expression of the gene) are useful predictors of the responsiveness of some tumors to alkylating agents (Esteller et al, 2000; Hegi et al, 2005). Potential opportunities exist to circumvent drug resistance

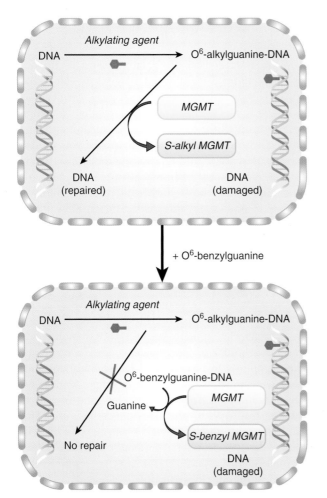

FIGURE 19–8 **Resistance mediated by repair of an alkylated guanine base by MGMT and inhibition of this repair by O^6-benzylguanine.** *Upper panel,* the DNA repair enzyme MGMT causes resistance by removing toxic adducts from the O^6 position of guanine in native DNA. It does this by transferring the alkyl group to a cysteine residue in the enzyme itself, resulting in auto-inactivation of enzyme; *lower panel,* in the presence of exogenous O^6-benzylguanine, MGMT is no longer available to repair the DNA and resistance is circumvented.

mediated by MGMT through the use of O^6-benzylguanine and related compounds. This relatively nontoxic agent can act as a noncompetitive substrate for MGMT, resulting in transfer of the benzyl group to the active site of the enzyme leading to irreversible inactivation (Fig. 19–8).

Bifunctional alkylating agents, such as cisplatin, as well as drugs targeting topoisomerase I and II, can cause the accumulation of DSBs, leading to cell death unless the breaks are repaired. Repair of DSBs can take place by either nonhomologous or homology-directed repair pathways, the relative contribution of which depends on a variety of different factors (see Chap. 5, Sec. 5.3). Many human cancers probably have impairment in DNA repair pathways that contributes to their genomic instability, and such tumors are likely to be more sensitive to DNA-damaging agents. Regaining the capacity for certain types of DNA repair is a potential mechanism by which tumor cells can acquire resistance to DNA targeting drugs. For example, exposure to cisplatin of ovarian tumor cells containing *BRCA2* mutations (which plays a crucial role in homologous recombination; see Chap. 5, Sec. 5.3.4) can select for drug-resistant cells, while additional mutations in *BRCA2* can result in partial restoration of BRCA2 function and thus drug sensitivity (Sakai et al, 2008).

DNA damage caused by chemotherapeutic agents can cause a delay in cell-cycle progression in order to allow time for the damage to be repaired. Cell-cycle delays result from changes in the level, localization, or posttranslational modification of one or more of the proteins involved in the checkpoint processes that regulate specific phases of the cell cycle, and have been linked to drug resistance. Included among these proteins are complexes of cyclins and cyclin-dependent kinases (CDKs), which can be regulated by CDK inhibitors such as p21 and p27 (see Chap. 5, Sec. 5.4 and Chap. 9, Sec. 9.3.1). Because disruption of the cell-cycle checkpoints interferes with DNA repair by homologous recombination, modulating the activity of one or more of the proteins involved in checkpoint processes has been proposed as a means by which drug sensitivity can be increased. For example, absent or aberrant cytoplasmic localization of the G_1-checkpoint proteins p21 (CDKN1A) and p27 (CDKN1B) has been linked to drug resistance in many in vitro cellular model systems (Abukhdeir and Park, 2009). Although convincing evidence of their relevance in clinical drug resistance is lacking, recent studies implicate both of them in resistance to the estrogen receptor modulator tamoxifen.

19.2.7 Resistance to Targeted Agents: The Tyrosine Kinase Inhibitors

The most widely used targeted drugs are small molecules, mostly derived from quinazoline, which act by inhibiting the kinase activity of oncogenes and/or growth factor receptors (see Chap. 17, Sec. 17.3.1). Other targeted agents include monoclonal antibodies with specificity for the external domain of cellular receptors, which thereby block binding of their endogenous ligands, and/or inhibit signaling from them. Thus agents that exploit mutations or amplification of the *cKIT* gene found in gastrointestinal stromal tumors, or the EGFR found in non–small cell lung cancers, or the *human epidermal growth receptor 2* (*HER2/NEU*) oncogene in breast cancer, or the BCR-ABL translocation protein product in chronic myelogenous leukemia (CML) have become important components in the therapy of these diseases (see Chap. 17, Secs. 17.3.1 and 17.3.3). Unfortunately, resistance to these drugs also occurs (Wheeler et al, 2010). For example, clinical resistance to imatinib, a small-molecule tyrosine kinase inhibitor, may result from point mutations that lead to diminished interaction of this drug with its target, the p210 BCR-ABL protein in CML (Milojkovic and Apperley, 2009). Resistance to imatinib in patients with CML is also associated with an increased copy number (amplification) of the *BCR-ABL* fusion gene (Gorre et al, 2001). Finally, imatinib is also a substrate of the P-glycoprotein and ABCG2/BCRP drug efflux pumps, which may limit the intracellular levels of imatinib that can be achieved (Dohse et al, 2010).

Response of lung cancer patients to the EGFR-targeted tyrosine kinase inhibitors erlotinib and gefitinib occurs in a subset of patients whose tumors have amplification of or mutations in the kinase domain of the *EGFR* gene (Gazdar, 2009). Subsequent studies led to the discovery of an *EGFR* mutation (T790M) that is associated with acquired resistance to these agents.

The limitations of imatinib and other small-molecule tyrosine kinase inhibitors directed against a single membrane receptor prompted the development of receptor tyrosine kinase inhibitors (eg, sorafenib and sunitinib) that target multiple receptors. These compounds do not rely on active transport by SLC proteins to enter the cell nor are they efficiently transported by the major ABC drug efflux pumps (Hu et al, 2009). Consequently, these agents are likely to be less affected by transporter-mediated alterations in drug levels and transporter-related resistance mechanisms. These agents are useful in treatment of metastatic kidney cancer, but as for other anticancer drugs, resistance develops with continued use, through mechanisms not yet fully defined.

Mechanisms underlying resistance to monoclonal antibodies that target growth factor receptor kinases are poorly understood (Wheeler et al, 2010). For example, although no mutations in *EGFR* have been identified that predict response to cetuximab, *KRAS* mutation (at least in colorectal cancer patients) is an important predictive biomarker for response to this agent (Lievre et al, 2006). Also, among breast cancer patients whose tumors contain multiple copies of *HER2* and respond initially to the monoclonal antibody trastuzumab, most experience disease progression within 1 year of initiation of treatment. The cause of resistance in the tumors of these women remains uncertain.

Resistance to all classes of tyrosine kinase inhibitors can also occur via activation of a parallel signaling pathway. For example, changes in the regulation of the signaling pathways downstream of the HER2 receptor have been implicated in trastuzumab resistance in breast cancer. Similarly, resistance to EGFR-targeted inhibitors may occur by a "bypass" mechanism mediated by amplification of the MET protooncogene,

which, when activated by hepatocyte growth factor (HGF), increases tumor cell survival (Pal et al, 2010).

19.2.8 Resistance to Apoptosis and Autophagy

Most of the mechanisms of drug resistance described in previous sections are those in which the interaction of the anticancer drug with its target has been modified such that the activation of the pathways that normally leads to tumor cell death may be diminished. However, differences in the sensitivity of tumor cells to anticancer drugs also occur because of changes in the pathways that mediate cell death and survival. Types of cell death that have been observed following treatment with anticancer drugs include apoptosis, necrosis, mitotic catastrophe, and senescence, whereas autophagy may act (paradoxically) to enhance either death or survival of the cell. The best studied of these, apoptosis, appears to be initiated by the mitochondrial cytochrome c/Apaf-1/caspase-9 pathway (see Chap. 9, Sec. 9.4.3) while signaling through the death receptor pathway by drug-induced FasL upregulation seems less important, except possibly for 5-FU-induced cytotoxicity (McLornan et al, 2010). The proapoptotic and antiapoptotic members of the bcl-2 family, the kinases and phosphatases that regulate their activity and subcellular localization, the initiator and effector caspases, the various inhibitors of apoptosis proteins (IAPs), as well as the presence of wild-type or mutant p53, are all examples of proteins that might influence the sensitivity of tumor cells to apoptotic cell death (Brown and Attardi, 2005).

Laboratory studies provide evidence that in some cell types, drug sensitivity (as measured by a colony-forming assay or effects on tumor growth) can be modulated by changing the expression and/or posttranslational modifications of proteins that are components of apoptotic signaling pathways. For example, decreases in APAF-1 have been reported to contribute to therapeutic resistance of melanomas (Soengas et al, 2003). In addition, in a murine lymphoma, transfection of the *bcl-2* gene led to increased resistance to multiple drugs (Schmitt et al, 2000), and the evidence for a contribution of blocked apoptosis to resistance of lymphomas/leukemias is quite convincing. However, several investigators have found little or no effect on drug sensitivity of solid tumors from modulating pathways of apoptosis (eg, Brown and Attardi, 2005). Markers of apoptosis such as an increase in TUNEL (terminal deoxynucleotidyl transferase-mediated deoxyuridine triphosphate-biotin nick-end labeling)-positive cells are observed commonly after treatment of malignant cells (or solid tumors) with anticancer drugs, but the clinical relevance of apoptotic pathways in determining drug sensitivity is not clear. Furthermore, studies of drug resistance in mice with conditionally mutated *p53* and *Brca1* as a model for hereditary breast cancer showed no changes in expression of *Bcl2*, *Apaf1*, or caspase genes after exposure to doxorubicin and paclitaxel. Rather, the major mechanism of resistance was upregulation of the P-glycoprotein drug efflux pump (see Sec. 19.2.3; Rottenberg et al, 2007). Similarly, exposure of these mice with

Brca1-associated breast cancer to the topoisomerase I inhibitor topotecan resulted in drug resistance caused by reduced levels of the topoisomerase I drug target and increased expression of the *Abcg2* drug efflux pump rather than changes in markers of apoptosis (Zander et al, 2010).

The *p53* gene plays a role in apoptosis, and normal wild-type *p53* can stimulate apoptosis of cells that have sustained damage to DNA (see Chap. 5, Sec. 5.3). A mutant *p53* gene, present in a substantial proportion of human cancers, may inhibit apoptosis. The p53 protein may influence response to anticancer drugs, and modification of apoptosis is probably one of several mechanisms of drug resistance that can be influenced by it. For example, when wild-type p53 was induced in colon cancer cells expressing a mutant p53 protein, sensitivity to 5-FU, camptothecin, and radiation was increased (Yang et al, 1996). In another study, restoration of p53 function led to regression of lymphomas and sarcomas in mice (Ventura et al, 2007). Loss of p53 function was also reported to confer high-level multidrug resistance in neuroblastoma cells (Xue et al, 2007). More recently, the chemosensitivity of human tumor cells, both in vitro and in mice, could be enhanced by using an adenovirus vector to increase p53 levels (and decrease p21 levels) (Idogawa et al, 2009). There is evidence that hypoxia in solid tumors can lead to a selective growth advantage for cells that express a mutant *p53* gene, leading to a drug-resistant population (see Sec. 19.3.2 and Chap. 12, Sec. 12.2.2). Finally, p53-related transcription factors p63 and p73 appear also to be involved in a microRNA-dependent circuit that mediates inducible drug resistance (Ory et al, 2011).

A key determinant of whether the process of apoptosis might be modified to influence drug sensitivity is whether it is primary in causing lethal damage to cells, or simply represents a pathway whereby cells that have already sustained lethal and nonrepairable damage undergo cellular lysis (Fig. 19–9; Brown and Attardi, 2005). It appears likely that this depends on both the drugs used and the cell type that is treated; ongoing efforts to evaluate therapeutic strategies that target proapoptotic

signaling pathways (see Chap. 9, Sec. 9.4.2) should help to distinguish between these possibilities.

There is growing interest in the role of autophagy in tumor development and response to cancer therapy (see Chap. 12, Sec. 12.3.7). Autophagy is a lysosomal degradation pathway for intracellular digestion of cellular macromolecules that maintains cellular metabolism in times of stress such as exposure to hypoxia or to cytotoxic drugs. When autophagy is activated, intracellular membrane vesicles form and engulf proteins, cytoplasm, organelles and protein aggregates, and these vesicles are then delivered to lysosomes where they and their contents are degraded. Autophagy-associated pathways can promote cell survival by limiting damage and conferring stress tolerance, especially under adverse conditions (White and DiPaola, 2009). The use of inhibitors of autophagy could therefore be a promising strategy for overcoming resistance. Hydroxychloroquine (HCQ) and proton pump inhibitors have been identified as inhibitors of autophagy because of their ability to block lysosomal acidification and autophagosome degradation (Marino et al, 2010). Several clinical trials of HCQ in combination with cytotoxic (docetaxel, temozolomide) and targeted (an HDAC inhibitor, a vascular endothelial growth factor receptor [VEGFR] inhibitor, gefitinib) agents are underway, based on the premise that inhibition of autophagy by HCQ should enhance the efficacy of these drugs. Inhibitors of autophagy with greater specificity than HCQ are also being developed.

It is important to gain a better understanding of the relative contributions of the signaling pathways and modes of cell death that result in resistance to anticancer drugs. Establishing the clinical relevance of these potential mechanisms of drug resistance will be crucial before effective strategies for their reversal can be implemented.

19.3 DRUG RESISTANCE IN VIVO

Many laboratory-based studies of drug-resistance mechanisms have followed an approach whereby cultured tumor cells at low density are exposed to repeated selection in increasing concentrations of the anticancer drug of interest. These studies have led to the characterization of multiple mechanisms of drug resistance, described in previous sections, many of which are relevant to human cancer. However, the selection of stable drug-resistant subpopulations, present because of mutation or gene amplification, provides an oversimplified model for drug resistance in human cancer. Drug resistance of human tumors often occurs without prior drug exposure or may emerge after brief exposure to a relatively low concentration of drugs that is achievable in human tissue. In contrast, the selection of genetically stable drug-resistant mutant cells in experimental systems is often difficult, and typically requires much higher selection pressures (eg, prolonged exposure to mutagens, higher doses, and longer duration of exposure to anticancer drugs) than may occur during the treatment of human tumors. Also, when human tumors relapse after initial chemotherapy,

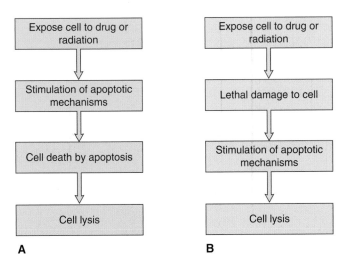

FIGURE 19–9 **Apoptosis as a primary or secondary mechanism of cell lysis after drug treatment.** (Adapted from Tannock and Lee, 2001.)

they may respond later to the same chemotherapy (Cara and Tannock, 2001), suggesting that at least in some instances, the resistant phenotype may be transient.

Clinical drug resistance may occur as a result of mechanisms that depend on the in vivo microenvironment. Tumors have a complex extracellular matrix (see Chap. 10, Sec. 10.2), and cells in common epithelial-derived tumors have close cellular contact. Solid tumors have a poorly formed vasculature, which leads to regions of hypoxia and extracellular acidity (see Chap. 12, Sec. 12.2), and a requirement that anticancer drugs penetrate over relatively long intercapillary distances (as compared to those in normal tissues) to reach the target tumor cells (Minchinton and Tannock, 2006; Trédan et al, 2007; Fig. 19–10). Variable concentration of nutrient metabolites in the extracellular environment, and other factors, lead to variable rates of cell proliferation before treatment, and of repopulation of surviving tumor cells after treatment, both of which influence drug sensitivity of experimental and clinical tumors.

Drug-resistance mechanisms that depend on the microenvironment may be explored by using model systems that maintain cellular interactions with other cells and with the extracellular matrix, thereby better reflecting how tumors in vivo are exposed to drugs. One model is provided by spheroids, in which malignant cells grow in contact with each other and with an extracellular matrix to form nodules in tissue culture (Durand, 1989; Hirschhaeuser et al, 2010; Fig. 19–11A). Alternatively, tumor cells can be grown on collagen-coated semiporous Teflon membranes to form multilayered cell cultures (MCCs) of relatively constant thickness to provide a useful model for studying drug penetration through tumor tissue (Hicks et al, 1997; Tannock et al, 2002; Fig. 19–11B; see

Sec. 19.3.3). Drug can then be added on one side of the MCC and its time-dependent concentration measured on the other (Fig. 19–11C) to quantify the penetration of drugs through the MCC as compared to that through the semipermeable membrane alone (Fig. 19–11D). Such model systems have allowed study of mechanisms of drug resistance that depend on the cellular environment, as well as metabolic factors such as hypoxia and acidity. They supplement direct studies of the relationship between drug concentration, activity, and microenvironment in solid tumors that are either transplanted or induced in experimental animals (Trédan et al, 2007).

19.3.1 Influence of Cell Contact and the Extracellular Matrix

Repeated drug treatment of solid tissue, either in the form of spheroids or tumor-bearing mice, may lead to drug resistance that is expressed only when the cells are grown in contact with one another. The tumor cells do not display drug resistance when grown without cell–cell contact as in dilute cell culture (Teicher et al, 1990; Kerbel et al, 1994). Further work suggests that drug resistance is correlated with the density of cell packing in spheroids, is dependent on integrin-mediated cell adhesion, and may be reversed by silencing of the gene encoding focal adhesion kinase (FAK), or by agents that inhibit adhesion between the cells (Chen et al, 2010; St Croix et al, 1996; Zutter, 2007; Chen et al, 2010). Integrin-mediated cell adhesion may influence multiple cellular properties, including cell proliferation, through regulation of cell-cycle checkpoints and upregulation of cell-cycle–inhibitory CDKs (Zutter, 2007; see Chap. 9, Sec. 9.2.2). Hence these effects may be mediated in part by a

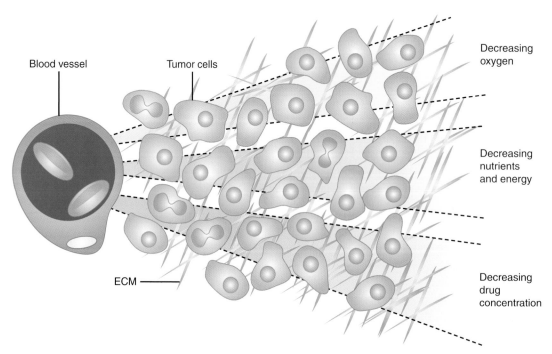

FIGURE 19–10 **Representation of gradients of oxygen and other metabolites, and of cell proliferation and death in relation to blood vessels in solid tumors.** ECM, extracellular matrix (Adapted from Minchinton and Tannock, 2006.)

Blood vessel

Tumor cells

Decreasing oxygen

Decreasing nutrients and energy

ECM

Decreasing drug concentration

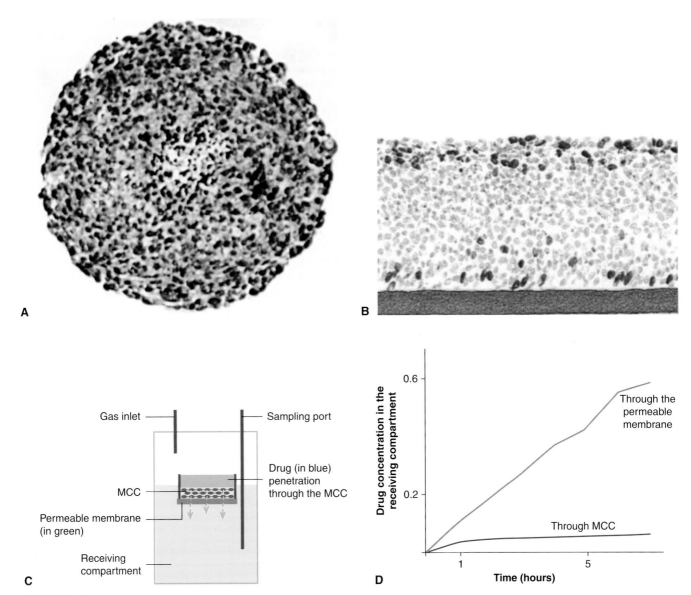

FIGURE 19–11 **Models used for study of drug resistance that depends on the microenvironment found in solid tumors.**
A) Multicellular tumor spheroid. The distribution of fluorescent compounds may be imaged directly. **B)** Multilayered cell culture (MCC) grown on a collagen-coated Teflon membrane. **C)** The MCC is floated on medium in a larger vessel and drug can be added to the upper compartment in dilute agar and sampled as a function of time in the stirred lower compartment, on the other side of the MCC, to evaluate. **D)** The time-dependent transport of drug through the MCC as compared to that through the semiporous membrane alone. (From Trédan et al, 2007.)

reduction in the rate of cell proliferation in the solid tissue environment, with consequent resistance to cycle-active drugs.

Many drugs have been tested against tumor cells in dilute tissue culture (eg, at a concentration of ~10^5 cells/mL) and there is an implicit assumption that relative cell kill will be similar at higher cell concentrations such as are found in solid tumors (10^8 to 10^9 cells/mL). This assumption of first-order kinetics is usually correct for drugs that are present in much higher concentration than their molecular targets, as is probably true for many anticancer drugs that kill cells by inducing a limited number of critical lesions in DNA. This assumption may not be correct for agents that must interact with a large number of cellular targets in order to be effective. For example, agents such as verapamil or cyclosporine, which reverse multidrug resistance caused by P-glycoprotein in dilute tissue culture, may lose their effect as the cell concentration in tissue culture increases (Tunggal et al, 1999); these agents have not been adequately evaluated against solid tumors in animals, and this effect may contribute to lack of efficacy of inhibitors of P-glycoprotein at cell concentrations that are observed in solid tumors (Yu et al, 2012). Inactivity at high cell concentrations could also be a problem for some other agents that are directed against targets on the cell surface, such as those that inhibit growth factor receptors, if there are a large number of targets per cell.

The drug sensitivity of tumor cells can be modulated by direct contact with other components of the tumor cell environment.

Thus both in vitro and in vivo studies show that contact with the extracellular matrix can provide tumor cells with protection against cell death mediated by anticancer drugs, described as cell-adhesion-mediated drug resistance (CAMDR; Shain and Dalton, 2001). CAMDR has been most studied in multiple myeloma, where myeloma cells interact with stroma in the bone marrow, leading to initiation of survival signals that are absent when the same cells are in suspension (Li and Dalton, 2006). Several strategies to circumvent this type of resistance have been proposed that target molecules in tumor cells and/ or in the extracellular matrix that are required for cell adhesion. The activity of the proteosome inhibitor bortezomib, which has led to improved prognosis in patients with multiple myeloma, appears to depend on its ability to inhibit CAMDR (Yanamandra et al, 2006; Noborio-Hatano et al, 2009).

19.3.2 Drug Resistance in Hypoxic Environments

Tumor vasculature is characterized by irregular blood flow and stasis, and by relatively large intercapillary distances in comparison to those in normal tissues (see Chap. 11, Sec. 11.5 and Chap. 12, Sec. 12.2). This leads to regions of tumors that are hypoxic, and, in turn, to regions where the extracellular pH is relatively low because of the production of lactic acid, and to poor clearance of this and other acidic products of metabolism (see Fig. 19–10). Hypoxia is widely recognized as a major factor leading to resistance of tumor cells to radiotherapy (see Chap. 16, Sec. 16.4), but several mechanisms may also cause cells in hypoxic regions to be resistant to anticancer drugs, as reviewed below.

Cells in nutrient-deprived regions of tumors tend to have a low rate of proliferation in comparison to cells situated close to functional blood vessels. Most anticancer drugs, including some molecular-targeted agents, are more toxic to proliferating than to nonproliferating cells (see Chap. 17, Sec. 17.5). Thus, even if the drugs achieve potentially cytotoxic concentrations in these regions, the level of cell kill may be limited. Surviving cells that were previously hypoxic may begin to proliferate following loss of killed cells closer to blood vessels, leading to improvement in the distribution of oxygen and nutrient metabolites, and therefore may allow regrowth of the tumor (see Sec. 19.3.4).

Hypoxia and extracellular acidity have direct effects on the activity and/or uptake of some anticancer drugs, independent of proliferative status. As for ionizing radiation, the toxicity of some drugs is dependent on the production of free radicals, and this process depends on availability of oxygen. Drugs that require active transport into cells are dependent on ATP, and anaerobic metabolism is much less efficient than oxidative phosphorylation in producing ATP. Drugs that are weak bases, such as doxorubicin, have a greater proportion of molecules in the charged form under acidic conditions, which decreases their ability to cross the plasma membrane and be taken up into the cell, leading to decreased activity. In contrast, extracellular acidity may enhance the uptake of drugs that are weak acids, such as chlorambucil or melphalan. In general, however, the direct effects of hypoxia and acidity on drug sensitivity are smaller than those on radiation sensitivity.

Hypoxia may influence genetically-based mechanisms of cellular drug resistance in at least 2 ways. Transient exposure to hypoxia, as may occur in tumors because of fluctuations in blood flow, may stimulate the amplification of genes, including those encoding DHFR, which leads to resistance to methotrexate (see Fig. 19–1; Rice et al, 1986; Sec. 19.2.5). Also, cells in many tumors do not express wild-type p53 (see Chap. 7, Sec. 7.6.1). Hypoxia has been found to provide a selective survival and growth advantage for cells lacking wild-type p53, because such cells show a diminished rate of apoptosis under hypoxic conditions (Graeber et al, 1996). This effect may help to explain why the presence of hypoxia in tumors is a poor prognostic factor after all types of management (including surgery). Following treatment with anticancer drugs that leads to selective killing of rapidly proliferating aerobic cells situated closer to tumor blood vessels, there may be selective repopulation of the tumor by p53(–/–) cells, which have survived hypoxic conditions, and which may be resistant to many therapeutic agents (see Sec. 19.2.8). The outgrowth of such p53(–/–) cells can confer resistance to treatment directed against tumor blood vessels, as well as to more conventional therapy (Yu et al, 2002).

Drugs are being developed that are selective for killing of hypoxic cells, and which might complement both radiotherapy and conventional chemotherapy. Hypoxia-activated prodrugs are inactive in their native form, but are activated by reduction under hypoxic conditions such as may occur in solid tumors, and may then kill tumor cells. The first agent to be tested clinically, tirapazamine, did not improve the activity of cisplatin and radiotherapy in randomized controlled trials, probably because it has poor diffusion characteristics into hypoxic regions. It also had toxicity to normal tissue (Rischin et al, 2010). Newer agents, such as PR-104 and TH-302, have more favorable properties and are under clinical development, although low levels of hypoxia in some normal tissues, including bone marrow, may lead to some normal-tissue toxicity.

19.3.3 Drug Access and Tumor Cell Resistance

Effective treatment of solid tumors requires both that the constituent cells be sensitive to the drug(s) that are used, and that the drugs achieve a sufficient concentration to exert lethal toxicity for all of the viable cells in the tumor. This depends on the efficient delivery of drugs through the vascular system of the tumor, and penetration of the drugs from tumor capillaries to reach tumor cells that are distant from them. Such cells will be in nutritionally deprived environments, as oxygen and other nutrients must gain access to the tumor by the same route, and may be relatively resistant to drugs for reasons described in the previous section (see Fig. 19–10).

The distribution of fluorescent or radiolabeled drugs in spheroids, and studies of their penetration through MCCs (see Fig. 19–11), indicate rather poor tissue penetration of multiple drugs, including doxorubicin, gemcitabine, taxanes, and methotrexate (Durand, 1989; Minchinton and Tannock, 2006). Smaller molecules distribute largely by diffusion, which depends on size, shape, charge, and solubility of the drug in the extracellular matrix, and "consumption" because of binding or metabolism by proximal cells. Larger molecules, such as therapeutic monoclonal antibodies, probably depend more on convection, which is inhibited by high levels of interstitial fluid pressure (Minchinton and Tannock, 2006). Both mechanisms depend on maintenance of a concentration gradient into tissue from tumor blood vessels, and distribution is therefore likely to be better for drugs with a prolonged lifetime within the circulation.

Drug distribution in relation to blood vessels in solid tumors can be quantified by using immunohistochemistry or autoradiography applied to tumor sections (Fig. 19–12). The blood vessels can be recognized by an antibody to an endothelial cell marker (eg, CD31), and patent vessels by an injected fluorescent marker, such as the carbocyanine dye DiOC7; hypoxic regions of tumors can be recognized by antibodies to injected markers of hypoxia such as pimonidazole or EF5. Drugs that are fluorescent, such as doxorubicin or mitoxantrone, can be recognized directly (Fig. 19–12A to C), while other agents (eg, monoclonal antibodies) can be recognized by fluorescent-tagged antibodies directed against them (Fig. 19–12D), or by autoradiography used to detect a radiolabeled form of the drug (as has been used to study the distribution of taxanes; Kuh et al, 1999). Pharmacodynamic markers of drug effect, such as changes in apoptosis (eg, activated

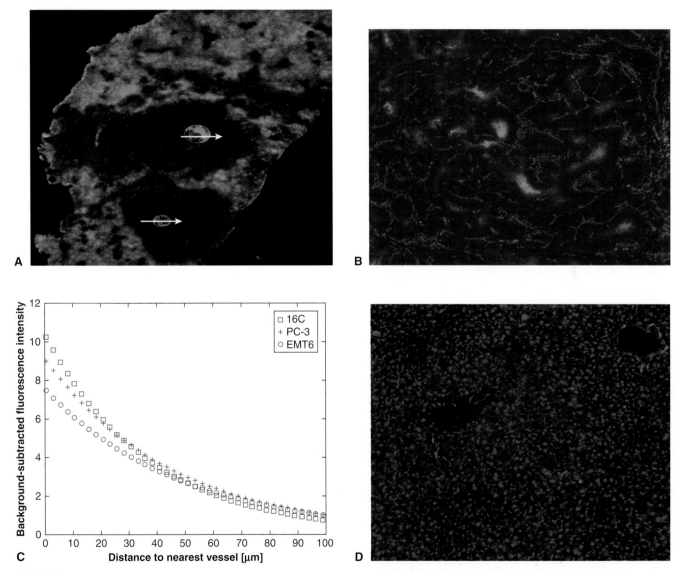

FIGURE 19–12 Drug distribution in tumor and normal tissue. A) Photomicrographs showing poor distribution of fluorescent mitoxantrone (green) into metastases (arrows) of a human breast carcinoma in the liver of a nude mice, as compared to normal liver. **B)** Distribution of doxorubicin (blue) in relation to blood vessels (red) and regions of hypoxia (green) in an experimental tumor. Note the perivascular distribution. **C)** Concentration of doxorubicin in relation to distance from blood vessels in 3 experimental tumors. **D)** Distribution of doxorubicin (blue) in relation to blood vessels (red) in normal mouse liver. (Parts B and C from Primeau et al, 2005.)

caspase-3), cell proliferation (eg, Ki67) or DNA damage (eg, γH2AX) may also be tracked by immunohistochemistry using fluorescent antibodies that recognize these biomarkers. Computerized image analysis programs can relate drug concentration (eg, as measured by fluorescence of doxorubicin), or a marker of drug effect, with distance from the nearest blood vessel or nearest region of hypoxia over the whole area of a tumor section.

Studies using the above techniques show that for drugs that can be visualized directly by their fluorescence, there is a sharply decreasing gradient of drug from functional blood vessels of tumors (including human breast cancers) such that cells distal from blood vessels have minimal exposure after a single injection, with little or no penetration of such drugs into hypoxic tumor regions (see Fig. 19–12A and B; Lankelma et al, 1999; Primeau et al, 2005). This contrasts with more uniform distribution of drugs in most normal tissues, which have an orderly and functional vascular system (see Fig. 19–12C), although the presence of P-glycoprotein, MRP4, and other membrane transporters in the blood–brain barrier leads to uniformly low drug concentrations in brain. Similar poor drug distributions have been reported for taxanes and gemcitabine (Kuh et al, 1999; Huxham et al, 2004). Although the distribution of anticancer drugs in solid tumors might improve with sequential courses of chemotherapy, failure of drugs to penetrate tumor tissue in sufficient concentrations to kill cells distal from functional blood vessels is likely to be a major cause of poor clinical response.

Several strategies might be used to either modify or complement the distribution of anticancer drugs in solid tumors to improve therapeutic efficacy (Trédan et al, 2007). Agents that lower interstitial fluid pressure would be expected to improve distribution of drugs that is mediated in part by convection. Using another strategy, we have shown that administration to mice of proton pump inhibitors such as pantoprazole can improve the distribution of doxorubicin in solid tumors and increase its antitumor activity. This may occur because pantoprazole raises the pH of intracellular compartments (as it does in the stomach when used to treat ulcers) thereby displacing basic drugs, such as doxorubicin, that are sequestered within them, allowing more drug both to interact with target DNA and to distribute to cells more distal from blood vessels. However, proton pump inhibitors also inhibit autophagy (Marino et al, 2010; see Sec. 19.2.8 and Chap. 12, Sec. 12.3.7), which may be a survival mechanism for poorly nourished cells distal from blood vessels. Agents that modify the stromal cells or extracellular matrix may also improve drug distribution. For example, Tuveson et al have generated a genetically engineered mouse model of human pancreatic cancer that has dense stromal tissue, poor vascular perfusion, high interstitial fluid pressure, and resistance to chemotherapy, similar to human pancreatic cancer (Olive et al, 2009). Both IPI-926, a drug that inhibits the Hedgehog signaling pathway (see Chap. 8, Sec. 8.4.3), and hyaluronidase, an enzyme that targets the extracellular matrix, are reported to deplete the dense stroma and to improve the distribution and activity of anticancer drugs in such tumors

(Olive et al, 2009; Provenzano et al, 2012); clinical trials evaluating such approaches are underway.

Hypoxia-activated prodrugs, described in the previous section, provide a potential method for complementing the action of conventional anticancer drugs that have limited penetration from tumor blood vessels, as they may act selectively against distal hypoxic cells that are exposed to low concentrations of the conventional agent. Once activated, some of these (hypoxia-dependent) drugs may also diffuse to kill cells in neighboring tumor regions.

19.3.4 Repopulation

Studies of the relationship between the probability of tumor control and duration of fractionated radiotherapy suggest that the proliferation of surviving tumor cells between daily doses of fractionated radiotherapy is an important cause of failure to achieve local tumor control (see Chap. 16, Sec. 16.6.2). Presumably this is a result of improving nutrition in the environment of surviving tumor cells as a result of killing of other cells in the tumor and better availability of nutrient metabolites and oxygen. For chemotherapy, the process of repopulation is likely to be more important because treatment courses are given typically at 3-week intervals, and in experimental studies a higher rate of proliferation (ie, of repopulation) has been reported after treatment of tumors by chemotherapy than in untreated control tumors (reviewed in Kim and Tannock, 2005). This process of tumor "recovery" may be analogous to repopulation of the bone marrow from stem cells that are stimulated to divide as a result of treatment. Few studies have assessed the rate of repopulation of human tumors following chemotherapy. This is problematic at early time intervals, because it is difficult or impossible to distinguish true surviving cells from lethally damaged cells that have yet to undergo the morphological changes that will precede their ultimate lysis, but less of a problem at longer intervals after drug treatment. There is evidence for accelerated repopulation and rapid regrowth of human tumors after completion of initial chemotherapy (Chen et al, 2011).

The possible effects of repopulation following chemotherapy have been modeled and are illustrated in Figure 19–13 (Kim and Tannock, 2005). If there is no change in the rate of repopulation, a human tumor may show net growth because of this process, even if each course of chemotherapy leads to killing of 70% of the viable tumor cells (Fig. 19–13A). However, a changing rate of repopulation can cause regrowth following initial tumor shrinkage (Fig. 19–13B), even if there is a delay in onset of repopulation after drug treatment caused by the immediate cytostatic effects of drugs on surviving cells (Fig. 19–13C). Tumor shrinkage or response followed by regrowth during continued treatment is observed commonly when chemotherapy is used to treat human tumors. The above modeling indicates that this can occur simply as a consequence of changes in the rate of repopulation of surviving cells after successive treatments and in the absence of any change in the intrinsic drug sensitivity of the constituent cells.

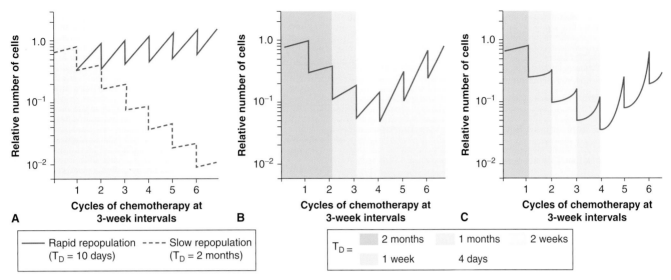

FIGURE 19–13 **Models of cell killing and repopulation during chemotherapy.** In (**A**) it is assumed that each 3-week course of treatment kills 70% of the tumor cells and repopulation is shown with a doubling time of 10 days (solid line) or 2 months (dashed line). In (**B**) the rate of repopulation increases between successive cycles of chemotherapy so that doubling time decreases from 2 months to 1 week. In (**C**) the model allows for initial cytostatic effects on surviving tumor cells after each dose of chemotherapy. *Note that shrinkage and regrowth of tumors, observed commonly in the clinic, may occur as a result of accelerating repopulation and without any selection of drug-resistant cells.* (From Davis and Tannock [2000].)

As for radiotherapy, there are strategies that might be used to inhibit repopulation between courses of chemotherapy, and thereby avoid the effective drug resistance that is observed. One method is to change the "fractionation" and to give lower doses of drugs more frequently or continuously. However, this is unlikely to be tumor specific, and may also lead to inhibition of cell proliferation in critical normal tissues such as bone marrow. Other approaches include inhibition of growth factor receptors that selectively stimulate tumor cell proliferation. Such agents will need to be short acting and discontinued just before the next cycle of chemotherapy, as anticancer drugs are likely to be more effective in killing cycling tumor cells.

19.3.5 Tumor Stem Cells and Drug Resistance

As described in Chapter 13, there is evidence that human tumors contain a small subpopulation of cells that have high potential to regenerate the tumor if they survive treatment, the putative human tumor stem cells, which are thus the important targets of treatment that aims to eradicate the tumor. Identification of specific proteins (markers) expressed on the cell surface have allowed for enrichment of this population in various types of tumors (eg, by using fluorescence-activated cell sorting after exposure to fluorescent-tagged monoclonal antibodies that recognize these markers), but it remains uncertain whether these markers truly characterize a stable population of stem cells, and how heterogeneity in their expression exists between cells within a tumor and between tumors. Studying the drug sensitivity of cells that bear stem cell markers is difficult because of their rarity within the tumor population and

the instability of their phenotype in cell culture. However, there is emerging evidence that such cells may be more resistant to chemotherapy than other cell populations in the tumor and therefore may selectively survive during drug treatment (Dean et al, 2005; Eyler and Rich, 2008). For example, treatment of human breast cancer with initial (neoadjuvant) chemotherapy is reported to lead to a population of surviving cells with an increased probability of expressing stem cell markers, indicating their relative resistance compared to other tumor cells in the population (Li et al, 2008; Tanei et al, 2009).

Automated high-throughput screens have been devised to select for agents that might have specific activity against human tumor stem cells; for example, salinomycin was reported to be much more active than clinically used paclitaxel against cultured human breast cancer cells that were induced to undergo epithelial-to-mesenchymal transition, a process that is associated with acquiring stem-like properties (see Chap. 13, Sec. 13.3). However, it is uncertain whether this type of model is relevant to treatment of stem-like cells in human cancer, and investigation of drug screens that may reflect more directly the sensitivity of human stem cells is underway.

The relative drug resistance of such stem cell populations results from a variety of different mechanisms, including an enhanced capacity for DNA damage repair and changes in key molecules involved in oncogenic signaling (Maugeri-Sacca et al, 2011). Differential expression of several ABC transporters also has been widely observed in stem cell enriched-cell populations from a variety of tumor types, with ABCG2 being the most frequently detected of these (see Sec. 19.2.3). Elevated levels of P-glycoprotein (ABCB1) have been detected in stem-like cells compared with non–stem-like cells in ovarian cancer cell lines and in primary patient ascites (Rizzo et al, 2011) but in this study, the histone methyltransferase EZH2 appears to play a more important role in determining chemoresistance.

The sensitivity of tumor stem cells within human tumors is also likely to depend on their proliferative state and on their microenvironment within solid tumors (Jinushi et al, 2011). Cancer stem cells may have a relatively low rate of cell proliferation, like stem cells in normal human bone marrow (see Chap. 12, Sec. 12.1.3); their proliferative state will determine, in part, their sensitivity to cell-cycle active drugs. The location of stem cells in relation to tumor blood vessels will determine the probable concentration of anticancer drugs that can be achieved within their microenvironment (see Sec. 19.3.3). There is evidence that stem cells may exist in perivascular niches in some types of cancer (eg, brain tumors; Calabrese et al, 2007), whereas other evidence suggests that stem cells may be enriched in hypoxic regions of tumors, and relatively protected from drug access (Mohyeldin et al, 2010). In such cases hypoxia-activated prodrugs might play an important role in eradication of tumor stem cells (see Sec. 19.3.2).

SUMMARY

- Drug resistance may occur because of mechanisms that are associated with individual tumor cells, or through mechanisms that relate to the microenvironment within tumors.
- Drug resistance of individual cells may occur because of mutation or amplification of genes, or because of epigenetic changes that lead to transient expression of cellular properties that are associated with drug resistance.
- Mechanisms that lead to resistance of individual cells include impaired drug uptake into cells, enhanced drug efflux from cells, changes in drug metabolism or in drug targets, repair of drug-induced damage (usually to DNA), or downregulation of cell death pathways.
- Several ABC proteins are expressed on the surface of cells, and can mediate enhanced efflux of multiple chemically unrelated drugs. Important members of this family that are expressed in human tumors include P-glycoprotein, MRP1, and ABCG2 (formerly known as BCRP). These proteins are also expressed in a polarized manner on cells in several normal tissues and influence the distribution of substrate drugs in the body.
- Drug resistance is observed during treatment with molecular-targeted agents, as well as with cytotoxic chemotherapy.
- Drug resistance may occur when cells are in contact as a result of interactions with other cells or with the extracellular matrix, even though the same cells are drug sensitive when separated in tissue culture.
- Drug distribution is often poor in solid tumors, such that cells distant from functional blood vessels are exposed to only a low concentration of drug. Such cells are often slowly proliferating and hence more resistant to cycle

active drugs. Agents that are activated under hypoxic conditions may have potential for overcoming this type of drug resistance.
- Repopulation of surviving tumor cells occurs between drug treatments, similar to repopulation of normal cells in bone marrow and other proliferating tissues. Accelerating repopulation during sequential courses of treatment may lead to tumor regrowth after an initial response, even if there is no selection of intrinsically drug resistant cells.
- Cells in human tumors with stem cell properties may be more resistant to certain drugs than other cell populations in the tumor.
- The complexity of mechanisms contributing to drug resistance requires a strategy for circumventing resistance in a clinical setting.

REFERENCES

Abukhdeir AM, Park BH. p21 and p27: roles in carcinogenesis and drug resistance. *Expert Rev Mol Med* 2009;10:e19.

Ashton LJ, Giffor AJ, Kwan E, et al. Reduced folate carrier and methylenetetrahydrofolate reductase gene polymorphisms: associations with clinical outcome in childhood acute lymphoblastic leukemia. *Leukemia* 2009;23:1348-1351.

Boni V, Bitarte N, Cristobal I, et al. miR-192/miR-215 influence 5-fluorouracil resistance through cell cycle-mediated mechanisms complementary to its post-transcriptional thymidylate synthase regulation. *Mol Cancer Ther* 2010;9:2265-2275.

Boumendjel A, Baubichon-Cortay H, Trompier D, et al. Anticancer multidrug resistance mediated by MRP1: recent advances in the discovery of reversal agents. *Med Res Rev* 2005;25:453-472.

Brown JM, Attardi LD. The role of apoptosis in cancer development and treatment response. *Nat Rev Cancer* 2005;5:231-237.

Burkhart CA, Watt F, Murray J, et al. Small-molecule multidrug resistance-associated protein 1 inhibitor reversan increases the therapeutic index of chemotherapy in mouse models of neuroblastoma. *Cancer Res* 2009;69:6573-6580.

Calabrese C, Poppleton H, Kocak M, et al. A perivascular niche for brain tumor stem cells. *Cancer Cell* 2007;11:69-82.

Cara S, Tannock IF. Retreatment of patients with the same chemotherapy: implications for clinical mechanisms of drug resistance. *Ann Oncol* 2001;12:23-27.

Chen CP, Weinberg VK, Jahan TM, Jablons DM, Yom SS. Implications of delayed initiation of radiotherapy: accelerated repopulation after induction chemotherapy for stage III non-small cell lung cancer. *J Thorac Oncol* 2011;6:1857-1864.

Chen Y, Wang Z, Chang P, et al. The effect of focal adhesion kinase gene silencing on 5-fluorouracil chemosensitivity involves an Akt/NF-kappaB signaling pathway in colorectal carcinomas. *Int J Cancer* 2010;127:195-206.

Cole SPC, Bhardwaj G, Gerlach JH, et al. Overexpression of a transporter gene in a multidrug-resistant human lung cancer cell line. *Science* 1992;258:1650-1654.

Cole SPC, Deeley RG. Transport of glutathione and glutathione conjugates by MRP1. *Trends Pharmacol Sci* 2006;27:438-446.

Davis AJ and Tannock JF. Repopulation of tumour cells between cycles of chemotherapy: a neglected factor. *Lancet Oncol* 2000; 1(2):86-93

Dean M, Allikmets R. Complete characterization of the human ABC gene family. *J Bioenerg Biomembr* 2001;33:475-479.

Dean M, Fojo T, Bates S. Tumour stem cells and drug resistance. *Nat Rev Cancer* 2005;5:275-284.

Deeley RG, Westlake C, Cole SPC. Transmembrane transport of endo- and xenobiotics by membrane ATP-binding cassette multidrug resistance proteins. *Physiol Rev* 2006;86:849-899.

DeGorter MK, Conseil G, Deeley RG, et al. Molecular modeling of the human multidrug resistance protein 1 (MRP1/ABCC1). *Biochem Biophys Res Commun* 2008;365:29-34.

Dohse M, Scharenberg C, Shukla S, et al. Comparison of ATP-binding cassette transporter interactions with the tyrosine kinase inhibitors imatinib, nilotinib, and dasatinib. *Drug Metab Dispos* 2010;38:1371-1380.

Doyle LA, Yang W, Abruzzo LV, et al. A multidrug resistance transporter from human MCF-7 breast cancer cells. *Proc Natl Acad Sci U S A* 1998;95:15665-15670.

Drori S, Jansen G, Mauritz R, et al. Clustering of mutations in the first transmembrane domain of the human reduced folate carrier in GW1843U89-resistant leukemia cells with impaired antifolate transport and augmented folate uptake. *J Biol Chem* 2000;275:30855-30863.

Dumontet C, Jordan MA. Microtubule-binding agents: a dynamic field of cancer therapeutics. *Nat Rev Drug Discov* 2010;9:790-803.

Durand RE. Distribution and activity of antineoplastic drugs in a tumor model. *J Natl Cancer Inst* 1989;81:146-152.

El-Sheikh AAK, van den Heuvel JJMW, Koenderink JB, et al. Interaction of nonsteroidal anti-inflammatory drugs with multidrug resistance protein (MRP) 2/ABCC2- and MRP4/ABCC4-mediated methotrexate transport. *J Pharmacol Exp Ther* 2007;320:229-235.

Esteller M, Garcia-Foncillas J, Andion E, et al. Inactivation of the DNA repair gene MGMT and the clinical response of gliomas to alkylating agents. *N Engl J Med* 2000;343:1350-1354.

Eyler CE, Rich JN. Survival of the fittest: cancer stem cells in therapeutic resistance and angiogenesis. *J Clin Oncol* 2008;26:2839-2845.

Ferlini C, Raspaglio G, Cicchillitti L, et al. Looking at drug resistance mechanisms for microtubule interacting drugs: does TUBB3 work? *Curr Cancer Drug Targets* 2007;7:704-712.

Gazdar AF. Activating and resistance mutations of EGFR in non-small-cell lung cancer: role in clinical response to EGFR tyrosine kinase inhibitors. *Oncogene* 2009;28 Suppl 1:S24-S31.

Goldie JH, Coldman AJ. The genetic origin of drug resistance in neoplasms: Implications for systemic therapy. *Cancer Res* 1984;44:3643-3653.

Gorre ME, Mohammed M, Ellwood K, et al. Clinical resistance to STI-571 cancer therapy caused by BCR-ABL gene mutation or amplification. *Science* 2001;293:876-880.

Gottesman MM, Fojo T, Bates SE. Multidrug resistance in cancer: role of ATP-dependent transporters. *Nat Rev Cancer* 2002;2:48-58.

Graeber TG, Osmanian C, Jacks T, et al. Hypoxia-mediated selection of cells with diminished apoptotic potential in solid tumours. *Nature* 1996;379:88-91.

Haber M, Smith J, Bordow SB, et al. Association of high-level MRP1 expression with poor clinical outcome in a large prospective study of primary neuroblastoma. *J Clin Oncol* 2006;24:1546-1553.

Hegi ME, Diserens AC, Gorlia T, et al. MGMT gene silencing and benefit from Temozolomide in glioblastoma. *N Engl J Med* 2005;352:997-1003.

Helleday T, Petermann E, Lundin C, et al. DNA repair pathways as targets for cancer therapy. *Nat Rev Cancer* 2008;8:193-204.

Hicks KO, Ohms SJ, van Zijl PL, et al. An experimental and mathematical model for the extravascular transport of a DNA intercalator in tumours. *Br J Cancer* 1997;76:894-903.

Hirschhaeuser F, Menne H, Dittfeld C, West J, Mueller-Klieser W, Kunz-Schughart LA. Multicellular tumor spheroids: an underestimated tool is catching up again. *J Biotechnol* 2010;148:3-15.

Hollenstein K, Dawson RJ, Locher KP. Structure and mechanism of ABC transporter proteins. *Curr Opin Struct Biol* 2007;17:412-418.

Howell SB, Safaei R, Larson CA, et al. Copper transporters and the cellular pharmacology of the platinum-containing cancer drugs. *Mol Pharmacol* 2010;77:887-893.

Hu S, Chen Z, Franke R, et al. Interaction of the multikinase inhibitors sorafenib and sunitinib with solute carriers and ATP-binding cassette transporters. *Clin Cancer Res* 2009;15:6062.

Humeniuk R, Menon LG, Mishra PJ, et al. Decreased levels of UMP kinase as a mechanism of fluoropyrimidine resistance. *Mol Cancer Ther* 2009;8:1037-1044.

Huxham LA, Kyle AH, Baker JH, et al. Microregional effects of gemcitabine in HCT-116 xenografts. *Cancer Res* 2004;64:6537-6541.

Idogawa M, Sasaki Y, Suzuki H, et al. A single recombinant adenovirus expressing p53 and p21-targeting artificial microRNAs efficiently induces apoptosis in human cancer cells. *Clin Cancer Res* 2009;15:3725-3732.

Ito K, Olsen SL, Qiu W, et al. Mutation of a single conserved tryptophan in multidrug resistance protein 1 (MRP1/ABCC1) results in loss of drug resistance and selective loss of organic anion transport. *J Biol Chem* 2001;276:15616-15624.

Jinushi M, Chiba S, Yoshiyama H, et al. Tumor-associated macrophages regulate tumorigenicity and anticancer drug responses of cancer stem/initiating cells. *Proc Natl Acad Sci U S A* 2011;108:12425-12430.

Kavallaris M. Microtubules and resistance to tubulin-binding agents. *Nat Rev Cancer* 2010;10:194-204.

Kelland L. The resurgence of platinum-based cancer chemotherapy. *Nat Rev Cancer* 2007;7:573-584.

Kelley SL, Basu A, Teicher BA, et al. Overexpression of metallothionein confers resistance to anticancer drugs. *Science* 1988;241:1813-1815.

Kerbel RS, Rak J, Kobayashi H, et al. Multicellular resistance: a new paradigm to explain aspects of acquired drug resistance of solid tumors. *Cold Spring Harb Symp Quant Biol* 1994;59:661-672.

Kim JJ, Tannock IF. Repopulation of cancer cells during therapy: an important cause of treatment failure. *Nat Rev Cancer* 2005;5:516-525.

Kimchi-Sarfaty C, Oh JM, Kim IW, et al. A "silent" polymorphism in the MDR1 gene changes substrate specificity. *Science* 2007;315:525-528.

Kondo Y, Woo ES, Michalska AE, et al. Metallothionein null cells have increased sensitivity to anticancer drugs. *Cancer Res* 1995;55:2021-2023.

Krishnamurthy P, Schwab M, Takenaka K, et al. Transporter-mediated protection against thiopurine-induced hematopoietic toxicity. *Cancer Res* 2008;68:4983-4989.

Kuh HJ, Jang SH, Wientjes MG, et al. Determinants of paclitaxel penetration and accumulation in human solid tumor. *J Pharmacol Exp Ther* 1999;290:871-880.

Kurz EU, Wilson SE, Leader KB, et al. The histone deacetylase inhibitor sodium butyrate induces DNA topoisomerase II alpha expression and confers hypersensitivity to etoposide in human leukemic cell lines. *Mol Cancer Ther* 2001;1:121-131.

Lagas JS, Vlaming MLH, Schinkel AH. Pharmacokinetic assessment of multiple ATP-binding cassette transporters: The power of combination knockout mice. *Mol Interv* 2009;9:136-145.

Lankelma J, Dekker H, Luque FR, et al. Doxorubicin gradients in human breast cancer. *Clin Cancer Res* 1999;5:1703-1707.

Leggas M, Adachi M, Scheffer GL, et al. Mrp4 confers resistance to topotecan and protects the brain from chemotherapy. *Mol Cell Biol* 2004;24:7612-7621.

Leslie EM, Deeley RG, Cole SPC. Multidrug resistance proteins in toxicology: role of P-glycoprotein, MRP1, MRP2 and BCRP (ABCG2) in tissue defense. *Toxicol Appl Pharmacol* 2005;204: 216-237.

Li X, Lewis MT, Huang J, et al. Intrinsic resistance of tumorigenic breast cancer cells to chemotherapy. *J Natl Cancer Inst* 2008;100: 672-679.

Li ZW, Dalton WS. Tumor microenvironment and drug resistance in hematologic malignancies. *Blood Rev* 2006;20:333-342.

Lievre A, Bachet JB, Le Corre D, et al. KRAS mutation status is predictive of response to cetuximab therapy in colorectal cancer. *Cancer Res* 2006;66:3992-3995.

Loe DW, Deeley RG, Cole SPC. Characterization of vincristine transport by the 190 kDa multidrug resistance protein, MRP: Evidence for co-transport with reduced glutathione. *Cancer Res* 1998;58:5130-5136.

Loo TW, Clarke DM. Recent progress in understanding the mechanism of P-glycoprotein-mediated drug efflux. *J Membr Biol* 2005;206:173-185.

Mano MS, Rosa DD, De Azambuja E, et al. The 17q12-q21 amplicon: Her2 and topoisomerase IIα and their importance to the biology of solid tumours. *Cancer Treat Rev* 2007;33:64-77.

Marino ML, Fais S, Djavaheri-Mergny M, et al. Proton pump inhibition induces autophagy as a survival mechanism following oxidative stress in human melanoma cells. *Cell Death Dis* 2010;1:e87.

Matsson P, Pedersen JM, Norinder U, et al. Identification of novel specific and general inhibitors of the three major human ATP-binding cassette transporters P-gp, BCRP and MRP2 among registered drugs. *Pharm Res* 2009;26:1816-1831.

Maugeri-Sacca M, Vigneri P, De Maria R. Cancer stem cells and chemosensitivity. *Clin Cancer Res* 2011;17:4942-4947.

McLornan DP, Barrett HL, Cummins R, et al. Prognostic significance of TRAIL signaling molecules in stage II and III colorectal cancer. *Clin Cancer Res* 2010;16:3442-3451.

Milojkovic D, Apperley J. Mechanisms of resistance to imatinib and second-generation tyrosine kinase inhibitors in chronic myeloid leukemia. *Clin Cancer Res* 2009;15:7519-7527.

Minchinton AI, Tannock IF. Drug penetration in solid tumours. *Nat Rev Cancer* 2006;6:583-592.

Mohyeldin A, Garzón-Muvdi T, Quiñones-Hinojosa A. Oxygen in stem cell biology: a critical component of the stem cell niche. *Cell Stem Cell* 2010;7:150-161.

Muller S, Kramer OH. Inhibitors of HDACs—effective drugs against cancer? *Curr Cancer Drug Targets* 2010;10:210-228.

Nies AT, Keppler D. The apical conjugate efflux pump ABCC2 (MRP2). *Pflugers Arch* 2007;453:643-659.

Nitiss JL. Targeting DNA topoisomerase II in cancer chemotherapy. *Nat Rev Cancer* 2009;9:338-350.

Noborio-Hatano K, Kikuchi J, Takatoku M, et al. Bortezomib overcomes cell-adhesion-mediated drug resistance through downregulation of VLA-4 expression in multiple myeloma. *Oncogene* 2009;28:231-242.

Olaussen KA, Dunant A, Fouret P, et al. DNA repair by ERCC1 in non–small cell lung cancer and cisplatin-based adjuvant chemotherapy. *N Engl J Med* 2006;355:983-991.

Olive KP, Jacobetz MA, Davidson CJ, et al. Inhibition of Hedgehog signaling enhances delivery of chemotherapy in a mouse model of pancreatic cancer. *Science* 2009;324:1457-1461.

Ory B, Ramsey MR, Wilson C, et al. A microRNA-dependent program controls p53-independent survival and chemosensitivity in human and murine squamous cell carcinoma. *J Clin Invest* 2011;121:809-820.

Pajic M, Murray J, Marshall GM, et al. ABCC1/G2012T single nucleotide polymorphism is associated with patient outcome in primary neuroblastoma and altered stability of the ABCC1 gene transcript. *Pharmacogenet Genomics* 2011;21:270-279.

Pal SK, Figlin RA, Reckamp K. Targeted therapies for non-small cell lung cancer: An evolving landscape. *Mol Cancer Ther* 2010;9: 1931-1944.

Pasello M, Michelacci F, Scionti I, et al. Overcoming glutathione S-transferase P1-related cisplatin resistance in osteosarcoma. *Cancer Res* 2008;68:6661-6668.

Pommier Y. DNA topoisomerase I inhibitors: chemistry, biology and interfacial inhibition. *Chem Rev* 2009;109:2894-2902.

Primeau AJ, Rendon A, Hedley D, et al. The distribution of the anticancer drug Doxorubicin in relation to blood vessels in solid tumors. *Clin Cancer Res* 2005;11:8782-8788.

Provenzano PP, Cuevas C, Chang AE, Goel VK, Von Hoff DD, Hingorani SR. Enzymatic targeting of the stroma ablates physical barriers to treatment of pancreatic ductal adenocarcinoma. *Cancer Cell* 2012;21:418-429.

Rappa G, Lorico A, Flavell RA, et al. Evidence that the multidrug resistance protein (MRP) functions as a co-transporter of glutathione and natural product toxins. *Cancer Res* 1997;57: 5232-5237.

Rice GC, Hoy C, Schimke RT. Transient hypoxia enhances the frequency of dihydrofolate reductase gene amplification in Chinese hamster ovary cells. *Proc Natl Acad Sci U S A* 1986;83: 5978-5982.

Rischin D, Peters LJ, O'Sullivan B, et al. Tirapazamine, cisplatin, and radiation versus cisplatin and radiation for advanced squamous cell carcinoma of the head and neck (TROG 02.02, HeadSTART): a phase III trial of the Trans-Tasman Radiation Oncology Group. *J Clin Oncol* 2010;28:2989-2995.

Rizzo S, Hersey JM, Mellor P, et al. Ovarian cancer stem cell-like side populations are enriched following chemotherapy and overexpress EZH2. *Mol Cancer Ther* 2011;10:325-335.

Rothnie A, Callaghan R, Deeley RG, et al. Role of GSH in estrone sulfate binding and translocation by the multidrug resistance protein 1 (MRP1, ABCC1). *J Biol Chem* 2006;281: 13906-13914.

Rottenberg S, Nygren AOH, Pajic M, et al. Selective induction of chemotherapy resistance of mammary tumors in a conditional mouse model for hereditary breast cancer. *Proc Natl Acad Sci U S A* 2007;104:12117-12122.

Russel FGM, Koenderink JB, Masereeuw R. Multidrug resistance protein 4 (MRP4/ABCC4): a versatile efflux transporter for drugs and signalling molecules. *Trends Pharmacol Sci* 2008; 29:200-207.

Sakai W, Swisher EM, Karlan BY, et al. Secondary mutations as a mechanism of cisplatin resistance in BRCA2-mutated cancer. *Nature* 2008;451:1116-1120.

Sarkadi B, Orban TI, Szakads G, et al. Evaluation of ABCG2 expression in human embryonic stem cells: Crossing the same river twice? *Stem Cells* 2010;28:174-176.

Sau A, Pillizzari Tregno F, Valentino F, et al. Glutathione transferases and development of new principles to overcome drug resistance. *Arch Biochem Biophys* 2010;500:116-122.

Schimke RT. Gene amplification, drug resistance, and cancer. *Cancer Res* 1984;44:1735-1742.

Schmitt CA, Rosenthal CT, Lowe SW. Genetic analysis of chemoresistance in primary murine lymphomas. *Nat Med* 2000;6:1029-1035.

Shain KH, Dalton WS. Cell adhesion is a key determinant in de novo multidrug resistance (MDR): new targets for the prevention of acquired MDR. *Mol Cancer Ther* 2001;1:69-78.

Sharma S, Kelly TK, Jones PA. Epigenetics in cancer. *Carcinogenesis* 2010;31:27-36.

Slot AJ, Molinski SV, Cole SPC. Mammalian multidrug-resistance proteins (MRPs). *Essays Biochem* 2011;50:179-207.

Slovak ML, Ho JP, Bhardwaj EU, et al. Localization of a novel multidrug resistance-associated gene in the HT1080/DR4 and H69AR human tumor cell lines. *Cancer Res* 1993;53:3221-3225.

Smitherman PK, Townsend AJ, Kute TE, et al. Role of multidrug resistance protein 2 (MRP2, ABCC2) in alkylating agent detoxification; MRP2 potentiates glutathione S-transferase A1-1-mediated resistance to chlorambucil cytotoxicity. *J Pharmacol Exp Ther* 2004;308:260-267.

Soengas MS, Lowe SW. Apoptosis and melanoma chemoresistance. *Oncogene* 2003;22:3138-3151.

St Croix B, Florenes VA, Rak JW, et al. Impact of the cyclin-dependent kinase inhibitor p27Kip1 on resistance of tumor cells to anticancer agents. *Nat Med* 1996;2:1204-1210.

Steele N, Finn P, Brown R, et al. Combined inhibition of DNA methylation and histone acetylation enhances gene re-expression and drug sensitivity in vivo. *Br J Cancer* 2009;100:758-763.

Sugano K, Kansy M, Artursson P, et al. Coexistence of passive and carrier-mediated processes in drug transport. *Nat Rev Drug Discov* 2010;9:597-614.

Tanei T, Morimoto K, Shimazu K, et al. Association of breast cancer stem cells identified by aldehyde dehydrogenase 1 expression with resistance to sequential Paclitaxel and epirubicin-based chemotherapy for breast cancers. *Clin Cancer Res* 2009;15:4234-4241.

Tannock IF, Lee C. Evidence against apoptosis as a major mechanism for reproductive cell death following treatment of cell lines with anti-cancer drugs. *Br J Cancer* 2001;84:100-105.

Tannock IF, Lee CM, Tunggal JK, et al. Limited penetration of anticancer drugs through tumor tissue: a potential cause of resistance of solid tumors to chemotherapy. *Clin Cancer Res* 2002;8:874-884.

Teicher BA, Herman TS, Holden SA, et al. Tumor resistance to alkylating agents conferred by mechanisms operative only in vivo. *Science* 1990;247:1457-1461.

Townsend DM, Tew KD. The role of glutathione-S-transferase in anti-cancer drug resistance. *Oncogene* 2003;22:7369-7375.

Trédan O, Galmarini CM, Patel K, Tannock IF. Drug resistance and the solid tumor microenvironment. *J Natl Cancer Inst* 2007;99:1441-1454.

Tunggal JK, Ballinger JR, Tannock IF. Influence of cell concentration in limiting the therapeutic benefit of P-glycoprotein reversal agents. *Int J Cancer* 1999;81:741-747.

Urasaki Y, Laco GS, Pourquier P, et al. Characterization of a novel topoisomerase I mutation from a camptothecin-resistant human prostate cancer cell line. *Cancer Res* 2001;61:1964-1969.

Ventura A, Kirsch DG, McLaughlin ME, et al. Restoration of p53 function leads to tumour regression in vivo. *Nature* 2007;445:661-665.

Vlaming ML, Lagas JS, Schinkel AH. Physiological and pharmacological roles of ABCG2 (BCRP): recent findings in Abcg2 knockout mice. *Adv Drug Deliv Rev* 2009;61:14-25.

Watson RG, Muhale F, Thorne LB, et al. Amplification of thymidylate synthetase in metastatic colorectal cancer patients pretreated with 5-fluorouracil-based chemotherapy. *Eur J Cancer* 2010;46:3358-3364.

Wheeler DL, Dunn EF, Harari PM. Understanding resistance to EGFR inhibitors—impact on future treatment strategies. *Nat Rev Clin Oncol* 2010;7:493-507.

White E, DiPaola RS. The double-edged sword of autophagy modulation in cancer. *Clin Cancer Res* 2009;15:5308-5316.

Wijnholds J, Evers R, Van Leusden MR, et al. Increased sensitivity to anticancer drugs and decreased inflammatory response in mice lacking the multidrug resistance-associated protein. *Nat Med* 1997;3:1275-1279.

Xue C, Haber M, Flemming C, et al. p53 determines multidrug sensitivity of childhood neuroblastoma. *Cancer Res* 2007;67:10351-10360.

Yanamandra N, Colaco NM, Parquet NA, et al. Tipifarnib and bortezomib are synergistic and overcome cell adhesion-mediated drug resistance in multiple myeloma and acute myeloid leukemia. *Clin Cancer Res* 2006;12:591-599.

Yang B, Eshlemen JR, Berger NA, et al. Wild-type p53 protein potentiates cytotoxicity of therapeutic agents in human colon cancer cells. *Clin Cancer Res* 1996;2:1649-1657.

Yang CG, Ciccolini J, Blesius A, et al. DPD-based adaptive dosing of 5-FU in patients with head and neck cancer: impact on treatment efficacy and toxicity. *Cancer Chemother Pharmacol* 2011;67:49-56.

Yee SW, Chen L, Giacomini KM. Pharmacogenomics of membrane transporters: past, present and future. *Pharmacogenomics* 2010;11:475-479.

Yu JL, Rak JW, Coomber BL, et al. Effect of p53 status on tumor response to anti-angiogenic therapy. *Science* 2002;295:1526-1528.

Yu M, Ocana A, Tannock IF. Reversal of ATP-binding-cassette drug transporter activity to modulate chemoresistance: why has it failed to provide clinical benefit? *Cancer Metastasis Rev* 2012 [epub ahead of print].

Zander SA, Kersbergen A, van der Burg E, et al. Sensitivity and acquired resistance of BRCA1;p53-deficient mouse mammary tumors to the topoisomerase I inhibitor topotecan. *Cancer Res* 2010;70:1700-1710.

Zhang J, Visser F, King KM, et al. The role of nucleoside transporters in cancer chemotherapy with nucleoside drugs. *Cancer Metastasis Rev* 2007;26:85-110.

Zutter MM. Integrin-mediated adhesion: tipping the balance between chemosensitivity and chemoresistance. *Adv Exp Med Biol* 2007;608:87-100.

CHAPTER

20

Hormones and Cancer

Paul S. Rennie, Eric Leblanc, and Leigh C. Murphy

20.1 INTRODUCTION

Breast and prostate cancers are the most commonly occurring cancers in Western society, and are the second leading cause of cancer death (next to lung cancer) in women and men, respectively. Both of these cancers arise in tissues that require steroid sex hormones (estrogens and androgens) for their development, growth, and function. Although human cancers occur in other hormone-dependent tissues, such as the uterus, ovary, and testis, this chapter focuses exclusively on breast and prostate cancer as models of hormone-dependent cancers.

The relationship between prostate enlargement and hormones produced by the testes has long been recognized.

Although the chemical nature of androgens was not known, it was reported in 1895 that castration of elderly men with prostate enlargement, presumably as a result of benign prostatic hyperplasia, resulted in rapid atrophy of prostatic tissue. Early anecdotal evidence regarding the testicular (ie, androgen) dependence of the human prostate is also derived from studies involving eunuchs from the Ottoman and Chinese courts, which indicated that prostates did not develop in prepubertal castrates. Following the isolation of "testosterone" as the most potent androgenic compound in the testes in 1935, Huggins and Hodges demonstrated the efficacy of surgical orchiectomy for the treatment of metastatic prostate cancer, for which Huggins received the Nobel Prize for Medicine in 1966. Similarly, a link between estrogen and breast cancer

469

growth was established at the end of the 19th century, when Beatson demonstrated that oophorectomy was useful in the treatment of metastatic breast cancer in some premenopausal women. However, a molecular basis for this observation was not forthcoming until the 1960s with the discovery of the estrogen receptor, followed by the demonstrated expression of estrogen receptors in some human breast tumors by Elwood Jensen.

Evidence for a direct link between the action of sex steroids, and a causal role in the carcinogenic process leading to breast and prostate tumors, was first provided by Robert Noble. He reported that prolonged exposure to estrogen, androgen, or combinations of the 2 led to breast and prostate cancers in rats. More recently, the successful use of the antiestrogen, tamoxifen, to reduce the incidence of breast cancer in high-risk women, supports a direct link between estrogen action and breast tumor formation. These hormones are fundamental not only to the development of normal mammary and prostate glands, but also to dysplastic and neoplastic processes that occur in these tissues.

In this chapter, relationships between hormones and cancers of the breast and prostate are explored in the context of basic mechanisms of hormone action, the natural history of the 2 diseases, and their treatment with hormonally based therapies.

20.2 BASIC MECHANISMS OF HORMONE ACTION

Hormones can be classified generally into 2 broad groups: (a) nonsteroidal (amino acids, peptides, and polypeptides), which usually require cell-membrane localized receptors that regulate second messenger molecules such as cyclic adenosine monophosphate (cAMP) to mediate their action (see Chap. 8, Sec. 8.2), and (b) steroidal, which bind directly to intracellular receptors to mediate their action. Breast and prostate cancer are dependent primarily on estrogen and androgen steroid hormones, respectively, for their growth and viability. Other examples of steroid hormones include glucocorticoids, mineralocorticoids, and progestins such as progesterone.

The bioavailability of steroid hormones at the site of action depends on several factors, including synthesis, transport via the blood, access to target tissue, metabolism in target tissue, and expression of receptors within the target cell.

20.2.1 Synthesis and Metabolism of Estrogens

As indicated in Figure 20–1, all steroids are synthesized from the common precursor, cholesterol. The primary site of synthesis of estrogens (eg, estrone and estradiol) in premenopausal women is the parafollicular region of the ovary. Ovarian steroid synthesis in premenopausal women is cyclical and regulated via the gonad–hypothalamus–pituitary feedback axis, as indicated in Figure 20–2A. Other sites of estrogen biosynthesis include mesenchymal cells in adipose tissue and skin;

these tissues become major sources for estrogen synthesis in postmenopausal women where adrenal androgens, in particular androstenedione, are converted to estrone by aromatase cytochrome P450 (Simpson, 2000). Some estrone molecules can then be converted to the more potent estradiol-17β by 17β-hydroxysteroid dehydrogenases (Miettinen et al, 2000). A large amount of estrone is converted by estrone sulfotransferase to estrone sulphate, which has a longer half-life in blood, and therefore can act as an estrogen reservoir, being converted back to estrone by the action of sulfatases (Miettinen et al, 2000). Aromatase activity has been detected in normal human breast tissue and in more than 50% of human breast tumors (Sasano and Harada, 1998). Estrone sulfotransferase, sulfatase and 17β-hydroxysteroid dehydrogenase type 1 have been detected in both normal and malignant human breast tissues (Miettinen et al, 2000) and the relative expression of these enzymes probably regulates the local availability of estrogens to target cells. Estrogen synthesis in postmenopausal women is not cyclical but serum and local tissue levels can differ between individuals because of a variety of environmental and genetic factors such as obesity and genetic variation/polymorphism in steroid metabolizing (biosynthetic and degrading) enzymes (Thompson and Ambrosone, 2000).

20.2.2 Synthesis and Metabolism of Androgens

The Leydig cells of the testes produce almost 90% of the body's androgens with the remainder being made mainly by the adrenal cortex. As illustrated in Figure 20–2B, the testes make primarily testosterone, whereas the major adrenal androgens are dehydroepiandrosterone (DHEA) and its derived sulfate, which although weak androgens, can be converted in other tissues to testosterone. The principal circulating androgen in man is testosterone (see Fig. 20–1). As with estrogen synthesis in the ovary, testosterone production in the testis is regulated by a negative feedback loop involving luteinizing hormone (LH) and luteinizing hormone-releasing hormone (LHRH) via the gonad–hypothalamus–pituitary feedback axis (see Fig. 20–2B). Although there are diurnal fluctuations of androgen secretion, their production does not follow a regular cyclical pattern. Also, there is no apparent equivalent to the menopause in men, although there is a progressive decrease in testosterone levels with age, which is accompanied by some degree of testicular failure.

There are 2 principal pathways through which testosterone can undergo metabolic conversion to more potent forms (see Fig. 20–1). The first involves the enzyme aromatase, which is present in many tissues (eg, adipose tissue, testis, brain) and which can convert approximately 0.5% of the daily production of testosterone to estradiol. Although this is a small proportion of the total amount, estradiol is a 200-fold more potent inhibitor of gonadotrophins than testosterone. The second major pathway is the conversion of testosterone to the more potent androgen dihydrotestosterone (DHT) by the enzyme 5α-reductase, which is present in many androgen

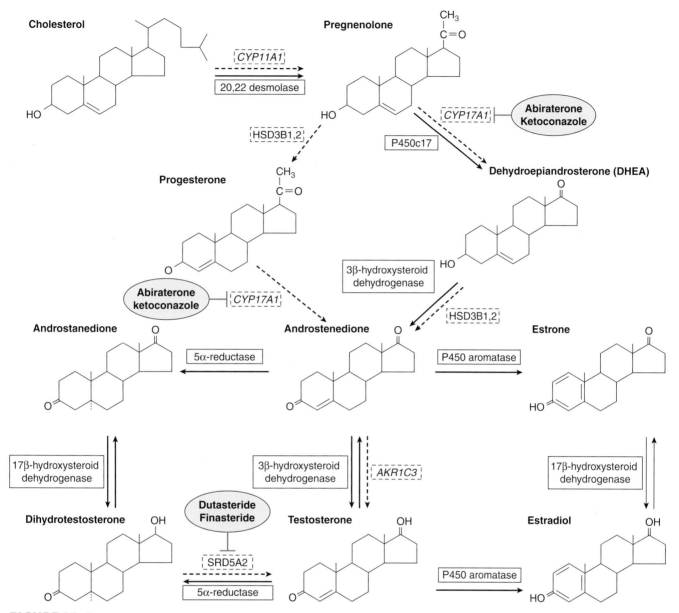

FIGURE 20–1 **The principal mammalian steroid biosynthetic pathways for estradiol, testosterone, and dihydrotestosterone are represented by solid arrows.** The enzymes that catalyze the reactions are shown in boxes. Although the main sites for steroid synthesis are the gonads and the adrenals, metabolic interconversions and activations occur in sex hormone target tissues, such as the prostate and breast, as well as other peripheral tissues, such as skin and adipose tissue. Dashed arrows and boxes represent the intratumoral androgen synthesis pathway. Inhibitors of enzymes are represented in blue ovals.

target tissues such as the prostate and skin. There are 2 isoforms of 5α-reductase, each with different kinetic properties and sensitivity to inhibitors, with the type II isoform predominating in human accessory sex tissue (Bruchovsky et al, 1988). The interaction of testosterone and DHT with the androgen receptor is different. Testosterone has a 2-fold lower affinity than DHT for the androgen receptor and is more effective in regulating differentiation. However, the dissociation rate of DHT from the receptor is 5-fold slower than testosterone, and it is a more potent androgen to induce growth and maintenance of the prostate gland (Grino et al, 1990).

20.2.3 Transport of Steroid Hormones in the Blood

As hydrophobic molecules in an aqueous environment, most steroid hormones are transported in the blood bound to proteins, predominantly sex hormone-binding globulin (SHBG) and albumin (as shown in Fig. 20–3). Only approximately 2% is in an unbound form, which is the biologically active fraction. SHBG also plays a role in permitting certain steroid hormones to act without entering the cell: estrogens and androgens bind with high affinity to SHBG, which, in turn,

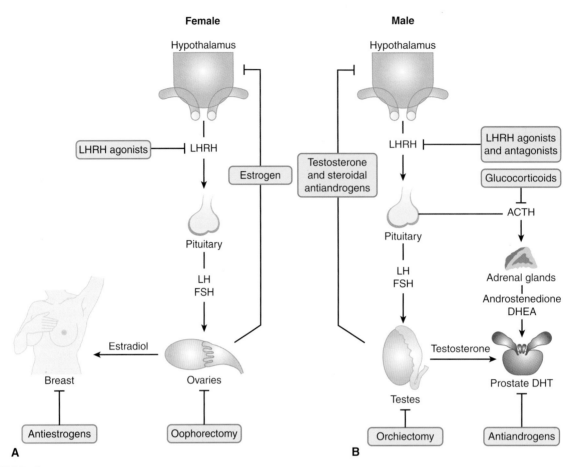

FIGURE 20–2 **The gonadal–hypothalamic–pituitary axis.** The pathways and feedback loops that regulate the production of estrogens in females (**A**) and androgens in males (**B**) and their target tissues are shown. The procedures and agents used for blocking the synthesis and activity of androgens and estrogens at the various steps in the pathway are highlighted. Note that luteinizing hormone-releasing hormone (LHRH) agonists initially stimulate release of luteinizing hormone (LH) followed by its inhibition. *ACTH*, adrenocorticotropic hormone; *FSH*, follicle-stimulating hormone; *DHEA*, dehydroepiandrosterone; *DHT*, dihydrotestosterone.

interacts with a specific, high-affinity receptor (SHBG-R) on cell membranes and transduces a signal via a G-protein/cAMP (Kahn et al, 2002). The steroid/SHBG-R/SHBG complex generates messages that have effects on the transcriptional activity of regular, intracellular receptors for steroid hormones. Hence, SHBG not only modulates the amount of ligand available to bind to these steroid receptors, but may also modulate their activity through interaction with the cell membrane. Factors that influence the levels of SHBG and albumin will affect the bioactivity of steroid hormones. For example, SHBG production is stimulated by both estrogens and by the antiestrogen tamoxifen, whereas androgens and progestins have been shown to suppress it. In addition, SHBG can be expressed inside the cytoplasm of prostate cells from de novo synthesis and, through binding to steroids such as DHT, can affect the intracellular concentration of free androgens (Kahn et al, 2002).

20.2.4 Steroid Hormone Receptors

An overview of how steroid hormones regulate growth and differentiation of their target cells is shown in Figure 20–3.

The majority of steroid hormone that enters the cell is derived from the small nonbound fraction in the circulation, which can enter by passive diffusion. Upon entry into the cell, the steroid or its metabolic derivative (eg, DHT) binds directly to a predominantly cytoplasmic (androgen receptor) or nuclear (estrogen receptor) steroid receptor protein. The steroid-receptor complex undergoes an activation step involving a conformational change and shedding of heat shock (including HSP70, HSP90, and HSP40) and other chaperone proteins, which are necessary to maintain the receptor in a competent ligand-binding state (Aranda and Pascual, 2001). After dimerization, and nuclear transport in the case of some steroid receptors like the androgen receptor, the activated receptor dimer complex binds to specific DNA motifs called hormone-responsive elements (HREs) found in the promoters of hormone-regulated genes (Aranda and Pascual, 2001). The receptor-DNA complexes, in turn, associate dynamically with coactivators and basal transcriptional components to enhance the transcription of genes, whose messenger RNAs (mRNAs) are translated into proteins that elicit specific biological responses. It is likely that receptors that are not bound to their ligands, or those

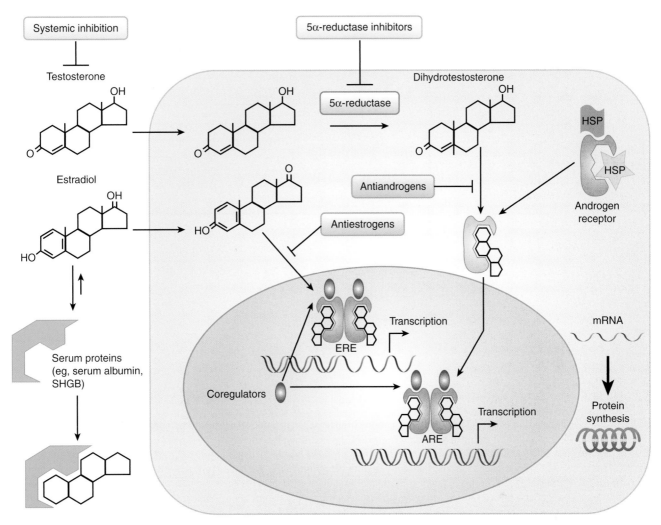

FIGURE 20–3 **Schematic pathways for the molecular action of testosterone and estradiol in hormone target cells.** A relatively simplistic overview of the key events in steroid hormone action with the sites at which the hormone signal can be inhibited, are indicated. Although the dynamics of estrogen and androgen action are similar, for full activity testosterone needs to be converted to dihydrotestosterone, which binds to a cytoplasmic form of the androgen receptor and is translocated into the nucleus, whereas estradiol binds directly to its receptor in the cell nucleus. *ARE*, androgen-responsive element; *ERE*, estrogen-responsive element; *HSP*, heat shock protein; *SHBG*, sex hormone-binding globulin.

bound to antagonists (Fig. 20–4), form complexes with corepressors to inhibit the transcription of specific genes (Perissi and Rosenfeld, 2005).

All steroid receptors are members of a so-called superfamily of more than 150 proteins. All are ligand-responsive transcription factors that share similarities with respect to their structural homology and functional properties. As shown in Figure 20–5, each member of the steroid receptor family possesses a modular structure composed of the following:

1. An N-terminal region containing ligand-independent transcriptional activating functions (collectively referred to as *a*ctivating *f*unction-1 or AF1);
2. A centrally located DNA binding domain of approximately 65 amino acids having 2 zinc fingers (see Chap. 8, Sec. 8.2.6);
3. A hinge region that contains signal elements for nuclear localization; and

4. A ligand-binding domain in the C-terminal region of the protein containing a ligand-dependent transcriptional activating function (called AF2).

AF1 and AF2 can function independently or synergistically, depending on the gene promoter and/or the cell type (Aranda and Pascual, 2001). Between members of the family of steroid receptors, the N-terminal region has the highest degree of amino acid sequence variability, whereas the DNA-binding domain has the most shared homology.

20.2.4.1 Androgen Receptors The androgen receptor (AR) is encoded on the X chromosome. As a single allele gene in males, it is susceptible to genetic defects whose phenotypes can range from minor undervirilization to a complete female phenotype known as *testicular feminization*. The normal, wild-type AR has a molecular weight of approximately 110 kDa, but truncated molecular variants have been observed in a variety

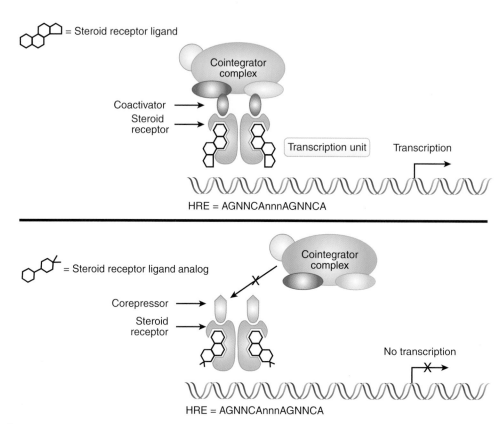

FIGURE 20–4 **Illustration of the role of coactivators and corepressor in regulation of steroid receptor action.** In the presence of agonistic ligands (eg, estradiol for estrogen receptor [ER] and DHT for androgen receptor [AR]), the steroid receptor-DNA complexes associate dynamically with coactivators, which, in turn, recruit other proteins, including cointegrator complexes, that contact and stabilize the basal transcription unit resulting in enhanced transcription of target genes. In the presence of antagonistic ligands (eg, tamoxifen for ER and flutamide for AR), the receptors are in a different conformational state (steroid receptor ligand analog) and the receptor-DNA complexes dynamically associate with corepressors (Co-R) which destabilize basal transcription units and result in reduced transcription of target genes. *HRE*, hormone-responsive element.

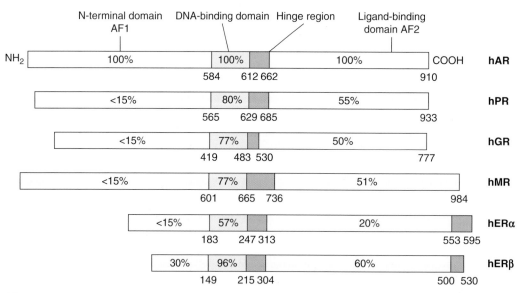

FIGURE 20–5 **The relative amino acid sequence homology within the functional domains of the principal members of the family of human (h) steroid hormone receptors.** The relative amino acid sequence homology (represented by the percentages indicated in boxes) for hERβ is in reference to hERα, whereas all the other receptors are relative to hAR. The numbers correspond to the amino acid positions from the N-terminus (NH₂), AF1 and AF2 refer to the transcriptional *a*ctivation *f*unction 1 and 2 that reside in the N-terminal and ligand-binding domains, respectively. *AR*, Androgen receptor; *ER*, estrogen receptor; *GR*, glucocorticoid receptor; *MR*, mineralocorticoid receptor; *PR*, progestin receptor.

of prostate cancers. These variants lack the ligand-binding domain of the AR but are still functional, even in the absence of androgen (Hu et al, 2009). In this chapter, AR refers only to the wild-type, 110-kDa form.

Relative to other steroid receptors, the AR has one of the largest N-terminal domains, which occupies more than half of the primary sequence of 919 amino acids (see Fig. 20–5). A unique feature of the AR relative to other members of this family is the occurrence of several stretches of the same amino acids (termed *homopolymeric*) in the N-terminal domain. These tracts include 17 to 29 repeating glutamine residues, starting approximately at amino acid 59, 9 proline residues at amino acid 372, and a 24-residue polyglycine stretch beginning at amino acid 449. These repeating tracts have been shown to modulate the folding and structural integrity of the N-terminal domain (Davies et al, 2008) and there is evidence of a reverse relationship between variations in their lengths and the transcription levels of mRNAs (Robins et al, 2008). Not surprisingly, these variations result in biological effects: for example, an abnormal extension of the polyglutamine tract to 40 or more residues is associated with neurodegenerative diseases such as X-linked spinal and bulbar muscular atrophy (La Spada et al, 1991). In contrast, a decreased size of these homopolymers may be linked with the development of prostate cancer (Robins et al, 2008), although there is no consensus on this relationship (Mir et al, 2002).

20.2.4.2 Estrogen Receptors
There are 2 estrogen receptor (ERs), ERα and ERβ, which, unlike AR isoforms, are encoded by separate genes (see Fig. 20–5). Several variant isoforms of each ER, generated by alternative RNA splicing, may also be expressed (Murphy et al, 1998). The centrally located DNA-binding domains for ERα and ERβ (see Fig. 20–5) are highly homologous (>95% identity). Their C-terminally located ligand-binding domains are approximately 60% identical. As with other steroid receptors, the ligand-binding domain contains a ligand-dependent dimerization function, and a ligand-dependent transactivation function, AF2. Similarly, a ligand-independent transactivation function, AF1, is present in the N-terminal domain. This latter domain is different in ERα and ERβ. In addition steroid receptors are subject to multiple posttranslational modifications such as phosphorylation, which can regulate receptor activity, transcriptional activity, DNA binding, protein turnover, and ligand sensitivity (Ward and Weigel, 2009).

20.2.5 Binding of Steroid Receptors to DNA

As transcription factors, steroid receptors modulate gene expression by first binding to specific DNA sequences in the promoter regions of hormone-regulated genes (see Fig. 20–4). The α-helix structure of the first zinc finger (see Chap. 8, Sec. 8.2.6) of the DNA-binding domain of a receptor is the primary discriminator for binding to different DNA sequence motifs of HREs (Aranda and Pascual, 2001). All members of the nuclear receptor family bind as dimers to pairs of a similar DNA sequence motif, AGNNCA (N = any nucleotide), which comprises the HRE found in the promoters of steroid regulated genes (Glass, 1994). Steroid receptors can bind to multiple HREs that are often hundreds of kilobase pairs distal to target gene promoters; furthermore steroid receptors and associated complexes bound at both distal and proximal HREs can interact, resulting in chromosome looping, to regulate target gene transcription (Fullwood et al, 2009). Nuclear receptors can be further subdivided on the basis of selection of the primary sequence of the core motif as either AGGTCA, for the ER and thyroid receptor subfamily, or AGAACA for the AR, glucocorticoid receptor (GR), or progestin receptor (PR). In general, 2 or more sets of interacting HREs in a gene promoter are required to elicit a steroid-mediated response (Klinge, 1999; Rennie et al, 1993).

The very high sequence homology of HREs has raised the question as to how steroid receptors govern hormone-specific responses. Although there is no definitive mechanism, the interaction with unique combinations of coregulators or other binding proteins is probably a major contributing factor to steroid-receptor specific gene regulation. Other parameters may also be important, such as the availability of receptor and ligand, the activity of proximal transcription factors, the cooperative binding of receptors to 2 or more DNA-binding sites, and altered DNA target motif recognition.

20.2.6 Interaction of Steroid Receptors with Coregulator Proteins

Important molecular mechanisms by which nuclear receptors regulate gene transcription involve not only direct interactions of steroid receptors with some of the basal transcription components, but also indirect interactions through recruitment of coregulator protein complexes to the promoters of target genes (Perissi and Rosenfeld, 2005; see Figs. 20–3 and 20–4). Coregulators fall into 2 main classes, coactivators and corepressors, which enhance or repress transcription, respectively (as illustrated in Fig. 20–4). There are many genes that encode coactivators, but the *steroid receptor coactivator* (SRC)/NCOA/p160 family are relatively specific for nuclear receptors and are the best studied (O'Malley and Kumar, 2009; Xu et al, 2009).

Although the auxiliary molecular components involved and the dynamics of their interactions remain to be established, a general pattern has emerged. The coactivators and corepressors are important for mediating both AF2 and AF1 activities of steroid receptors. Their mechanism of transcriptional activation is thought to involve 2 stages (Perissi and Rosenfeld, 2005). First, when recruited to the receptor by direct protein–protein binding, coregulators promote the local remodeling of chromatin structure through acetyltransferase or deacetylase activity and through their ability to recruit other proteins with chromatin remodeling activity (as outlined in Fig. 20–6). Second, the coactivators recruit and/or stabilize the basal transcription machinery by

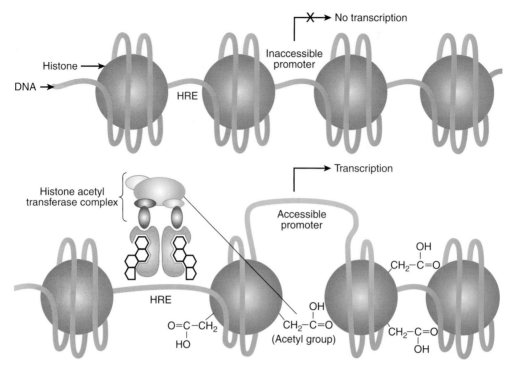

FIGURE 20–6 **Remodeling of chromatin and activation of transcription by steroid hormone receptors.** Steroid hormone receptors bind to hormone responsive elements (HREs) in the promoters of target genes and recruit coactivators (eg, SRC-1) and cointegrators (eg, CBP/p300), which have chromatin remodeling activity. Some coregulators and cointegrators have histone acetyltransferase (HAT) activity, which results in dynamic nucleosomal histone acetylation and increased access of basal transcription complexes (that include RNA polymerase II) to the promoters of target genes.

protein–protein interactions so as to enable efficient transcription of the target gene by RNA polymerase II (Perissi and Rosenfeld, 2005). The chromatin remodeling enables altered access of the promoter DNA to general transcription factors (Fig. 20–6).

It is uncertain as to which coactivators are necessary or sufficient for transcriptional activation. In MCF-7 breast cancer cells ERα and a number of coactivators associate rapidly with target promoters in a dynamic, cyclic fashion and the SRC/NCOA/p160 class of coactivators is sufficient for gene activation (Shang et al, 2000). It is likely that the relative availability of coregulators will vary in different tissues and may even be restricted to specific tissues. Also, although the occurrence of receptor-specific coregulators has not been confirmed, many coregulators bind preferentially to certain receptors (Leo and Chen, 2000). For example, a repressor of ER transcriptional activity, called *r*epressor of *e*strogen receptor *a*ctivity (REA) is active on ERα or ERβ, but not other steroid receptors (Montano et al, 1999). Its mechanism of action involves a competition with coactivators such as SRC-1 for binding to the ligand-binding domain of ER (Delage-Mourroux et al, 2000). Furthermore, a member of the SRC/NCOA family, SRC-3/NCOA3 or *a*mplified *i*n *b*reast *c*ancer 1 (AIB1) may have a role in breast cancer as it is amplified and overexpressed in some breast tumors and such overexpression has been correlated with tamoxifen resistance (Anzick et al, 1997; Xu et al, 2009).

20.2.7 Mechanisms for Transcriptional Regulation by Steroid Receptors

There are at least 3 different mechanisms by which steroid receptors regulate transcription of target genes:

1. Ligand-dependent and requiring direct binding of steroid receptors to HREs in promoter DNA (as described above and illustrated in Figs. 20–3 and 20–4);
2. Ligand-dependent but not requiring direct binding to DNA; and
3. Ligand-independent action.

Most hormone-regulated genes have ligand-dependent binding to HREs. Examples of target genes regulated in this fashion are prostate-specific antigen (PSA) and prostate-specific membrane antigen (PSMA). However, in some target genes, ligand-activated ER regulates transcription, without contacting the DNA directly, through protein–protein interaction with other transcription factors that are in direct contact with DNA via their own specific response elements. For example, ERα can interact with Sp1 and AP-1 transcription factors and regulate transcription of some genes.

Ligand-independent activation of ER and AR can occur through crosstalk with a variety of growth factor networks. Growth factors such as epidermal growth factor (EGF) and/or insulin-like growth factor (IGF)-I bind to their respective tyrosine kinase receptors located in the plasma membrane of target cells and activate signal transduction pathways involving activation of other kinases (see Chap. 8, Sec. 8.2); these events can lead to phosphorylation of steroid receptors. One enzyme activated by growth factor signaling that can phosphorylate directly both ERs as well as the AR is *mitogen activated protein kinase* (MAPK) (Ueda et al, 2002). Similarly, interleukin-6 and protein kinase A can activate AR and ERα directly in the absence of the appropriate steroid ligand. Interleukin-6 may bind to and influence AR activity without inducing phosphorylation of the AR (Ueda et al, 2002). Growth factor/phosphorylation pathways can also influence steroid hormone receptor pathways via their ability to modulate coactivators by phosphorylation (Han et al, 2009). These alternative pathways for regulation of ER and AR activity could have a profound influence on the emergence of hormone independence in tumors that have not lost their hormone receptors (see Sec. 20.5.5).

20.2.8 Nontranscriptional Actions of Steroid Receptors

There is evidence that not all effects of steroid hormones are mediated via the regulation of genomic or transcriptional events (Kelly and Levin, 2001). Transcription-independent effects of estrogen manifest themselves as rapid responses in target cells of the order of seconds to a few minutes. For estrogen, examples of nongenomic effects include modulation of calcium ion flux, effects on membrane channels in the central nervous system and peripheral excitable cells, membrane-associated interactions with growth factor receptors, and interactions with survival/apoptosis pathways. There is evidence that membrane-associated ERs coupled to G proteins or nitric oxide-generating systems mediate some of these actions. At least 2 categories of membrane-based receptors may exist: one related to the classical intracellular ERα or ERβ (Kelly and Levin, 2001), and the other distinct from them (Nadal et al, 2000). Other steroid hormones such as progesterone and testosterone may also influence cells via related mechanisms (Kousteni et al, 2001).

The importance of nontranscriptional actions of estrogen in breast cancer in relation to estrogen-dependent signaling is not known. There are multiple levels of estrogen interaction with growth factor receptor kinases and the signal transduction pathways that they regulate. Therefore, nongenomic and genomic actions of estrogen are likely to be integrated with and complementary to each other. Unravelling this molecular complexity has important implications with respect to new therapeutic combinations and approaches (Arpino et al, 2008).

20.2.9 Quantification of Steroid Hormone Receptors

ER and PR are biomarkers in breast cancer. In particular, they help to predict the likelihood of response to endocrine therapy. In an unselected group of breast cancer patients with advanced disease, 30% to 40% will respond to endocrine therapy. However, patients whose tumors are both ER and PR negative have less than 10% chance of responding to endocrine therapy

while in patients selected for the presence of both ER and PR in their primary breast tumor, the response rate to endocrine therapy is 70% to 80%.

Approximately 90% of unselected men with prostate cancer will respond to endocrine therapy: AR provides no prognostic or diagnostic value since almost all tumors usually possess a functioning AR, and almost all men respond initially to androgen withdrawal.

ER and PR are measured routinely in breast tumor biopsies by immunohistochemistry (IHC) using well characterized, specific monoclonal antibodies, as outlined in Figure 20–7A. IHC methods (Fitzgibbons et al, 2010; Hammond et al, 2010) can determine whether the detected receptor is within tumor cells, and can show receptor heterogeneity in tumor tissue. An example of ER heterogeneity within a breast tumor is shown in Figure 20–7B. Heterogeneity refers to the observation that both ER+ and ER– breast cancer cells can be present to varying degrees within any breast cancer biopsy sample, in addition to the presence of other types of cells (vascular cells, infiltrating cells of the immune system, normal stromal fibroblasts, normal breast adipocytes, and normal breast epithelial cells). Semiquantitative methods have been used to evaluate ER and PR by IHC, but positive results are generally reported when more than 1% of tumor nuclei stain positively (Hammond et al, 2010). There is a correlation between benefit and increasing ER level, which can be achieved by combining the level of staining intensity with the percentage of tumor cells positively stained to give H-scores or Allred scores (Hammond et al, 2010). Results can vary amongst laboratories, especially in the low to middle range of the receptor spectrum, and guidelines for standard operating procedures for tissue collection, assay validation, quality control, and interpretation have been published (Fitzgibbons et al, 2010; Hammond et al, 2010).

ER and PR can also be assayed by measuring their mRNA. This is currently being assessed as part of a 21-gene expression analysis, known as Oncotype DX, using reverse-transcription and quantitative polymerase chain reaction technology (see Chap. 2, Sec. 2.2.5). This evaluation is only carried out by the company that developed the assay, which generates a recurrence score (RS) that helps predict the benefit of adding chemotherapy to hormonal therapy in women with ER+ breast cancer (Paik et al, 2006; Albain et al, 2010). The clinical utility of the Oncotype DX assay and other multigene assays is still being evaluated in prospective clinical trials (TAILORx [Trial Assessing Individualized Options for Treatment for Breast Cancer]; MINDACT [Microarray in Node-Negative and 1-3 Node Positive Disease May Avoid Chemotherapy Trial]) (Cardoso et al, 2008).

20.3 NATURAL HISTORY OF BREAST AND PROSTATE CANCER

20.3.1 Risk Factors for Breast Cancer

Female gender and increasing age are the major risk factors for human breast cancer. Also, factors that increase the cumulative

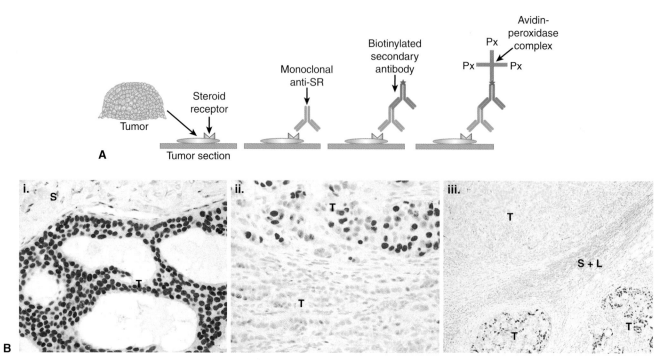

FIGURE 20-7 **Immunohistochemical–Avidin-biotin complex method. A)** Determination of hormone receptors in tumor tissue. Thin sections of tumor are cut from formalin-fixed, paraffin-embedded biopsy specimens. The section is next exposed to a monoclonal antibody specific for the steroid receptor (SR) being assessed. The section is then exposed to a second biotinylated antibody specific for the first antibody. Finally, avidin-peroxidase complex is added, followed by a chromogen, and color appears where the SR is located. **B)** Immunohistograms illustrating heterogeneity of human breast cancer biopsy samples. Brown staining represents ERα positivity. *T*, Invasive breast cancer; *S*, stromal and connective tissue elements; *L*, lymphocytes. (*i*) Homogenous expression of ERα within an invasive breast cancer, with negative adjacent vessels and stroma. (*ii*) Moderate heterogeneity of expression of ERα within an invasive breast cancer, with strong expression within solid nests of tumor cells in the upper field and weak or negative expression within less-cohesive clusters of tumor cells in the lower field. Stromal and lymphocytic elements are negative for ERα. (*iii*) Marked heterogeneity of expression of ERα within an invasive tumor metastatic to an axillary lymph node. In the upper part of the section one metastatic component is homogenously ERα –ve and in the lower part of the section the other component is moderate to highly ERα +ve. These 2 different elements are separated in this field of view by a band of fibrous stroma and infiltrating lymphocytes.

exposure and/or sensitivity of the breast epithelium to estrogen have been established as risk factors, including early menarche, late menopause, and obesity in postmenopausal women. Factors that reduce the cumulative exposure to estrogens, such as early first pregnancy, multiple full-term pregnancies, oophorectomy in premenopausal women, and physical activity, are associated with a reduced risk of breast cancer. Consistent with these observations, increased serum levels of estrogens are associated with postmenopausal breast cancer (Table 20–1). Use of hormone replacement therapies in menopausal women, particularly those that combine an estrogen and a progestin, also increase the risk of breast cancer (Banks et al, 2008).

Increased ER expression in normal breast epithelium is a risk factor for breast cancer (Khan et al, 1998), as is increased mammographic breast density (Martin et al, 2009) and increased circulating IGF-I levels (Key et al, 2010). These latter 2 factors are correlated and may be associated functionally (Becker and Kaaks, 2009). Estrogens have been shown to increase, and tamoxifen to decrease, mammographic density,

and the intimate association and crosstalk of the IGF-I signaling pathway with the ER signaling pathway in target cells may also play a role in the risk of breast cancer (Key et al, 2010).

Women with a family history of breast cancer are at increased risk of breast cancer and 2 genes, *BRCA1* and *BRCA2*, when carrying a germline mutation, are associated with an inherited predisposition to breast cancer (see Chap. 5, Sec. 5.3.4 and Chap. 7, Sec. 7.6.3). Only 5% of all breast cancer incidence can be attributed to inherited mutations in these genes and less than 10% of all breast cancer incidence can be attributed to an inherited predisposition. The importance of environmental factors is highlighted by the observation that the risk of breast cancer in Asian women rises over a few generations following migration to Western countries (Ziegler et al, 1993). Most breast cancers are sporadic, although polymorphisms in genes associated with the biosynthesis of estrogens (Thompson and Ambrosone, 2000) and factors that regulate ER activity such as AR (Giguere et al, 2001), may influence breast cancer development. Breast cancer risk is complex, probably because of the influence of multiple genes with the environment.

TABLE 20–1 Hormonally related epidemiological risk factors for breast cancer.

| Factor | Risk Group | | Relative Risk* |
	Low	High	
Sex	Male	Female	183
Oophorectomy	Age <35 y	No	2.5
Age at menarche	≥14 y	≤11 y	1.5
Age at first birth	<20 y	≥30 y	1.9
Parity	≥5 y	nulliparity	1.4
Age at natural menopause	<45 y	≥55 y	2.0
Obesity (BMI)[†]	<22.9	>30.7	1.6
Oral contraceptive use	Never	Ever	1.0
	Never	≥4 y before first pregnancy	1.7
Estrogen+ progestin replacement	Never	Ever >5 y	1.3
Dense mammogram[‡]	None	≥75% density	5.3

*Using low-risk group as a reference.
[†]Body mass index (kg/m^2).
[‡]Boyd et al, 2001.
Source: Adapted from Hulka et al, (1994).

The primary role of estrogen in breast cancer is thought to be because of its proliferative effect on breast epithelium. A complex interplay of steroid hormones, growth factors, extracellular matrix, and their respective receptors is likely involved. Genotoxic effects of steroids cannot be excluded, although the relative roles of the different mechanisms remain unclear (Lin et al, 2009; Pauklin et al, 2009).

20.3.2 Development of Breast Cancer

Some of the cellular events associated with the natural history of breast cancer are illustrated in Figure 20–8A. Most invasive breast cancers arise from the epithelial cells of the terminal duct lobular unit (TDLU). Histopathological studies have identified a series of premalignant breast lesions referred to as hyperplasia without atypia, usual ductal hyperplasia (UDH), atypical hyperplasia (AH), and ductal carcinoma in situ (DCIS). These lesions are associated with increasing risks of developing invasive breast cancer. For example, AH is associated with a 5-fold increased risk, and DCIS is associated with a 10-fold increased risk (Page et al, 2000). Comparisons between premalignant and/or preinvasive lesions in the same biopsy sample as invasive breast cancers have identified common genetic abnormalities, suggesting that the malignant lesions are clonally derived from the earlier lesions (Allred and Mohsin, 2000; Gong et al, 2001).

Although normal development of the mammary gland is dependent on the presence of ERα and only a rudimentary ductal remnant is present in "knockout" mice that do not have the ERα gene (Korach, 1994), only 7% to 17% of normal breast epithelial cells express ERα (Clarke et al, 1997). In contrast more than 70% of human breast tumors are ERα+, and often the level of ERα expression in tumor cells is higher than that found in normal breast luminal epithelial cells. Most hyperplastic lesions, with or without atypia, show increased expression of ERα and increased frequency of ER+ cells compared to normal epithelium, and more than 70% of DCIS are ERα+, similar to invasive breast cancer (Allred and Mohsin, 2000). In normal breast epithelial cells, ERα and Ki67, a marker of cell proliferation, are rarely, if ever, coexpressed (Anderson et al, 1998), suggesting that either ERα-expressing cells are incapable of proliferating or that ERα must be downregulated before normal breast epithelial cells can proliferate. This inverse relationship is maintained in UDH, but is lost in AH, DCIS, and ERα+ invasive breast cancer cells (Shoker et al, 1999). Thus an alteration in estrogen responsiveness and/or mechanism of estrogen action occurs during the development of breast cancer.

The second ER, ERβ, is also expressed in both normal and neoplastic human breast tissues (Leygue et al, 1998; Roger et al, 2001). Unlike ERα, ERβ does not play a pivotal role in development of the mammary gland as "knockout" mice for ERβ have normal development of the mammary gland (Couse and Korach, 1999). Expression of ERβ is much more frequent than ERα in normal human and rodent mammary glands, and its expression generally declines during breast cancer development (Leygue et al, 1998; Roger et al, 2001). Altered expression of several coregulators of ERα occurs during breast tumorigenesis (Murphy et al, 2000; Gojis et al, 2010) with a general trend toward increased expression of known coactivators and

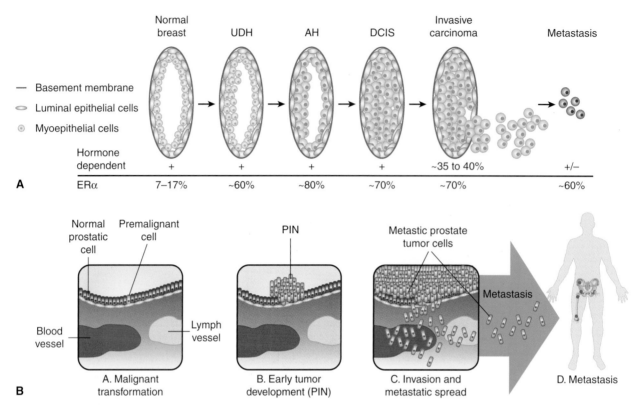

FIGURE 20-8   An overview of the natural history of cancers of the breast and the prostate. A) Normal breast epithelium can undergo a stepwise transition from a series of premalignant breast lesions referred to as hyperplasia without atypia/usual ductal hyperplasia (UDH), atypical hyperplasia (AH), and ductal carcinoma in situ (DCIS) leading to invasive carcinoma and metastasis (adapted from Myal et al, 2010). The relative hormonal dependency and receptor status at the various stages are indicated. **B)** A normal prostate epithelial cell can develop into a premalignant tumor cell that can give rise to prostatic intraepithelial neoplasia (PIN), and then become an invasive carcinoma.

decreased expression of known corepressors; this observation suggests that a marked upregulation of ERα signaling occurs during breast tumorigenesis.

Growth suppression pathways associated with transforming growth factor (TGF)-β (see Chap. 8, Sec. 8.4.4) are altered in some early lesions. For example TGF-β receptor type II is highly expressed in normal breast epithelium, but is downregulated in some UDH lesions and identifies a group of women at higher risk of developing breast cancer (Gobbi et al, 1999). Altered growth factor pathways that stimulate the cell cycle, for example overexpression of human epidermal growth receptor 2 (HER2) (neu/erbB-2) and cyclin D_1, and/or inactivation of tumor-suppressor genes such as p53, can be detected in some premalignant lesions such as DCIS (Allred and Mohsin, 2000; see Chap. 7, Secs. 7.5.3 and 7.6.1).

Breast cancer is extremely heterogeneous, as defined by the great variability that is seen in morphology, gene expression patterns, and behavior of individual tumor cells within any given tumor (Campbell and Polyak, 2007). The origin of this heterogeneity and the target cell(s) of origin of breast cancer are unknown, but 2 hypotheses that are not mutually exclusive have been suggested: the cancer stem or initiating cell and the clonal evolution hypotheses (see Chap. 13, Sec. 13.2). Substantial progress in defining the normal human mammary

stem cell and the mammary epithelial hierarchy has been made at the molecular and functional levels (Eirew et al, 2008; Visvader, 2009). Despite the importance of ERα signaling in human breast cancer and in the normal development of the mammary gland, normal mammary stem cells and/or populations enriched for stem cell repopulating characteristics, appear not to express ERα or PR, supporting the idea that at least in the normal mammary gland the effect of steroid hormones on proliferation is indirect. Expression of ERα seems to appear within the mammary epithelial hierarchy at the committed luminal progenitor stage (Visvader, 2009) and the expression of PR may occur earlier than this stage in the common-bipotent epithelial progenitor cells (Raouf et al, 2008). Support for the existence of a population of human breast cancer cells with cancer initiating/stem cell-like characteristics is emerging (Al-Hajj et al, 2003; Eirew et al, 2008; Lim et al, 2009; Korkaya et al, 2011; see Chap. 13, Sec. 13.4.5), but whether the target cell for breast cancer is the normal mammary stem cell or other cells along the mammary epithelial hierarchy is unknown. The use of molecular signatures from molecular expression analysis is helping to resolve such issues, as there are now data linking newly identified breast cancer subtypes (Fig. 20–9, discussed below) with their closest normal mammary epithelial counterpart based on similarities of

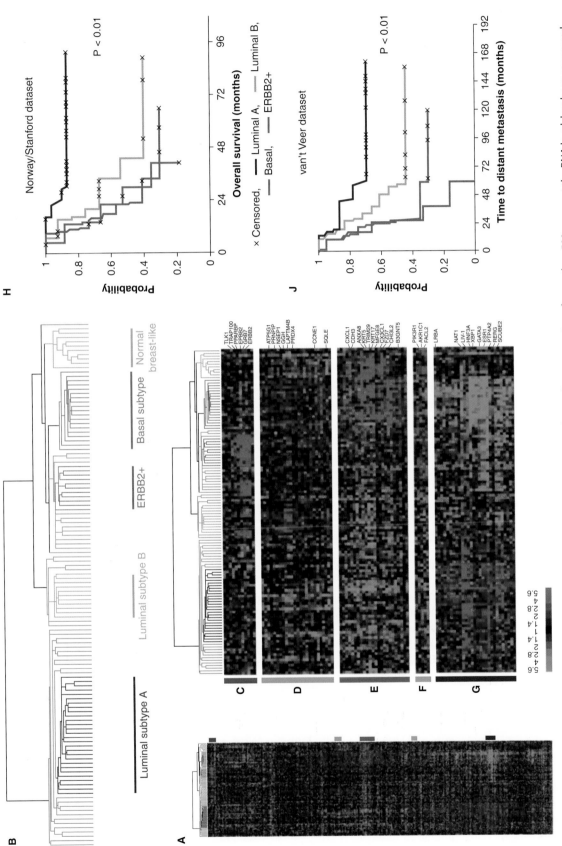

FIGURE 20–9 **Molecular subtypes of breast tumors. A)** Gene expression microarray analyses where expression of more than 500 genes, at the RNA level, has been measured in 122 different breast tissue samples (115 tumors, 7 non-malignant). Each column represents one breast sample, and each row represents the expression level of one gene. The scale bar represents the fold-change for any given gene relative to the median level of expression of all samples. Green is decreased and red is increased expression. **B)** Dendrogram of the heirarchical clustering of the tissues with respect to similarities in their gene expression patterns, into 5 subgroups shown by the different colors (*dark blue,* luminal A; *aqua-blue,* luminal B; *purple,* ERBB2+; *orange,* basal like; *green,* normal breast-like). Tumors with low correlations to these 5 subtypes are shown in gray. **C)** Gene cluster showing ERBB2 oncogene and co-expressed genes. **D)** Gene cluster associated with luminal subtype B. **E)** Gene cluster associated with the basal subtype. **F)** Gene cluster relevant for the normal breast-like group. **G)** Cluster of genes including the estrogen receptor (ESR1) highly expressed in luminal subtype A tumors. This classification is associated with different clinical outcomes as illustrated by Kaplan-Meier analyses from 2 different datasets shown in H and J where the colors of the survival curves correspond to those of the molecular subtypes. **H)** Overall survival for 72 patients with locally advanced breast cancer. **J)** Time to development of distal recurrence in 97 patients in another study (Adapted from Sorlie et al, 2003).

gene expression profiles (Visvader, 2009). However, it is also possible that cancer-initiating cells could be derived from mutation of tissue-specific progenitors or more differentiated cells which, because of mutation, acquire self-renewal capacity (Hershkowitz, 2010).

20.3.3 Progression of Invasive Breast Cancer

Amplification and upregulation of expression of several oncogenes, including those encoding growth factors such as EGF, TGF-α, IGF, and their receptor tyrosine kinases, for example, EGFR, HER2 (neu/erbB-2), and IGFR, together with inactivation or downregulation of tumor-suppressor genes, such as p53, Rb, or BRCA1, have been associated with breast cancer progression. The introduction of comparative genomic hybridization (CGH), fluorescence in situ hybridization (FISH), spectral karyotyping (SKY), DNA microarrays, and next-generation sequencing (Shah et al, 2009; see Chap. 2) is allowing a more global analysis of the molecular genetic alterations that occur during cancer progression.

Prognosis of patients with invasive breast cancer is related to lymph node involvement, tumor size, histological grade, and steroid receptor status. Approximately 70% of all primary invasive breast tumors are ER+, and in general, these tumors are more differentiated, less aggressive, and have lower levels of growth factor receptors compared to ER− tumors. In contrast, consistent evidence has accumulated to show that young patients (younger than age 40 years) with ER+ tumors have a worse prognosis than those with ER− tumors (Aebi, 2005).

Not only is ER status a prognostic factor, but it also is a marker of response to treatment, as is discussed subsequently. Until recently, the only molecular classifiers of breast cancers were ERα, PR, and HER2/ErbB2. ERα and overexpressed/amplified HER2 are the targets of endocrine therapies and the humanized antibody trastuzumab, respectively. HER2/ErbB2 is amplified and/or overexpressed in up to 20% of all breast tumors, and these tumors are aggressive with generally poor outcome, but the development of trastuzumab targeted to HER2 overexpressed protein has improved the outcome for these patients (Di Cosimo and Baselga, 2010). The advent of global molecular profiling technologies has led to a new way of classifying human breast cancer and is the basis of a more individualized approach to breast cancer prognostication and therapy. Most effort has focused on classification according to gene-expression profiling at the mRNA levels using microarray chip technology (Perou et al, 2000). However, a combination of transcriptomic, epigenetic, proteomic, and genomic analyses may be necessary to appreciate the true heterogeneity of breast cancer (Weigelt and Reis-Filho, 2009).

Despite the limitations outlined above, gene expression analysis has resulted in human breast tumors being classified into 5 different subtypes, with potentially a sixth recently identified (Visvader, 2009). The subtypes are called luminal A, luminal B, HER2 overexpressing, basal-like, normal breast-like (Sorlie, 2004) and, most recently, a claudin-low subtype has been described (Creighton et al, 2010). The different subtypes are clinically relevant as some are associated with different clinical outcomes (see Fig. 20–9). ERα and PR are only expressed in the luminal A and B subtypes, although about half of the HER2 overexpressing subtype also can express ERα. Furthermore, although alternative hypotheses cannot be excluded (Stingl and Caldas, 2007), the similarity of expression signatures to those represented in the mammary epithelial hierarchy may provide information concerning the cell of origin of the subtypes and identify the nature of the cancer-initiating cells such that new treatments can be designed to target them. However, these molecular classifications are research tools and are not used routinely in clinical practice, in contrast to the determination of ER, PR, and HER2 expression.

The triple negative (ERα-negative, PR-negative, and HER2-negative) group of tumors represents a challenge in breast cancer because of their lack of responsiveness to endocrine therapies and trastuzumab. These tumors are aggressive with increased risk of metastasis, but in some cases respond well to chemotherapy. The triple negative or basal-like subtype is itself heterogeneous, and a better understanding of the molecular heterogeneity of this subgroup is necessary to improve clinical outcome (Di Cosimo and Baselga, 2010). Most breast cancers arising from *BRCA1* mutation carriers are triple negative (Podo et al, 2010), whereas most breast cancers arising from *BRCA2* mutation carriers are ER+ and have a luminal molecular profile (Bane et al, 2007).

A proportion of all tumor subgroups, despite originally responding to treatment, will recur and progress, having acquired resistance to targeted therapies. Most ER+ tumors treated with endocrine therapies develop resistance despite the continued expression of ERα. Mechanisms of resistance to endocrine therapies are discussed below, but a challenge is to identify biomarkers that predict early resistance to endocrine therapy so that either more aggressive therapy can be used sooner, or a rational combination of therapies can be given. The use of new technologies that allow a more global analysis of the molecular and genetic alterations occurring in tumors holds promise with respect to achieving this goal (Wood et al, 2007).

20.3.4 Risk Factors for Prostate Cancer

Carcinogenesis of the prostate involves genetic and environmental influences with no obvious etiological agent. Risk factors include family history, age, and race (Hsing and Chokkalingam, 2006). First-degree male relatives of prostate cancer patients have an approximately 2.5-fold increase in risk, and the risk of prostate cancer appears to be higher for relatives of women with breast cancer. Men carrying a germline *BRCA2* mutation have increased risk of developing a more aggressive prostate cancer by 3.2-fold compared with noncarriers (Gallagher et al, 2010). However, hereditary factors most commonly affect men with early onset disease and are responsible for relatively few cases (<10%). Diet is probably important, with the predominantly vegetarian diet of Asians providing a protective influence, whereas the high intake of red meat associated with a typical American diet is likely related to increased risk (Denis et al, 1999). Epidemiological studies have linked obesity with a range of cancer types, although its role in the development and progression of prostate cancer has not been elucidated. The association of obesity with numerous hormonal changes that influence endocrine pathways may contribute to prostate cancer development and progression (Calle and Kaaks, 2004).

Prostate cancer is a disease of the elderly, with more than 75% of cancers diagnosed in men older than 65 years of age. However, microfoci of high-grade prostatic intraepithelial neoplasia (PIN), the presumed precursor of the disease, can be found in men in their third and fourth decade of life (see Fig. 20–8B). Most of the early tumors are microscopic, generally well to moderately differentiated, and tend to be multifocal. The frequency with which these neoplastic lesions are seen in autopsy material is similar among African Americans, white Americans, and Japanese men, but the incidence of clinical disease is higher in African American men and lower in Japanese men. In Japanese immigrants, the incidence of prostate cancer rises to levels near those of white Americans within 2 generations, suggesting the involvement of environmental factors. Collectively these observations suggest that the critical event in the natural history of prostate cancer is tumor promotion rather than tumor initiation, and that promotion and progression of this cancer are strongly influenced by epigenetic or adaptive processes.

20.3.5 Development of Prostate Cancer

Two pathological conditions that frequently coexist with latent and clinical prostate cancer are benign prostatic hyperplasia (BPH) and PIN. BPH shares many biological properties with prostate cancer, including androgen regulation of growth and increasing prevalence with advancing age. However, BPH is neither a premalignant lesion nor a precursor of invasive prostate cancer. A more likely candidate for this role is PIN, which is characterized by cytological atypia of proliferating luminal epithelium within preexisting acini and ducts with no penetration of the basement membrane (see Fig. 20–8B). Histologically, PIN is generally subdivided into low or high grade and autopsy studies reveal that high-grade PIN is found in association with cancer in 60% to 95% of malignant prostates and that a wide spectrum of molecular/genetic abnormalities are common to both high grade PIN and prostate cancer (Sakr and Partin, 2001). Specific chromosomal alterations (eg, loss of 8p, 10q, 16q, 18q, and gain of 7q31, 8q), amplification of the c-myc gene, along with changes in telomerase activity, cell-cycle status, and proliferative indices, suggest, collectively, that high-grade PIN is intermediate between benign epithelium and prostatic carcinoma (Sakr and Partin, 2001). A related staining profile for growth factors and for the AR has been demonstrated in the luminal epithelium of high-grade PIN and in carcinoma, with a tendency to higher expression of membrane EGFR, c-erbB-2, and cytoplasmic TGF-α, and

lower levels of fibroblast growth factor (FGF)-2, than in glands with low-grade PIN or BPH (Harper et al, 1998). In addition to being a precursor for prostate cancer, it is likely that PIN predates invasive cancer by at least a decade and thus may serve as a predictive marker for the disease.

Although uncertain, prostate and other cancers may arise as a consequence of genetic alterations in a stem cell population (Lawson and Witte, 2007). Indeed, their longevity makes stem cells more likely to develop genetic alterations over time that may eventually culminate in cancer. Moreover, unlike mature prostate cells, primitive stem cells can thrive under androgen depletion, and it has been shown that these cells can subsequently regenerate prostate tissues with androgen stimulation. These castration-resistant cells were found originally to be of basal origin (Mulholland et al, 2009); however, the recent finding in mice of a luminal stem cell population that displays castration-resistant characteristics during prostate regeneration (Wang et al, 2009) suggests that there may be at least 2 different cell types that play a role in the development of castration-resistant phenotypes. However, only a small proportion of cancer cells within a tumor may possess stem cell properties (see Chap. 13, Sec. 13.4). These findings may be of critical importance to identify novel therapeutic approaches for future clinical management.

20.3.6 Progression of Invasive Prostate Cancer

When organ confined, prostate cancer is potentially curable by prostatectomy or radiation therapy. The problem here is selecting patients who need such treatment, as many will never develop symptomatic disease, whereas others will have occult metastases. In men with locally advanced or metastatic disease, treatment is largely palliative with androgen withdrawal as first-line treatment. The clinical approaches used for androgen withdrawal are described below. Despite high initial response rates on the order of 80%, patients will inevitably progress to hormone-independent disease in a manner analogous to that seen following hormonal therapy for metastatic breast cancer. Response to androgen ablation therapies depends on the degree of retention by the tumor of the capacity for activation of apoptosis after androgen withdrawal. However, many so-called hormone-independent cancers may in fact still be dependent on androgens, but resistant to medical or surgical castration, hence the term *"castration-resistant"* prostate cancer (CRPC).

20.4 HORMONAL THERAPIES FOR BREAST AND PROSTATE CANCERS

20.4.1 Breast Cancer

Endocrine therapies for patients with breast cancer are aimed at inhibiting the proliferative effect of estrogen on breast cancer cells. As outlined in Figure 20–2A, this aim is generally achieved in 2 ways: decreasing the level of circulating and/or

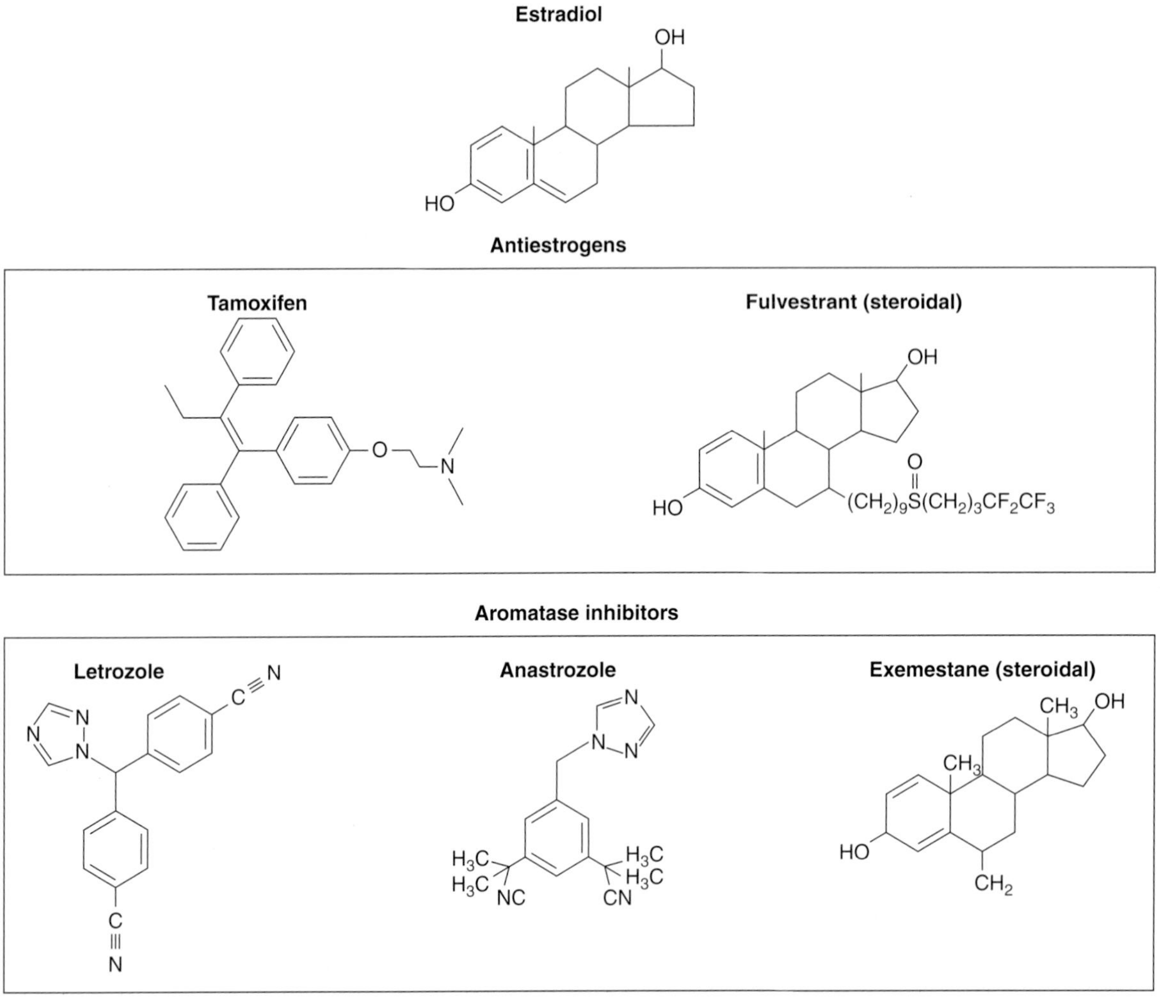

Estradiol

Antiestrogens

Tamoxifen

Fulvestrant (steroidal)

$(CH_2)_9S(CH_2)_3CF_2CF_3$

Aromatase inhibitors

Letrozole

Anastrozole

Exemestane (steroidal)

FIGURE 20–10 **Structures of antiestrogens and aromatase inhibitors.** The antiestrogens block estrogen binding to its receptor and the steroidal forms also increase turnover of the receptor protein. The aromatase inhibitors block the formation of estrogens from androgen precursors.

local estrogen, or blocking the action of estrogen on the target tissue. Only those breast tumors that express ER benefit from endocrine therapies.

Reduced levels of estrogen can be achieved surgically, by oophorectomy, and pharmacologically. In premenopausal women, options are surgical or radiation-induced oophorectomy, or the use of LHRH agonists, which initially stimulate and then block the LHRH receptor in the pituitary gland. This approach leads to a reduction in levels of gonadotrophins, which stimulate the ovary to synthesize estrogens.

In postmenopausal women, residual levels of estrogen can be reduced by selective aromatase inhibitors that inhibit the conversion of weak androgens to estrogens (see Fig. 20–1). As shown in Figure 20–10, aromatase inhibitors fall into 2 main classes—the steroidal (eg, exemestane) and the nonsteroidal (eg, anastrozole and letrozole). The 2 classes differ in their mechanism of action. The steroidal inhibitors compete with endogenous substrates for the active site of the enzyme, and are processed to intermediates that bind irreversibly to the active site, causing inhibition. The nonsteroidal inhibitors also compete with the endogenous substrates for the active site, but

form a strong, although reversible, coordinate bond with the heme iron atom, excluding endogenous substrates and oxygen from the enzyme. Removal of the nonsteroidal inhibitor results in reversal of enzyme inhibition. These agents are alternatives to tamoxifen (see below) as first-line treatment of postmenopausal women. Aromatase inhibitors are not effective alone in premenopausal women with ER+ breast cancer because the aromatase inhibitor-induced reduction in plasma estrogen increases follicle-stimulating hormone (FSH), which can override the block as a result of inhibition of aromatase, and eventually lead to increased estrogen from the ovary. Use of aromatase inhibitors, after oophorectomy or LHRH agonists have induced menopause, in premenopausal women is being evaluated (Di Cosimo and Baselga, 2010). Progestins, such as megestrol acetate, are useful as third-line endocrine therapies in breast cancer, and part of their mechanism of action could include the increased expression and/or activity of enzymes, which can metabolize strong estrogens into weaker compounds.

The nonsteroidal antiestrogen, tamoxifen has been the agent of choice for first-line endocrine therapy for the treatment of ER-positive and/or PR-positive breast cancer

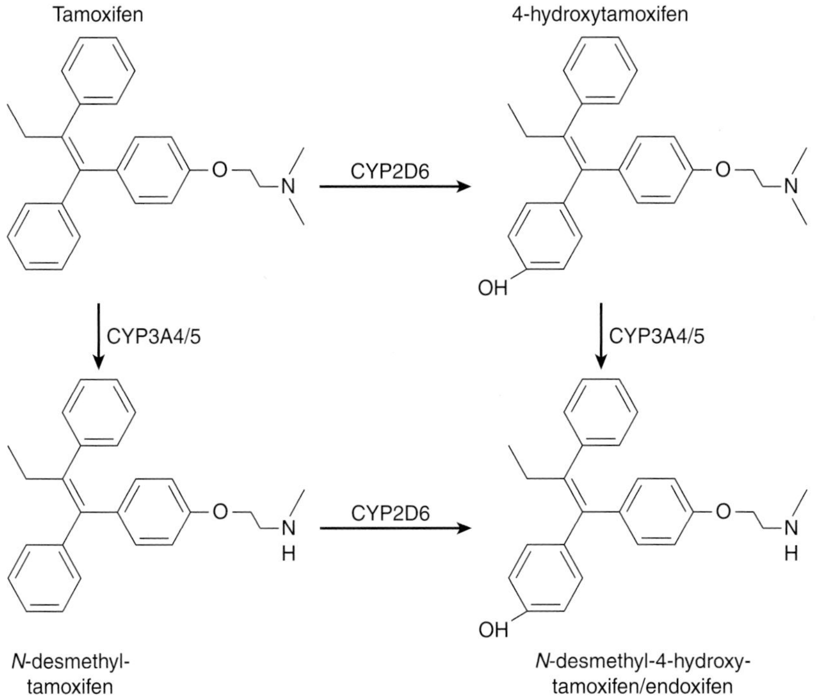

FIGURE 20–11 Metabolism of tamoxifen to more active metabolites such as 4-hydroxytamoxifen and *N*-desmethy-4-hydroxytamoxifen (endoxifen).

(see Fig. 20–10). It leads to improved survival when used as adjuvant therapy for women with receptor-positive breast cancer of all ages, and may decrease the incidence of breast cancer in groups of women at high risk for the disease. Tamoxifen and its more active metabolites, 4-hydroxy-tamoxifen and 4-hydroxy-desmethytamoxifen (endoxifen), competitively inhibit the binding of estradiol to the ligand-binding site of the ER in a dose-dependent manner (see Fig. 20–3). Because tamoxifen requires metabolism to more active metabolites, alterations in the activity of the enzymes responsible for its metabolism (Fig. 20–11) may affect an individual patient's responsiveness to tamoxifen. This possibility is discussed in more detail later.

When tamoxifen or similar compounds bind to the ER, they result in conformational changes that allow the inactive receptor to bind to DNA but not to activate transcription (see Fig. 20–4). X-ray crystallography studies of the ER ligand domain bound to either estradiol or 4-hydroxy-tamoxifen, show that estradiol binding causes formation of a hydrophobic cleft on the surface of this domain which serves as a docking site for coactivators. In contrast, antiestrogens displace part of the receptor, blocking this site, and therefore blocking coactivator access (Shiau et al, 1998). Compounds like tamoxifen have both estrogenic and antiestrogenic properties, depending on the cell type or the promoter of any particular target gene. Tamoxifen has estrogenic effects in bone and in cardiovascular tissue (which are desirable to prevent osteoporosis and cardiac disease) and in the uterus (which is undesirable, as it may stimulate proliferation and lead to a low incidence of uterine cancer). Compounds with different selectivity in their estrogenic and antiestrogenic properties are referred to collectively as selective estrogen receptor

modulators (SERMs). The basis of their differences is in the slightly different conformational changes that they induce in the ER, leading to differential abilities to interact with a variety of coregulators, whose expression and/or activation will vary between cell types and tissues, as illustrated in Figure 20–12 (McKenna and O'Malley, 2000). Because breast tumors often develop resistance to tamoxifen without loss of ER expression, and because tamoxifen has undesirable estrogenic properties in the uterus, other SERMs are being investigated for their usefulness in breast cancer treatment and prevention. For example, raloxifene is a SERM that has estrogenic effects on bone and the cardiovascular system, but is antiestrogenic in the breast and uterus (O'Regan and Jordan, 2001). A clinical trial (Study of Tamoxifen and Raloxifene [STAR]) has found it to have comparable efficacy to tamoxifen in breast cancer prevention in high risk women, without increasing the risk of endometrial cancer (Vogel et al, 2006).

Steroidal antiestrogens, such as fulvestrant (see Fig. 20–10), that show little if any estrogenic activity (in particular in the uterus) retain activity in some women whose breast cancers have acquired resistance to tamoxifen. The mechanism of action of these "pure" antiestrogens is distinct from the partial antiestrogens such as tamoxifen, in that they downregulate ER expression by increasing its degradation, as well as inactivate the ER complex (O'Regan and Jordan, 2001). Such compounds have been named selective estrogen receptor downregulators (SERDs). Because of its steroidal nature, fulvestrant is not suitable for oral administration and is administered by intramuscular injection, which is a disadvantage. High-dose progestin treatment that is used as a third-line endocrine treatment may also act partially by downregulating expression of the ER in breast tumors.

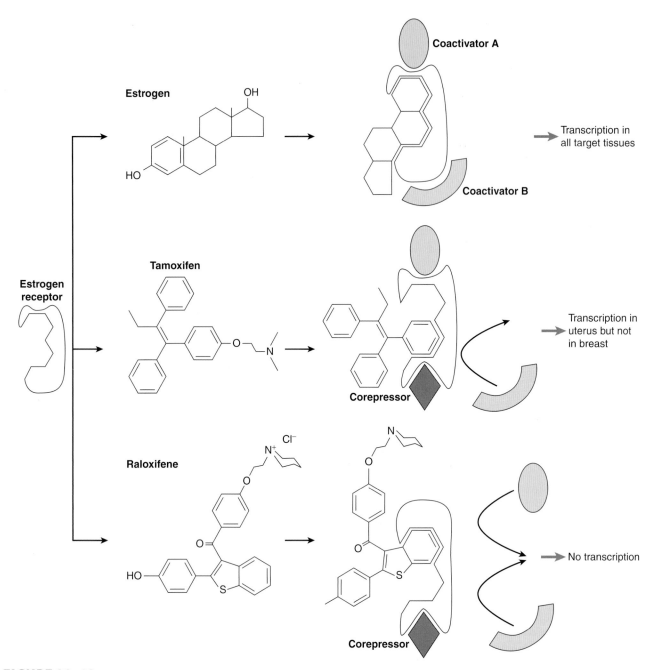

FIGURE 20–12 **Schematic of conformational changes induced by different SERMs (estrogen, tamoxifen, and raloxifene) resulting in differential recruitment of coregulators and differential activity.** Estrogen binds to the estrogen receptor (ER) causing a conformational change that leads to docking of appropriate coactivators (hypothetical coactivator A and coactivator B) with ER in all target tissues and resulting in enhanced transcription of target genes. Tamoxifen binds to ER giving rise to a different conformation such that it docks coactivator A and a hypothetical corepressor that in one tissue (breast) inhibits estrogen action, but in another tissue partially activates estrogen action (uterus). Another SERM called *raloxifene* binds to ER, resulting in a different conformation such that it only docks the corepressor and inhibits estrogen action in both target tissues.

20.4.2 Hormonal Therapy for Different Stages of Breast Cancer

Systemic adjuvant therapy given after surgical removal of the primary tumor is aimed at eliminating subclinical, micrometastatic cancer cell deposits that have spread from the original tumor site. Adjuvant hormonal therapies, such as tamoxifen or ovarian ablation in premenopausal women and tamoxifen or aromatase inhibitors (given for 5 years) in postmenopausal women with breast cancer, have been shown to increase both relapse-free and overall survival of women with ER+ early breast cancer, when used either alone, or following adjuvant chemotherapy (Early Breast Cancer Trialists' Collaborative Group, 2005). The hormonal therapies are also used to treat metastatic breast cancer, which is not curable, and the goals of therapy are to prolong survival and to maximize the quality of life of the patient. The hormonal treatments are often used in sequence, and women who respond to initial endocrine treatment have approximately a 50% chance of responding to a second agent, while other hormonal agents, including megestrol acetate and fulvestrant, may lead to further responses when used as third-line treatment in selected patients. Despite the responsiveness of advanced ER+ breast cancer to initial endocrine therapy, tumors eventually develop resistance to all forms of endocrine therapy. The multiple mechanisms thought to be involved in resistance to hormonal therapy are explored in Section 20.5.

Neoadjuvant (preoperative) endocrine therapy (with or without chemotherapy) is also used in some patients to reduce the size of the primary breast cancer, thereby increasing the possibility of breast-conserving surgery and allowing assessment of response to treatment in primary tumors.

20.4.3 New Approaches to Hormonal Treatment of Breast Cancer

Genomic molecular profiles (mutation and expression analyses) of human breast tumors can identify key activated pathways in ER+ tumors to provide a rational basis for using combinations of therapies in the most appropriate patients (Johnston, 2010). Several clinical trials of combinations of endocrine therapies with targeted biological agents are ongoing. The use of pharmacogenetics (see Chap. 18, Sec. 18.1.3) to identify those patients more likely to have adverse side effects or less likely to benefit from a particular treatment or combination of treatments is another important focus in cancer therapy. A more precise understanding of the mechanisms responsible for resistance to different endocrine therapies, may also lead to changes in sequencing and scheduling of treatment. For example, a potential mechanism for the development of resistance to aromatase inhibitors is upregulation of growth factor and survival pathways, and this resistance might be reversed by periods of time off treatment, in contrast to continuous treatment.

20.4.4 Prostate Cancer

Approximately 80% of patients with metastatic prostate cancer will respond to androgen withdrawal therapy, as indicated by a fall in the serum marker of the disease, PSA, and by an improvement in symptoms (most often pain caused by metastases in bone). Such treatment is associated with a median progression-free survival of 1 to 2 years and overall survival of 2 to 4 years. The failure to eradicate the entire malignant population by androgen withdrawal results in progression to castration resistance, as manifested by a rising serum PSA and/or clinical signs and symptoms. The goal of any form of androgen withdrawal therapy is to activate apoptosis or block cell proliferation in prostate tumor cells by inhibiting androgen-dependent signaling (see Fig. 20–2B). There are several methods for achieving androgen withdrawal, either by interfering with the synthesis or metabolic conversion of androgens or with their ability to interact with the AR. However, as most castration-resistant prostate tumors have normal or elevated levels of AR, there is no prognostic value in measuring these receptors.

Bilateral orchiectomy (castration) is the most direct way to block androgen stimulation of the prostate and has the advantages of low morbidity, low cost, and high compliance. However, the associated psychological problems have decreased its practice in favor of medical castration using LHRH agonists. LHRH agonists include goserelin, leuprolide, and buserelin, which can be administered as long-acting (3 to 4 months) formulations to block the secretion of LH by the pituitary gland and thereby inhibit the synthesis of testosterone by the testis (see Fig. 20–2B). Initially, LHRH agonists cause a rise in LH and testosterone that is termed a *"flare" response*; this effect is avoided by temporary coadministration of an antiandrogen to inhibit AR signaling in the tumor cell. A rising serum PSA level is usually the earliest manifestation of progression following initial endocrine therapy, often predating clinical evidence of progression by more than 6 months.

Antiandrogens, some of which are shown in Figure 20–13, act competitively with testicular or adrenal androgens to block AR activation within the prostate cell (see Fig. 20–3) and apart from transient use to prevent the flare associated with LHRH agonists, are usually added as second-line hormonal therapy at time of progression. Nonsteroidal antiandrogens, such as flutamide or bicalutamide (Fig. 20–13), have no gonadotropic or hypothalamic feedback activity to suppress circulating levels of testosterone, whereas steroidal antiandrogens such as cyproterone acetate do possess this feedback activity (see Fig. 20–2B). Approximately 30% of patients who have responded and then progressed after initial hormone therapy will respond to the subsequent addition of an antiandrogen. At the time of progression following this treatment, discontinuation of the antiandrogen leads to further response in approximately 20% of patients. The underlying molecular mechanism responsible for the antiandrogen withdrawal syndrome is not fully understood, but may relate to altered AR ligand specificity. A new, more potent nonsteroidal antiandrogen, called enzalutamide (MDV3100), has been developed. Enzalutamide binds the AR with greater affinity than bicalutamide, impairs its nuclear translocation, and may have negative effects on the binding of AR to androgen response elements and the recruitment of coactivators. The results of Phase II trials showed that enzalutamide had substantial antitumor effect in men who had progressed during or after treatment with first-generation antiandrogens, with few side effects (Tran et al, 2009; Scher et al, 2010). A randomized Phase III trial has shown that enzalutamide improves the survival of men with castrate-resistant prostate cancer, whose disease has progressed after receiving chemotherapy (Scher et al, 2012).

Other second- or third-line strategies include the use of ketoconazole to inhibit steroid synthesis in general, although this drug is likely to be replaced by abiraterone acetate, which is a more specific and potent inhibitor of androgen synthesis (see Fig. 20–13, see also Sec. 20.5.3). Abiraterone acetate has shown a

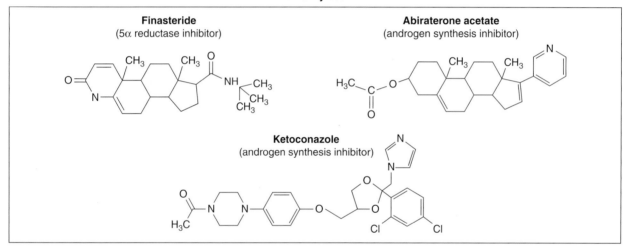

FIGURE 20-13 **Structures of antiandrogens and antienzymes that block androgen metabolism.** The antiandrogens block androgen binding to its receptor. The antienzymes inhibit the conversion of testosterone to the more active form dihydrotestosterone (5α reductase inhibitors) or block androgen synthesis (ketoconazole and abiraterone acetate).

substantial improvement in time to disease progression of men with metastatic castrate-resistant prostate cancer, and improved survival when used to treat men with late-stage metastatic prostate cancer, who had progressed after receiving chemotherapy (de Bono et al, 2011; Ryan et al, 2012). Glucocorticoids, such as prednisone and hydrocortisone, can inhibit production of adrenocorticotropic hormone (ACTH), which leads to decreased production of weak androgens by the adrenal gland, and can also lead to tertiary responses (see Fig. 20-2B). Estrogens have also been used to suppress LH and FSH by feedback effects on the pituitary; they have rare therapeutic effects in patients who have already received several hormonal treatments and may have direct effects on prostate cancer cells, which express both ERα and ERβ. Irrespective of the type of androgen withdrawal treatment used, the side effects can include hot flushes, loss of libido and sexual potency, gynecomastia, lethargy, depression,

loss of bone and muscle mass, and metabolic syndrome with increased diabetes and cardiac events.

Many patients have received treatment with "complete androgen blockade," which combines orchiectomy or an LHRH agonist with a nonsteroidal antiandrogen. Although a metaanalysis of several trials comparing complete androgen blockade with conventional medical or surgical castration showed no significant survival advantage (Prostate Cancer Trialists' Collaborative Group, 2000), the advent of new more potent antiandrogens, such as enzalutamide, may help to improve survival.

20.4.5 Intermittent Hormonal Therapy for Prostate Cancer

In addition to acting as mitogens to induce DNA synthesis and cell proliferation, estrogens and androgens are potent

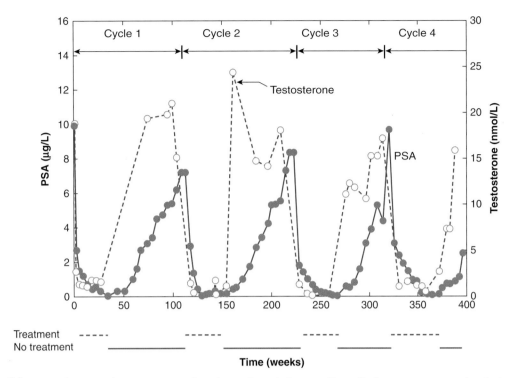

FIGURE 20–14 **Intermittent androgen suppression.** Approximately 8 years after radical prostatectomy and radiation treatment for positive surgical resection margins, the patient was started on a regimen of intermittent androgen suppression when his serum PSA had increased from a nadir of 0.6 μg/L to 10.4 μg/L. He was treated with a combination of antiandrogen (cyproterone acetate) and LHRH agonist (leuprolide acetate). The patient has undergone 4 cycles of androgen withdrawal and replacement over a period of more than 7 years. Open circles indicate serum testosterone values (nmol/L) and closed circles are serum levels of PSA (μg/L). (Used with permission from Dr. N. Bruchovsky.)

differentiating agents. In studies with castrated rodents, administration of small amounts of androgen was shown to induce markers of differentiation in the prostate without stimulating rounds of cell proliferation. This conditioning effect of androgens on surviving cells allowed them to retain desirable, hormone-regulated traits of differentiation, and the capacity to undergo apoptosis upon hormone withdrawal. Hence periodic exposure to hormones might maintain hormone responsiveness of prostate tumors. Figure 20–14 shows an idealized representation of how intermittent hormone suppression might regulate tumor growth.

The effectiveness of intermittent androgen suppression and replacement for delaying progression to androgen independence was first shown using the androgen-dependent Shionogi mouse mammary carcinoma (Akakura et al, 1993). With this tumor model, complete remissions are observed after androgen withdrawal, but invariably the disease recurs and is refractory to further hormonal manipulations. Because progression to androgen independence was linked to the cessation of androgen-induced differentiation of these stem cells, the effect of replacement of androgens at the end of a period of regression was tested by transplantation into noncastrated males (Akakura et al, 1993). This cycle of transplantation and castration-induced apoptosis was repeated and relative to one-time castration, intermittent androgen suppression approximately tripled the time to androgen independence. Other

experimental models of hormone-dependent prostate cancer have confirmed these effects.

Prospective clinical trials during the past 10 years have evaluated intermittent hormonal therapy and have found that intermittent treatment is at least as effective as continuous androgen suppression, while showing reduced treatment-related toxicity, lower cost, and improved quality of life, including recovery of sexual potency.

Androgen-deprivation therapy has been investigated before or after primary treatments for localized prostate cancer, such as prostatectomy or radiation therapy, or concurrent with radiation therapy. Initial hormone treatment can lead to a reduction in tumor size, but such therapy has not been shown to improve survival following radical surgery. However, the combination of radiation and hormonal therapy for locally advanced prostate cancer does prolong survival (Bolla et al, 2002; Warde et al, 2011).

20.4.6 New Hormone-Biological Therapies for Prostate Cancer

As described in Section 20.5.5, there may be a role for targeting those genes critical to cell survival (eg, TRPM-2, BCL-2, IGFBP-5) as enhancement of apoptotic cell kill might enhance the effects of androgen withdrawal and thereby delay time to recurrence and emergence of androgen independence.

Similarly, expression of the cell-survival protein clusterin is increased in prostate cancer in response to many treatments, including hormone ablation therapy, chemotherapy, and radiation therapy. Increased clusterin production is linked to faster rates of cancer progression, treatment resistance, shorter survival duration, and is closely correlated with increasing grade (ie, less differentiation), which is a strong prognostic factor for poor survival of patients with prostate cancer; thus clusterin is a possible target for tumor therapy. Several preclinical studies using androgen-regulated tumor models have demonstrated proof of principle that administration of antisense oligodeoxynucleotides is a viable approach to reducing activity of this and other survival factors, and these agents are being evaluated in clinical trials.

Understanding that progression to CRPC often occurs despite continued dependence on signaling from the AR (see Sec. 20.5) opens several doors to new therapeutic approaches, such as steroid enzyme inhibitors and more potent antiandrogens. Each enzyme involved in the androgen synthesis pathway, such as CYP17A1, may be a target for drug discovery. These agents could then be used in combination with existing AR antagonists and might increase the survival of patients.

20.4.7 Hormone and Chemoprevention Strategies for Prostate Cancer

Epidemiological studies of prostate cancer suggest that diet and lifestyle probably contribute more to prostate carcinogenesis than racial or familial factors. The observation that premalignant prostatic lesions (PIN) occur with almost equal frequency in different racial populations with both high and low risk of prostate cancer implies that a limiting step is progression from subclinical to locally invasive carcinoma. Also, there is considerable evidence that androgen stimulation over a long period of time is a necessary prerequisite for prostate cancer and therefore an obvious target in any chemoprevention strategy.

Clinical trials using tamoxifen as a chemopreventive agent for breast cancer in high-risk groups of women have provided a paradigm for using drugs that block androgen action and thereby prevent the emergence of prostate cancer. Drugs that show promise are the antiandrogen bicalutamide and the 5α-reductase inhibitors finasteride and its analog dutasteride (see Fig. 20–13), which block the intracellular metabolism of testosterone to the more potent DHT (see Fig. 20–3). The toxicity of antiandrogens such as bicalutamide (gynecomastia, gastrointestinal toxicity, etc) poses concerns for application in prevention studies, but the toxicity profiles of finasteride and dutasteride are more favorable. A Phase III trial of finasteride in 18,000 men older than 50 years of age has shown a cumulative reduction of 25% at 7 years of treatment in early stage, organ-confined, low-grade prostate cancer, but there was concern that use of finasteride was associated with increased prevalence of higher-grade disease (Thompson et al, 2003). A retrospective study of men involved in this study showed that finasteride may have contributed a bias toward the detection of high-grade disease by improving the performance characteristics of PSA and of prostate biopsies (Elliott et al, 2009). Similarly, a 4-year study showed that men receiving a daily dose of dutasteride reduced their incidence of developing cancer (although it did not reduce the development of the more lethal high-grade cancers) and improved the outcomes related to BPH (Andriole et al, 2010).

20.5 MECHANISMS FOR PROGRESSION TO HORMONE INDEPENDENCE AND DEVELOPMENT OF RESISTANCE TO HORMONAL THERAPIES

Cancer progression involves a series of changes in the malignant cell whereby its appearance and behavior inevitably evolve toward a more aggressive and poorly differentiated phenotype (see Fig. 20–8; see Chap. 10, Sec. 10.1). In breast and prostate cancer, the term *progression* is more commonly used in an endocrine sense to connote the process by which there is a change from hormone-dependent to the hormone-independent phenotype.

Resistance to hormonal therapies is of 2 types: de novo/intrinsic and acquired. Mechanisms responsible for de novo and acquired resistance to tamoxifen may differ because ER+ breast tumors with de novo tamoxifen resistance also are generally resistant to other forms of endocrine therapy. In contrast, tumors with acquired tamoxifen resistance are more likely to respond subsequently to second- and third-line endocrine therapy. This observation suggests that although some mechanisms of endocrine therapy resistance are general, there will be mechanisms specific for individual therapies (Musgrove and Sutherland, 2009). Less is known about resistance to aromatase inhibitors, but similar to tamoxifen resistance, multiple mechanisms are likely to be involved (Miller, 2010). Potential mechanisms include altered pharmacokinetics and pharmacogenetics of aromatase, decreased ER expression and/or activity together with increased activation of alternate signaling and survival pathways such as insulin-like growth factor receptor (IGFR) or EGFR (Johnston et al, 2009; Sabnis and Brodie, 2010). Interestingly, there seem to be some mechanisms common to aromatase inhibitors generally and others unique to individual aromatase inhibitors as crossresistance is not always seen and there are few clinical correlative data available to determine the relevance and/or frequency of such mechanisms in vivo (Miller, 2010). Figure 20–15A and B summarize potential mechanisms thought to be involved in resistance to tamoxifen and aromatase therapy, respectively.

20.5.1 Clonal Selection Versus Adaptation

Tumor progression is attributed usually to mutations, or to irreversible chromosomal rearrangements, losses, and

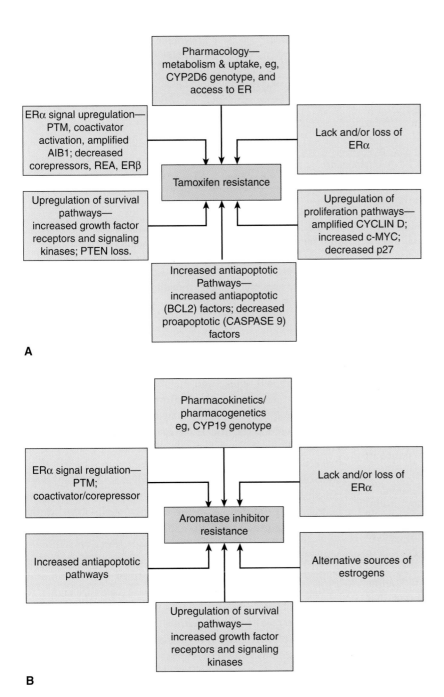

FIGURE 20–15 Summary of the multiple mechanisms of resistance to **(A)** tamoxifen and **(B)** aromatase inhibitors in human breast cancer. *REA*, repressor of ER activity; *PTM*, post-translational modifications

duplications, with selection of clones that have a growth or survival advantage. This widely accepted mechanism proposes that androgen or estrogen-independent tumor cells are present initially and that hormonal therapy kills all but this population of cells, which subsequently becomes the dominant phenotype of the tumor. There is evidence to support this mechanism in some animal tumor models whose rapid regrowth after androgen withdrawal implies the preexistence of androgen-independent clones (Gingrich et al, 1997). However, there is evidence to support alternative mechanisms, including heritable perturbations in regulatory pathways, that depend on interactions with inter- or intracellular

factors, and which may be in part a result of epigenetic/adaptive processes. Figure 20–16 outlines the 2 mechanisms for progression.

For breast cancer there are molecular data showing identical genetic abnormalities in synchronous premalignant, preinvasive, and invasive breast cancer lesions that support clonal selection in breast cancer progression. However, unlike prostate cancer where the vast majority of invasive prostate cancers are AR+, 2 biologically distinct groups of breast cancers exist, that is, ER+ and ER− tumors. Infrequent changes in ER status during tumor progression, suggest that the 2 tumor types are unlikely to be derived one from the

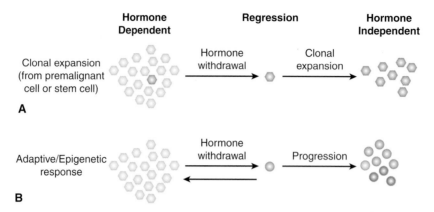

FIGURE 20–16 **Clonal selection and epigenetic/adaptive mechanisms for emergence of hormone independence in tumors.**
A) Upon hormone withdrawal, hormone-dependent cells are killed, leaving behind preexisting hormone-independent clones that repopulate the tumor. **B)** Upon hormone withdrawal, most cells are killed except for those expressing critical cell-survival genes. When reexposed to hormone, the pattern of gene expression reverts and the tumor regrows in response to hormone. However, through further adaptive changes in gene expression patterns, the cells no longer require hormone to sustain their growth.

other. Furthermore, when ER status has changed during progression, it has been impossible to distinguish between the suppression of ER expression due to promoter methylation, or that the original primary tumor was heterogeneous containing both ER+ and ER– breast cancer cells, with ER– cancer cells having a growth advantage. Most evidence suggests that progression to hormone independence and development of tamoxifen and/or aromatase inhibitor resistance in breast cancer is a result of epigenetic and adaptive mechanisms. However, discordance of receptor status between primary and metastatic breast cancer is frequent enough and has sufficient clinical implications to recommend biopsy and assessment of the receptor status of metastatic tumors where possible (Amir et al, 2012).

There are many molecular processes linked to prostate cancer progression that imply an epigenetic mechanism (Rennie and Nelson, 1998). Early experiments demonstrated that chronic administration of combinations of testosterone and estradiol to niobium (Nb) rats increased the incidence of prostate adenocarcinomas from less than 1% to greater than 18%. As neither estrogens nor androgens are mutagens, this finding suggests that prostate cancer can arise through an epigenetic mechanism. Furthermore, in this animal model, fractional replacement of estrogen by tamoxifen to keep the tumor in stasis (ie, neither regressing nor growing) delayed or prevented progression to hormone independence, implying that progression was also driven by epigenetic processes.

The extent to which the development or progression of breast and prostate cancer are driven by epigenetic or genetic mechanisms has important clinical implications. If progression occurs primarily as a consequence of preexisting genetic changes, perhaps in putative stem cells (see Chap. 13, Sec. 13.4), then options for prevention and treatment are limited. Conversely, if reversible adaptive or epigenetic processes are predominant, then breast and prostate cancer are potentially more amenable to therapeutic control, as indicated in Figure 20–16.

20.5.2 Altered Pharmacology

A possible mechanism for tamoxifen resistance in breast cancer is altered uptake and metabolism of tamoxifen by the tumor leading to reduced intratumoral drug concentrations. Because CYP2D6 is the major enzyme responsible for the generation of endoxifen, the active metabolite of tamoxifen (see Fig. 20–11), individuals with CYP2D6 gene polymorphisms that reduce enzymatic activity may have reduced benefit from tamoxifen (Hoskins et al, 2009; Kiyotani et al, 2010), although not all studies agree with this conclusion. Differences in the frequencies of mutations in the CYP2D6 gene occur in different ethnic groups and may influence the effectiveness of tamoxifen (Bernard et al, 2006). Also, selective serotonin reuptake inhibitors (SSRIs), and/or selective noradrenaline reuptake inhibitors (SNRIs) are prescribed quite commonly for depression or other reasons and these drugs are known to inhibit CYP2D6 activity (Hoskins et al, 2009). Altered availability of tamoxifen to ER within the tumor may also occur as a result of increased expression of binding proteins such as *anti*estrogen *b*inding *s*ites (AEBSs) that do not bind estrogen but would sequester tamoxifen away from ER. Data consistent with these mechanisms have been described both in some human breast tumors and in a model of tamoxifen-resistant human breast cancer where breast cancer cell lines are grown as xenografts in athymic mice (Clarke et al, 2001).

20.5.3 Alternative Signal Transduction Pathways and the Importance of Stroma

During progression to hormone independence, both autocrine and paracrine growth factor pathways may become dysregulated and growth factors may replace estrogens or androgens as primary growth regulators. Both normal and neoplastic epithelial cells exist in a complex 3D interaction with stromal cells (fibroblasts and adipocytes), blood vessels, and often immune cells within and surrounded by an extracellular matrix (ECM).

Cell–cell interactions may be mediated by growth factors or through interactions with the ECM via adhesion molecules called *integrins* located on the cell surface (see Chap. 10, Sec. 10.2). These interactions regulate signal transduction pathways and gene expression.

20.5.3.1 Alternate Pathways of Signal Transduction in Breast Cancer

In breast cancer, ligand-independent activation of the ER has been demonstrated frequently, and may contribute to hormone independence and antiestrogen resistance. Some of the more common alterations in breast tumors are upregulated and abnormally regulated growth factor pathways (EGFR, IGFR, HER2/NEU/ERBB-2) and/or their intracellular signal transduction molecules (RAS/RAF, MAPK, phophatidylinositol-3 kinase [PI3K], AKT; see Chap. 8, Sec. 8.2). Growth factors such as IGF-I, heregulin and EGF can activate ER in the absence or presence of estrogen through mechanisms involving phosphorylation of coregulators or of the ER itself (Musgrove and Sutherland, 2009). Similar phosphorylation mechanisms are almost certainly operational for the ligand-independent activation of ER by protein kinase A, protein kinase C, pp90rsk1, and protein kinase B (Ali and Coombes, 2000; Clarke et al, 2001). The expression and/or activity of many of these kinases are often increased in breast tumors compared to normal breast tissue, and specific phosphatases that deactivate these kinases are expressed at higher levels in some breast cancer cell lines with altered responses to estrogen. Thus an altered phosphorylation profile of the ER and/or its coregulators may underlie the progression to hormone independence and endocrine resistance (Xu et al, 2009; Skliris et al, 2010). The ability of tamoxifen to effect ligand-independent activation of ER is variable, which suggests that this is only one of several mechanisms that participate in the development of antiestrogen resistance (Clarke et al, 2001). For example, sustained activation of the PI3K/AKT pathway (see Chap. 8, Sec. 8.2.5) can protect breast cancer cells against tamoxifen-induced apoptosis. This is because of a positive feedback loop, whereby activated AKT activates ERα in a ligand-independent fashion, and ERα in the presence or absence of estrogen activates PI3K (Campbell et al, 2001; Sun et al, 2001). Because growth factors activate both the PI3K and MAPK pathways and both can impact ERα signaling, it seems that a marked amplification of ligand-independent ER signaling is inevitable.

Crosstalk between ER and other transcription factors or coregulator proteins may also play a role in progression to hormone independence. For example, crosstalk between ER and the transcription factor AP-1 takes several forms: estrogens can regulate the expression of the components of AP-1 transcription complexes; ER and AP-1 can interact directly by protein–protein interactions to regulate target gene expression; activation of AP-1 complexes can downregulate ER expression (Clarke et al, 2001). A mouse model of tamoxifen-resistant breast cancer has also shown an association of resistance with oxidative stress and increased AP-1 activity (Schiff et al, 2000). All of these mechanisms could influence the responsiveness of a breast cancer cell to tamoxifen as well

as to aromatase inhibitors, and there are some reports where altered AP-1 activity and/or levels of expression of AP-1 components can be correlated with acquired tamoxifen resistance. Thus multiple mechanisms may lead to progression to hormone independence and the development of resistance to endocrine therapies (see Fig. 20–15). Increasing knowledge of such mechanisms is leading to clinical trials evaluating endocrine therapy in combination with other therapies targeted to key molecules within signaling pathways known to be active within the patient's tumor (Di Cosimo and Baselga, 2010).

20.5.3.2 Alternate Pathways of Signal Transduction in Prostate Cancer

In prostate cancer, there is an increase in paracrine stimulation by growth factors produced in prostatic stroma with eventual autocrine production and stimulation by the prostate cancer epithelial cell (Rennie and Nelson, 1998). For example, in BPH, epithelial cells express EGFR but not its ligand TGF-α, whereas prostate stroma produces TGF-α but not EGFR. However, in many prostate epithelial tumor cells, coexpression of EGFR and TGF-α is observed, indicating a shift from paracrine to autocrine stimulation (Leav et al, 1998). Whether the molecular mechanisms responsible for the shift in this regulatory loop are a result of mutational or adaptive processes is unknown. However, by simply adapting the amount of the tyrosine kinase inhibitor genistein in the diet, the expression of EGFR in the EGFR/TGF-α system could be manipulated in a rat prostate cancer model (Dalu et al, 1998).

A similar shift from paracrine to autocrine regulation has been seen with the IGF regulatory network. In the normal prostate and in BPH, IGF-I, and IGF-II are produced and secreted by the stroma, and influence prostate epithelia in a paracrine fashion through IGF-I and IGF-II receptors. However, in prostate cancers, production of both types of IGF occurs in the tumor cells, which results in an autocrine loop for androgen-independent growth stimulation (Wang and Wong, 1998). Overall, as prostate cancer progresses, the stromal component tends to become redundant for controlling prostate growth.

There is evidence that intratumoral androgen synthesis occurs in men after chemical or surgical castration for prostate cancer (Fig. 20–17). Expression of genes mediating androgen synthesis in the prostate (eg, AKR1C2 and AKR1C1 involved, respectively, in the production of 3α-androstanediol and 3β-androstanediol from 5α-DHT), is elevated or modified in CRPC in contrast to primary tumors (Knudsen and Penning, 2010). In addition, testosterone levels in CRPC cells have been shown to be adequate for activation of androgen-dependent genes. Abiraterone acetate, an inhibitor of the CYP17A1 hydrolase involved in the transformation of progesterone to androstenedione, reduces the plasma level of testosterone in CRPC patients whose levels of circulating testosterone are already in the castrate range (Attard et al, 2008), and probably also inhibits testosterone synthesis in prostatic tissue. As indicated above, this drug leads to tumor response in a substantial proportion of men with metastatic CRPC, and improves their survival, indicating that nonlocalized tumors are often still dependent on androgens (Knudsen and Penning, 2010).

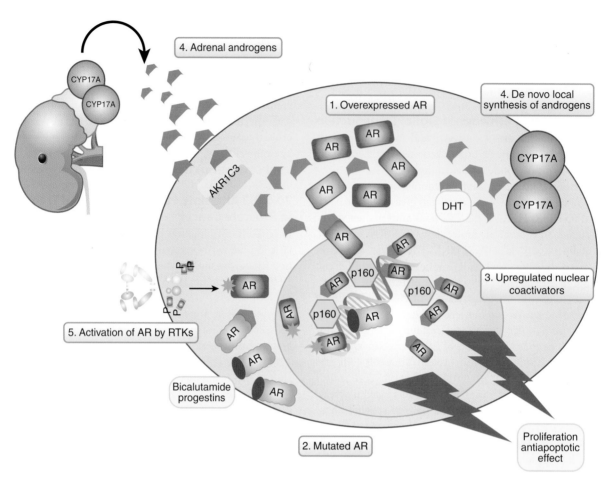

FIGURE 20–17 **Summary of the multiple mechanisms of castration-resistant prostate cancer.** Key regulatory proteins are the androgen receptor (AR), cytochrome P450 17A1 (CYP17A), p160 family members including SRC-1 and TIF2/SRC-2 (P160), aldo-keto reductase (AKR) 1C family member 3 (AKR1C3), and Receptor Tyrosine Kinase (RTK).

Many molecular alterations in prostate cancer have been discovered in recent years. Foremost among many are gene fusions involving E-twenty-six (*ETS*) genes, and especially the estrogen-regulated gene, *ERG*, and the androgen-regulated, prostate-specific, transmembrane protease serine 2 (*TMPRSS2*) gene, which can be found in approximately 50% of prostate cancers. In addition, several other *ETS* gene rearrangements have been discovered, including rearrangement of *ETV1*, *ETV4*, and *ETV5* with *TMPRSS2*, albeit at much lower frequencies than seen for *ERG*. *TMPRSS2* had previously been characterized as an androgen-regulated gene and thus its androgen-responsive regulatory element drives *ERG* overexpression in fusion-positive cases, promoting proliferation, invasion, and motility. It has been shown that androgen-dependent signaling induces proximity of the *TMPRSS2* and *ERG* genomic loci, facilitating the formation of the *TMPRSS2-ERG* gene fusion in response to genotoxic stress (Mani et al, 2009). Because prostate cancer is mainly driven by androgen signaling, this may explain why these types of fusions are apparently restricted to prostate cancer. Additional *ETS* gene rearrangements are being discovered, such as between the androgen-inducible tumor-suppressor *NDRG1* (*N-MYC*

downstream regulated gene 1) and *ERG*, while *TMPRSS2* rearrangements that do not involve known *ETS* genes have also been identified, suggesting that other androgen-response oncogenic elements may yet be discovered. These *ETS* fusions are being studied as biomarkers for prostate cancer initiation and/or progression, but correlation of their presence with clinical outcome remains controversial.

The critical genetic events associated with progression of breast and prostate cancer are still poorly understood, but owing to the development of approaches like gene microarrays, candidate genes are being discovered at a rapid rate. The current view is that the more likely mechanisms for progression of breast and prostate cancer involve ligand-independent activation of AR or ER via crosstalk with other transcription factors, signal transducers, and related pathways.

20.5.4 Estrogen Receptor and Androgen Receptor Amplifications and Mutations

In breast cancer, de novo hormone independence is often associated with absence of ER. However, a substantial proportion of ER+ breast tumors are either resistant de novo to endocrine therapy or acquire resistance after treatment with endocrine therapies despite the continued expression of ER. The presence of *ER* mutations and/or amplifications in breast cancer is infrequent. Although mutated *ERα* is quite rare in human breast cancers, variant ERs generated by alternative RNA splicing of both *ERα* and *ERβ* genes are common. Changes in expression of some of these variants have been documented in breast tumors, but only limited correlation with endocrine resistance has been reported (Shi et al, 2009).

Unlike breast cancer, androgen-independent human prostate cancer is seldom associated with absence of AR. Immunohistochemical analysis of AR in biopsies from virtually every stage and grade of prostate cancer show that AR is retained regardless of hormone sensitivity. Only in some multiply-passaged androgen-independent human prostate cancer cell lines, such as Du145 and PC3 cells, is there lack of detectable or functional AR. Because loss of AR expression is not normally associated with the malignant phenotype, attention has focused on more subtle mutational events in the *AR* gene that could give rise to alterations in AR activity (see Fig. 20–17).

Estimates of the incidence of somatic point mutations in the *AR* gene range from 0% to 30% of patients with CRPC and there is a tendency for the incidence of *AR* mutations to occur more frequently in advanced or metastatic disease. Also, patients treated with antiandrogens are more likely to have *AR* mutations as compared to patients treated solely by surgical castration or LHRH agonists (Taplin et al, 1999). Many *AR* mutations in the ligand-binding domain have been characterized, showing a range of effects from partial or complete loss of function as well as diverse transactivational activity (Shi et al, 2002). The well-characterized threonine-to-alanine (T877A) mutation in the *AR* ligand-binding domain of the LNCaP human prostate cancer cell line has been shown to alter androgen binding specificity, such that it can be activated by high concentrations of virtually any steroid or antiandrogen (Duff and McEwan, 2005). Similar types of mutations have been observed in some patients who manifest the antiandrogen withdrawal syndrome. Truncated forms of the AR expressed as alternatively spliced variants lacking a ligand-binding site are also constitutively active in some men with CRPC (Hu et al, 2009).

Amplification and overexpression of the wild-type *AR* gene are likely more common than mutations. Studies before and after androgen ablation have shown gene amplification of wild-type *AR* in approximately 30% of recurrent tumors. In *AR* gene-amplified tumors, PSA immunostaining appears to be about twice as high as in tumors with no amplification, indicating that *AR* gene amplification leads to upregulation of the PSA gene (and possibly other androgen-regulated genes). Thus patients with *AR* gene amplification may have elevated serum PSA concentrations without a clear correlation with tumor burden (Koivisto and Helin, 1999). The *AR* is the only gene consistently upregulated in tumor progression (Chen et al, 2004), and although androgen withdrawal is ineffective in most

castration-resistant prostate tumors, knockdown of *AR* using small interfering RNAs was able to decrease serum PSA and, in some cases, to cause tumor regression (Snoek et al, 2009).

20.5.5 Altered Receptor Structure and Function, Including Altered Coregulator Activity

The ability to recruit coactivators and/or corepressors to a promoter plays an important role in transcriptional regulation by a steroid hormone (see Fig. 20–4). Experimental alteration of the relative expression and/or activity of coactivator to corepressor suggests that such a mechanism can influence how a target cell interprets tamoxifen, either as an antiestrogen or an estrogen. Alterations of specific coactivators and corepressors of ER have been described in human breast tumors and correlations with resistance to tamoxifen have been reported (Osborne et al, 2003; Musgrove and Sutherland, 2009). Because coregulators are essential to ER signaling, altered expression and/or activity could theoretically affect sensitivity of tumors to aromatase inhibitors as a result of estrogen independence of growth and survival pathways. Growth factor/phosphorylation pathways can also influence steroid hormone receptor pathways via their ability to modulate coactivators by phosphorylation (Han et al, 2009) and may influence on the emergence of hormone independence.

In prostate cancer, overexpression of coactivators might lower the ligand threshold of the AR such that physiological concentrations of adrenal androgens are then adequate to drive androgen-regulated responses, such as PSA expression (Chmelar et al, 2007). Indeed, immunohistochemical evaluation of human prostate cancer samples demonstrated overexpression of the coactivator SRC-1 in approximately half of nontreated prostate cancers, as well as high levels of both SRC-1 and SRC-2 in the majority of castration-resistant tumors (Gregory et al, 2001). Other coactivators that are involved in prostate cancer progression and in the development of a castration-resistant state are the thyroid hormone receptor-associated protein mediator complex (MEDI/TRAP220), which is involved in AR-mediated transcription of the PSA gene, and AR chaperones such as heat shock protein (HSP) 27 and cell division cycle (CDC) 37. Chaperones have an essential role in stabilizing AR interaction with DHT. Interestingly, *MED1/TRAP220* is overexpressed in both AR-positive and -negative prostate cancer cell lines, as well as in clinically localized prostate cancers, suggesting that MED1/TRAP220 hyperactivity might promote prostate tumor formation.

20.5.6 Changes in Gene Expression

The inappropriate upregulation of cell-survival genes is another potential mechanism whereby cancer cells become treatment-resistant. Recently, genome-wide analyses and the generation of gene expression signatures have added support to experimental data that deregulation of proliferation and survival pathways plays an important role in resistance to both tamoxifen and aromatase inhibitors (Musgrove and Sutherland, 2009).

The *BCL* family of genes has been implicated in progression of breast cancer and *BCL-2* is an estrogen-inducible gene in ER+ breast cancer cell lines. Other survival pathways, such as the AKT (protein kinase B) pathway, may also be important in progression of human breast cancer. As described above, AKT is activated by ligand-bound EGFR and IGFR, and can phosphorylate coactivators as well as ERα (Musgrove and Sutherland, 2009), and can activate ER in a ligand-independent fashion. Furthermore, overexpression of AKT in breast cancer cell lines leads to upregulation of BCL-2 and protects breast cancer cells from tamoxifen-induced apoptosis (Campbell et al, 2001). There appears to be a positive feedback loop involved in this network whereby ERα in the presence or absence of estrogen can activate the regulatory subunit of PI3K, which, in turn, activates AKT (see also Sec. 20.5.3.1).

Tumor-suppressor genes, such as Rb (retinoblastoma) and p53, are inactivated in many tumor types, including breast and the late stages of prostate cancer. E-cadherin and other cell-adhesion genes, which have been characterized as suppressors of the metastatic phenotype, are frequently inactivated or downregulated during progression to advanced prostate cancer and are associated with poor clinical outcome (Bussemakers, 1999).

In prostate cancer, elevated expression of the antiapoptotic gene *BCL-2* is found in virtually all CRPC and overexpression confers resistance to androgen withdrawal by blocking the normal apoptotic signals (McDonnell et al, 1997). The antiapoptotic protein clusterin (also known as TRPM-2 or SGP-2) is also upregulated with disease progression in prostate cancer; it confers resistance to hormonal therapy when overexpressed in prostate tumor cell lines (Steinberg et al, 1997).

SUMMARY

- Breast and prostate cancer share many common epidemiological and biological features. Many factors contribute to their etiology, but a western-type diet appears to be a major factor associated with high incidence.
- Both breast and prostate cancer require long-term exposure to sex-steroid hormones to develop. A direct causal link to overstimulation with estrogens and androgens has been demonstrated in animal tumor models; conversely, a protective effect has been observed from treatments that block the action of these hormones (eg, prepubertal castration or administration of antihormonal drugs).
- Estrogens and androgens share many features in their mechanism of action: both are synthesized from common precursors (eg, cholesterol); both are carried mainly by the same protein in the blood (ie, SHGB [sex hormone-binding globulin]); and both bind to structurally related intracellular receptors. Both types of hormone-receptor complexes, in turn, bind to comparable regulatory DNA sequences in the promoters of genes and interact with similar sets of coregulator proteins to activate or repress gene expression.

- Approximately 70% of breast carcinomas are ER+ and approximately 50% of these will respond to endocrine therapy, giving an overall response rate of approximately 35% to 40%. By comparison, most prostate cancers are AR+ and most (~90%) respond to hormonal therapy. Therefore, ER assays are performed routinely in women with breast cancer and only ER+ tumors are hormonally treated, whereas no receptor-based selection process is applied to prostate tumors.
- Treatment modalities used to kill hormone-dependent breast or prostate tumor cells are based on the same principles of either blocking the synthesis of the steroid hormone or blocking their activity in the target cell. Unfortunately, endocrine therapy for locally advanced or metastatic disease is not curative as the tumors progress from hormone-dependence to hormone-independence.
- Potential mechanisms leading to hormone independence include ascendancy of alternative signal transduction pathways; receptor gene mutations or amplifications; ligand-independent receptor crosstalk with growth factors or kinases; autocrine synthesis of androgens; and upregulation of cell-survival genes. Whether the hormone-independent phenotype is caused by the outgrowth of preexisting clones with these genetic abnormalities or by adaptive/epigenetic changes is unknown.
- There are no proven treatments to delay or prevent progression to hormone independence in either prostate or breast cancer. However, there are several ongoing prospective clinical trials to test the efficacy of intermittent androgen suppression on delay of progression in men with prostate cancer.
- Increased understanding of steroid hormone action and the use of techniques such as DNA and protein microarrays are driving the development of better markers for the prediction of treatment response, the risk of developing invasive cancer, and the identification of alternative targets for the treatment and prevention of breast and prostate cancers.

ACKNOWLEDGMENT

The authors would like to thank Dr. Jason Read for his help in preparing the figures for this chapter.

REFERENCES

Aebi S. Special issues related to the adjuvant therapy in very young women. *Breast* 2005;14:594-599.

Akakura K, Bruchovsky N, Goldenberg SL, et al. Effects of intermittent androgen suppression on androgen-dependent tumors. Apoptosis and serum prostate-specific antigen. *Cancer* 1993;71:2782-2790.

Al-Hajj M, Wicha MS, Benito-Hernandez A, et al. Prospective identification of tumorigenic breast cancer cells. *Proc Natl Acad Sci U S A* 2003;100:3983-3988.

Albain KS, Barlow WE, Shak S, et al. Prognostic and predictive value of the 21-gene recurrence score assay in postmenopausal women with node-positive, oestrogen-receptor-positive breast cancer on chemotherapy: a retrospective analysis of a randomised trial. *Lancet Oncol* 2010;11:55-65.

Ali S, Coombes RC. Estrogen receptor alpha in human breast cancer: occurrence and significance. *J Mammary Gland Biol Neoplasia* 2000;5:271-281.

Allred DC, Mohsin SK. Biological features of premalignant disease in the human breast. *J Mammary Gland Biol Neoplasia* 2000;5:351-364.

Amir E, Miller N, Geddie W, et al. Prospective study evaluating the impact of tissue confirmation of metastatic disease in patients with breast cancer. *J Clin Oncol* 2012;30:587-592.

Anderson E, Clarke RB, Howell A. Estrogen responsiveness and control of normal human breast proliferation. *J Mammary Gland Biol Neoplasia* 1998;3:23-35.

Andriole GL, Bostwick DG, Brawley OW, et al. Effect of dutasteride on the risk of prostate cancer. *N Engl J Med* 2010;362:1192-1202.

Anzick SL, Kononen J, Walker RL, et al. AIB1, a steroid receptor coactivator amplified in breast and ovarian cancer. *Science* 1997;277:965-968.

Aranda A, Pascual A. Nuclear hormone receptors and gene expression. *Physiol Rev* 2001;81:1269-1304.

Arpino G, Wiechmann L, Osborne CK, Schiff R. Crosstalk between the estrogen receptor and the HER tyrosine kinase receptor family: molecular mechanism and clinical implications for endocrine therapy resistance. *Endocr Rev* 2008;29:217-233.

Attard G, Reid AH, Yap TA, et al. Phase I clinical trial of a selective inhibitor of CYP17, abiraterone acetate, confirms that castration-resistant prostate cancer commonly remains hormone driven. *J Clin Oncol* 2008;26:4563-4571.

Bane AL, Beck JC, Bleiweiss I, et al. BRCA2 mutation-associated breast cancers exhibit a distinguishing phenotype based on morphology and molecular profiles from tissue microarrays. *Am J Surg Pathol* 2007;31:121-128.

Banks E, Canfell K, Reeves G. HRT and breast cancer: recent findings in the context of the evidence to date. *Womens Health (Lond Engl)* 2008;4:427-431.

Becker S, Kaaks R. Exogenous and endogenous hormones, mammographic density and breast cancer risk: can mammographic density be considered an intermediate marker of risk? *Recent Results Cancer Res* 2009;181:135-157.

Bernard S, Neville KA, Nguyen AT, Flockhart DA. Interethnic differences in genetic polymorphisms of CYP2D6 in the U.S. population: clinical implications. *Oncologist* 2006;11:126-135.

Bolla M, Collette L, Blank L, et al. Long-term results with immediate androgen suppression and external irradiation in patients with locally advanced prostate cancer(an EORTC study): a phase III randomised trial. *Lancet* 2002;360:103-106.

Boyd NF, Martin LJ, Stone J, et al. Mammographic densities as a marker of human breast cancer risk and their use in chemoprevention. *Curr Oncol Rep* 2001;3:314-321.

Bruchovsky N, Rennie PS, Batzold FH, et al. Kinetic parameters of 5 alpha-reductase activity in stroma and epithelium of normal, hyperplastic, and carcinomatous human prostates. *J Clin Endocrinol Metab* 1988;67:806-816.

Bussemakers MJ. Changes in gene expression and targets for therapy. *Eur Urol* 1999;35:408-412.

Calle EE, Kaaks R. Overweight, obesity and cancer: epidemiological evidence and proposed mechanisms. *Nat Rev Cancer* 2004;4:579-591.

Campbell LL, Polyak K. Breast tumor heterogeneity: cancer stem cells or clonal evolution? *Cell Cycle* 2007;6:2332-2338.

Campbell RA, Bhat-Nakshatri P, Patel NM, et al. Phosphatidylinositol 3-kinase/AKT-mediated activation of estrogen receptor alpha: a new model for anti-estrogen resistance. *J Biol Chem* 2001;276:9817-9824.

Cardoso F, Van't Veer L, Rutgers E, et al. Clinical application of the 70-gene profile: the MINDACT trial. *J Clin Oncol* 2008;26:729-735.

Chen CD, Welsbie DS, Tran C, et al. Molecular determinants of resistance to antiandrogen therapy. *Nat Med* 2004;10:33-39.

Chmelar R, Buchanan G, Need EF, et al. Androgen receptor coregulators and their involvement in the development and progression of prostate cancer. *Int J Cancer* 2007;120:719-733.

Clarke R, Leonessa F, Welch JN, Skaar TC. Cellular and molecular pharmacology of antiestrogen action and resistance. *Pharmacol Rev* 2001;53:25-71.

Clarke RB, Howell A, Potten CS, Anderson E. Dissociation between steroid receptor expression and cell proliferation in the human breast. *Cancer Res* 1997;57:4987-4991.

Couse JF, Korach KS. Estrogen receptor null mice: what have we learned and where will they lead us? *Endocr Rev* 1999;20:358-417.

Creighton CJ, Chang JC, Rosen JM. Epithelial-mesenchymal transition (EMT) in tumor-initiating cells and its clinical implications in breast cancer. *J Mammary Gland Biol Neoplasia* 2010;15:253-260.

Dalu A, Haskell JF, Coward L, Lamartiniere CA. Genistein, a component of soy, inhibits the expression of the EGF and ErbB2/Neu receptors in the rat dorsolateral prostate. *Prostate* 1998;37:36-43.

Davies P, Watt K, Kelly SM, et al. Consequences of poly-glutamine repeat length for the conformation and folding of the androgen receptor amino-terminal domain. *J Mol Endocrinol* 2008;41:301-314.

de Bono JS, Logothetis CJ, Molina A, et al. Abiraterone and increased survival in metastatic prostate cancer. *N Engl J Med* 2011;364:1995-2005.

Delage-Mourroux R, Martini PG, Choi I, et al. Analysis of estrogen receptor interaction with a repressor of estrogen receptor activity (REA) and the regulation of estrogen receptor transcriptional activity by REA. *J Biol Chem* 2000;275:35848-35856.

Denis L, Morton MS, Griffiths K. Diet and its preventive role in prostatic disease. *Eur Urol* 1999;35:377-387.

Di Cosimo S, Baselga J. Management of breast cancer with targeted agents: importance of heterogenicity. *Nat Rev Clin Oncol* 2010;7:139-147.

Duff J, McEwan IJ. Mutation of histidine 874 in the androgen receptor ligand-binding domain leads to promiscuous ligand activation and altered p160 coactivator interactions. *Mol Endocrinol* 2005;19:2943-2954.

Early Breast Cancer Trialists' Collaborative Group. Effects of chemotherapy and hormonal therapy for early breast cancer on recurrence and 15-year survival: an overview of the randomised trials. *Lancet* 2005;365:1687-1717.

Eirew P, Stingl J, Raouf A, et al. A method for quantifying normal human mammary epithelial stem cells with in vivo regenerative ability. *Nat Med* 2008;14:1384-1389.

Elliott CS, Shinghal R, Presti JC Jr. The influence of prostate volume on prostate-specific antigen performance: implications for the prostate cancer prevention trial outcomes. *Clin Cancer Res* 2009;15:4694-4699.

Fitzgibbons PL, Murphy DA, Hammond ME, et al. Recommendations for validating estrogen and progesterone receptor immunohistochemistry assays. *Arch Pathol Lab Med* 2010;134:930-935.

Fullwood MJ, Liu MH, Pan YF, et al. An oestrogen-receptor-alpha-bound human chromatin interactome. *Nature* 2009;462:58-64.

Gallagher DJ, Gaudet MM, Pal P, et al. Germline BRCA mutations denote a clinicopathologic subset of prostate cancer. *Clin Cancer Res* 2010;16:2115-2121.

Giguere Y, Dewailly E, Brisson J, et al. Short polyglutamine tracts in the androgen receptor are protective against breast cancer in the general population. *Cancer Res* 2001;61:5869-5874.

Gingrich JR, Barrios RJ, Kattan MW, et al. Androgen-independent prostate cancer progression in the TRAMP model. *Cancer Res* 1997;57:4687-4691.

Glass CK. Differential recognition of target genes by nuclear receptor monomers, dimers, and heterodimers. *Endocr Rev* 1994;15:391-407.

Gobbi H, Dupont WD, Simpson JF, et al. Transforming growth factor-beta and breast cancer risk in women with mammary epithelial hyperplasia. *J Natl Cancer Inst* 1999;91:2096-2101.

Gojis O, Rudraraju B, Gudi M, et al. The role of SRC-3 in human breast cancer. *Nat Rev Clin Oncol* 2010;7:83-89.

Gong G, DeVries S, Chew KL, et al. Genetic changes in paired atypical and usual ductal hyperplasia of the breast by comparative genomic hybridization. *Clin Cancer Res* 2001;7:2410-2414.

Gregory CW, He B, Johnson RT, et al. A mechanism for androgen receptor-mediated prostate cancer recurrence after androgen deprivation therapy. *Cancer Res* 2001;61:4315-4319.

Grino PB, Griffin JE, Wilson JD. Testosterone at high concentrations interacts with the human androgen receptor similarly to dihydrotestosterone. *Endocrinology* 1990;126:1165-1172.

Hammond ME, Hayes DF, Dowsett M, A, et al. American Society of Clinical Oncology/College of American Pathologists guideline recommendations for immunohistochemical testing of estrogen and progesterone receptors in breast cancer. *Arch Pathol Lab Med* 2010;134:907-922.

Han SJ, Lonard DM, O'Malley BW. Multi-modulation of nuclear receptor coactivators through posttranslational modifications. *Trends Endocrinol Metab* 2009;20:8-15.

Harper ME, Glynne-Jones E, Goddard L, et al. Expression of androgen receptor and growth factors in premalignant lesions of the prostate. *J Pathol* 1998;186:169-177.

Herschkowitz JI. Breast cancer stem cells: initiating a new sort of thinking. *Dis Model Mech* 2010;3:257-258.

Hoskins JM, Carey LA, McLeod HL. CYP2D6 and tamoxifen: DNA matters in breast cancer. *Nat Rev Cancer* 2009;9:576-586.

Hsing AW, Chokkalingam AP. Prostate cancer epidemiology. *Front Biosci* 2006;11:1388-1413.

Hu R, Dunn TA, Wei S, et al. Ligand-independent androgen receptor variants derived from splicing of cryptic exons signify hormone-refractory prostate cancer. *Cancer Res* 2009;69:16-22.

Hulka BS, Liu ET, Lininger RA. Steroid hormones and risk of breast cancer. *Cancer* 1994;74:1111-24.

Johnston S, Pippen J Jr, Pivot X, et al. Lapatinib combined with letrozole versus letrozole and placebo as first-line therapy for postmenopausal hormone receptor-positive metastatic breast cancer. *J Clin Oncol* 2009;27:5538-5546.

Johnston SR. New strategies in estrogen receptor-positive breast cancer. *Clin Cancer Res* 2010;16:1979-1987.

Kahn SM, Hryb DJ, Nakhla AM, et al. Sex hormone-binding globulin is synthesized in target cells. *J Endocrinol* 2002;175:113-120.

Kelly MJ, Levin ER. Rapid actions of plasma membrane estrogen receptors. *Trends Endocrinol Metab* 2001;12:152-156.

Key TJ, Appleby PN, Reeves GK, Roddam AW. Insulin-like growth factor 1 (IGF1), IGF binding protein 3 (IGFBP3), and breast cancer risk: pooled individual data analysis of 17 prospective studies. *Lancet Oncol* 2010;11:530-542.

Khan SA, Rogers MA, Khurana KK, et al. Estrogen receptor expression in benign breast epithelium and breast cancer risk. *J Natl Cancer Inst* 1998;90:37-42.

Kiyotani K, Mushiroda T, Imamura CK, et al. Significant effect of polymorphisms in CYP2D6 and ABCC2 on clinical outcomes of adjuvant tamoxifen therapy for breast cancer patients. *J Clin Oncol* 2010;28:1287-1293.

Klinge CM. Estrogen receptor binding to estrogen response elements slows ligand dissociation and synergistically activates reporter gene expression. *Mol Cell Endocrinol* 1999;150:99-111.

Knudsen KE, Penning TM. Partners in crime: deregulation of AR activity and androgen synthesis in prostate cancer. *Trends Endocrinol Metab* 2010;21:315-324.

Koivisto PA, Helin HJ. Androgen receptor gene amplification increases tissue PSA protein expression in hormone-refractory prostate carcinoma. *J Pathol* 1999;189:219-223.

Korach KS. Insights from the study of animals lacking functional estrogen receptor. *Science* 1994;266:1524-1527.

Korkaya H, Liu S, Wicha MS. Breast cancer stem cells, cytokine networks, and the tumor microenvironment. *J Clin Invest* 2011;121:3804-3809.

Kousteni S, Bellido T, Plotkin LI, et al. Nongenotropic, sex-nonspecific signaling through the estrogen or androgen receptors: dissociation from transcriptional activity. *Cell* 2001;104:719-730.

La Spada AR, Wilson EM, Lubahn DB, et al. Androgen receptor gene mutations in X-linked spinal and bulbar muscular atrophy. *Nature* 1991;352:77-79.

Lawson DA, Witte ON. Stem cells in prostate cancer initiation and progression. *J Clin Invest* 2007;117:2044-2050.

Leav I, McNeal JE, Ziar J, Alroy J. The localization of transforming growth factor alpha and epidermal growth factor receptor in stromal and epithelial compartments of developing human prostate and hyperplastic, dysplastic, and carcinomatous lesions. *Hum Pathol* 1998;29:668-675.

Lee CJ, Dosch J, Simeone DM. Pancreatic cancer stem cells. *J Clin Oncol* 2008;26:2806-2812.

Leo C, Chen JD. The SRC family of nuclear receptor coactivators. *Gene* 2000;245:1-11.

Leygue E, Dotzlaw H, Watson PH, Murphy LC. Altered estrogen receptor alpha and beta messenger RNA expression during human breast tumorigenesis. *Cancer Res* 1998;58:3197-3201.

Lim E, Vaillant F, Wu D, et al. Aberrant luminal progenitors as the candidate target population for basal tumor development in BRCA1 mutation carriers. *Nat Med* 2009;15:907-913.

Lin C, Yang L, Tanasa B, et al. Nuclear receptor-induced chromosomal proximity and DNA breaks underlie specific translocations in cancer. *Cell* 2009;139:1069-1083.

Mani RS, Tomlins SA, Callahan K, et al. Induced chromosomal proximity and gene fusions in prostate cancer. *Science* 2009;326:1230.

Martin LJ, Minkin S, Boyd NF. Hormone therapy, mammographic density, and breast cancer risk. *Maturitas* 2009;64:20-26.

McDonnell TJ, Navone NM, Troncoso P, et al. Expression of bcl-2 oncoprotein and p53 protein accumulation in bone marrow metastases of androgen independent prostate cancer. *J Urol* 1997;157:569-574.

McKenna NJ, O'Malley BW. An issue of tissues: divining the split personalities of selective estrogen receptor modulators. *Nat Med* 2000;6:960-962.

Miettinen M, Isomaa V, Peltoketo H, et al. Estrogen metabolism as a regulator of estrogen action in the mammary gland. *J Mammary Gland Biol Neoplasia* 2000;5:259-270.

Miller WR. Aromatase inhibitors: prediction of response and nature of resistance. *Expert Opin Pharmacother* 2010;11:1873-1887.

Mir K, Edwards J, Paterson PJ, et al. The CAG trinucleotide repeat length in the androgen receptor does not predict the early onset of prostate cancer. *BJU Int* 2002;90:573-578.

Montano MM, Ekena K, Delage-Mourroux R, et al. An estrogen receptor-selective coregulator that potentiates the effectiveness of antiestrogens and represses the activity of estrogens. *Proc Natl Acad Sci U S A* 1999;96:6947-6952.

Mulholland DJ, Xin L, Morim A, et al. Lin-Sca-1+CD49fhigh stem/progenitors are tumor-initiating cells in the Pten-null prostate cancer model. *Cancer Res* 2009;69:8555-8562.

Murphy LC, Dotzlaw H, Leygue E, et al. The pathophysiological role of estrogen receptor variants in human breast cancer. *J Steroid Biochem Mol Biol* 1998;65:175-180.

Murphy LC, Simon SL, Parkes A, et al. Altered expression of estrogen receptor coregulators during human breast tumorigenesis. *Cancer Res* 2000;60:6266-6271.

Musgrove EA, Sutherland RL. Biological determinants of endocrine resistance in breast cancer. *Nat Rev Cancer* 2009;9:631-643.

Myal Y, Leygue E, Blanchard AA. Claudin 1 in breast tumorigenesis: revelation of a possible novel"claudin high" subset of breast cancers. *J Biomed Biotechnol* 2010;2010:956897 (epub).

Nadal A, Ropero AB, Laribi O, et al. Nongenomic actions of estrogens and xenoestrogens by binding at a plasma membrane receptor unrelated to estrogen receptor alpha and estrogen receptor beta. *Proc Natl Acad Sci U S A* 2000;97:11603-11608.

O'Malley BW, Kumar R. Nuclear receptor coregulators in cancer biology. *Cancer Res* 2009;69:8217-8222.

O'Regan RM, Jordan VC. Tamoxifen to raloxifene and beyond. *Semin Oncol* 2001;28:260-273.

Osborne CK, Bardou V, Hopp TA, et al. Role of the estrogen receptor coactivator AIB1 (SRC-3) and HER-2/neu in tamoxifen resistance in breast cancer. *J Natl Cancer Inst* 2003;95:353-361.

Page DL, Jensen RA, Simpson JF, Dupont WD. Historical and epidemiologic background of human premalignant breast disease. *J Mammary Gland Biol Neoplasia* 2000;5:341-349.

Paik S, Tang G, Shak S, et al. Gene expression and benefit of chemotherapy in women with node-negative, estrogen receptor-positive breast cancer. *J Clin Oncol* 2006;24:3726-3734.

Pauklin S, Sernandez IV, Bachmann G, et al. Estrogen directly activates AID transcription and function. *J Exp Med* 2009;206:99-111.

Perissi V, Rosenfeld MG. Controlling nuclear receptors: the circular logic of cofactor cycles. *Nat Rev Mol Cell Biol* 2005;6:542-554.

Perou CM, Sorlie T, Eisen MB, et al. Molecular portraits of human breast tumours. *Nature* 2000;406:747-752.

Podo F, Buydens LM, Degani H, et al. Triple-negative breast cancer: present challenges and new perspectives. *Mol Oncol* 2010;4:209-229.

Prostate Cancer Trialists' Collaborative Group. Maximum androgen blockade in advanced prostate cancer: an overview of the randomised trials. *Lancet* 2000;355:1491-1498.

Raouf A, Zhao Y, To K, et al. Transcriptome analysis of the normal human mammary cell commitment and differentiation process. *Cell Stem Cell* 2008;3:109-118.

Rennie PS, Bruchovsky N, Leco KJ, et al. Characterization of two cis-acting DNA elements involved in the androgen regulation of the probasin gene. *Mol Endocrinol* 1993;7:23-36.

Rennie PS, Nelson CC. Epigenetic mechanisms for progression of prostate cancer. *Cancer Metastasis Rev* 1998;17:401-409.

Robins DM, Albertelli MA, O'Mahony OA. Androgen receptor variants and prostate cancer in humanized AR mice. *J Steroid Biochem Mol Biol* 2008;108:230-236.

Roger P, Sahla ME, Makela S. Decreased expression of estrogen receptor beta protein in proliferative preinvasive mammary tumors. *Cancer Res* 2001;61:2537-2541.

Ryan CJ, Smith MR, De Bono JS, et al. Abiraterone in metastatic prostate cancer without previous chemotherapy. *N Engl J Med* 2012;Dec 10 [epub].

Sabnis G, Brodie A. Adaptive changes results in activation of alternate signaling pathways and resistance to aromatase inhibitor resistance. *Mol Cell Endocrinol* 2011;340:142-147.

Sakr WA, Partin AW. Histological markers of risk and the role of high-grade prostatic intraepithelial neoplasia. *Urology* 2001;57:115-120.

Sasano H, Harada N. Intratumoral aromatase in human breast, endometrial, and ovarian malignancies. *Endocr Rev* 1998;19:593-607.

Scher HI, Beer TM, Higano CS, et al. Antitumour activity of MDV3100 in castration-resistant prostate cancer: a phase 1-2 study. *Lancet* 2010;375:1437-1446.

Scher HI, Fizazi K, Saad F, et al. Increased survival with enzalutamide in prostate cancer after chemotherapy. *N Engl J Med* 2012;367:1187-1197.

Schiff R, Reddy P, Ahotupa M, et al. Oxidative stress and AP-1 activity in tamoxifen-resistant breast tumors in vivo. *J Natl Cancer Inst* 2000;92:1926-1934.

Shah SP, Morin RD, Khattra J, et al. Mutational evolution in a lobular breast tumour profiled at single nucleotide resolution. *Nature* 2009;461:809-813.

Shang Y, Hu X, DiRenzo J, et al. Cofactor dynamics and sufficiency in estrogen receptor-regulated transcription. *Cell* 2000;103:843-852.

Shi L, Dong B, Li Z, et al. Expression of ER-{alpha}36, a novel variant of estrogen receptor {alpha}, and resistance to tamoxifen treatment in breast cancer. *J Clin Oncol* 2009;27:3423-3429.

Shi XB, Ma AH, Xia L, et al. Functional analysis of 44 mutant androgen receptors from human prostate cancer. *Cancer Res* 2002;62:1496-1502.

Shiau AK, Barstad D, Loria PM, et al. The structural basis of estrogen receptor/coactivator recognition and the antagonism of this interaction by tamoxifen. *Cell* 1998;95:927-937.

Shoker BS, Jarvis C, Sibson DR, et al. Oestrogen receptor expression in the normal and pre-cancerous breast. *J Pathol* 1999;188: 237-244.

Simpson ER. Biology of aromatase in the mammary gland. *J Mammary Gland Biol Neoplasia* 2000;5:251-258.

Skliris GP, Nugent ZJ, Rowan BG, et al. A phosphorylation code for oestrogen receptor-alpha predicts clinical outcome to endocrine therapy in breast cancer. *Endocr Relat Cancer* 2010;17:589-597.

Snoek R, Cheng H, Margiotti K, et al. In vivo knockdown of the androgen receptor results in growth inhibition and regression of well-established, castration-resistant prostate tumors. *Clin Cancer Res* 2009;15:39-47.

Sorlie T. Molecular portraits of breast cancer: tumour subtypes as distinct disease entities. *Eur J Cancer* 2004;40:2667-2675.

Sorlie T, Tibshirani R, Parker J, et al. Repeated observation of breast tumor subtypes in independent gene expression data sets. *Proc Natl Acad Sci USA* 2003;100(14):8418-8423.

Steinberg J, Oyasu R, Lang S, et al. Intracellular levels of SGP-2 (clusterin) correlate with tumor grade in prostate cancer. *Clin Cancer Res* 1997;3:1707-1711.

Stingl J, Caldas C. Molecular heterogeneity of breast carcinomas and the cancer stem cell hypothesis. *Nat Rev Cancer* 2007;7: 791-799.

Subramanian J, Simon R. What should physicians look for in evaluating prognostic gene-expression signatures? *Nat Rev Clin Oncol* 2010;7:327-334.

Sun M, Paciga JE, Feldman RI, et al. Phosphatidylinositol-3-OH Kinase (PI3K)/AKT2, activated in breast cancer, regulates and is induced by estrogen receptor alpha (ERalpha) via interaction between ERalpha and PI3K. *Cancer Res* 2001;61:5985-5991.

Taplin ME, Bubley GJ, Ko YJ, et al. Selection for androgen receptor mutations in prostate cancers treated with androgen antagonist. *Cancer Res* 1999;59:2511-2515.

Thompson IM, Goodman PJ, Tangen CM, et al. The influence of finasteride on the development of prostate cancer. *N Engl J Med* 2003;349:215-224.

Thompson PA, Ambrosone C. Molecular epidemiology of genetic polymorphisms in estrogen metabolizing enzymes in human breast cancer. *J Natl Cancer Inst Monogr* 2000;27:125-134.

Tran C, Ouk S, Clegg NJ, et al. Development of a second-generation antiandrogen for treatment of advanced prostate cancer. *Science* 2009;324:787-790.

Ueda T, Bruchovsky N, Sadar MD. Activation of the androgen receptor N-terminal domain by interleukin-6 via MAPK and STAT3 signal transduction pathways. *J Biol Chem* 2002;277: 7076-7085.

Visvader JE. Keeping abreast of the mammary epithelial hierarchy and breast tumorigenesis. *Genes Dev* 2009;23:2563-2577.

Vogel VG, Costantino JP, Wickerham DL, et al. Effects of tamoxifen vs raloxifene on the risk of developing invasive breast cancer and other disease outcomes: the NSABP Study of Tamoxifen and Raloxifene (STAR) P-2 trial. *JAMA* 2006;295:2727-2741.

Wang X, Kruithof-de Julio M, Economides KD, et al. A luminal epithelial stem cell that is a cell of origin for prostate cancer. *Nature* 2009;461:495-500.

Wang YZ, Wong YC. Sex hormone-induced prostatic carcinogenesis in the noble rat: the role of insulin-like growth factor-I (IGF-I) and vascular endothelial growth factor (VEGF) in the development of prostate cancer. *Prostate* 1998;35:165-177.

Ward RD, Weigel NL. Steroid receptor phosphorylation: assigning function to site-specific phosphorylation. *Biofactors* 2009;35: 528-536.

Warde P, Mason M, Ding K, et al. Combined androgen deprivation therapy and radiation therapy for locally advanced prostate cancer: a randomised phase III trial. *Lancet* 2011;378:2104-2111.

Weigelt B, Reis-Filho JS. Histological and molecular types of breast cancer: is there a unifying taxonomy? *Nat Rev Clin Oncol* 2009;6:718-730.

Wood LD, Parsons DW, Jones S, et al. The genomic landscapes of human breast and colorectal cancers. *Science* 2007;318: 1108-1113.

Xu J, Wu RC, O'Malley BW. Normal and cancer-related functions of the p160 steroid receptor co-activator (SRC) family. *Nat Rev Cancer* 2009;9:615-630.

Ziegler RG, Hoover RN, Pike MC, et al. Migration patterns and breast cancer risk in Asian-American women. *J Natl Cancer Inst* 1993;85:1819-1827.

The Immune System and Immunotherapy

Linh T. Nguyen, Evan F. Lind, and Pamela S. Ohashi

21.1 INTRODUCTION TO THE IMMUNE SYSTEM

One feature that is common to all organisms is the ability to defend themselves against challenges in the environment in which they live. Mammals have a complex phalanx of defenses against bacteria, viruses, and parasites, which comprise the immune system. The immune system can be very broadly characterized as having 2 major arms: *innate immunity* and *adaptive immunity*. The innate immune system is the "first line of defense" against pathogens, and includes macrophages and dendritic cells that function in part to present antigens to the cells in the adaptive immune system. The adaptive arm of the immune system is mediated by lymphocytes and responds with higher specificity to pathogens. Key cells of the adaptive immune system are helper T cells (Th) that express a marker known as CD4, cytotoxic T lymphocytes (CTL) that are distinguished by the CD8 marker, and B cells that produce antibodies. The molecular components of pathogens that are recognized by T and B cells are broadly referred to as antigens.

The adaptive immune system has evolved to respond to an initial encounter with a variety of foreign pathogens as well as a potential secondary encounter with the same pathogen. These challenges have shaped the development of the immune system to have the properties of diversity, specificity, and memory. Diversity enables an individual to respond to a broad array of possible pathogens, while at the same time generating exquisite specificity to elements of specific pathogens, ensuring a focused response to a given pathogen while minimizing collateral damage to the host tissues. Memory is the ability of the immune system to respond rapidly to a pathogen that has previously been encountered, thus avoiding sickness and quickly clearing the offending organism without damaging the host.

Another feature of the immune system is that it generally does not attack the host's own tissues. This recognition of "self" versus "non-self" and the ability to avoid attacking self-tissues is referred to as *self-tolerance*. Although these mechanisms of tolerance are critical to avoid autoimmunity, they are impediments that need to be overcome in antitumor immunity.

21.2 INNATE IMMUNITY

21.2.1 Antigen Presentation

One of the main functions of the innate immune system is to present antigens to the adaptive immune system to orchestrate

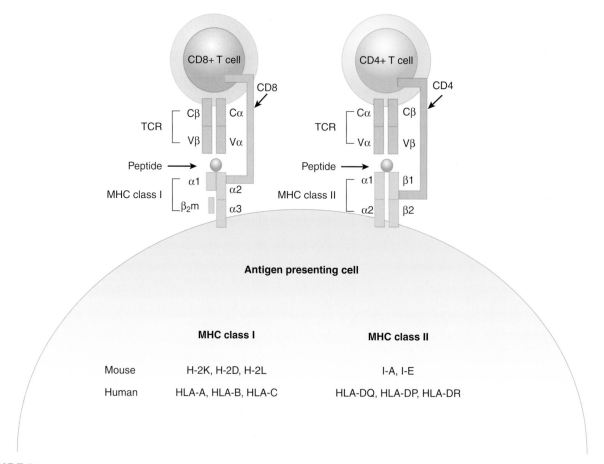

FIGURE 21–1 **T-cell recognition of antigens in the context of MHC molecules.** The α/β dimer of the T-cell receptor (TCR) recognizes peptide fragments on the surface of antigen-presenting cells (APCs). The TCR on CD4+ T cells binds MHC class II molecules bearing an antigenic peptide. This interaction is stabilized by the CD4 coreceptor from the surface of the CD4+ T-cell binding to the MHC class II molecule. The TCR on CD8+ T cells binds MHC class I molecules bearing an antigenic peptide. This interaction is stabilized by the CD8 coreceptor. The nomenclature of MHC alleles in human and mouse is listed at the bottom of the figure. β_2m, β_2-microglobulin.

a functional immune response. Dendritic cells (DCs) are highly specialized and efficient antigen-presenting cells (APCs). One key function that differentiates DCs from other "professional" APCs, such as macrophages and B cells, is their ability to activate naïve T cells. Antigens are presented to T cells by major histocompatibility complex (MHC) molecules. The MHC consists of a series of proteins encoded by highly polymorphic codominantly expressed genes. As a result, each individual expresses a particular combination of MHC alleles that is different between individuals, and a huge diversity exists in populations. There are 2 main types of MHC molecules. MHC class I molecules are expressed on almost all cells. MHC class II molecules are expressed primarily on APCs such as macrophages, DCs and B cells, or can be induced to be expressed on cells only in the case of inflammation. The mouse MHC class I molecules are referred to as H-2K, H-2D, and H-2L; the mouse MHC class II molecules are I-A and I-E. The human MHC is comprised of 3 class I molecules, HLA-A, HLA-B, and HLA-C and 3 class II molecules, HLA-DQ, HLA-DP, and HLA-DR. Class I heterodimers comprise a transmembrane α-chain noncovalently bound to the nonpolymorphic β_2-microglobulin

protein (β_2m). The class II MHC molecule is expressed on the cell surface as an α and β heterodimer. A schematic of MHC class I and II molecules is depicted in Figure 21–1.

The functions of MHC class I and II molecules are to bind and display peptide fragments for T-cell recognition. These peptides may be derived from self proteins or foreign proteins. The peptide binding cleft of MHC molecules contains the regions of highest polymorphism within the molecule and has an impact on the array of peptides that may be bound. Class I and class II differ in the size of peptides that can bind the cleft. MHC class I binds smaller peptide fragments (8 to 11 amino acids) whereas class II presents larger fragments of proteins (15 to 18 amino acids).

The 3 major pathways by which peptides can be processed and loaded into the binding cleft of MHC molecules are referred to as the exogenous, endogenous, and cross-presentation pathways. These pathways are depicted in Figure 21–2. The exogenous pathway is the predominant pathway for class II loading, whereas the proteins processed through the endogenous and cross-presentation pathways result in class I loading. The endogenous pathway occurs in most cells, whereas the

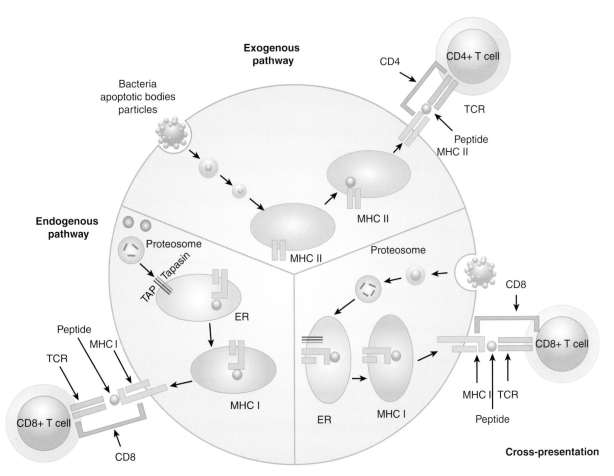

FIGURE 21-2 Antigen-processing pathways in the APC. There are 3 pathways of antigen processing by the APC: exogenous, endogenous, and cross-presentation. The exogenous pathway processes proteins produced outside the APC and places their peptides on MHC class II for recognition by CD4+ T cells. Proteins derived from apoptotic bodies, bacteria, and particulate antigens are processed into peptides by the exogenous pathway. The exogenous pathway occurs in phagocytic cells, including B cells, macrophages, and dendritic cells. The endogenous pathway places cell-produced peptides into the peptide-binding groove of MHC class I for recognition by CD8+T cells. The endogenous pathway is responsible for immune recognition of viral peptides or self peptides. Peptides are cleaved from proteins in the cytosol by the proteasome. They then enter the endoplasmic reticulum (ER) in a process dependent on the transporter associated with antigen processing (TAP) and are loaded onto MHC class I, which is then shuttled to the cell surface. This pathway occurs in most cells, not just APCs, allowing sensing of viral infection in all cell types. The cross-presentation pathway also loads peptides onto MHC class I for recognition by CD8+T cells, but the proteins that are processed are not cell-intrinsic, and are instead taken up from the surrounding environment. This pathway is important for detecting viruses that infect cells other than APCs and tumor antigens taken up in the form of tumor apoptotic bodies. The cross-presentation pathway is most efficient in dendritic cells.

other 2 pathways (exogenous and cross-presentation) occur primarily in APCs.

The exogenous pathway of protein processing begins when an APC acquires material from outside the cell by phagocytosis or receptor-mediated endocytosis. This exogenous material is processed initially in an acidified early endosome by pH-sensitive proteases. The endosome containing the fragmented protein finally fuses with a vesicle containing newly formed MHC class II molecules where the peptides then bind in the cleft of the MHC molecule. MHC class II is produced in the endoplasmic reticulum. When the protein is produced a chaperone protein known as the invariant chain initially occupies the peptide-binding groove. As the MHC/invariant complex leaves the Golgi apparatus, the invariant chain targets

the complex to enter the endosomal pathway where proteases known as cathepsins digest the invariant chain until only a small fragment known as CLIP (class II-associated invariant chain-derived peptide) remains in the binding cleft. The MHC II-CLIP complex next associates with proteins that aid in the release of CLIP, freeing the peptide-binding groove for occupancy by the extrinsically obtained peptides. After this peptide exchange, the complex is shuttled to the cell membrane where it is available to be recognized by CD4+ Th cells (Bryant and Ploegh, 2004; Trombetta and Mellman, 2005).

The endogenous pathway is responsible for loading cell-intrinsic proteins in the binding cleft of MHC class I molecules. Proteins are digested by a large macromolecular complex known as the proteasome (see Chap. 8, Fig. 8-9 and Chap. 9,

Fig. 9–4). The proteosome normally processes self proteins but when a cell is exposed to inflammatory cytokines, such as interferon-γ (IFN-γ) or tumor necrosis factor (TNF)-α the structure of the proteosome is altered into a structure known as the *immunoproteosome*, which is more efficient at processing peptides with high binding efficiency to the MHC class I peptide-binding cleft. Self proteins are cleaved into short fragments by the proteosome in the cytoplasm and are then shuttled into the endoplasmic reticulum by the TAP protein complex. As the peptides are guided into the ER by the TAP transporter, they are loaded onto empty MHC class I molecules, which are held close to the TAP complex by the protein Tapasin. In the case of viral infections, peptides derived from the virus will be processed and loaded onto the MHC class I molecule resulting in viral detection by CD8+ T cells. In the case of tumor cells, proteins derived from the tumor cell will be processed and loaded onto MHC class I via the cross-presentation pathway (Pamer and Cresswell, 1998).

Efficient activation of T cells depends upon the acquisition of antigens by APCs and the subsequent presentation of selected peptides in combination with MHC molecules on the cell surface for recognition by T cells. Because MHC class I-restricted peptides are derived from proteins produced intrinsically by the cell, a conundrum arises as to how a T-cell response can be initiated against viruses or bacteria that infect cell types other than APCs. A process known as cross-presentation can occur where cell-exogenous proteins can be taken up by DCs and presented on MHC class I molecules (see Fig. 21–2). This pathway is critical to activation of tumor-specific T cells, as the tumor cells are not usually APCs. The presence of measurable T-cell responses to many tumors implies that at one point a DC may have acquired tumor-derived proteins and processed them into MHC class I-restricted peptides, resulting in the activation of naïve tumor-reactive CD8+ T cells (Shen and Rock, 2006).

21.2.2 Maturation of Antigen-Presenting Cells

APCs can exist in an immature state or a mature (ie, activated) state (Fig. 21–3). Maturation of APCs occurs via specialized cell-surface receptors or intracellular receptors that recognize pathogen associated-molecular patterns (PAMPs). These receptor classes include Toll-like receptors (TLRs), nucleotide binding domain and leucine-rich repeat receptors (NLRs), the retinoic acid-inducible gene-like receptors (RLRs), and c-type lectins (Iwasaki and Medzhitov, 2010). The best-studied receptors are the TLR family of proteins (Takeda and Akira, 2005). The ligands for TLRs include viral/bacterial DNA and RNA, bacterial lipids and endogenously derived molecules, such as heat shock proteins and uric acid crystals that alert the immune system to tissue damage. There are at least 11 identified TLRs in mammals, 9 of which are conserved between human and mouse (TLR1 to TLR9). TLR4 is one of the best-characterized TLRs; the pathogen-associated ligand for TLR4 is lipopolysaccharide (LPS), a molecule found on the outer membrane of Gram-negative bacteria. Several TLR

- Low costimulatory molecule levels
- Low MHC expression
- Highly phagocytic
- Found in peripheral tissue

- Upregulate costimulatory molecules
- Upregulate MHC
- Produce proinflammatory cytokines
- Migrate to spleen/lymph nodes

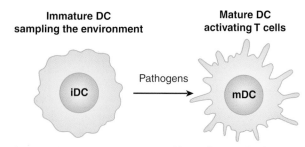

FIGURE 21–3 DC maturation and migration. The DC is the most effective sentinel for the immune system, migrating throughout peripheral tissues seeking damage or infection. The immature DC (iDC) has low expression of costimulatory molecules and MHC. This limits inappropriate activation of T cells in the absence of infection or tissue damage. The iDC is highly phagocytic, sampling the local environment for antigens. Upon encounter with a maturation signal such as ligands for the Toll-like receptor (TLR) family molecules or ligation of the CD40 molecule, the iDC increases levels of costimulatory molecules and MHC and migrates to the local draining lymph node where it can interact with and activate T cells. *mDC*, Mature dendritic cell.

stimuli are being investigated for use as immune adjuvants in humans. For example, the drug imiquimod (see Sec. 21.3.3), that is used as a treatment for warts, activates TLR7. Signaling through TLR7 either by drugs such as imiquimod, or from viral infection, results in production of interferon-α. TLR9 recognizes unmethylated CpG (cytosine phosphate guanine) DNA structures (Hemmi et al, 2000), that are plentiful in bacterial DNA but rare in mammals. Activation of TLR9 by CpG DNA results in production of the cytokines interleukin (IL)-12 and TNF-α which contribute to the induction of cell-mediated immunity.

The NOD-like and RIG-I-like families of proteins (NLRs and RLRs) detect the presence of bacteria and viruses, respectively. NLR proteins sense bacterial products in the cytoplasm by interacting with the C-terminal leucine-rich repeat regions (LRR). Bacterially-derived products bind to the LRR, resulting in a conformational change in intracellular NOD proteins. This change activates the NOD proteins resulting in recruitment of signaling kinases and activation of Caspase (CASP)-1 through binding to caspase recruitment domains (CARDs). This activation results in both de novo cytokine transcription via activation of the nuclear factor-kappa B (NF-κB) and AP1 transcription factors (see Chap. 8, Sec. 8.2.6) and activation of IL-1 through CASP-1 activity (Franchi et al, 2009). RLRs are also localized in the cytoplasm but bind viral-derived RNA sequences. The RLR family contains several members, such as RIG-I, MDA-5, and LGP2. These proteins bind modifications found in the 5′ end of virally produced RNAs that are not found in mammalian RNA. Detection of viral RNA in the cytoplasm results in activation of NF-κB and IRF3 (interferon regulatory factor 3), thereby inducing inflammatory cytokine and type-1 interferon production by the infected cell (Kawai and Akira, 2008).

After the detection of pathogens via these different receptor families, the APC becomes mature and upregulates expression of MHC class II and other costimulatory molecules that contribute to the activation of T cells (see Fig. 21–3). In addition, mature APCs are induced to secrete cytokines and chemokines that promote immune function in a variety of ways. Signaling through TLRs also induces a change in migration of the APC. DCs will change their responsiveness to chemokine signals and migrate out of the peripheral tissues and localize ("home") to lymph nodes, thus increasing their chances of encountering a T cell with specificity to the pathogen that activated the DC. Monocytes and macrophages will migrate in the opposite pattern, entering the infected or damaged tissue where they take part in pathogen clearance or tissue repair, at the same time acting as local APCs to maintain activation of T cells at the site of infection.

21.3 ADAPTIVE IMMUNITY

21.3.1 Generation of Lymphocyte Diversity

B cells and T cells express highly specific receptors that recognize antigen. The B-cell receptor (BCR) and T-cell receptor (TCR) are generated uniquely in each cell as the consequence of genomic DNA rearrangements. The BCR is a membrane-bound form of the soluble immunoglobulin (antibody) that will be produced by that cell upon activation, as a consequence of the ability to bind a specific antigen. BCRs can bind to antigens in their native form, so that the B cell can detect unprocessed antigens. In contrast, the TCR is not secreted and stimulation via the TCR may lead to the activation of the T-cell response. Antigen recognition by T cells is also different from antigen recognition by B cells. T cells do not react to antigen in its unprocessed form, but rather recognize peptide fragments bound in the MHC of APCs (as described above; see also Fig. 21–1). These differences allow B and T cells to defend the host in 2 different ways: by directly recognizing the pathogen and by recognizing cells infected by the pathogen.

The TCR is composed of 2 protein chains joined together by disulfide bonds (Fig. 21–4A). This dimer can be composed of either α and β chains or γ and δ chains. The αβ TCR is present on the majority of mature T cells found in the blood and lymphoid organs while γδ TCR-bearing T cells are found primarily in skin and intestine. The TCR is expressed at the cell surface in a molecular complex that includes proteins that have intracellular signaling domains (immunoreceptor tyrosine activation motifs; ITAMs): CD3δε, CD3γε, and TCRζζ. Once the TCR is bound by specific peptide/MHC complexes, the ITAMs in the CD3 and TCR molecules aggregate together and initiate an intracellular signaling cascade.

The TCR chains are not encoded as single transcripts; rather, they are the result of genomic DNA rearrangements that bring together different gene segments and splice them into a combined exon (Davis, 1990; see Fig. 21–4B). This genomic splicing is dependent on an enzyme known as *recombination activation gene recombinase* (*RAG* recombinase) that is expressed exclusively in developing T and B cells (Krangel, 2009). The TCRα chain is comprised of 2 separate rearranged gene segments brought together during recombination. Variable (V) gene segments undergo rearrangement with joining (J) gene segments and are expressed together with constant (C) regions, forming the α chain of the TCR. The β chain has 3 rearranged gene segments: variable, diversity (D), and joining regions that undergo rearrangement and are expressed with the constant region of the β locus. The large number of possible combinations of VJ in the α chain and VDJ in the β chain results in enormous diversity among T-cell populations, especially as each mature T cell will rearrange its own TCR independently (Krangel, 2009; see Fig. 21–4B). In addition, a strategy called "N region diversity" occurs that generates additional nucleotides during the rearrangement process, which increases the repertoire of antigens that can be recognized by each TCR. The specificity of the TCR for a defined peptide bound in the groove of an MHC molecule is determined by regions of the TCR called complementary determining regions (CDRs). Interactions of the CDR with the peptide/MHC complex are a result of the combination of the V chains expressed, as well as the diversity generated by pairing of the VJ and VDJ gene segments.

21.3.2 T-cell Activation

The functional status of a mature T cell depends on whether it expresses a receptor that can bind to a peptide/MHC molecule expressed by a mature APC. T cells can exist in a *naïve* or resting state, or they can be *effector* T cells, which means that they have engaged a mature DC cell bearing their cognate antigen and have differentiated subsequently into functional T cells. Alternatively, they can be *memory* T cells, which are previously activated antigen-specific cells that persist after the pathogen has been eliminated. These 3 states (naïve, effector, and memory) impart quite different phenotypic and functional properties (Fig. 21–5). These stages of development have been studied most extensively in the CD8+ MHC class I-restricted lineage of T cells, and thus much of the following information will refer to CD8+ T cells; however, they also broadly apply to CD4+ T cells.

Most T-cell responses can be subdivided into 3 phases: activation (also known as priming), expansion, and contraction (Fig. 21–6). A naïve T cell has a high threshold for activation, which means that when a mature T cell encounters its cognate antigen/MHC complex for the first time, it is slow to respond and requires several signals to initiate proliferation and acquisition of effector function. The DC is the main cell responsible for T-cell activation. During priming, a DC acquires antigen and matures at the site of infection and travels to the draining lymph node where it enters the T-cell area and interacts with the T cells resident there. An "integrin" receptor-ligand interaction occurs between leukocyte function-associated antigen

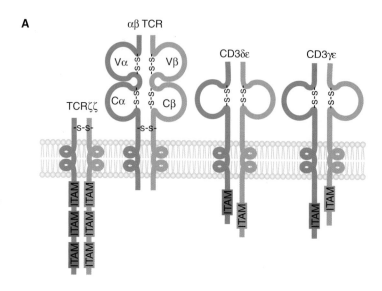

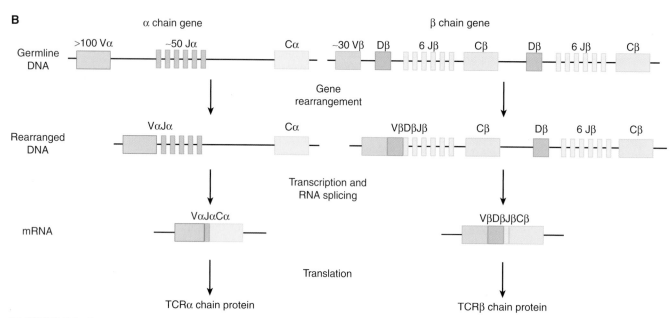

FIGURE 21–4 **The TCR. A)** The TCR is composed of 2 chains, α and β, each containing 2 immunoglobulin domains formed by an intrachain disulfide bond. The TCR is associated with the dimeric proteins CD3δε, CD3γε, and TCRζζ, and together with the αβ TCR, they comprise the TCR complex. *ITAM*, Immunoreceptor tyrosine-based activation motifs. **B)** The variable (V), diversity (D), joining (J), and constant (C) domains of the TCR are encoded by corresponding gene segments that undergo somatic rearrangement to generate the αβTCR heterodimer. In the mouse, the α chain consists of more than 100 V, approximately 50 J, and 1 C gene segments. The β chain consists of approximately 30 V regions and 2 clusters each of 1 D, 6 J, and 1 C gene segments. Following V(D)J gene rearrangement and transcription, the RNA is spliced to the C gene segment. The resulting messenger RNA (mRNA) encodes the TCR chains that dimerize to form the complete TCR protein.

(LFA)-1 and LFA-2 on the T cell and intercellular adhesion molecule (ICAM) expressed on the DC. These interactions initially slow migration of the DC past the naïve T cell and then help bring the 2 cell membranes into close proximity, allowing MHC/TCR interactions (Dustin and Cooper, 2000; Fig. 21–6). If a mature DC presents a peptide on its MHC molecules that is recognized by the specific TCR on the T cell, a signal will be sent into the T cell. This antigen-specific recognition, together with other receptor ligand interactions, promotes a functional T-cell response. One of the well-studied molecules that leads

to optimal T-cell activation is CD28. The ligands of CD28 are CD80 (B7-1) and CD86 (B7-2), which are upregulated on the surface of mature DCs. This CD28 costimulatory signal results in the production of IL-2, a cytokine critical for T-cell proliferation and survival (Fig. 21–6). T-cell activation also results in the increased expression of several other molecules, including CD154, which is the ligand for the TNF family member CD40 that is present on the surface of the DC. The binding of CD40 on the DC results in the upregulation of costimulatory molecules, cytokines, and increased DC survival, allowing for

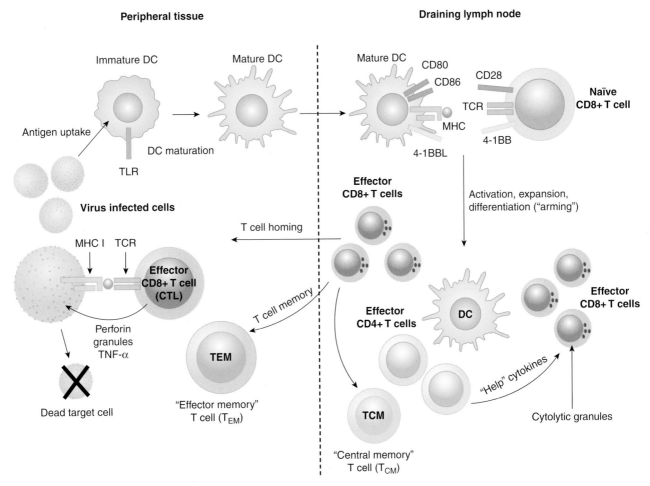

Peripheral tissue

Draining lymph node

Immature DC

Mature DC

Mature DC   CD80

CD86   CD28

TCR

MHC

4-1BBL   4-1BB

Naïve CD8+ T cell

Antigen uptake

DC maturation

TLR

Virus infected cells

Activation, expansion, differentiation ("arming")

Effector CD8+ T cells

T cell homing

MHC I   TCR

Effector CD8+ T cell (CTL)

T cell memory

Effector CD4+ T cells

DC

Effector CD8+ T cells

"Help" cytokines

Perforin granules TNF-α

TEM

Cytolytic granules

Dead target cell

"Effector memory" T cell (T$_{EM}$)

TCM

"Central memory" T cell (T$_{CM}$)

FIGURE 21–5 **The stages of a cytotoxic T-cell response.** CD8+ T-cell immune responses begin when a DC is activated by a pathogen or inflammatory signal in the periphery. Antigens are picked up by the DC and processed into peptides and placed onto MHC class I molecules via the cross-presentation pathway. Mature DCs migrate to T-cell areas in the lymph nodes, where they interact with naïve T cells. The T cell recognizes its cognate peptide bound to MHC class I on the DC, resulting in activation of the T cell. If the TCR signal is followed by costimulation by CD28 on the T cell interacting with CD80 and CD86 on the DC, the T cell will begin to proliferate, expanding the clone of the T cell that has specificity to the antigen. The CD8+ T cell will become armed by exposure to cytokines resulting in cytolytic granule formation. The T cell then exits the lymph node and traffics to sites of inflammation to engage and kill cells that present the cognate antigenic peptide on their MHC class I molecules.

prolonged antigen presentation (Quezada et al, 2004). The positive feedback loop between T cells and the DC results in expansion of antigen-specific T-cell clones. These expanded T cells are now functional effector T cells that change their chemokine and integrin expression patterns; they leave the lymph nodes and home to sites of inflammation.

21.3.3 T-cell Memory

After the pathogen that initiated a T-cell response has been cleared, the effector T cells that responded to that pathogen disappear, leaving only a small pool of specialized T cells behind, known as *memory T cells*. These cells respond rapidly upon a re-encounter with the appropriate antigen, and thus offer protection from subsequent infections with the same pathogen. Memory T cells are CD8+ and can be subdivided into 2 categories: T effector memory (T$_{EM}$) and T central memory (T$_{CM}$) cells. These subsets can be defined by their localization,

surface molecule expression, and function. The T$_{CM}$ cells are found in secondary lymphoid tissues. These cells express the chemokine receptor CCR7, express high levels of CD62L, and do not have preformed lytic granules. T$_{CM}$ cells most likely represent a pool of antigen-specific CD8+ T cells that are ready to expand again upon a second encounter with their cognate antigen. The T$_{EM}$ cells are found in nonlymphoid tissues: these cells have preformed cytolytic granules and are ready to act immediately at the sites of pathogen entry. T$_{EM}$ cells are identified by virtue of the profile CD8+, CD62 low, and CCR7−. The maintenance of memory CD8+ T cells is dependent in part on 2 cytokines, IL-7 and IL-15 (Kalia et al, 2006).

21.3.4 T-cell Subsets

CTLs are CD8+ T cells that possess the ability to kill target cells directly if the TCR is specific for peptides presented by MHC class I molecules expressed by the target cell. Differentiation of

A

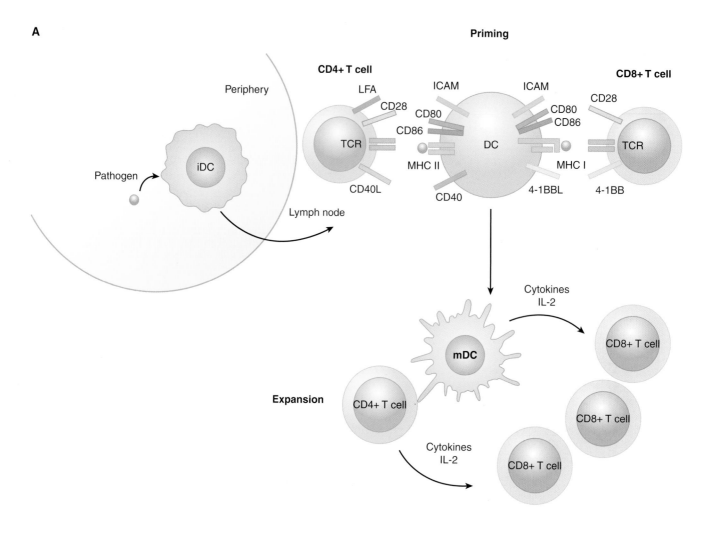

B

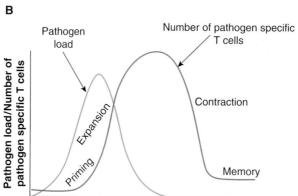

FIGURE 21-6 **T-cell activation: priming, expansion, and contraction. A)** After sensing tissue damage or infection in a peripheral tissue, the DC bearing antigen migrates to the T-cell area of a draining lymph node. DCs and T cells mingle in the lymph node, adhering to one another through interactions between LFA (lymphocyte function-associated antigen) on the T cell and ICAM (intercellular adhesion molecule) on the DC. A T cell with a TCR that is specific for the antigen obtained at the site of infection will interact with the DC and signal through the antigen-specific TCR. At the same time, CD28 on the T cell will bind to CD80 and CD86 on the DC. This signal is referred to as *costimulation*. CD4+ T cells will express CD40 ligand (CD154) that binds to CD40 on the DC, promoting the antigen-bearing DC's survival and increasing cytokine production. Antigen-specific CD8+ and CD4+ T cells that receive these signals will then begin to divide. These expanded antigen-specific T cells then travel to the peripheral tissues to clear the infection. **B)** The T-cell immune response can be divided into several phases. Priming occurs when an antigen is first presented to naïve T cells and they are induced to expand for the first time. As the levels of antigen wane because of clearance by the immune system, contraction of the antigen-specific T-cell clones occurs. After contraction, a greater number of specific T cells remain than before the infection. These cells are referred to as memory T cells and have properties that allow them to react rapidly to reinfection with the same pathogen.

the CD8+ T cell from a resting naïve T cell into a mature CTL includes the formation of cytolytic granules (see Fig. 21–5). The cytolytic granules contain the molecules Perforin and proteases of the Granzyme family. After TCR engagement on the CTL, the cytolytic granules fuse quickly with the cell membrane, releasing Perforin and Granzymes. Perforin forms pores in the target cell membrane allowing the Granzyme proteases to enter. Granzymes initiate cleavage of proteins inside the target cell, and the result is apoptosis.

Th cells express the CD4 coreceptor and recognize peptides presented by MHC class II molecules. Th cells can be divided into several subgroups that are defined by their functional properties and/or their ability to produce a defined cytokine profile (Fig. 21–7). The first identified Th cell subsets were termed *Th1* and *Th2* and represented 2 discrete pathways of CD4+ mature T-cell differentiation. Th1 cells express the transcription factor T-BET (Szabo et al, 2000); they produce high levels of the cytokines IL-2, TNF-α, and IFN-γ, and induce IL-12 production by APCs. A Th1 cell augments primarily a CD8+ CTL-type response focused on elimination of intracellular pathogens, such as viruses and intracellular bacteria. Th2 cells mediate humoral (antibody) responses that are directed generally against extracellular pathogens and parasites. The Th2 T cell produces IL-4 among other cytokines: binding of IL-4 to its receptor on CD4+ T cells results in signal transducers and activators of transcription 6 (STAT6) activation and transcription of GATA3, which is the master transcription factor (see Chap. 8, Sec. 8.3.1) required for Th2 cell function (Zheng and Flavell, 1997).

A newly identified Th subset is named Th17 for the ability to produce the cytokine IL-17, which is believed to act on local tissues to promote inflammation (McGeachy and Cua,

2008). These cells are required for many types of autoimmune diseases (Gutcher and Becher, 2007), and their possible role in antitumor responses is of great interest (Ji and Zhang, 2010).

Regulatory T cells (Tregs) represent another CD4+ T-cell population that has the ability to inhibit immune responses. This subset is key for preventing autoimmune diseases. In the mouse, they have been shown to express the markers CD25 and FoxP3, and their presence is dependent on the transcription factor FoxP3. There are 2 major sources of Tregs. One subset develops during thymic selection and is called natural T reg (nTreg). The second group of Tregs originates from mature peripheral CD4+ T cells that are converted into regulatory cells through signals in their environment; they are referred to as induced Tregs (iTregs) (Jonuleit and Schmitt, 2003; Josefowicz and Rudensky, 2009; Sakaguchi et al, 2008).

21.3.5 Suppression of T-cell Activation

Activation of T cells is required and desirable to resolve many infections, but uncontrolled T-cell activation may result in damage to the surrounding tissues. A balance between costimulatory activators and inhibitory molecules enables inhibition of a T-cell response when appropriate. Two of these inhibitory molecules are cytotoxic T-lymphocyte antigen (CTLA)-4 and programmed death (PD)-1. CTLA-4 is upregulated after TCR engagement on T cells, although it is constitutively found on Tregs. CTLA-4 competes with CD28 for binding with CD80 and CD86. Studies show that CTLA-4 has a higher affinity than CD28 for CD80 and CD86. Clustering of CD80/86 on the surface of APCs sends a signal to the APC to activate an enzyme called indoleamine 2,3-deoxygenase (IDO), which, in turn, metabolizes tryptophan and inhibits T-cell proliferation.

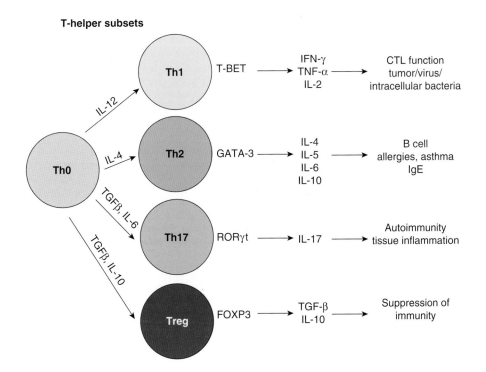

T-helper subsets

FIGURE 21–7 Th cell subsets. Th cells express the CD4 coreceptor and recognize peptides presented on MHC class II molecules of APCs. After activation through TCR engagement the T cell goes down 1 of 4 differentiation pathways, resulting in different effector functions. These pathways begin when a naïve CD4+ T cell (Th0) is activated in the presence of different cytokine and signaling conditions. The differentiation pathways have been identified to rely on transcriptional patterns enforced by specific transcription factors. After differentiation the subsets produce signature sets of cytokines that characterize their final effector function.

Signaling through CTLA-4 into the T cell recruits the Src homology domain-containing phosphatase (SHP)-1 and interrupts the TCR signal. The critical role of CTLA-4 in inhibiting T-cell responses is evident in mice that have been genetically manipulated to lack the CTLA-4 protein (CTLA-4 "knockout" mice), as these mice develop severe autoimmunity (Fife and Bluestone, 2008).

PD-1, like CTLA-4, is expressed on activated CD4+ and CD8+ T cells, but is always present on Tregs. There are 2 known ligands for PD-1. PD-L1 (B7-H1) exhibits broad expression; it is found on many nonhematopoietic cells, as well as immune cells, including APCs. The expression of PD-L2 is restricted mainly to APCs. Expression of PD-L1 has been found on many tumors and correlates with poor prognosis. Signaling though PD-1 blocks the function and survival of effector T cells. Tregs have been shown to express both PD-1 and PD-L1 (Fife and Bluestone, 2008).

21.3.6 T-cell Tolerance

Because the rearrangements of the TCR are random, inevitably combinations will arise that are specific for self antigens. One of the main roles of the thymus is the production of functional, but not autoreactive T cells. This process can be broken down into 2 major events (Sebzda et al, 1999). First, a T cell must express a TCR that is able to interact with self MHC molecules. This process is known as *positive selection* and is important for selecting only those T cells that express receptors that recognize self MHC, as all foreign peptides are presented by self MHC. As a consequence of positive selection, each T cell in the repertoire is selected for recognition of the different MHC molecules in a given host; selection is based on weak interactions between the TCR and MHC presenting self peptide. Cells that essentially cannot bind to self MHC do not receive any signal through their TCR and undergo apoptosis ("no selection"). In contrast, T cells that have TCRs with high avidity to self peptides presented by the MHC are deleted; this process is referred to as "negative selection." Alternatively, some high avidity, self-reactive thymocytes are rendered tolerant by a process called *anergy*, which results in T-cell inactivation. Finally, T cells with high avidity to self peptides may also differentiate into Tregs, which play a critical role in the maintenance of peripheral tolerance (Sakaguchi et al, 2003). A schematic of the model of thymocyte selection is shown in Figure 21–8.

Some autoreactive T cells escape negative selection in the thymus and enter the periphery. It is likely that this process occurs when some self antigens are not expressed in the thymus and therefore potentially self-reactive T cells cannot be rendered tolerant. The mechanisms involved in preventing these T cells with self-specificity from becoming activated either can be intrinsic to the T cell or a result of immune regulation by other cells.

Intrinsic mechanisms of peripheral tolerance include *deletion* and *anergy*, which are similar to the self-tolerance mechanisms that occur in the thymus. DCs have the ability

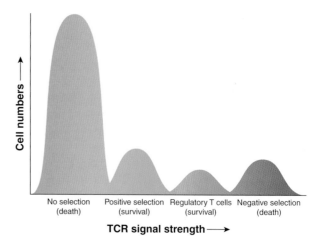

FIGURE 21–8 **Thresholds of T-cell selection.** T cells are selected during development in the thymus for their ability to bind peptides in the context of self-MHC molecules but at the same will not be activated by self-peptides to become effector cells. Random genomic re-arrangements of the TCR genes result in receptors with various affinities for self-peptides bound by MHC. T cells that essentially cannot bind to self-MHC do not receive any signal through their TCR and undergo apoptosis ("no selection"). Cells that bind self-MHC, but do not react strongly to self-peptides, finish development and enter the periphery as naïve T cells ("positive selection"). T cells with intermediate affinity to self-peptides will differentiate into regulatory T cells (Tregs). Finally, T cells that develop high-affinity TCRs, which would result in strong affinity to "self," are deleted ("negative selection").

to imprint the "fate" of deletion or anergy of mature self-reactive T cells. DCs can display self antigen that has been acquired from tissues and, if the DC is in a resting state, it renders T cells tolerant to these self antigens. However, as described in Section 21.2.2, DCs also have the ability to activate the immune system. The distinction that permits the induction of T-cell tolerance or T-cell immunity is the "functional status" of the DC: resting or steady state DCs present peptide/MHC complexes that can lead to induction of tolerance, whereas mature or activated DCs induce immunity (Steinman et al, 2003).

There are certain thresholds or concentrations of self antigen/MHC complexes that are required to induce tolerance (Ohashi, 1994). If tissue-specific antigens are not presented at an immunologically detectable level, T-cell ignorance is the result. In this situation, self-reactive T cells exist in the T-cell repertoire in a naïve or ignorant state. However, if these cells encounter antigen in an immune-stimulatory setting, these cells can be activated to destroy self-tissues. This scenario has been demonstrated experimentally in many models, including a mouse model of multiple sclerosis where myelin fragments are injected with a powerful immune stimulator (complete Freund adjuvant [CFA]). These myelin antigens are presented to naïve self-reactive T cells in the context of local inflammation induced by the CFA. The myelin-specific T cells then become activated and attack the myelin sheaths in the nervous system (Mendel et al, 1995).

Tregs are critical for the maintenance of peripheral immune tolerance in both mouse and man. Mice lacking Treg expression because of a mutation in the *foxp3* gene (the transcription factor that is required for Tregs), succumb to severe multiorgan autoimmune disease. In humans, mutations impairing Treg development or function are correlated with the fatal autoimmune disease immune dysregulation, polyendocrinopathy, enteropathy, X-linked (IPEX; Wildin and Freitas, 2005). Current models propose that Tregs are antigen specific, but suppress in a nonspecific manner. This duality implies that to function properly they need to encounter self antigen and subsequently suppress the function of other T cells with various antigen specificities in their area. This phenomenon is known as "bystander suppression." Tregs function in various ways, including cell contact- and soluble factor-mediated mechanisms. Activated Tregs possess the ability to kill directly both T cells and APCs in their local environment by producing Granzyme B that can enter surrounding cells and induce apoptosis (Gondek et al, 2005). This targeted elimination can reduce the quantity of activated T cells in an inflammatory site and terminate antigen presentation. Tregs have also been shown to inhibit killing by CTL by impairing granule exocytosis (Mempel et al, 2006). The high levels of CTLA-4 present on Tregs will bind to CD80 and CD86 on APCs resulting in increased intracellular levels of the tryptophan metabolizing enzyme IDO (Orabona et al, 2004). These high IDO levels then cause depletion of tryptophan from the local environment, thereby inhibiting T cell proliferation (Munn and Mellor, 2007). Tregs also express high levels of the IL-2 receptor CD25, and as a consequence, Tregs bind IL-2 more rapidly than other T cells in the local area. Thus, Tregs may function in part by limiting the amount of this T-cell growth factor available to effector cells nearby. Activated Tregs have also been shown to secrete the antiinflammatory cytokines IL-10 and transforming growth factor (TGF)-β (Sakaguchi et al, 2009); TGF-β also has antiproliferative functions and may contribute to limiting immune responses.

21.4 TUMOR IMMUNOLOGY

As described above, the immune system is equipped to recognize and eliminate foreign threats such as bacteria and viruses. However, studies demonstrate clearly that the immune system is also capable of recognizing tumors and mounting an immune response against our own "self" tissues. Many strategies that activate or enhance the immune response to tumors have been devised over the last few decades as therapies for cancer.

21.4.1 Tumor-Associated Antigens

One fundamental aspect that was critical to move the field of tumor immune therapy forward was the identification of tumor-associated antigens (TAAs). TAAs are intracellular or extracellular proteins that are expressed preferentially by tumor cells, but often can be expressed by normal cells. These proteins are processed and presented on MHC class I and II

molecules in a similar manner to proteins of nontumor origin (eg, self proteins, or viral or bacterial proteins), as described above. Therefore, specific T cells can recognize TAAs through their TCRs. The identification of TAAs was important for tumor immunology and immunotherapy as it allowed for the detection and characterization of T cells that can recognize specific TAAs. It also allows for the design of immunotherapy that specifically activates TAA-specific T cells, for example by vaccination against specific TAAs.

21.4.1.1 Identification of Tumor-Associated Antigens
The first TAA was identified by Boon and colleagues (van der Bruggen et al, 1991). Using a panel of CTL clones isolated from a patient with metastatic melanoma in combination with various sublines of melanoma tumor cells derived from the same patient, the authors identified a gene whose product was targeted by a particular CTL clone. This gene was not expressed in normal tissues. Furthermore, T cells from the original patient could recognize melanoma cell lines established from other human leukocyte antigen (HLA)-A–matched patients that also expressed the same TAA. Through this approach the MAGE, BAGE, and GAGE families of TAAs were identified.

Other approaches have successfully identified many TAAs. One method is referred to as SEREX (*s*erological analysis of *r*ecombinant cDNA *ex*pression libraries; Sahin et al, 1995). Serum samples taken from cancer patients were postulated to contain antibodies that recognize TAAs. Expression libraries composed of complementary DNAs (cDNAs) isolated from autologous tumor cells were cloned into prokaryotic expression vectors. These libraries were used to bind antibodies and clones that were bound by antibodies were isolated and sequenced. The TAA recognized by the antibody was then identified based on the DNA sequence. Confirmation of the identified protein as a TAA was established in various ways, including evaluating protein expression in normal and malignant tissues. Important TAAs, such NY-ESO-1, were thus identified using the SEREX approach. Other methods to identify TAAs include the acid-elution of MHC-bound peptides from tumor cells and subsequent screening of peptide fractions for recognition by T cells from cancer patients, and, more recently, gene expression microarray analyses (see Chap. 2, Sec. 2.2.12) of tumor cells compared with normal cells. These approaches are depicted in Figure 21–9.

Once a TAA has been identified, it is important to identify the peptide sequences in that protein that can be recognized by various TCRs. One common approach is to identify peptides that can be presented by HLA-A*0201 molecules and recognized by human T cells (Kawashima et al, 1998). HLA-A*0201 is prevalent in Caucasians and is often the focus of studies involving unique peptides that bind this HLA molecule. First, peptides that contained amino acid motifs that would be predicted to bind the HLA-A*0201 molecule were identified. The ability to bind HLA-A*0201 was verified using MHC-binding assays. These peptides were then tested for their ability to expand peptide-specific T cells from the peripheral blood

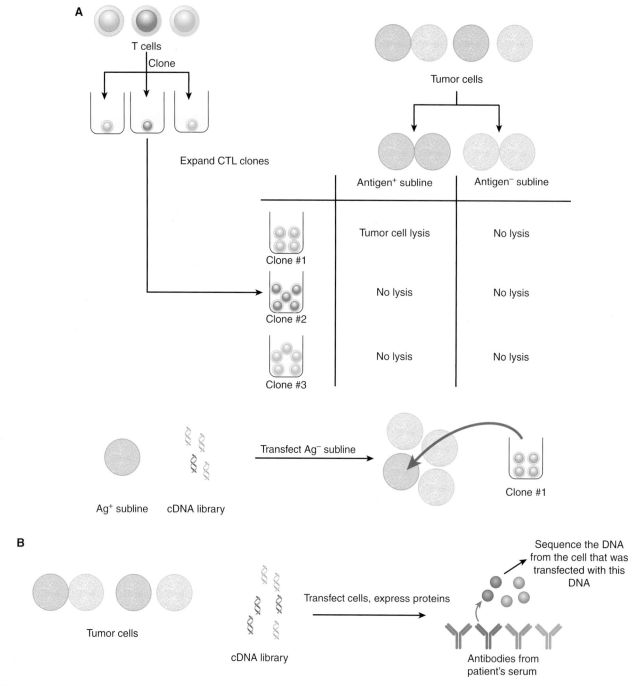

FIGURE 21–9 Approaches for identifying TAAs. A) CTLs from a cancer patient are cloned by plating them at 1 cell per well and expanding each clone. Autologous tumor cells are cultured in vitro and various sublines are obtained, some of which are "antigen-loss" variants. The CTL clones are tested for their ability to lyse the tumor cell sublines. If a clone is able to lyse one subline, but not another, the antigen expressed by the former is identified by transfecting antigen-negative target cells with cDNA libraries derived from the antigen-positive tumor cells. The DNA encoding the target antigen (the TAA) is isolated based on the ability of the CTL clone to lyse the target cell that was transfected with the TAA. **B)** In the SEREX approach, expression libraries composed of cDNAs isolated from autologous tumor cells are cloned into prokaryotic expression vectors. Serum samples from cancer patients (which should contain antibodies that recognize TAAs) are used to screen these libraries. Clones that are bound by antibodies are then isolated and sequenced. *(Continued on next page)*

T-cell population of HLA-A*0201-positive donors. These expansions were achieved by stimulating T cells with autologous DCs that had been exposed to the peptide of interest. After multiple rounds of peptide stimulation, the expanded T cells were tested for their ability to lyse peptide-coated target cells. Using this approach, multiple immunogenic peptides for the MAGE-A2, MAGE-A3, carcinoembryonic antigen (CEA), and human epidermal growth receptor (HER)-2/neu proteins were identified. A database of immunogenic TAA-derived peptides is available at www.cancerimmunity.org.

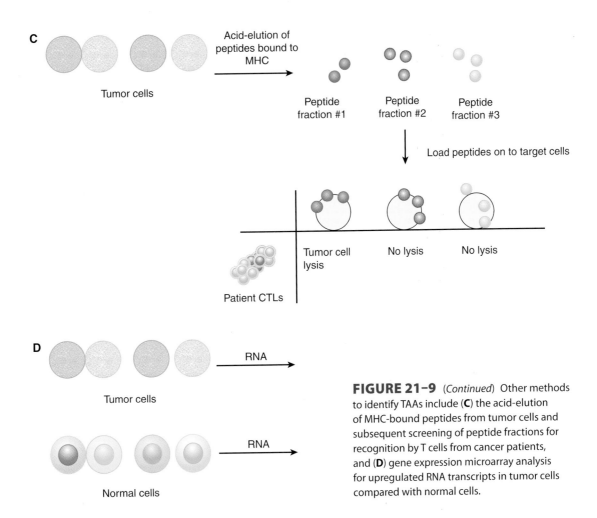

FIGURE 21–9 (*Continued*) Other methods to identify TAAs include (**C**) the acid-elution of MHC-bound peptides from tumor cells and subsequent screening of peptide fractions for recognition by T cells from cancer patients, and (**D**) gene expression microarray analysis for upregulated RNA transcripts in tumor cells compared with normal cells.

21.4.1.2 Types of Tumor-Associated Antigens

TAAs can be classified into several broad categories: (a) mutation antigens, (b) cancer-testis antigens, (c) differentiation antigens, (d) overexpressed antigens, (e) viral antigens, and (f) antigens with unique posttranslational modifications (Fig. 21–10).

Mutation antigens are generally proteins that harbor mutations that are unique to an individual patient, although some mutations are common to a subset of patients. For example, approximately 2% of solid tumors and 40% to 60% of melanomas express a mutant form of the oncogenic protein B-RAF (see Chap. 7, Sec. 7.5.5). The overwhelming majority of patients have a valine → phenylalanine amino acid substitution at position 600. Mutated antigens are not necessarily recognized as unique by T cells, but they can serve as targets for other therapeutic approaches (eg, protein kinase inhibitors).

The expression of cancer-testis antigens is restricted to tumor cells and normal placental trophoblasts and testicular germ cells, and therefore represent appealing targets for immunotherapy. Cancer-testis antigens include the MAGE, BAGE, and GAGE proteins, as well as the commonly expressed NY-ESO-1.

Differentiation antigens are proteins that are expressed on both normal tissues and tumors derived from a particular tissue. For example, Melan-A/MART-1 is expressed on normal melanocytes, as well as malignant melanoma. CEA is expressed on normal colonic epithelium, as well as many carcinomas of the gut. Other differentiation antigens include gp100 (melanoma), tyrosinase (melanoma), and prostate-specific antigen (PSA-prostate cancer). Differentiation antigens also include oncofetal antigens, such as α-fetoprotein, which are expressed in various tissues during fetal development and are reexpressed on tumors.

Overexpressed TAAs are expressed on various normal tissues, as well as tumor cells but with higher expression on tumor cells. For example, Wilms tumor-1 (WT-1) is expressed in a proportion of breast cancers, lung cancers, and other tumor cells.

Viral TAAs are expressed by tumors that are induced by viral transformation. This includes Epstein-Barr virus (EBV)-induced tumors such as some lymphomas and nasopharyngeal carcinoma, and human papilloma virus (HPV)-induced cervical neoplasias (see Chap. 6).

Another class of TAAs consists of proteins where posttranslational modification occurs differently in normal cells compared with tumor cells. T cells are able to distinguish between the same peptide with different posttranslational modifications, such as differential glycosylation levels. For example, mucin-1 (MUC-1) proteins in tumor cells are generally

Normal cell   Tumor cell

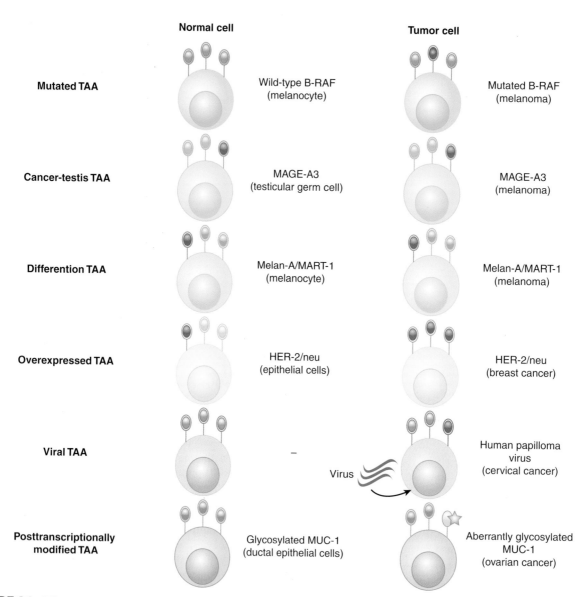

Mutated TAA   Wild-type B-RAF   Mutated B-RAF
                        (melanocyte)   (melanoma)

Cancer-testis TAA   MAGE-A3   MAGE-A3
                        (testicular germ cell)   (melanoma)

Differention TAA   Melan-A/MART-1   Melan-A/MART-1
                        (melanocyte)   (melanoma)

Overexpressed TAA   HER-2/neu   HER-2/neu
                        (epithelial cells)   (breast cancer)

Viral TAA   –   Virus   Human papilloma
                                                 virus
                                                 (cervical cancer)

Posttranscriptionally   Glycosylated MUC-1   Aberrantly glycosylated
modified TAA   (ductal epithelial cells) MUC-1
                                                 (ovarian cancer)

FIGURE 21–10 **Types of tumor-associated antigens (TAAs).** Various classes of TAAs are depicted and an example of each type of TAA is given. Expression on a normal cell and a tumor cell is shown. TAAs are depicted in red.

hypoglycosylated in tumor cells compared with normal cells. Furthermore, the sugar moieties on tumor-associated MUC-1 tend to be shorter.

21.4.2 Tumor-Associated Antigen-Specific T cells in Humans

The development of MHC/peptide multimer reagents has enabled the direct detection of T cells specific for various TAAs. This reagent generally consists of soluble MHC class I molecules (eg, HLA-A*0201) folded together with a peptide of interest (eg, a peptide derived from a tumor-associated protein that is known to bind that particular HLA allele) (Fig. 21–11). Each MHC molecule is tagged covalently with a molecule of biotin. Multiple MHC/peptide complexes are then aggregated together using streptavidin, which possesses

4 biotin-binding sites. The multimeric nature of the reagent allows for higher avidity binding of specific TCRs, and any bound cells can be detected by flow cytometric analysis of the fluorochrome-conjugated streptavidin moiety. The first reported multimers were synthesized using HIV and influenza A-derived peptides (Altman et al, 1996). Although MHC/peptide multimers have also been constructed using MHC class II molecules and class II-binding peptides, they are generally not as robust as MHC class I-derived multimers (Vollers and Stern, 2008).

Early studies using HLA-A*0201 MHC/peptide multimers were able to identify the presence of peripheral T cells that could recognize melanoma-associated antigens. These tumor-specific T cells could be detected directly ex vivo, without the need for in vitro stimulation or expansion using specific peptides. T cells specific for the melanoma-associated

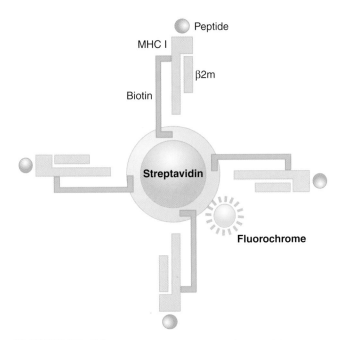

FIGURE 21–11   Structure of an MHC/peptide multimer.
An MHC/peptide tetramer is depicted, where 4 MHC class I/peptide complexes are complexed together. Each MHC class I molecule is biotinylated; each biotinylated MHC class I/peptide complex is bound via the biotin molecule to a streptavidin molecule, and the streptavidin molecule is conjugated to a fluorochrome. These reagents are helpful for monitoring tumor specific T-cell responses.

antigens Melan-A/MART-1 and tyrosinase were detected by ex vivo staining of tumor-infiltrated lymph nodes (Romero et al, 1998). MHC/peptide multimers were also used to isolate specific T cells by fluorescence-activated cell sorting (FACS), and these cells were found to be functional, as they could lyse autologous melanoma tumor cells in vitro (Romero et al, 1998).

The presence and function of tumor-specific T cells have also been demonstrated for other cancers. Numerous studies have demonstrated that some women with breast cancer have preexisting immunity against breast TAAs. In one study, 7 of 13 breast cancer patients had detectable tumor-specific T-cell responses at the time of diagnosis (Rentzsch et al, 2003). This response was demonstrated by evaluating the induction of IFN-γ RNA transcripts in response to stimulation with peptides derived from several common antigens expressed by breast cancers: MUC-1, HER-2/neu, CEA, NY-ESO-1, and SSX-2. HER-2/neu is expressed by a variety of cancers and preexisting immunity to HER-2/neu has been demonstrated in patients whose cancers expressed HER-2/neu (breast, ovarian, lung, colorectal, prostate) (Sotiropoulou et al, 2003). After a brief restimulation of peripheral blood T cells ex vivo with HER-2/neu peptide-exposed DCs, effector function of the restimulated T cells was evaluated by enzyme-linked immunospot (ELISPOT) assay (production of IFN-γ on a per-cell basis) and CTL assay (ability to kill target cells).

Clearly, immune tolerance against tumors is incomplete, as TAA-specific T cells can be detected in cancer patients. Whether these tumor-specific T cells can mediate antitumor activity, and how they might be induced to do so by therapeutic intervention, is a major challenge for successful development of immunotherapy.

21.4.3 Immune Surveillance

Historically, the concept of "immune surveillance," where the immune system surveys the body and targets tumor cells even in the absence of therapeutic intervention, has not always been accepted. Early studies that argued against immune surveillance examined tumor development in mice that carried the "nude" mutation and lacked a thymus and were considered immunodeficient (Stutman, 1974, 1979). It was found that nude mice developed both carcinogen (methylcholanthrene [MCA])-induced and spontaneous tumors at similar frequencies to wild-type mice, and it was concluded that the immune system does not play a role in inhibiting tumor progression. Several factors that could influence the interpretation of this model have been identified. Firstly, it is now known that nude mice still have some intact immune cells. Secondly, the importance of the innate immune system (which is intact in nude mice) in antitumor immunity has been established. Thirdly, the genetic background of the nude mice used in the above studies (CBA/H background) express a particular isoform of the enzyme that metabolizes MCA. Therefore, nude mice could be more resistant to MCA-induced tumor formation, which could mask any consequences related to an impaired immune response.

Numerous studies provide strong evidence in support of cancer immunosurveillance (Dunn et al, 2004). That the immune system eliminates tumor cells was shown using various immunodeficient mice: (a) mice deficient in the Rag protein and therefore lacking all T and B cells, (b) mice deficient in the receptor for the immunostimulatory cytokine interferon-γ (IFN-γ receptor 1 knockout mice), and (c) mice deficient in the key intracellular signaling molecule downstream of IFN-γ receptor signaling (*Stat1* knockout mice). These immunodeficient mice developed MCA-induced and spontaneous tumors at a higher frequency and with faster kinetics compared with immunocompetent mice (Kaplan et al, 1998; Shankaran et al, 2001). A model has been proposed to describe the role of the immune response during various stages of tumor progression, which includes three phases: elimination, equilibrium, and escape (Dunn et al, 2004) (Fig. 21–12).

During the elimination phase of immunosurveillance, the immune system recognizes tumor cells and mounts a response against the tumor. During the equilibrium phase, the immune system and the tumor are in dynamic equilibrium, where the combination of the genomic instability of tumor cells and selective pressure exerted by the antitumor immune response results in editing, or "sculpting" of the tumor cell population. The elimination of certain tumor cells by the immune system results in the selection of less

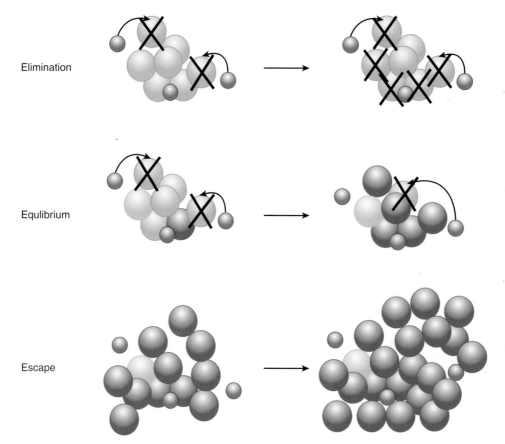

FIGURE 21–12 **The three Es of cancer immunoediting.** In the model proposed by Dunn et al (2004), immunoediting is comprised of 3 main phases. During the *elimination phase*, the immune system recognizes tumor cells and mediates their elimination. During the *equilibrium phase*, the immune system and the tumor are in dynamic equilibrium, where the combination of genomic instability of tumor cells and selective pressure exerted by the antitumor immune response results in editing, or "sculpting" of the tumor cell population. The elimination of certain tumor cells by the immune system results in the selection of less immunogenic tumors. During the *escape phase*, enough tumor cell variants arise that the tumor can escape elimination by the immune system. *Blue*, immune cell; *orange/green/red*, tumor cells.

immunogenic tumors. During the escape phase, enough tumor cell variants arise that the tumor can escape elimination by the immune system. Escape may be partly a result of reduced immunogenicity of tumor cells, such as reduced expression of TAAs, or downregulation of MHC class I, but there are many mechanisms whereby the tumor can evade the immune system. These mechanisms include negative regulatory immune cell types, immunosuppressive factors produced by tumor cells, and surface receptors that dampen the T-cell response.

21.4.4 T-cell Infiltration and Disease Prognosis

The importance of T-cell immunity in reducing clinical tumor burden in humans is highlighted in part by studies evaluating tumor tissues for infiltration by immune cells. In many studies where immunohistochemical or gene expression analyses of tumor tissue are performed, the data show an association between immune cell (especially T-cell) infiltration and better prognosis (eg, Galon et al, 2006; Tuthill et al, 2002; Zhang et al, 2003).

In an example of this type of study, genomic analysis for RNA expression was performed for 75 colorectal tumors (Galon et al, 2006). Expression levels of a cluster of Th1-related genes showed a statistically significant inverse correlation with tumor recurrence, thus implicating the Th1 response in dampening progression of human tumors. In the same study, immunohistochemistry for immune cell infiltration in paraffin-embedded tissue microarrays constructed from 415 colorectal tumors was also performed. High densities of CD3+ T cells, CD8+ T cells, Granzyme B (a cytotoxic granule produced by lytic T cells), and CD45RO (a T-cell activation marker) were found in patients without recurrence compared to patients with recurrence. In a multivariate analysis, the density of CD3+ cells in tumors was shown to be an independent prognostic factor, and these T-cell markers proved to be a better predictor of patient survival than standard histopathologically based staging methods.

21.4.5 Barriers That Inhibit Antitumor Immunity

Despite the evidence that the immune system can respond to tumor cells, it is difficult to estimate the relative importance of antitumor immunity in tumor progression. However, it is clear that when tumors do develop, the immune response is unable to control tumor growth. Various mechanisms can lead to failure of immune-mediated tumor control; many of them are the same mechanisms that prevent autoimmunity and thereby suppress immune responses against self-tissues. Various mechanisms of peripheral T-cell tolerance are discussed above (see Sec. 21.3.7): T-cell deletion, T-cell anergy, and the function of negative regulatory cells and molecules have all been demonstrated to possess a negative impact on the immune response to tumors in various models. In addition, factors produced by tumor cells, or by tumor-infiltrating immune cells are known to suppress antitumor T-cell responses. Two examples of tumor-related immunosuppressive factors are TGF-β and IDO.

TGF-β is produced by tumor-associated macrophages, tumor cells, and Tregs. It exerts immunosuppressive effects on multiple cell types, including DCs and effector T cells. TGF-β signaling in DCs results in the downregulation of MHC class II, CD40, CD80, and CD86, as well as the inhibition of the proinflammatory cytokines IL-12, interferon (IFN)-α and tumor necrosis factor (TNF)-α. Thus, TGF-β induces a tolerogenic phenotype in DCs. These tolerogenic DCs themselves have been shown to secrete TGF-β leading to the induction of Tregs in mouse and human models. The immune suppressive effect of TGF-β on T cells is also well-established. TGF-β signaling results in suppression of Granzyme A, Granzyme B, and FAS ligand in CTLs. In addition, iTregs can be generated by TGF-β.

Clinical trials for various agents aimed at blocking the effect of TGF-β have been conducted (Flavell et al, 2010). Blocking strategies include small molecule inhibitors, delivery of antisense molecules, and the use of blocking antibodies. Clinical responses have been limited, but further investigation into the immunological effect of these strategies and combination of TGF-β blockade with other immunotherapeutic strategies might lead to improved responses.

IDO is an important immunosuppressive mediator (Munn and Mellor, 2007). IDO is an enzyme involved in oxidative catabolism of tryptophan, and since tryptophan is important for T-cell proliferation and activation, depletion of tryptophan by IDO inhibits T-cell responses. IDO-secreting DCs have been found in patients with various cancers, including melanoma, breast cancer, and colon cancer (Munn et al, 2002). IDO-secreting DCs have also been found in tumor-draining lymph nodes and, furthermore, these IDO-secreting DCs can induce anergy of tumor-specific T cells in vivo. Immunohistological detection of IDO in tumor-draining lymph nodes of melanoma patients revealed that IDO expression correlated with poor prognosis (Lee et al, 2005; Munn et al, 2004). Tumor cells can also secrete IDO.

Understanding the mechanisms by which tumor-specific T cells fail to control tumor growth may form the basis for designing therapeutic strategies. For example, unresponsive tumor-specific T cells may need to be rescued ex vivo and then reinfused; negative regulatory molecules may need to

be blocked; or deleted tumor-specific T cells may need to be replenished. Immunosuppressive molecules present in the tumor microenvironment may also need to be inhibited. It is likely that a combination of these approaches will lead to the most effective approaches to immunotherapy.

21.5 IMMUNOTHERAPY

21.5.1 Introduction to Immunotherapeutic Approaches

Our improved understanding of tumor immunology has led to a growing list of immunotherapeutic agents being approved for use against cancer. One broad category of agents consists of monoclonal antibodies (mAbs). Although the mechanisms of action of various mAbs are not always related to the antitumor T-cell response that is discussed above—many function in a manner completely independent of T cells—they are, nevertheless, important players in cancer therapy.

Immunotherapy that is aimed at augmenting antitumor T-cell immunity can be broadly categorized into (a) nonspecific immunotherapy, (b) specific immunotherapy, and (c) adoptive cell therapy. Each category encompasses many different strategies—some investigational and some approved for therapy. The small number of these strategies selected for discussion in this chapter are listed in Table 21–1.

Nonspecific immunotherapy refers to strategies that augment general T-cell responses, in a "nonspecific" or "polyclonal" manner. Nonspecific immunotherapy includes the use of cytokines (eg, INF-α, IL-2), immunological adjuvants (Imiquimod), and agents that target immunomodulatory molecules (anti–CTLA-4 antibody). Specific immunotherapy focuses on the activation and enhancement of the number of T cells that can recognize TAAs by using vaccine strategies. Although the induction of an immune response by vaccination often refers to a prophylactic strategy, such as that used to limit viral infection, vaccination may also refer to therapy aimed at eliciting antitumor immune responses to eliminate established cancers. The field of prophylactic cancer vaccines will not be addressed in this chapter but is reviewed in Lollini et al (2006). Common vaccine approaches include the use of TAAs or peptides derived from TAAs. Other approaches are based on vaccination using whole tumor cells (autologous or allogeneic) that have been irradiated prior to infusion to prevent their proliferation following infusion. In adoptive cell therapy, autologous immune cells such as DCs and T cells are manipulated ex vivo and then reinfused.

21.5.2 Monoclonal Antibodies for Cancer Therapy

Monoclonal antibodies (mAbs) bind specifically to their target protein and can block the target protein's function, trigger signaling downstream of the target protein, or deliver conjugated

TABLE 21–1 Selected approaches to cancer immunotherapy.

Monoclonal antibody therapies	(See Table 21–2)
Nonspecific immunotherapies	Bacillus of Calmette and Guérin (BCG)*
	Interferon-α*
	Interleukin-2*
	Imiquimod*
	Anti-CTLA-4 blockade (Ipilimumab)*
Specific immunotherapies (vaccination)	Vaccination with:
	Tumor-associated proteins
	Tumor-associated peptides
	Irradiated tumor cells
Adoptive cell therapies	Dendritic cells
	Sipuleucel-T*
	T-cell clones
	Tumor-infiltrating lymphocytes

*Currently FDA approved.

toxins to cells expressing the target protein. Current Food and Drug Administration (FDA)-approved mAbs include those that target antigens expressed by tumor cells (eg, CD20 on non-Hodgkin lymphoma and chronic lymphocytic leukemia), molecules that promote tumor growth (eg, epidermal growth factor receptor), or angiogenic molecules (eg, vascular endothelial growth factor). Table 21–2 lists examples of antibodies approved for cancer therapy.

21.5.2.1 Production of Monoclonal Antibodies A mAb that recognizes a given protein target is derived from an antibody molecule that was produced by a single B cell. Originally, mAbs were produced by fusing B cells from the spleen of an animal that had been immunized with the target protein, with a myeloma cell line that was selected for the inability to produce immunoglobulin. Primary spleen cells cannot survive ex vivo in unsupplemented culture medium. The myeloma cell line was also selected for a deficiency in an enzyme (hypoxanthine-guanine phosphoribosyltransferase [HGPRT]) that renders the cells unable to grow in culture medium containing hypoxanthine, aminopterin, and thymidine (HAT). Successful cell fusions between spleen cells (expressing HGPRT) and myeloma cells could therefore be selected by culturing in HAT-containing medium. Fused cells were then cloned: Cells were plated at limiting numbers and individual cells were expanded separately. These fused cells (called *hybridomas*) were then screened for secretion of antibodies that could bind the target protein of interest. Once a hybridoma with the desired antibody specificity is identified, large batches of antibodies can be produced by expanding the hybridoma in culture, or expanding the hybridoma in the peritoneal cavity of animals (mice, rabbits)

TABLE 21–2 Table of monoclonal antibodies approved for cancer therapy.

Monoclonal Antibody	Cancer Targeted	Target Molecule	Type of mAb
Alemtuzumab	CLL	CD52	Humanized IgG$_1$
Bevacizumab	Colorectal, lung cancer	VEGF	Humanized IgG$_1$
Cetuximab	Colorectal cancer	EGFR	Chimeric IgG$_1$
Gemtuzumab	AML	CD33	Humanized IgG$_4$
Ibritumomab tiuxetan	NHL	CD20	Mouse
Ofatumumab	CLL	CD20	Human IgG$_1$
Panitumumab	Colorectal cancer	EGFR	Human IgG$_2$
Rituximab	NHL, CLL	CD20	Chimeric IgG$_1$
Tositumomab	NHL	CD20	Mouse
Trastuzumab	Breast cancer	HER-2/neu	Humanized IgG$_1$

Abbreviations: ADCC, Antibody-dependent cell-mediated cytotoxicity; *AML,* acute myelogenous leukemia; *CLL,* chronic lymphocytic leukemia; *EGFR,* epidermal growth factor receptor; *IgG,* immunoglobulin G; *NHL,* non-Hodgkin lymphoma; *VEGF,* vascular endothelial growth factor.

and harvesting the ascites. A schematic of this classical method of antibody production, and an example of a current method based on a genetic approach, described below, are depicted in Figure 21–13.

21.5.2.2 Types of Therapeutic Antibodies Antibodies that recognize human proteins were generated initially by immunization of animals (eg, mice) with human proteins and isolation of specific antibodies, as described in the hybridoma

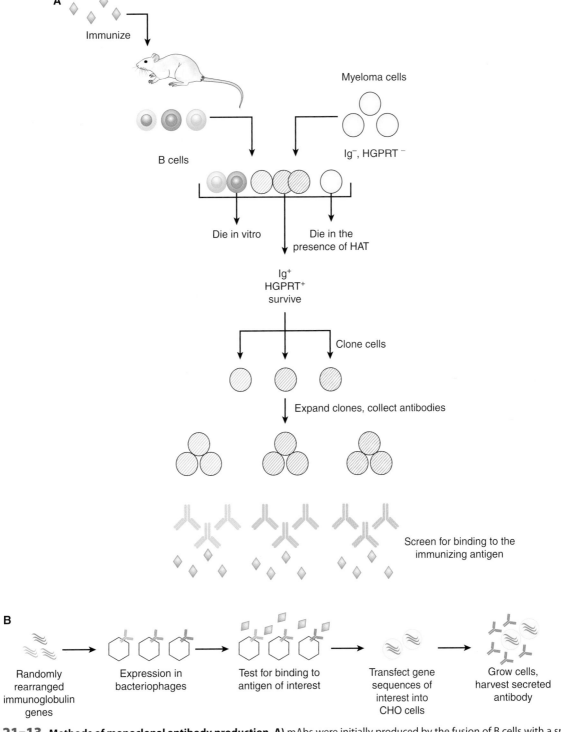

FIGURE 21–13 **Methods of monoclonal antibody production. A)** mAbs were initially produced by the fusion of B cells with a specialized myeloma cell line. Fused cells were cloned and then the clone that produced the antibody of interest was selected for antibody production. Further details are provided in the text. **B)** Other methods are based on recombinant technologies, where the desired antibody genes are transfected into cells such as Chinese hamster ovary (CHO) cells and antibodies are harvested from culture supernatants. In this example, the antibody genes of interest are identified by screening bacteriophages for binding to the antigen of interest. The bacteriophages have been engineered to express antibodies that are the product of random rearrangement of immunoglobulin genes.

approach above. However, mouse antibodies have limited therapeutic value for several reasons. First, mouse Fc domains (which are the "constant" domain of an antibody that is conserved amongst all antibodies of a particular class) are not recognized as efficiently as human Fc domains by human immune cells, and such recognition is required for some of the mechanisms of action of antibody therapy, described below. Also, mouse antibodies are recognized as foreign proteins by the human immune system and thus repetitive antibody administration would result in an immune response against the therapeutic antibody. One solution has been the generation of *chimeric antibodies,* which are engineered to contain the variable (Fv) region from a mouse antibody and the human constant (Fc) regions. An alternate approach is to generate *humanized antibodies* where the hypervariable regions of the variable antigen-binding domain (Fv) is derived from a mouse antibody and the rest of the Fv and the entire Fc region is derived from human sequences. To completely circumvent neutralizing antibodies with xenogeneic sequences, many current therapeutic antibodies are fully human. These antibodies can be isolated from mice that have been engineered to express only human antibodies, or they can be isolated by a phage display approach, where libraries of random recombinations of human antibody genes are expressed in bacteriophages. The antibody-expressing phages are then screened for the ability to bind the target protein. Recombinant antibodies are often produced by transfecting Chinese hamster ovary (CHO) cells with the desired antibody genes, as CHO cells grow well in suspension culture. Figure 21–14 illustrates these types of antibodies.

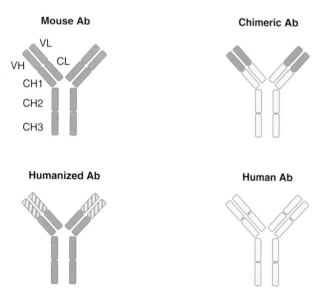

FIGURE 21–14   Chimeric and humanized antibodies. In chimeric antibodies, the variable fragment (Fv) of the antibody molecule is of mouse origin and the constant regions (Fc) is of human origin. In humanized antibodies, only the hypervariable region of the Fv is of mouse origin; the rest of the antibody molecule is of human origin.

21.5.2.3 Mechanisms of Action of Antibodies

Antibodies that bind to receptors on the cell surface can block receptor signaling (by steric blockade of ligand binding) or can trigger receptor signaling (by aggregation of multiple receptors). Antibodies can also lead to lysis of cells that express the molecule targeted by the antibody. Target-cell lysis can occur by activation of the complement protein cascade or initiation of antibody-dependent cell-mediated cytotoxicity (ADCC) (Fig. 21–15). The complement cascade is initiated by binding of the Fc domain of immunoglobulin (Ig)G to a complement protein, which then leads to a cascade of cleavage of various complement system proteins. The end result of this cascade is the formation of a protein complex called the membrane attack complex (MAC) on the target cell (in this case, the tumor cell) that leads to pore formation and lysis of the target cell. Other proteins activated by the complement cascade are able to mediate chemoattraction of various immune cells to the site of tumor. ADCC, on the other hand, is initiated upon binding of the Fc region of antibodies by Fc receptors (FcRs). FcRs are expressed on various innate immune cell types, and the activation of FcRs leads to activation of cytotoxic activity against target cells. For example, FcγRIIIA is expressed by natural killer (NK) cells, and binding of this receptor by the Fc region of an IgG molecule activates NK cell-mediated lysis of the target cell. Trastuzumab (Herceptin), which is principally thought to bind and inhibit signaling through the HER-2/neu growth receptor (see Chap. 7, Sec. 7.5.3 and Chap. 20, Sec. 20.3.3), also has been shown to mediate antitumor activity via ADCC (Clynes et al, 2000). Because ADCC is a potentially important mechanism mediating the action of therapeutic antibodies, the most effective antibodies should be engineered or selected to bind well to activating FcRs and to bind poorly to the inhibitory FcγIIB (Nimmerjahn and Ravetch, 2008).

Antibodies may also lead to enhanced T-cell priming. In the natural course of tumor progression or during antibody-mediated lysis of tumor cells, fragments of dying tumor cells can be recognized and bound by TAA-specific antibodies (see Fig. 21–15). These complexes can then be recognized by FcRs expressed on DCs, internalized, and the TAA-derived peptides presented to tumor-specific T cells via cross-presentation. The relative contribution of each of these different mechanisms for various antibodies is unclear.

21.5.2.4 Modified Antibodies

Antibodies can be modified in various ways in order to alter their therapeutic function. For example, bispecific T-cell engager (BiTE) molecules consist of 2 Fv fragments, each with different specificities, linked together with a flexible linker (Wolf et al, 2005). For example, a BiTE has been generated that is specific for CD3 and epithelial cell adhesion molecule (EpCAM). The EpCAM-specific component binds tumor cells expressing this common tumor adhesion molecule and the CD3-specific component functions to recruit T cells to EpCAM-expressing tumor cells. Another example is Blinatumomab, which has been shown to mediate regression of non-Hodgkin B-cell lymphomas

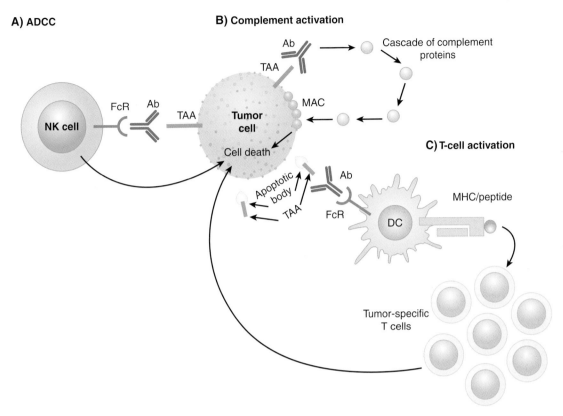

FIGURE 21–15 Tumor-specific antibodies can promote tumor regression by multiple mechanisms. In addition to either blocking or triggering cell-surface receptors, antibodies can lead to immune-mediated elimination of tumor cells. **A)** ADCC is induced when antibodies bound to tumor antigens (TAA) on the surface of tumor cells are then bound by Fc receptors expressed by natural killer (NK) cells. Triggering of the Fc receptors activates the cytolytic activity of NK cells. **B)** Complement activation is induced by binding of complement proteins to the Fc domain of antibody/antigen complexes. One of the end results of the complement cascade is the formation of the membrane attack complex (MAC) in the cell membrane of target cells, leading to cell death. **C)** Antibodies can also bind to tumor antigens present on apoptotic bodies formed when tumor cells undergo apoptosis during the normal cycle of proliferation and cell death. By this route, tumor antigens are taken up by DCs via Fc receptors. Tumor antigens can be processed by the DCs and presented as peptide/MHC complexes to T cells. Tumor-specific T cells can then be activated and mediate antitumor activities including cytotoxic activity against tumor cells.

(Bargou et al, 2008). This agent is specific for CD19 (expressed on non-Hodgkin lymphoma cells) and CD3 (to recruit T cells to tumor cells).

Three FDA-approved antibodies for cancer have been modified to deliver toxic or radioactive molecules to tumor cells. Gemtuzumab is fused to the toxin ozogamicin, Ibritumomab tiuxetan is conjugated to yttrium-90, and Tositumomab is conjugated to iodine-131 (Bross et al, 2001; Fisher et al, 2005; Witzig et al, 2002).

21.5.3 Nonspecific Immune Modulators

21.5.3.1 Bacillus Calmette-Guérin
Bacillus Calmette-Guérin (BCG) is a live-attenuated strain of *Mycobacterium bovis* and is effective in preventing the recurrence of superficial bladder carcinoma. BCG is administered intravesically, and its mechanism of action is related to its immunostimulatory activity (Patard et al, 1998).

After instillation in the bladder, BCG is processed and presented locally by APCs. These APCs then stimulate CD4 and CD8 T-cell responses. In addition, upregulation of MHC class I and II on urothelial cells is observed. During BCG treatment, levels of various cytokines are found in the urine: IL-1, IL-6, IL-8, and IL-10 early during treatment, and IL-2, TNF-α, and IFN-γ later during treatment. Infiltration of T cells into the bladder wall is also observed after treatment. Overall, BCG instillation leads to a local T-cell response, which appears to have features of a Th1-type response. The mechanism whereby tumor cells are eliminated is unclear. It is possible that mycobacteria-specific T cells are activated and lyse tumor cells that have been infected with the mycobacteria. It is also possible that the immune stimulation induced by BCG promotes the activation of T cells specific for bladder tumor antigens and that these T cells kill tumor cells.

21.5.3.2 Interferon-α
IFN-α is produced by many cell types, including cells of the immune system such as T cells, B cells, NK cells, DCs, and macrophages, and has direct antitumor effects, as well as a role in immunomodulation (Dunn et al, 2006). IFN-α can directly inhibit proliferation of tumor cells,

downregulate expression of oncogenes, and induce tumor-suppressor genes. It also possesses antiangiogenic activity.

IFN-α therapy induces responses in more than 90% of patients with hairy cell leukemia, although most patients will relapse within 2 years. IFN-α also shows some activity in patients with other hematological cancers, such as chronic myelogenous leukemia, myeloma, and low-grade non-Hodgkin lymphoma. Although approved by the FDA for patients with melanoma and renal cell carcinoma, the overall clinical response rate in these patients to IFN-α therapy is relatively low. Furthermore, high-dose IFN-α therapy is associated with severe toxicities, including hypotension, vomiting, fever, and diarrhea (Kirkwood et al, 1996; Motzer et al, 2002).

Although the utility of IFN-α therapy is limited, IFN-α is an important enhancer of antitumor immunity. IFN-α induces upregulation of MHC class I and contributes to maturation of DCs. It also is important for promoting CD8 T-cell survival and enhances migration of T cells into tissues. For example, mice treated with an IFN-α receptor-blocking antibody could not reject MCA-induced sarcomas that could be rejected in untreated mice. In addition, IFN-α receptor 1-deficient mice were more susceptible to MCA-induced tumor formation (Dunn et al, 2006). IFN-α may have a therapeutic role in combination with other types of immunotherapy. For example, in a murine model of colon carcinoma, combination therapy using an immunostimulatory antibody (agonistic anti-CD137 mAb) and IFN-α resulted in synergistic antitumor immunity (Dubrot et al, 2011).

21.5.3.3 Interleukin-2

IL-2 is a well-characterized cytokine that acts primarily to stimulate proliferation of T cells and NK cells. High-dose IL-2 therapy is an approved treatment for renal cell carcinoma and melanoma, but the clinical response rate for this therapy is only in the range of 15% for both cancer types (Atkins et al, 1999; Fyfe et al, 1995). High-dose IL-2 therapy is also associated with substantial toxicity, including cardiac arrhythmias, capillary leak syndrome leading to hypotension, central nervous system toxicity leading to confusion and gastrointestinal toxicity such as diarrhea (Rosenberg et al, 1989). Although IL-2 promotes effector T-cell responses and can function to reverse anergy of effector T cells, IL-2 may not represent an ideal agent to promote immunity because it also promotes the expansion of Tregs.

21.5.3.4 Imiquimod

Imiquimod is a synthetic compound that triggers the TLR7 molecule. TLRs are a family of molecules that are stimulated by conserved molecular motifs that are present on various microorganisms (Akira et al, 2006; see also Sec. 21.2.2). For example, the natural ligand for TLR7 is single-stranded RNA, which is present in some viruses. The TLRs are expressed by many cell types, including cells of the innate immune system such as macrophages and DCs. Interactions between TLRs and corresponding ligands lead to activation of innate immune cells, which promote elimination of the microorganism through various mechanisms, including production of interferons and proinflammatory cytokines.

Because TLRs activate APCs such as DCs, they can enhance the ability of DCs to stimulate antitumor T-cell responses. Various TLR ligands are under investigation in animal models and early clinical trials for cancer immunotherapy. These agents are often used in combination with vaccination strategies to enhance T-cell responses induced by vaccination.

Imiquimod is approved for use in the treatment of superficial basal cell carcinoma, and for treatment of genital warts and actinic keratosis. Treatment is generally effective for superficial basal cell carcinoma, with complete clearance rates of approximately 75% or higher (compared to a few percent in placebo-treated groups). Imiquimod has been shown to induce proinflammatory mediators such as IFN-α, TNF-α, and IL-6 by various innate immune cell types, including macrophages and a specialized subset of DCs called *plasmacytoid DCs*. Imiquimod also upregulates costimulatory molecules and chemokine receptors on plasmacytoid DCs, thus enhancing their ability to activate T cells and home to sites of T-cell activation, respectively. Histological studies have shown an increase in infiltration of tumor lesions with T cells and DCs following Imiquimod treatment, further supporting its immunological mechanism of action.

21.5.4 Other Approaches to Immunotherapy

21.5.4.1 Dendritic Cell Vaccines

Mature DCs are highly efficient APCs and therefore are central players in the induction of T-cell responses. Therefore, adoptive cell therapy using DCs that present TAAs to induce antitumor T cells in vivo is of major interest (Tacken et al, 2007). In general, these DCs are obtained by in vitro differentiation of bone marrow progenitor cells (for mice) or peripheral blood monocytes (for humans). Granulocyte macrophage-colony stimulating factor (GM-CSF) and IL-4 are commonly used to stimulate differentiation. Figure 21–16 outlines the generation of DCs for infusion. Some of the methods for loading DCs with TAAs include loading peptides derived from TAAs into surface MHC molecules, incubating DCs with whole TAA proteins, and transfecting or transducing DCs with DNA encoding TAAs. TAA-loaded DCs may also be exposed to a variety of maturation stimuli in order to enhance their immunogenicity. These stimuli include agonistic anti-CD40 antibody, various TLR ligands (eg, CpG oligodeoxynucleotides, poly I:C, LPS), and cytokine cocktails (eg, a cocktail of IL-1β, IL-6, TNF, and prostaglandin E2).

Clinical trials based on DC vaccination have demonstrated that this approach is associated with minimal toxicity, and there is some evidence for clinical effectiveness (Tacken et al, 2007; Palucka et al, 2012).

21.5.4.2 Sipuleucel-T

Sipuleucel-T was the first autologous cellular therapy for cancer to receive FDA approval. The therapeutic product is produced by leukapheresis from a patient with prostatic cancer. The leukapheresis product is transported to a central facility where the cells are processed and incubated with a fusion protein of a prostate TAA

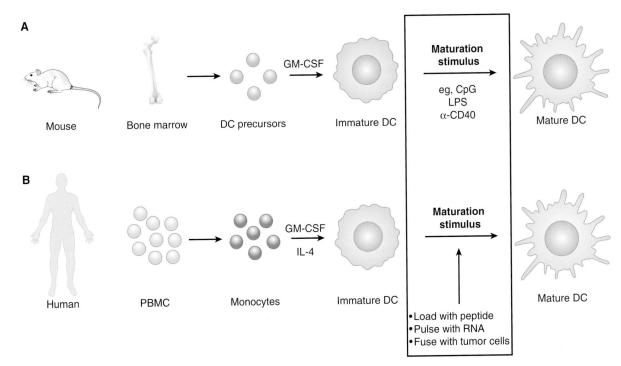

FIGURE 21–16 Generating DCs for therapy. Common methods for generating DCs for vaccination are shown. **A)** For mouse studies, DC precursors are obtained from bone marrow cells and differentiated into immature DCs in vitro using GM-CSF. (B) For human studies, monocytes are obtained from peripheral blood mononuclear cells by a variety of methods, including elutriation, plastic adherence, or isolation of CD14+ cells. Monocytes are then differentiated into immature DCs in vitro using GM-CSF and IL-4. For both mouse and human studies, immature DCs are manipulated to present tumor-associated antigens. This can be done by a variety of approaches, including exposing them to peptides or RNA, or fusing the DCs with tumor cells. DC maturation is induced by stimuli such as TLR ligands (eg, LPS or CpG oligodeoxynucleotides) or agonistic anti-CD40 antibody. Mature DCs presenting TAAs are then ready for infusion.

(prostatic acid phosphatase [PAP]) and the cytokine GM-CSF (Small et al, 2000). The cellular product is then reinfused into the same patient. The premise of this therapy is APCs, such as DCs, will take up the fusion protein. The PAP will be processed and presented by MHC molecules on the surface of APCs and will thus be able to stimulate PAP-specific T cells to mediate antitumor activity. The functions of GM-CSF include promoting the differentiation of DCs. Presentation of a prostate TAA by efficient APCs such as DCs should activate endogenous prostate-specific T cells upon reinfusion. However, it remains unclear how the other cell types present in the leukapheresis product may contribute to the effectiveness of the treatment. In vitro biological potency tests as well as clinical trial data indicate that the activity can be attributed to the cell fraction expressing CD54, which is a cell adhesion molecule expressed on a variety of cell types, including APCs. An integrated analysis of 2 Phase III trials showed a survival benefit for advanced prostate cancer patients treated with sipuleucel-T compared to placebo (Higano et al, 2009), with a 23.2-month median survival in the Sipuleucel-T arms and an 18.9-month median survival in the placebo arms. Common adverse events included chills, pyrexia, and headache, and were mostly low grade. An additional double-blind, multicenter Phase III trial showed similar results. In this trial, 512 men with metastatic castration-resistant prostate cancer were randomized at a 2:1 ratio to receive Sipuleucel-T or placebo (Kantoff et al, 2010).

Interestingly, the time to objective disease progression was similar in both arms, but the relative risk of death was reduced by 22% in the Sipuleucel-T arm compared to the placebo arm, leading to a 4-month improvement in median survival. However, this trial has been criticized because the leukapheresis procedure was used in control patients (but leukocytes were not re-infused into all of the control patients), and loss of white cells might be harmful, particularly to older adults, leading (in part) to a difference in survival because of poorer outcome in controls (Huber et al, 2012).

21.5.4.3 CTLA-4 Blockade CTLA-4 is expressed on activated T cells and also Treg cells. Initial experiments in animal models demonstrated that blockade of CTLA-4 induces tumor regression. Two therapeutic anti–CTLA-4 blocking antibodies have been developed. One is a fully human IgG_2 antibody (Tremelimumab) (Ribas, 2008), the other is a fully human IgG_1 antibody (Ipilimumab) (Weber, 2008). These agents have been tested mainly in patients with metastatic melanoma.

The clinical activity of these agents, when assessed initially using objective response (ie, tumor shrinkage) to evaluate clinical responses, appeared to be relatively low. However, this type of immunomodulatory agent may induce unconventional response patterns, such as tumor progression that precedes regression, or mixed responses of different lesions but with overall decreases in tumor burden (Wolchok et al, 2009).

Indeed, a Phase III randomized trial in patients with unresectable Stage III or IV melanoma demonstrated that patients that received Ipilimumab had a significantly longer median overall survival (10.0 months) compared with patients not receiving anti–CTLA-4 blockade (6.4 months) (Hodi et al, 2010). Because anti–CTLA-4 blockade is not an antigen-targeted approach, it is associated with some grade 3 or 4 autoimmune toxicities, the most common being colitis. In 2010, Ipilimumab received FDA approval for treatment of patients with unresectable or metastatic melanoma.

Although the negative regulatory role of CTLA-4 signaling is well established, the mechanism(s) whereby anti–CTLA-4 blockade induces antitumor T-cell immunity remains under investigation. There remains some debate whether the predominant target of anti–CTLA-4 blockade is to "release the brakes" on effector T cells or to inhibit the suppressive activity of Tregs. CTLA-4 blockade is thought to enhance effector T cells by the following mechanisms: Anti–CTLA-4 antibodies may prevent the interaction of CD80 and CD86 with CTLA-4, thereby allowing for prolonged interaction of CD80 and CD86 with the positive costimulatory receptor CD28. In addition, CTLA-4 blockade may inhibit the CTLA-4–mediated negative intracellular signals that shut down effector T cells. There is also strong evidence that CTLA-4 suppresses effector T cells in a non–cell-autonomous fashion, that is, by inhibiting the suppressive activity of Tregs (Bachmann et al, 1999; Read et al, 2000). Evidence suggests that the effects of CTLA-4 on both effector T cells and Tregs contribute to its ability to enhance antitumor immune responses (Peggs et al, 2009).

21.5.4.4 Adoptive T-cell Therapy

Infusion of T cells that can recognize and destroy tumor cells is a major area of interest for immunotherapy. That transferred T cells can mediate potent antitumor effects has been conclusively demonstrated by donor lymphocyte infusions (DLIs), which are the standard treatment for patients with relapsed leukemia following allogeneic bone marrow transplantation. For therapy using DLI, lymphocytes from allogeneic bone marrow transplantation donors are stored in a sample bank. If the leukemia patient relapses following a bone marrow transplantation, then the lymphocytes from the same donor are infused into the patient. These lymphocytes mediate regression of the relapsed leukemia (a so-named graft-versus-leukemia effect). For patients with relapsed chronic myelogenous leukemia, 70% of patients treated with DLI experience complete remission (Kolb et al, 2004). This approach demonstrates that T cells have the potential to mediate antitumor activity.

Adoptive T-cell therapy is based on ex vivo expansion and manipulation of patient-derived tumor specific T cells followed by reinfusion in an autologous manner. General approaches to generate T cells for adoptive cell therapy are depicted in Figure 21–17 and described below.

21.5.4.4.1 Adoptive Cell Therapy with T-cell Clones

One source of T cells for adoptive cell therapy is expanded T-cell clones from the peripheral blood of cancer patients. This approach is advantageous in that the peptide specificity of the transferred T cells is well defined, and peripheral blood T cells have not been subjected to immunosuppressive factors present within the tumor microenvironment and therefore may be more responsive. Potential drawbacks for this approach include the possibility that these T cells may not home to the tumor site. It is also possible that tumor cells do not express the peptide recognized by the T-cell clones and will escape detection by the T cells.

The general approach to generating T-cell clones for therapy involves stimulation of bulk peripheral blood T cells with peptides derived from TAAs of interest. The most well-studied TAA-derived peptides are those that bind the HLA-A*0201 MHC molecule, and therefore trials of adoptive cell therapy using clones are generally limited to HLA-A*0201–positive patients. Peptide-stimulated T cells are then cultured under limiting dilution conditions in order to expand a population of T cells derived from a single clone. All T cells expanded from a single T cell will express identical TCRs and therefore can be considered clones. CD8+ T-cell clones and, more recently, CD4+ T-cell clones have been used in early phase clinical trials that have demonstrated this approach is associated with low toxicity (Yee, 2010).

21.5.4.4.2 Adoptive Cell Therapy with Tumor-Infiltrating Lymphocytes

Many solid tumors are infiltrated with T cells. Because, under normal circumstances, T cells do not infiltrate tissues, the presence of tumor-infiltrating T cells (TILs) suggests that an antitumor response is occurring and the T-cell infiltrate is likely enriched for those that can recognize TAAs. Therefore, TILs represent a source of tumor-specific T cells for use in therapy. TILs can be obtained following dissociation of tumor tissue and expansion of TILs can be undertaken ex vivo in the presence of various T-cell growth factors such as IL-2. Adoptive transfer of bulk populations of TILs has been performed in trials for various cancers, including melanoma, ovarian cancer, renal cell carcinoma, and non–small cell lung cancer. Collectively, these trials demonstrate that adoptive transfer of TILs is associated with minimal toxicity and some of these studies provide evidence that TILs are clinically active.

High clinical response rates have been observed when patients with metastatic melanoma were treated with TIL-based protocols in a particular series of trials. In these protocols, patients were given nonmyeloablative lymphodepleting chemotherapy (cyclophosphamide and fludarabine) immediately prior to infusion of TILs (10^{10} to 10^{11} cells) and high-dose IL-2 therapy. Using this protocol, the objective clinical response rate by RECIST (Response Evaluation Criteria in Solid Tumors) criteria was approximately 50% (21/43 patients) (Dudley et al, 2002, 2005). When total body irradiation was added to the treatment protocol, a trend to higher clinical response rates with increasing intensity of lymphodepletion was observed (Dudley et al, 2008). Therefore the combination of TIL transfer with other therapeutic interventions has the potential to improve disease outcomes, although this has not yet been tested in Phase III trials.

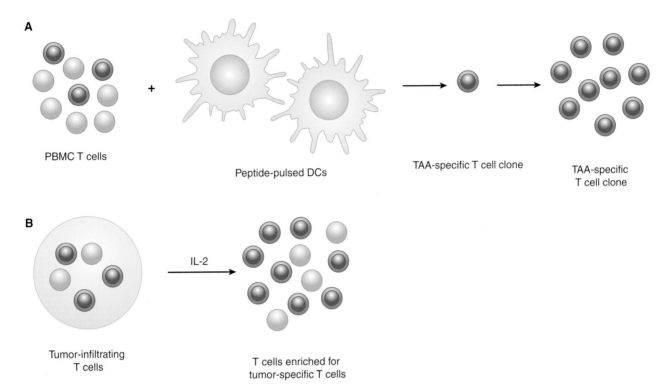

A

PBMC T cells

\+

Peptide-pulsed DCs

TAA-specific T cell clone

TAA-specific
T cell clone

B

Tumor-infiltrating
T cells

IL-2

T cells enriched for
tumor-specific T cells

FIGURE 21–17 Generating T cell clones or tumor-infiltrating lymphocytes (TILs) for adoptive cell therapy. A) To generate T-cell clones, peripheral blood mononuclear cells are isolated and the bulk T-cell population is stimulated with DCs that have been exposed to peptides derived from tumor-associated antigens. Through successive rounds of stimulation and expansion, tumor-specific T cells are selectively expanded. These T cells are cultured under "limiting dilution" conditions to generate cultures originating from 1 parent cell (a "clone") consisting of T cells with the same T-cell receptor. **B)** To generate TILs, tumor tissue is dissociated and the bulk population of TILs is expanded in vitro using a T-cell growth factor (eg, IL-2). In theory, the resulting T-cell population is enriched for tumor-specific T cells.

SUMMARY

The Immune System

- The two arms of the immune system are innate immunity and adaptive immunity. One of the functions of the innate immune system is to detect the presence of pathogens and present antigens to cells of the adaptive immune system. Dendritic cells (DCs) are efficient antigen-presenting cells (APCs). When DCs encounter pathogens, they differentiate from an immature to a mature state. Mature DCs have the ability to efficiently activate T cells.

- Antigens are presented to T cells by major histocompatibility complex (MHC) molecules. The antigens presented by MHC molecules are peptide fragments that can be derived from self or foreign proteins. There are 2 main types of MHC molecules: MHC class I and MHC class II. In general, MHC class I molecules present antigens from intracellular proteins ("endogenous pathway"), and MHC class II molecules present antigens from extracellular proteins ("exogenous pathway"). The exception to this paradigm is a pathway called "cross-presentation," where MHC class I molecules can present antigens derived from exogenous sources.

- B cells recognize antigens in their native form via a B cell receptor (BCR). The BCR is a membrane-bound form of the soluble immunoglobulin (antibody) that will be produced by that B cell upon activation. T cells recognize antigens as peptide fragments that are presented by MHC molecules via the T-cell receptor (TCR). The TCR is expressed on the surface of T cells and is not secreted. The diversity of BCR and TCR specificities is partly a result of a DNA rearrangement process called V(D)J rearrangement. In this process, selected gene segments from a large number of possible gene segments are spliced into a combined exon.

- A T-cell response is induced when TCRs are engaged by their cognate peptide/MHC ligand. Productive T-cell activation also requires signaling through costimulatory molecules (eg, CD28). T-cell activation leads to proliferation of the T cell as well as the acquisition of effector functions. After T-cell activation, most of the activated T cells disappear, leaving only a small pool of memory T cells behind. T-cell responses are subject to suppression by various mechanisms, including down-regulation via molecules such as cytotoxic T-lymphocyte antigen (CTLA)-4 and programmed death (PD)-1.

- There are various types of T cells. Cytotoxic T lymphocytes (CTLs) can kill target cells and generally express the CD8 co-receptor and recognize peptides presented by MHC class I molecules. T helper cells (Th cells) secrete various cytokines depending on their particular Th cell subtype (Th1, Th2, Th17, etc). T helper cells express the CD4 co-receptor and recognize peptides presented by MHC class II molecules.
- Various mechanisms help to establish T-cell tolerance to self antigens. For example, during T-cell development in the thymus, T cells that strongly recognize self antigens are eliminated. Self-reactive T cells that escape thymic development can be suppressed by various peripheral tolerance mechanisms including regulatory T cells (Tregs).

Tumor Immunology and Immunotherapy

- Tumor-associated antigens (TAAs) are proteins that are expressed preferentially (or uniquely) by tumor cells. Types of TAAs include mutated self proteins, cancer-testis antigens, proteins normally expressed during differentiation, overexpressed self proteins, and viral antigens. They may also have unique post-translational modifications. Some TAA-derived peptides can be recognized by T cells. Peptide/MHC multimer reagents can aid in the detection of TAA-specific T cells.
- The immune system can survey the body for tumor cells and eliminate them, a concept termed "cancer immune surveillance". Immune surveillance was in part demonstrated in studies where immunodeficient mice developed tumors at a higher frequency and with faster kinetics than did immunocompetent mice. A current model for tumor progression and the relationship with the immune system includes three phases: elimination, equilibrium, and escape. The importance of the immune system in controlling tumor growth is in part demonstrated by studies that show a correlation between T-cell infiltration in tumors and good prognosis.
- Barriers that inhibit the T-cell response against tumors include the tolerance mechanisms that also inhibit the T-cell response against self antigens. In addition, immunosuppressive factors in the tumor microenvironment may be present such as transforming growth factor (TGF)-β and indolamine 2,3-dioxygenase (IDO).
- Monoclonal antibodies (mAbs) bind specifically to their target protein. The classical method of mAb production involves the generation of hybridomas. Monoclonal Abs can be completely of animal origin (eg, mouse) or can be chimeric, humanized, or fully human. Monoclonal Ab therapy has various possible mechanisms of action: blockade of receptor signaling, triggering of receptor signaling, activation of the complement cascade leading to target cell lysis, or target cell lysis via antibody-dependent cell-mediated cytotoxicity. In addition, mAb therapy may enhance T-cell priming due to enhanced uptake and presentation of antigens.

- Approved immunotherapies for cancer include Bacillus Calmette-Guerin for superficial bladder cancer, interferon-α for some hematological cancers, interleukin-2 for renal cell carcinoma and melanoma, Imiquimod for superficial basal cell carcinoma, and Ipilimumab (a monoclonal antibody that blocks the negative regulation of T-cell responses) for metastatic melanoma. These are "nonspecific" approaches that augment T-cell responses in a polyclonal manner.
- Other immunotherapeutic approaches are at various stages of development. Vaccination with DCs involves the in vitro production of autologous DCs. Generally, these DCs are loaded with TAA-derived peptide(s) and matured with various stimuli before administration. The first autologous cellular therapy for cancer to receive FDA approval was Sipuleucel-T for prostate cancer. Other types of adoptive cell therapies under investigation include immunotherapy with tumor-specific T cell clones or with tumor-infiltrating lymphocytes.

REFERENCES

Akira S, Uematsu S, Takeuchi O. Pathogen recognition and innate immunity. *Cell* 2006;124:783-801.

Altman JD, Moss PA, Goulder PJ, et al. Phenotypic analysis of antigen-specific T lymphocytes. *Science* 1996;274:94-96.

Atkins MB, Lotze MT, Dutcher JP, et al. High-dose recombinant interleukin 2 therapy for patients with metastatic melanoma: analysis of 270 patients treated between 1985 and 1993. *J Clin Oncol* 1999;17:2105-2116.

Bachmann MF, Kohler G, Ecabert B, et al. Cutting edge: lymphoproliferative disease in the absence of CTLA-4 is not T cell autonomous. *J Immunol* 1999;163:1128-1131.

Bargou R, Leo E, Zugmaier G, et al. Tumor regression in cancer patients by very low doses of a T cell-engaging antibody. *Science* 2008;321:974-977.

Bross PF, Beitz J, Chen G, et al. Approval summary: gemtuzumab ozogamicin in relapsed acute myeloid leukemia. *Clin Cancer Res* 2001;7:1490-1496.

Bryant P, Ploegh H. Class II MHC peptide loading by the professionals. *Curr Opin Immunol* 2004;16:96-102.

Clynes RA, Towers TL, Presta LG, et al. Inhibitory Fc receptors modulate in vivo cytotoxicity against tumor targets. *Nat Med* 2000;6:443-446.

Davis M. T cell receptor gene diversity and selection. *Annu Rev Biochem* 1990;59:475-496.

Dubrot J, Palazon A, Alfaro C, et al. Intratumoral injection of interferon-alpha and systemic delivery of agonist anti-CD137 monoclonal antibodies synergize for immunotherapy. *Int J Cancer* 2011;128:105-118.

Dudley ME, Wunderlich JR, Robbins PF, et al. Cancer regression and autoimmunity in patients after clonal repopulation with antitumor lymphocytes. *Science* 2002;298:850-854.

Dudley ME, Wunderlich JR, Yang JC, et al. Adoptive cell transfer therapy following non-myeloablative but lymphodepleting chemotherapy for the treatment of patients with refractory metastatic melanoma. *J Clin Oncol* 2005;23:2346-2357.

Dudley ME, Yang JC, Sherry R, et al. Adoptive cell therapy for patients with metastatic melanoma: evaluation of intensive myeloablative chemoradiation preparative regimens. *J Clin Oncol* 2008;26:5233-5239.

Dunn GP, Koebel CM, Schreiber RD. Interferons, immunity and cancer immunoediting. *Nat Rev Immunol* 2006;6: 836-848.

Dunn GP, Old LJ, Schreiber RD. The three Es of cancer immunoediting. *Annu Rev Immunol* 2004;22:329-360.

Dustin ML, Cooper JA. The immunological synapse and the actin cytoskeleton: molecular hardware for T cell signaling. *Nat Immunol* 2000;1:23-29.

Fife BT, Bluestone JA. Control of peripheral T-cell tolerance and autoimmunity via the CTLA-4 and PD-1 pathways. *Immunol Rev* 2008;224:166-182.

Fisher RI, Kaminski MS, Wahl RL, et al. Tositumomab and iodine-131 tositumomab produces durable complete remissions in a subset of heavily pretreated patients with low-grade and transformed non-Hodgkin's lymphomas. *J Clin Oncol* 2005;23:7565-7573.

Flavell RA, Sanjabi S, Wrzesinski SH, et al. The polarization of immune cells in the tumour environment by TGFbeta. *Nat Rev Immunol* 2010;10:554-567.

Franchi L, Warner N, Viani K, et al. Function of Nod-like receptors in microbial recognition and host defense. *Immunol Rev* 2009;227:106-128.

Fyfe G, Fisher RI, Rosenberg SA, et al. Results of treatment of 255 patients with metastatic renal cell carcinoma who received high-dose recombinant interleukin-2 therapy. *J Clin Oncol* 1995;13:688-696.

Galon J, Costes A, Sanchez-Cabo F, et al. Type, density, and location of immune cells within human colorectal tumors predict clinical outcome. *Science* 2006;313:1960-1964.

Gondek DC, Lu LF, Quezada SA, et al. Cutting edge: contact-mediated suppression by CD4+CD25+ regulatory cells involves a granzyme B-dependent, perforin-independent mechanism. *J Immunol* 2005;174:1783-1786.

Gutcher I, Becher B. APC-derived cytokines and T cell polarization in autoimmune inflammation. *J Clin Invest* 2007;117:1119-1127.

Hemmi H, Takeuchi O, Kawai T, et al. A toll-like receptor recognizes bacterial DNA. *Nature* 2000;408:740-745.

Higano CS, Schellhammer PF, Small EJ, et al. Integrated data from 2 randomized, double-blind, placebo-controlled, phase 3 trials of active cellular immunotherapy with sipuleucel-T in advanced prostate cancer. *Cancer* 2009;115:3670-3679.

Hodi FS, O'Day SJ, McDermott DF, et al. Improved survival with ipilimumab in patients with metastatic melanoma. *N Engl J Med* 2010;363:711-723.

Huber ML, Haynes L, Parker C, Iversen P. Interdisciplinary critique of sipuleucel-T as immunotherapy in castration-resistant prostate cancer. *J Natl Cancer Inst* 2012;104:1-7.

Iwasaki A, Medzhitov R. Regulation of adaptive immunity by the innate immune system. *Science* 2010;327:291-295.

Ji Y, Zhang W. Th17 cells: positive or negative role in tumor? *Cancer Immunol Immunother* 2010;59:979-987.

Jonuleit H, Schmitt E. The regulatory T cell family: distinct subsets and their interrelations. *J Immunol* 2003;171:6323-6327.

Josefowicz SZ, Rudensky A. Control of regulatory T cell lineage commitment and maintenance. *Immunity* 2009;30:616-625.

Kalia V, Sarkar S, Gourley TS, et al. Differentiation of memory B and T cells. *Curr Opin Immunol* 2006;18:255-264.

Kantoff PW, Higano CS, Shore ND, et al. Sipuleucel-T immunotherapy for castration-resistant prostate cancer. *N Engl J Med* 2010;363:411-422.

Kaplan DH, Shankaran V, Dighe AS, et al. Demonstration of an interferon gamma-dependent tumor surveillance system in immunocompetent mice. *Proc Natl Acad Sci U S A* 1998;95: 7556-7561.

Kawai T, Akira S. Toll-like receptor and RIG-I-like receptor signaling. *Ann N Y Acad Sci* 2008;1143:1-20.

Kawashima I, Hudson SJ, Tsai V, et al. The multi-epitope approach for immunotherapy for cancer: identification of several CTL epitopes from various tumor-associated antigens expressed on solid epithelial tumors. *Hum Immunol* 1998;59:1-14.

Kirkwood JM, Strawderman MH, Ernstoff MS, et al. Interferon alfa-2b adjuvant therapy of high-risk resected cutaneous melanoma: the Eastern Cooperative Oncology Group Trial EST 1684. *J Clin Oncol* 1996;14:7-17.

Kolb HJ, Schmid C, Barrett AJ, et al. Graft-versus-leukemia reactions in allogeneic chimeras. *Blood* 2004;103:767-776.

Krangel MS. Mechanics of T cell receptor gene rearrangement. *Curr Opin Immunol* 2009;21:133-139.

Lee JH, Torisu-Itakara H, Cochran AJ, et al. Quantitative analysis of melanoma-induced cytokine-mediated immunosuppression in melanoma sentinel nodes. *Clin Cancer Res* 2005;11:107-112.

Lollini PL, Cavallo F, Nanni P, et al. Vaccines for tumour prevention. *Nat Rev Cancer* 2006;6:204-216.

McGeachy MJ, Cua DJ. Th17 cell differentiation: the long and winding road. *Immunity* 2008;28:445-453.

Mempel TR, Pittet MJ, Khazaie K, et al. Regulatory T cells reversibly suppress cytotoxic T cell function independent of effector differentiation. *Immunity* 2006;25:129-141.

Mendel I, Kerlero dR, Ben Nun A. A myelin oligodendrocyte glycoprotein peptide induces typical chronic experimental autoimmune encephalomyelitis in H-2b mice: fine specificity and T cell receptor V beta expression of encephalitogenic T cells. *Eur J Immunol* 1995;25:1951-1959.

Motzer RJ, Bacik J, Murphy BA, et al. Interferon-alfa as a comparative treatment for clinical trials of new therapies against advanced renal cell carcinoma. *J Clin Oncol* 2002;20:289-296.

Munn DH, Mellor AL. Indoleamine 2,3-dioxygenase and tumor-induced tolerance. *J Clin Invest* 2007;117:1147-1154.

Munn DH, Sharma MD, Hou D, et al. Expression of indoleamine 2,3-dioxygenase by plasmacytoid dendritic cells in tumor-draining lymph nodes. *J Clin Invest* 2004;114:280-290.

Munn DH, Sharma MD, Lee JR, et al. Potential regulatory function of human dendritic cells expressing indoleamine 2,3-dioxygenase. *Science* 2002;297:1867-1870.

Nimmerjahn F, Ravetch JV. Fcgamma receptors as regulators of immune responses. *Nat Rev Immunol* 2008;8:34-47.

Ohashi PS. Ignorance is bliss. *Immunologist* 1994;2:87-92.

Orabona C, Grohmann U, Belladonna ML, et al. CD28 induces immunostimulatory signals in dendritic cells via CD80 and CD86. *Nat Immunol* 2004;5:1134-1142.

Palucka K, Banchereau J. Cancer immunotherapy via dendritic cells. *Nat Rev Cancer* 2012;12:265-277.

Pamer E, Cresswell P. Mechanisms of MHC class I—restricted antigen processing. *Annu Rev Immunol* 1998;16:323-358.

Patard JJ, Saint F, Velotti F, et al. Immune response following intravesical bacillus Calmette-Guerin instillations in superficial bladder cancer: a review. *Urol Res* 1998;26:155-159.

Peggs KS, Quezada SA, Chambers CA, et al. Blockade of CTLA-4 on both effector and regulatory T cell compartments contributes to the antitumor activity of anti-CTLA-4 antibodies. *J Exp Med* 2009;206:1717-1725.

Quezada SA, Jarvinen LZ, Lind EF, et al. CD40/CD154 interactions at the interface of tolerance and immunity. *Annu Rev Immunol* 2004;22:307-328.

Read S, Malmstrom V, Powrie F. Cytotoxic T lymphocyte-associated antigen 4 plays an essential role in the function of CD25(+) CD4(+) regulatory cells that control intestinal inflammation. *J Exp Med* 2000;192:295-302.

Rentzsch C, Kayser S, Stumm S, et al. Evaluation of pre-existent immunity in patients with primary breast cancer: molecular and cellular assays to quantify antigen-specific T lymphocytes in peripheral blood mononuclear cells. *Clin Cancer Res* 2003;9: 4376-4386.

Ribas A. Overcoming immunologic tolerance to melanoma: targeting CTLA-4 with tremelimumab (CP-675,206). *Oncologist* 2008;13(suppl 4):10-15.

Romero P, Dunbar PR, Valmori D, et al. Ex vivo staining of metastatic lymph nodes by class I major histocompatibility complex tetramers reveals high numbers of antigen-experienced tumor-specific cytotoxic T lymphocytes. *J Exp Med* 1998;188:1641-1650.

Rosenberg SA, Lotze MT, Yang JC, et al. Experience with the use of high-dose interleukin-2 in the treatment of 652 cancer patients. *Ann Surg* 1989;210:474-484.

Sahin U, Tureci O, Schmitt H, et al. Human neoplasms elicit multiple specific immune responses in the autologous host. *Proc Natl Acad Sci U S A* 1995;92:11810-11813.

Sakaguchi S, Hori S, Fukui Y, et al. Thymic generation and selection of CD25+CD4+ regulatory T cells: implications of their broad repertoire and high self-reactivity for the maintenance of immunological self-tolerance. *Novartis Found Symp* 2003;252: 6-16; discussion 16-23.

Sakaguchi S, Wing K, Onishi Y, et al. Regulatory T cells: how do they suppress immune responses? *Int Immunol* 2009;21: 1105-1111.

Sakaguchi S, Yamaguchi T, Nomura T, et al. Regulatory T cells and immune tolerance. *Cell* 2008;133:775-787.

Sebzda E, Mariathasan S, Ohteki T, et al. Selection of the T cell repertoire. *Annu Rev Immunol* 1999;17:829-874.

Shankaran V, Ikeda H, Bruce AT, et al. IFNgamma and lymphocytes prevent primary tumour development and shape tumour immunogenicity. *Nature* 2001;410:1107-1111.

Shen L, Rock KL. Priming of T cells by exogenous antigen cross-presented on MHC class I molecules. *Curr Opin Immunol* 2006;18:85-91.

Small EJ, Fratesi P, Reese DM, et al. Immunotherapy of hormone-refractory prostate cancer with antigen-loaded dendritic cells. *J Clin Oncol* 2000;18:3894-3903.

Sotiropoulou PA, Perez SA, Iliopoulou EG, et al. Cytotoxic T-cell precursor frequencies to HER-2 (369-377) in patients with HER-2/neu-positive epithelial tumours. *Br J Cancer* 2003;89: 1055-1061.

Steinman RM, Hawiger D, Nussenzweig MC. Tolerogenic dendritic cells. *Annu Rev Immunol* 2003;21:685-711.

Stutman O. Chemical carcinogenesis in nude mice: comparison between nude mice from homozygous matings and heterozygous matings and effect of age and carcinogen dose. *J Natl Cancer Inst* 1979;62:353-358.

Stutman O. Tumor development after 3-methylcholanthrene in immunologically deficient athymic-nude mice. *Science* 1974;183:534-536.

Szabo SJ, Kim ST, Costa GL, et al. A novel transcription factor, T-bet, directs Th1 lineage commitment. *Cell* 2000;100: 655-669.

Tacken PJ, de Vries IJ, Torensma R, et al. Dendritic-cell immunotherapy: from ex vivo loading to in vivo targeting. *Nat Rev Immunol* 2007;7:790-802.

Takeda K, Akira S. Toll-like receptors in innate immunity. *Int Immunol* 2005;17:1-14.

Trombetta ES, Mellman I. Cell biology of antigen processing in vitro and in vivo. *Annu Rev Immunol* 2005;23:975-1028.

Tuthill RJ, Unger JM, Liu PY, et al. Risk assessment in localized primary cutaneous melanoma: a Southwest Oncology Group study evaluating nine factors and a test of the Clark logistic regression prediction model. *Am J Clin Pathol* 2002;118: 504-511.

van der Bruggen P, Traversari C, Chomez P, et al. A gene encoding an antigen recognized by cytolytic T lymphocytes on a human melanoma. *Science* 1991;254:1643-1647.

Vollers SS, Stern LJ. Class II major histocompatibility complex tetramer staining: progress, problems, and prospects. *Immunology* 2008;123:305-313.

Weber J. Overcoming immunologic tolerance to melanoma: targeting CTLA-4 with ipilimumab (MDX-010). *Oncologist* 2008;13(suppl 4):16-25.

Wildin RS, Freitas A. IPEX and FOXP3: clinical and research perspectives. *J Autoimmun* 2005;25(suppl):56-62.

Witzig TE, Gordon LI, Cabanillas F, et al. Randomized controlled trial of yttrium-90-labeled ibritumomab tiuxetan radioimmunotherapy versus rituximab immunotherapy for patients with relapsed or refractory low-grade, follicular, or transformed B-cell non-Hodgkin's lymphoma. *J Clin Oncol* 2002;20:2453-2463.

Wolchok JD, Hoos A, O'Day S, et al. Guidelines for the evaluation of immune therapy activity in solid tumors: immune-related response criteria. *Clin Cancer Res* 2009;15:7412-7420.

Wolf E, Hofmeister R, Kufer P, et al. BiTEs: bispecific antibody constructs with unique anti-tumor activity. *Drug Discov Today* 2005;10:1237-1244.

Yee C. Adoptive therapy using antigen-specific T-cell clones. *Cancer J* 2010;16:367-373.

Zhang L, Conejo-Garcia JR, Katsaros D, et al. Intratumoral T cells, recurrence, and survival in epithelial ovarian cancer. *N Engl J Med* 2003;348:203-213.

Zheng W, Flavell RA. The transcription factor GATA-3 is necessary and sufficient for Th2 cytokine gene expression in CD4 T cells. *Cell* 1997;89:587-596.

Guide to Clinical Studies

Eitan Amir and Ian F. Tannock

22.1 INTRODUCTION

To select the optimal treatment for patients, clinical oncologists need to be skilled at critically evaluating data from clinical studies and interpreting these appropriately. Clinicians should also be proficient in the application of diagnostic tests, assessment of risk, and the estimation of prognosis. Equally, scientists involved in translational research should be aware of the problems and pitfalls in undertaking clinical studies. This chapter provides a critical overview of methods used in clinical research.

22.2 TREATMENT

22.2.1 Purpose of Clinical Trials

Clinical trials are used to assess the effects of specific interventions on the health of individuals. Possible interventions include treatment with drugs, radiation, or surgery; modification of diet, behavior, or environment; and surveillance with physical examination, blood tests, or imaging tests. This section focuses on trials of treatment.

Clinical trials may be separated conceptually into *explanatory* trials, designed to evaluate the biological effects of treatment, and *pragmatic* trials, designed to evaluate the practical effects of treatment (Schwartz et al, 1980). This distinction is crucial, because treatments that have desirable biological effects (eg, the ability to kill cancer cells and cause tumor shrinkage) may not have desirable effects in practice (ie, may not lead to improvement in duration or quality of life). Table 22–1 lists the major differences between explanatory and pragmatic trials.

The evaluation of new cancer treatments usually involves progression through a series of clinical trials. Phase I trials are designed to evaluate the relationship between dose and toxicity and aim to establish a tolerable schedule of administration. Phase II trials are designed to screen treatments for their antitumor effects in order to identify those worthy of further evaluation. Phase I and Phase II trials are explanatory—they assess the biological effects of treatment on host and tumor in small numbers of subjects to guide decisions about further research. Randomized Phase III trials are designed to determine the usefulness of new treatments in the management of patients, and are therefore pragmatic. Randomization is the process of assigning participants to experimental and control

TABLE 22–1 Classification of clinical trials.

Characteristic	Explanatory (Phase I and Phase II Trials)	Pragmatic (Phase III Trials)
Purpose	To guide further research and not to formulate treatment policy	To select future treatment policy
Treatment and dosing	To assist in selecting a schedule and to define the maximal tolerated dose (Phase I) and to seek evidence of biological activity (Phase II)	Choose treatment schedule and dose that is tolerated for the target population based on earlier trials
Assessment criteria	Criteria that give biological information (such as inhibition of intended target), tumor response, and dose-dependent toxicity	Should reflect benefit to patients, such as overall survival, quality of life, and toxic effects
Choice of patients	Patients most likely to demonstrate an effect	Patients representative of those to whom the treatment will be applied
Entry criteria	Idealized conditions: exclude patients with conditions that might decrease chance of showing an effect	Real-life conditions: include patients who are expected to receive treatment at end of trial

(existing) therapy, with each participant having a pre-specified (usually equal) chance of being assigned to any group.

Phase I trials are used commonly to define the maximum tolerable dose of a new drug, with a focus on the relationship between dosage and toxicity and on pharmacokinetics (see Chap. 18, Sec. 18.1). Small numbers of patients are treated at successively higher doses until the maximum acceptable degree of toxicity is reached. Many variations have been used; a typical design is to use a low initial dose, unlikely to cause severe side effects, based on tolerance in animals. A *modified Fibonacci sequence* is then used to determine dose escalations: Using this method, the second dose level is 100% higher than the first, the third is 67% higher than the second, the fourth is 50% higher than the third, the fifth is 40% higher than the fourth, and all subsequent levels are 33% higher than the preceding levels. Three patients are treated at each level until any potentially dose-limiting toxicity is observed. Six patients are treated at any dose where such dose-limiting toxicity is encountered. The maximum tolerated dose (MTD) is defined as the maximum dose at which dose-limiting toxicity occurs in fewer than one-third of the patients tested. This design is based on experience that few patients have life-threatening toxicity and on the assumption that the MTD is also the most effective anticancer dose. It has been criticized because most patients receive doses that are well below the MTD and are therefore participating in a study where they have little chance of therapeutic response. Adaptive trials using accelerated titration where fewer patients are treated at the lowest doses, and Bayesian dose-finding designs where the magnitude of dose increments is determined by toxicity observed at lower doses, have been suggested as methods to address this limitation (Simon et al, 1997; Yin et al, 2006). Furthermore, it has been suggested that for molecular-targeted agents, use of MTD is less meaningful. First, MTD generally defines acute toxicity. The use of targeted agents is usually chronic and chronic tolerability is often independent of acute tolerability. Second, early clinical trials of biological agents demonstrated that maximal beneficial effects could be seen at doses lower than the MTD. This led to the concept of the optimal biological dose, which is defined as the dose that produces the maximal beneficial

effects with the fewest adverse events (Herberman, 1985). However, difficulties in determination of the optimal biological dose mean that it only rarely forms the basis of dose selection of targeted agents (Parulekar and Eisenhauer, 2004).

Phase II trials are designed to determine whether a new treatment has sufficient anticancer activity to justify further evaluation, although particularly when evaluating targeted agents, they should ideally provide some information about target inhibition and, hence, mechanism of action. They usually include highly selected patients with a given type of cancer and may use a molecular biomarker to define patients most likely to respond (eg, expression of the estrogen receptor in women with breast cancer when evaluating a hormonal agent; see Chap. 20, Sec. 20.4.1). Phase II studies usually exclude patients with "nonevaluable" disease, and use the proportion of patients whose tumors shrink or disappear (response rate) as the primary measure of outcome. Their sample size is calculated to distinguish active from inactive therapies according to whether response rate is greater or less than some arbitrary or historical level. The resulting sample size is inadequate to provide a precise estimate of activity. For example, a Phase II trial with 24 patients and an observed response rate of 33% has a 95% confidence interval of 16% to 55%. Tumor response rate is a reasonable end point for assessing the anticancer activity of a cytotoxic drug and can predict for eventual success of a randomized Phase III trial. However, response rate is a suboptimal end point in trials evaluating targeted agents, which can modify time to tumor progression without causing major tumor shrinkage (El-Maraghi and Eisenhauer, 2008). Furthermore, it is not a definitive measure of patient benefit. Phase II trials are suitable for guiding decisions about further research but are rarely suitable for making decisions about patient management. There are 2 dominant designs to Phase II trials: single-arm and randomized. Single-arm Phase II trials are simple, easy to execute, and require small sample sizes. They are also able to restrict false-positive and false-negative rates to reasonable levels. However, results usually need to be compared to historical controls. In contrast, randomized Phase II designs are more complex, require up to 4-fold more patients as compared with single-arm trials, but do provide more robust preliminary evidence of comparative efficacy. Single-arm trials may be preferred for single agents with tumor response end points. They may also be preferable in less common tumor sites where accrual may be more challenging. Randomized designs may be favorable for trials of combination therapy and with time to event end points (Gan et al, 2010). The literature is confusing, however, because Phase II trials, especially those with randomized designs have sometimes been reported and interpreted as if they did provide definitive answers to questions about patient management.

Phase III trials are designed to answer questions about the usefulness of treatments in patient management. Questions about patient management are usually comparative, as they involve choices between alternatives—that is, an experimental versus the current standard of management. The current standard may include other anticancer treatments or may be "best supportive care" without specific anticancer therapy. The aim of a Phase III trial is to estimate the difference in outcome associated with a difference in treatment, sometimes referred to as the *treatment effect.* Ideally, alternative treatments are compared by administering them to groups of patients that are equivalent in all other respects, that is, by randomization of suitable patients between the current standard and the new experimental treatment. Randomized controlled Phase III trials are currently regarded as the best, and often only, reliable means of determining the usefulness of treatments in patient management. Phase III drug trials are often conducted in order to register drug treatment for particular indications, which requires approval by agencies such as the United States Food and Drug Administration (FDA) or the European Medicines Agency (EMA). Their end points should reflect patient benefit, such as duration and quality of survival. Most randomized Phase III clinical studies are designed to show (or exclude) statistically significant improvements in overall survival, although many cancer trials use surrogate end points such as disease-free survival (DFS) or progression-free survival (PFS) as the primary end point. The use of a surrogate end point is only clinically meaningful if it has been validated as predicting for improvement in overall survival or quality of life (see below). The following discussion focuses on randomized controlled Phase III trials.

One criticism of the structure of clinical trials is that it takes a long time for drugs to go from initial (Phase I) testing to regulatory approval (based on results of Phase III trials). More recently, more adaptive designs have been introduced to try to speed up drug development. The multiarm, multistage trial design (Royston et al, 2003) is a new approach for conducting randomized trials. It allows several agents or combinations of agents to be assessed simultaneously against a single control group in a randomized design. Recruitment to research arms that do not show sufficient promise in terms of an intermediate outcome measure may be discontinued at interim analyses. In contrast, recruitment to the control arm and to promising research arms continues until sufficient numbers of patients have been entered to assess the impact in terms of the definitive primary outcome measure. By assessing several treatments

in one trial, this design allows the efficacy of drugs to be tested more quickly and with smaller numbers of patients compared with a program of separate Phase II and Phase III trials.

Another criticism is that in an era of molecular-targeted therapy, treatments are often provided on an empirical basis with few trials assessing novel methods for enriching participants for those most likely to benefit from the experimental therapy. Trials with biomarkers selecting patients for benefit have needed smaller sample size to detect similar levels of benefit to those not using biomarkers to select a probable drug-sensitive population (Amir et al, 2011). Some agents (eg, imatinib for the treatment of patients with gastrointestinal stromal tumors [GISTs]) did not need randomized Phase III trials to detect substantial benefits. There are 2 broad ways to select patients for targeted drugs based on biomarkers. In the enrichment approach, all patients are assessed prospectively for presence of the biomarker, and only those with the biomarker are included in the trial (eg, trastuzumab in human epidermal growth factor receptor 2 [HER2]-positive breast cancer). In the retrospective approach the presence or absence of a biomarker is determined in all treated patients and related to the probability of response to a targeted agent (eg, panitumumab in colorectal cancer in relation to K-ras mutations). The enrichment approach leads to greater economic value across the drug development pathway and could reduce both the time and costs of the development process (Trusheim et al, 2011).

22.2.2 Sources of Bias in Clinical Trials

Important characteristics of the patients enrolled in a clinical trial include demographic data (eg, age and gender), clinical characteristics (the stage and pathological type of disease), general well-being, and activities of daily life (performance status), as well as other prognostic factors. Phase III trials are most likely to have positive outcomes if they are applied to homogenous populations. Consequently, most usually have multiple exclusion criteria, such that patients with selected comorbidities and use of some concomitant medications are often excluded. For this and other unknown reasons, patients enrolled in clinical trials often have better outcomes (even if receiving standard treatment) than patients who are seen in routine practice (Chua and Clarke, 2010). The selection of subjects and inclusion and exclusion criteria must be described in sufficient detail for clinicians to judge the degree of similarity between the patients in a trial and the patients in their practice. Treatments, whether with drugs, radiation, or surgery, must be described in sufficient detail to be replicated. Because not all patients may receive the treatment as defined in the protocol, differences between the treatment specified in the protocol and the treatment actually received by the patients should be reported clearly. Although patients in randomized trials may differ from those seen in clinical practice, this difference does not usually detract from the primary conclusion of a randomized trial, although the selection of patients may limit the ability to generalize results to an unselected population.

Treatment outcomes for patients with cancer often depend as much on their initial prognostic characteristics as on their subsequent treatment, and imbalances in prognostic factors can have profound effects on the results of a trial. The reports of most randomized clinical trials include a table of baseline prognostic characteristics for patients assigned to each arm. The *p*-values often reported in these tables are misleading, as any differences between the groups, other than the treatment assigned, *are known* to have arisen by chance. The important question as to whether any such imbalances influence the estimate of treatment effect is best answered by an analysis that is adjusted for any imbalance in prognostic factors (see Sec. 22.4).

Compliance refers to the extent to which a treatment is delivered as intended. It depends on the willingness of physicians to prescribe treatment as specified in the protocol and the willingness of patients to take treatment as prescribed by the physician. Patient compliance with oral medication is variable and may be a major barrier to the delivery of efficacious treatments (Hershman et al, 2010).

Contamination occurs when people in one arm of a trial receive the treatment intended for those in another arm of the trial. This may occur if people allocated to placebo obtain active drug from elsewhere, as has occurred in trials of treatments for HIV infection. This type of contamination is rare in trials of anticancer drugs but common in trials of dietary treatments, vitamin supplements, or other widely available agents. The effect of contamination is to blur distinctions between treatment arms.

Crossover is a related problem that influences the interpretation of trials assessing survival duration. It occurs when people allocated to one treatment subsequently receive the alternative treatment when their disease progresses. Although defensible from pragmatic and ethical viewpoints, crossover changes the nature of the question being asked about survival duration. In a 2-arm trial without crossover, the comparison is of treatment A versus treatment B, whereas with crossover, the comparison is of treatment A followed by treatment B versus treatment B followed by treatment A.

Cointervention occurs when treatments are administered that may influence outcome but are not specified in the trial protocol. Examples are blood products and antibiotics in drug trials for acute leukemia, or radiation therapy in trials of systemic adjuvant therapy for breast cancer. Because cointerventions are not allocated randomly, they may be distributed unequally between the groups being compared and can contribute to differences in outcome.

22.2.3 Importance of Randomization

Well-conducted randomized trials provide a high level of evidence about the value of a new treatment (Table 22–2). The ideal comparison of treatments comes from observing their effects in groups that are otherwise equivalent, and randomization is the only effective means of achieving this. Comparisons between historical controls, between concurrent but nonrandomized controls, or between groups that are allocated

TABLE 22-2 Hierarchy of evidence.

Level	Study Methods
High	Systematic review/metaanalysis
	Randomized controlled trial
	Cohort study
	Case-control study
	Case series
	Case report
	Expert Opinion
Low	Laboratory data

Source: Data from Guyatt et al, 2000.

to different treatments by clinical judgment, are almost certain to generate groups that differ systematically in their baseline prognostic characteristics. Important factors that are measurable can be accounted for in the analysis; however, important factors that are poorly specified—such as comorbidity, a history of complications with other treatments, the ability to comply with treatment, or family history—cannot. Comparisons based on historical controls are particularly prone to bias because of changes over time in factors other than treatment, including altered referral patterns, different criteria for selection of patients, and improvements in supportive care. These changes over time are difficult to assess and difficult to adjust for in analysis. Such differences tend to favor the most recently treated group and to exaggerate the apparent benefits of new treatments.

Stage migration causes systematic variation (Fig. 22–1), and occurs when patients are assigned to different clinical stages because of differences in the precision of staging rather than differences in the true extent of disease. This can occur if patients staged very thoroughly as part of a research protocol are compared with patients staged less thoroughly in the course of routine clinical practice, or if patients staged with newer more-accurate tests are compared with historical controls staged with older, less-accurate tests. Stage migration is important because the introduction of new and more sensitive diagnostic tests produces apparent improvements in outcome for each anatomically defined category of disease in the absence of any real improvement in outcome for the disease overall (Feinstein et al, 1985). This paradox arises because, in general, the patients with the worst prognosis in each category are reclassified as having more advanced disease. As illustrated in Figure 22–1, a portion of those patients initially classified as having localized disease (stage I) may be found to have regional spread if more sensitive imaging is used, and a portion of those initially classified as having only regional spread (stage II) will be found to have systemic spread (stage III). With more-sensitive testing, fewer patients classified as having localized disease will actually have regional spread, making the measured outcome of the localized group appear

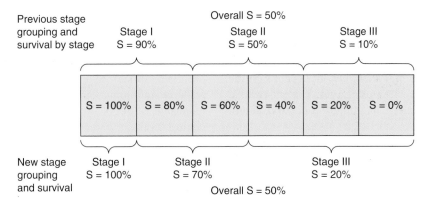

FIGURE 22–1 Stage migration. The diagram illustrates that a change in staging investigations may lead to the apparent improvement of results within each stage without changing the overall results. In the hypothetical example, patients are divided into 6 equal groups, each with the indicated survival. Introduction of more-sensitive staging investigations moves patients into higher-stage groups, as shown, but the overall survival of 50% remains unchanged. (Adapted from Bush, 1979.)

improved. Similarly, the outcome of patients newly classified as having regional disease will be better than that of those with larger volumes of regional disease seen on less-sensitive tests, thereby improving the outcomes of the regional disease group. The same applies for patients moving from the regional to the systemic category. As a consequence, the prognosis of each category of disease improves in the absence of any real improvement in the prognosis of the disease overall.

The major benefit of randomization is the unbiased distribution of *unknown* and *unmeasured* prognostic factors between treatment groups. However, it is only ethical to allocate patients to treatments randomly when there is uncertainty about which treatment is best. The difficulty for clinicians is that this uncertainty, known as *equipoise*, usually resides among physicians collectively rather than within them individually.

Random allocation of treatment does not ensure that the treatment groups are equivalent, but it does ensure that any differences in baseline characteristics are a result of chance. Consequently, differences in outcome must be a result of either chance or treatment. Standard statistical tests estimate the probability (*p* value) that differences in outcome, as observed, might be a result of chance alone. The lower the *p* value, the less plausible is the *null hypothesis* that the observed difference is a result of chance, and the more plausible is the *alternate hypothesis* that the difference is a result of treatment.

Imbalances in known prognostic factors can be reduced or avoided by *stratifying* and *blocking* groups of patients with similar prognostic characteristics during the randomization procedure. For example, in a trial of adjuvant hormone therapy for breast cancer, patients might be stratified according to the presence or absence of lymph node involvement, hormone receptor levels, and menopausal status. *Blocking* ensures that treatment allocation is balanced for every few patients within each defined group (strata). This is practical only for a small number of strata. Randomization in multicenter trials is often blocked and stratified by treatment center to account for differences between centers; however, this carries the risk

that when there is almost complete accrual within a block the physicians may know the arm to which the next patient(s) will be assigned, creating the possibility of selection bias (see below). An alternative approach to adjust for imbalances in prognostic factors is to use multivariable statistical methods (see Sec. 22.4.1 and Chap. 3, Sec 3.3.3).

For randomization to be successfully implemented and to reduce bias, the randomization sequence must be adequately concealed so that the investigators, involved health care providers, and subjects are not aware of the upcoming assignment. The absence of adequate allocation concealment can lead to selection bias, one of the very problems that randomization is supposed to eliminate. Historically, allocation concealment was achieved by the use of opaque envelopes, but in multicenter studies, centralized or remote telephone-based, computer-based, or internet-based allocation systems are now used.

If feasible, it is preferable that both physicians and patients be unaware of which treatment is being administered. This optimal double-blind design prevents bias. Evidence for bias in nonblinded randomized trials comes from the observation that they lead more often to apparent improvements in outcome from experimental treatment than blinded trials and that assignment sequences in randomized trials have sometimes been deciphered (Chalmers et al, 1983; Wood et al, 2008).

22.2.4 Choice and Assessment of Outcomes

The measures used to assess a treatment should reflect the goals of that treatment. Treatment for advanced cancer is often given with palliative intent—to prolong survival or reduce symptoms without realistic expectation of cure. Survival duration has the advantage of being an unequivocal end point that can be unambiguously measured, but if a major end point is improved quality of life, then appropriate methods should be used to measure quality of life. Anti-cancer treatments may prolong survival through toxic effects on the cancer or may shorten survival through toxic effects on the host. Similarly, anticancer treatments may improve quality of life by reducing cancer-related symptoms or may worsen quality of life by adding toxicity due to treatment. Patient benefit depends on the trade-off between these positive and negative effects, which can be assessed only by measuring duration of survival and quality of life directly.

Surrogate or indirect measures of patient benefit, such as tumor shrinkage, DFS, or PFS, can sometimes provide an early indication of efficacy, but they are not substitutes for more direct measures of patient benefit. For example, the use of DFS rather than overall survival in studies of adjuvant treatment requires fewer subjects and shorter follow-up but ignores what happens following the recurrence of disease. Surrogate measures can be used if they have been validated as predicting for benefit in clinically relevant end points such as the use of DFS as a surrogate for overall survival in patients with colorectal cancer receiving fluorouracil-based treatment (Sargent et al, 2005). Higher tumor response rates or improvements in DFS do not always translate into longer overall survival or better quality of life (Ng et al, 2008). Changes in the concentration of tumor markers in serum, such as prostate-specific antigen (PSA) for prostate cancer or cancer antigen 125 (CA125) in ovarian cancer, have been used as outcome measures in certain types of cancer. Levels of these markers may reflect tumor burden in general, but the relationship is quite variable; there are individuals with extensive disease who have low levels of a tumor marker in serum. The relationship between serum levels of a tumor marker and outcome is also variable. In men who have received local treatment for early stage prostate cancer, the reappearance of PSA in the serum indicates disease recurrence. In men with advanced prostate cancer, however, baseline levels of serum PSA may not be associated with duration of survival, and changes in PSA following treatment are not consistently related to changes in symptoms.

It is essential to assess outcomes for all patients who enter a clinical trial. It is common in cancer trials to exclude patients from the analysis on the grounds that they are "not evaluable." Reasons for nonevaluability vary, but may include death soon after treatment was started or failure to receive the full course of treatment. It may be permissible to exclude patients from analysis in explanatory Phase II trials that are seeking to describe the biological effects of treatment; these trials indicate the effect of treatment in those who were able to complete it. It is seldom appropriate to exclude patients in randomized trials, which should reflect the conditions under which the treatment will be applied in practice. Such trials test a policy of treatment, and the appropriate analysis for a pragmatic trial is by *intention to treat*: patients should be included in the arm to which they were allocated regardless of their subsequent course.

For some events (eg, death) there is no doubt as to whether the event has occurred, but assignment of a particular cause of death (eg, whether it was cancer related) may be subjective, as is the assessment of tumor response, recognition of tumor recurrence, and therefore determination of DFS. The

compared groups should be followed with similar types of evaluation so that they are equally susceptible to the detection of outcome events such as recurrence of disease. Whenever the assessment of an outcome is subjective, variation between observers should be examined. Variable criteria of tumor response and imprecise tumor measurement have been documented as causes of variability when this end point is used in clinical trials.

22.2.5 Survival Curves and Their Comparison

Subjects may be recruited to clinical trials over several years, and followed for an additional period to determine their time of death or other outcome measure. Subjects enrolled early in a trial are observed for a longer time than subjects enrolled later and are more likely to have died by the time the trial is analyzed. For this reason, the distribution of survival times is the preferred outcome measure for assessing the influence of treatment on survival. Survival duration is defined as the interval from some convenient "zero time," usually the date of enrollment or randomization in a study, to the time of death of any cause. Subjects who have died provide actual observations of survival duration. Subjects who were alive at last follow-up provide *censored* (incomplete) observations of survival duration; their eventual survival duration will be at least as long as the time to their last follow-up. Most cancer trials are analyzed before all subjects have died, so a method of analysis, which accounts for censored observations, is required.

Actuarial survival curves provide an estimate of the eventual distribution of survival duration (when everyone has died), based on the observed survival duration of those who have died and the censored observations of those still living. Actuarial survival curves are preferred to simple cross-sectional measures of survival because they incorporate and describe all of the available information. Table 22–3 illustrates the *life-table method* for construction of an actuarial survival curve. The period of follow-up after treatment is divided into convenient short intervals—for example, weeks or months. The probability of dying in a particular interval is estimated by dividing the number of people who died during that interval by the number of people who were known to be alive at its beginning ($E = C/B$ in Table 22–3). The probability of surviving a particular interval, having survived to its beginning, is the complement of the probability of dying in it ($F = 1 - E$). The actuarial estimate of the probability of surviving for a given time is calculated by cumulative multiplication of the probabilities of surviving each interval until that time (Fig. 22–2).

The Kaplan-Meier method of survival analysis, also known as the *product limit method*, is identical to the actuarial method except that the calculations are performed at each death rather than at fixed intervals. The Kaplan-Meier survival curve is depicted graphically with the probability of survival on the *y*-axis and time on the *x*-axis: vertical drops occur at each death. The latter part of a survival curve is often the focus of most interest, as it estimates the probability of long-term

TABLE 22–3 Calculation of actuarial survival.

Follow-up Interval (A)	Number at Risk (B)	Number Dying (C)	Number Withdrawn Alive (D)	Probability of Dying During Interval (E)	Probability of Surviving During Interval (F)	Overall Probability of Survival (G)
0	100	—	—	—	—	1
1	100	8	2	0.080	0.920	0.920
2	90	3	2	0.033	0.967	0.890
3	85	1	0	0.012	0.988	0.879
4	84	3	1	0.036	0.964	0.847
5	80	7	3	0.088	0.912	0.773
6	70	6	4	0.086	0.914	0.706
7	60	5	5	0.083	0.917	0.648
8	50	1	4	0.020	0.980	0.635
9	45	1	2	0.022	0.978	0.621
10	42	1	1	0.024	0.976	0.606

Note: A. Follow-up intervals may be of any convenient size; usually days, weeks, or months. B. Number at risk means number of patients alive at the start of the interval. C. Number dying is number of patients dying during each interval. D. Number withdrawn alive refers to patients alive who have not been followed longer than the interval after randomization. E. Probability of dying during each interval is number of patients dying (C) divided by the number at risk (B). F. Probability of survival during each interval is the complement (1 − E) of the probability of dying. G. Overall probability of survival is the cumulative product of the probabilities in (F). The numbers in this column may be plotted against time as an actuarial survival curve.

survival; however, it is also the least-reliable part of the curve, because it is based on fewer observations and therefore more liable to error. The validity of all actuarial methods depends on the time of censoring being independent of the time of death; that is, those who have been followed for a short period of time or who are lost to follow-up are assumed to have similar probability of survival as those who have been followed longer. The most obvious violation of this assumption occurs if subjects are lost to follow-up because they have died or are too sick to attend clinics.

Overall survival curves do not take into account the cause of death. Cause-specific survival curves are constructed by considering only death from specified causes; patients dying from other causes are treated as censored observations at the time of their death. The advantage of cause-specific survival curves is that they focus on deaths because of the cause of interest.

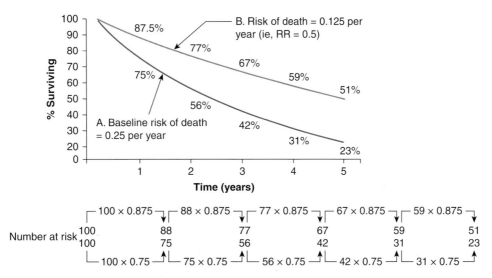

FIGURE 22–2 **Hypothetical survival curves for 2 patient groups.** In a 1-year interval, patients in group A have a 25% probability of dying, while those in group B have a 12.5% probability of dying (ie, relative risk [RR] = 0.5). At the end of 5 years 77% of patients in group A have died (survival rate = 23%). Note that although the hazard rate of death in group B = 0.5, by the end of 5 years, the cumulative risk of death is 49%, not 0.5 × 77% (= 38.5%).

However, they may be influenced by uncertainty about the influence of cancer or its treatment on death because of apparently unrelated causes. Deaths from cardiovascular causes, accidents, or suicides, for example, may all occur as an indirect consequence of cancer or its treatment.

The first step in comparing survival distributions is visual inspection of the survival curves. Ideally, there will be indications of both the number of censored observations and the number of people at risk at representative time points, often indicated beneath the curve (see Fig. 22–2). Curves that cross are difficult to interpret, because this means that short-term survival is better in one arm, whereas long-term survival is better in the other. Two questions must be asked of any observed difference in survival curves: (a) whether it is clinically important and (b) whether it is likely to have arisen by chance. The first is a value judgment that will be based on factors such as absolute magnitude of the observed effect, toxicity, baseline risk, and cost of the treatment (see Sec. 22.2.10). The second is a question of statistical significance, which, in turn, depends on the size of the difference, the variability of the data, and the sample size of the trial.

The precision of an estimate of survival is conveniently described by its *95% confidence interval*. Confidence intervals are closely related to *p*-values: a 95% confidence interval that excludes a treatment effect of zero indicates a *p*-value of less than 0.05. The usual interpretation of the 95% confidence interval is that there is a 95% probability that the true value of the measurement (hazard ratio, odds ratio, risk ratio) lies within the interval. The *statistical significance* of a difference in survival distributions is expressed by a *p*-value, which is the probability that a difference as large as or larger than that observed would have arisen by chance alone. Several statistical tests are available for calculating the *p*-value for differences in survival distributions. The *log-rank test* (also known as the Mantel-Cox test) and the *Wilcoxon test* are the most commonly used methods for analyzing statistical differences in survival curves. Both methods quantify the difference between survival curves by comparing the difference between the observed number of deaths and the number expected if the curves were equivalent. Because the Wilcoxon test gives more weight to early follow-up times when the number of patients is greater, it is less sensitive than the log-rank test to differences between survival curves that occur later in follow-up.

Survival analyses can be adjusted, in principle, for any number of prognostic variables. For example, a trial comparing the effects of 2 regimens of adjuvant chemotherapy on the survival of women with early stage breast cancer might include women with or without spread to axillary lymph nodes and with or without hormone-receptor expression. An unadjusted analysis would compare the survivals of the 2 treatment groups directly. The estimate of the treatment effect can be adjusted for any imbalances in these prognostic factors by including them in a multivariable analysis. Although simple parametric tests such as the Kaplan-Meier method can account for categorical variables, in order to assess for continuous or time-dependent variables, the more complex *Cox proportional hazards model* is preferred (Tibshirani, 1982; see Sec. 22.4.1 and Chap. 3, Sec. 3.3.3). In large randomized trials, such adjustments rarely affect the conclusions, because the likelihood of major imbalances is small.

Differences in the distribution of survival times for 2 treatments compared in a randomized trial may be summarized in several ways:

1. The absolute difference in the median survival or in the proportion of patients who are expected to be alive at a specified time after treatment (eg, at 5 or 10 years).
2. The hazard ratio (ratio of the probability of mortality over a specific time interval) between the 2 arms.
3. The number of patients who would need to be treated to prevent 1 death over a given period of time.

Differences in data presentation may create substantially different impressions of the clinical benefit derived from a new treatment. For example, a substantial reduction in hazard ratio may correspond to only a small improvement in absolute survival and a large number of patients who would need to be treated to save 1 life. These values depend on the expected level of survival in the control group. For example, a 25% relative improvement in overall survival has been found for use of adjuvant combination chemotherapy in younger women with breast cancer (Early Breast Cancer Trialists Collaborative Group, 2005). If this treatment effect is applied to node-positive women with a control survival at 10 years of less than 50%, it will lead to an absolute increase in survival of approximately 12%; between 8 and 9 women would need to be treated to save 1 life over that 10-year period. The same 25% reduction in hazard ratio would lead to approximately a 6% increase in absolute survival at 10 years for node-negative women where control survival at 10 years is around 75%. This corresponds to 1 life saved over 10 years for every 17 women treated. When presented with different summaries of trials, physicians may select the experimental treatment on the basis of what appears to be a substantial reduction in hazard or odds ratio, but reject treatment on the basis of a smaller increase in absolute survival or a large number of patients that need to be treated to save 1 life, even though these represent different expressions of the same effect (Chao et al, 2003). Note also that over a long time interval, the cumulative risk of death in one group cannot be determined simply by multiplying the hazard ratio by the cumulative risk of death in the baseline group. Because the number of patients at risk changes with time, the absolute gain in survival does not equal the product of this calculation (see Fig. 22–2).

22.2.6 Statistical Issues

The number of subjects required for a randomized clinical trial where the primary end point is duration of survival depends on several factors:

1. The minimum difference in survival rates that is considered clinically important: the smaller the difference, the larger the number of subjects required.

TABLE 22–4 Number of patients required to detect or exclude an improvement in survival. Data assume $\alpha = 0.05$; power, $1 - \beta = 0.90$

		Expected Survival in Experimental Group										
		0	0.1	0.2	0.3	0.4	0.5	0.6	0.7	0.8	0.9	1.0
	0		150	75	50	35	30	25	20	15	15	10
	0.1			430	140	75	50	35	25	20	15	15
	0.2				625	185	90	55	40	30	20	15
	0.3					755	210	100	60	40	25	20
	0.4						815	215	100	55	35	25
Expected survival in control group	0.5							815	210	90	50	30
	0.6								755	185	75	35
	0.7									625	140	50
	0.8										430	75
	0.9											150
	1.0											

2. The number of deaths expected with the standard treatment used in the control arm: a smaller number of subjects is required when the expected survival is either very high or very low (see Table 22–4).

3. The probability of (willingness to accept) a false-positive result (alpha, or type I error): the lower the probability, the larger the number of subjects required.

4. The probability of (willingness to accept) a false-negative result (beta, or type II error): the lower the probability, the larger the number of subjects required.

The minimum difference that is clinically important is the smallest difference that would lead to the adoption of a new treatment. This judgment will depend on the severity of the condition being treated and the feasibility, toxicity, and cost of the treatment(s). Methods are available to help quantify such judgments. For example, the practitioners who will be expected to make decisions about treatment based on the results of the trial can be asked what magnitude of improvement would be sufficient for them to change their practice by adopting the new treatment. Based on such information, the required number of patients to be entered into a trial can be estimated from tables similar to Table 22–4. The acceptable values for the error probabilities are matters of judgment. Values of 0.05 for alpha (false-positive error) and 0.1 or 0.2 for beta (false-negative error) are well-entrenched. There are good arguments for using lower (more stringent) values, although perhaps even more important is that trials should be repeated by independent investigators before their results are used to change clinical practice.

In a trial assessing survival duration, it is the number of deaths rather than the number of subjects that determines the reliability of its conclusions. For example, a trial with 1000 subjects and 200 deaths will be more reliable than a trial with 2000 subjects and 150 deaths. From a statistical point of view, this means that it is more efficient to perform trials in subjects who are at a higher risk of death than at a lower risk of death. It also explains the value of prolonged follow-up—longer follow-up means more deaths, which produce more reliable conclusions.

22.2.6.1 Power The power of a trial refers to its ability to detect a difference between treatments when in fact they do differ. The power of a trial is the complement of beta, the type II error (power = 1 – beta). Table 22–4 shows the relationship between the expected difference between treatments and the number of patients required. A randomized clinical trial that seeks to detect an absolute improvement in survival of 20%, compared with a control group receiving standard treatment whose expected survival is 40%, will require approximately 108 patients in each arm at $\alpha = 0.05$ and a power of 0.9. This means that a clinical trial of this size has a 90% chance of detecting an improvement in survival of this magnitude. Detection of a smaller difference between treatments—for example, a 10% absolute increase in survival—would require approximately 410 patients in each arm. A substantial proportion of published clinical trials are too small to detect clinically important differences reliably. This may lead to important deficiencies in the translation of clinical research into practice. If an underpowered study finds "no statistically significant difference" associated with the use of a given treatment, the results may mask a clinically important therapeutic gain that the trial was unable to detect. If there are insufficient patients to have an 80% to 90% chance of detecting a worthwhile difference in survival, then a trial should probably not be undertaken. In contrast some trials, especially those sponsored by pharmaceutical companies, have become so large that they can detect very small differences in survival, which are statistically significant but may not be clinically meaningful. For example, in the National Cancer Institute of Canada PA3 trial, investigators reported a statistically significant improvement in overall survival. However, in absolute terms this amounted to an improvement in median survival of around 11 days and came at the cost of increased toxicity and treatment-related death (Moore et al, 2007).

22.2.7 Metaanalysis

Metaanalysis is a method by which data from individual randomized clinical trials that assess similar treatments (eg, adjuvant chemotherapy for breast cancer versus no chemotherapy) are combined to give an overall estimate of treatment effect. Metaanalysis can be useful because (a) the results of individual trials are subject to random error and may give misleading results, and (b) a small effect of a treatment (eg, approximately 5% improvement in absolute survival for node-negative breast cancer from use of adjuvant chemotherapy) may be difficult to detect in individual trials. Detection of such a small difference will require several thousand patients to be randomized, yet it may be sufficiently meaningful to recommend adoption of the new treatment as standard.

Metaanalysis requires the extraction and combination of data from trials addressing the question of interest. The preferred method involves collection of data on individual patients (date of randomization, date of death, or date last seen if alive) that were entered in individual trials, although literature-based approaches are also recognized. The trials will, in general, compare related strategies of treatment to standard management (eg, radiotherapy with or without chemotherapy for stage III non–small cell lung cancer) but may not be identical (eg, different types of chemotherapy might be used).

Metaanalysis is typically a 2-stage process. First, summary statistics (such as risk or hazard ratios) are calculated for individual studies. Then a summary (pooled) effect estimate is calculated as a weighted average of the effects of the intervention in the individual studies. There are 2 models for weighting studies in the pooled estimate. If each study is assumed to estimate the same relative outcome such that there is no interstudy heterogeneity, then any error is derived from measurement error within individual studies, and studies are weighted by their sample size. In studies not all estimating the same outcome, it is assumed that interstudy variability is more significant than intrastudy variability and a random-effects metaanalysis is carried out, which weights most studies equally regardless of their size. All methods of metaanalysis should incorporate a test of heterogeneity—an assessment of whether the variation among the results of the separate studies is compatible with random variation, or whether it is large enough to indicate inconsistency in the effects of the intervention across studies (interaction).

Data are presented typically in forest plots as in Figure 22–3, which illustrates the comparison of a strategy (in this example, ovarian ablation as adjuvant therapy for breast cancer) used alone versus no such treatment (upper part of figure) and a related comparison where patients in both arms also receive chemotherapy (lower part of figure). Here, each trial

included in the metaanalysis is represented by a symbol, proportional in area to the number of patients on the trial, and by a horizontal line representing its confidence interval. A vertical line represents the null effect, and a diamond beneath the individual trials represents the overall treatment effect and confidence interval. If this diamond symbol does not intersect the vertical line representing the null effect, a significant result is declared.

The potential for bias and methodological quality can be assessed in a metaanalysis. A funnel plot is a simple scatter plot in which a measure of each study's size or precision is plotted against a measure of the effect of the intervention. Symmetrical funnel plots suggest, but do not confirm absence of bias and high methodological quality. Sources of asymmetry in funnel plots include selection biases (such as publication bias: that is, the tendency for preferential and earlier publication of positive studies, and selective reporting of outcomes), poor methodological quality leading to spuriously inflated effects in smaller studies, inadequate analysis, or fraud.

Metaanalysis is an expensive and time-consuming procedure. Important considerations are as follows:

1. Attempts should be made to include the latest results of all trials; unpublished trials should be included to avoid publication bias.
2. Because of publication bias and other reasons, metaanalyses obtained from reviews of the literature tend to overestimate the effect of experimental treatment as compared with a metaanalysis based on data for individual patients obtained from the investigators (Stewart and Parmar, 1993).
3. Because metaanalysis may combine trials with related but different treatments (eg, less-effective and more-effective chemotherapy), the results may underestimate the effects of treatment that could be obtained under optimal conditions.

There is extensive debate in the literature about the merits and problems of metaanalyses and their advantages and disadvantages as compared with a single, large, well-designed trial (Parmar et al, 1996; Buyse et al, 2000; Noble, 2006). A well-performed metaanalysis uses all the available data, recognizes that false-negative and false-positive trials are likely to be common, and may limit the inappropriate influence of individual trials on practice.

22.2.8 Patient-Reported Outcomes

Physician-evaluated performance status and patient reported outcomes such as quality of life are correlated, but are far from identical, and both can provide independent prognostic information in clinical trials (see Sec. 22.4.3). Patient-reported outcomes include symptom scales (eg, for pain or fatigue) and measures of quality of life. Physicians and other health professionals are quite poor in assessing the level of symptoms of their patients, and simple methods for grading symptoms by patients, such as the Functional Assessment of Cancer Therapy (FACT) Scale or the Edmonton Symptom Assessment Scale (Cella et al, 1993; Nekolaichuk et al, 1999) can give valuable information

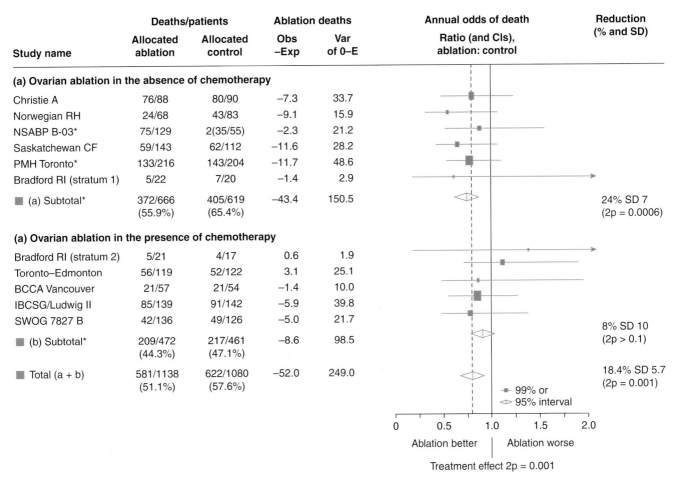

| | Deaths/patients | | Ablation deaths | | Annual odds of death | Reduction |
Study name	Allocated ablation	Allocated control	Obs −Exp	Var of 0−E	Ratio (and Cls), ablation: control	(% and SD)
(a) Ovarian ablation in the absence of chemotherapy						
Christie A	76/88	80/90	−7.3	33.7		
Norwegian RH	24/68	43/83	−9.1	15.9		
NSABP B-03*	75/129	2(35/55)	−2.3	21.2		
Saskatchewan CF	59/143	62/112	−11.6	28.2		
PMH Toronto*	133/216	143/204	−11.7	48.6		
Bradford RI (stratum 1)	5/22	7/20	−1.4	2.9		
■ (a) Subtotal*	372/666 (55.9%)	405/619 (65.4%)	−43.4	150.5		24% SD 7 (2p = 0.0006)
(a) Ovarian ablation in the presence of chemotherapy						
Bradford RI (stratum 2)	5/21	4/17	0.6	1.9		
Toronto–Edmonton	56/119	52/122	3.1	25.1		
BCCA Vancouver	21/57	21/54	−1.4	10.0		
IBCSG/Ludwig II	85/139	91/142	−5.9	39.8		
SWOG 7827 B	42/136	49/126	−5.0	21.7		
■ (b) Subtotal*	209/472 (44.3%)	217/461 (47.1%)	−8.6	98.5		8% SD 10 (2p > 0.1)
■ Total (a + b)	581/1138 (51.1%)	622/1080 (57.6%)	−52.0	249.0		18.4% SD 5.7 (2p = 0.001)

■ 99% or
◇ 95% interval

0   0.5   1.0   1.5   2.0

Ablation better | Ablation worse

Treatment effect 2p = 0.001

FIGURE 22–3 Presentation of results of a metaanalysis in a forest plot. Each trial is represented by a square symbol, whose area is proportional to the number of patients entered, and by a horizontal line. These represent the mean and 95% confidence interval for the ratio of annual odds of death in the experimental and standard arms. A vertical line drawn through odds ratio 1.0 represents no effect. The trials are separated into those asking a simple question (in this example, ovarian ablation versus no adjuvant treatment for early breast cancer) and a related but more complex question (ovarian ablation plus chemotherapy versus chemotherapy alone). Diamonds represent overall mean odds ratios and their 95% confidence intervals for the 2 subsets of trials and for overall effect. The vertical dashed line represents mean reduction in annual odds of death for all trials. (Adapted from Early Breast Cancer Trialists Collaborative Group, 1996.)

about palliative (or toxic) effects on patients with cancer who are participating in clinical trials. Quality of life is an abstract, multidimensional concept reflecting physical, psychological, spiritual, and social aspects of life that includes but is not limited to the concept of health. It reflects an individual's perception of and response to his or her unique circumstances. This definition gives primacy to the individual's views and self-assessment is essential. *Instruments* (questionnaires) addressing differing aspects of quality of life from a variety of perspectives are now available. Questionnaires range from generic instruments designed for people with a variety of conditions or diseases to instruments designed for patients with a specific type and stage of cancer. The FACT–General (FACT-G), developed for people receiving cancer treatments (Cella et al, 1993); and the European Organization for Research and Treatment of Cancer Core Quality of Life Questionnaire (EORTC QLQ-C30), developed for people with cancer participating in international clinical trials (Aaronson et al, 1993) are used most often to evaluate

people with cancer. Both combine a core questionnaire relevant to most patients with cancer, as well as an increasing number of subscales that allow subjects to evaluate additional disease or symptom-specific items.

The *validity* of an instrument refers to the extent to which it measures what it is supposed to measure. The validity of a quality-of-life instrument is always open to question, as there is no objective, external gold standard for comparison. Instead, a variety of indirect methods are used to gauge the validity of quality-of-life instruments (Aaronson et al, 1993). Examples include *convergent validity*, the degree of correlation between instruments or scales purporting to measure similar attributes; and *discriminant validity* or the degree to which an instrument can detect differences between different aspects of quality of life. *Face validity* and *content validity* refer to the extent to which an instrument addresses the issues that are important. *Responsiveness* refers to the detection of changes in quality of life with time, such as those caused by effective treatment, while *predictive validity* refers to the prognostic information of a quality-of-life scale in predicting an outcome such as duration of survival. Validated quality-of-life scales are often strong predictors of survival (see Sec. 22.4.3).

Validity is *conditional*—it cannot be judged without specifying for what and for whom it is to be used. Good validity of a questionnaire in symptomatic men with advanced hormone-resistant prostate cancer does not guarantee good validity in men with earlier-stage prostate cancer, for whom pain might be less important and sexual function more important. Even within the same population of subjects, differences between interventions, such as toxicity profiles, might influence validity. For example, nausea and vomiting might be important in a trial of cisplatin-based chemotherapy, whereas sexual function might be more important in a trial of hormonal therapy. The context in which an instrument is to be used and the context(s) in which its validity was assessed must be reexamined for each application. Furthermore, it is important that an a priori hypothesis for palliative end points is defined and preferable that the proportion of patients with palliative response is reported (Joly et al, 2007).

There are methodological challenges to using patient-reported outcomes such as quality-of-life data. There is little evidence to inform the optimal timing for assessment and the intervals at which assessments should be repeated. Attrition because of incomplete data collection remains a challenge and can confound quality-of-life analysis (patients with poor quality of life are less likely to complete questionnaires). Patient perceptions of their quality of life can change over time (eg, "good quality of life" may be quite different for a patient who has lived with cancer for several years as compared to someone without the disease; this is known as response-shift). Psychological defenses also tend to conserve perception of good quality of life even in the presence of worsening symptoms (Sprangers, 1996).

22.2.9 Health Outcomes Research

Outcomes research seeks to understand the *end results* of various factors on patients and populations. It can be used to assess prognostic factors, such as the effect of socioeconomic status on cancer survival (Booth et al, 2010), studies that compare different approaches to the management of specific medical conditions, studies that examine patients' and clinicians' decision making, studies describing geographic variations in clinical practice, and studies to develop or test practice guidelines. Outcomes research usually addresses the interrelated issues of cost and quality of health care, and public and private sector interest. The availability of computer methods to link large data bases (eg, cancer incidence and mortality data from cancer registries and treatment data from hospital records) has facilitated the ability of health outcomes research to address important clinical questions.

Various methodological designs are utilized in outcomes research. These include cohort studies, case-control studies, and studies of the uptake and outcome of new evidence-based

treatment for management (also called phase 4 studies). These studies can be undertaken prospectively or retrospectively. End points in outcomes research are usually clinical, economic, or patient-centered. Clinical outcomes include mortality or medical events as a result of an intervention. Economic outcomes include direct health costs (eg, costs of medical care, see Sec. 22.2.10), direct nonhealth costs (eg, cost of care providers), indirect costs (eg, productivity costs) and intangible costs (eg, pain and suffering). Patient-centered outcomes include quality of life and patient satisfaction. In most studies, the focus is on clinical outcomes. A major difference between outcomes research and randomized trials is that outcomes research lacks the controls and highly structured and artificial environment. An example of the utility of outcomes research comes from the Prostate Cancer Outcomes Study. In this project, the Surveillance, Epidemiology, and End Results (SEER) database of the United States National Cancer Institute was used to assess the outcomes of approximately 3500 men who had been diagnosed with primary invasive prostate cancer. Unlike many randomized trials, this study included a substantial number of men of different ethnic origins and socioeconomic groups, who had been treated in a variety of settings. This methodology enabled investigators to assess racial differences in stage at diagnosis and in treatment to help explain the significantly higher mortality rates from prostate cancer among black men in the United States (Hoffman et al, 2001).

The gold standard for assessing a medical intervention remains the randomized trial. However, randomized trials are not feasible in all settings and such trials tend to be conducted in highly selected populations and their results are not always applicable to the general population. Outcomes research aims to bridge the transition from research that is designed to assess the efficacy and safety of medical interventions to research that is undertaken under real-world conditions to evaluate their effectiveness in normal clinical practice. Health outcomes research has a number of advantages over traditional controlled trials, such as a lack of selection bias and the ability to generalize results to the real world. These advantages make outcomes research more helpful in assessing societal benefit from medical intervention than controlled trials. Disadvantages to outcomes research include lack of randomized comparisons and the likelihood that causality may be attributed to several interventions, not only the one of interest. An example of this is the exploration of screening mammography for breast cancer. Outcomes data show improved outcomes after the introduction of screening in many populations. Unfortunately, it remains unclear whether the improved outcomes can be associated with mammography alone or a combination of mammography, improvements in treatment and patient awareness and the establishment of multidisciplinary teams (Welch, 2010).

22.2.10 Cost-Effectiveness

Pharmacoeconomic evaluations play an integral role in the funding decisions for cancer drugs. The basic premise of the evaluation of cost-effectiveness is to compare the costs and consequences of alternative interventions, and to determine which treatment offers best value for limited resources. There are several methods available to evaluate economic efficiency, including cost minimization, cost benefit, and cost effectiveness analysis (Canadian Agency for Drugs and Technology in Health, 2006; Shih and Halpern, 2008). With respect to anticancer drugs, cost utility analysis (a type of cost-effectiveness analysis) is the preferred method because it considers differences in cost, survival, and quality of life between 2 competing interventions. In its most common form, a new strategy is compared to a reference standard to calculate the incremental cost-effectiveness ratio (ICER):

$$\text{ICER} = \frac{Cost\ (new) - Cost\ (old)}{Effectiveness\ (new) - Effectiveness\ (old)} \quad \text{[Eq. 22.1]}$$

In Equation 22.1, the ICER may be expressed as the increased cost per life-year gained, which can be estimated from differences in survival when the new treatment is compared with the standard treatment in a randomized controlled led trial. The increase in survival can be adjusted for differences in quality of survival by multiplying the median survival with each treatment by the "utility" of the survival state, where "utility" is a factor between zero and 1 that is a measure of the relative quality of life of patients following each treatment (as compared to perfect health) (Shih and Halpern, 2008). The ICER is then expressed as the increased cost to gain 1 quality-adjusted life-year (QALY); in practice, utility is often difficult to estimate, and in the absence of major differences in toxicity between new and standard treatment, the simpler increase in cost-per-life-year gained is often used.

If the ICER falls below a predefined threshold, the new treatment is considered cost-effective, otherwise it is considered cost-ineffective. A major challenge in the use of pharmacoeconomic modeling for estimating drug cost is in establishing the threshold for value. For example, the National Institute for Clinical Excellence in the United Kingdom has established a threshold ICER of £30,000 (~US$50,000) per QALY gained (Devlin and Parkin, 2004). In many other jurisdictions, a similar US$50,000 threshold has been used (Laupacis et al, 1992). There remains no consensus as to what threshold is appropriate, but by convention, cutoffs of $50,000 to $100,000 per QALY are often used for public funding of new treatments in developed countries; much lower costs per QALY can be supported in the developing world (Sullivan et al, 2011).

In principle, the added costs per QALY gained can be used by public health systems to make choices between funding quite different health interventions. For example, a health jurisdiction might compare the cost effectiveness ratio from extending the use of coronary artery bypass surgery to that from introduction of a new anticancer drug, and select that which provides the lower cost for a given increase in QALYs or life-years.

22.3 DIAGNOSIS AND SCREENING

22.3.1 Diagnostic Tests

Diagnostic tests are used to screen for cancer in people who are symptom free, establish the existence or extent of disease in those suspected of having cancer, and follow changes in the extent and severity of the disease during therapy or follow-up. Diagnostic tests are used to distinguish between people with a particular cancer and those without it. Test results may be expressed quantitatively on a continuous scale or qualitatively on a categorical scale. The results of serum tumor marker tests, such as PSA, are usually expressed quantitatively as a concentration, whereas the results of imaging tests, such as a computed tomography (CT) scan, are usually expressed qualitatively as normal or abnormal. To assess how well a diagnostic test discriminates between those with and without disease, it is necessary to have an independent means of classifying those with and without disease—a "gold standard." This might be the findings of surgery, the results of a biopsy, or the clinical outcome of patients after prolonged follow-up. If direct confirmation of the presence of disease is not possible, the results of a range of different diagnostic tests may be the best standard available.

Simultaneously classifying the subjects into diseased (D+) and nondiseased (D−) according to the gold-standard test and positive (T+) or negative (T−) according to the diagnostic test being assessed defines 4 subpopulations (Fig. 22–4). These are true-positives (TPs: people with the disease in whom the test is positive), true-negatives (TNs: people without the disease in whom the test is negative), false-positives (FPs: people without the disease in whom the test is positive), and false-negatives (FNs: people with the disease in whom the test is negative).

	Disease status	
	Disease present (D+)	Disease absent (D−)
Test positive (T+)	True positive (TP) T+D+	False positive (FP) T+D−
Test negative (T+)	False negative (FN) T−D+	True negative (TN) T−D−

"Vertical properties" calculated from columns:

Sensitivity	=	TP/(TP+FN)
Specificity	=	TN/(TN+FP)
False-negative rate	=	FN/(FN+TP)
False-positive rate	=	FP/(FP+TN)

"Horizontal properties" calculated from rows:

Positive predictive value	=	TP/(TP+FP)
Negative predictive value	=	TN/(TN+FN)

FIGURE 22−4 Selection of a cutoff point for a diagnostic test defines 4 subpopulations as shown. Predictive values (but not sensitivity and specificity) depend on the prevalence of disease in the population tested.

Test performance can be described by indices calculated from the 2 × 2 table shown in Figure 22–4. "Vertical" indices are calculated from the columns of the table and describe the frequency with which the test is positive or negative in people whose disease status is known. These indices include sensitivity (the proportion of people with disease who test positive) and specificity (the proportion of people without disease who test negative). These indices are characteristic of the particular test and do not depend on the prevalence of disease in the population being tested. The sensitivity and specificity of a test can be applied directly to populations with differing prevalence of disease.

"Horizontal" indices are calculated from the rows of the table and describe the frequency of disease in individuals whose test status is known. These indices indicate the predictive value of a test—for example, the probability that a person with a positive test has the disease (positive predictive value) or the probability that a person with a negative test does not have the disease (negative predictive value). These indices depend on characteristics of both the test (sensitivity and specificity) and the population being tested (prevalence of disease in the study population). The predictive value of a test cannot be applied directly to populations with differing prevalence of disease.

Figure 22–5 illustrates the influence of disease prevalence on the performance of a hypothetical test assessed in populations with high, intermediate, and low prevalence of disease. Sensitivity and specificity are constant, as they are independent of prevalence. As the prevalence of disease declines, the positive predictive value of the test declines. This occurs because, although the *proportions* of TP results among diseased subjects and FP results among nondiseased subjects remain the same, the *absolute numbers* of TP and FP results differ. In Figure 22–5, in the high-prevalence population, the absolute number of false positives (10) is small in comparison with the absolute number of true positives (80): a positive result is 8 times

more likely to come from a subject with disease than a subject without disease, and the positive predictive value of the test is relatively high. In the low-prevalence population, the absolute number of false positives (1000) is large in comparison with the absolute number of true positives (80): a positive result is 12.5 times more likely to come from a subject without disease, and the positive predictive value is relatively low. For this reason, diagnostic tests that may be useful in patients where there is already suspicion of disease (high-prevalence situation) may not be of value as screening tests in a less selected population (low-prevalence situation; see Sec. 22.3.3).

If a quantitative test is to be used to distinguish subjects with or without cancer, then a cutoff point must be selected that distinguishes positive results from negative results. Quantitative test results are often reported with a normal or reference range. This is the range of values obtained from some arbitrary proportion, usually 95%, of apparently healthy individuals; the corollary is that 5% of apparently healthy people will have values outside this range. Diagnostic test results are rarely conclusive about the presence or absence of diseases such as cancer; more often, they just raise or lower the likelihood that it is present.

Figure 22–6 shows the effects of choosing different cutoff points for a diagnostic test. A cutoff point at level A provides some separation of subjects with and without cancer, but because of overlap, there is always some misclassification. If the cutoff point is increased to level C, fewer subjects without cancer are wrongly classified (ie, the specificity increases) but more people with cancer fall below the cutoff and will be incorrectly classified (ie, the sensitivity decreases). A lower cutoff point at level B has the opposite effect: More subjects with cancer are correctly classified (sensitivity increases), but at the cost of incorrectly classifying larger numbers of people without cancer (specificity decreases). This trade-off between sensitivity and specificity is a feature of all diagnostic tests.

The 2 × 2 table and the indices derived from it (see Fig. 22–4) provide a simple and convenient method for describing test performance at a single cutoff point, but they give no indication of the effect of using different cutoff points. A receiver operating characteristic (ROC) curve provides a method for summarizing the effects of different cutoff points

High prevalence (50%)

	D⁺	D⁻		
T⁺	80	10	Sensitivity	80%
			Specificity	90%
T⁻	20	90	Predictive value (+)	89%

Intermediate prevalence (~9%)

	D⁺	D⁻		
T⁺	80	100	Sensitivity	80%
			Specificity	90%
T⁻	20	900	Predictive value (+)	44%

Low prevalence (~1%)

	D⁺	D⁻		
T⁺	80	1000	Sensitivity	80%
			Specificity	90%
T⁻	20	9000	Predictive value (+)	7.4%

FIGURE 22–5 Test properties and disease prevalence. Examples of application of a diagnostic test to populations in which disease has high, intermediate, or low prevalence. The predictive value of the test decreases when there is a low prevalence of disease.

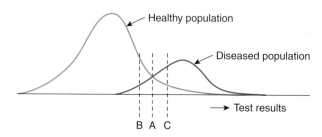

FIGURE 22–6 Interpretation of a diagnostic test (eg, PSA for prostate cancer) requires the selection of a cutoff point that separates negative from positive results. The position of the cutoff point (which might be set at A, B, or C) influences the proportion of patients who are incorrectly classified as being healthy or having disease.

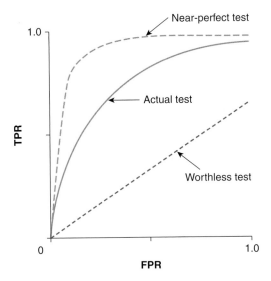

FIGURE 22-7 Curves showing ROCs in which the true-positive rate (TPR) is plotted against the false-positive rate (FPR) of a diagnostic test as the cutoff point is varied. The performance of the test is indicated by the shape of the curve, as shown.

TABLE 22-5 Factors that may distort the estimated performance of a diagnostic test.

Spectrum of patients for evaluation of the test
Clinical spectrum: Should include patients with a wide range of features of the disease
Comorbid spectrum: Should include patients with a wide range of other diseases
Pathologic spectrum: Should include patients with a range of histological types of disease
Potential sources of bias in test evaluation
Exclusion of equivocal cases
Work-up bias: Results of the test influence the choice of subsequent tests that confirm or refute diagnosis
Test review bias: Results of the test influence the interpretation of subsequent tests to establish diagnosis
Diagnostic review bias: Knowledge of the disease influences the interpretation of the test
Incorporation bias: Test information is used as a criterion to establish diagnosis

on sensitivity, specificity, and test performance. Figure 22–7 shows examples of ROC curves. The ROC curve plots the true-positive rate (TPR; which equals sensitivity) against the false-positive rate (FPR; which equals 1 − specificity) for different cutoff values. The "best" cutoff point is the one that offers the best compromise between TPR and FPR. This is represented by the point on the ROC curve closest to the upper left-hand corner. Statistically, ROC curves represent the balance between sensitivity and specificity with the area under the ROC curve (AUC; also known as the C-statistic) showing a model's discriminatory accuracy. An AUC of 0.5 is no better than a flip of a coin, whereas an AUC of 1.0 represents a perfect test. Realistically, an AUC of 0.7 or 0.8 is consistent with good discriminatory accuracy.

22.3.2 Sources of Bias in Diagnostic Tests

The performance of a diagnostic test is usually evaluated in a research study to estimate its usefulness in clinical practice. Differences between the conditions under which a test is evaluated, and the conditions under which it will be used, may produce misleading results. Important factors relating both to the people being tested and the methods being used are summarized in Table 22–5 (see also Jaeschke et al, 1994, and Scales et al, 2008). If a test is to be used to identify patients with colon cancer, then the study sample should include people with both localized and advanced disease (a wide clinical spectrum). The sample should also include people with other clinical conditions that might be mistaken for colon cancer (eg, diverticular disease) in order to evaluate the ability of the test to distinguish between these conditions, or to detect colon cancer in its presence (comorbidity). If there are different histological types of a cancer, then the test should be evaluated in a sample of patients that have these different histological types.

The evaluation of diagnostic test performance requires subjects to be classified by both disease status (diseased or nondiseased) and test status (positive or negative). For the evaluation to be valid, the 2 acts of classification must be independent. If either the classification of disease status is influenced by the test result or the interpretation of the test result is influenced by disease status, then there will be an inappropriate and optimistic estimate of test performance (see below and Table 22–5).

Work-up bias arises if the results of the diagnostic test under evaluation influence the choice of other tests used to determine the subject's disease status. For example, suppose that the performance of a positron emission tomographic (PET) scan is to be evaluated as an indicator of spread of hitherto regional lung cancer by comparing it with the results of mediastinal lymph node biopsy. Work-up bias will occur if only patients with abnormal PET scans are selected for mediastinoscopy, because regional spread in patients with normal PET scans will remain undetected. This leads to an exaggerated estimate of the predictive value of PET scanning.

Test-review bias occurs when the subjective interpretation of one test is influenced by knowledge of the result of another test. For example, a radiologist's interpretation of a PET scan might be influenced by knowledge of the results of a patient's CT scan. Using the CT scan to help interpret the results of an ambiguous PET scan may lead to a systematic overestimation of the ability of PET scan to identify active tumor. The most obvious violation of independence of the test and the method used to establish diagnosis arises when the test being evaluated is itself incorporated into the classification of disease status.

Diagnostic-review bias occurs when the reference test results are not definitive and the study test results affect or influence how the final diagnosis is established (Begg and McNeil, 1988).

22.3.3 Tests for Screening of Disease

Diagnostic tests are often used to screen an asymptomatic population to detect precancerous lesions or early cancers that are more amenable to treatment than cancers detected without screening. There are factors that influence the value of a screening program other than the sensitivity and specificity of the screening test. First, the cancer must pass through a pre-clinical phase that can be detected by the screening test. Slowly growing tumors are more likely to meet this criterion. Second, treatment must be more effective for screen-detected patients than for those treated after symptoms develop: If the outcome of treatment is uniformly good or bad regardless of the time of detection, then screening will be of no benefit. Third, the prevalence of disease in the population must be sufficient to warrant the cost of a screening program. Finally, the screening test must be acceptable to the target population: painful and inconvenient tests are unlikely to be accepted as screening tools by asymptomatic individuals.

The primary goal of a screening program is to reduce *disease-specific mortality,* that is, the proportion of people in a population who die of a given cancer in a specified time. For disease-specific mortality, the denominator is the whole population; it is therefore independent of factors that influence the time of diagnosis of disease. Other end points often reported in screening studies include stage of diagnosis and *case fatality rate* (the proportion of patients with the disease who die in a specified period). However, these intermediate end points are affected by several types of bias, particularly length-time bias and lead-time bias.

Length-time bias is illustrated in Figure 22–8. The horizontal lines in the figure represent the length of time from inception of disease to the time it produces clinical signs or symptoms and would be diagnosed in the absence of screening. Long lines indicate slowly progressing disease and short

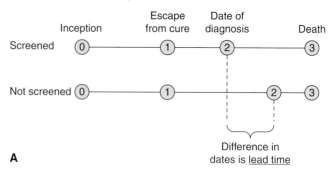

Comparison of date marks

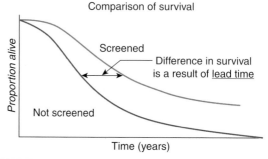

A

FIGURE 22–9 Illustration of lead-time bias. A) Application of a test may lead to earlier diagnosis without changing the course of disease. **B)** There is an improvement in survival when measured from time of diagnosis.

lines indicate rapidly progressing disease. A single examination, such as screening for breast cancer with mammography (represented in the figure by the dashed vertical line), will intersect (detect) a larger number of long lines (people with indolent disease) than short lines (people with aggressive disease). Thus, a screening examination will selectively identify those people with slowly progressing disease.

Lead-time bias is illustrated in Figure 22–9. The purpose of many diagnostic tests, and of all tests that are used to screen healthy people, is to allow clinicians to identify disease at an earlier stage in its clinical course than would be possible without the test. Four critical time points in the clinical course of the disease are indicated in Figure 22–9: the time of disease inception (0), the time at which the disease becomes incurable (1), the time of diagnosis (2), and the time of death (3). Many patients with common cancers are incurable by the time their disease is diagnosed, and the aim of a screening test is to advance the time of diagnosis to a point where the disease is curable. Even if the cancer is incurable despite the earlier time of diagnosis, survival will appear to be prolonged by early detection because of the additional time (the lead-time) that the disease is known to be present (Fig. 22–9). In screening for breast cancer with mammography, the lead-time is estimated to be approximately 2 years. Advancing the date of diagnosis may be beneficial if it increases the chance of cure. However, if it does not increase the chance of cure, then advancing the date of diagnosis may be detrimental, because patients spend a longer time with the knowledge that they have incurable disease.

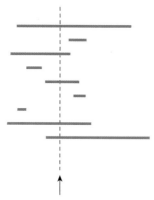

Point of application of screening test

Horizontal lines represent the length of time that disease is present prior to the death of the patient.

FIGURE 22–8 Illustration of length-time bias in a screening test. The test is more likely to detect disease that is present for a long time (ie, slowly growing disease). Horizontal lines represent the length of time that disease is present prior to clinical diagnosis.

The strongest study design for evaluating the impact of a diagnostic or screening test involves the randomization of people to have the test or to be followed in the usual way without having the test. The most important outcome measures that are assessed in such a trial include overall survival, disease-specific survival, and quality of life. Both randomized trials and those using health outcomes methods have demonstrated reductions in mortality rates as a result of breast cancer associated with mammographic screening in postmenopausal women (Kalager et al, 2010) and with fecal occult blood testing for colorectal carcinoma (Towler et al, 1998). However, an overview of the quality of trials of screening mammography has questioned whether there is a true reduction in mortality (Olsen and Gotzsche, 2001). Also, there has been a decrease in disease-specific mortality, but an increase in death rate from all causes in some trials (Black et al, 2002). Some screening procedures might be harmful in that they lead to investigations with some associated morbidity and mortality. Randomized trials have demonstrated a small benefit associated with screening people at high risk for lung cancer using spiral CT scans (National Lung Screening Trial, 2010), while trials evaluating the value of PSA screening for prostate cancer have either shown no benefit or a small decrease in disease-specific mortality (Andriole et al, 2009; Schröder et al, 2009).

22.3.4 Diagnostic Tests During Follow-up of Treated Tumors

Among patients who have had a complete response to treatment, most follow-up tests can be viewed as a form of screening for local or metastatic recurrence. Consequently, many of the requirements for an effective screening test described above also apply to follow-up tests. Because most recurrent cancers are not curable (particularly metastatic recurrences), it is uncommon that early intervention to treat asymptomatic recurrence will produce a true improvement in mortality due to disease. Studies of follow-up tests that report improvement in case-fatality rates usually suffer from lead-time bias. As with screening studies, randomized trials provide the best methodology to compare the utility of alternative approaches to follow-up. Four randomized, controlled clinical trials involving 3055 women with breast cancer, found no difference in overall survival or DFS between patients observed with intensive radiological and laboratory testing and those observed with clinical visits and mammography (Rojas et al, 2005). These findings demonstrate that for follow-up tests to improve survival, they must detect recurrences for which curative treatment is available; unfortunately, for most common tumors in adults such treatment is rarely available.

22.3.5 Bayes Theorem and Likelihood Ratios

The results of diagnostic tests are rarely conclusive about the presence or absence of disease and prognostic tests are rarely definitive about the course of disease. The utility of these tests is that they raise or lower the probability of observing a particular disease or prognosis (Jaeschke et al, 1994). This concept is embodied in the *Bayes theorem*. This theorem allows an initial estimate of a probability to be adjusted to take account of new information from a diagnostic or prognostic test, thus producing a revised estimate of the probability. The initial estimate is referred to as the *prior* or *pretest probability*; the revised estimate is the *posterior* or *posttest probability*.

For example, the pretest probability of breast cancer in a 45-year-old American woman presenting for screening mammography is approximately 3 in 1000 (the prevalence of disease in women of this age). If her mammogram is reported as "suspicious for malignancy," then her posttest probability of having breast cancer rises to approximately 300 in 1000, whereas if the mammogram is reported as "normal," then her posttest probability of having breast cancer falls to approximately 0.4 in 1000 (Kerlikowske et al, 1996).

Bayes theorem describes the mathematical relationship between the new posttest probability, the former prior probability (ie, the prevalence of disease in the tested population), and the additional information provided by a test (or clinical trial). This relationship can be expressed with 2 formulas that look different but are logically equivalent. For a diagnostic test with the characteristics defined in Figure 22–4, *the probability form of Bayes' theorem* can be expressed as

$$\text{Posttest probability} = \frac{\text{sensitivity} \times \text{prevalence}}{(\text{sensitivity} \times \text{prevalence}) + (1 - \text{specificity})(1 - \text{prevalence})}$$

[Eq. 22.2]

The alternative form of the Bayes theorem is expressed in terms of a likelihood ratio and is much easier to use. The *likelihood ratio* is a useful concept that for any test result represents the ratio of the probability that disease is present to the probability that it is absent. For a positive diagnostic test, the likelihood ratio is the likelihood that the positive test represents a true positive rather than a false positive:

$$\textit{Likelihood Ratio of a positive test result} = \frac{sensitivity}{1 - specificity} = \frac{true\ positive\ rate}{false\ positive\ rate}$$

[Eq. 22.3]

For a negative diagnostic test, the likelihood ratio is the likelihood that the negative result represents a false negative rather than a true negative (ie, *false negative rate/true negative rate*). A good diagnostic test has a high likelihood ratio for a positive test (ideally >10) and a low likelihood ratio for a negative test (ideally <0.1).

22.4 PROGNOSIS

A prognosis is a forecast of expected course and outcome for a patient with a particular stage of disease. It may apply to the unique circumstances of an individual or to the general circumstances of a group of individuals. People with apparently similar types and stages of cancer live for different lengths of time, have different patterns of progression, and respond differently to the same treatments. Variables associated with the outcome of a disease that can account for some of this heterogeneity are known as *prognostic factors,* and they may relate to the tumor, the host, or the environment. An increasing number of tumor-related factors, including various gene signatures (see Sec. 22.5; Chap. 2, Sec. 2.7.2), have been found to convey prognostic information.

Differences in prognostic characteristics often account for larger differences in outcome than do differences in treatment. For example, in women with primary breast cancer, differences in survival according to lymph node status are much greater than differences in survival according to treatment. Imbalances in the distribution of such important prognostic factors in clinical trials, which compare different treatments, may produce biased results by either obscuring true differences or creating spurious ones. Furthermore, the effects of treatment may be different in patients with differing prognostic characteristics. For example, the prognosis of hormone receptor-negative breast cancer is worse than that of hormone receptor-positive disease; however, the benefit from adjuvant chemotherapy for hormone receptor-negative patients is greater.

A *predictive test* evaluates the probability of outcome after some form of treatment. Prognostic factors (eg, for overall survival) may or may not predict the likelihood of benefit to a particular treatment. An example is the recurrence score of the 21-gene predictor, Oncotype DX in breast cancer. This test provides both prognostic and predictive information. For instance, adjuvant endocrine therapy (eg, tamoxifen) is highly effective in the treatment of hormone receptor-positive breast cancer and the additional benefit of chemotherapy is not well defined. The predictive roles of the Oncotype DX assay were assessed in patients with node-negative, estrogen-receptor-positive tumors. Tamoxifen was most effective when the recurrence score was low, whereas patients whose primary tumors had a high recurrence score derived more benefit from adjuvant chemotherapy (Paik et al, 2006).

22.4.1 Identification of Prognostic Factors

Two stages are often used in the characterization of prognostic factors. In an initial exploratory analysis, apparent patterns and relationships are examined, and are used to generate hypotheses. In a confirmatory analysis, the level of support for a prespecified hypothesis is examined critically using a different set of data. Most studies evaluate a number of "candidate" prognostic factors with varying levels of prior support.

In univariable analysis, the strength of association between each candidate prognostic factor and the outcome is assessed separately. Univariable analyses are simple to perform, but they do not indicate whether different prognostic factors are providing the same or different information. For example, in women with breast cancer, lymph node status and hormone receptor status are both found to be associated with survival duration in univariable analysis; however, they are also found

to be associated with one another. Univariable analysis will not provide a clear indication as to whether measuring both factors provides more prognostic information than measuring either factor alone. Multivariable analyses are more complex, but adjust for the simultaneous effects of several variables on the outcome of interest (see also Chap. 3, Sec. 3.3.3). Variables that are significant when included together in a multivariable model provide independent prognostic information.

Cox proportional hazards regression is a commonly used form of multivariable modeling of potential prognostic factors. Cox regression can be used to model time-to-relapse or time-to-death in a cohort of patients who have been followed for different lengths of time. The method models the "hazard function" of the event, which is defined as the rate at which the event (eg, relapse) occurs. The effect of the prognostic factor on the event rate, called the *hazard ratio* or *relative risk*, represents the change in risk caused by the presence or absence of the prognostic factor. For example, if the outcome of interest is tumor recurrence, a hazard ratio of 2 represents a 2-fold increase in the risk of recurrence (negative effect) as a result of the presence of the prognostic factor. A hazard ratio of 1 implies that the prognostic factor does not have an effect. The greater (or smaller) the value of the hazard ratio above or below 1 the larger the negative (or positive) effect of the prognostic factor.

The Cox proportional hazards method assumes that the relative effect of a given prognostic factor compared to the "baseline" is constant throughout the patient's follow-up period (ie, there is a constant "proportional hazard"). For many factors of clinical interest, this assumption may be incorrect, and the Cox model may then provide misleading estimates of prognostic value. A Cox model may also assume "linearity," meaning that a given absolute increase in the level of a factor is assumed to have the same prognostic significance throughout the range of its measured values. For example, if PSA is modeled as a continuous linear variable (as is often done) when studying the association between pretreatment PSA level and relapse rate, an increase from 5 ng/mL to 15 ng/mL is assumed to have the same prognostic significance as an increase from 100 ng/mL to 110 ng/mL. Because this is not likely to be true (considering that cell populations tend to grow exponentially), adjustment of the model can be undertaken to account for the nonlinear association between PSA on outcome (eg, by using *ln* [PSA] in the model). Finally, variables may "interact" with each other biologically, and such interaction will not be accounted for in a Cox model unless a specific "interaction term" is included. For example, compared to hormone receptor-negative breast cancer, hormone receptor-positive disease is associated with better prognosis in those age 35 years or older and a worse prognosis in those younger than age 35 years. Consequently, a Cox model will more accurately indicate the relationship between hormone receptor positivity and outcome if it includes an "interaction term" between hormone receptor positivity and age.

Recursive partitioning is a "tree-based" form of modeling that can be used to group patients with similar prognoses according to different levels of the prognostic factors of interest. The outcome of interest may be measured on a binary (eg, relapse/no relapse), ordinal, or continuous scale. Recursive partitioning has several advantages. The method more easily accounts for interaction between prognostic variables, without the necessity of explicit inclusion of interaction terms, as is required for Cox models. This is especially advantageous when analyzing complex data with substantial interaction between prognostic variables (eg, performance status, age, and mental status among patients with malignant glioma). Also, recursive partitioning yields transparent and easily interpretable clinical categories that can be used to predict prognosis. The major disadvantage of recursive partitioning is "overfitting" of the data, such that small changes in the characteristics of the patients used to create the tree may create substantial changes in the results. This can reduce the predictive power of the recursive partitioning tree if it is not "pruned" by excluding some variables and then tested in a confirmatory study on a cohort of patients different from that used to create the tree. Also, an important prognostic variable may be excluded from the tree if it is highly correlated (colinear) with other variables in the tree, thereby "masking" its significance.

22.4.2 Evaluation of Prognostic Factor Studies

Methods of classifying cancer are based on factors known to influence prognosis, such as anatomic extent and histology of the tumor. The widely used TNM system for staging cancers is based on the extent of the primary tumor (T), the presence or absence of regional lymph node involvement (N), and the presence or absence of distant metastases (M). Other attributes of the tumor that have an influence on outcome, such as the estrogen-receptor concentration in breast cancer, are also included as prognostic factors in the analysis and reporting of therapeutic trials. The identification of novel prognostic factors using the methods of molecular biology is an area of active investigation. Guidelines for selecting useful prognostic factors have been suggested by Levine et al (1991). The utility of a prognostic factor depends on the accuracy with which it can be measured. For example, the size and extent of the primary tumor are important prognostic factors in men with early prostate cancer, but there is substantial variability between observers in assessing these attributes. This variation between observers contributes to the variability in outcome among patients assigned to the same prognostic category by different observers.

Several factors may diminish the validity of studies that report the discovery of a "significant" prognostic factor. Prognostic studies usually report outcomes for patients who are referred to academic centers and/or who participate in clinical studies. These patients may differ systematically from patients with similar malignancies in the community as they are selected for better performance status and fewer comorbidities, consequently leading to *referral bias*. Also, patients who participate in clinical trials may have better outcomes than those who do not participate in clinical trials, even if they receive similar treatment (Peppercorn et al, 2004; Chua and Clarke, 2010). Thus population-based data—for example, data from cancer registries—may provide more pertinent information regarding overall prognosis than data from highly selected patients referred to academic centers or enrolled in clinical trials. However, the *relative* influence of a prognostic factor is less likely to be affected by referral bias than the *absolute* influence on prognosis for that disease. For example, if hormone-receptor status influences survival irrespective of treatment administered, then it is likely to influence survival within each center, even if the absolute survival of patients may differ between centers. Ideally, a prognostic study should include all identified cases within a large, geographically defined area.

Objective criteria, independent of knowledge of the patients' initial prognostic characteristics, must be used to assess the relevant outcomes such as disease recurrence or cause of death in studies of prognosis. *Work-up bias, test-review bias*, and *diagnostic-review bias*, discussed in Section 22.3.2, have their counterparts in studies of prognosis. For example, a follow-up bone scan in a patient with breast cancer that is equivocal may be more likely to be read as positive (ie, indicating recurrence of disease) if it is known that the patient initially had extensive lymph node involvement or that she subsequently developed proven bone metastases. To avoid these biases, all patients should be assessed with the same frequency, using the same tests, interpreted with the same explicit criteria and without knowledge of the patient's initial characteristics or subsequent course.

Several deficiencies in statistical analysis are common in prognostic factor studies. Typically, a large number of candidate prognostic factors are assessed in univariable analyses, and those factors exhibiting some degree of association, often defined in terms of a p value less than 0.05, are included in a starting set of variables for the multivariable analysis. The final multivariable model reported usually contains only the subset of these variables that remain significant when simultaneously included in the same model. Consequently, a multivariable model reported in a study that contains 10 prognostic variables may be the result of hundreds of different statistical comparisons. Because the probability of detecting spurious associations as a result of chance increases dramatically with the number of comparisons, the conventional interpretation of a p value as the probability of detecting an association if none existed is inappropriate in this setting. The large numbers of comparisons frequently performed generally make the p-values provided with most multivariable prognostic models invalid unless the model is prespecified before analysis begins. Similarly, for a factor that is measured on a continuous or ordinal scale, it is not valid to identify an "optimal" cutpoint using the study cohort, and then demonstrate that the factor is associated with prognosis in the same cohort. Such results usually will not be applicable to other groups of patients. Cutpoints should be defined prior to analysis and, ideally, the prognostic model should be developed in a "training set" of patients, with the robustness of the results tested in a separate "validation set."

Prognostic factor studies need to assess sufficient patients to allow detection of potentially significant effects. A rough but widely accepted guideline is that a minimum of 10 outcome events should have occurred for each prognostic factor assessed. Thus in a study assessing prognostic factors for survival in 200 patients of whom 100 have died, no more than 10 candidate prognostic factors should be assessed.

Studies of new biological markers often correlate the presence of the marker with known prognostic factors (eg, tumor grade). Although this might provide insight into biology of the tumor, it does not indicate the prognostic value of the marker. Furthermore, even if a multivariable analysis adds the new marker preferentially into a prognostic model and excludes a recognized prognostic factor, this does not necessarily indicate the superior prognostic value of the marker in clinical practice. This is because the analysis of models that are used to include and exclude variables that are associated with each other will depend on the data set used; the results may not give the same preference between the 2 markers for other cohorts of patients with minor differences in outcome. Also, because conventional prognostic factors are generally easier to measure than novel biological markers, the practical question is whether the new marker provides clinically important *additional* prognostic information after controlling for known prognostic factors, rather than whether the new marker can replace an old one.

Prognostic classifications based solely on attributes of the tumor ignore patient-based factors known to affect prognosis such as performance status, quality of life, and the presence of other illnesses (comorbidity). Performance status, a measure of an individual's physical functional capacity, is one of the most powerful and consistent predictors of prognosis across the spectrum of malignant disease (Weeks, 1992). Studies in individual cancers, as well as a systematic review (Viganò et al, 2000), have consistently demonstrated strong, independent associations between simple measures of quality of life, obtained by patients completing validated questionnaires (see Sec. 22.2.8), and survival. Incorporation of these measures in clinical studies can reduce the heterogeneity that remains after accounting for attributes of the tumor.

22.4.3 Predictive Markers

Predictive markers are characteristics that are associated with treatment response. Mechanistically, they are involved in a synergistic or antagonistic relationship with treatment. Statistically they are associated with an interaction effect with treatment. In contrast, prognostic tests are associated with improved outcomes independently of treatment (Fig. 22–10).

Predictive tests for the selection of cancer drugs are intuitively simple and mirror the routine use of cultures of bacteria causing infections in testing for sensitivity to antibiotics. Testing of anticancer drugs, in which tumor biopsies or cells derived from them are exposed to the drugs in tissue culture, followed by a test that evaluates killing of the tumor cells, has been described for several decades. Initial success was limited, but advances in methods and data acquisition have improved predictive accuracy (Schrag et al, 2004). Despite this, cell-based testing remains a research tool and is not recommended in clinical practice guidelines.

Predictive assays that are in routine clinical use include analysis of estrogen (ER) and/or progesterone receptor (PgR) expression (see Chap. 20, Sec. 20.4.1). This is the most established predictive test in oncology and most oncologists would not consider endocrine therapy for women with breast cancer in the absence of a positive test for tumor cell expression of ER and/or PgR. Another established predictive test is the analysis of HER2 overexpression for the use of trastuzumab or lapatinib. Despite their routine use, validation of these tests is suboptimal. The tests are prone to methodological problems with interobserver and interlaboratory variation occurring in up to 20% of the patients.

More recently, research has focused on predictive factors for activity of inhibitors of the epidermal growth factor receptor (EGFR; see Chap. 7, Sec. 7.5.3 and Chap. 17, Sec. 17.3). The efficacy of drugs targeting the EGFR signaling pathway has been associated with specific mutations in the EGFR gene, increased EGFR gene copy number, absence of *K-ras* mutations and high expression of genes for endogenous EGFR ligands (Tsao et al, 2005; Lièvre et al, 2006).

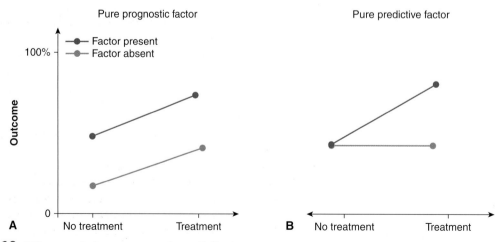

FIGURE 22–10 **Differences between prognostic predictive tests.** (From Hayes et al, 1998.)

Molecular techniques will likely lead to rapid progress in the development of predictive tests. The antitumor activity of an increasing number of targeted therapeutics is based on the presence of specific biomarkers. This has created a need for real-time detection of such genetic aberrations. Some cancer mutations occur at similar DNA bases in tumors from different patients (recurrent mutations). It is therefore possible to use assays that test for single bases (a process referred to as *mutation genotyping*) to detect these aberrations (Tran et al, 2012). Currently, there are only a few clinically validated recurrent mutations. However, the repertoire of recurrent mutations is increasing, and there is interest in testing these to evaluate their role as predictive mutations for the numerous molecular targeted agents in development. A paradigm shift in the development and use of cancer drugs may be necessary to translate this to patient benefit. Assessment of drug activity in intact tumor cells, and tumor cell gene expression signatures, have potential for the development of versatile predictive tests (Nygren et al, 2008).

22.5 CANCER GENOMICS

The field of cancer genomics is growing rapidly as a result of advances in DNA sequencing technologies (see Chap. 2, Sec. 2.2.10). Two main methods are available to study the cancer genome:

1. *Whole-genome sequencing (WGS)* is the backbone technology that supports the in-depth sequencing the entire human genome (Metzker, 2009).
2. *Targeted genome sequencing* refers to strategies that enrich for DNA regions potentially involved in tumor biology. This includes the whole exome or the cancer genome (Robison, 2010).

High-throughput genotyping platforms such as microarrays, have been successfully used for genotyping clinical samples (Thomas et al, 2007). The development of DNA microarray technology holds promise for improvements in the diagnosis, prognosis, and tailoring of treatment. The technical aspects of creating gene expression profiles are described in Chapter 2, Section 2.6. The ability to investigate the transcription of thousands of genes concurrently by using DNA microarrays poses a variety of analytical challenges. Microarray datasets are commonly very large and can be affected by numerous variables. Challenges to microarray analysis include methods for taking into account the effects of background noise (known as normalization of the data), and removal of poor-quality and low-intensity data, as well as choice of a statistical test for determination of significant differences between tumor and control samples (see Chap. 2, Sec. 2.7).

A variety of tests for the identification of statistically significant changes are utilized. These include a spectrum from simple tests such as t-test or analysis of variance (ANOVA), 2 nonparametric smoothing analyses or Bayesian methods. These should be tailored to the specific microarray dataset, and should take into account multiple comparisons. When applied in repeated testing, the standard P-value is conceptually associated with the specificity of a test. Use of a P-value cutoff of less than 0.05 means that false-positive rates will be approximately 5%, but this level of false positivity is too high for microarray data. Consequently, there has been a shift from the use of P-values to the false-discovery rate (FDR; see Chap. 2, Sec. 2.7.2), which is defined as the expected proportion of false positives among the declared significant results.

Cluster analysis is frequently performed to identify genes with similar expression patterns, which are grouped together using either *supervised* or *unsupervised analysis.* Supervised analysis involves using samples with 2 or more known characteristics (eg, malignant or benign cells) and developing a gene-expression classification scheme to identify these characteristics. For example, Golub et al (1999), created a classification scheme that was able to distinguish acute myelogenous leukemia from acute lymphoid leukemia based on the expression of 50 genes in 38 samples. This classification method was subsequently able to categorize correctly 29 of 34 test samples. Several alternative methods of classification have been described, including logistic regression, neural networks, and linear discriminant analysis (see Brazma and Vilo, 2000, for explanation of these methods). In unsupervised analysis genes and/or samples with similar properties are clustered together, without reference to predefined sample characteristics. Again, several different algorithms have been developed to perform such cluster analysis. For example, a hierarchical algorithm has been used to cluster different samples of diffuse large B-cell lymphoma with similar gene expression profiles. Two distinct forms with gene expression profiles indicative of different phases of B-cell development were identified. These different clusters could not be identified on the basis of traditional histological features, and could only be distinguished by the gene expression profiles; moreover, the 2 different clusters differed in prognosis (Alizadeh et al, 2000).

The analysis of gene expression profiles is evolving rapidly, and several methodological issues surrounding the use of microarrays in prognostic or other studies are yet to be resolved (see also Chap. 2, Sec 2.7).

1. There is minimal standardization, and researchers have not successfully compared results from different laboratories using different microarray technologies. There is also a lack of rigorous standards for data collection, analysis, and validation.
2. There is little information about measuring the reliability of gene expression levels in microarray experiments. Every measurement has a margin of error. Most clinicians are familiar with the concept of the "confidence interval," which is used to quantify the uncertainty with which different estimates (eg, of 5-year survival) are made. There are data suggesting that "false-positive" overexpression or "false-negative" underexpression of genes may occur if microarray experiments are not replicated (Ioannidis et al, 2009).

3. DNA microarrays allow one to assess the association between prognosis and the expression of thousands of different genes. The vast amount of DNA expression data obtained from tumor samples from a series of cancer patients virtually ensures that some constellation of gene expression can be found to be associated with prognosis (Petronis, 2010), if that is the goal. Consequently, it is vital that a "prognostic" gene expression profile developed on a training set of tumor samples be validated in an independent and external set of samples to ensure reproducibility of the results.

4. The quality and amount of RNA remains a major challenge in microarray experiments. The amount of tissue obtained and the complexity of the tissue sample can limit the quality and quantity of RNA that can be isolated. Efforts are under way to reduce the amount of sample required for analysis, and newer technologies can analyze samples with only nanogram amounts of tissue.

SUMMARY

- The evaluation of new treatments in clinical trials remains the backbone of clinical research in oncology, but only a small proportion of the interventions provided to cancer patients have been tested in Phase III trials.
- The continued publication of underpowered trials provides an ongoing need for metaanalyses to detect clinically meaningful outcomes.
- Increasing use of health outcomes research, based on analysis of registries or other large databases will help in assessing the impact of health interventions at a societal level.
- Although tumor relapse and duration of survival are important outcomes and are easily measured in trials, they are often not the most relevant measures of treatment success. In many cases, treatment is offered to reduce symptoms, or there may be a choice between different treatments with apparently equivalent antitumor activity. In such trials, symptom control and quality of life is important.
- As diagnostic technologies and treatments continue to advance, oncologists must be able to conduct, evaluate, and interpret studies to define the best use of them. Although the methodological principles that define valid, high-quality studies have been established, enthusiasm to adopt new technology often leads to studies that are subject to well-described biases, and do not aid the rational use of the studied test.
- As our understanding of tumor biology improves, so, too, will our ability to predict tumor response and patient outcome based on biological parameters. The large amount of biological data becoming available will lead to the development and refinement of new methods for recognizing and analyzing prognostic information from the expression profiles of thousands of genes.

REFERENCES

Aaronson NK, Ahmedzai S, Bergman B, et al. The European Organisation for Research and Treatment of Cancer QLQ-C30: a quality of life instrument for use in international clinical trials in oncology. *J Natl Cancer Inst* 1993;85:365-376.

Alizadeh AA, Eisen MB, Davis RE, et al. Distinct types of diffuse large B-cell lymphoma identified by gene expression profiling. *Nature* 2000;403:503-511.

Amir E, Seruga B, Martinez-Lopez J, et al. Oncogenic targets, magnitude of benefit, and market pricing of antineoplastic drugs. *J Clin Oncol* 2011;29:2543-2549.

Andriole GL, Crawford ED, Grubb RL 3rd, et al. Mortality results from a randomized prostate-cancer screening trial. *N Engl J Med* 2009;360:1310-1319.

Begg CB, McNeil BJ. Assessment of radiologic tests: control of bias and other design considerations. *Radiology* 1988;167:565-569.

Black WC, et al. All-cause mortality in randomized trials of cancer screening. *J Natl Cancer Inst* 2002;94:369-375.

Booth CM, Li G, Zhang-Salomons J, Mackillop WJ. The impact of socioeconomic status on stage of cancer at diagnosis and survival: a population-based study in Ontario, Canada. *Cancer* 2010;116:4160-4167.

Brazma A, Vilo J. Gene expression data analysis. *FEBS Lett* 2000;480:17-24.

Bush RS. Cancer of the ovary: natural history. In: Peckham MJ, Carter RL, eds. *Malignancies of the Ovary, Uterus and Cervix: The Management of Malignant Disease, Series #2,* London, England: Edward Arnold; 1979:26-37.

Buyse M, Piedbois P, Piedbois Y, Carlson RW. Meta-analysis: methods, strengths, and weaknesses. *Oncology (Williston Park)* 2000;14:437-443.

Canadian Agency for Drugs and Technology in Health. *Guidelines for the Economic Evaluation of Health Technologies.* 3rd ed. Ottawa, Canada; 2006. http://www.cadth.ca/media/pdf/186_EconomicGuidelines_e.pdf. Accessed November 8, 2010.

Cella DF, Tulsky DS, Gray G, et al. The functional assessment of cancer therapy scale: development and validation of the general measure. *J Clin Oncol* 1993;11:570-579.

Chalmers TC, Celano P, Sacks HS, Smith H Jr. Bias in treatment assignment in controlled clinical trials. *N Engl J Med* 1983;309:1358-1361.

Chao C, Studts JL, Abell T, et al. Adjuvant chemotherapy for breast cancer: how presentation of recurrence risk influences decision-making. *J Clin Oncol* 2003;21:4299-4305.

Chua W, Clarke SJ. Clinical trial information as a measure of quality cancer care. *J Oncol Pract* 2010;6:170-171.

De Haes JCJM, Zittoun RA. Quality of life. In: Peckham M, Pinedo HM, Veronesi V, eds. *Oxford Textbook of Oncology.* Oxford, England: Oxford University Press; 1995:2400-2408.

Detsky AS, Naglie IG. A clinicians guide to cost-effectiveness analysis. *Ann Intern Med* 1990;113:147-154.

Devlin N, Parkin D. Does NICE have a cost-effectiveness threshold and what other factors influence its decisions? A binary choice analysis. *Health Econ* 2004;13:437-452.

Dillman RO, Herndon J, Seagreen SL, et al. Improved survival in stage III non-small cell lung cancer: seven-year follow-up of Cancer and Leukemia Group B (CALGB) 8433 trial. *J Natl Cancer Inst* 1996;88:1210-1215.

Doyle C, Stockler M, Pintilie M, et al. Resource implications of palliative chemotherapy for ovarian cancer. *J Clin Oncol* 1997;15:1000-1007.

Early Breast Cancer Trialists Collaborative Group (EBCTCG). Effects of chemotherapy and hormonal therapy for early breast cancer on recurrence and 15 years survival: an overview of the randomised trials. *Lancet* 2005;365:1687-1717.

Early Breast Cancer Trialists' Collaborative Group. Ovarian ablation in early breast cancer: Overview of the randomised trials. *Lancet* 1996;348:1189-1196.

El-Maraghi RH, Eisenhauer EA. Review of phase II trial designs used in studies of molecular targeted agents: outcomes and predictors of success in phase III. *J Clin Oncol* 2008;26: 1346-1354.

Feinstein AR. Clinical *Epidemiology: The Architecture of Clinical Research*. Philadelphia, PA: Saunders; 1985.

Feinstein AR, Sosin DM, Wells CK. The Will Rogers phenomenon: stage migration and new diagnostic techniques as a source of misleading statistics for survival in cancer. *N Engl J Med* 1985;312:1604-1608.

Freedman LS. Tables of the number of patients required in clinical trials using the log rank test. *Stat Med* 1982;1:121-129.

Gan HK, Grothey A, Pond GR, Moore MJ, Siu LL, Sargent D. Randomized phase II trials: inevitable or inadvisable? *J Clin Oncol* 2010;28:2641-2647.

Golub TR, Slonim DK, Tamayo P, et al. Molecular classification of cancer: class discovery and class prediction by gene expression monitoring. *Science* 1999;286:531-537.

Gøtzsche PC, Olsen O. Is screening for breast cancer with mammography justifiable? *Lancet* 2000;355:129-134.

Guyatt GH, Haynes RB, Jaeschke RZ, et al. Users' Guides to the Medical Literature: XXV. Evidence-based medicine: principles for applying the Users' Guides to patient care. Evidence-Based Medicine Working Group. *JAMA* 2000;284: 1290-1296.

Guyatt GH, Sackett DL, Sinclair JC, Hayward R, Cook DJ, Cook RJ. Users' guides to the medical literature. IX. A method for grading health care recommendations. *JAMA* 1995;274:1800-1804.

Hayes DF, Trock B, Harris AL. Assessing the clinical impact of prognostic factors: when is "statistically significant" clinically useful? *Breast Cancer Res Treat* 1998;52:305-319. http://www.ncbi.nlm.nih.gov/pubmed/10066089.

Herberman RB. Design of clinical trials biological response modifiers. *Cancer Treat Rep* 1985;69:1161-1164.

Hershman DL, Kushi LH, Shao T, et al. Early discontinuation and nonadherence to adjuvant hormonal therapy in a cohort of 8,769 early-stage breast cancer patients. *J Clin Oncol* 2010; 28:4120-4128.

Hillner BE, Smith TJ. Efficacy and cost-effectiveness of adjuvant chemotherapy in women with node-negative breast cancer: A decision analysis model. *N Engl J Med* 1991;324:160-168.

Hoffman RM, Gilliland FD, Eley JW, et al. Racial and ethnic differences in advanced-stage prostate cancer: the Prostate Cancer Outcomes Study. *J Natl Cancer Inst* 2001;93:388-395.

Ioannidis JP, Allison DB, Ball CA, et al. Repeatability of published microarray gene expression analyses. *Nat Genet* 2009;41:149-155.

Jaeschke R, Guyatt GH, Sackett DL, for the Evidence-Based Medicine Working Group. Users' guides to the medical literature: III. How to use an article about a diagnostic test. *JAMA* 1994;271:389-391, 703-707.

Joly F, Vardy J, Pintilie M, Tannock IF. Quality of life and/or symptom control in randomized clinical trials for patients with advanced cancer. *Ann Oncol* 2007;18:1935-1942.

Kalager M, Zelen M, Langmark F, Adami HO. Effect of screening mammography on breast-cancer mortality in Norway. *N Engl J Med* 2010;363:1203-1210.

Kerlikowske K, Grady D, Barclay J, et al. Likelihood ratios for modern screening mammography: Risk of breast cancer based on age and mammographic interpretation. *JAMA* 1996;276:39-43.

Laupacis A, Feeny D, Detsky AS, Tugwell PX. How attractive does a new technology have to be to warrant adoption and utilization? Tentative guidelines for using clinical and economic evaluations. *CMAJ* 1992;146:473-481.

Laupacis A, Wells G, Richardson S, et al, for the Evidence-Based Medicine Working Group. Users' guides to the medical literature: V. How to use an article about prognosis. *JAMA* 1994;272: 234-237.

Levine MN, Browman GP, Gent M, et al. When is a prognostic factor useful? A guide for the perplexed. *J Clin Oncol* 1991;9: 348-356.

Lièvre A, Bachet J-B, Le Corre D, et al. KRAS mutation status is predictive of response to cetuximab in colorectal cancer. *Cancer Res* 2006;66:3992-3995.

Mason J, Drummond M, Torrance G. Some guidelines on the use of cost-effectiveness league tables. *BMJ* 1993;306:570-572.

Metzker ML. Sequencing technologies: The next generation. *Nat Rev Genet* 2009;11:31-46.

Moore MJ, Goldstein D, Hamm J, et al. Erlotinib plus gemcitabine compared with gemcitabine alone in patients with advanced pancreatic cancer: a phase III trial of the National Cancer Institute of Canada Clinical Trials Group. *J Clin Oncol* 2007;25:1960-1966.

Moore MJ, O'Sullivan B, Tannock IF. How expert physicians would wish to be treated if they had genitourinary cancer. *J Clin Oncol* 1988;6:1736-1745.

National Lung Screening Trial. Press release: Lung cancer trial results show mortality benefit with low-dose CT. National Cancer Institute. http://www.cancer.gov/newscenter/pressreleases/ NLSTresultsRelease, Accessed November 1, 2010.

Nekolaichuk CL, Maguire TO, Suarez-Almazor M, et al. Assessing the reliability of patient, nurse, and family caregiver symptom ratings in hospitalized advanced cancer patients. *J Clin Oncol* 1999;17:3621-3630.

Ng R, Pond GR, Tang PA, et al. Correlation of changes between 2-year disease-free survival and 5-year overall survival in adjuvant breast cancer trials from 1966 to 2006. *Ann Oncol* 2008;19:481-486.

Noble JH Jr. Meta-analysis: methods, strengths, weaknesses, and political uses. *J Lab Clin Med* 2006;147:7-20.

Nygren P, Larsson R. Predictive tests for individualization of pharmacological cancer treatment. *Expert Opin Med Diagn* 2008;2:349-360.

Olsen O, Gotzsche PC. Cochrane review on screening for breast cancer with mammography. *Lancet* 2001;358:1340-1342.

Paik S, Shak S, Tang G, et al. A multigene assay to predict recurrence of tamoxifen-treated, node negative, estrogen receptor positive breast cancer. *J Clin Oncol* 2006;24:3726-3734.

Parmar MKB, Stewart LA, Altman DG. Meta-analyses of randomised trials: when the whole is more than just the sum of the parts. *Br J Cancer* 1996;74:496-501.

Parulekar WR, Eisenhauer EA. Phase I trial design for solid tumor studies of targeted, non-toxic agents: theory and practice. *J Natl Cancer Inst* 2004;96:990-997.

Peppercorn JM, Weeks JC, Cook EF, et al. Comparison of outcomes in cancer patients treated within and outside clinical trials: conceptual framework and structured review. *Lancet* 2004;363:263-270.

Petronis A. Epigenetics as a unifying principle in the aetiology of complex traits and diseases. *Nature* 2010;465:721-727.

Robison K. Application of second-generation sequencing to cancer genomics. *Brief Bioinform* 2010;11:524-534.

Rojas MP, Telaro E, Russo A, et al. Follow-up strategies for women treated for early breast cancer. *Cochrane Database Syst Rev* 2005;(1):CD001768.

Royston P, Parmar MK, Qian W. Novel designs for multi-arm clinical trials with survival outcomes with an application in ovarian cancer. *Stat Med* 2003;22:2239-2256.

Sargent DJ, Wieand HS, Haller DG, et al. Disease-free survival versus overall survival as a primary end point for adjuvant colon cancer studies: individual patient data from 20,898 patients on 18 randomized trials. *J Clin Oncol* 2005;23:8664-8670.

Scales CD Jr, Dahm P, Sultan S, et al. How to use an article about a diagnostic test. *J Urol* 2008;180:469-476.

Schrag D, Garewal HS, Burstein HJ, et al. American Society of Clinical Technology Assessment: chemotherapy sensitivity and resistance assays. *J Clin Oncol* 2004;22:3631-3638.

Schröder FH, Hugosson J, Roobol MJ, et al. Screening and prostate-cancer mortality in a randomized European study. *N Engl J Med* 2009;360:1320-1328.

Schwartz D, Flamant R, Lellouch J. *Clinical Trials.* London, UK: Academic Press; 1980.

Shih YC, Halpern MT. Economic evaluations of medical care interventions for cancer patients: how, why, and what does it mean? *CA Cancer J Clin* 2008;58:231-244.

Simon R, Freidlin B, Rubinstein L, Arbuck SG, Collins J, Christian MC. Accelerated titration designs for phase I clinical trials in oncology. *J Natl Cancer Inst* 1997;89:1138-1147.

Sprangers MAG. Response-shift bias: a challenge to the assessment of patients' quality of life in cancer clinical trials. *Cancer Treat Rev* 1996;22(Suppl A):55-62.

Stewart LA, Parmar MKB. Meta-analysis of the literature or of individual patient data: is there a difference? *Lancet* 1993;341:418-422.

Sullivan R, Peppercorn J, Sikora K, et al. Delivering affordable cancer care in high-income countries. *Lancet Oncol* 2011;12:933-980.

Thomas RK, Baker AC, Debiasi RM, et al. High-throughput oncogene mutation profiling in human cancer. *Nat Genet* 2007;39:347-351.

Tibshirani R. A plain man's guide to the proportional hazards model. *Clin Invest Med* 1982;5:63-68.

Torrance GW. Utility approach to measuring health-related quality of life. *J Chronic Dis* 1987;40:593-600.

Towler B, Irwig L, Glasziou P, et al. A systemic review of the effects of screening for colorectal cancer using the faecal occult blood test, hemoccult. *BMJ* 1998;317:559-565.

Tran B, Dancey JE, Kamel-Reid S, et al. Cancer genomics: technology, discovery, and translation. *J Clin Oncol* 2012;30:647-660.

Trusheim MR, Burgess B, Hu SX, et al. Quantifying factors for the success of stratified medicine. *Nat Rev Drug Discov* 2011;10:817-833.

Tsao M-S, Sakurada A, Cutz JC, et al. Erlotinib in lung cancer—molecular and clinical predictors of outcome. *N Engl J Med* 2005;353:133-144.

Viganò A, Dorgan M, Buckingham J, et al. Survival prediction in terminal cancer patients: a systematic review of the medical literature. *Palliat Med* 2000;14:363-374.

Walter S. In defense of the arcsine approximation. *Statistician* 1979;28:219-222.

Weeks J. Performance status upstaged? *J Clin Oncol* 1992;10:1827-1829.

Welch HG. Screening mammography—a long run for a short slide? *N Engl J Med* 2010;363:1276-1278.

Wood L, Egger M, Gluud LL, et al. Empirical evidence of bias in treatment effect estimates in controlled trials with different interventions and outcomes: meta-epidemiological study. *BMJ* 2008;336:601-605.

Yin G, Li Y, Ji Y. Bayesian dose-finding in phase I/II clinical trials using toxicity and efficacy odds ratios. *Biometrics* 2006;62:777-784.

BIBLIOGRAPHY

Crowley J. *Handbook of Statistics in Clinical Oncology.* New York, NY: Dekker; 2001.

Fletcher RH, Fletcher SW. *Clinical Epidemiology: The Essentials.* Baltimore, MD: Lippincott Williams & Wilkins; 2005.

Hulley SB. *Designing Clinical Research.* Philadelphia, PA: Lippincott Williams & Wilkins; 2007.

Sackett DL, Haynes RB, Guyatt GH, Tugwell P. *Clinical Epidemiology: A Basic Science for Clinical Medicine.* Boston, MA: Little, Brown; 1991.

Index

Page numbers followed by *f* or *t* indicate figures or tables, respectively.